Quantitative Imaging in the Thorax

Ritu Gill • Prabhakar Rajiah
Editors

Quantitative Imaging in the Thorax

Springer

Editors
Ritu Gill
Radiology
Columbia University Medical Center
New York, NY, USA

Prabhakar Rajiah
Radiology
Mayo Clinic
Rochester, MN, USA

ISBN 978-3-032-14102-6 ISBN 978-3-032-14103-3 (eBook)
https://doi.org/10.1007/978-3-032-14103-3

This Springer imprint is published by the registered company Springer Nature Switzerland AG
The registered company address is: Gewerbestrasse 11, 6330 Cham, Switzerland

*To **U. Joseph Schoepf, MD (1969–2025)**—a visionary pioneer in cardiovascular and thoracic imaging. His passion, mentorship, and innovation continue to inspire the pursuit of precision in quantitative imaging in the thorax.*

Foreword

The field of cardiothoracic imaging has entered an extraordinary era. Advances in imaging technology, computational analytics, and artificial intelligence are transforming how we evaluate and manage heart and lung disease. What was once limited to descriptive interpretation is now evolving into a quantitative, data-driven discipline, where measurable features from images can guide diagnosis, prognostication, and personalized therapy.

Quantitative Imaging in the Thorax is a landmark contribution to this rapidly evolving field. The editors have brought together a truly global team of experts, each contributing their knowledge and experience across the spectrum of cardiothoracic imaging—from cardiac MRI and CT to nuclear medicine, AI applications, and thoracic imaging of the lungs, pleura, and mediastinum. This book provides not only the technical principles behind quantitative imaging but also the clinical context that makes these methods meaningful and actionable.

What sets this volume apart is its emphasis on integration. The chapters demonstrate how quantitative imaging can bridge the gap between radiology, clinical cardiology, pulmonology, and computational science. The result is a resource that is at once rigorous, practical, and forward-looking—a text that equips readers to translate complex imaging data into actionable clinical insights.

For trainees, clinicians, radiologists, and researchers, this book offers both a foundation and a roadmap. It illustrates how to harness the power of quantitative metrics, radiomics, and AI to improve patient outcomes, while also highlighting current challenges and opportunities for future innovation. The global perspectives and collaborative spirit of this work reflect the very essence of modern medicine: interdisciplinary, evidence-driven, and patient-centered.

It is my hope that this book inspires its readers as much as it informs them, providing the knowledge and vision necessary to advance the practice of cardiothoracic imaging in the era of precision medicine.

CUIMC
New York, NY, USA

Jay Leb,

Preface

Cardiothoracic imaging is in a transformative era. What was once primarily qualitative and interpretive is now rapidly evolving into a field grounded in quantitative, data-driven insights. The ability to extract measurable features from images—ranging from cardiac MRI and CT to thoracic CT and nuclear medicine—enables clinicians and researchers to assess disease with unprecedented precision. These quantitative tools are shaping the future of personalized medicine, allowing patient-specific risk stratification, prognostication, and therapeutic guidance.

Quantitative Imaging in the Thorax was conceived to provide a comprehensive, practical, and authoritative reference for this dynamic field. It brings together the expertise of global leaders in radiology, cardiology, and data science, offering a roadmap for integrating quantitative imaging into clinical and research workflows. From foundational principles to advanced applications in AI and machine learning, this book covers the full spectrum of cardiothoracic imaging, emphasizing both technical rigor and clinical relevance.

The text is organized into 27 chapters, reflecting the breadth of the field:

- Foundational concepts, including the principles of quantitative imaging
- Quantitative cardiac imaging, spanning MRI, CT, myocardial perfusion, valvular heart disease, structural interventions, electrophysiology, and cardio-oncology
- Thoracic imaging, including lungs, pulmonary hypertension, embolism, airway diseases, interstitial lung disease, lung nodules, masses, pleura, mediastinum, and sarcopenia
- Advanced applications, including artificial intelligence and machine learning, radiomics, and nuclear medicine approaches

Each chapter is authored by international experts, providing readers with insights into best practices, current challenges, and emerging innovations. The collaborative nature of this work highlights the global effort to advance quantitative imaging, reflecting a diversity of perspectives, experience, and expertise.

This book is intended for a wide audience: radiologists, cardiologists, pulmonologists, trainees, and data scientists alike. Whether you are beginning your journey in quantitative imaging or seeking advanced guidance, the goal of this text is to provide clarity, depth, and inspiration—bridging the gap between imaging science, clinical application, and computational innovation.

We are profoundly grateful to the authors whose scholarship and dedication made this volume possible. We also thank our readers, whose curiosity and commitment to advancing cardiothoracic imaging will drive the next generation of innovation. It is our hope that this book serves as a foundation, a guide, and a source of inspiration for all who seek to harness the power of quantitative imaging to improve patient care.

New York, NY, USA — Ritu Gill
Rochester, MN, USA — Prabhakar Rajiah

Acknowledgments

We sincerely thank all the contributing authors, editors, and reviewers whose expertise and dedication made this book possible.

We are also grateful to our families and colleagues for their support and encouragement throughout this project.

Contents

Contributors

Charalambos Antoniades Acute Multidisciplinary Imaging and Interventional Centre, Radcliffe Department of Medicine, Division of Cardiovascular Medicine, University of Oxford, Oxford, UK

Benjamin Auer Joint Program in Nuclear Medicine, Department of Radiology, Brigham and Women's Hospital, Harvard Medical School, Boston, MA, USA

Georgina Bailey Department of Radiology, The Royal Brompton Hospital, London, UK

Dhiraj Baruah Medical University of South Carolina, Charleston, SC, USA

Estelle Blanc-Autran Hôpital Marie Lannelongue, Nuclear Medicine Department, Le Plessis-Robinson, France

Scott M. Bugenhagen Mallinckrodt Institute of Radiology, Department of Radiology, Washington University School of Medicine, St. Louis, MO, USA

Caroline Caramella Hôpital Marie Lannelongue, Radiology Department, Le Plessis-Robinson, France

Julia Cha Department of Diagnostic Radiology, Beth Israel Deaconess Medical Center, Harvard Medical School, Boston, MA, USA

Hyuk-Jae Chang Yonsei University, Severance Cardiovascular Hospital, Seodaemun, Seoul, South Korea

Su Min Chang Department of Cardiovascular Imaging, The Houston Methodist Hospital, Houston, TX, USA

Ming-fang Chao Department of Cardiovascular Imaging, The Houston Methodist Hospital, Houston, TX, USA

Ming Hui Chen Boston Children's Hospital, Boston, MA, USA

Harvard Medical School, Boston, MA, USA

Dana-Farber Cancer Institute, Boston, MA, USA

Shane M. Crilly Department of Radiology, St. Vincent's University Hospital, Dublin, Ireland

Ariel Hernán Curiale Applied Chest Imaging Laboratory, Department of Radiology, Brigham and Women's Hospital, Harvard Medical School, Somerville, MA, USA

Wojciech Cytawa Department of Nuclear Medicine, Medical University of Gdańsk, Gdańsk, Poland

Constance de Margerie-Mellon Hôpital Saint-Louis APHP, Radiology Department, Paris, France

INSERM UMR_S970, PARCC, Université Paris Cité, Paris, France

Aneesh Dhore-Patil Department of Cardiovascular Imaging, The Houston Methodist Hospital, Houston, TX, USA

Marcelo Fernando Di Carli Division of Nuclear Medicine and Molecular Imaging, Cardiovascular Imaging Department of Radiology, Brigham and Women's Hospital, Harvard Medical School, Boston, MA, USA

Raquelle El Alam Brigham and Women's Hospital, Department of Radiology, Boston, MA, USA

Sonia F. Epstein Boston Children's Hospital, Boston, MA, USA

Antonio Esposito Experimental Imaging Center, IRCCS San Raffaele Scientific Institute, Milan, Italy

School of Medicine, Vita-Salute University, Milan, Italy

Raúl San José Estépar Applied Chest Imaging Laboratory, Department of Radiology, Brigham and Women's Hospital, Harvard Medical School, Somerville, MA, USA

Jadwiga Fijałkowska 2nd Department of Radiology, Medical University of Gdańsk, Gdańsk, Poland

Fai Wang Fong Department of Diagnostic Radiology, School of Clinical Medicine, Li Ka Shing Faculty of Medicine, The University of Hong Kong, Pok Fu Lam, Hong Kong

Christopher Francois Department of Radiology, Mayo Clinic, Rochester, MN, USA

Elisa Franquet Division of Nuclear Medicine and Molecular Imaging, Department of Radiology, University of Massachusetts Medical Health, UMass Chan Medical School, Worcester, MA, USA

Thomas Frauenfelder University Hospital Zurich, Institute of Diagnostic and Interventional Radiology, Zurich, Switzerland

Ritu R. Gill Department of Radiology, Columbia University Medical Center, New York, NY, USA

Chiara Gnasso Experimental Imaging Center, IRCCS San Raffaele Scientific Institute, Milan, Italy

School of Medicine, Vita-Salute University, Milan, Italy

Jonathan M Goldstein Department of Radiology, Columbia University Medical Center, New York, NY, USA

Jin Mo Goo Department of Radiology, Seoul National University Hospital, Seoul National University College of Medicine, Seoul, South Korea

Deepa Gopalan Department of Radiology, Hammersmith Hospital, Imperial College Healthcare NHS Trust, London, UK

Mark M. Hammer Brigham and Women's Hospital, Department of Radiology, Boston, MA, USA

Shaun Hinen Medical University of South Carolina, Charleston, SC, USA

Eui Jin Hwang Department of Radiology, Seoul National University Hospital, Seoul National University College of Medicine, Seoul, South Korea

Fangchao Jiang Center for Systems Biology, Massachusetts General Hospital, Harvard Medical School, Boston, MA, USA

Ismail Kabakus Medical University of South Carolina, Charleston, SC, USA

Desmond Killick Department of Radiology, St. Vincent's University Hospital, Dublin, Ireland

Aparna Komarraju Department of Radiology, Beth Israel Deaconess Medical Center, Harvard Medical School, Boston, MA, USA

Neha Kwatra Joint Program in Nuclear Medicine, Department of Radiology, Brigham and Women's Hospital, Harvard Medical School, Boston, MA, USA

Division of Nuclear Medicine and Molecular Imaging, Department of Radiology, Boston Children's Hospital, Harvard Medical School, Boston, MA, USA

Hui Chong Lau Cardiology, Massachusetts General Hospital, Harvard Medical School, Boston, MA, USA

Cardiovascular Imaging Research Center, Massachusetts General Hospital, Harvard Medical School, Boston, MA, USA

Meghavi Mashar Beth Israel Deaconess Medical Center, Boston, MA, USA

Michail C. Mavrogiannis Radcliffe Department of Medicine, Division of Cardiovascular Medicine, University of Oxford, Oxford, UK

Vivek Modi Department of Cardiovascular Imaging, The Houston Methodist Hospital, Houston, TX, USA

Sedra Mohammadi Division of Nuclear Medicine and Molecular Imaging, Department of Radiology, Massachusetts General Hospital, Harvard Medical School, Boston, MA, USA

David J. Murphy Department of Radiology, St. Vincent's University Hospital, Dublin, Ireland

School of Medicine University College Dublin, Dublin, Ireland

Pietro Nardelli Applied Chest Imaging Laboratory, Department of Radiology, Brigham and Women's Hospital, Harvard Medical School, Somerville, MA, USA

Ming-Yen Ng Department of Diagnostic Radiology, School of Clinical Medicine, Li Ka Shing Faculty of Medicine, The University of Hong Kong, Pok Fu Lam, Hong Kong

Thomas S. C. Ng Division of Nuclear Medicine and Molecular Imaging, Department of Radiology, Massachusetts General Hospital, Harvard Medical School, Boston, MA, USA

Joint Program in Nuclear Medicine, Department of Radiology, Brigham and Women's Hospital, Harvard Medical School, Boston, MA, USA

Center for Systems Biology, Massachusetts General Hospital, Harvard Medical School, Boston, MA, USA

Julia Niemierko Department of Radiology, Medical University Hospital of Gdańsk, Gdańsk, Poland

Masahiko Nomura Department of Diagnostic Radiology, Fujita Health University School of Medicine, Toyoake, Aichi, Japan

Joint Research Laboratory of Advanced Medical Imaging, Fujita Health University School of Medicine, Toyoake, Aichi, Japan

Yoshiharu Ohno Department of Diagnostic Radiology, Fujita Health University School of Medicine, Toyoake, Aichi, Japan

Joint Research Laboratory of Advanced Medical Imaging, Fujita Health University School of Medicine, Toyoake, Aichi, Japan

Yoshiyuki Ozawa Department of Diagnostic Radiology, Fujita Health University School of Medicine, Toyoake, Aichi, Japan

Anna Palmisano Experimental Imaging Center, IRCCS San Raffaele Scientific Institute, Milan, Italy

School of Medicine, Vita-Salute University, Milan, Italy

Hyung-Bok Park Catholic Kwandong University, International St. Mary's Hospital, Seoul, Incheon, South Korea

Hena Patel Department of Medicine, University of Chicago, Chicago, IL, USA

Prabhakar Shantha Rajiah Department of Radiology, Cardiovascular Radiology Division, Mayo Clinic, Rochester, MN, USA

Carole A. Ridge Department of Radiology, The Royal Brompton Hospital, London, UK

National Heart and Lung Institute, Imperial College London, London, UK

Dipan Shah Department of Cardiovascular Imaging, The Houston Methodist Hospital, Houston, TX, USA

Katarzyna Sienkiewicz Department of Radiology, Medical University Hospital of Gdańsk, Gdańsk, Poland

Aparna Singh Brigham and Women's Hospital, Department of Radiology, Boston, MA, USA

Jadranka Stojanovska Grossman School of Medicine, New York University, New York, NY, USA

Roberto Storelli Department of Diagnostic and Interventional Radiology, University Hospital Freiburg, Freiburg im Breisgau, Baden-Württemberg, Germany

Logan Sun Department of Radiology, The Royal Brompton Hospital, London, UK

Daisuke Takenaka Department of Diagnostic Radiology, Fujita Health University School of Medicine, Toyoake, Aichi, Japan

Yalynska Tetyana University Hospital Zurich, Institute of Diagnostic and Interventional Radiology, Zurich, Switzerland

Takahiro Ueda Department of Diagnostic Radiology, Fujita Health University School of Medicine, Toyoake, Aichi, Japan

Laetitia Vercellino Hôpital Saint-Louis APHP, Nuclear Medicine Department, Paris, France

INSERM UMR_S942, Université Paris Cité, Paris, France

Haonan Wang GE HealthCare, Waukesha, WI, USA

Takeshi Yoshikawa Department of Diagnostic Radiology, Fujita Health University School of Medicine, Toyoake, Aichi, Japan

Eddy D. Zandee van Rilland Department of Radiology, Stanford University Medical Center, Palo Alto, CA, USA

Merissa N. Zeman Division of Nuclear Medicine and Molecular Imaging, Department of Radiology, Massachusetts General Hospital, Harvard Medical School, Boston, MA, USA

Joint Program in Nuclear Medicine, Department of Radiology, Brigham and Women's Hospital, Harvard Medical School, Boston, MA, USA

Principles of Quantitative Imaging

1

Julia Cha and Ritu R. Gill

Introduction

The core concept behind radiomics is that images captured by machines contain a wealth of information that is not visible to the human eye but can be interpreted by algorithms in other machines [33]. For instance, a tumor with "rough borders" on a clinical report could be analyzed more accurately by an algorithm that extracts and quantifies various textural features, providing a multidimensional understanding of the tumor's texture. The methods used by these algorithms have been under development since the early twentieth century, alongside the rise of computer science and artificial intelligence (Figs. 1.1 and 1.2).

X-rays were discovered in 1895, followed by the introduction of PET, CT, and MRI scans in the 1960s and 1970s. During the same period, computer science and artificial intelligence were rapidly advancing. In 1963, computer-aided diagnosis (CAD) was introduced, allowing physicians to move from qualitative to quantitative imaging [36]. Shannon's 1948 paper on information theory, titled *A Mathematical Theory of Communication*, explored how information is transmitted and extracted, proposing that communication involved sending data through a "noisy channel" and that minimizing distortions and errors during this process could be achieved by coding. In 1973, Haralick introduced the use of a gray-level co-occurrence matrix (GLCM) to quantify the spatial relationships between pixels [20]. In 1975, Galloway expanded on this concept by using gray-level run lengths to quantify texture features [40]. Although these developments influenced numerous fields, texture analysis was first applied to medical imaging in 1972 when Sutton and Hall used it to automatically classify pulmonary diseases based on chest radiographs [33, 41].

The term "radiomics" was introduced by Lambin in 2012. Lambin proposed that advanced imaging techniques could reveal genomic and proteomic information crucial for diagnosis and tailored treatment, as imaging-guided biopsies have shown different spatial resolutions linked to distinct proteomic signatures [35]. For example, Kuo et al. demonstrated that CT-derived phenotypes of hepatocellular carcinoma were associated with drug response transcriptional profiles, establishing the concept of radiogenomics [27]. Similarly, Diehn et al. compared MRI neuroimaging with DNA microanalysis to show that tumor contrast enhancement and mass effect could predict specific gene expression patterns and hypoxia. By combining imaging with immu-

J. Cha
Department of Diagnostic Radiology, Beth Israel Deaconess Medical Center, Harvard Medical School, Boston, MA, USA

R. R. Gill (✉)
Department of Radiology, Columbia University Medical Center, New York, NY, USA
e-mail: Rg3675@cumc.columbia.edu

R. Gill, P. Rajiah (eds.), *Quantitative Imaging in the Thorax*,
https://doi.org/10.1007/978-3-032-14103-3_1

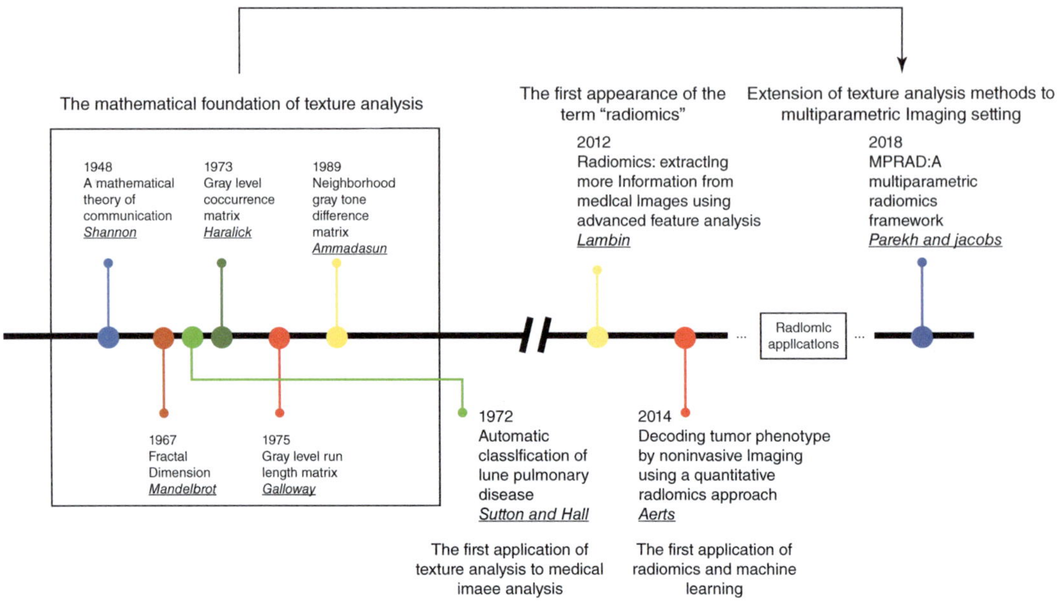

Fig. 1.1 Timeline of radiomics history [11]

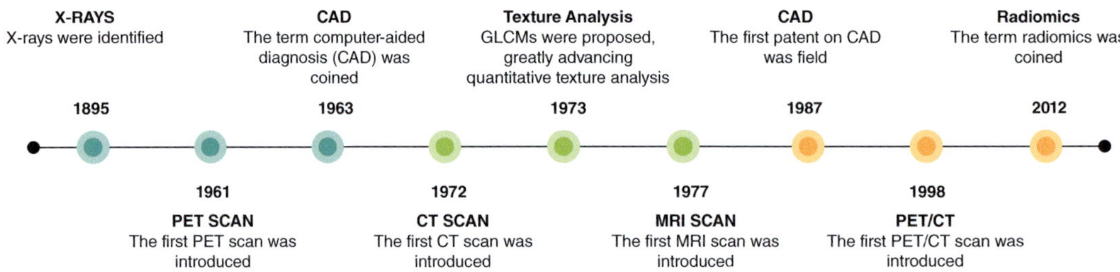

Fig. 1.2 Timeline of radiology [36]

nohistochemistry, they also showed that specific imaging phenotypes could predict EGFR overexpression [18]. These findings position radiomics as a promising noninvasive approach to personalize treatment, as patients with similar imaging diagnoses may have distinct genomic signatures and responses to treatment.

Detailed Description of Radiomics Steps

The radiomics process involves several steps. First, images are obtained using MRI, CT, or PET scans, with parameters selected based on the imaging goal (diagnostic or treatment) and the type of tissue. Next, the images undergo preprocessing to make them compatible with the algorithm. Afterward, the region of interest is segmented either manually or automatically. A range of features, determined through statistical and morphological analysis, are then extracted [39]. The final step is the analysis of these extracted features. User-defined high-interest features then train a machine learning algorithm, which creates a predictive model [1, 35]. The following section will discuss each of these steps in greater detail (Fig. 1.3).

Image Acquisition

The first step in radiomics involves inherent variability, as it depends on image acquisition and

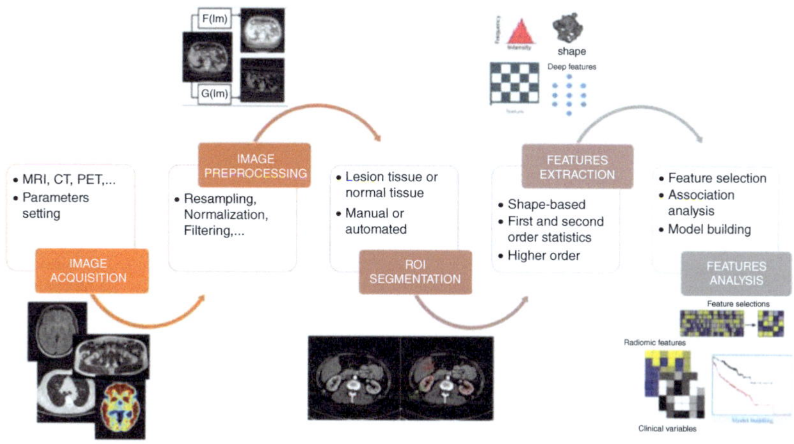

Fig. 1.3 Flow of radiomics [1]

reconstruction parameters, which are influenced by the imaging modality (such as X-ray, computed tomography, magnetic resonance imaging, or positron emission tomography). Additionally, factors such as the technique and equipment used, along with potential human error, can affect the quality of the acquired images. To address the challenge of non-standardized acquisition methods, the Quantitative Imaging Biomarkers Alliance (QIBA) was created by the Radiological Society of North America [1]. These initiatives are focused on improving the replicability and reliability of radiomics in the future.

Image Processing

After images are acquired, they undergo reconstruction and preprocessing to ensure they are in a standardized format that can be interpreted by an algorithm. The reconstruction process includes filtering with mathematical kernels to reduce image noise, normalizing and quantizing gray levels, correcting for motion, and resampling the pixel count. As René Magritte's 1929 painting *The Treachery of Images* illustrated, a medical image is merely a representation of a patient's anatomy, not the anatomy itself. The goal of this step is to create a representation as close to raw data as possible, minimizing human or technical distortions. For instance, image normalization distributes gray pixels evenly within a standardized range to eliminate bias or outliers, which is particularly important in multicenter studies where methods may vary. Additionally, filters such as Laplacian, Gaussian, and edge filters are used to detect intensity changes, smooth noisy areas, and enhance edges, respectively (Table 1.1) [1].

Segmentation

The segmentation of the region of interest (ROI), which can be either two-dimensional (e.g., X-ray) or three-dimensional (e.g., volumetric CT), can be performed manually, semiautomatically, or automatically. Manual segmentation, a technique in use since the early days of imaging, remains a critical step in the planning of radiation therapy. However, despite its widespread use, it is inherently subjective, resulting in less reproducible data. Several software tools, such as 3D Slicer, employ deep learning neural networks to perform automatic segmentation [1, 35, 36].

Feature Extraction

Once the ROI is defined, relevant features are extracted using mathematical methods. Since radiomics is a data-driven approach, clinical interpretation is not incorporated during this stage. First-order statistics focus on the distribution of individual voxels. Features identified through first-order statistics, referred to as first-

Table 1.1 Preprocessing algorithms and filters [1]

Preprocessing step	Description
Resampling	Adjusts image resolution using interpolation methods (e.g., linear, polynomial, and spline)
Intensity normalization	Standardizes pixel intensities to correct for bias, scaling differences, and outliers
Gray-level quantification	Reduces the number of gray levels to simplify image representation
Motion correction	Minimizes motion artifacts and confounding factors
Noise filtering/enhancement Laplacian filter Gaussian filter Edge filters Law filters Wavelet transform	Highlights areas of rapid intensity change; used for edge detection Smooths the image and reduces noise Enhances edges by approximating horizontal and vertical gradients Extracts texture features like spots, ripples, waves, and oscillations Decomposes image to enhance textures at multiple scales; allows for tailored wavelet functions per application
Inhomogeneity correction (MRI)	Corrects intensity variation from magnetic field inhomogeneities and RF coil imperfections not resolved by normalization

order features, include total energy, entropy, standard deviation, variance, kurtosis, and skewness. Higher-order statistics, introduced by Haralick in 1973, provide insight into the spatial relationships between pairs of pixels, using various types of gray-level matrices. For example, gray-level co-occurrence matrices (GLCM) quantify the conditional probabilities of pixel intensities based on their spatial distribution [1], while gray-level dependence matrices (GLDM) compare each voxel to its central voxel [11]. The application of multiple filters or transformations to an image can yield more complex, higher-order features [20].

Feature Analysis

There are numerous machine learning models available to analyze extracted features, with deep learning (DL) models currently being the predominant choice. Deep learning models, specifically convolutional neural networks (CNNs), directly analyze features from a segmented image without requiring a separate extraction phase. CNNs process imaging data as arrays, passing through multiple hidden layers [7]. These layers first perform convolution to extract relevant features, followed by classification and identification, culminating in the final output. While deep radiomics offers a more streamlined approach compared to traditional methods, it requires larger datasets for training and presents interpretative challenges due to its "black box" nature [1, 11, 36].

Applications

Tumors exhibit a spectrum of spatial and temporal heterogeneity, driven by variations in vascularization, genomics, and metabolism. Growing evidence suggests that repeated, noninvasive, holistic sampling through imaging may offer superior diagnostic and therapeutic benefits compared to invasive biopsies taken from random locations. In fact, tumor tissue heterogeneity may also manifest phenotypically in imaging [5]. This section will explore the diverse clinical applications of radiomics in lung cancer, including tumor classification, prognostication, treatment outcome prediction, and genomic characterization [13, 19, 34].

Lung cancer is the second most common cancer and the leading cause of cancer-related deaths in the United States, accounting for one in five cancer deaths. In 2023, the American Cancer Society estimates that there will be 238,340 new cases and 127,070 deaths from lung cancer. Approximately 85% of these cases are non-small cell lung cancer (NSCLC), while around 15% are small cell lung cancer (SCLC). In response to these alarming statistics, efforts have intensified to use low-dose chest CT for lung cancer screening.

The National Lung Screening Trial (NLST) and the Dutch-Belgian Lung Cancer Screening Trial (NELSON) were pivotal studies that demonstrated that low-dose CT screening in high-risk populations can reduce mortality by as much as 60%. The NLST followed 53,454 high-risk patients across 33 US medical centers. Participants underwent three annual screenings between 2002 and 2004, using either low-dose CT or an anterior-posterior chest X-ray, with data on lung cancer incidence and mortality collected through 2009. The study concluded that low-dose CT screening reduced relative mortality from lung cancer by 20% [37]. This substantial reduction in mortality was further confirmed by the NELSON trial during a 10-year follow-up [38].

Given the pivotal role that imaging plays in early detection, treatment planning, and reducing overall mortality in lung cancer, radiomics is a valuable tool for segmenting pulmonary nodules. Radiomic features such as nodule size, texture, and heterogeneity are more easily characterized with this approach. For example, the volume doubling time (VDT) of a nodule has demonstrated predictive value for malignancy [31]. In the NELSON trial, nodules with a VDT of less than 400 days had a 9.7% likelihood of being malignant, compared to 4.1% for nodules with a VDT between 400 and 600 days [38].

Detection and Classification

The first comprehensive study applying radiomics to lung cancer was conducted in 2014, involving 1019 patients, including 788 with NSCLC and 231 with head and neck cancers. The patients were divided into 7 cohorts, from which 440 radiomic features were extracted. A survival prognostic algorithm, trained on 1 cohort of 422 lung cancer patients, was validated using the remaining cohorts. Additionally, gene expression analysis revealed a correlation between radiomic features and gene expression. These findings demonstrated that radiomics could be used to determine a prognostic lung cancer phenotype from a single CT scan [10].

In 2016, a study examined 127 indeterminate pretreatment lung nodules and extracted 583 features related to nodule intensity, texture, and heterogeneity. A diagnostic model trained on this data was able to distinguish malignant from benign nodules with a specificity of 80%, compared to 56.9% for experienced radiologists [22]. Another study performed quantitative analysis on imaging data from the NLST, focusing on two matched cohorts: one with screen-detected lung cancer and the other with benign pulmonary nodules. The radiomics model trained on these cohorts could predict which nodules would become cancerous in 1 or 2 years, achieving accuracies of 80% and 79%, respectively, surpassing the performance of Lung-RADS and volume scores [26].

Persistent subsolid nodules are at a higher risk of malignancy compared to transient or solid nodules [24]. Lee et al. studied 47 persistent subsolid nodules in 46 patients, alongside 39 transient subsolid nodules in 31 patients. They identified radiomic features, such as higher mean attenuation and lower skewness, that significantly differentiated persistent from transient nodules. When combined with clinical eosinophilia, lesion size, multiplicity, and other clinical features, these radiomic features proved to be more effective than CT and clinical features alone in identifying persistent subsolid nodules [42].

Histopathological Prediction

Several studies have suggested that radiomics classifiers can predict NSCLC histopathology. The two most common subtypes of NSCLC, adenocarcinoma and squamous cell carcinoma, have distinct histological patterns. Adenocarcinoma, typically found in the peripheral lung, is characterized by glandular organization, while squamous cell carcinoma, located centrally in the lung, exhibits individual cell keratinization. These subtypes also differ in glycolysis and hypoxia-related markers, leading to contrasting prognoses and treatment responses. Radiomics has the potential to distinguish between these subtypes, providing valuable insights for personalized treatment strategies.

While invasive biopsy remains the standard method for histopathological diagnosis, radiomics has shown promise as a potentially superior alternative. Wu et al. extracted 440 radiomic features from pretreatment CT images of 350 NSCLC patients, identifying 53 features significantly associated with histological subtype prediction, yielding an AUC of 0.72 [17]. In another study, 45 quantitative features were extracted from a cohort of 85 patients with primary lung tumors, resulting in an AUC of 0.88 for histopathological prediction [9]. Given the substantial heterogeneity of lung cancers, precise classification is essential. Among invasive lung adenocarcinoma subtypes—lepidic, acinar, solid, papillary, and micropapillary—the latter is associated with a poor prognosis. Song et al. performed quantitative CT analysis on 339 patients undergoing resection for lung adenocarcinoma, incorporating features such as histogram, size and shape, GLCM, and intensity variance. They identified that lower minimum pixel values and reduced positive pixel variance were predictive of micropapillary structures within lung adenocarcinoma [21]. These studies collectively indicate that radiomics can noninvasively provide comprehensive histopathological insights, aiding in diagnosis and treatment planning.

Cancer Genetics

The genetic profile of cancers significantly influences prognosis and treatment decisions, often necessitating multiple biopsies at different time points. One retrospective study evaluated the CT scans of 298 patients with surgically resected lung adenocarcinomas, extracting 219 features, 59 of which were independent. Significant differences in 11 radiomic features were observed between EGFR mutant and wild-type groups, with 5 radiomic features—related to CT attenuation energy, tumor direction, and texture—able to predict EGFR mutation status. Adding these radiomic features to a clinical model improved predictive power (AUC increased from 0.667 to 0.709) [28]. Another study on 48 early-stage NSCLC cases identified that positive skewness and lower kurtosis were strongly associated with K-ras mutations, with kurtosis serving as a significant predictor of overall and disease-free survival, where lower kurtosis values indicated poorer survival [23]. Additionally, mutations in the anaplastic lymphoma kinase (ALK) gene, particularly the EML4-ALK fusion, have been implicated in NSCLC pathogenesis and associated with positive responses to crizotinib treatment [16]. A radiogenomic predictor for ALK+ status, derived from a cohort of 59 NSCLC patients, found significant associations between ALK+ status and central tumor location, absence of pleural tail, and large pleural effusion. These CT traits demonstrated strong discriminatory power, with a sensitivity of 83.3% and accuracy of 78.8%. Furthermore, disorganized vessel patterns were linked to shorter progression-free survival in crizotinib-treated patients [3]. These studies underscore the potential of radiomics in providing valuable genetic insights that can significantly impact prognosis, treatment planning, and response.

Tumor Staging

The TNM staging system (tumor, lymph node invasion, and distant metastasis) is the cornerstone of cancer risk stratification and treatment planning. However, this method primarily assesses tumor resectability, while increasing numbers of cancer patients opt for chemoradiation therapy first. Consequently, radiomics has emerged as a more informative staging method. In one of the pioneering radiomics studies in lung cancer, the combination of radiomics and TNM staging outperformed TNM staging alone [10]. Another study demonstrated the ability of radiomics to predict distant metastases in lung cancer. By analyzing the pretreatment CTs of 348 patients, 485 radiomic features were extracted, yielding an AUC of 72.84% for distant metastasis prediction, which increased to 89.09% when combined with clinical data [15]. These findings were corroborated in another study that associated quantitative CT features with both distant and nodal metastases, with AUCs of 0.92 and 0.84, respectively [9].

In early-stage lung cancer, the presence or absence of nodal metastasis influences the surgical approach. Preoperative PET-CT is often used to evaluate nodal metastasis, but studies have shown its limitations. A comparison of preoperative 18F-FDG PET-CT with postoperative pathology in 113 patients with 120 resected NSCLC cases showed a sensitivity of 53.8%, specificity of 76.6%, and a false-positive rate of 61.1% [25]. Consequently, more accurate imaging methods are necessary. In a retrospective study of 649 pre-surgical patients with stage IA NSCLC, 396 radiomic features were extracted from contrast-enhanced CT scans, and a model combining clinical and radiomic data predicted lymph node metastasis in early NSCLC. Both the radiomics-only and combined models outperformed the clinical model alone (AUC of 0.614), achieving AUCs of 0.851 and 0.860, respectively [14].

Treatment Response and Prognosis

Tumor staging is traditionally used to define prognosis, but even patients with the same staging can experience widely varying treatment responses and outcomes. Radiomics has the potential to provide individualized prognostic and treatment stratification. Hosny et al. analyzed CT scans of 1194 NSCLC patients treated with surgery or radiotherapy and found that deep learning networks were significantly more effective at stratifying patients into low and high mortality risk groups based on 2-year overall survival [12]. In another study, a radiomic signature based on 107 features from 378 patients with resected stage I NSCLC successfully stratified patients into high- and low-risk groups for resection-free survival [32].

Radiomics has also been applied to predict treatment response. A study on 127 patients with locally advanced NSCLC found that radiomic data from pretreatment CT scans predicted the response to neoadjuvant chemoradiation. Seven radiomic features were predictive of pathological residual disease (AUC >0.6), while conventional volumetric features were not predictive (AUC <0.6) [29]. In a study of 92 SCLC patients receiving standard etoposide and cisplatin treatment, a radiomic signature based on CT scans performed both before and after therapy outperformed a clinicopathological model in predicting response (AUC 0.797 vs. 0.670) [4]. Additionally, combining radiomic and clinical data demonstrated strong predictive power for pathological complete response and gross residual disease in 85 patients with resectable stage II–III NSCLC [30].

In the era of immunotherapy, radiomics holds promise in personalizing treatment. A 2020 study created a CT-based radiomic signature to predict progression-free survival in stage IV ALK+ NSCLC patients treated with crizotinib. The signature successfully stratified patients into rapid versus slow progression groups, and the model outperformed one based on clinical attributes [8]. Radiomics could also serve as a valuable tool in clinical trials. A study by Sun et al. used CT images and RNA sequencing data from 135 patients with advanced solid tumors enrolled in PD-1/PD-L1 therapy trials to create a radiomic signature that predicted tumor immune phenotype, distinguishing between inflamed and immune desert tumors. This signature predicted objective responses and overall survival in patients treated with anti-PD-1 and PD-L1 therapies [2]. These findings suggest the growing potential of radiomics in predicting disease progression and treatment outcomes.

Limitations, Challenges, and Future Directions

Despite its promising potential, radiomics faces several challenges. One significant limitation is the variability across imaging data sets and the absence of a standardized dataset for machine learning algorithms. Current models rely on data from different centers, acquired using varied protocols, contributing to the "black box" phenomenon in radiomics analysis [6, 36]. Efforts to mitigate this variability include the development of the Quantitative Imaging Biomarkers Alliance (QIBA) Profile for FDG PET/CT imaging. The QIBA profile aims to standardize the measurement of tumor glycolytic activity (SUV) in PET/CT imaging to improve reliability and reduce variability.

References

1. Scapicchio C, Gabelloni M, Barucci A, Cioni D, Saba L, Neri E. A deep look into radiomics. Radiol Med. 2021;126(10):1296–311.
2. Sun R, et al. A radiomics approach to assess tumour-infiltrating CD8 cells and response to anti-PD-1 or anti-PD-L1 immunotherapy: an imaging biomarker, retrospective multicohort study. Lancet Oncol [Internet]. [cited 2023 Mar 1]. Available from: https://www.thelancet.com/journals/lanonc/article/PIIS1470-2045(18)30413-3/fulltext.
3. Yamamoto S, Korn RL, Oklu R, Migdal C, Gotway MB, Weiss GJ, et al. ALK molecular phenotype in non-small cell lung cancer: CT radiogenomic characterization. Radiology. 2014;272(2):568–76.
4. Wei H, Yang F, Liu Z, Sun S, Xu F, Liu P, et al. Application of computed tomography-based radiomics signature analysis in the prediction of the response of small cell lung cancer patients to first-line chemotherapy. Exp Ther Med. 2019;17(5):3621–9.
5. Tunali I, Gillies RJ, Schabath MB. Application of radiomics and artificial intelligence for lung cancer precision medicine. Cold Spring Harb Perspect Med. 2021;11(8):a039537.
6. Yip SSF, Aerts HJWL. Applications and limitations of radiomics. Phys Med Biol [Internet]. [cited 2023 Feb 26]. Available from: https://www.ncbi.nlm.nih.gov/pmc/articles/PMC4927328/.
7. Davies ER. Chapter 15—Deep-learning networks. In: Davies ER, editor. Computer vision. 5th ed. Academic Press; 2018. p. 453–93. Available from: https://www.sciencedirect.com/science/article/pii/B9780128092842000150.
8. Li H, Zhang R, Wang S, Fang M, Zhu Y, Hu Z, et al. CT-based radiomic signature as a prognostic factor in stage IV ALK-positive non-small-cell lung cancer treated with TKI Crizotinib: a proof-of-concept study. Front Oncol. 2020;10:57.
9. Ferreira-Junior JR, Koenigkam-Santos M, Magalhães Tenório AP, Faleiros MC, Garcia Cipriano FE, Fabro AT, et al. CT-based radiomics for prediction of histologic subtype and metastatic disease in primary malignant lung neoplasms. Int J Comput Assist Radiol Surg. 2020;15(1):163–72.
10. Aerts HJWL, Velazquez ER, Leijenaar RTH, Parmar C, Grossmann P, Cavalho S, et al. Decoding tumour phenotype by noninvasive imaging using a quantitative radiomics approach. Nat Commun. 2014;5:4006.
11. Parekh VS, Jacobs MA. Deep learning and radiomics in precision medicine. Expert Rev Precis Med Drug Dev. 2019;4(2):59–72.
12. Hosny A, Parmar C, Coroller TP, Grossmann P, Zeleznik R, Kumar A, et al. Deep learning for lung cancer prognostication: a retrospective multi-cohort radiomics study. PLoS Med. 2018;15(11):e1002711.
13. Chen B, Zhang R, Gan Y, Yang L, Li W. Development and clinical application of radiomics in lung cancer. Radiat Oncol. 2017;12:154.
14. Cong M, Feng H, Ren JL, Xu Q, Cong L, Hou Z, et al. Development of a predictive radiomics model for lymph node metastases in pre-surgical CT-based stage IA non-small cell lung cancer. Lung Cancer. 2020;139:73–9.
15. Zhou H, Dong D, Chen B, Fang M, Cheng Y, Gan Y, et al. Diagnosis of distant metastasis of lung cancer: based on clinical and radiomic features. Transl Oncol. 2017;11(1):31–6.
16. Shaw AT, Yeap BY, Solomon BJ, Riely GJ, Gainor J, Engelman JA, et al. Effect of crizotinib on overall survival in patients with advanced non-small-cell lung cancer harbouring ALK gene rearrangement: a retrospective analysis. Lancet Oncol. 2011;12(11):1004–12.
17. Wu W, Parmar C, Grossmann P, Quackenbush J, Lambin P, Bussink J, et al. Exploratory study to identify radiomics classifiers for lung cancer histology. Front Oncol. 2016;6:71.
18. Diehn M, et al. From the cover: identification of noninvasive imaging surrogates for brain tumor gene-expression modules. Proc Natl Acad Sci USA. 2008;105(13):5213–8. Available from: https://www.ncbi.nlm.nih.gov/pmc/articles/PMC2278224/.
19. Ding H, et al. Radiomics in oncology: a 10-year bibliometric analysis [Internet]. Front Oncol. 11:689802. Available from: https://www.frontiersin.org/articles/10.3389/fonc.2021.689802/full.
20. Löfstedt T, et al. Gray-level invariant Haralick texture features. PLoS One [Internet]. 2019;14:e0212110. Available from: https://journals.plos.org/plosone/article?id=10.1371/journal.pone.0212110.
21. Song SH, Park H, Lee G, Lee HY, Sohn I, Kim HS, et al. Imaging phenotyping using radiomics to predict micropapillary pattern within lung adenocarcinoma. J Thorac Oncol. 2017;12(4):624–32.
22. Ma J, Wang Q, Ren Y, Hu H, Zhao J. Automatic lung nodule classification with radiomics approach. In: Medical imaging 2016: PACS and imaging informatics: next generation and innovations, vol. 9789. SPIE; 2016. p. 26–31.
23. Weiss GJ, Ganeshan B, Miles KA, Campbell DH, Cheung PY, Frank S, et al. Noninvasive image texture analysis differentiates K-ras mutation from pan-wildtype NSCLC and is prognostic. PLoS One. 2014;9(7):e100244.
24. Godoy MCB, Naidich DP. Overview and strategic management of subsolid pulmonary nodules. J Thorac Imaging. 2012;27(4):240–8.

25. de Castro ABG, Ferreirós Domínguez J, Delgado Bolton R, Fernández Pérez C, Cabeza Martínez B, García García-Esquinas M, et al. PET-CT in presurgical lymph node staging in non-small cell lung cancer: the importance of false-negative and false-positive findings. Radiologia. 2017;59(2):147–58.
26. Hawkins S, Wang H, Liu Y, Garcia A, Stringfield O, Krewer H, et al. Predicting malignant nodules from screening CTs. J Thorac Oncol. 2016;11(12):2120–8.
27. Kuo MD, Gollub J, Sirlin CB, Ooi C, Chen X. Radiogenomic analysis to identify imaging phenotypes associated with drug response gene expression programs in hepatocellular carcinoma. J Vasc Interv Radiol. 2007;18(7):821–31.
28. Liu Y, Kim J, Balagurunathan Y, Li Q, Garcia AL, Stringfield O, et al. Radiomic features are associated with EGFR mutation status in lung adenocarcinomas. Clin Lung Cancer. 2016;17(5):441–448.e6.
29. Coroller TP, Agrawal V, Narayan V, Hou Y, Grossmann P, Lee SW, et al. Radiomic phenotype features predict pathological response in non-small cell lung cancer. Radiother Oncol. 2016;119(3):480–6.
30. Coroller TP, Agrawal V, Huynh E, Narayan V, Lee SW, Mak RH, et al. Radiomic-based pathological response prediction from primary tumors and lymph nodes in NSCLC. J Thorac Oncol. 2017;12(3):467–76.
31. Wilson R, Devaraj A. Radiomics of pulmonary nodules and lung cancer. Transl Lung Cancer Res. 2017;6(1):86. Available from: https://pubmed.ncbi.nlm.nih.gov/28331828/.
32. Wang T, Deng J, She Y, Zhang L, Wang B, Ren Y, et al. Radiomics signature predicts the recurrence-free survival in stage I non-small cell lung cancer. Ann Thorac Surg. 2020;109(6):1741–9.
33. Parekh V, Jacobs MA. Radiomics: a new application from established techniques. Expert Rev Precis Med Drug Dev. 2016;1(2):207–26.
34. Chen B, Yang L, Zhang R, Luo W, Li W. Radiomics: an overview in lung cancer management—a narrative review. Ann Transl Med. 2020;8(18):1191.
35. Lambin P, et al. Radiomics: extracting more information from medical images using advanced feature analysis. Eur J Cancer. 2012;48(4):441–6. Available from: https://www.ncbi.nlm.nih.gov/pmc/articles/PMC4533986/.
36. Rogers W, et al. Radiomics: from qualitative to quantitative imaging. Br J Radiol. 2020;93(1108):20190948. Available from: https://www.ncbi.nlm.nih.gov/pmc/articles/PMC7362913/.
37. The National Lung Screening Trial Research Team. Reduced lung-cancer mortality with low-dose computed tomographic screening. N Engl J Med. 2011;365(5):395–409. Available from: https://www.ncbi.nlm.nih.gov/pmc/articles/PMC4356534/.
38. de Koning HJ, et al. Reduced lung-cancer mortality with volume CT screening in a randomized trial. N Engl J Med. 2020;382:503–13. Available from: https://www.nejm.org/doi/10.1056/NEJMoa1911793?url_ver=Z39.88-2003&rfr_id=ori:rid:crossref.org&rfr_dat=cr_pub%20%20 0pubmed.
39. Wu G, Jochems A, Refaee T, Ibrahim A, Yan C, Sanduleanu S, et al. Structural and functional radiomics for lung cancer. Eur J Nucl Med Mol Imaging. 2021;48(12):3961–74
40. Galloway MM. Texture analysis using gray level run lengths. Comput Graph Image Process. 1975;4(2):172–9. Available from: https://www.sciencedirect.com/science/article/abs/pii/S0146664X75800086.
41. Sutton RN, Hall EL. Texture measures for automatic classification of pulmonary disease. IEEE Trans Comput. 1972;C-21(7):667–76. Available from: https://ieeexplore.ieee.org/document/1672165.
42. Lee SH, Lee SM, Goo JM, Kim KG, Kim YJ, Park CM. Usefulness of texture analysis in differentiating transient from persistent part-solid nodules (PSNs): a retrospective study. PLoS One. 2014;9(1):e85167.

Quantitative Techniques in Cardiac MRI

2

Vivek Modi, Aneesh Dhore-Patil, Ming-fang Chao, Su Min Chang, and Dipan Shah

Cardiac Magnetic Resonance

Evaluation of cardiac function is crucial for diagnosis, prognosis, and management in patients with cardiovascular diseases. Cardiac magnetic resonance imaging (CMR) provides high spatial and temporal resolution in the assessment of cardiac function for accurate and reproducible quantitative measurements. This has enabled CMR to become the clinical and research gold standard for quantitative functional assessment. Ventricular functional assessment by CMR is also an area of active research with many emerging sequences and quantitative parameters each with a promise of improving efficiency and granularity. This chapter provides an overview of various techniques used in the acquisition and interpretation of CMR for quantitative cardiac functional assessment.

Technical Aspects of Image Acquisition

It is important to acquire high-quality images for the assessment of systolic function. Various technical considerations for image acquisition are described below.

Gating

Cardiac cine images are generated by synchronizing image acquisition with an electrocardiogram called gating. The duration of the cardiac cycle as it extends between an R-R interval is divided into multiple time intervals called phases. A set of k-space lines are acquired to produce a still image at each phase of the cardiac cycle. As the duration of a phase in a single cardiac cycle is usually not enough to acquire all lines of k-space, it is segmented such that a subset of k-space lines is acquired in each cardiac cycle and the entire image set representing a phase is actually acquired over several cardiac cycles.

The types of gating are as follows (Fig. 2.1):

1. Retrospective gating: It is the preferred gating strategy. The image acquisition and ECG signal are continuously recorded. During image reconstruction, the acquired data is sorted and allocated to specific cardiac phases based on the ECG signal recorded during the scan. This allows for complete coverage of the cardiac

V. Modi · A. Dhore-Patil · M.-f. Chao · S. M. Chang · D. Shah (✉)
Department of Cardiovascular Imaging, The Houston Methodist Hospital, Houston, TX, USA
e-mail: adhore@houstonmethodist.org; cmin-fang@houstonmethodist.org; smchang@houstonmethodist.org; djshah@houstonmethodist.org

R. Gill, P. Rajiah (eds.), *Quantitative Imaging in the Thorax*,
https://doi.org/10.1007/978-3-032-14103-3_2

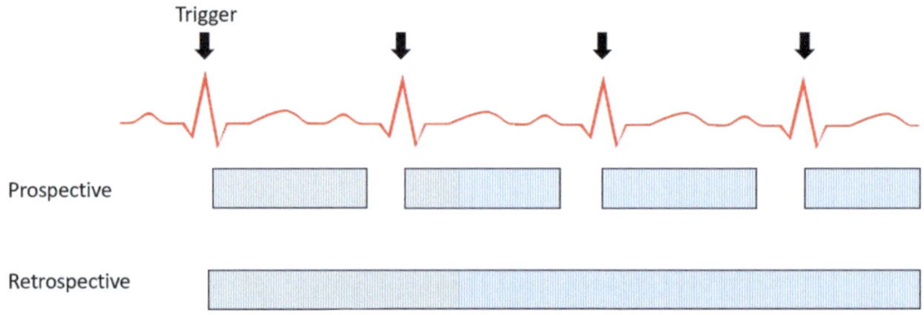

Fig. 2.1 Gating: In the prospective gating, the acquisition is triggered by the R-wave for a set period. No image is acquired at the end of each cardiac cycle. In retrospective gating images are acquired continuously throughout multiple cardiac cycles and reconstructed using ECG data

cycle but is susceptible to artifacts from irregular heart rhythms.

2. Prospective gating: The image acquisition is triggered at the onset of an R wave on the ECG signal. Acquisition continues for a prespecified period. The image acquisition time window is set long enough to allow for adequate coverage of the cardiac cycle but kept shorter than usual R-R variation to ensure consistent triggering into the next cycle. This gating strategy is useful in the presence of arrhythmias but comes at the cost of incomplete coverage of the cardiac cycle.

Temporal and Spatial Resolution

The image of a given phase is the average cardiac activity for the duration of the phase. Therefore, shorter phases lead to better temporal resolution. Spatial resolution depends on the number of k-space lines per image. In general, an improvement in either spatial resolution, temporal resolution, or breath-hold time can only be made at the expense of one of the other parameters. Therefore, careful consideration must be given to balancing these factors based on the specific clinical goals and constraints of the cardiac MRI study. Usually, a temporal resolution of up to 45 ms and an in plane spatial resolution of up to 3 mm can be tolerated without significantly affecting cardiac functional parameters [1, 2].

Sequences

There are two main sequences used for cine imaging.

1. Steady-state free precession (SSFP): Steady-state free precession is the preferred sequence for cine imaging. It uses repeated excitation pulses to generate a freely precessing constant magnetization [3]. The steady state of transverse magnetization allows for rapid continuous readout for faster image acquisition during gating. The images generated are T2 over T1-weighted resulting in a bright signal for blood and a dark signal for myocardium. Therefore, this sequence provides excellent contrast between the blood and myocardium and has a high signal-to-noise ratio. The limitation of SSFP includes its susceptibility to field inhomogeneity and motion, which can lead to image blurring or ghosting.
2. Spoiled gradient echo (GRE): Spoiled gradient echo uses repeated radiofrequency (RF) excitation pulses with a spoiler gradient to generate a T1-weighted image. This sequence has a lower signal-to-noise ratio. While it also results in bright blood signal, it has a lower contrast between blood and myocardium and is susceptible to slow flow artifact. Also, the acquisition time of each k-space line using GRE is longer than SSFP. It is however less sensitive to field inhomogeneity compared to SSFP and can be useful to obtain diagnostic images in the presence of a cardiac implantable electronic device [4].

Acceleration Techniques

Acceleration techniques are methods used to speed up image acquisition while maintaining adequate temporal and spatial resolution. These techniques are particularly useful for patients who struggle with breath holding. Commonly used acceleration techniques are described below:

1. Parallel imaging (PI): Parallel imaging utilizes multiple radiofrequency receiver coils and the spatial sensitivity information they provide to accelerate image acquisition. This technique allows for faster imaging by undersampling k-space data while using the sensitivity information from the coils to reconstruct the full image [5]. SENSE (sensitivity encoding) and GRAPPA (GeneRalized Autocalibrating Partially Parallel Acquisitions) are two popular PI techniques. SENSE uses a calibration scan to estimate the coil sensitivities and reconstruct images with reduced acquisition time, while GRAPPA estimates the missing k-space data based on the correlation between adjacent coil elements. PI may predispose to higher image noise and artifacts, particularly in areas far from the coil elements or regions with poor coil sensitivity.
2. Compressed sensing (CS): Compressed sensing is a mathematical technique that exploits the sparsity or compressibility of the image data to reduce the amount of acquired data while still maintaining image quality. Similar to PI, CS-MRI speeds up the acquisition process by undersampling k-space data and is also susceptible to noise and artifacts due to data undersampling of k-space. Additionally, CS adds computational requirements during the image reconstruction process. A meta-analysis comparing traditional segmented cine acquisition with accelerated image acquisition using compressed sensing showed comparable LV mass and volumes with only a slight underestimation of ejection fraction but with a significant reduction in breath hold time (33%–67%) and total scan time [6].
3. Partial Fourier: Partial Fourier exploits the fact that k-space is symmetric, and only a fraction of the k-space data needs to be acquired to reconstruct the full image. This technique also leads to a reduced signal-to-noise ratio and may introduce artifacts due to undersampling.
4. Non-cartesian k-space acquisition: Usually k-space is acquired along rectilinear grides, but non-cartesian k-space acquisition methods sample k-space along nonlinear trajectories. Common non-cartesian trajectories include radial and spiral sampling patterns. These non-cartesian sampling trajectories allow for faster image acquisition but require more sophisticated image reconstruction algorithms and hardware configurations that are not always readily available.

   Real-time imaging: As opposed to traditional segmented k-space acquisition across multiple cardiac cycles, real-time imaging techniques aim to acquire and reconstruct cardiac images in a single heartbeat. Maintaining adequate temporal resolution during real-time imaging invariably leads to undersampling of k-space requiring the use of various acceleration techniques such as parallel imaging or compressed sensing to reconstruct images with adequate spatial resolution.

   Real-time imaging can provide diagnostic quality images for patients with significant arrhythmia, motion, or issues with breath-holding [7].

Assessment of Volumes, Mass, and Function

Quantitative assessment of systolic function starts with an assessment of cardiac volumes and mass. Cardiac MRI is the gold standard in the assessment of systolic function due to its ability to obtain accurate and reproducible cardiac volumes.

Slice selection: Multiple regularly spaced short-axis slices are selected to cover the entire myocardium from base to apex (Fig. 2.2). These slices are typically acquired in a stack fashion, with each slice acquired during a separate breath-hold to minimize motion artifacts. In addition, four-chamber, two-chamber, and three-chamber views are commonly acquired for qualitative

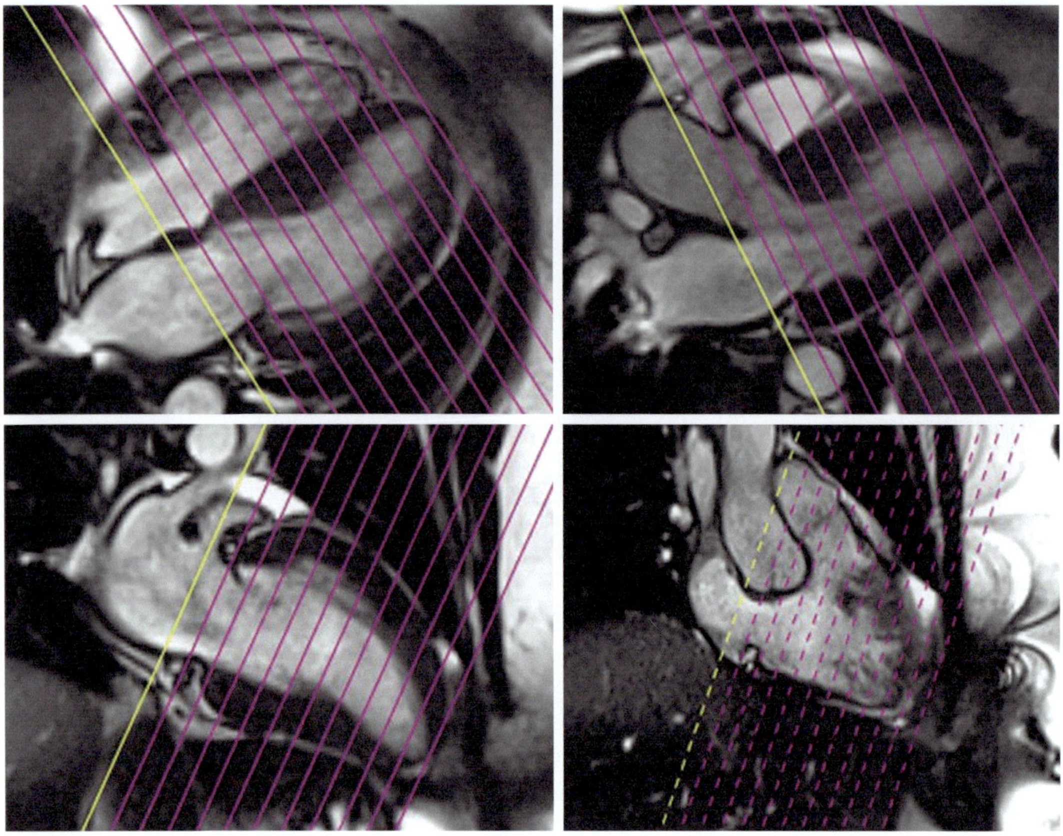

Fig. 2.2 A stack of short-axis slices is acquired to cover the entire myocardium and ventricular cavities from base to apex

assessment of regional wall motion abnormalities and global cardiac function.

Phase selection: Short-axis and long-axis cine images are visually assessed to choose the correct end-diastolic phase when the global ventricular volumes are largest and the end-systolic phase when the global ventricular volumes are smallest for analysis (Fig. 2.3). Choosing the incorrect phase can lead to an underestimation of end-diastolic volume (EDV) and an overestimation of end-systolic volume (ESV); thus, resulting in underestimation of ventricular stroke volume.

Planimetry: Planimetry of biventricular endocardial and left ventricular epicardial borders is performed on each short-axis slice at both end-diastole and end-systole using specialized software tools (Fig. 2.3). Care must be taken in planimetry of basal slices as mitral and aortic valves can make it challenging to accurately delineate the endocardial borders. In addition, the base of the heart descends during systole so the systolic basal most slice is usually more apical than the diastolic basal most slice (Fig. 2.4). A simple strategy to follow during planimetry of the basal slices is to planimeter the endocardium wherever ventricular muscle is seen. Left ventricular outflow tract should be included in the LV cavity. LV trabeculae and papillary muscles should ideally be excluded from the cavity. It is especially important in cases with LV hypertrophy [8]. This approach leads to a lower LV EDV, ESV, and a higher EF [9]. However, not all post-processing software provide semiautomated or automated delineation of the trabeculae and papillary muscles. In these cases, laboratories may choose to include them in the cavity to avoid time exhaustive manual planimetry. It is important to consult reference values derived from a similar

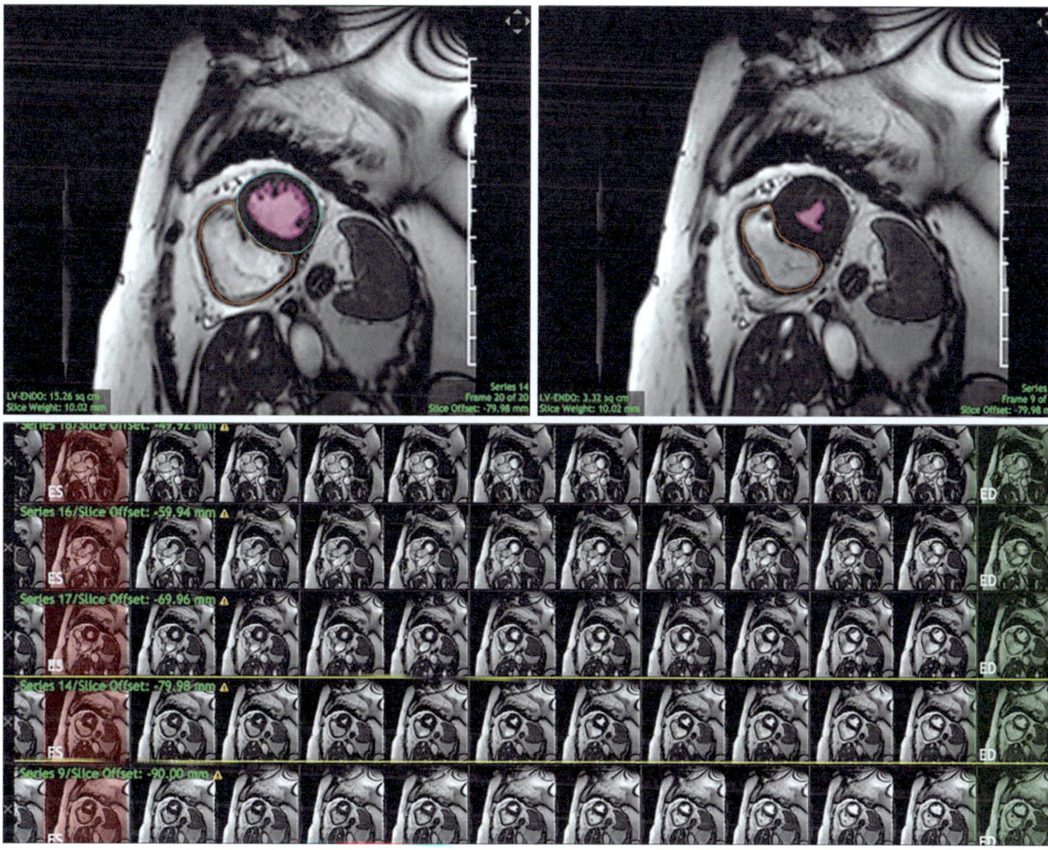

Fig. 2.3 End-diastolic (largest cavity size) and end-systolic (smallest cavity size) frames are selected for each short-axis slice. Endocardial borders are planimetered for both ventricles. Epicardial borders are planimetered for the left ventricle. As shown in the figure, we exclude papillary muscles from the left ventricular cavity

post-processing strategy during image interpretation [10].

Volume calculation: Once the planimetry of the endocardial and epicardial borders is complete at end-diastole and end-systole for each individual slice, modified Simpson's rule is commonly used to calculate the volumes and LV mass (Fig. 2.5). In this method the planimetered area from each slice is multiplied by the sum of slice thickness and the interslice distance to obtain the volume of each slice. All the slice volumes are summed to obtain total EDV and ESV.

Mass calculation: To calculate LV mass, LV epicardial and endocardial tracings along with slice thickness are used by the software to obtain myocardial volumes. These volumes are then multiplied by the density of the myocardial tissue to calculate myocardial mass.

$$\text{LV mass} = \text{LV myocardial volume} \times \text{myocardial density}\left(1.05\text{g}/\text{ml}\right)$$

EF calculation: Left ventricular ejection fraction is calculated by dividing the difference between EDV and ESV by EDV. The formula is as follows:

$$\text{EF} = \text{EDV} - \text{ESV}/\text{EDV}$$

Internal checks: Quantitatively derived EF should be compared with a visual assessment of global ventricular function to ensure the accuracy and reliability of the measurements. In addition, the stroke volume derived from quantitative ventricular volumes should be comparable to inde-

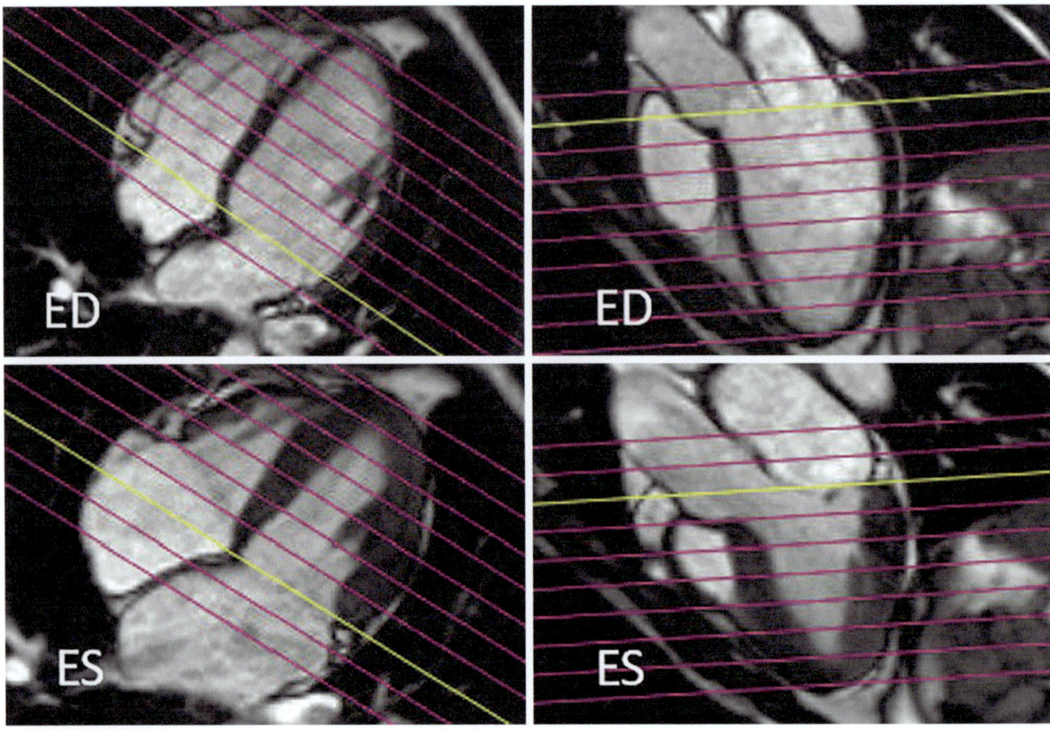

Fig. 2.4 Annular descent causes the systolic basal most slice to shift toward the apex compared to the diastolic basal most slice. *ED* end-diastole, *ES* end-systole

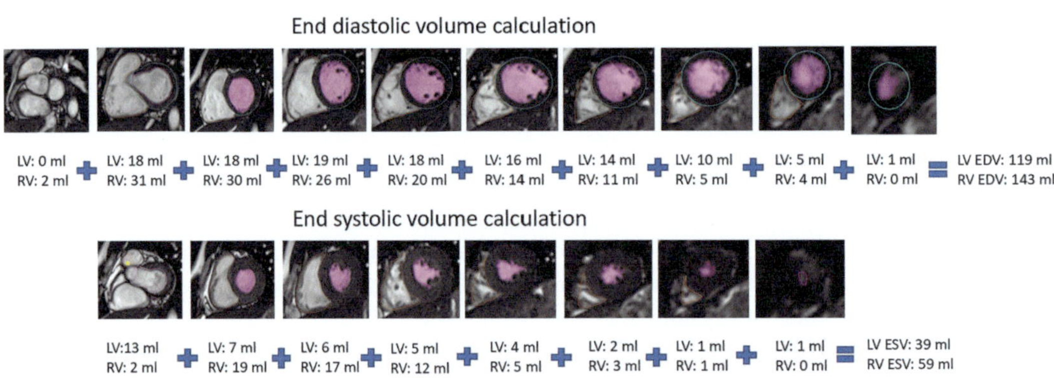

Fig. 2.5 Simpson's rule: Planimetered area from each slice is multiplied by the slice thickness to obtain the volume for each slice. All the slice volumes are summed to obtain total enddiastolic volumes (EDV) and end-systolic volumes (ESV) for the left ventricle (LV) and the right ventricle (RV)

pendently derived stroke volume from phase-contrast MRI. It is recommended that all MRI laboratories incorporate data from ten healthy individuals without valvular regurgitation and shunts into their validation process. By achieving comparable calculated LV and RV stroke volumes with phase-contrast MRI measurements of aortic and pulmonary flows, respectively, laboratories can ensure the accuracy of their assessments.

Regional Function

Short-axis and long-axis cine images are visually assessed for thickening. A 16-segment model of

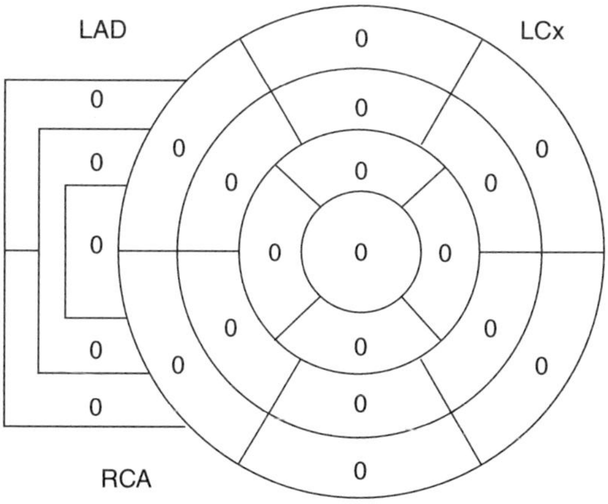

Fig. 2.6 Polar plot for visual representation of regional wall motion using a 17-segment model

the heart is used to assign a wall motion score to each segment based on thickening. Scores of 0, 1, 2, and 3 are assigned for normokinesis, hypokinesis, akinesis, and dyskinesis, respectively. A polar plot is displayed for a visual representation of the regional score for each segment (Fig. 2.6). The regional score of each segment is summed to obtain the total regional wall motion score (RWMS). Higher scores represent a worse cardiac function while lower scores represent good function.

Special Circumstances

1. Cardiac implantable electronic device: The presence of a device can affect the accuracy of cardiac MRI measurements, as it can cause artifacts and hinder visualization of certain structures including endocardial and epicardial borders (Fig. 2.7). A simple maneuver of raising the arm ipsilateral to the device can sometimes reduce the artifact by increasing the distance between the device and the heart. Additionally, field inhomogeneity in the presence of a CIED can cause significant artifact in SSFP cine images, in which case GRE sequence can be used to obtain diagnostic cine images [4].
2. Arrhythmia: In the presence of arrhythmia, ECG gating may be challenging and can result in unreliable measurements of LV volumes and mass and therefore EF. It is important to carefully monitor and assess the ECG signal during the imaging acquisition to identify any arrhythmia that may affect gating. Arrhythmia rejection can be employed at the cost of prolonged breath hold time during retrospective gating to avoid gating artifacts, alternatively, prospective ECG-triggered acquisitions can be considered. With significant R-R variations such as in atrial fibrillation with variable rate, it may be necessary to use real-time imaging sequence.
3. Inability to breath hold: Respiratory motion can affect the accuracy of cardiac MRI measurements. Oftentimes it may not be possible for the patients to hold their breath due to morbidity. Motion artifacts can lead to misalignment of the imaging planes and distortions in the myocardial borders during gating, affecting the accuracy of volume and mass calculations. Abovementioned acceleration techniques can be employed to expedite image acquisition and mitigate the effects of patient motion. If acceleration techniques are unable to provide diagnostic gated cine images real-time imaging can be tried.

Strengths of Cardiac MRI

1. Accuracy: The key strength of MRI in the calculation of LV volumes and mass compared to other noninvasive techniques is its nonreliance on geometric assumptions. This allows for more accurate and reliable measurements, particularly in the presence of structural abnormalities or distorted ventricular geometry. This is especially important in assessing right ventricular (RV) function due to its complex geometry [11, 12]. Validation studies that used cardiac phantoms, animal models, and comparisons with autopsy measurements have shown excellent agreement between MRI-derived volumes and actual volumes [13–16].
2. Reproducibility: Multiple studies have shown small intra-observer, inter-observer, and interstudy variability in the assessment of cardiac volumes and ejection fraction with cardiac

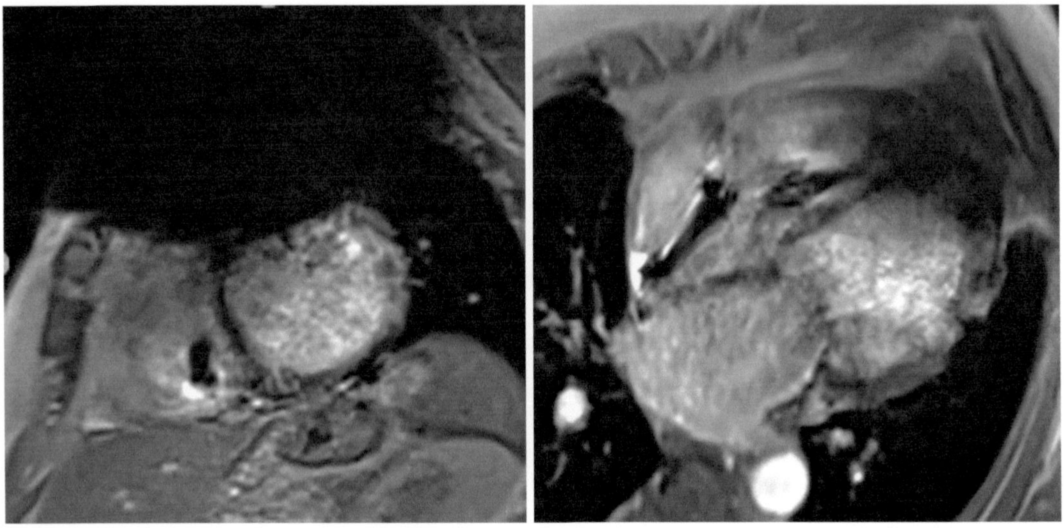

Fig. 2.7 Signal void caused by an implantable cardioverter-defibrillator obscuring part of ventricular myocardium and ventricular cavity

MRI [12, 17, 18]. Reproducibility allows for reliable assessment of disease progression or treatment response over time. Additionally, it translates to smaller sample size requirements to assess for clinically meaningful change of volumes and EF in research studies, making cardiac MRI a cost-effective tool for clinical trials and longitudinal studies [19, 20].

3. Quality: Cardiac MRI provides excellent spatial and temporal resolution along with the ability to visualize the entire heart in multiple planes to avoid foreshortening. This provides high-quality images to assess asymmetrical wall thickening and regional wall motion abnormalities.

Reference Values

Cardiac MRI-derived reference values for left and right ventricular volumes and mass exhibit variability across populations. This heterogeneity stems from several key factors, including age, sex, body surface area, and methodological variations in tracing, such as the inclusion or exclusion of papillary muscles. Recognizing this inter-group variability is important for the accurate interpretation of individual patient measurements. These reference values can be found in a recently published SCMR-endorsed document [21]. However, some key reference values from the document are presented (Tables 2.1, 2.2 and 2.3).

Diastolic Function

Evaluation of diastolic function using CMR is an active area of research [22]. One of the key challenges is the lack of standardized and widely accepted parameters. Some notable techniques and parameters are described below:

1. Phase contrast CMR (PC-CMR): This retrospectively gated sequence utilizes velocity encoding to obtain flow and velocity data. A plane is proscribed perpendicular to the transmitral flow yielding an en-face view of the mitral orifice during diastole. By outlining the valve, *E* (early diastolic filling) and *A* (late diastolic filling) velocities, as well as their ratio (*E*/*A*), can be obtained. PC-CMR can also be used to measure tissue velocity at the basal septum (*E′*). Although CMR's temporal resolution (30–40 ms) lags behind echocardiography (10 ms), small studies suggest a

Table 2.1 Left ventricular parameters in the adult for men and women (ages 18–83), papillary muscles included in left ventricular mass [21]

	Men				Women			
Parameter	*n*	Mean	SD	LL–UL[a]	*n*	Mean	SD	LL–UL[a]
LVEDV (ml)	464	155	30	95–215	485	123	22	78–167
LVEDV/BSA (ml/m²)	875	79	15	50–108	931	73	12	50–96
LVESV (ml)	464	55	15	25–85	485	43	11	21–64
LVESV/BSA (ml/m²)	875	29	9	11–47	931	25	7	10–40
LVSV (ml)	410	103	21	61–145	432	83	16	52–114
LVSV/BSA (ml/m²)	701	52	10	33–72	758	49	8	33–64
LVEF (%)	875	64	8	49–79	931	66	7	52–79
LVM (g)	464	121	28	66–176	485	83	21	41–125
LVM/BSA (g/m²)	805	62	11	39–85	861	49	10	30–68
LVCO (l/min)	91	5.6	1.1	3.4–7.8	89	4.5	0.9	2.7–6.3
LVCI (l/min/m²)	91	3.0	0.6	1.8–4.2	89	2.9	0.5	1.9–3.9
LVM/LVEDV (g/ml)	287	0.7	0.1	0.4–0.9	327	0.6	0.1	0.3–0.8

n number of study subjects included in the weighted mean values, *mean* pooled weighted mean, *SD* pooled standard deviation, *LL* lower limit, *UL* upper limit, *LV* left ventricular, *EDV* end-diastolic volume, *ESV* end-systolic volume, *SV* stroke volume, *EF* ejection fraction, *LVM* left ventricular mass, *CO* cardiac output, *CI* cardiac index, *BSA* body surface area

[a]Calculated as mean ± 2 × SD

Table 2.2 Right ventricular parameters for adult men by age group, papillary muscles included in right ventricular volume [21]

	20–29 years		30–39 years		40–49 years		50–59 years	
Parameter	*n*	Mean ± SD (LL–UL)[a]	*n*	Mean ± SD (LL–UL)[a]	*n*	Mean ± SD (LL–UL)[a]	*n*	Mean ± SD (LL–UL)[a]
RVEDV/BSA (ml/m²)	47	78 ± 12 (55–101)	51	76 ± 12 (51–100)	46	74 ± 14 (46–102)	46	69 ± 13 (42–95)
RVESV/BSA (ml/m²)	47	33 ± 12 (10–56)	51	31 ± 8 (15–48)	46	29 ± 8 (13–45)	46	28 ± 8 (11–44)
RVSV/BSA (ml/m²)	37	46 ± 9 (28–63)	33	45 ± 12 (22–69)	35	47 ± 11 (24–69)	37	42 ± 10 (22–62)
RVEF (%)	47	56 ± 11 (34–78)	51	58 ± 9 (39–77)	46	60 ± 8 (44–76)	46	61 ± 8 (44–78)

n number of study subjects included in the weighted mean values, *mean* pooled weighted mean, *SD* pooled standard deviation, *LL* lower limit, *UL* upper limit, *RV* right ventricular, *EDV* end-diastolic volume, *ESV* end-systolic volume, *SV* stroke volume, *EF* ejection fraction, *BSA* body surface area

[a]Calculated as mean ± 2 × SD

good correlation between CMR-derived *E*/*A* and *E*/*E'* ratios with echocardiographic values [23, 24].

2. Myocardial tagging: This technique involves applying specialized markers or "tags" to the myocardium to track its motion throughout the cardiac cycle. These tags are created and tracked using a specialized sequence called complementary spatial modulation of magnetization (CSPAMM). Myocardial tagging enables the quantification of several parameters relevant to diastolic function, including early diastolic peak strain rate, time to peak diastolic strain, and the diastolic twisting/untwisting motion (torsion) of the heart. Notably, a sub-study within the MESA population revealed that CMR-derived diastolic assessment through myocardial tagging provides a predictive model for identifying patients at high risk of developing heart failure and atrial fibrillation within 8 years [25].
3. Feature tracking CMR (FT CMR): FT MRI is a post-processing technique applied to cine CMR images using image registration

Table 2.3 Right ventricular parameters for adult women by age group, papillary muscles included in right ventricular volume [21]

Parameter	20–29 years n	20–29 years Mean ± SD (LL–UL)[a]	30–39 years n	30–39 years Mean ± SD (LL–UL)[a]	40–49 years n	40–49 years Mean ± SD (LL–UL)[a]	50–59 years n	50–59 years Mean ± SD (LL–UL)[a]
RVEDV/BSA (ml/m^2)	47	78 ± 12 (55–101)	51	76 ± 12 (51–100)	46	74 ± 14 (46–102)	46	69 ± 13 (42–95)
RVESV/BSA (ml/m^2)	47	33 ± 12 (10–56)	51	31 ± 8 (15–48)	46	29 ± 8 (13–45)	46	28 ± 8 (11–44)
RVSV/BSA (ml/m^2)	37	46 ± 9 (28–63)	33	45 ± 12 (22–69)	35	47 ± 11 (24–69)	37	42 ± 10 (22–62)
RVEF (%)	47	56 ± 11 (34–78)	51	58 ± 9 (39–77)	46	60 ± 8 (44–76)	46	61 ± 8 (44–78)

n number of study subjects included in the weighted mean values, weighted mean, standard deviation, *LL* lower limit, *UL* upper limit, *RV* right ventricular, *EDV* end-diastolic volume, *ESV* end-systolic volume, *SV* stroke volume, *EF* ejection fraction, *BSA* body surface area

[a]Calculated as mean ± 2 × SD

algorithms to track prominent myocardial features usually at the blood myocardium interface and calculate strain. This technique can be used to obtain regional and atrial strain values and can provide additional insights into regional diastolic function [26].

Other advanced MRI techniques that can be used to assess tissue deformation and strain include SENC (strain encoding) and DENSE (displacement encoding with stimulated echoes). Additionally, promising new techniques are under development. Four-dimensional flow CMR is an advanced technique that allows detailed visualization of three-dimensional blood flow patterns during diastole, providing new perspectives on hemodynamics during diastole.

Although the research into the validation of a reliable and practical parameter to assess diastolic function is ongoing, the modality's current strength lies in its unparalleled ability to (1) delineate cardiac structure to reveal potential structural contributors to diastolic dysfunction and (2) Characterize myocardial tissue using techniques such as T1 mapping and late gadolinium enhancement to refine diagnosis in patients with established diastolic dysfunction.

Computed Tomography

In routine practice, cardiac computed tomography (CCT) is used for assessment of ventricular volumes and function primarily in cases where CMR is not feasible like patients with left ventricular assist devices or in patients undergoing cardiac CT for other indications (e.g., transcatheter aortic valve implantation evaluation or selected congenital heart disease evaluations or patients with severe claustrophobia).

Image Acquisition Protocol

For volumetric analysis with CT, two approaches can be used depending on the type of scanner.

1. Conventional CT: Conventional CT scanners, use rotating X-ray tubes and detectors with a conventional fan-beam based projection. They have narrower detector arrays with shorter *z*-axis coverage (up to 4 cm); hence, they require acquisitions from multiple heartbeats to cover the heart. To acquire multiple heartbeats, various ECG gating methods can be used, but retrospective ECG gating is the most used method.

2. Wide-detector CT: Wide-detector volume CT scanners employ a flat panel detector and conebeam-based projection. This allows greater *z*-axis coverage up to 16 cm, resulting in a single beat volume acquisition of the entire heart. This comes with the advantage of avoiding step artifacts and shorter breath hold time for the patient. The caveats of this approach are ensuring that the heart is in the center of the image as due to the divergence of the conebeam, the peripheries of the image have incomplete sampling and may result in decreased spatial resolution. ECG gating is still used for image acquisition, but only prospective gating is used as acquisition of images occurs in a single heartbeat.

Gating

1. Retrospective gating: In conventional CT scanners, retrospective ECG gating CT is essential in ascertaining accurate EDV and ESV. It involves simultaneous acquisition of ECG signal along with constant X-ray emission during a slow-pitch spiral/helical scan acquisition. The ECG signal is used to retrospectively determine the exact phase of the cardiac cycle, allowing for reconstruction of multiple images corresponding to different phases. These images are then used for volumetric assessment of the ventricles. The constant, high radiation exposure results in oversampled datasets and high temporal resolution. This comes at the expense of high radiation exposure for relatively small area of coverage in the *z*-axis (10–15 cm for a normal adult heart).
2. Prospective ECG gating with padding: This technique entails prospective ECG-triggered data acquisition during desired time periods corresponding to end-systole and end-diastole along with additional low-dose scan during flanking portions of cardiac cycle (padding) to obtain adequate coverage of entire cardiac cycle but with a lower radiation dose. This method provides sufficient coverage of systole and diastole to derive ESV and EDV. However, a study by Plass et al. has shown that padding may lead to similar radiation exposure when compared to retrospective gating [27].
3. ECG gating with dose modulation: This technique is performed to reduce radiation exposure and involves radiation dose modulation during acquisition. A large portion of the cardiac cycle is acquired at a low radiation dose (20%) and selective portions of interest are acquired at full radiation dose (e.g., end-systole 35%–45% and end-diastole 65%–75%). The X-ray tube can be turned off between heartbeats as well. This can be done with prospective gating or retrospective gating. With prospective gating in a small cohort of patients, this approach has been shown to provide comparable volumetric measurements when compared to CMR with minimal radiation exposure [28].

ECG editing: ECG editing can be utilized in retrospective gating alone to improve the accuracy of CT for volumetric assessment. It involves the manual adjustment of the ECG signal to correct for irregular heart rhythms or ectopic beats, ensuring that the reconstructed images correspond to the desired phases of the cardiac cycle. This is particularly important in patients with arrhythmias or irregular heartbeats, as inaccurate ECG signals can lead to misalignment of images and result in erroneous measurements of ventricular volumes. However, manual removal of ectopic beats may lead to data loss and corruption of images and hence inaccuracies with EDV and ESV measurements.

Premedication: Lowering the heart rate with medications such as beta blockers and calcium channel blockers is ideal for coronary assessment, but when utilizing cardiac CT for ejection fraction assessment, the use of these agents may have a negative ionotropic impact on the ventricular function and may affect the clinically applicability of volumetric assessment. Ivabradine, a medication which selectively inhibits I-f current in the sinoatrial node, reduces heart rate without affecting ventricular function and contractility maybe an effective alternative if the patient has a high baseline heart rate and ventricular assessment by CT is desired. However, currently, the cost of the medication limits routine use in cardiac CT.

Spatial and Temporal Resolution

Spatial resolution: The spatial resolution of image acquisition is a function of the detector size and the number of detector elements. Spatial resolution of a CT image depends on scanner geometry and cannot be changed as in CMR. Modern CT scanners acquire data with a fixed spatial resolution of 0.5–0.6 mm, which allows for highly accurate isotropic voxel reconstruction that can be used for accurate multiplanar reformatting of images. This enables accurate visualization of endocardial borders and precise assessment of anatomical structures in various planes.

Temporal resolution: The temporal resolution is dependent on the gantry rotation time of the CT scanner which is the time taken for the gantry of a CT scanner to complete 180° rotation around the patient. It is dependent on the scanner's ability to capture images quickly and accurately. In dual source scanners, gantry rotation time is essentially halved, resulting in improved temporal resolution for cardiac imaging. With dual source CT scanners, temporal resolution can be as low as 66 ms, whereas with wide-detector single-source CT scanners it is approximately 120 ms. This worse temporal resolution of CT (when compared to CMR and echo) can lead to higher ESV measurement [29]. In patients with heart rates ranging in between 60 and 70 bpm, the temporal resolution of cardiac CT is sufficient for accurate assessment of ventricular volumes. However, in patients with higher heart rates or arrhythmias, the accuracy of ventricular volume assessment is suboptimal. To ensure every phase of the cardiac cycle is captured, acquisition time can be lengthened to sample multiple heart beats and increase the accuracy of ventricular volume assessment, but this comes at the expense of greater radiation exposure.

Assessment of Volumes and Mass

1. Segmentation: Threshold and contour-based algorithms use attenuation thresholds defined as the differences in attenuation between the blood pool and myocardium, enabling the digital separation of these structures. Following this, contour detection algorithms are utilized to outline the endocardial borders, providing accurate measurements of the ventricular volumes. The reliability of this technique is dependent on adequate contrast opacification of the LV cavity; hence, contrast optimization in terms of dose and timing of the scan is imperative. Adequate contrast threshold for accurate segmentation is at least 150–200 HU within the LV cavity. Similarly, volumes can be defined for other cardiac chambers (Fig. 2.8). High attenuation materials like dense contrast, intracardiac metallic devices (e.g., pacemakers and mechanical valves) can introduce error in measurement (Fig. 2.9).
   While these automated or semiautomated methods significantly reduce the manual labor involved in contouring, there are nuances in the threshold selection and contour initiation, which may introduce variability in the measurements. It is crucial for the clinical user to

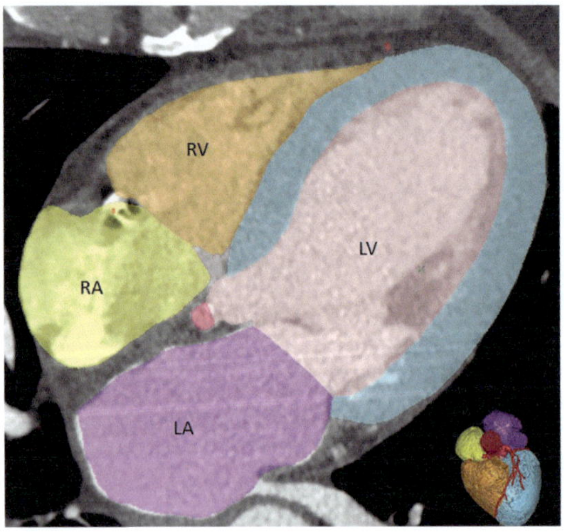

Fig. 2.8 Thresholding and contouring applied to other cardiac structures (*RA* right atrium, *LA* left atrium, *RV* right ventricle, and *LV* left ventricle)

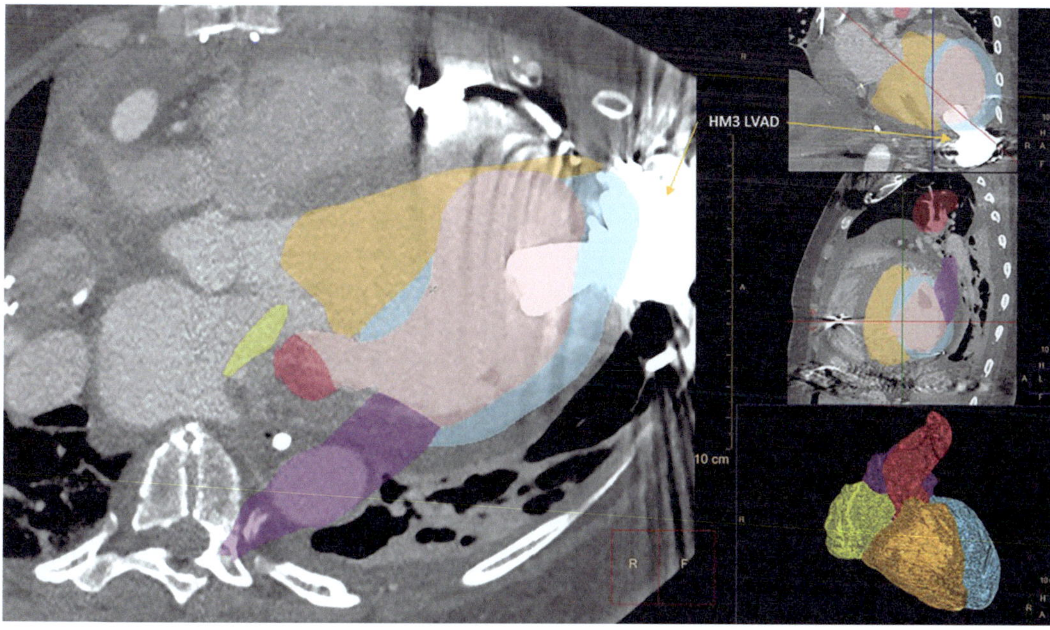

Fig. 2.9 Errors in automated segmentation as a result of poor contrast opacification and the presence of a metallic device (LVAD). In these cases, manual contouring can be performed to correctly identify endocardial borders (*HM3 LVAD* HeartMate 3™ left ventricular assist device)

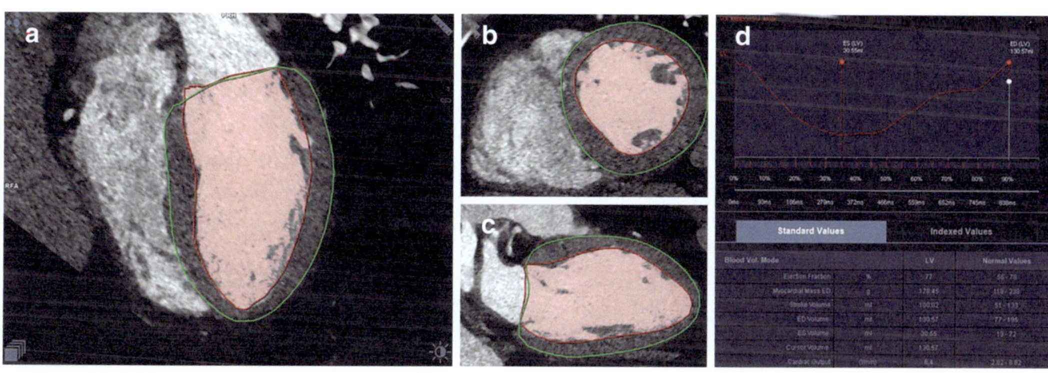

Fig. 2.10 Automated thresholding and contouring performed on post-processing software. Figures (**a–c**) represent the left ventricular four-chamber view, short-axis view, and two-chamber view, respectively. With multiplanar reconstruction, multiple planes can be reconstructed to verify the accuracy of contours. Figure (**d**) represents the calculated volumes and mass with a time-volume curve representing volume over all phases of the cardiac cycle

review and adjust these automated delineations as needed to ensure accuracy and consistency in the volumetric assessment (Fig. 2.10). For example, in some softwares, the mitral annular plane (LV inlet) needs to be reviewed for accurate delineation of the LV from the left atrium. Depending on if thresholding is done alone or combined with contouring, papillary muscles can be excluded or included in LV volume assessment. As with CMR, consistency in either exclusion or inclusion is vital for reproducibility.

In recent years, there have been advancements in deep-learning segmentation techniques that have shown strong agreement with manual segmentation in adults with coronary heart disease [30]. Currently, it is being used for coronary disease assessment but can improve the workflow and accuracy of ventricular volume assessment.

2. Calculation of ventricular volumes: As data is reconstructed into isotropic voxels, volumetric assessment by CT is done by multiplying the number of voxels within the segmented volume by the volume of each voxel. For example, if the LV cavity in the end systolic phase consists of 500 voxels acquired at a spatial resolution of 0.5 mm, the volume can be calculated as 500 voxels × $(0.5\ \text{mm})^3$ = 62.5 ml. The accuracy of volume assessment by CT depends on the spatial resolution of the acquired data and the proper delineation of the region of interest. The highest possible spatial resolution allows for accurate endocardial border definition and minimum partial volume averaging at the blood-pool myocardial interface. Utilization of the time volume curve constructed from the calculated volume of each phase can be correlated with ECG changes to assess for arrhythmic artifacts (Figs. 2.11 and 2.12).
3. Calculation of ventricular mass: Thresholding and contouring are also used in accurate epicardial and endocardial border definition yielding myocardial volume by multiplying the number of myocardial voxels with individual voxel volume. Like CMR, myocardial mass is calculated by multiplying the myocardial volume by myocardial density.

Diastolic Function

Diastolic function assessment by CT is still evolving and not used outside of research. Using time volume curves, changes in LV volume can be tracked across the phases of the cardiac cycle to derive trans mitral velocities (Fig. 2.11) [31]. Left atrial and left ventricular strain can also be tracked using CT with comparable results with 2D echocardiography [32].

Comparison of Modalities

When directly compared CT-derived volumes and ejection fraction correlate well with CMR-derived measurements (Table 2.4) [29, 33–37]. The 2D echocardiography (2DE)-derived volumes and ejection fraction, on the other hand, tend to underestimate the true values and can be limited by foreshortening and poor acoustic windows. The 3D echocardiography (3DE)- and contrast echocardiography-derived volumes and ejection fraction show better agreement with cardiac MRI measurements compared to 2D echocardiography. In 1 meta-analysis of 23 studies, the pooled biases ±2 standard deviations for 3DE

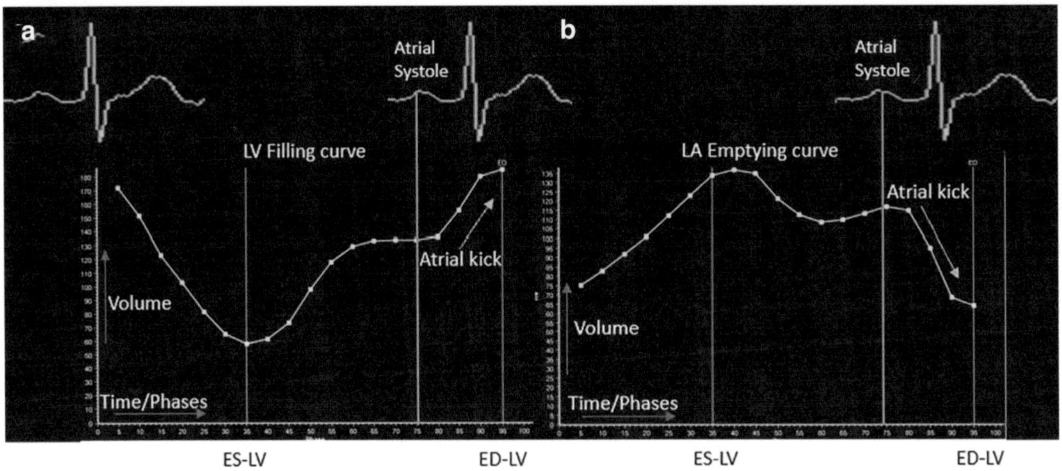

Fig. 2.11 (**a**) ECG correlation with the time volume curve of LV filling in the retrospectively gated study. In normal sinus rhythm, the atrial kick is clearly seen which can help in the accuracy of ESV and EDV assessment. (**b**) LA emptying curve in the same patient. This can be used in the assessment of diastolic function by CT (*LV* left ventricle, *LA* left atrium)

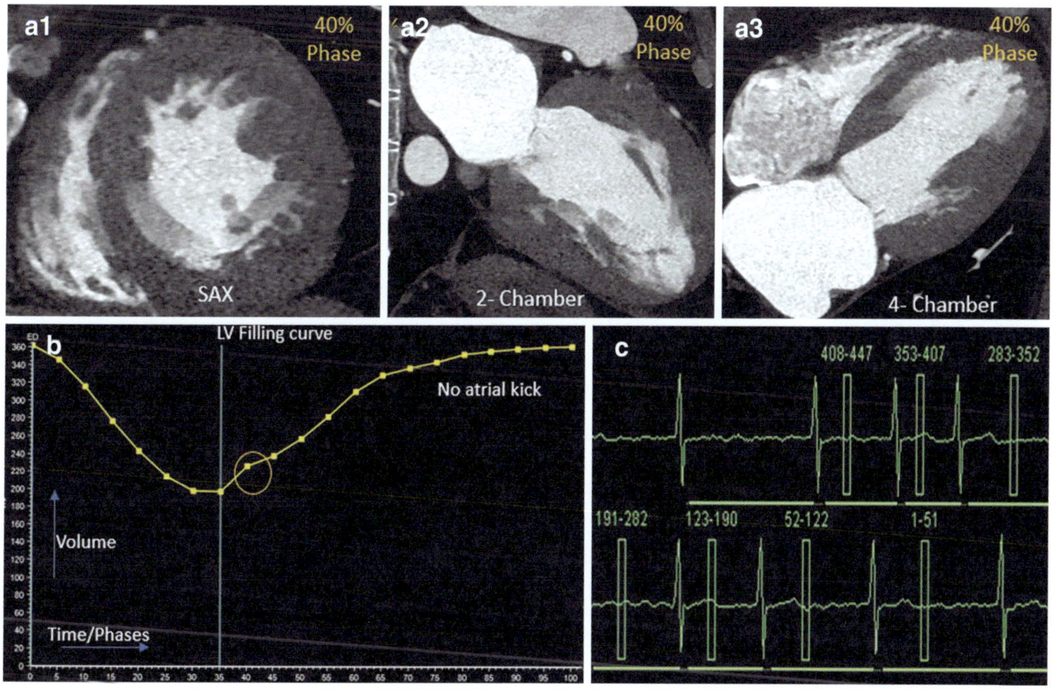

Fig. 2.12 (**a1** **3**) demonstrate artifact from irregular heart rhythm on the 40% phase of the cardiac cycle. Automated endocardial border tracing can be inaccurate in these cases. (**b**) The time-volume curve in the same patient, notice the lack of atrial kick which alludes to the presence of atrial fibrillation. (**c**) ECG for the same patient confirming atrial fibrillation (*LV* left ventricle)

Table 2.4 Studies comparing cardiac coronary tomography (CT) and cardiac magnetic resonance (CMR) in the assessment of cardiac function [29, 33–37]

Title	First author (et al.)	Year	Number of patients	Conclusion
Evaluating global and regional left ventricular function in patients with reperfused acute myocardial infarction by 64-slice multidetector CT	Sarwar et al.	2009	21	64-slice CT (MDCT) provides an accurate and reproducible measurement of regional and global LV function in patients with reperfused acute myocardial infarction
Multi-detector row cardiac computed tomography accurately quantifies right and left ventricular size and function compared with cardiac magnetic resonance	Raman et al.	2006	26	Cardiac CT accurately quantifies LV size and function, with strong correlation with CMR measurements over a wide range of left ventricular function
Quantitative assessment of left ventricular size and function: Side-by-side comparison of real-time three-dimensional echocardiography and computed tomography with magnetic resonance reference	Sugeng et al.	2006	31	CT significantly overestimated end-diastolic and end-systolic volumes compared to CMR, resulting in a small but significant bias in ejection fraction

(continued)

Table 2.4 (continued)

Title	First author (et al.)	Year	Number of patients	Conclusion
Left ventricular functional analysis using 64-slice multidetector row computed tomography: Comparison with left Ventriculography and cardiovascular magnetic resonance	Wu et al.	2007	41	64-slice CT shows excellent correlation with CMR in left ventricular function assessment and is a clinically acceptable method for LV function evaluation
Quantitative assessment of right ventricular function and pulmonary regurgitation in surgically repaired tetralogy of Fallot using 256-slice CT	Yamasaki et al.	2014	33	256-slice CT correlates highly with CMR in assessing right ventricular function and pulmonary regurgitant fraction in patients with repaired tetralogy of Fallot
Head-to-head comparison of left ventricular function assessment with 64-row computed tomography, biplane left cineventriculography, and both two- and three-dimensional transthoracic echocardiography: Comparison with magnetic resonance imaging as the reference standard	Greupner et al.	2012	36	64-row CT may be more accurate than CVG, 2D echo, and 3D echo in comparison with MRI as the reference standard for assessment of global LV function

MDCT multidetector computed tomography, *CVG* cardiac ventriculography

were −19.1 ± 34.2 ml, −10.1 ± 29.7 ml, and −0.6% ± 11.8% for LV EDV, ESV, and EF, respectively while studies including data from 2DE showed pooled biases of −48.2 ± 55.9 ml, −27.7 ± 45.7 ml, and 0.1% ± 13.9% for LV EDV, ESV, and EF, respectively [38]. The negative bias of echocardiography compared to CMR in the assessment of volumes may be due to its inability to resolve trabeculations [39].

References

1. Miller S, Simonetti OP, Carr J, Kramer U, Finn JP. MR imaging of the heart with cine true fast imaging with steady-state precession: influence of spatial and temporal resolutions on left ventricular functional parameters. Radiology. 2002;223:263–9. https://doi.org/10.1148/radiol.2231010235.
2. Kramer CM, Barkhausen J, Flamm SD, Kim RJ, Nagel E. Standardized cardiovascular magnetic resonance imaging (CMR) protocols, society for cardiovascular magnetic resonance: board of trustees task force on standardized protocols. J Cardiovasc Magn Reson. 2008;10:35. https://doi.org/10.1186/1532-429X-10-35.
3. Bieri O, Scheffler K. Fundamentals of balanced steady state free precession MRI. J Magn Reson Imaging. 2013;38:2–11. https://doi.org/10.1002/jmri.24163.
4. Schwitter J. Image quality of cardiac magnetic resonance imaging in patients with an implantable cardioverter defibrillator system designed for the magnetic resonance imaging environment. Circ Cardiovasc Imaging. 2016;9(5):e004025. https://pubmed.ncbi.nlm.nih.gov/27151268/. Accessed 20 Jan 2024.
5. Deshmane A, Gulani V, Griswold MA, Seiberlich N. Parallel MR imaging. J Magn Reson Imaging. 2012;36:55–72. https://doi.org/10.1002/jmri.23639.
6. Craft J, Li Y, Nashta NF, Weber J. Comparison between compressed sensing and segmented cine cardiac magnetic resonance: a meta-analysis. BMC Cardiovasc Disord. 2023;23:473. https://doi.org/10.1186/s12872-023-03426-1.
7. Nayak KS, Lim Y, Campbell-Washburn AE, Steeden J. Real-time magnetic resonance imaging. J Magn Reson Imaging. 2022;55:81–99. https://doi.org/10.1002/jmri.27411.
8. Sherrid MV, Bernard S, Tripathi N, Patel Y, Modi V, Axel L, et al. Apical aneurysms and mid–left ventricular obstruction in hypertrophic cardiomyopathy. JACC Cardiovasc Imaging. 2023;16:591–605. https://doi.org/10.1016/j.jcmg.2022.11.013.
9. Riffel JH, Schmucker K, Andre F, Ochs M, Hirschberg K, Schaub E, et al. Cardiovascular magnetic resonance of cardiac morphology and function: impact of different strategies of contour drawing and indexing. Clin Res Cardiol. 2019;108:411–29. https://doi.org/10.1007/s00392-018-1371-7.
10. Schulz-Menger J, Bluemke DA, Bremerich J, Flamm SD, Fogel MA, Friedrich MG, et al. Standardized image interpretation and post-processing in cardiovascular magnetic resonance—2020 update. J

Cardiovasc Magn Reson. 2020;22:19. https://doi.org/10.1186/s12968020-00610-6.
11. Rudski LG, Lai WW, Afilalo J, Hua L, Handschumacher MD, Chandrasekaran K, et al. Guidelines for the echocardiographic assessment of the right heart in adults: a report from the American Society of Echocardiography endorsed by the European Association of Echocardiography, a registered branch of the European Society of Cardiology, and the Canadian Society of Echocardiography. J Am Soc Echocardiogr. 2010;23:685–13; quiz 786–8. https://doi.org/10.1016/j.echo.2010.05.010.
12. Pattynama PM, Lamb HJ, Van Der Velde EA, Van Der Wall EE, De Roos A. Left ventricular measurements with cine and spin-echo MR imaging: a study of reproducibility with variance component analysis. Radiology. 1993;187:261–8. https://doi.org/10.1148/radiology.187.1.8451425.
13. Bloomgarden D, Fayad Z, Ferrari V, Chin B, Sutton MGSJ, Axel L. Global cardiac function using fast breath-hold MRI: validation of new acquisition and analysis techniques. Magn Reson Med. 1997;37:683–92. https://doi.org/10.1002/MRM.1910370510.
14. Heusch A, Koch J, Krogmann O, Korbmacher B, Bourgeois M. Volumetric analysis of the right and left ventricle in a porcine heart model: comparison of three-dimensional echocardiography, magnetic resonance imaging and angiocardiography. Eur J Ultrasound. 1999;9(3):245–55. https://doi.org/10.1016/S0929-8266(99)00032-4.
15. Koch J, Poll L, Godehardt E, Korbmacher B, Mödder U. Right and left ventricular volume measurements in an animal heart model in vitro: first experiences with cardiac MRI at 1.0 T. Eur Radiol. 2000;10:455–8. https://doi.org/10.1007/s003300050075.
16. Bloomgarden D, Fayad Z, Chang C-N, Ferrari V, Young A, Axel L. 929-64 global cardiac function using active contour models with fast breath-hold MRI. J Am Coll Cardiol. 1995;25:113A. https://doi.org/10.1016/0735-1097(95)91923-L.
17. Semelka RC, Tomei E, Wagner S, Mayo J, Caputo G, O'Sullivan M, et al. Interstudy reproducibility of dimensional and functional measurements between cine magnetic resonance studies in the morphologically abnormal left ventricle. Am Heart J. 1990;119:1367–73. https://doi.org/10.1016/s0002-8703(05)80187-5.
18. Stratemeier EJ, Thompson R, Brady TJ, Miller SW, Saini S, Wismer GL, et al. Ejection fraction determination by MR imaging: comparison with left ventricular angiography. Radiology. 1986;158:775–7. https://doi.org/10.1148/radiology.158.3.3945753.
19. Strohm O, Schulz-Menger J, Pilz B, Osterziel KJ, Dietz R, Friedrich MG. Measurement of left ventricular dimensions and function in patients with dilated cardiomyopathy. J Magn Reson Imaging. 2001;13:367–71. https://doi.org/10.1002/jmri.1052.
20. Bellenger N, Davies LC, Francis J, Coats A, Pennell D. Reduction in sample size for studies of remodeling in heart failure by the use of cardiovascular magnetic resonance. J Cardiovasc Magn Reson. 2000;2(4):271–8. https://doi.org/10.3109/10976640009148691.
21. Kawel-Boehm N, Hetzel SJ, Ambale-Venkatesh B, Captur G, Francois CJ, Jerosch-Herold M, Salerno M, Teague SD, Valsangiacomo-Buechel E, Van der Geest RJ, Bluemke DA. Reference ranges ("normal values") for cardiovascular magnetic resonance (CMR) in adults and children: 2020 update. J Cardiovasc Magn Reson. 2020;22:87. https://jcmronline.biomedcentral.com/articles/10.1186/s12968-020-00683-3. Accessed 4 Jan 2024.
22. Rajiah PS, Moore A, Broncano J, Anand V, Kolluri N, Shah DJ, et al. Diastology with cardiac MRI: a practical guide. Radiographics. 2023;43:e220144. https://doi.org/10.1148/rg.220144.
23. Buss SJ, Krautz B, Schnackenburg B, Abdel-Aty H, Santos MFB, Andre F, et al. Classification of diastolic function with phase-contrast cardiac magnetic resonance imaging: validation with echocardiography and age-related reference values. Clin Res Cardiol. 2014;103:441–50. https://doi.org/10.1007/s00392-014-0669-3.
24. Paelinck BP, de Roos A, Bax JJ, Bosmans JM, van Der Geest RJ, Dhondt D, et al. Feasibility of tissue magnetic resonance imaging: a pilot study in comparison with tissue Doppler imaging and invasive measurement. J Am Coll Cardiol. 2005;45:1109–16. https://doi.org/10.1016/j.jacc.2004.12.051.
25. Ambale-Venkatesh B, Armstrong AC, Liu C-Y, Donekal S, Yoneyama K, Wu CO, et al. Diastolic function assessed from tagged MRI predicts heart failure and atrial fibrillation over an 8-year follow-up period: the multi-ethnic study of atherosclerosis. Eur Heart J Cardiovasc Imaging. 2014;15:442–9. https://doi.org/10.1093/ehjci/jet189.
26. Schuster A, Hor KN, Kowallick JT, Beerbaum P, Kutty S. Cardiovascular magnetic resonance myocardial feature tracking: concepts and clinical applications. Circ Cardiovasc Imaging. 2016;9:e004077. https://doi.org/10.1161/CIRCIMAGING.115.004077.
27. Feuchtner G, Goetti R, Plass A, Baumueller S, Stolzmann P, Scheffel H, et al. Dual-step prospective ECG-triggered 128-slice dual-source CT for evaluation of coronary arteries and cardiac function without heart rate control: a technical note. Eur Radiol. 2010;20:2092–9. https://doi.org/10.1007/s00330-010-1794-7.
28. Fink C, Krissak R, Henzler T, Lechel U, Brix G, Takx RAP, et al. Radiation dose at coronary CT angiography: second-generation dual-source CT versus single-source 64-MDCT and FirstGeneration dual-source CT. Am J Roentgenol. 2011;196:W550–7. https://doi.org/10.2214/AJR.10.5153.
29. Sugeng L, Mor-Avi V, Weinert L, Niel J, Ebner C, Steringer Mascherbauer R, et al. Quantitative assessment of left ventricular size and function: side-by side comparison of real-time three-dimensional echocardiography and computed tomography

with magnetic resonance reference. Circulation. 2006;114:654–61. https://doi.org/10.1161/CIRCULATIONAHA.106.626143.
30. Chen C, Qin C, Qiu H, Tarroni G, Duan J, Bai W, et al. Deep learning for cardiac image segmentation: a review. Front Cardiovasc Med. 2020;7:25. https://doi.org/10.3389/fcvm.2020.00025.
31. Boogers MJ, van Werkhoven JM, Schuijf JD, Delgado V, El-Naggar HM, Boersma E, et al. Feasibility of diastolic function assessment with cardiac CT: feasibility study in comparison with tissue Doppler imaging. JACC Cardiovasc Imaging. 2011;4:246–56. https://doi.org/10.1016/j.jcmg.2010.11.017.
32. Szilveszter B, Nagy AI, Vattay B, Apor A, Kolossváry M, Bartykowszki A, et al. Left ventricular and atrial strain imaging with cardiac computed tomography: validation against echocardiography. J Cardiovasc Comput Tomogr. 2020;14:363–9. https://doi.org/10.1016/j.jcct.2019.12.004.
33. Sarwar A, Shapiro MD, Nasir K, Nieman K, Nomura CH, Brady TJ, et al. Evaluating global and regional left ventricular function in patients with reperfused acute myocardial infarction by 64-slice multidetector CT: a comparison to magnetic resonance imaging. J Cardiovasc Comput Tomogr. 2009;3:170–7. https://doi.org/10.1016/j.jcct.2009.05.002.
34. Raman SV, Shah M, McCarthy B, Garcia A, Ferketich AK. Multi-detector row cardiac computed tomography accurately quantifies right and left ventricular size and function compared with cardiac magnetic resonance. Am Heart J. 2006;151:736–44. https://doi.org/10.1016/j.ahj.2005.04.029.
35. Wu Y-W, Tadamura E, Kanao S, Yamamuro M, Okayama S, Ozasa N, et al. Left ventricular functional analysis using 64-slice multidetector row computed tomography: comparison with left ventriculography and cardiovascular magnetic resonance. Cardiology. 2008;109:135–42. https://doi.org/10.1159/000105555.
36. Yamasaki Y, Nagao M, Yamamura K, Yonezawa M, Matsuo Y, Kawanami S, et al. Quantitative assessment of right ventricular function and pulmonary regurgitation in surgically repaired tetralogy of Fallot using 256-slice CT: comparison with 3-Tesla MRI. Eur Radiol. 2014;24:3289–99. https://doi.org/10.1007/s00330-014-3344-1.
37. Greupner J, Zimmermann E, Grohmann A, Dübel H-P, Althoff TF, Borges AC, et al. Head-to-head comparison of left ventricular function assessment with 64-row computed tomography, biplane left cineventriculography, and both 2- and 3-dimensional transthoracic echocardiography: comparison with magnetic resonance imaging as the reference standard. J Am Coll Cardiol. 2012;59:1897–907. https://doi.org/10.1016/j.jacc.2012.01.046.
38. Dorosz JL, Lezotte DC, Weitzenkamp DA, Allen LA, Salcedo EE. Performance of 3-dimensional echocardiography in measuring left ventricular volumes and ejection fraction: a systematic review and meta-analysis. J Am Coll Cardiol. 2012;59:1799–808. https://doi.org/10.1016/j.jacc.2012.01.037.
39. Mor-Avi V, Jenkins C, Kühl HP, Nesser H-J, Marwick T, Franke A, et al. Real-time 3Dimensional echocardiographic quantification of left ventricular volumes. JACC Cardiovasc Imaging. 2008;1:413–23. https://doi.org/10.1016/j.jcmg.2008.02.009.

3 Quantitative CT Imaging in Coronary Artery Disease

Hyung-Bok Park and Hyuk-Jae Chang

Clinical Value of Coronary Artery Disease Quantification

Evaluating coronary artery disease (CAD) involves two types of assessments: qualitative and quantitative. Qualitative assessments are advantageous in quickly assessing the severity of CAD and making informed decisions. However, they are subjective and have limitations in risk assessment, standardization, and treatment monitoring due to inter- and intra-observer variability. On the other hand, quantitative assessments provide a higher level of objectivity compared to qualitative assessments. They allow for the precise evaluation of lesions and contribute to a comprehensive understanding of the disease's extent and severity. This approach facilitates more accurate risk assessment, effective treatment monitoring, improved communication, and the development of a comprehensive long-term management plan, ultimately enhancing personalized patient care [1, 2]. Nevertheless, variations in the results of quantitative assessments can occur depending on the types of tools used, the operator's expertise, and the interpretation of processing conditions, which may vary depending on vendors and circumstances. In other words, higher image quality guarantees more reliable results, while lower image quality renders the results of quantitative measurements unreliable. Hence, the automated quantification method is essential for a quantitative evaluation of CAD [1].

Coronary artery calcification (CAC) is a widely used diagnostic tool for asymptomatic and symptomatic patients because it is noninvasive, involves minimal radiation exposure, and does not require contrast agents [3, 4]. The CAC score, developed by Dr. Agatston and measured through a standardized protocol for accuracy, not only aids in predicting future cardiovascular events and screening for coronary artery disease (CAD) but is also employed in pretest probability metrics for symptomatic patients [3–5].

However, despite its utility, coronary computed tomography angiography (CCTA) is primarily recommended for qualitative assessment in clinical applications, mainly due to spatial resolution constraints in quantitative coronary analysis and the emphasis on qualitative assessment of high-risk plaque (HRP) features [6–8]. The updated Coronary Artery Disease Reporting and Data System (CAD-RADS) now incorporates a grading scale for plaque burden, albeit relying on qualitative assessment [9]. There is a pressing need to establish and implement standardized protocols for quantitative evaluation in clinical settings to enhance patient management.

H.-B. Park
Catholic Kwandong University, International St. Mary's Hospital, Seoul, Incheon, South Korea

H.-J. Chang (✉)
Yonsei University, Severance Cardiovascular Hospital, Seodaemun, Seoul, South Korea
e-mail: HJCHANG@yuhs.ac

R. Gill, P. Rajiah (eds.), *Quantitative Imaging in the Thorax*,
https://doi.org/10.1007/978-3-032-14103-3_3

Quantification of Coronary Artery Calcium by Calcium Scan

Coronary Atherosclerosis and Calcification

Atherosclerotic plaques in the coronary arteries are formed due to a chronic inflammatory process involving lipid deposition in the arterial wall, occurring in the presence of cardiovascular risk factors such as dyslipidemia, diabetes, and hypertension [10]. Coronary calcification begins with microcalcifications near the internal elastic lamina of the endothelium, due to apoptosis of smooth muscle cells or macrophage apoptosis (the latter often observed in thin-cap fibroatheromas [TFCA]); these coalesce into larger aggregates, forming speckled patterns or fragments and eventually evolving into calcified plaques and sheets or plates. These can lead to nodular calcifications with fibrin deposition upon fracturing, sometimes protruding into the lumen or media, and potentially causing acute thrombosis in 2%–7% of cases [10]. However, calcification areas ranging in size from 1.03 to 1.37 mm^2 can be observed in vivo through CT imaging, meaning that microcalcifications are not detected on CT scans; only nodular calcifications located at the intimal medial border can be observed [4, 10, 11].

The Definition of the CAC Score

The CAC score is a method for detecting coronary calcification, utilizing electrocardiography (ECG)-gated electron-beam computed tomography (EBCT) with a 3-mm slice thickness. Developed by Arthur Agatston and his team, who also named it the Agatston score, this method is widely recognized in the field [4, 5]. In CT imaging, calcification is defined as areas with CT attenuation of more than 130 Hounsfield units (HU) and an area greater than $1 mm^2$ to minimize confusion with noise [4]. The Agatston score is calculated by multiplying the area of voxels corresponding to the calcified lesion by a weighting factor [4, 12]. The weighting factor is determined by the maximum HU value of the voxel area: 1 for 130–199 HU, 2 for 200–299 HU, 3 for 300–399 HU, and 4 for over 400 HU [12]. The total CAC score is the sum of the Agatston scores for each lesion [12]. Calcium scoring categories are standardized, with a score of 0 indicating no detected calcified plaque, 1 to 10 suggesting minimal plaque, 11 to 100 denoting mild plaque, 101 to 400 indicating moderate plaque, and any score above 400 signifying severe plaque accumulation as shown in Table 3.1 [13].

The Standardized Measurement and Quantification Process of the Calcium Score

The Agatston score, calculated using specific imaging protocols on EBCT which typically employ a 130-kVp voltage, 639-mA current, and a 512 × 512 voxel matrix, may vary based on the image acquisition protocol and is occasionally refined by normalizing the slice increment to the slice thickness [12]. The advent of multi-detector computed tomography (MDCT) in clinical settings has led to a decrease in EBCT use for cal-

Table 3.1 Clinical interpretation of CAC score

CAC score (Agatston score)	Plaque burden	Coronary artery disease	Framingham risk score	10-year event rate (%)
0	None	Very low, <5%	Very low	1.1–1.7
1–10	Minimal	Unlikely, <10%	Low	2.3–5.9
11–100	Mild	Mild or minimal disease		
101–400	Moderate	Moderate nonobstructive disease, obstructive disease possible	Intermediate	12.8–16.4
>400	Extensive	High likelihood of significant coronary disease	High	22.5–28.6
>1000			Very high	37.0

cium scans; however, historical research often relies on CAC scores from EBCT, which offers higher temporal resolution but is surpassed by MDCT's superior spatial resolution, enabling detection of smaller calcified lesions yet precluding the identification of microcalcifications [10]. Regarding radiation dose, EBCT is associated with doses ranging from 0.7 to 1.3 mSv, while MDCT typically involves slightly higher doses, from 1.0 to 1.9 mSv [11, 13]. However, studies have shown that both MDCT and EBCT offer equivalent reproducibility and are currently recognized in clinical practice without a preference for one over the other [11].

Nevertheless, the Agatston score exhibits inherent inter-scan variability because its weighting factor is based on the maximum HU within the calcium voxel area, with significant HU variation within the calcification area posing challenges to accurately representing the entire area's calcification density [5, 12]. Additionally, if the HU is close to the threshold of a weighting factor cutoff, this can result in a weighting factor difference of two, with the actual HU potentially falling within the margin of error during measurement [12]. Despite the inability to always ensure a linear relationship between the quantity of calcium and the Agatston score, its widespread adoption in clinical practice is attributed to the vast amount of clinical data collected across various demographics and the risk stratification studies conducted using this data [14].

Recognizing the complexity and nonlinearity of the Agatston score between calcium amount and score, Callister and his team proposed the volume score to improve reproducibility, calculated by multiplying the number of voxels above 130 HU by each voxel's volume, treating all calcium above this threshold equally, resulting in less variability between scans than the Agatston score but potentially leading to overestimation of very dense calcifications and underestimation of less dense ones due to the partial volume effect [15]. To further reduce inter-scan variability and more accurately determine the actual mass of calcium, the mass score has been introduced, which involves using CT calibration phantoms with varying concentrations of calcium hydroxyapatite (CaHA) placed under the patient's thorax during CT imaging to calculate the total calcium mass based on the mineral concentration density within the phantom [16]. However, this calcium mass score has not been widely used due to the complexity of scanning and post-processing procedures, as well as the scarcity of clinical research data regarding its usefulness. According to a study, the mean inter-scan variability for the Agatston, volume, and mass scores was reported to be 20.4%, 13.9%, and 9.3%, respectively [17].

Coronary Calcium and Cardiovascular Risk

The CAC score serves as a crucial marker for both the unseen and evident forms of atherosclerosis. Individuals are identified as having high-risk or premature atherosclerosis when their age-, gender-, and ethnicity-adjusted CAC score percentile exceeds the 75th percentile in a symptom-free population [4].

The Multi-Ethnic Study of Atherosclerosis (MESA), involving 6722 individuals, demonstrated significant gender and ethnicity impacts on calcium levels [18]. Typically, Caucasian and Hispanic men, along with Caucasian women, have higher CAC scores, contrasting with African Americans and young individuals of Chinese descent who generally have lower scores, except for older Chinese women who show increased scores, yet regardless of these demographic variations, higher CAC scores, particularly those ranging between 101 and 300 or exceeding 300, consistently indicated a notably higher risk of coronary events over a 3.8-year period compared to a score of 0 [18]. In a study conducted by Yeboah and his team, integrating the CAC score with the Framingham risk score was found to significantly increase its accuracy in a subset of the MESA involving intermediate-risk individuals without diabetes, with the AUC improving from 0.623 to 0.784, thereby surpassing other markers such as carotid intima-media thickness and C-reactive protein [19]. The findings of this study contributed to the ACC/AHA 2013 guidelines, which now recommend CAC scoring for more accurate risk evaluation in people at intermediate risk.

Furthermore, the MESA dataset's 10-year follow-up confirmed a strong correlation between CAC scores and the risk of developing atherosclerotic cardiovascular disease (ASCVD), with those having a CAC score above 100 facing a risk exceeding 7.5%, and each doubling of the CAC score associated with a 14% increase in ASCVD risk, consistent across all ages, genders, and ethnicities, and unaffected by variables like age, gender, ethnicity, or initial use of lipid-lowering drugs [20]. In another related study using the MESA cohort, Budoff et al. found that in 5682 adults tracked for coronary heart disease (CHD) events over a median period of 7.7 years, the rate of CAC score progression, measured through follow-up scans about 2.5 years apart, significantly influenced CHD incidence, remaining below 10% for those with less than 100 units annual increase in CAC scores but exceeding 30% for individuals with annual increases of more than 300 units [21].

The Coronary Artery Risk Development in Young Adults (CARDIA) study, focusing on cardiovascular disease risk in adults aged 32–46 and tracking participants for 12.5 years using CAC scanning, found that the presence of CAC increased the risk of CHD events fivefold and ASCVD events threefold, with the risk of CHD events rising with varying CAC scores, evidenced by hazard ratios (HR) of 2.6 for scores of 1–19, 5.8 for 20–99, and 9.8 for 100+, and importantly, a CAC score above 100 was linked to early mortality, highlighting heightened cardiovascular and mortality risks in adults under 50 [22]. The Walter Reed Cohort study, which examined 23,637 subjects free from cardiovascular disease (CVD), confirmed the significant role of CAC scoring in predicting CVD outcomes, regardless of age and other risk factors [23]. Moreover, the CAC Consortium study revealed that women exhibit a lower prevalence and severity of CAC compared to men, yet despite having similar ASCVD mortality rates to men at a CAC score of 0, women with any CAC level face a 1.3-fold higher mortality risk than men [24]. On the other hand, the 6-year follow-up of the Coronary CT Angiography Evaluation For Clinical Outcomes: An International Multicenter (CONFIRM) registry suggested that CCTA does not enhance cardiovascular risk prediction beyond traditional factors and the CAC score, resulting in recommendations against using CCTA for cardiovascular risk assessment in asymptomatic individuals, considering the CAC score [25].

Coronary Artery Calcium and Coronary Stenoses

The CAC score demonstrates a strong correlation with the total coronary plaque burden and the severity of CAD, but only a modest correlation with coronary stenoses [10]. While the CAC score shows high sensitivity, its specificity in detecting obstructive CAD characterized by more than 50% luminal stenosis is relatively low [11]. In a study of 1851 symptomatic patients who underwent EBCT, researchers found that the overall sensitivity for identifying obstructive CAD via invasive coronary angiography (ICA) using any CAC score was 96%, with a specificity of 40%, the sensitivity for predicting stenosis decreased to 90%, 79%, and 76% for calcium scores above 20, 80, and 100, respectively, whereas the specificity increased to 58%, 72%, and 75% [26]. Another extensive study, involving 1764 patients referred for ICA due to suspected CAD who underwent EBCT, showed that a CAC score of 100 had high diagnostic accuracy for detecting obstructive CAD, with sensitivities of 93% in men and 82% in women and specificities of 75% in men and 76% in women [27]. Even in the symptomatic population from the CONFIRM registry during the MDCT era, a CAC score of 100 demonstrated the ability to predict both the presence and severity of CAD [25], as shown in Fig. 3.1. Research suggests using higher CAC score thresholds of 300 or 400 for screening obstructive CAD [28, 29]. Meta-analysis data indicates that for CAC scores over 100, sensitivity and specificity for obstructive CAD were 96.5% (95% confidence interval (CI) 94–98) and 55.5% (95% CI 44–66), respectively, and for scores over 400, these values altered to

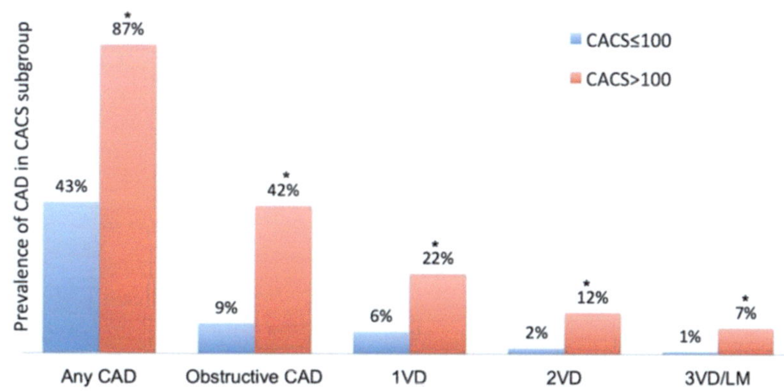

	Any CAD	Obstructive CAD	Subgroup of obstructive CAD		
			1VD	2VD	3VD/LM
CACS≤100	1017 (42.5%)	204 (8.5%)	147 (6.1%)	39 (1.6%)	18 (0.8%)
CACS>100	716 (86.8%)	342 (41.5%)	185 (22.4%)	96 (11.6%)	61 (7.4%)

* *P*<0.001 compared with CACS≤100

Fig. 3.1 Prevalence of CAD according to a CAC score of 100. Number and percentage (%). Any CAD includes both obstructive and nonobstructive forms of CAD; CACS, coronary artery calcium score; CCTA, coronary computed tomography angiography; LM, left main disease; VD, vessel disease

97.5% (95% CI 95–99) and 42% (95% CI 28–56), demonstrating a decrease in specificity with increasing CAC scores while maintaining high sensitivity [30].

The Power of Zero Calcium Score

A zero CAC score strongly indicates the absence of coronary atherosclerosis, especially in individuals with a low pretest probability of CAD and fewer cardiovascular risk factors [31], as shown in Fig. 3.2. A zero CAC score is widely recognized as a marker of significantly low cardiac event risk. Large registries and clinical trials have consistently demonstrated low cardiovascular risk in people with a zero CAC score, with annual event rates ranging between 0.11% and 0.13% [18, 32–34]. Moreover, a multicenter study of 19,898 asymptomatic individuals with a zero CAC score confirmed a 10-year all-cause mortality rate of less than 1%, highlighting the predictive value of a zero CAC score for lower cardiac event risk and mortality in asymptomatic individuals [33].

This trend is evident in symptomatic patients as well. For example, the CONFIRM registry indicates that symptomatic patients with a zero CAC score experienced a mere 0.4% mortality rate over an average follow-up of 2.1 years [35]. The PROMISE (Prospective Multicenter Imaging Study for Evaluation of Chest Pain) trial observed similar outcomes, with a 0.6% rate of cardiovascular death or myocardial infarction in patients with stable chest pain or dyspnea and an intermediate pretest probability for obstructive coronary artery disease [36]. Similarly, an observational cohort study involving 1978 patients with stable chest pain and a zero CAC score noted an exceptionally low annual mortality rate of 0.3%, with no coronary event-related deaths during an average follow-up of 5.2 years [37]. These observations reaffirm the role of a zero CAC score in indicating a lower likelihood of serious coronary incidents and death in both asymptomatic and symptomatic individuals.

However, the incidence of obstructive CAD in patients with a zero CAC score varies in different studies. In symptomatic patients, reported incidence rates vary, with some studies indicating 19% ($n = 291$) [38], 7% ($n = 231$) [39], and 0.9% ($n = 447$) [40]. The CONFIRM registry, which included 4738 symptomatic patients without known CAD who underwent both CAC scoring and CCTA, identified a 5.1% incidence of obstructive CAD in those with a zero CAC score [35]. Additionally, a recent pooled analysis revealed a 4.4% incidence of obstructive CAD identified by CT coronary angiography in symptomatic patients without CAC [41]. In the asymp-

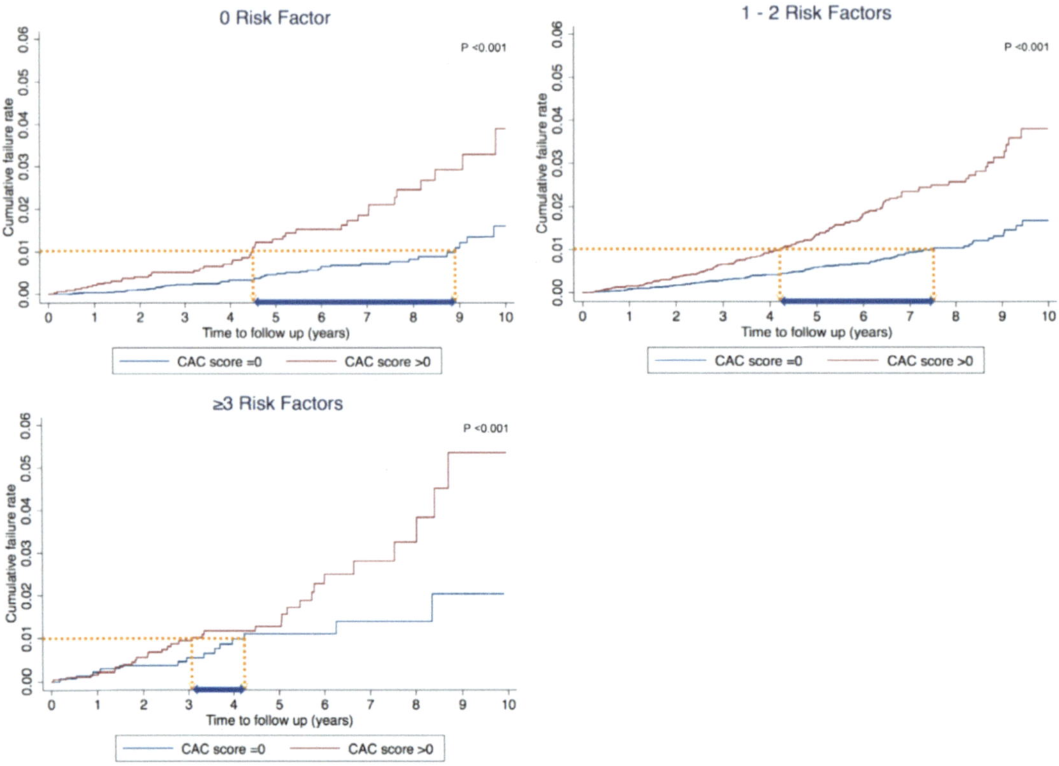

Fig. 3.2 Warranty period differences for CAC score 0 vs. CAC score > 0 based on the risk factor burden. Overall, subjects with a zero CAC score exceeded a 1% all-cause mortality rate in 9 years, significantly longer than those with a non-zero CAC score, and Kaplan-Meier analysis showed a more favorable warranty period for zero CAC scores across all pre-specified risk factor groups, especially in the absence of any risk factors; CAC, coronary artery calcium

tomatic population, different cohorts have reported incidence rates of 6% ($n = 972$) [42], 5% ($n = 1000$) [43], and 0.7% ($n = 6531$) [44]. While a zero CAC score strongly indicates low risk and aids in ruling out obstructive CAD, its absence should not be completely discounted in both symptomatic and asymptomatic individuals, particularly in the presence of risk factors and among younger populations.

Artificial Intelligence-Based Automatic CAC Scoring

With the advancement of artificial intelligence technology, a fully automated coronary artery calcification (CAC) scoring method was introduced. Initially, a feature-based model was developed, which extracted all coronary calcification candidates using HU-threshold without considering coronary anatomical structural information, and then classified them as coronary calcifications using a specific set of features [45, 46]. However, this method had a high false positive rate and required operator manipulation for accurate classification. In contrast, the atlas-based model, designed to standardize heart volumes among patients and extract coronary artery areas and segments, showed inferior performance compared to the feature-based model [47]. To overcome previous methods' limitations, a multi-atlas approach was developed, merging the benefits of feature-based and atlas-based techniques by collecting spatial data via the pairwise alignment of ten atlas images, although it was limited by lengthy execution times due to heavy computation [48].

Recently, deep learning-based methods using convolutional neural networks for classifying calcium candidate objects were introduced; however, these methods neglected coronary anatomical information and other surrounding structures, leading to a higher false positive rate [49]. To overcome these issues, a multistep deep-learning model was proposed that identifies coronary artery, aorta, aortic valve, and mitral valve regions, classifies coronary calcification, and significantly reduces computation time [50, 51]. Recent studies have demonstrated the clinical utility of this deep learning-based method, showing high levels of correlation and agreement with manual analysis [52, 53]. This advanced deep-learning model is expected to be implemented in clinical practice soon.

Quantification of Coronary Artery Disease by CCTA

Diagnostic Accuracy and Prognostic Value of CCTA

Since the introduction of 64-slice CCTA in 2005, and particularly after 3 pivotal multicenter trials in 2008 evaluated its effectiveness in detecting obstructive CAD, CCTA has gained recognition as a highly reliable diagnostic tool for assessing chest pain when compared to ICA [54–56], as shown in Fig. 3.3. Numerous subsequent studies have consistently highlighted its high diagnostic accuracy, with detection rates ranging from 88% to 96%, a sensitivity of 95%–99%, and a specific-

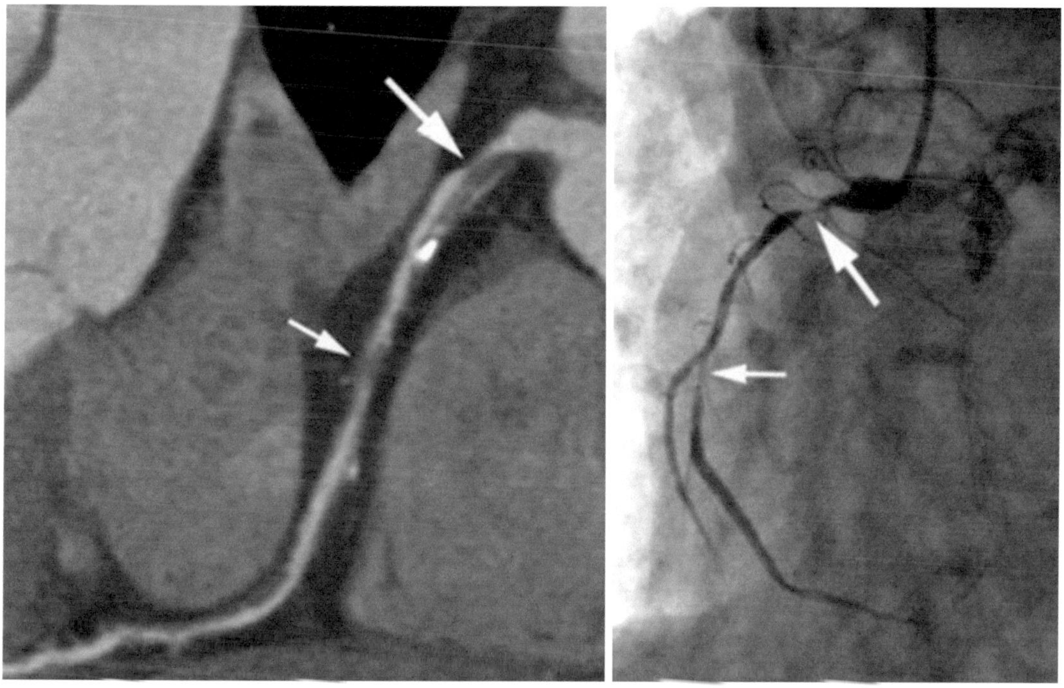

Fig. 3.3 Diagnostic accuracy of CCTA compared to ICA. The left panel displays a severe stenosis lesion at the proximal and mid RCA, while the right panel confirms its presence through ICA; CCTA, coronary computed tomography angiography; ICA, invasive coronary angiography; RCA, right coronary artery

ity of 68%–93% [57]. Consequently, current guidelines now endorse CCTA as the primary diagnostic approach for patients with an intermediate to high pretest probability of CAD [58, 59].

The prognostic impact of CCTA was assessed by extensively analyzing the CONFIRM registry data, which included 27,125 consecutive participants from 12 clusters across 6 countries in North America, Europe, and Asia [60]. In a primary analysis of the CONFIRM registry involving 23,854 patients without prior coronary artery disease, CCTA facilitated risk stratification by assessing the severity of coronary stenosis and plaque extent, uncovering distinct risk profiles for various age and sex groups over a 2.3-year monitoring period (Fig. 3.4) [61]. In a separate analysis of 13,966 patients over a median follow-up of 22.5 months, CCTA proved to be more effective than traditional clinical risk factors, including left ventricular ejection fraction measured by echocardiography, in predicting all-cause mortality [62]. However, for the asymptomatic population in the CONFIRM registry, including 7590 individuals without chest pain syndrome, CCTA showed no additional risk-predictive benefit over the CAC score, leading to recommendations against its use for risk assessment in these individuals [25].

In 2015, two pivotal prospective trials, the Prospective Multicenter Imaging Study for Evaluation of Chest Pain (PROMISE) and the Scottish Computed Tomography of the Heart (SCOT-HEART), were conducted to assess the prognostic impact of CCTA compared to functional or conventional modalities [63, 64]. In the PROMISE study of 10,003 symptomatic patients, participants were randomly assigned to either initial CCTA or various functional tests (exercise ECG, nuclear stress testing, or stress echocardiography), and over 25 months, the CCTA group did not show superior MACE reduction (3.3% vs. 3.0%, $p = 0.75$) compared to the functional test group, where only 10.2% underwent exercise ECG and 67.3% had nuclear stress imaging, suggesting CCTA's comparable prognostic performance to nuclear stress testing but with lower radiation doses and costs [63].

Conversely, in the SCOT-HEART trial featuring a practical design, 2073 patients were each randomly assigned to either standard care plus CCTA or standard care alone, where in the latter, 85% underwent exercise ECG and 9% nuclear stress tests; after 1.7 years, the CCTA group saw a 38% reduction in fatal and nonfatal myocardial infarction (HR 0.62, $p = 0.0527$), although this did not reach statistical significance [64]. However, a post hoc landmark analysis showed that CCTA significantly reduced the incidence of fatal and nonfatal myocardial infarctions by 50% compared to standard care (HR 0.50, $p = 0.020$)

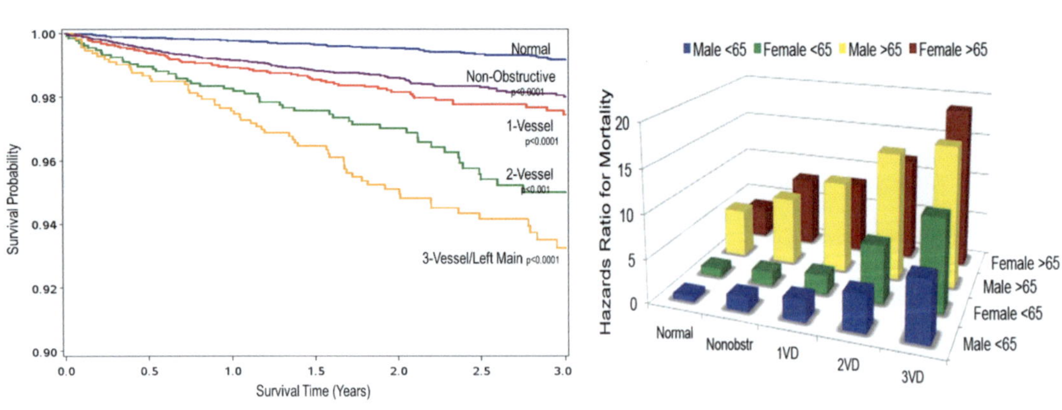

Fig. 3.4 Prognostic value of CCTA based on CAD extent and severity. The left panel displays a 3-year Kaplan-Meier survival graph unadjusted for all causes, illustrating the dose-response relationship between mortality and the increasing number of vessels with obstructive CAD as detected by CCTA. The right panel presents multivariable-adjusted hazard ratios for all-cause mortality, stratified by age and sex; CAD, coronary artery disease; CCTA, coronary computed tomography angiography

[65]. Furthermore, in a 5-year clinical outcomes analysis of SCOT-HEART, CCTA demonstrated long-term benefits in patients with stable chest pain, reducing the rate of death from coronary heart disease or nonfatal myocardial infarction by 41% without increasing the rate of coronary angiography or revascularization, as shown in Fig. 3.5. (HR 0.59, p = 0.004) [66]. The DISCHARGE (Diagnostic Imaging Strategies for Patients with Stable Chest Pain and Intermediate Risk of Coronary Artery Disease) trial recently compared CCTA's effectiveness to ICA as an initial diagnostic tool for stable chest pain patients. The study included 3561 patients and found that the CCTA group demonstrated similar rates of MACE over 3.5 years, confirming its safety as a primary diagnostic modality [67]. These findings further solidify CCTA's role as the recommended primary diagnostic modality for stable chest pain in guidelines.

Qualitative (or Semiquantitative) Coronary Artery Stenosis Grading: CAD-RADS

With the increasing use of CCTA, now established as the first-line diagnostic imaging test for patients with stable chest pain and low to intermediate risk, there is still notable variability in CCTA reporting systems and how referring physicians interpret these reports. This variability stems from the absence of a standardized method for communicating CCTA findings and associated management recommendations. To address this issue, in 2016, multiple societies from the radiology and cardiology communities introduced the Coronary Artery Disease Reporting and Data System (CAD-RADS) as a collaborative effort [68]. CAD-RADS is similar to other radiology reporting systems like BI-RADS for breast imaging, LI-RADS for the liver, Lung-RADS for the lungs, and PI-RADS for the prostate. The aim of CAD-RADS is to establish a standardized classification method for CAD to improve communication between interpreting and referring clinicians, thereby facilitating decision-making regarding patient management. Additionally, it contributes to the creation of a consistent patient database for use in clinical research, quality assurance of tests, patient education, and ultimately, the improvement of the quality of care [68].

In 2022, CAD-RADS was updated to version 2.0, incorporating new CCTA technical developments in ischemia detection like CT-fractional flow reserve (CT-FFR) and myocardial CT perfusion (CTP), as well as to reflect the growing evi-

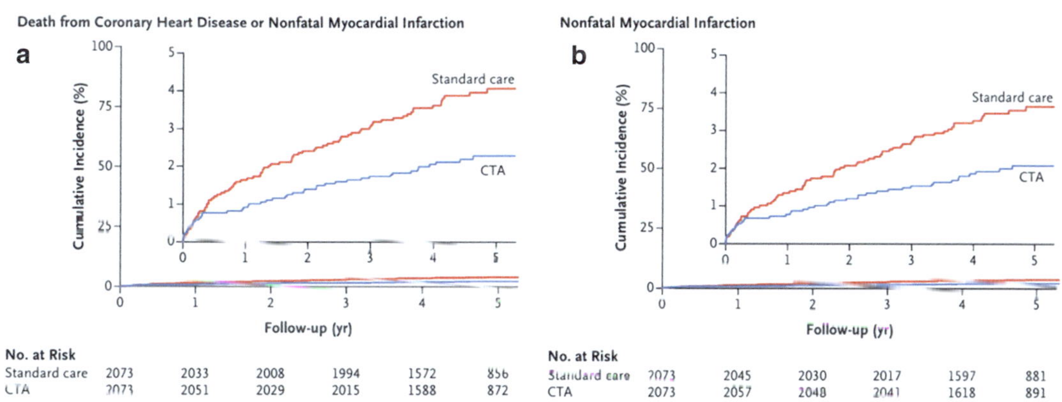

Fig. 3.5 Long-term clinical outcomes of CTA compared to standard care. Panel (**a**) displays the cumulative incidence curves for the primary outcome, which includes death due to coronary heart disease or nonfatal myocardial infarction, comparing patients who received CTA along with standard care to those who only received standard care. Panel (**b**) illustrates the cumulative likelihood of nonfatal myocardial infarction for each group. Additionally, an inset in each panel presents these data with an expanded y-axis for clearer visualization; CTA, coronary computed tomography angiography

dence of the relationship between the amount of coronary plaque burden and a worse prognosis [9]. The CAD-RADS system categorizes CAD based on the degree of maximal coronary stenosis and plaque burden grading, with classifications such as "CAD-RADS 2/P2" being detailed in Tables 3.2 and 3.3 [9].

In evaluating stable chest pain, CAD-RADS 0 indicates the absence of CAD, CAD-RADS 1 denotes minimal nonobstructive CAD, and CAD-RADS 2 signifies mild nonobstructive CAD. These classifications suggest that no further cardiac investigation is needed, and physicians should consider non-atherosclerotic causes of symptoms. To accurately determine the degree of stenosis, especially in calcified plaque, setting the proper window level and width is crucial due to calcium blooming artifacts, which can make the stenosis appear much more severe than it is, as illustrated in Fig. 3.6.

For CAD-RADS 2 with plaque grades P1 or P2, it is recommended to consider risk factor modification and initiate preventive pharmacotherapy. Conversely, for plaque grades P3 or P4, more aggressive risk factor modification and pharmacotherapy are advised. An example image of CAD-RADS 2 can be found in Fig. 3.7. CAD-RADS 3 indicates moderate stenosis and necessitates a functional assessment; aggressive risk factor modification and preventive pharmacotherapy are recommended regardless of plaque burden, in addition to guideline-directed care. The "I+" modifier suggests ICA may be needed in cases with persistent symptoms despite guideline-directed medical therapy. CAD-RADS 4, denoting severe stenosis, is subdivided into 4A (70%–99% stenosis) and 4B (left main ≥50% or three-vessel obstructive disease ≥70%), with ICA or functional assessment considered for 4A and ICA recommended for 4B. CAD-RADS 5 indicates total or near-total occlusion, where ICA, functional, or viability assessment may be considered, depending on the clinical scenario of acute or chronic occlusion. CAD-RADS N represents a nondiagnostic study, necessitating additional or alternative evaluation as obstructive CAD cannot be excluded. Additionally, six

Table 3.2 CAD-RADS 2.0 grading scale for stenosis severity, plaque burden, and ischemia

Degree of luminal diameter stenosis	*Terminology*
0%	No visible stenosis
1%–24%	Minimal stenosis
25%–49%	Mild stenosis
50%–69%	Moderate stenosis
70%–99%	Severe stenosis
100%	Occluded
Grading scale for plaque burden: terminology	*Overall plaque burden*
P1	Mild amount of plaque
P2	Moderate amount of plaque
P3	Severe amount of plaque
P4	Extensive amount of plaque
Grading scale for ischemia detection: terminology	*Meaning*
Modifier I	Indicates that CT ischemia test was performed either with CT-FFR or myocardial CTP
I+	Indicates that CT-FFR or CTP demonstrates lesion specific ischemia or reversible perfusion defect
I−	Indicates that CT-FFR or CTP is negative for lesion specific ischemia or reversible ischemia[a]
I±	Indicates that CT-FFR or CTP is borderline

[a]Patients who have experienced a prior myocardial infarction and exhibit fixed perfusion defects, yet show no signs of myocardial ischemia according to CTP, should be categorized as I−

Table 3.3 Various methods for assessing the grade of overall plaque burden

	Overall amount of coronary plaque	CAC	SIS[a]	Visual[b]
P1	Mild	1–100	≤2	1–2 vessels with mild amount of plaque
P2	Moderate	101–300	3–4	1–2 vessels with moderate amount 3 vessels with mild amount of plaque
P3	Severe	301–999	5–7	3 vessels with moderate amount 1 vessel with severe amount of plaque
P4	Extensive	>1000	≥8	2–3 vessels with severe amount of plaque

Please be aware that categories might not align consistently across various scoring systems. In cases of discrepancy, consider utilizing coronary artery calcium (CAC) or total plaque burden quantification when accessible
SIS segment involvement score
[a]Please note that CAD-RADS 0 signifies the absence of both stenosis and plaque, therefore, the P0 classification is unnecessary
[b]Since there is no universally mandated method for quantifying the overall plaque amount, CAD-RADS advises imagers to choose the technique deemed most suitable within their specific institution

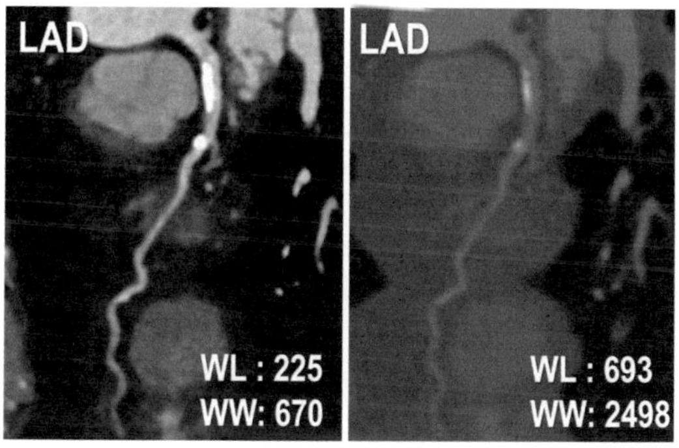

Fig. 3.6 An example of CAD-RADS 1/P2 after proper window setting. The left panel displays moderate stenosis (50%–69%) in CAD using a window level of 225 and a window width of 670, whereas the right panel demonstrates the same lesion, reclassified as minimal stenosis (1%–24%), after adjustment to a window level of 693 and a window width of 2498; LAD, left anterior descending artery; WL, window level; WW, window width

modifiers exist within the system: N (nondiagnostic), HRP (high-risk plaque), I (ischemia), S (stent), G (graft), and E (exceptions). Modifier E encompasses non-atherosclerotic causes of coronary abnormalities, such as coronary dissection, anomalous coronary artery origins, coronary artery aneurysm or pseudoaneurysm, vasculitis, coronary artery fistula, extrinsic coronary artery compression, arteriovenous malformation, and other causes.

Clinical Value of Coronary Atherosclerotic Plaque Evaluation by CCTA

Over 30% of patients with CAD experience acute myocardial infarction as their first symptom [69]. Statistically, in the USA, 1 in 9 men and 1 in 40 women are at risk of sudden cardiac death before reaching 70 years of age, underscoring CAD's unpredictability [70]. Several postmortem studies reveal that most myocardial infarctions result from nonobstructive or subclinical atherosclerosis [71].

This finding underscores the importance of understanding plaque vulnerability, as extensively documented in pathological studies. Vulnerable plaques are characterized by a high plaque burden with positive remodeling, lipid-rich composition with a necrotic core, TCFA, macrophage infiltration, intraplaque hemorrhage, and spotty calcification [71]. Recent studies have demonstrated that these characteristics of vulnerable plaques can lead to sudden and rapid plaque progression, resulting in plaque rupture and acute coronary syndrome (ACS) [72, 73].

The primary goal of CCTA in evaluating atherosclerotic plaque is to identify subclinical atherosclerosis, which carries an increased risk of plaque rupture and is often asymptomatic in the

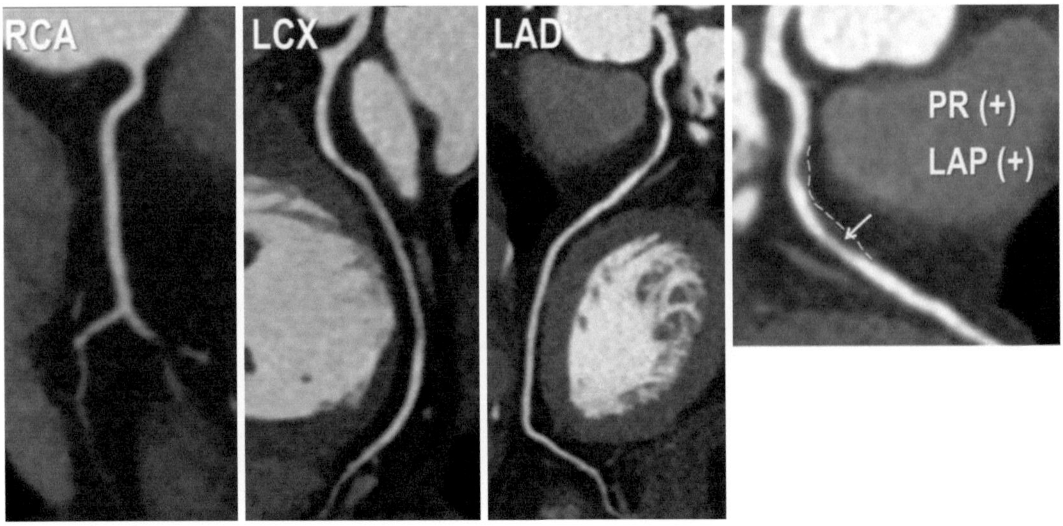

Fig. 3.7 An example of CAD-RADS 2/P2/HRP. There are no significant stenoses in the RCA and LCX, but mild stenosis (25%–49%) lesions are observed in the mid LAD; HRP, high-risk plaque; LAD, left anterior descending artery; LCX, left circumflex artery; LAP, low attenuation plaque; PR, positive remodeling; RCA, right coronary artery

initial stages, and to monitor the effects of treatment on the plaque.

Qualitative (or Semiquantitative) Atherosclerotic Plaque Evaluation

The initial in vivo assessment of atherosclerotic plaques, focusing on understanding the progression of these high-risk lesions, was conducted using grayscale intravascular ultrasonography (IVUS) [74]. This modality efficiently analyzes both the cross-sectional area and burden of plaques, as well as the longitudinal length of lesions and vessel remodeling. Furthermore, the utilization of advanced radiofrequency analysis of ultrasound signals has led to the development of IVUS-derived virtual histology (VH-IVUS), which provides detailed insights into plaque morphology and quantitatively assesses plaque composition [74].

Notably, the PROSPECT (Providing Regional Observations to Study Predictors of Events in the Coronary Tree) study demonstrated that TCFA identified by VH-IVUS are associated with an increased risk of major adverse cardiovascular events (HR 3.35, $p < 0.001$), even in non-culprit lesions, and that lesions with a plaque burden of ≥70% (HR 5.03, $p < 0.001$) or a minimal luminal area of ≤4.0 mm^2 (HR 3.21, $p = 0.001$) also showed heightened risk, crucially indicating that ACS caused by vulnerable plaques do not necessarily align with the degree of angiographic stenosis at the lesion site [75].

CCTA, an in vivo method, effectively and noninvasively identifies atherosclerotic plaques surrounding luminal stenosis [7]. Initially, plaques were categorized based on CT density into calcified, noncalcified, or mixed plaques [76]. Hoffmann et al. introduced a novel concept in CCTA by characterizing atherosclerotic plaques in ACS patients and comparing them to stable lesions, discovering that culprit lesions in ACS typically had larger plaque areas and higher remodeling indexes than stable lesions, along with a more frequent presence of noncalcified plaques [77].

Motoyama et al. identified HRP features visible on CCTA, including positive remodeling (PR), low-attenuation noncalcified plaque (LAP; <30 HU), and spotty calcification (SC), and found in their study that these features were more frequently present in culprit lesions of ACS patients ($n = 38$) compared to stable lesions ($n = 33$) [78]. Expanding their study to include over 1000 patients, they investigated the prospective relationship between adverse plaque characteristics and ACS over a 27-month follow-up period, concluding that lesions with two high-risk features, such as PR and larger plaque volumes with LAP, were significantly associated with acute coronary events, suggesting that such lesions with two high-risk features could be considered potentially vulnerable, whereas those without could be considered potentially stable [79].

Another significant HRP identified on CCTA, through integrative research with pathological studies, is the napkin-ring sign (NRS), characterized by a ring-like enhancement pattern surrounding large low-attenuation plaques, potentially indicative of TCFA [80]. Histological examinations of ACS culprit lesions frequently revealed the presence of NRS, which was also validated in prospective trials as being closely associated with future ACS events, independent of PR and LAP presence [80, 81]. Currently, four HRP features have been established on CCTA: PR, LAP, SC, and NRS, as shown in Fig. 3.8. The presence of more than two of these features can define a plaque as high-risk or vulnerable.

Quantitative Atherosclerotic Plaque Evaluation

In 2001, Schroeder et al. set a precedent in the field of quantitative atherosclerotic plaque evaluation by comparing the accuracy of coronary lesion configuration using CCTA with IVUS, revealing that soft plaques had an average density of 14 ± 26 HU (ranging from −42 to +47 HU), intermediate plaques 91 ± 21 HU (ranging from 61 to 112 HU), and calcified plaques 419 ± 194 HU (ranging from 126 to 736 HU) [82]. Building on this research, Leber et al. used CCTA to distinguish coronary plaque composition in lesions associated with myocardial infarction from stable ones, finding that myocardial infarction lesions predominantly had noncalcified plaques, along with increased stenosis and a higher total plaque burden compared to stable lesions [76]. Achenbach and his team pioneered the segmental quantification of coronary atherosclerotic plaque volume using CCTA, comparing it with IVUS in patients with nonobstructive coronary stenoses; they measured plaque volume in each coronary segment by producing contiguous 1-mm-thick cross-sectional images, viewing them under a fixed setting (700-HU window width, 200-HU window level), and manually delineating plaque areas to calculate their volumes, highlighting CCTA's potential in quantifying atherosclerotic plaque, though it tends to undervalue the volume of noncalcified plaques [83]. Prior to the introduction of semiautomated plaque quantification software, manually tracing lumen and vessel contours to calculate plaque volume and percent aggregate plaque volume was laborious and lacked reproducibility. However, these quantitative analyses have revealed interesting correlations between plaque volume and lesion-specific ischemia [84]. With the advent of semiautomated quantification software, plaque quantification has

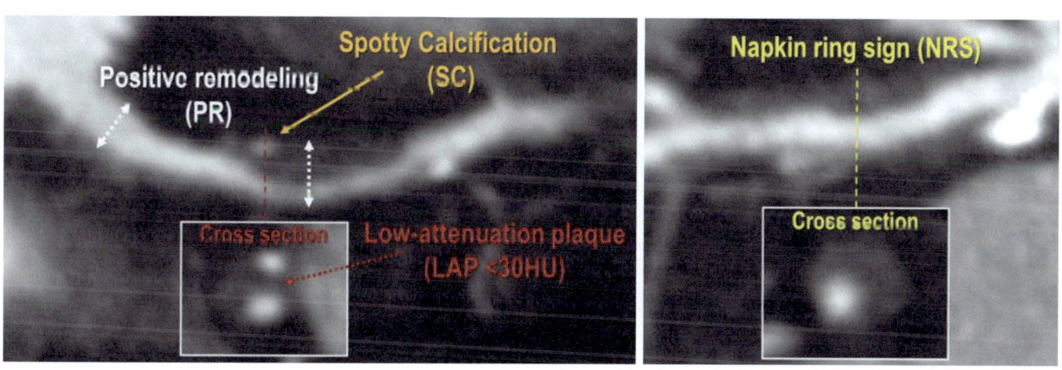

Fig. 3.8 Illustrations of four high-risk plaque features identified on CCTA

become more efficient, spurring further investigations into its practicality, particularly when compared with IVUS.

Voros et al., in their study employing a conventional dedicated workstation (Vitrea 2.0, Vital Images, Minnetonka, Minnesota) for three-dimensional standardized quantitative analysis of CCTA and coregistering results with VH-IVUS in 50 lesions from 50 patients, found that CCTA tends to overestimate diameter stenosis and minimal lumen area while underestimating minimal lumen diameter, yet demonstrated a strong correlation in both area stenosis and percentage of atheroma volume, with low-density noncalcified plaque corresponding to necrotic core plus fibro-fatty tissue on VH-IVUS, suggesting CCTA's utility in population-based studies despite broad limits of agreement [85]. Conversely, Dey and colleagues used their AUTOPLAQ (APQ) software for noncalcified plaque quantification, comparing it with IVUS in 22 atherosclerotic plaques from 20 patients, and demonstrated excellent correlation between noncalcified plaque volumes quantified with APQ, IVUS, and manual CCTA tracing, suggesting an automated approach to plaque quantification [86].

QAngio CT (QAngio CT 1.1, Medis medical imaging systems, Leiden, the Netherlands), a specialized automated quantitative software, provides automated contouring for both the lumen and vessel wall, with manual adjustment capabilities, and features a unique 3D registration algorithm facilitating automatic fusion of quantitative computed tomography (QCT) and IVUS images [87], as illustrated in Fig. 3.9.

Boogers et al. conducted a comparative analysis with QCT on 146 lesions from 51 patients, aligning these with images from a dedicated IVUS system (Volcano Corporation, Rancho Cordova, CA, USA), and found strong correlations for minimal lumen area (MLA) ($r = 0.75$) and mean plaque burden ($r = 0.64$), as well as a moderate correlation for the remodeling index ($r = 0.56$), but noted that QCT significantly tends to overestimate lumen area stenosis and plaque burden at MLA compared to IVUS, with its accuracy being image quality dependent, and demonstrated excellent reproducibility for these parameters, with intra-class correlation coefficients ranging between 0.84 and 0.92 [87].

Furthermore, in a cross-correlation comparison of QCT with VH-IVUS involving 108 lesions from 57 patients, QCT evaluated not only per lesion stenosis parameters and plaque volumes but also assessed four different types of plaque volumes—necrotic core (NC), dense calcium (DC), fibrotic (FI), and fibro-fatty tissue (FF)—using predefined HU thresholds, showing an excellent overall plaque volume correlation ($r = 0.928$) with VH-IVUS, particularly for FF ($r = 0.714$) and DC ($r = 0.736$), and modest correlations for FI ($r = 0.695$) and NC ($r = 0.523$),

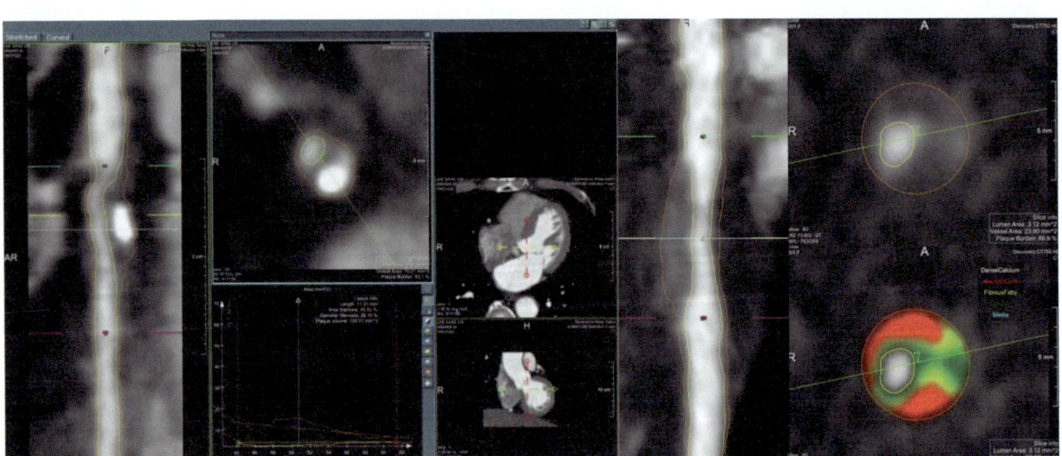

Fig. 3.9 Examples of quantitative computed tomography analysis

thereby demonstrating the feasibility of tissue characterization using QCT [88].

A study using the advanced QAngio CT Research Edition (v2.02) compared 2D and 3D parameters of 150 segments from 142 patients, analyzed by expert, nonexpert, and automatic groups, correlating findings with IVUS; despite QCT's user-friendly interface, challenges in reproducibility and significant operator-dependence were noted, with correlation coefficients (r) between QCT (expert/nonexpert/automatic) and IVUS reported as 0.94, 0.79, and 0.84 for plaque volume and 0.91, 0.73, and 0.84 for mean plaque burden, respectively, as shown in the example analyses in Fig. 3.10 [89]. The study found that nonexpert QCT overestimated calcified plaque volume while automatic QCT underestimated noncalcified and mixed plaque volumes, highlighting the limitations of fully automated plaque quantification, particularly with suboptimal image quality or artifacts, while also emphasizing the need for a skilled operator for accurate quantification, which, however, imposes constraints on reproducibility, a factor particularly significant in the context of using QCT for serial CCTA analyses to monitor therapeutic effects [89].

Extensive analyses to improve QCT plaque quantification accuracy initially focused on optimal boundary detection methods, comparing two lumen contouring methods—one with no gap and another with a 0.3-mm gap, based on histopathology of the intima and media—and found the 0.3-mm gap method more accurate for 51 lesions using both CCTA and IVUS; additionally, three window settings were evaluated, a fixed HU with a window width and level of 740/220, an adjusted HU based on 155% and 65% of mean luminal

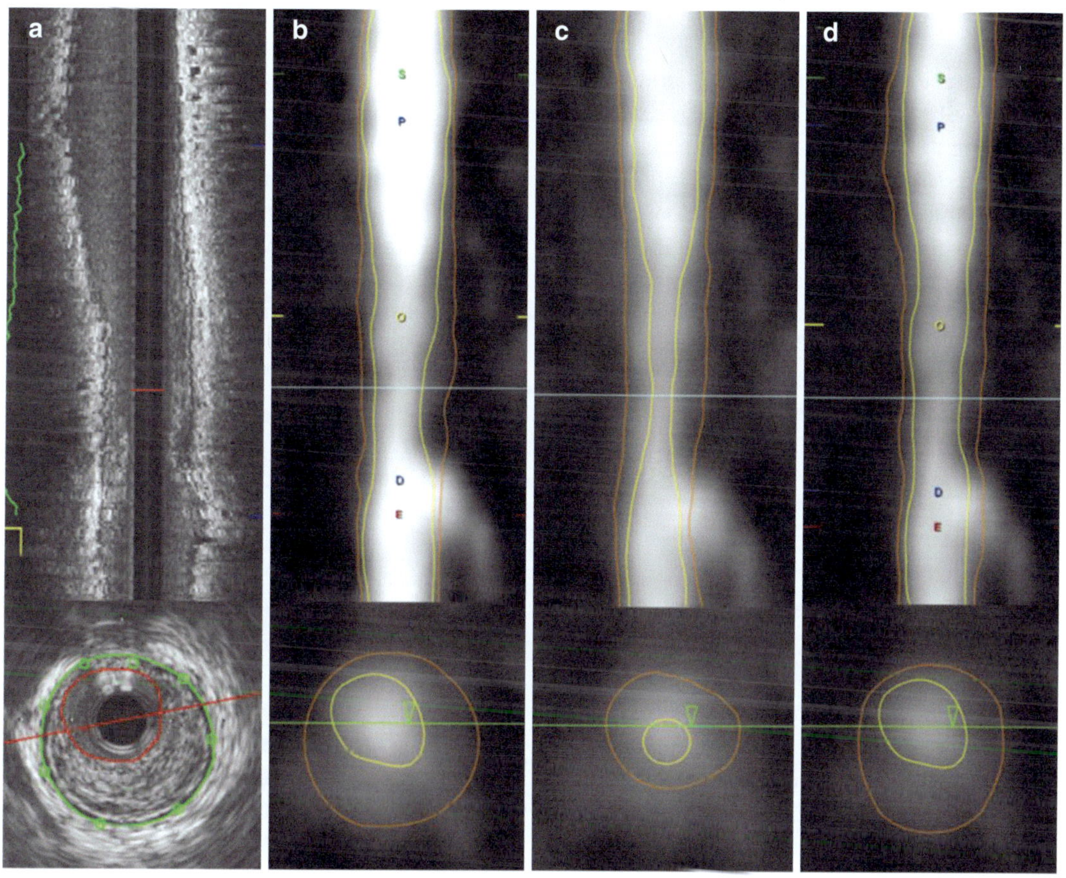

Fig. 3.10 IVUS (**a**) vs. expert (**b**), nonexpert (**c**), and automatic (**d**) QCT plaque analysis

intensity from a disease-free proximal reference level, and an aorta-adjusted HU based on 155% and 65% of the mean luminal intensity of the aortic root, with the fixed HU setting (740/220) showing highest accuracy compared to IVUS, while the aorta-adjusted settings significantly underestimated plaque volumes [90].

A study assessing the reproducibility and reliability of serial QCT quantitative analysis analyzed paired CT scans within a 90-day interval, including 847 segment pairs and 130 lesion pairs from 95 patients with consistent tube voltages (kVp), plus 210 segment pairs and 36 lesion pairs from 24 patients with varying kVp between initial and follow-up scans; evaluations of total plaque volumes and subtypes of plaque volumes with consistent kVp between index and follow-up CCTA showed no significant differences in per-patient, per-segment, and per-lesion analyses, and this consistency was maintained even with different tube voltages used between index and follow-up CCTA across all analysis levels [91].

These results demonstrate the reproducibility and reliability of QCT's quantitative analysis, suggesting that CCTA is viable for serial quantitative assessment of CAD progression, independent of variations in image acquisition protocol, leading to the establishment of the PRADIGM registry focused on serial CCTA, under which numerous studies have been conducted to assess clinical implications of HRPs, monitor plaque progression, evaluate the therapeutic effects of statin treatment, and explore the interrelationships between various risk factors and the progression or regression of plaque and plaque subtypes [92].

Quantitative Coronary Plaque Tracking by Serial CCTA

Motoyama et al. previously showed in a large-scale cohort study ($n = 3158$) with an average follow-up of 3.9 years that plaque progression, along with HRP features, significantly influences prognosis, with consistent findings regardless of the baseline degree of stenosis; notably, even in cases of significant stenosis (defined as ≥70%), the event rate was only 2.6% in the absence of high-risk plaque, but this rate escalated to 14.9% when HRP was present, irrespective of the degree of stenosis, and among the 449 patients who underwent follow-up CT scans, those with both plaque progression and HRP had the highest event rate (27.6%), while the event rate was a mere 0.3% in patients without plaque progression, regardless of initial HRP [93]. However, it should be noted that in this study, plaque progression was defined as either an elevation in stenosis by at least one grade or an increase in the remodeling index ratio exceeding 1.1, a definition that lacks a quantitative measurement of 3D plaque volume or overall plaque burden [93].

The dynamics of plaque characteristics and volume in high-risk groups have been thoroughly investigated using invasive techniques such as IVUS and VH-IVUS. In Kubo et al.'s study, over a 12-month follow-up period, nearly half (4%) of all baseline lesions with TCFA, representing 9% of cases identified in VH-IVUS, stabilized, while 6% of new TCFAs developed from previously stable lesions, as observed in 216 lesions in a serial VH-IVUS study [94]. In addition, Puri et al. conducted a meta-analysis of eight serial IVUS datasets and found that coronary percent atheroma volume (PAV) and calcium indices changes were affected by statin intensity [95]. High-intensity statin therapy resulted in more significant plaque regression compared to low-intensity therapy, with plaque progression noted in the no-statin group, and the highest increase in calcium indices in the intensive statin group led to the "calcium paradox" theory, suggesting that statin therapy may stabilize vulnerable plaques by enhancing calcium density, thus lowering the risk of plaque rupture [95, 96].

Numerous invasive studies have advocated for targeting LDL cholesterol levels below 70 mg/dL to achieve plaque regression [97]. Similarly, non-invasive studies using QCT analysis have shown that for low to intermediate-risk populations, an LDL cholesterol target of 70 mg/dL is effective, with individuals maintaining levels below this threshold showing smaller annual plaque volume changes compared to those above 70 mg/dL (12.7 ± 38.2 mm^3 vs. 44.2 ± 73.6 mm^3) [98].

The PARADIGM (Progression of Atherosclerotic Plaque Determined by Computed Tomographic Angiography Imaging) registry, the most extensive serial CCTA dataset to date, includes over 2000 patients from 13 sites across 7 countries, with an interscan interval of at least 2 years [92]. A primary analysis of 3576 lesions in 1255 patients revealed that statin therapy is associated with a 21% reduction in the annual progression of total plaque area volume (PAV) and a 35% decrease in high-risk plaque (HRP) development, also reaffirming the accelerated progression of calcified PAV under statin therapy, which supports the concept of the calcium paradox [99], as shown in Fig. 3.11.

Similarly, in a study of mild CAD (25%–49% of diameter stenosis) involving 1432 lesions in 613 patients, statin therapy led to a 37% decrease in the annual progression of PAV (0.97 ± 2.02 vs. 1.55 ± 2.22, $p = 0.038$), as well as reductions in necrotic core volume and increases in dense calcium volume, compared to those not receiving statins, indicating that aggressive statin treatment may be particularly effective in mild CAD, especially with the presence of multiple HRPs [100].

Another study from the PARADIGM registry on plaque progression identified "rapid plaque progressors" as patients with an annual plaque burden increase over 0.33% and found they had worse outcomes like cardiac death, nonfatal myocardial infarction, and coronary revascularization compared to slower plaque progressors, underscoring the importance of quantitative CCTA in predicting CAD progression and related events, thereby suggesting a shift in focus from luminal stenosis to overall atherosclerotic burden [101], as shown in Fig. 3.12.

Various studies from the PARADIGM registry have brought to light specific patterns in diverse population groups. In diabetic patients, there was a noted increase in both plaque progression and the development of new HRPs compared to non-diabetics [102]. Obesity was also found to influence plaque progression, as indicated by baseline body mass index (BMI) assessments, although BMI reduction did not consistently halt plaque progression [103]. Sex differences in plaque composition were noted, with women generally having more calcified plaque components and men more noncalcified components; despite similar annual plaque progression rates between sexes, men were found to have a higher susceptibility to developing new HRPs [104].

Further analysis of calcium score progression in statin-treated patients revealed differing outcomes between the statin and non-statin groups; despite similar increases in calcium scores, the statin group experienced less total plaque progression, marked by increased calcified and decreased noncalcified plaque volume, whereas in the no-statin group, both calcified and noncalcified plaque volumes increased, challenging the

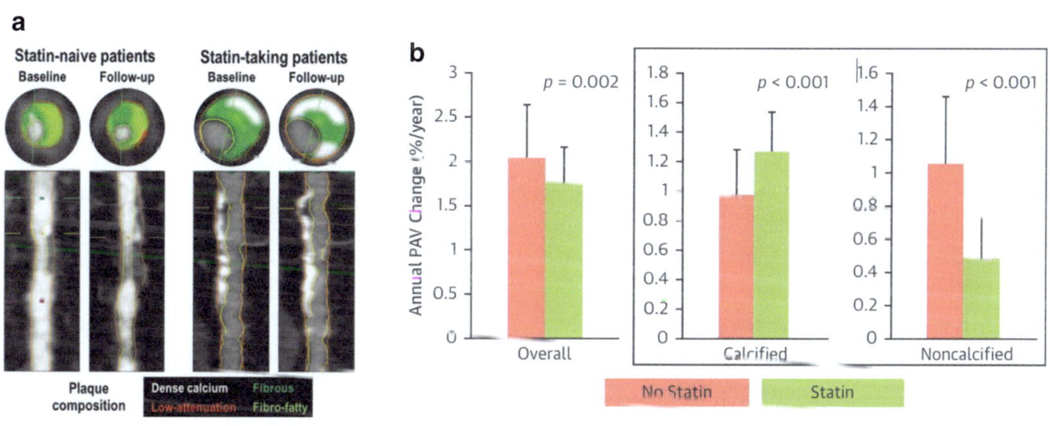

Fig. 3.11 Changes over time in the composition of noncalcified plaque volumes with statin use. (**a**) Representative QCT analysis of lesions at baseline and follow-up. (**b**) Annualized PAV change and PAV by composition according to statin

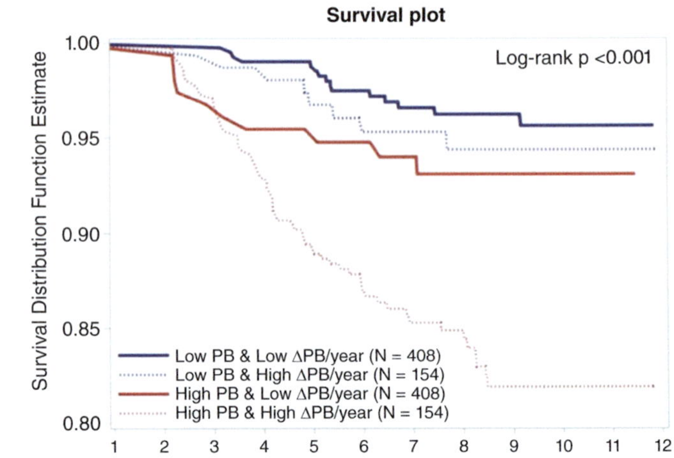

	1	2	3	4	5	6	7	8	9	10	11	12
Low PB & Low ΔPB/year	408	408	408	402	385	344	297	255	177	56	13	0
Low PB & Low ΔPB/year	154	154	153	151	143	131	117	95	62	20	4	0
High PB & Low ΔPB/year	154	154	149	147	140	126	106	87	64	28	6	0
High PB & Low ΔPB/year	408	408	395	378	350	293	233	185	111	38	9	0

Fig. 3.12 Outcomes in patients with various cross-sectional and longitudinal quantitative indices. When patients were stratified into four groups based on baseline plaque burden (PB) and annual progression rate of PB, patients who had both high PB and rapid progression rate experienced the worst clinical outcomes. ΔPB/y, annual progression of plaque burden

established correlation between calcium score progression and adverse outcomes and suggesting that such progression in statin-treated patients might not necessarily signal a worsening condition [105].

A recent study exploring statin nonresponders discovered that a high baseline plaque burden, including HRP features, strongly predicted statin nonresponse, defined as an absolute increase in PAV of 1.0% or more per year, emphasizing the necessity for additional therapies to lower risk in these patients and highlighting the importance of screening to identify potential statin nonresponders [106].

Predicting ACS Through Quantitative Analysis of Coronary Plaques

The ICONIC (Incident Coronary Syndromes Identified by Computed Tomography) registry, the largest case-control study nested within the CONFIRM registry to date, included 234 adjudicated patients who experienced ACS events and propensity-matched controls without such events [107]. The main analysis of 234 ACS cases and their controls revealed that over 65% of patients with ACS had nonobstructive CAD at baseline, 52% HRPs, and factors such as % diameter stenosis (%DS), cross-sectional plaque burden (PB), and volumes of fibrofatty and necrotic core, especially when combined with HRPs, significantly increased the risk of ACS [107]. A subanalysis on preventive plaque characteristics showed that "1K plaques" (dense calcified plaques with density over 1000 HU) were less common in lesions preceding ACS (*n* = 189) compared to the most stenotic lesions in the control group (*n* = 189), suggesting that 1 K plaques might be associated with a lower risk of future ACS and support the idea of plaque stability at both individual and lesion-specific levels [108]. The registry's examination of atherosclerosis patterns in ACS, considering age and sex, showed that older patients had higher total and calcified plaque volumes than younger ones; no significant sex differences were found in calcified plaque, but females had lower noncalcified plaque volumes than males, suggesting similar prognostic values of HRP presence and characteristics for both sexes, irrespective of age [109]. Moreover, the registry's examination of coronary plaque instability before an ACS incident revealed that patients with early ACS (≤90 days) had greater maximal %DS, maximal cross-sectional PB, and larger total, fibrous, fibrofatty, and necrotic core volumes compared to those with late ACS (>90 days), suggesting that a higher burden of noncalcified plaque on CCTA is strongly linked to imminent plaque instability and increased ACS risk [110].

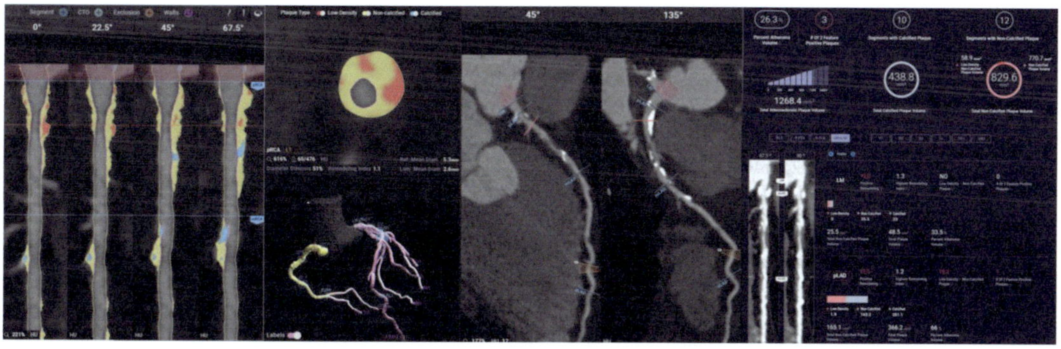

Fig. 3.13 Automated plaque quantification using artificial intelligence

Furthermore, the ICONIC registry revealed that nonobstructive HRP lesions, though less prevalent than obstructive lesions, pose a comparable risk to obstructive lesions without HRPs, highlighting the need for clinical reporting of HRPs even in nonobstructive CAD cases [111]. This case-control result was validated by a prospective post hoc analysis from the SCOT-HEART study, which followed 1769 patients for 5 years and showed that patients with nonobstructive disease and HRPs had similar outcomes to those with obstructive disease without HRPs, suggesting that CAD assessment should encompass both luminal severity and plaque characteristics, as well as overall plaque burden [112].

Artificial Intelligence-Based Automatic Plaque Quantification

Although quantitative coronary atherosclerosis evaluation shows promise, as numerous well-designed studies have highlighted its potential benefits for clinical practice, its wide adoption is hindered by the labor and time-intensive nature of the process and the high level of expertise required, even with user-friendly semiautomated software. Previous studies have indicated that mechanical approaches based on CT intensity thresholds in conventional automatic algorithms often fail to accurately detect optimal lumen or vessel borders, particularly in the presence of artifacts such as motion or calcium blooming. In these situations, manual adjustments or informed estimations for optimal borders become necessary, resulting in significant inter- and intra-operator variability [89].

This variability underscores the need for high expertise in this field, particularly for whole-heart quantitative CCTA analysis, rather than just specific lesion assessment. However, recent advancements in deep learning-based imaging analysis could address this challenge by appropriately assuming border detection in various situations, thereby mimicking expert decision-making without the inter- and intra-operator variability. In addition to plaque quantification, this technology can automatically grade stenosis, label coronary segments, detect high-risk plaques (HRPs), and generate reports, performing these tasks at a level comparable to human experts [113–116], as illustrated in Fig. 3.13.

References

1. Williams MC, Earls JP, Hecht H. Quantitative assessment of atherosclerotic plaque, recent progress and current limitations. J Cardiovasc Comput Tomogr. 2022;16(2):124–37. https://doi.org/10.1016/j.jcct.2021.07.001.
2. Mezquita AJV, Biavati F, Falk V, Alkadhi H, Hajhosseiny R, Maurovich-Horvat P, et al. Clinical quantitative coronary artery stenosis and coronary atherosclerosis imaging: a consensus statement from the quantitative cardiovascular imaging study group. Nat Rev Cardiol. 2023;20(10):696–714. https://doi.org/10.1038/s41569-023-00880-4.
3. Hisamatsu T, Kinuta M. Coronary artery calcium in assessment of atherosclerotic cardiovascular disease risk and its role in primary prevention. J Atheroscler Thromb. 2023;30(10):1289–302. https://doi.org/10.5551/jat.RV22009.

4. Hecht HS. Coronary artery calcium scanning: past, present, and future. JACC Cardiovasc Imaging. 2015;8(5):579–96. https://doi.org/10.1016/j.jcmg.2015.02.006.
5. Agatston AS, Janowitz WR, Hildner FJ, Zusmer NR, Viamonte M Jr, Detrano R. Quantification of coronary artery calcium using ultrafast computed tomography. J Am Coll Cardiol. 1990;15(4):827–32. https://doi.org/10.1016/0735-1097(90)90282-t.
6. Kwan AC, Cater G, Vargas J, Bluemke DA. Beyond coronary stenosis: coronary computed tomographic angiography for the assessment of atherosclerotic plaque burden. Curr Cardiovasc Imaging Rep. 2013;6(2):89–101. https://doi.org/10.1007/s12410-012-9183-z.
7. Maurovich-Horvat P, Ferencik M, Voros S, Merkely B, Hoffmann U. Comprehensive plaque assessment by coronary CT angiography. Nat Rev Cardiol. 2014;11(7):390–402. https://doi.org/10.1038/nrcardio.2014.60.
8. Serruys PW, Hara H, Garg S, Kawashima H, Norgaard BL, Dweck MR, et al. Coronary computed tomographic angiography for complete assessment of coronary artery disease: JACC state-of-the-art review. J Am Coll Cardiol. 2021;78(7):713–36. https://doi.org/10.1016/j.jacc.2021.06.019.
9. Cury RC, Leipsic J, Abbara S, Achenbach S, Berman D, Bittencourt M, et al. CAD-RADS 2.0-2022 coronary artery disease-reporting and data system: an expert consensus document of the Society of Cardiovascular Computed Tomography (SCCT), the American College of Cardiology (ACC), the American College of Radiology (ACR), and the North America Society of Cardiovascular Imaging (NASCI). JACC Cardiovasc Imaging. 2022;15(11):1974–2001. https://doi.org/10.1016/j.jcmg.2022.07.002.
10. Otsuka F, Sakakura K, Yahagi K, Joner M, Virmani R. Has our understanding of calcification in human coronary atherosclerosis progressed? Arterioscler Thromb Vasc Biol. 2014;34(4):724–36. https://doi.org/10.1161/ATVBAHA.113.302642.
11. Alani A, Budoff MJ. Coronary calcium scoring and computed tomography angiography: current indications, future applications. Coron Artery Dis. 2014;25(6):529–39. https://doi.org/10.1097/MCA.0000000000000147.
12. Alluri K, Joshi PH, Henry TS, Blumenthal RS, Nasir K, Blaha MJ. Scoring of coronary artery calcium scans: history, assumptions, current limitations, and future directions. Atherosclerosis. 2015;239(1):109–17. https://doi.org/10.1016/j.atherosclerosis.2014.12.040.
13. Lehker A, Mukherjee D. Coronary calcium risk score and cardiovascular risk. Curr Vasc Pharmacol. 2021;19(3):280–4. https://doi.org/10.2174/1570161118666200403143518.
14. Thomas DM, Divakaran S, Villines TC, Nasir K, Shah NR, Slim AM, et al. Management of coronary artery calcium and coronary CTA FINDINGS. Curr Cardiovasc Imaging Rep. 2015;8(6):18. https://doi.org/10.1007/s12410-015-9334-0.
15. Callister TQ, Cooil B, Raya SP, Lippolis NJ, Russo DJ, Raggi P. Coronary artery disease: improved reproducibility of calcium scoring with an electron-beam CT volumetric method. Radiology. 1998;208(3):807–14. https://doi.org/10.1148/radiology.208.3.9722864.
16. Hoffmann U, Siebert U, Bull-Stewart A, Achenbach S, Ferencik M, Moselewski F, et al. Evidence for lower variability of coronary artery calcium mineral mass measurements by multi-detector computed tomography in a community-based cohort--consequences for progression studies. Eur J Radiol. 2006;57(3):396–402. https://doi.org/10.1016/j.ejrad.2005.12.027.
17. Hong C, Bae KT, Pilgram TK. Coronary artery calcium: accuracy and reproducibility of measurements with multi-detector row CT—assessment of effects of different thresholds and quantification methods. Radiology. 2003;227(3):795–801. https://doi.org/10.1148/radiol.2273020369.
18. Detrano R, Guerci AD, Carr JJ, Bild DE, Burke G, Folsom AR, et al. Coronary calcium as a predictor of coronary events in four racial or ethnic groups. N Engl J Med. 2008;358(13):1336–45. https://doi.org/10.1056/NEJMoa072100.
19. Yeboah J, McClelland RL, Polonsky TS, Burke GL, Sibley CT, O'Leary D, et al. Comparison of novel risk markers for improvement in cardiovascular risk assessment in intermediate-risk individuals. JAMA. 2012;308(8):788–95. https://doi.org/10.1001/jama.2012.9624.
20. Budoff MJ, Young R, Burke G, Jeffrey Carr J, Detrano RC, Folsom AR, et al. Ten-year association of coronary artery calcium with atherosclerotic cardiovascular disease (ASCVD) events: the multi-ethnic study of atherosclerosis (MESA). Eur Heart J. 2018;39(25):2401–8. https://doi.org/10.1093/eurheartj/ehy217.
21. Budoff MJ, Young R, Lopez VA, Kronmal RA, Nasir K, Blumenthal RS, et al. Progression of coronary calcium and incident coronary heart disease events: MESA (multi-ethnic study of atherosclerosis). J Am Coll Cardiol. 2013;61(12):1231–9. https://doi.org/10.1016/j.jacc.2012.12.035.
22. Carr JJ, Jacobs DR Jr, Terry JG, Shay CM, Sidney S, Liu K, et al. Association of coronary artery calcium in adults aged 32 to 46 years with incident coronary heart disease and death. JAMA Cardiol. 2017;2(4):391–9. https://doi.org/10.1001/jamacardio.2016.5493.
23. Mitchell JD, Paisley R, Moon P, Novak E, Villines TC. Coronary artery calcium and long-term risk of death, myocardial infarction, and stroke: the Walter reed cohort study. JACC Cardiovasc Imaging. 2018;11(12):1799–806. https://doi.org/10.1016/j.jcmg.2017.09.003.
24. Shaw LJ, Min JK, Nasir K, Xie JX, Berman DS, Miedema MD, et al. Sex differences in calcified

plaque and long-term cardiovascular mortality: observations from the CAC consortium. Eur Heart J. 2018;39(41):3727–35. https://doi.org/10.1093/eurheartj/ehy534.

25. Cho I, Chang HJ, Hartaigh BO, Shin S, Sung JM, Lin FY, et al. Incremental prognostic utility of coronary CT angiography for asymptomatic patients based upon extent and severity of coronary artery calcium: results from the COronary CT angiography EvaluatioN for clinical outcomes InteRnational multicenter (CONFIRM) study. Eur Heart J. 2015;36(8):501–8. https://doi.org/10.1093/eurheartj/ehu358.
26. Budoff MJ, Diamond GA, Raggi P, Arad Y, Guerci AD, Callister TQ, Berman D. Continuous probabilistic prediction of angiographically significant coronary artery disease using electron beam tomography. Circulation. 2002;105(15):1791–6. https://doi.org/10.1161/01.cir.0000014483.43921.8c.
27. Haberl R, Becker A, Leber A, Knez A, Becker C, Lang C, et al. Correlation of coronary calcification and angiographically documented stenoses in patients with suspected coronary artery disease: results of 1,764 patients. J Am Coll Cardiol. 2001;37(2):451–7. https://doi.org/10.1016/s0735-1097(00)01119-0.
28. Descalzo M, Vidal-Perez R, Leta R, Alomar X, Pons-Llado G, Carreras F. Usefulness of coronary artery calcium for detecting significant coronary artery disease in asymptomatic individuals. Rev Clin Esp. 2014;214(5):235–41. https://doi.org/10.1016/j.rce.2014.01.005.
29. Ahn SJ, Kang DK, Sun JS, Yoon MH. Accuracy and predictive value of coronary computed tomography angiography for the detection of obstructive coronary heart disease in patients with an Agatston calcium score above 400. J Comput Assist Tomogr. 2013;37(3):387–94. https://doi.org/10.1097/RCT.0b013e318282d61c.
30. Abdulla J, Pedersen KS, Budoff M, Kofoed KF. Influence of coronary calcification on the diagnostic accuracy of 64-slice computed tomography coronary angiography: a systematic review and meta-analysis. Int J Cardiovasc Imaging. 2012;28(4):943–53. https://doi.org/10.1007/s10554-011-9902-6.
31. Lee JH, Han D, B OH, Rizvi A, Gransar H, Park HB, et al. Warranty period of zero coronary artery calcium score for predicting all-cause mortality according to cardiac risk burden in asymptomatic Korean adults. Circ J. 2016;80(11):2356–61. https://doi.org/10.1253/circj.CJ-16-0731.
32. Raggi P, Callister TQ, Cooil B, He ZX, Lippolis NJ, Russo DJ, et al. Identification of patients at increased risk of first unheralded acute myocardial infarction by electron-beam computed tomography. Circulation. 2000;101(8):850–5. https://doi.org/10.1161/01.cir.101.8.850.
33. Blaha M, Budoff MJ, Shaw LJ, Khosa F, Rumberger JA, Berman D, et al. Absence of coronary artery calcification and all-cause mortality. JACC Cardiovasc Imaging. 2009;2(6):692–700. https://doi.org/10.1016/j.jcmg.2009.03.009.
34. Arad Y, Goodman KJ, Roth M, Newstein D, Guerci AD. Coronary calcification, coronary disease risk factors, C-reactive protein, and atherosclerotic cardiovascular disease events: the St. Francis heart study. J Am Coll Cardiol. 2005;46(1):158–65. https://doi.org/10.1016/j.jacc.2005.02.088.
35. Villines TC, Hulten EA, Shaw LJ, Goyal M, Dunning A, Achenbach S, et al. Prevalence and severity of coronary artery disease and adverse events among symptomatic patients with coronary artery calcification scores of zero undergoing coronary computed tomography angiography: results from the CONFIRM (coronary CT angiography evaluation for clinical outcomes: an international multicenter) registry. J Am Coll Cardiol. 2011;58(24):2533–40. https://doi.org/10.1016/j.jacc.2011.10.851.
36. Budoff MJ, Mayrhofer T, Ferencik M, Bittner D, Lee KL, Lu MT, et al. Prognostic value of coronary artery calcium in the PROMISE study (prospective multicenter imaging study for evaluation of chest pain). Circulation. 2017;136(21):1993–2005. https://doi.org/10.1161/CIRCULATIONAHA.117.030578.
37. Mittal TK, Pottle A, Nicol E, Barbir M, Ariff B, Mirsadraee S, et al. Prevalence of obstructive coronary artery disease and prognosis in patients with stable symptoms and a zero-coronary calcium score. Eur Heart J Cardiovasc Imaging. 2017;18(8):922–9. https://doi.org/10.1093/ehjci/jex037.
38. Gottlieb I, Miller JM, Arbab-Zadeh A, Dewey M, Clouse ME, Sara L, et al. The absence of coronary calcification does not exclude obstructive coronary artery disease or the need for revascularization in patients referred for conventional coronary angiography. J Am Coll Cardiol. 2010;55(7):627–34. https://doi.org/10.1016/j.jacc.2009.07.072.
39. Rubinshtein R, Gaspar T, Halon DA, Goldstein J, Peled N, Lewis BS. Prevalence and extent of obstructive coronary artery disease in patients with zero or low calcium score undergoing 64-slice cardiac multidetector computed tomography for evaluation of a chest pain syndrome. Am J Cardiol. 2007;99(4):472–5. https://doi.org/10.1016/j.amjcard.2006.08.060.
40. Koulaouzidis G, Charisopoulou D, Jenkins PJ, Koulaouzidis A, McArthur T. Prevalence of noncalcified coronary plaque in patients with calcium score of 0: the silent enemy. Angiology. 2013;64(3):205–10. https://doi.org/10.1177/0003319712440618.
41. Koopman MY, Willemsen RTA, van der Harst P, van Bruggen R, Gratama JWC, Braam R, et al. The diagnostic and prognostic value of coronary calcium scoring in stable chest pain patients: a narrative review. RöFo. 2022;194(3):257–65. https://doi.org/10.1055/a-1662-5711.
42. Park HB, Jeong H, Lee JH, Suh Y, Hwang ES, Cho YH, Cho DK. Predictors of severe or moderate

coronary artery disease in asymptomatic individuals with extremely low coronary calcium scores. Yonsei Med J. 2019;60(7):619–25. https://doi.org/10.3349/ymj.2019.60.7.619.
43. Choi EK, Choi SI, Rivera JJ, Nasir K, Chang SA, Chun EJ, et al. Coronary computed tomography angiography as a screening tool for the detection of occult coronary artery disease in asymptomatic individuals. J Am Coll Cardiol. 2008;52(5):357–65. https://doi.org/10.1016/j.jacc.2008.02.086.
44. Lee MS, Chun EJ, Kim KJ, Kim JA, Yoo JY, Choi SI. Asymptomatic subjects with zero coronary calcium score: coronary CT angiographic features of plaques in event-prone patients. Int J Cardiovasc Imaging. 2013;29(Suppl 1):29–36. https://doi.org/10.1007/s10554-013-0257-z.
45. Isgum I, Rutten A, Prokop M, van Ginneken B. Detection of coronary calcifications from computed tomography scans for automated risk assessment of coronary artery disease. Med Phys. 2007;34(4):1450–61. https://doi.org/10.1118/1.2710548.
46. Kurkure U, Chittajallu DR, Brunner G, Le YH, Kakadiaris IA. A supervised classification-based method for coronary calcium detection in non-contrast CT. Int J Cardiovasc Imaging. 2010;26(7):817–28. https://doi.org/10.1007/s10554-010-9607-2.
47. Brunner G, Chittajallu DR, Kurkure U, Kakadiaris IA. Toward the automatic detection of coronary artery calcification in non-contrast computed tomography data. Int J Cardiovasc Imaging. 2010;26(7):829–38. https://doi.org/10.1007/s10554-010-9608-1.
48. Shahzad R, van Walsum T, Schaap M, Rossi A, Klein S, Weustink AC, et al. Vessel specific coronary artery calcium scoring: an automatic system. Acad Radiol. 2013;20(1):1–9. https://doi.org/10.1016/j.acra.2012.07.018.
49. van Velzen SGM, Lessmann N, Velthuis BK, Bank IEM, van den Bongard D, Leiner T, et al. Deep learning for automatic calcium scoring in CT: validation using multiple cardiac CT and chest CT protocols. Radiology. 2020;295(1):66–79. https://doi.org/10.1148/radiol.2020191621.
50. Martin SS, van Assen M, Rapaka S, Hudson HT Jr, Fischer AM, Varga-Szemes A, et al. Evaluation of a deep learning-based automated CT coronary artery calcium scoring algorithm. JACC Cardiovasc Imaging. 2020;13(2 Pt 1):524–6. https://doi.org/10.1016/j.jcmg.2019.09.015.
51. Zhang N, Yang G, Zhang W, Wang W, Zhou Z, Zhang H, et al. Fully automatic framework for comprehensive coronary artery calcium scores analysis on non-contrast cardiac-gated CT scan: total and vessel-specific quantifications. Eur J Radiol. 2021;134:109420. https://doi.org/10.1016/j.ejrad.2020.109420.
52. Lee JG, Kim H, Kang H, Koo HJ, Kang JW, Kim YH, Yang DH. Fully automatic coronary calcium score software empowered by artificial intelligence technology: validation study using three CT cohorts. Korean J Radiol. 2021;22(11):1764–76. https://doi.org/10.3348/kjr.2021.0148.
53. Ihdayhid AR, Lan NSR, Williams M, Newby D, Flack J, Kwok S, et al. Evaluation of an artificial intelligence coronary artery calcium scoring model from computed tomography. Eur Radiol. 2023;33(1):321–9. https://doi.org/10.1007/s00330-022-09028-3.
54. Miller JM, Rochitte CE, Dewey M, Arbab-Zadeh A, Niinuma H, Gottlieb I, et al. Diagnostic performance of coronary angiography by 64-row CT. N Engl J Med. 2008;359(22):2324–36. https://doi.org/10.1056/NEJMoa0806576.
55. Budoff MJ, Dowe D, Jollis JG, Gitter M, Sutherland J, Halamert E, et al. Diagnostic performance of 64-multidetector row coronary computed tomographic angiography for evaluation of coronary artery stenosis in individuals without known coronary artery disease: results from the prospective multicenter ACCURACY (assessment by coronary computed tomographic angiography of individuals undergoing invasive coronary angiography) trial. J Am Coll Cardiol. 2008;52(21):1724–32. https://doi.org/10.1016/j.jacc.2008.07.031.
56. Meijboom WB, Meijs MF, Schuijf JD, Cramer MJ, Mollet NR, van Mieghem CA, et al. Diagnostic accuracy of 64-slice computed tomography coronary angiography: a prospective, multicenter, multivendor study. J Am Coll Cardiol. 2008;52(25):2135–44. https://doi.org/10.1016/j.jacc.2008.08.058.
57. Nielsen LH, Ortner N, Norgaard BL, Achenbach S, Leipsic J, Abdulla J. The diagnostic accuracy and outcomes after coronary computed tomography angiography vs. conventional functional testing in patients with stable angina pectoris: a systematic review and meta-analysis. Eur Heart J Cardiovasc Imaging. 2014;15(9):961–71. https://doi.org/10.1093/ehjci/jeu027.
58. Knuuti J, Wijns W, Saraste A, Capodanno D, Barbato E, Funck-Brentano C, et al. 2019 ESC guidelines for the diagnosis and management of chronic coronary syndromes. Eur Heart J. 2020;41(3):407–77. https://doi.org/10.1093/eurheartj/ehz425.
59. Gulati M, Levy PD, Mukherjee D, Amsterdam E, Bhatt DL, Birtcher KK, et al. 2021 AHA/ACC/ASE/CHEST/SAEM/SCCT/SCMR guideline for the evaluation and diagnosis of CHEST pain: a report of the American College of Cardiology/American Heart Association joint committee on clinical practice guidelines. Circulation. 2021;144(22):e368–454. https://doi.org/10.1161/CIR.0000000000001029.
60. Min JK, Dunning A, Lin FY, Achenbach S, Al-Mallah MH, Berman DS, et al. Rationale and design of the CONFIRM (COronary CT angiography EvaluatioN for clinical outcomes: an InteRnational multicenter) registry. J Cardiovasc Comput Tomogr. 2011;5(2):84–92. https://doi.org/10.1016/j.jcct.2011.01.007.

61. Min JK, Dunning A, Lin FY, Achenbach S, Al-Mallah M, Budoff MJ, et al. Age- and sex-related differences in all-cause mortality risk based on coronary computed tomography angiography findings results from the international multicenter CONFIRM (coronary CT angiography evaluation for clinical outcomes: an international multicenter registry) of 23,854 patients without known coronary artery disease. J Am Coll Cardiol. 2011;58(8):849–60. https://doi.org/10.1016/j.jacc.2011.02.074.
62. Chow BJ, Small G, Yam Y, Chen L, Achenbach S, Al-Mallah M, et al. Incremental prognostic value of cardiac computed tomography in coronary artery disease using CONFIRM: COroNary computed tomography angiography evaluation for clinical outcomes: an InteRnational multicenter registry. Circ Cardiovasc Imaging. 2011;4(5):463–72. https://doi.org/10.1161/CIRCIMAGING.111.964155.
63. Douglas PS, Hoffmann U, Patel MR, Mark DB, Al-Khalidi HR, Cavanaugh B, et al. Outcomes of anatomical versus functional testing for coronary artery disease. N Engl J Med. 2015;372(14):1291–300. https://doi.org/10.1056/NEJMoa1415516.
64. Investigators S-H. CT coronary angiography in patients with suspected angina due to coronary heart disease (SCOT-HEART): an open-label, parallel-group, multicentre trial. Lancet. 2015;385(9985):2383–91. https://doi.org/10.1016/S0140-6736(15)60291-4.
65. Williams MC, Hunter A, Shah ASV, Assi V, Lewis S, Smith J, et al. Use of coronary computed tomographic angiography to guide management of patients with coronary disease. J Am Coll Cardiol. 2016;67(15):1759–68. https://doi.org/10.1016/j.jacc.2016.02.026.
66. Investigators S-H, Newby DE, Adamson PD, Berry C, Boon NA, Dweck MR, et al. Coronary CT angiography and 5-year risk of myocardial infarction. N Engl J Med. 2018;379(10):924–33. https://doi.org/10.1056/NEJMoa1805971.
67. Group DT, Maurovich-Horvat P, Bosserdt M, Kofoed KF, Rieckmann N, Benedek T, et al. CT or invasive coronary angiography in stable chest pain. N Engl J Med. 2022;386(17):1591–602. https://doi.org/10.1056/NEJMoa2200963.
68. Cury RC, Abbara S, Achenbach S, Agatston A, Berman DS, Budoff MJ, et al. Coronary artery disease—reporting and data system (CAD-RADS): an expert consensus document of SCCT, ACR and NASCI: endorsed by the ACC. JACC Cardiovasc Imaging. 2016;9(9):1099–113. https://doi.org/10.1016/j.jcmg.2016.05.005.
69. Lerner DJ, Kannel WB. Patterns of coronary heart disease morbidity and mortality in the sexes: a 26-year follow-up of the Framingham population. Am Heart J. 1986;111(2):383–90. https://doi.org/10.1016/0002-8703(86)90155-9.
70. Bogle BM, Ning H, Mehrotra S, Goldberger JJ, Lloyd-Jones DM. Lifetime risk for sudden cardiac death in the community. J Am Heart Assoc. 2016;5(7):e002398. https://doi.org/10.1161/JAHA.115.002398.
71. Falk E, Shah PK, Fuster V. Coronary plaque disruption. Circulation. 1995;92(3):657–71. https://doi.org/10.1161/01.cir.92.3.657.
72. Yokoya K, Takatsu H, Suzuki T, Hosokawa H, Ojio S, Matsubara T, et al. Process of progression of coronary artery lesions from mild or moderate stenosis to moderate or severe stenosis: a study based on four serial coronary arteriograms per year. Circulation. 1999;100(9):903–9. https://doi.org/10.1161/01.cir.100.9.903.
73. Ahmadi A, Leipsic J, Blankstein R, Taylor C, Hecht H, Stone GW, Narula J. Do plaques rapidly progress prior to myocardial infarction? The interplay between plaque vulnerability and progression. Circ Res. 2015;117(1):99–104. https://doi.org/10.1161/CIRCRESAHA.117.305637.
74. Nair A, Kuban BD, Tuzcu EM, Schoenhagen P, Nissen SE, Vince DG. Coronary plaque classification with intravascular ultrasound radiofrequency data analysis. Circulation. 2002;106(17):2200–6. https://doi.org/10.1161/01.cir.0000035654.18341.5e.
75. Stone GW, Maehara A, Lansky AJ, de Bruyne B, Cristea E, Mintz GS, et al. A prospective natural-history study of coronary atherosclerosis. N Engl J Med. 2011;364(3):226–35. https://doi.org/10.1056/NEJMoa1002358.
76. Leber AW, Knez A, White CW, Becker A, von Ziegler F, Muehling O, et al. Composition of coronary atherosclerotic plaques in patients with acute myocardial infarction and stable angina pectoris determined by contrast-enhanced multislice computed tomography. Am J Cardiol. 2003;91(6):714–8. https://doi.org/10.1016/s0002-9149(02)03411-2.
77. Hoffmann U, Moselewski F, Nieman K, Jang IK, Ferencik M, Rahman AM, et al. Noninvasive assessment of plaque morphology and composition in culprit and stable lesions in acute coronary syndrome and stable lesions in stable angina by multidetector computed tomography. J Am Coll Cardiol. 2006;47(8):1655–62. https://doi.org/10.1016/j.jacc.2006.01.041.
78. Motoyama S, Kondo T, Sarai M, Sugiura A, Harigaya H, Sato T, et al. Multislice computed tomographic characteristics of coronary lesions in acute coronary syndromes. J Am Coll Cardiol. 2007;50(4):319–26. https://doi.org/10.1016/j.jacc.2007.03.044.
79. Motoyama S, Sarai M, Harigaya H, Anno H, Inoue K, Hara T, et al. Computed tomographic angiography characteristics of atherosclerotic plaques subsequently resulting in acute coronary syndrome. J Am Coll Cardiol. 2009;54(1):49–57. https://doi.org/10.1016/j.jacc.2009.02.068.
80. Maurovich-Horvat P, Schlett CL, Alkadhi H, Nakano M, Otsuka F, Stolzmann P, et al. The napkin-ring sign indicates advanced atherosclerotic lesions in coronary CT angiography. JACC Cardiovasc Imaging. 2012;5(12):1243–52. https://doi.org/10.1016/j.jcmg.2012.03.019.

81. Otsuka K, Fukuda S, Tanaka A, Nakanishi K, Taguchi H, Yoshikawa J, et al. Napkin-ring sign on coronary CT angiography for the prediction of acute coronary syndrome. JACC Cardiovasc Imaging. 2013;6(4):448–57. https://doi.org/10.1016/j.jcmg.2012.09.016.
82. Schroeder S, Kopp AF, Baumbach A, Meisner C, Kuettner A, Georg C, et al. Noninvasive detection and evaluation of atherosclerotic coronary plaques with multislice computed tomography. J Am Coll Cardiol. 2001;37(5):1430–5. https://doi.org/10.1016/s0735-1097(01)01115-9.
83. Achenbach S, Moselewski F, Ropers D, Ferencik M, Hoffmann U, MacNeill B, et al. Detection of calcified and noncalcified coronary atherosclerotic plaque by contrast-enhanced, submillimeter multidetector spiral computed tomography: a segment-based comparison with intravascular ultrasound. Circulation. 2004;109(1):14–7. https://doi.org/10.1161/01.CIR.0000111517.69230.0F.
84. Nakazato R, Shalev A, Doh JH, Koo BK, Gransar H, Gomez MJ, et al. Aggregate plaque volume by coronary computed tomography angiography is superior and incremental to luminal narrowing for diagnosis of ischemic lesions of intermediate stenosis severity. J Am Coll Cardiol. 2013;62(5):460–7. https://doi.org/10.1016/j.jacc.2013.04.062.
85. Voros S, Rinehart S, Qian Z, Vazquez G, Anderson H, Murrieta L, et al. Prospective validation of standardized, 3-dimensional, quantitative coronary computed tomographic plaque measurements using radiofrequency backscatter intravascular ultrasound as reference standard in intermediate coronary arterial lesions: results from the ATLANTA (assessment of tissue characteristics, lesion morphology, and hemodynamics by angiography with fractional flow reserve, intravascular ultrasound and virtual histology, and noninvasive computed tomography in atherosclerotic plaques) I study. JACC Cardiovasc Interv. 2011;4(2):198–208. https://doi.org/10.1016/j.jcin.2010.10.008.
86. Dey D, Schepis T, Marwan M, Slomka PJ, Berman DS, Achenbach S. Automated three-dimensional quantification of noncalcified coronary plaque from coronary CT angiography: comparison with intravascular US. Radiology. 2010;257(2):516–22. https://doi.org/10.1148/radiol.10100681.
87. Boogers MJ, Broersen A, van Velzen JE, de Graaf FR, El-Naggar HM, Kitslaar PH, et al. Automated quantification of coronary plaque with computed tomography: comparison with intravascular ultrasound using a dedicated registration algorithm for fusion-based quantification. Eur Heart J. 2012;33(8):1007–16. https://doi.org/10.1093/eurheartj/ehr465.
88. de Graaf MA, Broersen A, Kitslaar PH, Roos CJ, Dijkstra J, Lelieveldt BP, et al. Automatic quantification and characterization of coronary atherosclerosis with computed tomography coronary angiography: cross-correlation with intravascular ultrasound virtual histology. Int J Cardiovasc Imaging. 2013;29(5):1177–90. https://doi.org/10.1007/s10554-013-0194-x.
89. Park HB, Lee BK, Shin S, Heo R, Arsanjani R, Kitslaar PH, et al. Clinical feasibility of 3D automated coronary atherosclerotic plaque quantification algorithm on coronary computed tomography angiography: comparison with intravascular ultrasound. Eur Radiol. 2015;25(10):3073–83. https://doi.org/10.1007/s00330-015-3698-z.
90. Heo R, Park HB, Lee BK, Shin S, Arsanjani R, Min JK, Chang HJ. Optimal boundary detection method and window settings for coronary atherosclerotic plaque volume analysis in coronary computed tomography angiography: comparison with intravascular ultrasound. Eur Radiol. 2016;26(9):3190–8. https://doi.org/10.1007/s00330-015-4121-5.
91. Lee SE, Park HB, Xuan D, Lee BK, Hong MK, Jang Y, Chang HJ. Consistency of quantitative analysis of coronary computed tomography angiography. J Cardiovasc Comput Tomogr. 2019;13(1):48–54. https://doi.org/10.1016/j.jcct.2018.09.012.
92. Lee SE, Chang HJ, Rizvi A, Hadamitzky M, Kim YJ, Conte E, et al. Rationale and design of the progression of AtheRosclerotic PlAque DetermIned by computed TomoGraphic angiography IMaging (PARADIGM) registry: a comprehensive exploration of plaque progression and its impact on clinical outcomes from a multicenter serial coronary computed tomographic angiography study. Am Heart J. 2016;182:72–9. https://doi.org/10.1016/j.ahj.2016.09.003.
93. Motoyama S, Ito H, Sarai M, Kondo T, Kawai H, Nagahara Y, et al. Plaque characterization by coronary computed tomography angiography and the likelihood of acute coronary events in mid-term follow-up. J Am Coll Cardiol. 2015;66(4):337–46. https://doi.org/10.1016/j.jacc.2015.05.069.
94. Kubo T, Maehara A, Mintz GS, Doi H, Tsujita K, Choi SY, et al. The dynamic nature of coronary artery lesion morphology assessed by serial virtual histology intravascular ultrasound tissue characterization. J Am Coll Cardiol. 2010;55(15):1590–7. https://doi.org/10.1016/j.jacc.2009.07.078.
95. Puri R, Nicholls SJ, Shao M, Kataoka Y, Uno K, Kapadia SR, et al. Impact of statins on serial coronary calcification during atheroma progression and regression. J Am Coll Cardiol. 2015;65(13):1273–82. https://doi.org/10.1016/j.jacc.2015.01.036.
96. Ferencik M, Chatzizisis YS. Statins and the coronary plaque calcium "paradox": insights from noninvasive and invasive imaging. Atherosclerosis. 2015;241(2):783–5. https://doi.org/10.1016/j.atherosclerosis.2015.05.021.
97. Tsujita K, Sugiyama S, Sumida H, Shimomura H, Yamashita T, Yamanaga K, et al. Impact of dual lipid-lowering strategy with ezetimibe and atorvastatin on coronary plaque regression in patients with percutaneous coronary intervention: the multicenter randomized controlled PRECISE-IVUS trial. J Am Coll Cardiol. 2015;66(5):495–507. https://doi.org/10.1016/j.jacc.2015.05.065.
98. Shin S, Park HB, Chang HJ, Arsanjani R, Min JK, Kim YJ, et al. Impact of intensive LDL choles-

terol lowering on coronary artery atherosclerosis progression: a serial CT angiography study. JACC Cardiovasc Imaging. 2017;10(4):437–46. https://doi.org/10.1016/j.jcmg.2016.04.013.
99. Lee SE, Chang HJ, Sung JM, Park HB, Heo R, Rizvi A, et al. Effects of statins on coronary atherosclerotic plaques: the PARADIGM study. JACC Cardiovasc Imaging. 2018;11(10):1475–84. https://doi.org/10.1016/j.jcmg.2018.04.015.
100. Park HB, Arsanjani R, Sung JM, Heo R, Lee BK, Lin FY, et al. Impact of statins based on high-risk plaque features on coronary plaque progression in mild stenosis lesions: results from the PARADIGM study. Eur Heart J Cardiovasc Imaging. 2023;24(11):1536–43. https://doi.org/10.1093/ehjci/jead110.
101. Lee SE, Sung JM, Rizvi A, Lin FY, Kumar A, Hadamitzky M, et al. Quantification of coronary atherosclerosis in the assessment of coronary artery disease. Circ Cardiovasc Imaging. 2018;11(7):e007562. https://doi.org/10.1161/CIRCIMAGING.117.007562.
102. Kim U, Leipsic JA, Sellers SL, Shao M, Blanke P, Hadamitzky M, et al. Natural history of diabetic coronary atherosclerosis by quantitative measurement of serial coronary computed tomographic angiography: results of the PARADIGM study. JACC Cardiovasc Imaging. 2018;11(10):1461–71. https://doi.org/10.1016/j.jcmg.2018.04.009.
103. Won KB, Lee SE, Lee BK, Park HB, Heo R, Rizvi A, et al. Longitudinal quantitative assessment of coronary plaque progression related to body mass index using serial coronary computed tomography angiography. Eur Heart J Cardiovasc Imaging. 2019;20(5):591–9. https://doi.org/10.1093/ehjci/jey192.
104. Lee SE, Sung JM, Andreini D, Al-Mallah MH, Budoff MJ, Cademartiri F, et al. Sex differences in compositional plaque volume progression in patients with coronary artery disease. JACC Cardiovasc Imaging. 2020;13(11):2386–96. https://doi.org/10.1016/j.jcmg.2020.06.034.
105. Lee SE, Sung JM, Andreini D, Budoff MJ, Cademartiri F, Chinnaiyan K, et al. Differential association between the progression of coronary artery calcium score and coronary plaque volume progression according to statins: the progression of AtheRosclerotic PlAque DetermIned by computed TomoGraphic angiography imaging (PARADIGM) study. Eur Heart J Cardiovasc Imaging. 2019;20(11):1307–14. https://doi.org/10.1093/ehjci/jez022.
106. van Rosendael SE, van den Hoogen IJ, Lin FY, Andreini D, Al-Mallah MH, Budoff MJ, et al. Clinical and coronary plaque predictors of atherosclerotic nonresponse to statin therapy. JACC Cardiovasc Imaging. 2023;16(4):495–504. https://doi.org/10.1016/j.jcmg.2022.10.017.
107. Chang HJ, Lin FY, Lee SE, Andreini D, Bax J, Cademartiri F, et al. Coronary atherosclerotic precursors of acute coronary syndromes. J Am Coll Cardiol. 2018;71(22):2511–22. https://doi.org/10.1016/j.jacc.2018.02.079.
108. van Rosendael AR, Narula J, Lin FY, van den Hoogen IJ, Gianni U, Al Hussein Alawamlh O, et al. Association of high-density calcified 1K plaque with risk of acute coronary syndrome. JAMA Cardiol. 2020;5(3):282–90. https://doi.org/10.1001/jamacardio.2019.5315.
109. Conte E, Dwivedi A, Mushtaq S, Pontone G, Lin FY, Hollenberg EJ, et al. Age- and sex-related features of atherosclerosis from coronary computed tomography angiography in patients prior to acute coronary syndrome: results from the ICONIC study. Eur Heart J Cardiovasc Imaging. 2021;22(1):24–33. https://doi.org/10.1093/ehjci/jeaa210.
110. van den Hoogen IJ, Stuijfzand WJ, Gianni U, van Rosendael AR, Bax AM, Lu Y, et al. Early versus late acute coronary syndrome risk patterns of coronary atherosclerotic plaque. Eur Heart J Cardiovasc Imaging. 2022;23(10):1314–23. https://doi.org/10.1093/ehjci/jeac114.
111. Ferraro RA, van Rosendael AR, Lu Y, Andreini D, Al-Mallah MH, Cademartiri F, et al. Non-obstructive high-risk plaques increase the risk of future culprit lesions comparable to obstructive plaques without high-risk features: the ICONIC study. Eur Heart J Cardiovasc Imaging. 2020;21(9):973–80. https://doi.org/10.1093/ehjci/jeaa048.
112. Williams MC, Moss AJ, Dweck M, Adamson PD, Alam S, Hunter A, et al. Coronary artery plaque characteristics associated with adverse outcomes in the SCOT-HEART study. J Am Coll Cardiol. 2019;73(3):291–301. https://doi.org/10.1016/j.jacc.2018.10.066.
113. Singh G, Al'Aref SJ, Van Assen M, Kim TS, van Rosendael A, Kolli KK, et al. Machine learning in cardiac CT: basic concepts and contemporary data. J Cardiovasc Comput Tomogr. 2018;12(3):192–201. https://doi.org/10.1016/j.jcct.2018.04.010.
114. Dey D, Slomka PJ, Leeson P, Comaniciu D, Shrestha S, Sengupta PP, Marwick TH. Artificial intelligence in cardiovascular imaging: JACC state-of-the-art review. J Am Coll Cardiol. 2019;73(11):1317–35. https://doi.org/10.1016/j.jacc.2018.12.054.
115. Choi AD, Marques H, Kumar V, Griffin WF, Rahban H, Karlsberg RP, et al. CT evaluation by artificial intelligence for atherosclerosis, stenosis and vascular morphology (CLARIFY): a multi-center, international study. J Cardiovasc Comput Tomogr. 2021;15(6):470–6. https://doi.org/10.1016/j.jcct.2021.05.004.
116. Jonas R, Patel T, Crabtree TR, Jennings RS, Heo R, Park HB, et al. Relation of gender to atherosclerotic plaque characteristics by differing angiographic stenosis severity. Am J Cardiol. 2023;204:276–83. https://doi.org/10.1016/j.amjcard.2023.07.004.

CT Fractional Flow Reserve in Coronary Artery Disease

4

Shaun Hinen, Dhiraj Baruah, and Ismail Kabakus

Introduction

With ischemic heart disease being the leading cause of death worldwide, the imperative for efficient and effective diagnostic tools in the evaluation process cannot be overstated. Coronary computed tomography angiography (CCTA) has proven to be an important asset during the screening process for patients with low to moderate pre-test probability for coronary artery disease (CAD) with high accuracy and high negative predictive values [1]. This has proven to be an important gatekeeper to invasive cardiac catheterization which has served as the gold standard for identifying hemodynamically significant obstructive lesions that could require intervention. Through the late twentieth century and early twenty-first century, this has been accomplished using fractional flow reserve (FFR) calculation during invasive coronary angiography (ICA) in which the ratio of flow through a stenotic lesion compared to the hypothetical flow without obstruction can be expressed by pressure measured distal to the stenosis divided by the pressure proximal to stenosis during maximum hyperemia [2]. Reduced FFR values below 0.8 would imply hemodynamically significant lesions that could benefit from percutaneous coronary intervention (PCI) [2, 3].

S. Hinen · D. Baruah (✉) · I. Kabakus
Medical University of South Carolina, Charleston, SC, USA
e-mail: baruah@musc.edu

Within the past decade, the development of computed tomography (CT)-derived FFR which can emulate this process has expanded the capability of CCTA to be used as a first-line test in chest pain workup. Now, CCTA with FFR does not only address the presence of disease but also enhances specificity for stenotic lesions, enabling a more precise identification of patients who could benefit from invasive intervention [4].

Technique

CT FFR is a noninvasive imaging modality which can simulate the invasive measurement of FFR values to determine physiologically significant coronary artery stenoses. This process is applied to standard coronary CT angiography series first by creating a three-dimensional model of the coronary artery anatomy. Next a physiologic model of the coronary circulation is derived from set boundaries for inflow and outflow, and hemodynamic conditions such as resting myocardial blood flow are determined from myocardial mass, while microvascular resistance is modeled by the size of the epicardial arteries. These conditions are then used to estimate maximal hyperemia mimicking administration of adenosine without the need for actual administration. This is performed by computations using the Navier-Stokes equations which dictate the laws of fluid dynamics by off-site super computers to calcu-

R. Gill, P. Rajiah (eds.), *Quantitative Imaging in the Thorax*,
https://doi.org/10.1007/978-3-032-14103-3_4

late coronary flow, velocity, and pressure at rest and during hyperemia [5, 6]. The final FFR values are then masked over the 3D model of the coronary tree allowing FFR values to be viewed at each point throughout each coronary artery [5]. The only United States Food and Drug Administration (FDA)-approved application to accomplish this task is HeartFlow thus making it the most widely used service [6].

To accomplish this modeling, there must be a standardized approach to acquiring coronary CTA images as these estimates cannot be made on artifact and motion degraded examinations. These parameters should be met on state-of-the-art CT systems with fast gantry rotations at most rotating 350 ms. The minimum detector requirement is 64 slices with widths of 0.625 mm or less [7]. High injection rates should be achieved at 4–7 cc/s, and bolus tracking/test bolus protocols may be acceptable. Scans are typically obtained at 100–120 kVp with potential and tube current modulation techniques favorable to achieve reduced radiation exposure while preserving image quality. Prospectively electrocardiogram (ECG) triggered axial acquisition is recommend as first choice for coronary CTA with alternative such as high-pitch spiral acquisition and retrospectively ECG-gated helical or spiral acquisition possible [7]. Scan ranges should include the carina to the apex of the heart with a field of view centered on the heart (usually a FOV of 200–250 mm), and axial images should be reconstructed with a slice width less than 1.0 mm, and minimal slice thickness should be obtained, typically 0.5–0.6 mm^2. A semi-sharp reconstruction kernel should also be used with sharp kernels used to help reduce blooming artifacts. Multiple phases of the cardiac cycle should be reconstructed typically with mid-diastolic standstill serving as the optimal time point for well controlled heart rates and end systolic phase for faster heart rates [7]. With that, oral and intravenous beta blocker use is routinely used to achieve a heart rate less than 60 beats per minute, and the use of sublingual versus spray nitrate is recommended to maximally dilate the coronary arteries [7]. HeartFlow provides scanner-specific parameters and protocol recommendations in greater detail as adequate diagnostic image quality is paramount to CT-FFR generation.

Recommended CCTA technical parameters	
Minimum detector row	64 slices with width of 0.625 mm
Gantry rotation time	350 ms
Injection rate	4–7 ml/s
Tube potential	100–120 kVp
Scan range	Carina to the bottom of the heart
FOV	20–25 cm
Reconstruction slice thickness	0.6 mm or less
Reconstruction kernel strength level	40
Medication	Nitro and beta blockers (to achieve HR < 60)

Patient Selection

Coronary Artery Disease Reporting and Data System (CAD-RADS) is a standardized reporting system for patients receiving coronary CTA which is the product of an expert consensus of several societies including the American College of Cardiology (ACC) and American College of Radiology (ACR). This classification system is determined by the most severe coronary luminal stenosis per patient with CAD-RADS 0 representing absence any coronary lesion, while CAD-RADS 5 indicates total occlusion with categories in between representing different degrees of stenosis represented as a percentage, and each category has corresponding management recommendations which range from no further workup for low-risk anatomy to ICA for higher severity disease [8]. The updated 2022 CAD-RADS document includes recommendations pertaining to CT FFR which states that CT FFR may be considered and be the most useful for further evaluation beginning with CAD-RADS 3 lesions which reflect moderate stenosis (50–69%) and intermediate risk of ischemia particularly if it would change management or there is persistent stable or acute chest pain despite medical therapy [6, 8]. CAD-RADS 4 is the next most severe classification which is divided into two separate categories (A and B), and the recommendations can vary depending upon the involvement of the left main coronary artery and the presence of severe (70–99%) three-vessel disease. CT FFR is also specifically listed as a consideration for CAD-RADS 4A which indicates the case of single vessel or two vessels severe stenosis whereas ICA is generally recommended for CAD-RADS 4B which indicates at least 50% stenosis of the left main coronary artery or three vessel severe stenosis [8]. For category 4 lesions, CT FFR may be particularly useful for helping guide revascularization planning especially with multivessel disease [6]. Furthermore, in line with the 2021 Chest Pain Guidelines issued by the American Heart Association and the American College of Cardiology, CT FFR may be helpful for acute chest pain patients with intermediate risk and inconclusive stenosis or those with more than 50% stenosis on CCTA. Additionally, CT FFR may prove beneficial for stable chest pain patients, whether or not they have known CAD, exhibiting 40–90% stenosis on CCTA. It's worth noting that the guidelines highlight the importance of considering turnaround times for FFR CT, as delays could impact timely clinical care decisions (PMID: 34709879) [9].

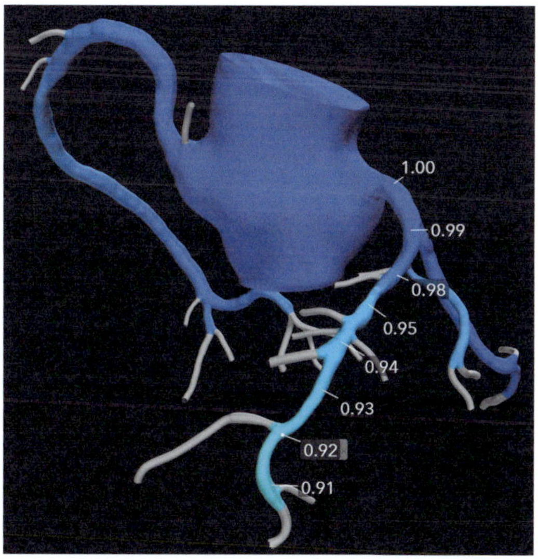

Fig. 4.1 Illustration depicting the decline in normal CT FFR values along the course of a vessel, attributed to the natural tapering phenomenon

How to Interpret

Firstly, the initial interpretation of CT FFR values should be specifically correlated to the original coronary CTA with focus on location and severity of stenosis. The CT FFR values decline along the course of a vessel due to their natural tapering (Fig. 4.1), and serial lesions become additive in their pressure loss; thus, interpretation must be made on a lesion-by-lesion basis [4]. The FFR values range from 0 to 1 with values greater than 0.8 being normal, values between 0.76 and 0.8 being borderline, and values less than or equal to 0.75 being abnormal, and HeartFlow displays a color-coded overlay on the 3D model of the coronary tree which is interactable allowing for individual FFR values to be examined at each segment of the coronary arteries [4, 6]. Studies have shown that FFR values measured 1–2 cm distal to the questioned lesion allow for the greatest specificity for ischemia associated with that lesion [4, 6]. A modifier is also included in the updated version of CAD-RADS to incorporate this functional assessment for ischemia with the modifier, "I" [8]. For values greater than 0.8 which imply that the lesion is not hemodynamically significant, a "I−" (negative ischemia) modifier would be used, and deferral of ICA with medical optimization would be sufficient (Fig. 4.2). Borderline values between 0.76 and 0.8 would receive "I+/−" corresponding to indeterminate value with decisions regarding further workup depending upon several factors such as lesion location, clinical factors such as symptom severity/stability, and delta CT FFR values (trans-lesional values) [8]. Finally, a "I+" designation would be appropriate for hemodynamically significant lesions with values less than or equal to 0.75, and ICA should generally be considered in large enough vessels for PCI (Figs. 4.3 and 4.4) [8].

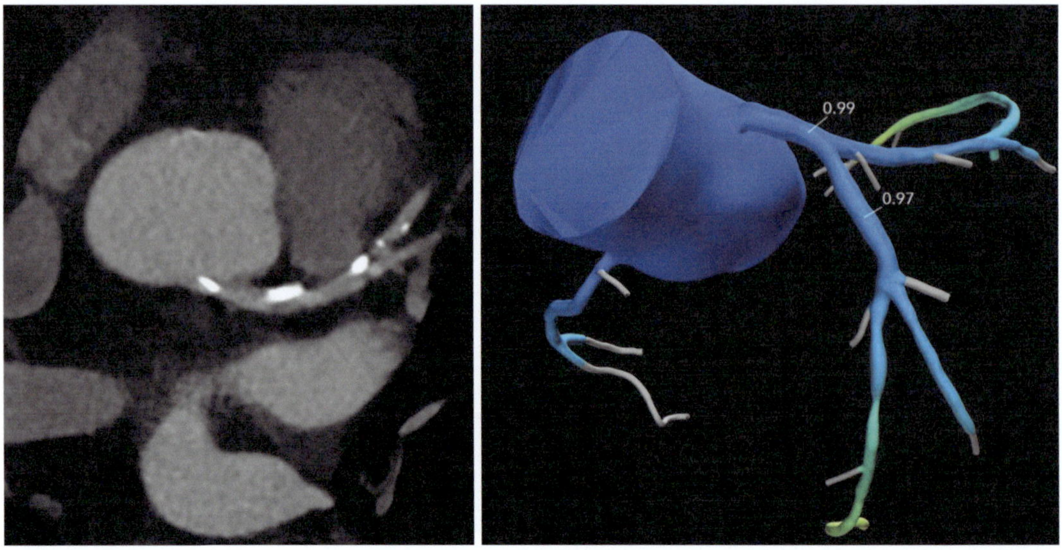

Fig. 4.2 Visualization of a patient with moderate stenosis in proximal LAD segment. CT FFR analysis indicates no ischemia, supporting invasive coronary angiography deferral coupled with medical treatment optimization

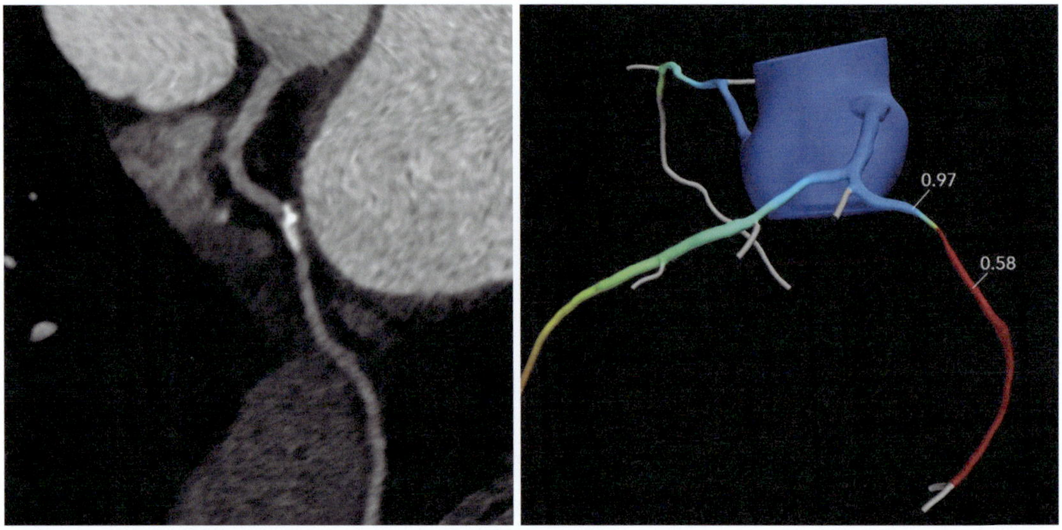

Fig. 4.3 Visualization of a patient with moderate stenosis in LCx. CT FFR analysis indicates ischemia, supporting invasive coronary angiography

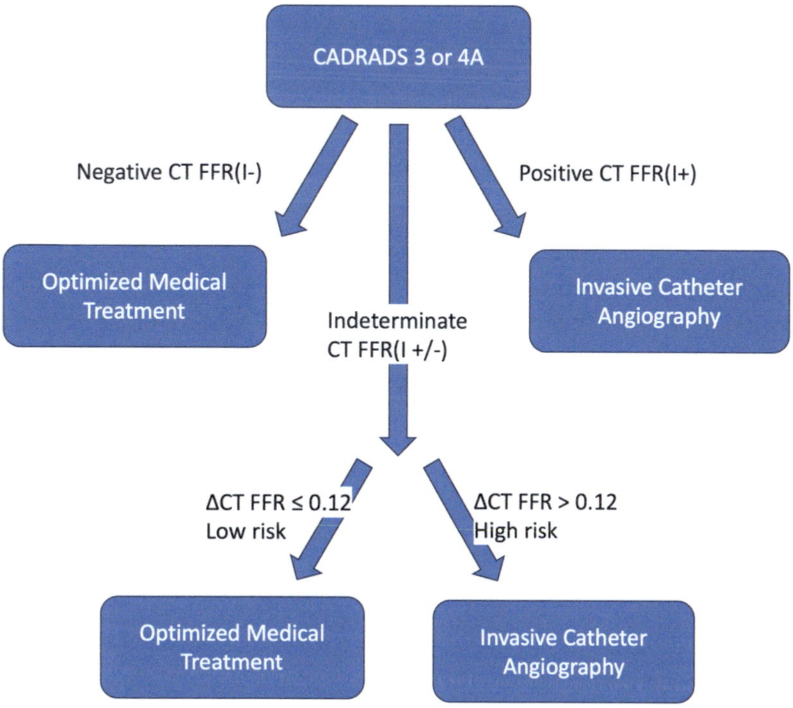

Fig. 4.4 Decision tree outlining the considerations based on CADRADS and CT FFR results

Nuance of Borderline Values

Recommendations for cases yielding a borderline or indeterminate FFR value (0.76–0.8) should be tailored based upon several additional factors with the aim of identifying patients who would be at a higher risk of cardiovascular event who could benefit from earlier invasive assessment. These include things such as high-risk plaque features (low attenuation, positive remodeling, napkin-ring sign, and spotty calcification), stenosis location (proximal over distal or main versus side-branch), vessel territory, degree of plaque burden, and number of vessels involved [4, 6]. In the case of higher risk features, invasive testing may be appropriately recommended, whereas outpatient medical therapy may be considered in those groups without high-risk features [6]. CAD-RADS also recommends consideration of delta CT FFR to help guide which patients may benefit from ICA referral in borderline categories stating that a trans-lesion gradient greater than 0.12 may be hemodynamically significant [8]. This delta CT FFR value would be represented as the pressure loss 1–2 cm proximal to the stenosis compared to 1–2 cm distal to the stenosis [8]. Some groups have suggested assigning all indeterminate patients to outpatient medical therapy for 3 months, and if symptoms persist at 3 months, then ICA referral may be appropriate [6]. In any case, this category group should always be assessed with careful consideration of additional imaging features and clinical parameters to help guide additional follow-up as these cases will often be highly specific to each patient.

Discordance

Discrepancy in values obtained between CTA and CT FFR do occur and can be expected given that anatomical alterations do not have a linear relationship with hemodynamic changes. Multiple different factors may account for this occurrence particularly where a low FFR value is seen despite only seeing a mildly stenotic lesion, and things to consider when interpreting these results should include minimal luminal diameter, length and shape of the stenotic lesion, location of the lesion (particularly proximal versus distal), main versus side branch involvement, and myocardial mass [6]. All these factors may lead to decreased FFR values especially if a stenosis is seen in a larger vessel supplying a larger area of myocardium such as the proximal LAD. On the other end of the spectrum, severe stenosis can have normal FFR values which can be accounted for by good collateralization distally, or if the lesion is located distally, then that vessel may only supply a relatively small volume of myocardium [8]. For this reason, cases of severe stenosis could be appropriately managed medically. Consensus on how to manage abnormal CT FFR values without significant stenosis varies, but these imaging characteristics as well as the clinical context should be considered to help guide recommendations [6]. CAD-RADS addresses this topic stating that lesions with abnormal FFR without concordant lesion should be given an "I−" (ischemia negative) modifier if the interpreter is confident that the FFR value is a false positive which can occur secondary to modeling errors, whereas an indeterminate modifier can be utilized if there is questionable interpretation of both CTA and FFR findings [8].

Diffuse Disease and Serial Lesions

There is a natural tendency for FFR values to decrease as you progress distally along the coronary tree which can be attributed to the natural tapering of the coronary vessels with myocardial mass and diffuse atherosclerotic disease/serial lesion also increasing the overall pressure drop distally [6] (Fig. 4.5). For this reason, evaluation of distal-most FFR results should be performed with the context of lesion location and severity of stenosis as abnormal values may be the reflection of summative effects of diffuse disease or multiple lesions. This understanding signifies the importance of measuring FFR values within 1–2 cm distal to a lesion to provide lesion-specific hemodynamic contributions [4, 6]. Assessing the individual contribution of each lesion in the case of serial stenoses has proven to be challenging as studies in the past have shown that change in FFR across each lesion by invasive and noninvasive techniques have underestimated the contribution of individual stenosis to ischemia [6]. This has been thought to be due to complex interactions in flow dynamics which make it difficult to achieve maximal hyperemia in the setting of multiple

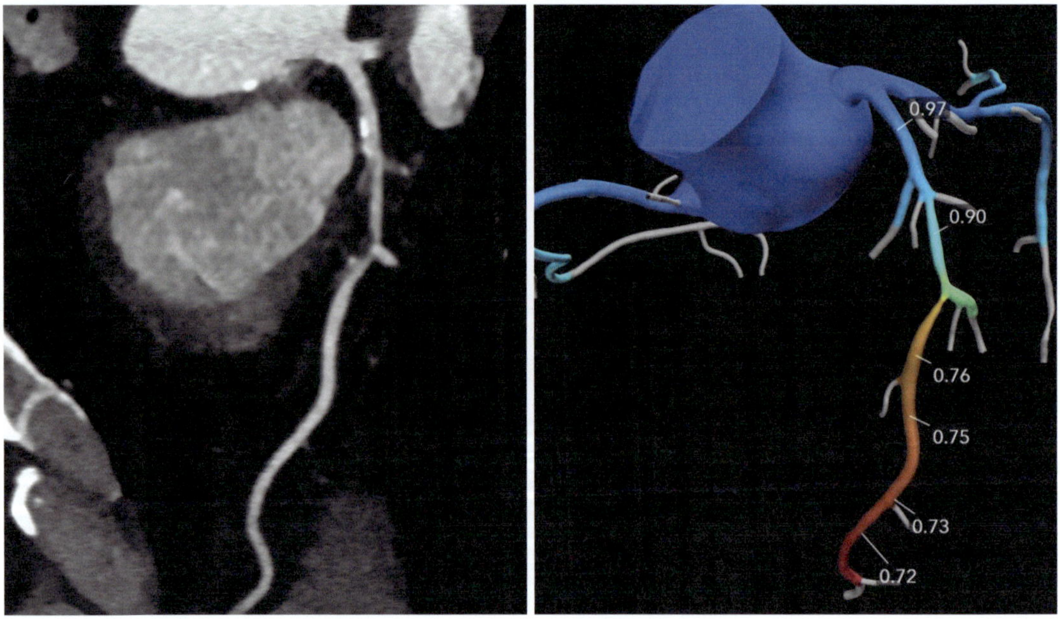

Fig. 4.5 Visualization of a patient with diffuse atherosclerotic disease/serial lesions in LAD. CT FFR analysis reveals ischemia at the distal LAD attributed to the cumulative effect of these lesions

resistance modifying lesions [6]. Despite this limitation, recent studies have shown that a CT FFR based revascularization planner based upon CT geometric information may more accurately display which lesions provide the greatest improvements in flow following revascularization by simulating new FFR values [10].

Pitfalls

One should be aware that correlation between the 3D model and native coronary CTA is paramount as modeling errors can occur altering the overall downstream FFR values and final interpretation. Careful attention should be made to ensure that the questioned stenosis is relatively well modeled in the resulting 3D coronary tree as motion artifact may artificially worsen the severity of stenosis on the CT FFR imaging. Similarly, some severe stenoses may not be appropriately represented in the final model, and sometimes anatomic areas especially side-branches can be excluded from the resultant model [6]. These potential pitfalls underline the importance of ensuring an efficient and standardized scanning protocol as producing high-quality diagnostic coronary CTA will help reduce these potential pitfalls. Additional pitfalls of CT FFR have been well outlined above including but not limited to gradual decreases in FFR values (which can be normal or attributed to diffuse disease/serial stenosis), low values in distal most vessels without focal lesions, and discordant FFR values.

Other Considerations

With the advent of CT FFR, there has been much emphasis placed on comparing its accuracy and reproducibility compared to invasive FFR, and some have even investigated its ability to simulate post PCI FFR values. The latter measurement has been explored as post-PCI FFR values have a prognostic indication with low FFR values after intervention portending a poorer prognosis than those with high values (greater than 0.8) [11]. This measurement can be obtained using a CT FFR Planner tool, also available through HeartFlow, which can simulate the placement of a stent of a selected length across a specified lesion providing a calculated FFR after intervention, and this information could prove useful to help decide which lesions may benefit most from treatment. A recent study demonstrated that CT FFR Planner was just as accurate and precise as conventional measurement of FFR post-PCI (mean difference only differing by 0.02 ± 0.07 unit) [11]. Additional explorations have also shown that CT FFR following stent placement can be just as accurate as invasive techniques to identify in-stent restenosis with an accuracy of 86% [12]. While many studies have supported that CT FFR is comparable to traditional standards, some newer research has suggested that CT FFR has its limitations with room for further improvement. A recent randomized clinical trial in 2023 examined the use of on-site machine learning-based CT FFR against standard of care that included CTA plus functional stress testing; while the rate of patients with stable chest pain without obstructive lesions had decreased revascularization, the overall number of patients receiving revascularization was increased compared to the control without any improvement of symptoms, quality of life, or reducing major cardiovascular events [13]. The FORECAST study showed that employing a strategy of CCTA with selective CT FFR in patients with stable angina did not exhibit significant differences in clinical outcomes when compared to standard clinical care pathways. However, it did result in a slight increase in total costs (though not statistically significant) and a reduction in the utilization of invasive coronary angiography [14]. A meta-analysis revealed that there was no significant difference in the risk of all-cause mortality between patients with obstructive CAD and those with nonobstructive CAD as identified by CT FFR. However, it was found that obstructive lesions were linked to an increased risk of morbidity related to revascularization procedures. It is important to note that machine-based learning CT FFR represents a distinct methodology compared to the off-site computational fluid dynamics used by HeartFlow. This distinction necessitates further long-term studies to evaluate the impact these differing approaches have on accuracy and overall patient outcomes, particularly in terms of morbidity and mortality.

Conclusion

Originally, coronary CTA was proven to be a helpful screening tool in the workup for patients presenting with chest pain owing to their high sensitivity for detecting the presence of coronary lesions. An early limitation was that the positive predictive value related to degree of stenosis was relatively poor, thus making it difficult to discern which patients would benefit most from invasive coronary evaluation for potential PCI placement. The advent of CT FFR modeling has drastically altered coronary CTA as a diagnostic tool as it improved specificity by providing accurate simulation of FFR values compared to invasive testing providing a noninvasive means of quantifying which lesions could benefit most from revascularization when identified. An understanding of normal, indeterminate, and abnormal FFR values is required with measurement of FFR values 1–2 distal to the questioned stenosis key. Moreover, interpretating physician should remain vigilant about potential pitfalls encountered while assessing CT FFR results. A thorough correlation with anatomic features and clinical context becomes imperative, emphasizing the need for a customized approach in each case.

References

1. Maroules CD, Rajiah P, Bhasin M, Abbara S. Current evidence in cardiothoracic imaging: growing evidence for coronary computed tomography angiography as a first-line test in stable chest pain. J Thorac Imaging. 2019;34(1):4–11. https://doi.org/10.1097/RTI.0000000000000357.
2. Mathew RC, Gottbrecht M, Salerno M. Computed tomography fractional flow reserve to guide coronary angiography and intervention. Interv Cardiol Clin. 2018;7(3):345–54. https://doi.org/10.1016/j.iccl.2018.03.008.
3. Frobert O, Gotberg M. Fractional flow reserve-dichotomous decisions in myocardial ischemia. Circ Cardiovasc Interv. 2022;15(2):e011787. https://doi.org/10.1161/CIRCINTERVENTIONS.122.011787.
4. Norgaard BL, Fairbairn TA, Safian RD, et al. Coronary CT angiography-derived fractional flow reserve testing in patients with stable coronary artery disease: recommendations on interpretation and reporting. Radiol Cardiothorac Imaging. 2019;1(5):e190050. https://doi.org/10.1148/ryct.2019190050.
5. Tesche C, De Cecco CN, Albrecht MH, et al. Coronary CT angiography-derived fractional flow reserve. Radiology. 2017;285(1):17–33. https://doi.org/10.1148/radiol.2017162641.
6. Rajiah P, Cummings KW, Williamson E, Young PM. CT fractional flow reserve: a practical guide to application, interpretation, and problem solving. Radiographics. 2022;42(2):340–58. https://doi.org/10.1148/rg.210097.
7. Abbara S, Blanke P, Maroules CD, et al. SCCT guidelines for the performance and acquisition of coronary computed tomographic angiography: a report of the society of Cardiovascular Computed Tomography Guidelines Committee: endorsed by the North American Society for Cardiovascular Imaging (NASCI). J Cardiovasc Comput Tomogr. 2016;10(6):435–49. https://doi.org/10.1016/j.jcct.2016.10.002.
8. Cury RC, Leipsic J, Abbara S, et al. CAD-RADS 2.0 – 2022 coronary artery disease – reporting and data system an expert consensus document of the Society of Cardiovascular Computed Tomography (SCCT), the American College of Cardiology (ACC), the American College of Radiology (ACR) and the North America Society of Cardiovascular Imaging (NASCI). Radiol Cardiothorac Imaging. 2022;4(5):e220183. https://doi.org/10.1148/ryct.220183.
9. Gulati M, Levy PD, Mukherjee D, et al. AHA/ACC/ASE/CHEST/SAEM/SCCT/SCMR guideline for the evaluation and diagnosis of chest pain: a report of the American College of Cardiology/American Heart Association Joint Committee on clinical practice guidelines. Circulation. 2021;144(22):e368–454. https://doi.org/10.1161/CIR.0000000000001029.
10. Modi BN, Sankaran S, Kim HJ, et al. Predicting the physiological effect of revascularization in serially diseased coronary arteries. Circ Cardiovasc Interv. 2019;12(2):e007577. https://doi.org/10.1161/CIRCINTERVENTIONS.118.007577.
11. Matteucci A, Massaro G, Mamas MA, Biondi-Zoccai G. Expanding the role of fractional flow reserve derived from computed tomography (FFR(CT)) for the non-invasive imaging of patients with coronary stents: rise of the machines? Eur Radiol. 2021;31(9):6589–91. https://doi.org/10.1007/s00330-021-07974-y.
12. Sonck J, Nagumo S, Norgaard BL, et al. Clinical validation of a virtual planner for coronary interventions based on coronary CT angiography. JACC

Cardiovasc Imaging. 2022;15(7):1242–55. https://doi.org/10.1016/j.jcmg.2022.02.003.
13. Yang J, Shan D, Wang X, et al. On-site computed tomography-derived fractional flow reserve to guide management of patients with stable coronary artery disease: the TARGET randomized trial. Circulation. 2023;147(18):1369–81. https://doi.org/10.1161/CIRCULATIONAHA.123.063996.
14. Curzen N, Nicholas Z, Stuart B, et al. Fractional flow reserve derived from computed tomography coronary angiography in the assessment and management of stable chest pain: the FORECAST randomized trial. Eur Heart J. 2021;42(37):3844–52. https://doi.org/10.1093/eurheartj/ehab444.

CT Myocardial Perfusion Imaging

5

Roberto Storelli

Basic Principles of CT-MPI

CT-MPI is a noninvasive imaging technique that utilizes computed tomography (CT) to visualize and assess myocardial perfusion dynamics. It relies on the intravenous injection of iodinated contrast agents, allowing the visualization of blood flow patterns within the myocardium.

The basic principle of CT-MPI involves acquiring CT images during the first pass of the contrast agent through the myocardium under stress conditions. By analyzing the contrast density in the myocardium, information about myocardial blood flow and perfusion can be obtained (Fig. 5.1).

General Consideration *To differentiate between reversible and fixed myocardial perfusion defects, the examination should include both rest and stress acquisition protocols* [2]:

During the stress scan, a vasodilator medication (i.e., adenosine or regadenoson) is used to increase blood flow to the heart, which simulates physical stress. Then a contrast agent is injected intravenously, and a CT scanner captures images of the heart, ideally at the time of maximum myocardial contrast enhancement. The rest scan is a repeat scan with a second contrast bolus using the same imaging acquisition parameters as for the stress scan but without stress medication. It provides a baseline comparison of myocardial enhancement.

By comparing the images from both scans, the imaging physician can evaluate differences in contrast enhancement reflecting blood flow patterns. Areas with reduced blood flow indicate perfusions deficits, which can be indicative of hemodynamically relevant epicardial coronary artery disease or other cardiac pathologies (Fig. 5.2).

Reduced perfusion only during stress and not at rest suggests vital myocardium with stress-induced ischemia, indicating a relevant stenosis in the corresponding coronary artery perfusion territory (Fig. 5.3).

However, if perfusion is reduced both at stress and rest, it indicates a persistent perfusion deficit, which may indicate either an infarction or a high-grade stenosis/subtotal occlusion with resting ischemia.

An additional delayed enhancement CT scan may be performed 5–10 min after vascular contrast washout, which can help to detect myocardial scar, allowing for better differentiation from vital myocardium with a perfusion deficit.

R. Storelli (✉)
Department of Diagnostic and Interventional Radiology, University Hospital Freiburg, Freiburg im Breisgau, Baden-Württemberg, Germany
e-mail: roberto.storelli@uniklinik-freiburg.de

R. Gill, P. Rajiah (eds.), *Quantitative Imaging in the Thorax*,
https://doi.org/10.1007/978-3-032-14103-3_5

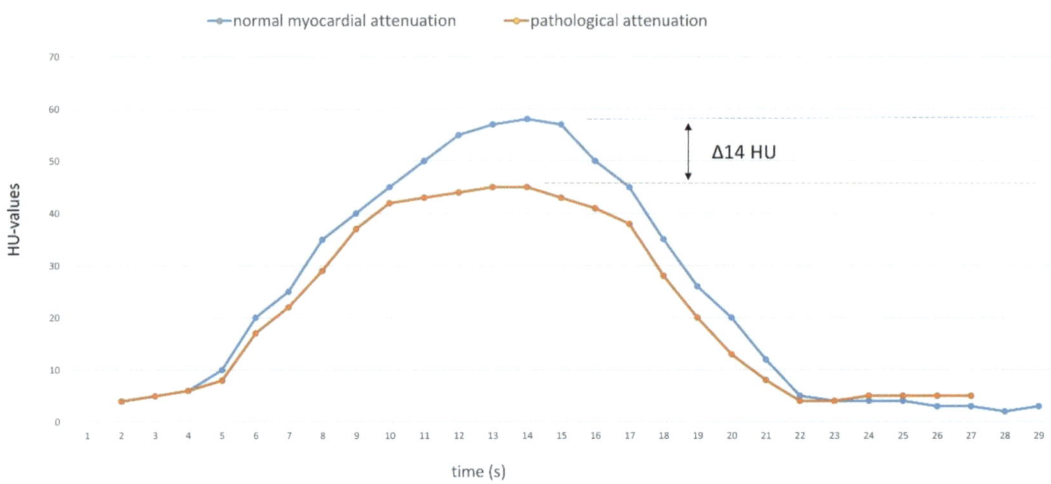

Fig. 5.1 Chart shows the time attenuation curve in normal myocardium (blue) after injecting contrast medium compared to pathological attenuation (orange). The difference between peak attenuation levels in the myocardium is small but lasts for a while

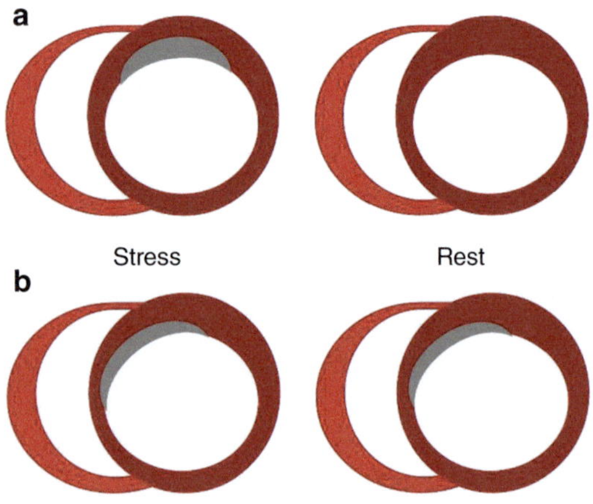

Fig. 5.2 Each showing a perfusion deficit in LAD perfusion territory with the following: (**a**) Stress inducible ischemia by a relevant coronary artery stenosis with perfusion deficit only at stress conditions. (**b**) Infarction consecutive to a coronary artery occlusion with perfusion deficit at stress and rest

Imaging Techniques

To prevent an insufficient effect of stress medication, a patient should avoid influencing substances before the examination such as caffeine for around 12 h and nicotine for 3 h.

Several techniques and imaging protocols have been developed for CT-MPI. In the following we describe the two main acquisition techniques:

Static CT-MPI

Description: In static CT-MPI, images are typically acquired at one or more specific time points during the cardiac cycle, often at rest and stress phases.

Timing: The imaging is synchronized to specific phases of the cardiac cycle, capturing images when the heart is at rest and when it is under stress (induced by medications or exercise) at the moment of maximum myocardial enhancement.

Purpose: Static CT-MPI is useful for assessing perfusion defects and identifying areas of the myocardium with reduced blood flow. It provides a snapshot of the blood distribution in the heart at one specific moment and allows for qualitative and semiquantitative perfusion evaluation.

Dynamic CT-MPI Image Acquisition

Description: Dynamic CT-MPI creates a series of images capturing the contrast passage through the myocardium over time.

Timing: The imaging is not limited to specific phases but covers the entire time that the contrast agent is flowing through the myocardium, allowing for the assessment of the contrast kinetics and myocardial perfusion dynamics.

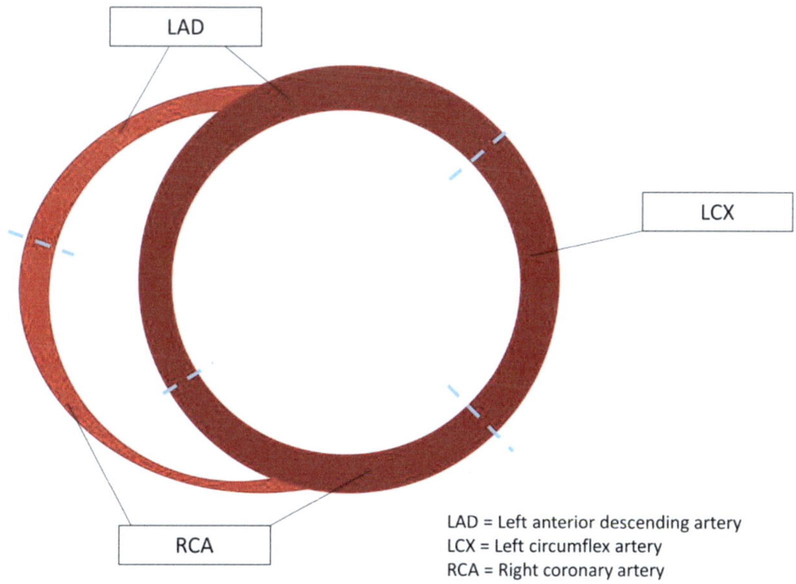

Fig. 5.3 Schematic illustration of coronary artery perfusion territories

Purpose: Dynamic CT-MPI provides information on the temporal evolution of contrast enhancement in the myocardium. It can be valuable in evaluating not only perfusion defects but also the flow patterns and timing of contrast arrival and washout. At this point it is important to mention that quantitative perfusion evaluation with determination, e.g., of the myocardial blood flow (MBF), will be only possible using dynamic CT-MPI and not using static CT-MPI—in this regard we refer to section "Quantitative Parameters".

Temporal Resolution

One scan is performed every 2–3 s, with a total of 10–15 time points or "frames" acquired over a 20–30-s period. This allows for capturing dynamic changes in contrast distribution over time.

In summary, the main difference lies in the timing and purpose of image acquisition (Fig. 5.4). Static CT MPI captures specific moments during the cardiac cycle for a snapshot analysis, while dynamic CT-MPI continuously records images to assess the temporal dynamics of myocardial perfusion. The choice between static and dynamic approaches depends on the clinical questions and objectives of the imaging study. Both techniques are compared in Table 5.1.

Scanner Requirements for Dynamic CT-MPI

Dynamic perfusion imaging requires a CT system capable of capturing repeated images covering the entire myocardium in one breath hold (20–30 s). High temporal resolution is crucial to minimize motion artifacts during stress or breath hold. Second— and third-generation dual-source CT, as well as later single-source CT systems, fulfill these requirements. The z-axis coverage depends on detector rows. This is why there are limitations in 64-detector and first-gen dual-source CT-scanners. Higher slice systems provide whole heart coverage but may have lower temporal resolution.

Scan-Timing and Frequency of Temporal Sampling

Dynamic perfusion imaging involves accurately measuring the arrival, peak, and washout of contrast in the myocardium over time.

Repeated images at different time points (1–3 s apart) create a dynamic dataset, generating time-attenuation curves (TAC) in each myocardial voxel (tissue) and an arterial input function in the aorta. Crucial time points include a pre-contrast baseline frame, frames defining upslope, peak, and early downslope of time-attenuation curves (Fig. 5.4).

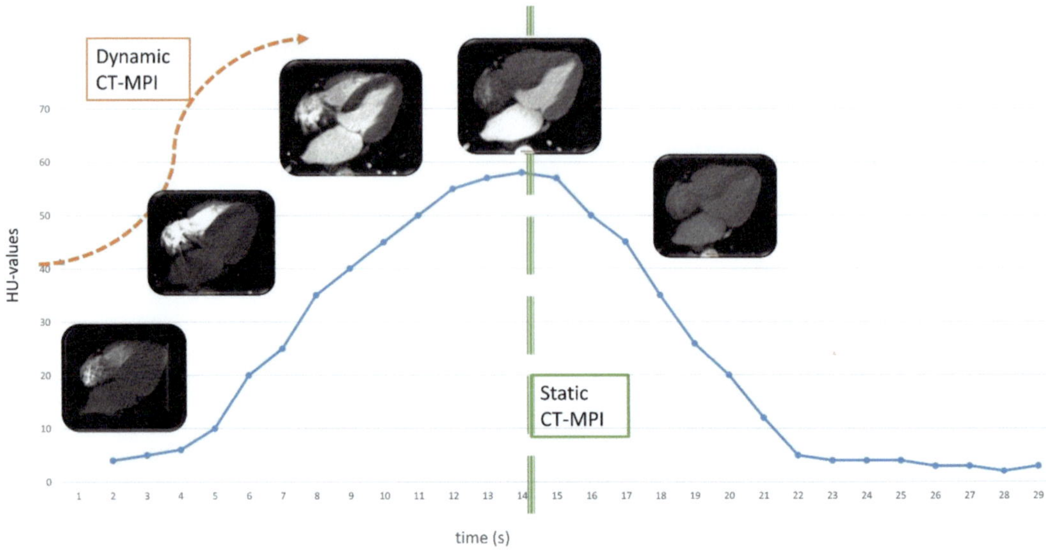

Fig. 5.4 Image acquisition in times in dynamic and static CT-MPI

Table 5.1 Comparison of static and dynamic CT-MPI techniques

	Static CT-MPI: single scan acquired at peak myocardial perfusion	Dynamic CT-MPI: repeated scans over time to create time attenuation curves (TAC's)
Advantages	Shorter breath holding More modest radiation dose	Quantification of myocardial perfusion is possible Able to detect balanced and microvascular ischemia
Disadvantages	No quantification of myocardial perfusion.	May require shuttle mode Higher radiation exposure

Differences in Single-Source and Dual-Source CT

Dual-Source CT

Lacking full heart coverage, dual-source CT uses a "shuttling" technique where the patient moves back and forth during image acquisition. This allows data collection at two table positions, covering the entire myocardium, e.g., in the end-systolic phase.

Second- and third-generation dual-source technology permits dynamic perfusion imaging at every heartbeat, with temporal sampling of 2–3 s under stress conditions. This technique enables the estimation and fitting of time-attenuation curves (TAC) while minimizing radiation exposure. It facilitates double temporal sampling for constructing the arterial input function and provides sufficient time points for TAC construction in the left ventricle, aorta, and each myocardial voxel (tissue). Usually, the scan typically acquires 10–15 whole myocardial volumes corresponding to 10–15 time points (or frames) over 20–30 s [3].

Single-Source CT

Larger coverage scanners, like the 320-rows-detector CT, image the entire heart in one rotation without table motion, providing up to 16 cm coverage. This allows rapid acquisition within a single heartbeat, ensuring homogeneous contrast attenuation and avoiding reconstruction artifacts. However, if there is smaller (<8 cm) coverage, single-source CT also uses the "shuttling" technique, similar to dual-source CT, but may lack the temporal resolution for complete TAC data points.

Injectables

Adenosine

Adenosine is used as pharmacologic stressor, which induces coronary vasodilation. Adenosine has a short half-life. Nevertheless, the specific contraindications for adenosine must be considered (Table 5.2).

Contrast Agents

Nonionic contrast agents are applied intravenously with precautions to general contraindications [1]. The following injection protocol has been tested in studies: a 45-mL contrast bolus at 5.5 mL/s (iopromide, Bayer) (370 mg/mL), followed by 40-mL saline, with minor modification [1].

Perfusion imaging at both single- and dual-source scanners may be performed using dual-energy (DE) techniques. DE imaging provides enhanced iodine contrast and may improve delineation of myocardial perfusion deficit. As this topic is beyond the scope of the article, we recommend referring to dedicated literature for more in-depth information [3, 4].

Protocol with Strategy

Typically, CT perfusion protocols involve both rest and stress CT scans. The rest portion allows for coronary anatomy assessment and evaluation of rest myocardial perfusion. The sequence of scans (rest first versus stress first) has not been definitively determined. Each order has pros and cons. The different sequences are schematized in the following:

Performing the rest scan first including coronary CT angiography (CCTA) is recommended in patients with low to intermediate pretest probability of CAD (Fig. 5.5).

If CCTA excludes relevant coronary stenosis (<50%), stress CT-MPI may be omitted. However, initiating with coronary CT angiography (CCTA) may result in myocardial saturation with contrast agent. That means, residual contrast enhancement in the myocardium could mask areas of reduced myocardial perfusion on stress CT-MPI images. Therefore, a delay of 10–20 min between rest and stress CT acquisitions is recommended to minimize contrast agent contamination [3]. There is also the problem that combining adenos-

Table 5.2 Contraindications for adenosine

Second- or third-degree AV block (except in patients with a functioning artificial pacemaker)
Sinus node disease, such as sick sinus syndrome or symptomatic bradycardia (except in patients with a functioning artificial pacemaker)Known or suspected bronchoconstrictive or bronchospastic lung disease (e.g., asthma)
Known hypersensitivity to adenosine injection

To complete, compare with Table 5.3

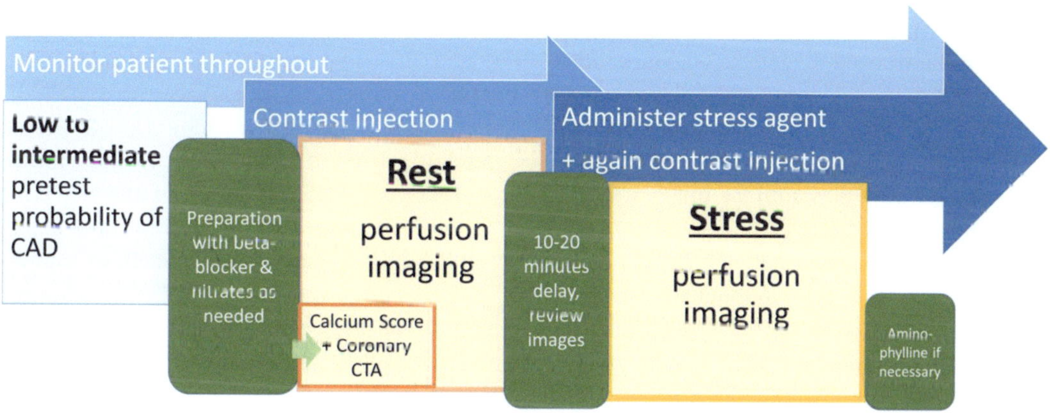

Fig. 5.5 Sequence of image acquisition in rest-stress protocol. (Modified from Patel et al. [3])

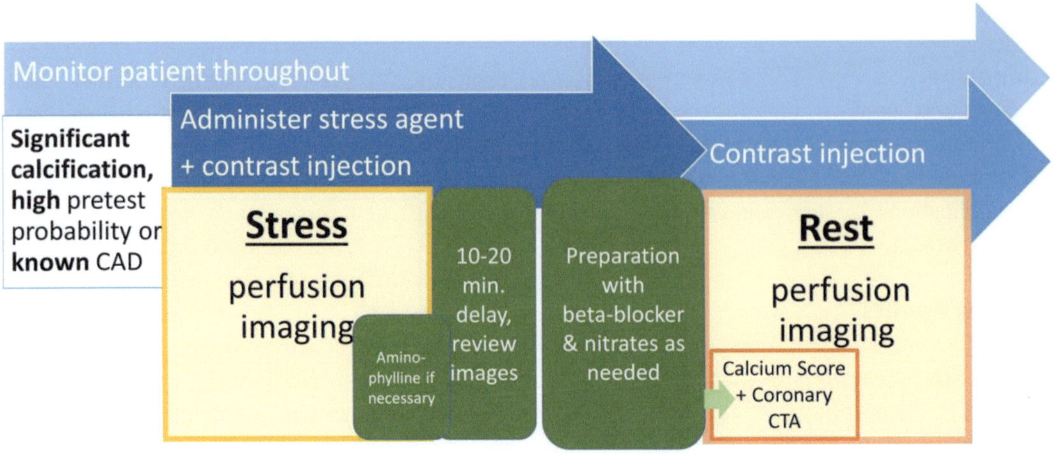

Fig. 5.6 Sequence of image acquisition in stress-rest protocol. (Modified from Patel et al. [3])

ine and nitroglycerine can lead to dangerous drop in blood pressure. It is therefore recommended to wait after initial nitroglycerin administration before considering adenosine to avoid a cumulative, potentially harmful effect.

When stress CT imaging is done first, it may be easier to detect ischemia as there is no residual contrast in the myocardium from an earlier injection (Fig. 5.6). Beta blockers are administered before the resting scan to improve image quality of CCTA. The challenge is to reduce the pulse rate after the stress phase.

Image Reconstruction

Depending on acquisition parameters, images can be analyzed in systolic and/or diastolic phases. For improved diagnostic accuracy, additional reconstructions at multiple phases of the cardiac cycle can be beneficial, usually at 5%–10% intervals. It's advisable to keep the raw CTA and CTP data files until the image interpretation is finished.

To ensure proper interpreting CTP, the workstations should meet the same standards as those used for standard coronary CTA interpretation. Additionally, if dynamic CTP is conducted, the software must allow visualization of myocardial enhancement over time.

An appropriate image reconstruction is in 3.0-mm-thick slices with 2.0-mm overlap.

Imaging Interpretation and Analysis

Concomitant interpretation of coronary CTA and CT-MPI is recommended.

Qualitative Assessment of CT-MPI

It mainly involves subjective interpretation of the images to evaluate myocardial perfusion characteristics (Figs. 5.7 and 5.8). Here are some key aspects of qualitative assessment:

Perfusion Defects

Location: Radiologists assess the presence and location of perfusion defects. These defects can indicate areas of the myocardium with reduced blood flow; perfusion abnormalities can lead to uneven or patchy patterns.

Severity: The degree of perfusion impairment is often categorized as mild, moderate, or severe based on the extent and intensity of the perfusion defect.

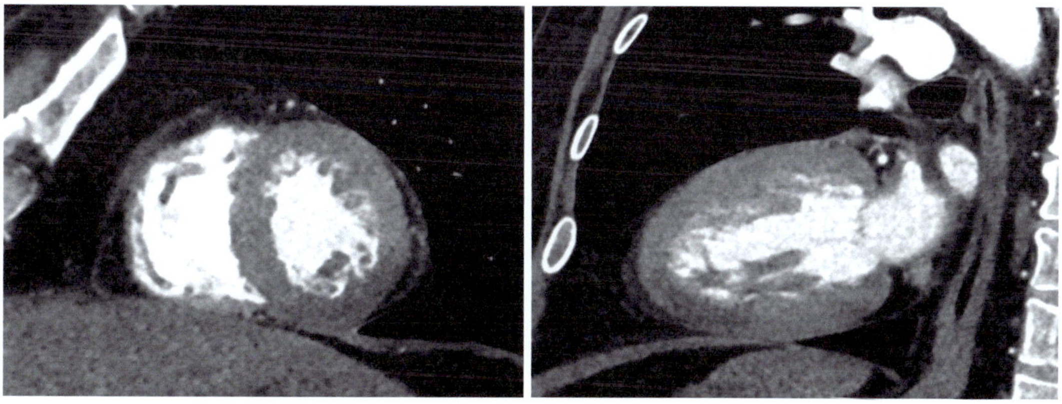

Fig. 5.7 Static CT-MPI: visual assessment of a stress CT perfusion axial image reveals a low-density area in the left ventricular posterior wall. It corresponded to a high-grade stenosis of the left posterolateral branch of the left circumflex artery. (With permissions from Dr. M. Soschynski, University Hospital Freiburg)

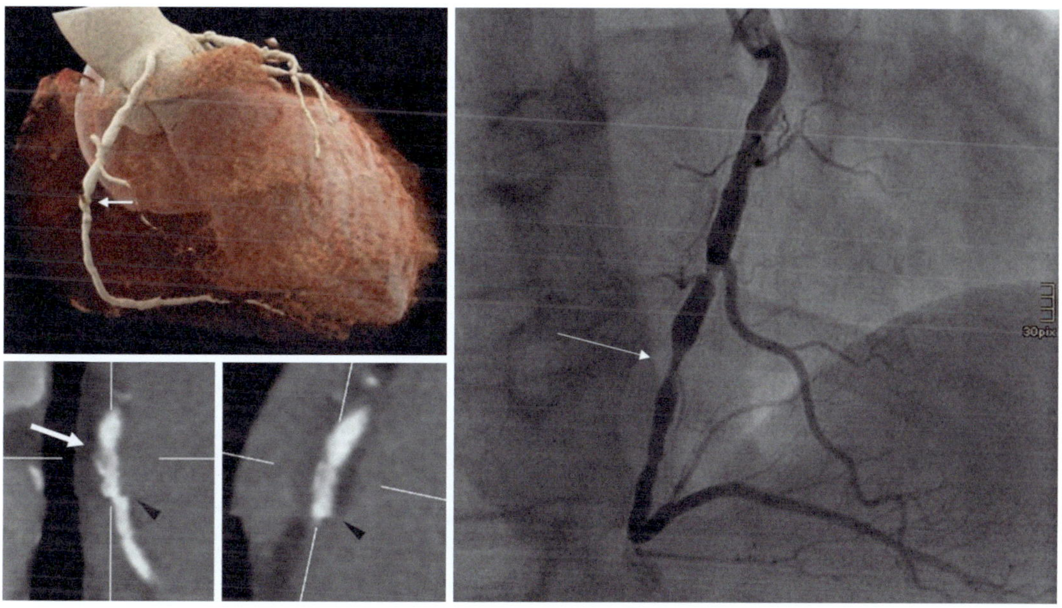

Fig. 5.8 CCTA (left bottom) displays a visual stenosis in right coronary artery (white arrow). Note the step-artifacts (black arrowheads) on both the 3D reconstructed heart (top left) and in CCTA just distal to the stenosis (white arrow). Invasive coronary angiography (right) confirms intermediate stenosis of 50%–60%. (With permissions from Dr. M. Soschynski, University Hospital Freiburg)

Transmural Extent

Full thickness vs. subendocardial defects: The assessment includes determining whether the perfusion defect involves the full thickness of the myocardium (transmural) or only the inner layers (subendocardial). Transmural defects are often associated with more severe ischemia.

Correlation with Anatomic Findings

Coronary artery territories: Radiologists correlate perfusion defects with the coronary artery territories to identify the vessel causing the perfusion abnormality.

Artifact Recognition

Motion artifacts: Assessment includes identifying motion artifacts, which can affect the interpretation of perfusion images.

With sequential image acquisition, the so-called step artifacts may occur, which can be identified on multiplanar reconstructions of the CT images.

Clinical Context

Integration with clinical information: Qualitative assessment is done in conjunction with clinical history, symptoms, and other diagnostic findings to provide a comprehensive interpretation.

Quantitative Assessment of CT-MPI

Once the images are acquired, specialized software is used to analyze them quantitatively [5]. This software employs advanced algorithms to calculate parameters related to myocardial perfusion [6]. The most common parameters are myocardial blood flow (MBF), myocardial perfusion reserve (MPR), and time to peak (TTP) enhancement. They are explained in the next section. Quantitative parameters are visualized by generating color-coded maps that depict the magnitude and temporal dynamics of blood flow distribution across different regions of the heart.

Quantitative Parameters

I. Myocardial blood flow (MBF)
   Absolute MBF represents the volume of blood flowing through the myocardium per unit of time. It is typically measured in milliliters per minute per gram of myocardial tissue (mL/100 g/min). To determine absolute MBF, the software measures the density changes in specific regions of interest within the myocardium over time. By comparing these density changes with known values, it can estimate the amount of blood flowing through those regions.Relative MBF compares blood flow ratios between myocardial regions and is calculated per vessel territory, as the absolute MBF divided by the reference MBF.An example of an MBF map in Fig. 5.9.
II. Myocardial perfusion reserve (MPR)
   MPR is a ratio that compares myocardial blood flow during stress (induced by medication or exercise) to rest conditions. It reflects the ability of the coronary arteries to dilate and increase blood flow when demand is higher. A reduced MPR indicates impaired

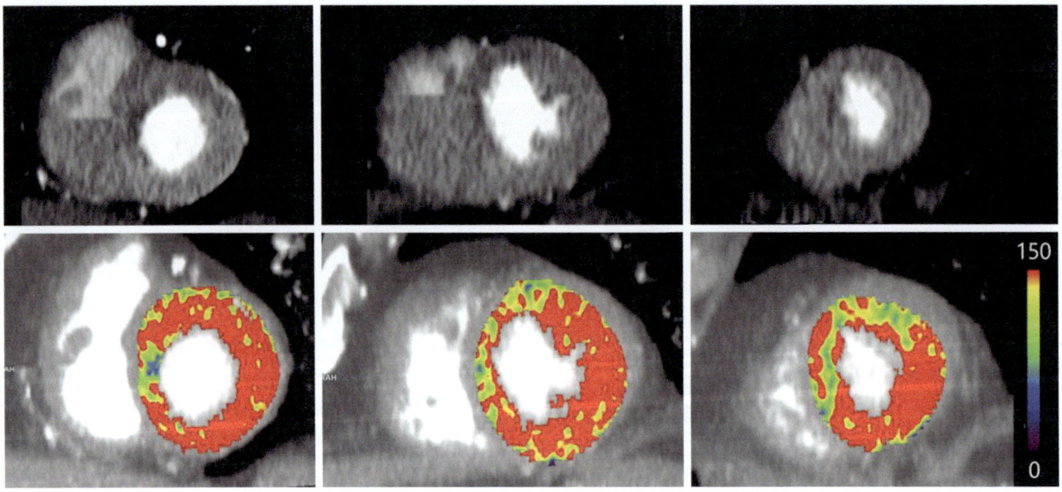

Fig. 5.9 Quantification of myocardial blood flow (MBF absolute). Dynamic CT-MPI demonstrates a notable perfusion reduction (yellow-blue) in the interventricular septum and in the anterior wall, indicating ischemia. Absolute myocardial blood flow in ml/100 ml myocardium/min (MBF). Relative myocardial blood flow = MBF (local)/MBF (global ref.). (With permissions from Dr. Martin Soschynski, University Hospital Freiburg)

vasodilator capacity and may be an early indicator of coronary artery disease.

III. Time to peak enhancement (TTP): TTP (in seconds) refers to the time taken for contrast agent to reach its maximum concentration within the myocardium after injection (Fig. 5.10).
Prolonged TTP indicates contrast delay, which could be associated with stenotic or occluded coronary arteries.

Challenges and Limitations in Imaging Interpretation

I. Image Artifacts
Reliability of the obtained images can be compromised by various artifacts. These are the following:
- *Motion artifacts*, induced by patient movement during scanning, present a significant hurdle in cardiac imaging. Although CT-MPI is less focused on coronary arteries, it can still affect diagnostic accuracy, emphasizing the need for distinguishing them from genuine perfusion defects based on their characteristics across cardiac cycle phases and coronary territories. Motion artifacts can be reduced by *multisector reconstruction*. Raw data is subdivided into sectors based on cardiac phases, which minimizes the impact of motion artifacts, ensuring clearer representations of the myocardium.
- *Beam-hardening artifacts*, resulting from the preferential absorption of lower-energy X-ray photons, introduce streaks or shading artifacts that can impede accurate assessments of contrast-enhanced regions. Beam-hardening artifacts are notably in the basal inferolateral wall and can create false positive perfusion defects, and while reconstruction algorithms aim to correct for this, it remains problematic.

Timing scans during systole minimizes contrast agent volume in the cavities, addressing both beam hardening artifacts and optimizing contrast for more precise myocardial perfusion assessment. Utilizing a soft kernel with a 2–3 mm thickness enhances image quality by reducing noise. These refinements can be combined with advanced reconstruction methods [3].

II. Diagnostic issues: balanced ischemia
Balanced ischemia in three-vessel CAD has been reported as a rare cause of false-negative myocardial perfusion scans [7].

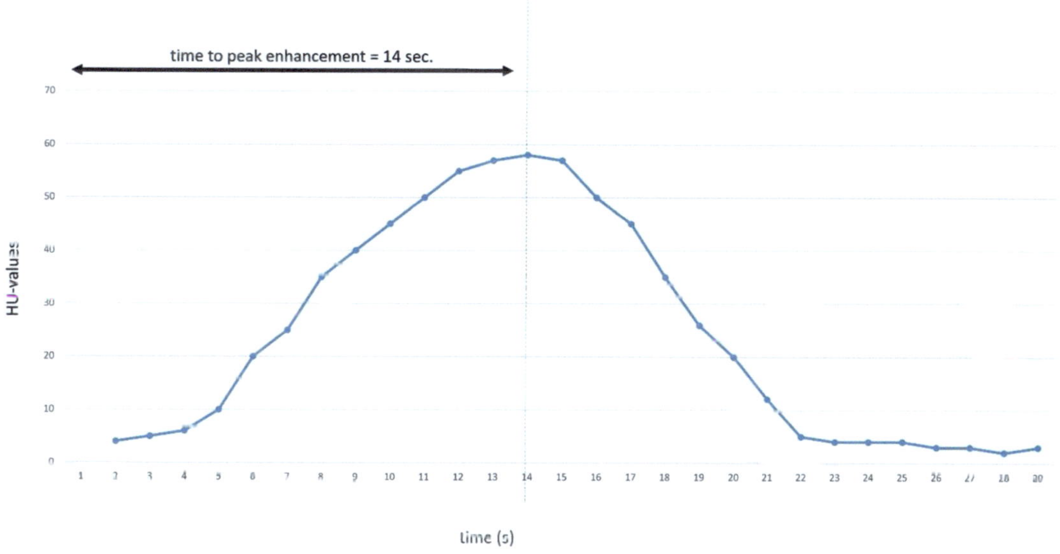

Fig. 5.10 Time to peak enhancement, in this physiological example relatively short with 14 s

The perfusion deficit may be overlooked with a purely qualitative analysis, as all subendocardial wall layers equally (poorly) enhance and no regionally lower attenuation can be identified. Quantitative analysis can objectively demonstrate a reduced absolute MBF in certain wall sections in hemodynamically relevant three-vessel CAD. It can therefore possibly detect a perfusion deficit even in the presence of balanced ischemia [8].

Clinical Applications of CT-MPI

Indication in Coronary Artery Disease (CAD)

Several studies already showed that dynamic CT perfusion imaging allowed for the identification of hemodynamically significant coronary artery stenosis [9].According to the 2020 CTP consensus document by the Society of Cardiac Computed Tomography (SCCT) [3], adding dynamic coronary computed tomography perfusion (CTP) is recommended alongside coronary CT angiography (CTA) for patients with a high likelihood of coronary artery disease (CAD), known CAD, prior coronary interventions, or significant coronary calcifications. For patients with acute chest pain, negative troponins, and low to intermediate CAD risk, coronary CTA alone is typically sufficient. However, if moderate stenosis (50%–69% maximal coronary stenosis CAD-RADS 3) is found, incorporating dynamic CT-MPI along with coronary CTA can enhance the detection of flow-limiting coronary lesions and significantly improve specificity [10].

Role of CT-MPI in Diagnosis, Treatment Decisions, and for Prognosis

CT-MPI has shown promise in various clinical scenarios:

I. Diagnosis of coronary artery disease (CAD)
CT-MPI had a high sensitivity and specificity for detecting CAD when compared to invasive coronary angiography (ICA) as the reference standard [10].

II. Risk stratification and prognosis
By quantitatively assessing ischemia, CT-MPI can provide valuable information for risk stratification of patients with suspected or known CAD, enabling more personalized treatment strategies. The extent and severity of myocardial ischemia evaluated through CT-MPI are associated with future cardiovascular events, enabling prognostication and long-term patient management.
Some studies advocate MBF as a prime risk-stratification parameter in suspected CAD patients: MBF, indicating ischemia severity, proves superior to other morphological criteria an independent predictor for MACE. It captures microvascular dysfunction, enhancing risk stratification beyond epicardial vessel assessment. MBF also surpasses high-risk plaque features in prognostic evaluation, offering potent risk estimates. Calcium score (CACS) complements MACE prediction, aligning with its association with decreased MBF and subsequent revascularization. CACS provides valuable screening, and a combined dynamic CT-MPI and CCTA approach is preferable for comprehensive assessment [11].
There have been several registry reports on the prognostic value of CT-MPI. Nakamura et al. could show that a summed stress score based on normalized MBF by CT-MPI predicted a composite endpoint of cardiac death, nonfatal myocardial infarction, unstable angina, or hospitalization for congestive heart failure, with an incremental prognostic value on CTA-based coronary stenosis [12].

III. Treatment guidance
In clinical practice, CT-MPI can be used following a positive CCTA to assess the functional severity of coronary lesions.
CT-MPI helps guide treatment decisions, such as revascularization procedures (e.g., percutaneous coronary intervention or coronary artery bypass grafting), by identifying regions of reversible ischemia that could benefit from intervention.
The CRESCENT II trial demonstrated that a tailored cardiac CT approach, including

Table 5.3 Absolute and relative contraindications to pharmacologic stress myocardial CT perfusion

Absolute contraindications		Relative contraindications
High-risk unstable angina pectoris	Acute myocarditis/pericarditis	Left main coronary stenosis > 50%
Decompensated congestive heart failure	Aortic dissection	Hypertrophic obstructive cardiomyopathy (HOCM), and other forms of outflow tract obstruction
Uncontrolled hypertension	Severe pulmonary hypertension	Significant tachyarrhythmias or bradyarrhythmias
Hypotension	Acute myocardial infarction	Recent stroke
Known allergy to contrast medium	Renal insufficiency (GFR < 30 ml/min)	Recent seizures
Allergy to stress agent	High-degree AV block	Moderate renal insufficiency (GFR 30–60 ml/min)
Uncontrolled arrhythmias		Obesity (BMI > 40)
Symptomatic aortic stenosis		
Bronchospastic lung disease		
Acute pulmonary embolism		
Cardiovascular accident		

dynamic CT-MPI, resulted in a higher rate of severe CAD requiring revascularization compared to standard stress testing, without increasing overall invasive catheterization rates [13]. The CATCH trial, which randomized patients with acute chest pain, found that combining CCTA with CT-MPI decreased catheterization referral rates without affecting long-term outcomes [14].

Radiation Dose Consideration

In dynamic CT, which requires continuous imaging throughout the passage of contrast, the radiation dose is typically higher than in static CT-MPI, which only includes a single point of time. Advances in CT technology, including dose reduction techniques and improved image reconstruction algorithms, aim to mitigate radiation concerns while providing clinically valuable information. Although the later generation scanners are preferred to reduce the radiation dose, the radiation exposure in dynamic CTP varies among protocols and vendors. The range varies between an effective dose of 4.6 and 12.8 mSv [10]. Effective radiation dose can be lower with third-generation DSCT compared to second-generation DSCT [15].

Contraindications

Although stress CT-MPI is safe, there are some circumstances where it should avoided altogether or only used with caution. Absolute and relative CT-MPI contraindications in general are listed in Table 5.3.

Comparative Analysis with Other Imaging Modalities

Comparison with Nuclear Myocardial Perfusion Imaging (MPI)

Single-photon emission computed tomography (SPECT) relies on radioactive tracers to provide information on myocardial perfusion. SPECT is a well-established technique with longstanding experience. However, its limitations lie in lower spatial resolution, prolonged acquisition times, and exposure to ionizing radiation [16]. CT-MPI offers high-resolution anatomical coronary images alongside perfusion data in shorter acquisition times. In studies, diagnostic accuracy of CT-MPI was comparable to that of PET and is superior to that of SPECT [17].

Comparison with Magnetic Resonance Imaging (MRI)

Patients with a history of myocardial infarction typically undergo cardiac magnetic resonance (CMR) imaging due to its superior ability to depict infarcts. However, in cases where CMR is contraindicated, computed tomography (CT) can be considered as an alternative with similar sensitivity and specificity for perfusion deficits [17].

Conclusion and Summary

Conclusion

CT myocardial perfusion imaging (CT-MPI) has emerged as a promising tool for the qualitative and quantitative assessment of myocardial ischemia. When combined with coronary CT angiography, both anatomical and functional information are provided. With ongoing technological advancements, continued research, and clinical validation, CT-MPI has the potential to play a leading role in the comprehensive evaluation and management of patients with suspected or known ischemia, contributing to improved patient outcomes and enhanced cardiovascular care.

Recapitulation of Main Points Discussed in the Chapter

1. CT-MPI imaging utilizes two types of CT acquisitions: static and dynamic. Static CT-MPI captures a snapshot of the entire heart at a single time-point of contrast enhancement, typically using the same parameters as coronary CTA. Dynamic CT-MPI involves acquiring multiple CT datasets during the passage of contrast through the myocardium. The key advantage of dynamic CT-MPI is the ability to calculate absolute MBF for both ischemic and healthy myocardium.
   This allows quantification of myocardial blood flow (MBF) to assess myocardial status in known coronary artery disease (CAD).
2. Choosing patients for CT-MPI: If a patient has no significant coronary artery disease (CAD) or only mild stenosis (<50%), a coronary CTA may be enough.
   But if there's uncertainty about stenosis' impact or severe calcification, adding CT-MPI is helpful.
3. Whether you prefer following the stress-rest or the rest-stress protocol depends on the pretest probability of the patient.
4. Advantage of systolic gating: Systolic gating is preferred due to less beam hardening artifacts during systole, also for fewer motion artifacts at high heart rates (HF). However, most studies have traditionally been diastolic.
5. While cardiac magnetic resonance (CMR) remains the preferred method to visualize myocardial changes as a result of myocardial infarction (MI), a CT-based exam can serve as an alternative, particularly in patients with contraindications for CMR.
   Conceptually, CT-MPI is a well-established method and can offer similar benefits, all with reduced acquisition time compared to CMR.
6. Stress CT-MPI is safe for most, but in some cases precautions must be taken to avoid adverse drug reactions (e.g. from stress agents).

Acknowledgments Many thanks to Prof. Dr. Bamberg together with publisher Springer Nature for making this transcript possible. Also many thanks to Dr. Soschynski for providing the image examples and for the final proofread.

References

1. Nous FMA, Geisler T, Kruk MBP, Alkadhi H, Kitagawa K, Vliegenthart R, Hell MM, Hausleiter J, Nguyen PK, Budde RPJ, Nikolaou K, Kepka C, Manka R, Sakuma H, Malik SB, Coenen A, Zijlstra F, Klotz E, van der Harst P, Artzner C, Dedic A, Pugliese F, Bamberg F, Nieman K. Dynamic myocardial perfusion CT for the detection of hemodynamically significant coronary artery disease. JACC Cardiovasc Imaging. 2022;15(1):75–87. https://doi.org/10.1016/j.jcmg.2021.07.021. Epub 2021 Sept 15.
2. Meinel FG, De Cecco CN, Schoepf UJ, Nance JW, Silverman JR, Flowers BA, Henzle T. First-arterial-pass dual-energy CT for assessment of myocardial

blood supply: do we need rest, stress, and delayed acquisition? Comparison with SPECT. Radiology. 2014;270(3):708–16. https://doi.org/10.1148/radiol.13131183.

3. Patel AR, Bamberg F, Branch K, Carrascosa P, Chen M, Cury RC, Ghoshhajra B, Ko B, Nieman K, Pugliese F, Schoepf J, Blankstein R. Society of cardiovascular computed tomography expert consensus document on myocardial computed tomography perfusion imaging. J Cardiovasc Comput Tomogr. 2020;14(1):87–100. https://doi.org/10.1016/j.jcct.2019.10.003.
4. Jin KN, De Cecco CN, Caruso D, Tesche C, Spandorfer A, Varga-Szemes A, Schoepf UJ. Myocardial perfusion imaging with dual energy CT. Eur J Radiol. 2016;85:1914–21. https://doi.org/10.1016/j.ejrad.2016.06.023.
5. Ebersberger U, Marcus RP, Schoepf UJ, Lo GG, Wang Y, Blanke P, Geyer LL, Gray JC III, AD MQ, Cho YJ, Scheuering M. Dynamic CT myocardial perfusion imaging: performance of 3D semi-automated evaluation software. Eur Radiol. 2014;24:191–9. https://doi.org/10.1007/s00330-013-2997-5.
6. Kim Y-C, Choe YH. Automated identification of myocardial perfusion defects in dynamic cardiac computed tomography using deep learning. Phys Med. 2023;107:102555. https://doi.org/10.1016/j.ejmp.2023.102555.
7. Aarnoudse WH, Botman KJ, Pijls NH. False-negative myocardial scintigraphy in balanced three-vessel disease, revealed by coronary pressure measurement. Int J Cardiovasc Interv. 2003;5(2):67–71. https://doi.org/10.1080/14628840310003244. PMID: 12745861.
8. Collet J-P, Thiele H, Barbato E, et al. 2020 ESC guidelines for the management of acute coronary syndromes in patients presenting without persistent ST-segment elevation: the task force for the management of acute coronary syndromes in patients presenting without persistent ST-segment elevation of the European Society of Cardiology (ESC). Eur Heart J. 2021;42:1289–367.
9. Bamberg F, Becker A, Schwarz F, et al. Detection of hemodynamically significant coronary artery stenosis: incremental diagnostic value of dynamic CT-based myocardial perfusion imaging. Radiology. 2011;260:689–69.
10. Sliwicka O, Sechopoulos I, Baggiano A, et al. Dynamic myocardial CT perfusion imaging—state of the art. Eur Radiol. 2023;33:5509–25. https://doi.org/10.1007/s00330-023-09550-y
11. Yu L, Lu Z, Dai X, Shen C, Zhang L, Zhang J. Prognostic value of CT-derived myocardial blood flow, CT fractional flow reserve and high-risk plaque features for predicting major adverse cardiac events. Cardiovasc Diagn Ther. 2021;11(4):956–66. https://doi.org/10.21037/cdt-21-219.
12. Nakamura S, Kitagawa K, Goto Y, Omori T, Kurita T, Yamada A, Takafuji M, Uno M, Dohi K, Sakuma H. Incremental prognostic value of myocardial blood flow quantified with stress dynamic computed tomography perfusion imaging. JACC Cardiovasc Imaging. 2019;12(7 Pt 2):1379–87. https://doi.org/10.1016/j.jcmg.2018.05.021. Epub 2018 July 18.
13. Lubbers M, Coenen A, Kofflard M, Bruning T, Kietselaer B, Galema T, Kock M, Niezen A, Das M, van Gent M, van den Bos EJ. Comprehensive cardiac CT with myocardial perfusion imaging versus functional testing in suspected coronary artery disease: the multicenter, randomized CRESCENT-II trial. JACC Cardiovasc Imaging. 2018;11(11):1625–36. https://doi.org/10.1016/j.jcmg.2017.10.010.
14. Sørgaard MH, Linde JJ, Kühl JT, Kelbæk H, Hove JD, Fornitz GG, Jørgensen TBS, Heitmann M, Kragelund C, Hansen TF, Abdulla J, Engstrøm T, Jensen JS, Wiegandt YT, Høfsten DE, Køber LV, Kofoed KF. Value of myocardial perfusion assessment with coronary computed tomography angiography in patients with recent acute-onset chest pain. JACC Cardiovasc Imaging. 2018;11(11):1611–21. https://doi.org/10.1016/j.jcmg.2017.09.022.
15. Takafuji M, Kitagawa K, Ishida M, Goto Y, Nakamura S, Nagasawa N, Sakuma H. Myocardial coverage and radiation dose in dynamic myocardial perfusion imaging using third-generation dual-source CT. Korean J Radiol. 2020;21(1):58–67. https://doi.org/10.3348/kjr.2019.0323. PMID: 31920029; PMCID: PMC6960309.
16. Limone B, et al. Diagnostic accuracy of cardiac positron emission tomography versus single photon emission computed tomography for coronary artery disease: a bivariate meta-analysis. Circ Cardiovasc Imaging. 2012;5(6):700–707.
17. Yang K, Yu SQ, Lu MJ, Zhao SH. Comparison of diagnostic accuracy of stress myocardial perfusion imaging for detecting hemodynamically significant coronary artery disease between cardiac magnetic resonance and nuclear medical imaging: a meta-analysis. Int J Cardiol. 2019;293:278–85. https://doi.org/10.1016/j.ijcard.2019.06.054

Quantitative Stress Perfusion Cardiac Magnetic Resonance

6

Fai Wang Fong, Haonan Wang, Hena Patel, and Ming-Yen Ng

Introduction

Stress perfusion by cardiac magnetic resonance (CMR) is increasingly utilized as a precise and noninvasive alternative in clinical evaluation of coronary artery disease (CAD) regarding the severity of stenosis and hemodynamic significance, as compared to longer established imaging modalities like nuclear myocardial perfusion imaging. Contrast-enhanced stress perfusion CMR examinations use a fast multi-slice imaging sequence [1–4]. These fast multi-slice perfusion images are assessed qualitatively. When reviewed by experts, stress-induced perfusion defects can be identified to confirm the presence of obstructive CAD. Occasionally, coronary microvascular disease (CMD) can be identified with the appearance of circumferential perfusion defects. However, CMD can also be present without an appreciable perfusion defect [5].

A new development in stress CMR is the advent of fully quantitative perfusion (QP). Quantitative stress CMR represents a cutting-edge technology. It has significant advantages over traditional qualitative stress CMR. Firstly, it provides confirmation of the visual interpretation by providing perfusion maps, allowing this technology to be opened up to less experienced readers. It has also shown better performance than expert readers performing qualitative analysis in a recent publication [6]. Secondly, it confirms the adequacy of stress. Lastly, it provides an objective measurement to diagnose CMD which was previously based on visual assessment. Currently, CMD is underdiagnosed and there is no effective treatment for CMD [7]. Therefore, this ability to diagnose CMD also lends itself to opening up a new avenue of research and patient follow-up with the benefit of magnetic resonance imaging (MRI) being a nonionizing radiation technique.

Performing Stress-Induced Cardiac MRI

Basic Rationale of Stress-Induced Cardiac MRI

Stress-induced cardiac MRI works on the basis that a patient's heart is "stressed" using pharmacological agents such as adenosine, regadenoson, dipyridamole, or adenosine triphosphate (ATP).

F. W. Fong · M.-Y. Ng (✉)
Department of Diagnostic Radiology, School of Clinical Medicine, Li Ka Shing Faculty of Medicine, The University of Hong Kong, Pok Fu Lam, Hong Kong
e-mail: u3569755@connect.hku.hk; myng2@hku.hk

H. Wang
GE HealthCare, Waukesha, WI, USA
e-mail: haonan.wang@gehealthcare.com

H. Patel
Department of Medicine, University of Chicago, Chicago, IL, USA
e-mail: hena.patel@bsd.uchicago.edu

R. Gill, P. Rajiah (eds.), *Quantitative Imaging in the Thorax*,
https://doi.org/10.1007/978-3-032-14103-3_6

These agents act by causing vasodilatation which causes the patient's heart rate to rise >10 beats/min (bpm) and blood pressure to drop >10 mmHg with or without symptoms similar to exercise (e.g., shortness of breath). In obstructive CAD, blood will flow preferentially into the nonobstructive coronary arteries creating a coronary steal phenomenon. This reduced flow in the territory of the obstructive coronary artery causes a dark stress-induced perfusion defect which resolves at rest (see Fig. 6.3).

Choice of Stress Agents

Cardiac stress can be achieved by vasodilators such as adenosine, dipyridamole, ATP, or regadenoson [8]. However, in the context of quantitative stress CMR, adenosine and regadenoson have been the agents most frequently used [5, 9–12]. There is a paucity in the literature on the use of dipyridamole and ATP for quantitative stress perfusion. Dipyridamole has been shown to produce a lower vasodilatory effect than regadenoson and adenosine [13]. Adenosine and regadenoson have been the agents of choice in many sites due to their faster onset of action with ATP and dipyridamole taking longer to achieve adequate stress [14, 15]. In addition, in a meta-analysis adenosine has been shown to have a higher diagnostic accuracy than dipyridamole [16].

Principle, Computational Algorithm, and Interpretation of QP

In order to quantify myocardial blood flow (MBF) using quantitative perfusion, two approaches can be utilized: a model-independent or model-dependent approach. We will briefly summarize these approaches; however, more detail can be found in a review by Jerosch-Herold [17]. In the model independent approach, the Indicator-dilution/Central Volume principle is utilized, without specifying the physiologic functional model of the tissue structure, the movement of tracers through these spaces as well as the permeability between these spaces. The MBF is calculated based on knowing the concentrations at the arterial inlet and venous outlet, the mass of tracer in the region, and the rate of change with time [18, 19].

In contrast to model independent approach, specific physiologic models have also been employed to describe the tracer movements, permeability of the vasculature within the tissue structure. Models such as the two compartments and distributed parameter model have been utilized to calculate MBF [20, 21].

Regardless of the model-based method or the model independent method, to accurately quantify MBF, the blood and tissue enhancement data needs to be measured accurately. However, the contrast enhancement in the blood pool has a nonlinear relation with contrast concentration, especially at high concentration. With concentration increase, due to T2* effects, the signal intensity would even start to plateau above a certain contrast level.

Two solutions have been proposed to avoid these signal saturation effects. The first is the dual bolus technique. The second is dual sequence in which a dedicated perfusion sequence acquires both high-temporal-low-spatial-resolution images and high-spatial-resolution images within a single bolus injection. The high-temporal-low-spatial images are acquired at the base of the left ventricle to determine the arterial input function. The two techniques have been shown to produce significantly different stress/rest MBF results but good correlation between stress/rest MBF and MPR [22].

Dual Bolus

To overcome the saturation effects, the dual bolus approach utilizes a lower contrast dosage, which is usually a 10% contrast bolus, to calculate the arterial input function. This is then followed by a 100% contrast bolus to complete the myocardial perfusion calculation. The perfusion sequences used for the 10% and 100% bolus are the same and has the benefit of being able to utilize standard perfusion sequences to calculate the stress/

rest myocardial blood flow and myocardial perfusion reserve index [23, 24]. This technique results in a longer procedural time due to the requirement to acquire an additional set of images for the arterial input function. Importantly, during the dual bolus acquisition, it is crucial that adenosine injection continues so that the patient is under stress during the acquisition. Recently dual bolus has shown to have prognostic significance for major adverse cardiovascular events [25].

Dual Sequence

Dual-sequence refers to the acquisition of two different perfusion sequences concurrently comprising an arterial input function (AIF) sequence which comprises of a low-resolution spoiled gradient echo with short saturation preparation time in the basal region and the three standard high-resolution perfusion images acquired in the short-axis oblique position of the left ventricular base, mid-ventricle, and apex. Recently, dual sequence has shown better prognostic significance than the dual bolus technique for major adverse cardiovascular events [25].

Semiquantitative Perfusion CMR

Semiquantitative techniques in CMR are different to fully quantitative methods in that traditional perfusion sequences are utilized with standard contrast injection techniques. Signal intensity-time curves are generated and are utilized to derive the myocardial perfusion reserve (MPR) and maximum upslope stress to rest ratio. These measures are also derived from the signal intensity-time curve (see Figs. 6.1 and 6.2) in which the myocardial contrast enhancement on stress and rest images are contoured. This allows the signal intensity of the myocardium to be calculated. In addition, the blood pool is also con-

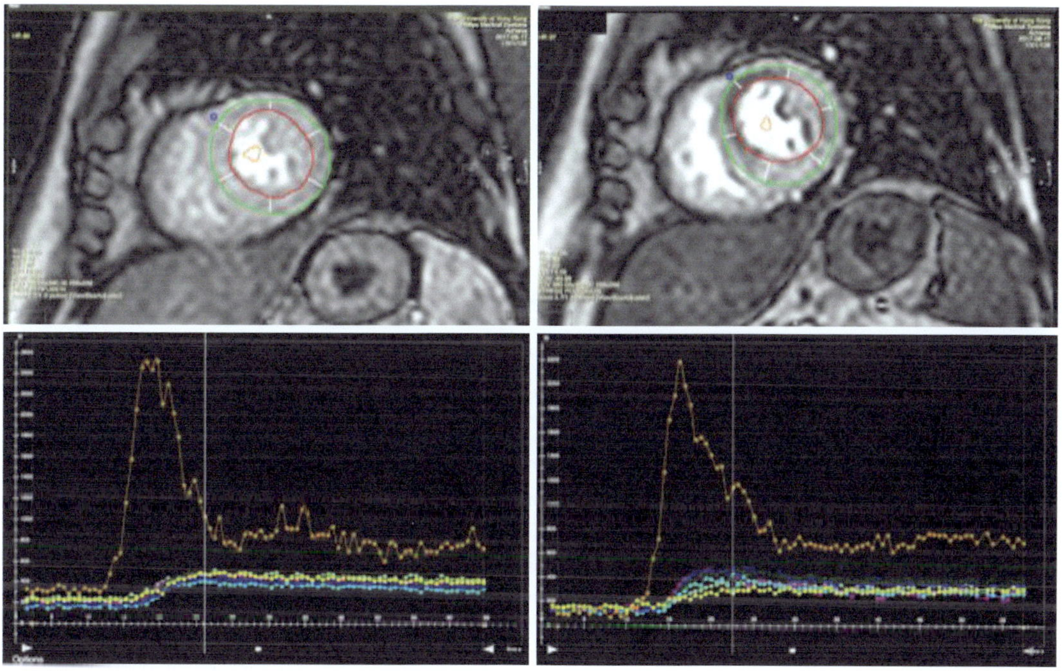

Fig. 6.1 Workstation screenshot of semiquantitative perfusion assessment on stress cardiac magnetic resonance. The top row of images are short axis oblique images of the left ventricle. The green and red contours delineate the epicardial and endocardial borders which are drawn manually. The orange contour in the left ventricular (LV) cavity measures the contrast flow into the LV cavity (i.e., arterial input function). The bottom row of images represent contrast flow into the LV cavity (orange line) and contrast enhancement of the myocardium (lines of different colors). The maximum slope ratio and myocardial perfusion reserve index is calculated by the software automatically

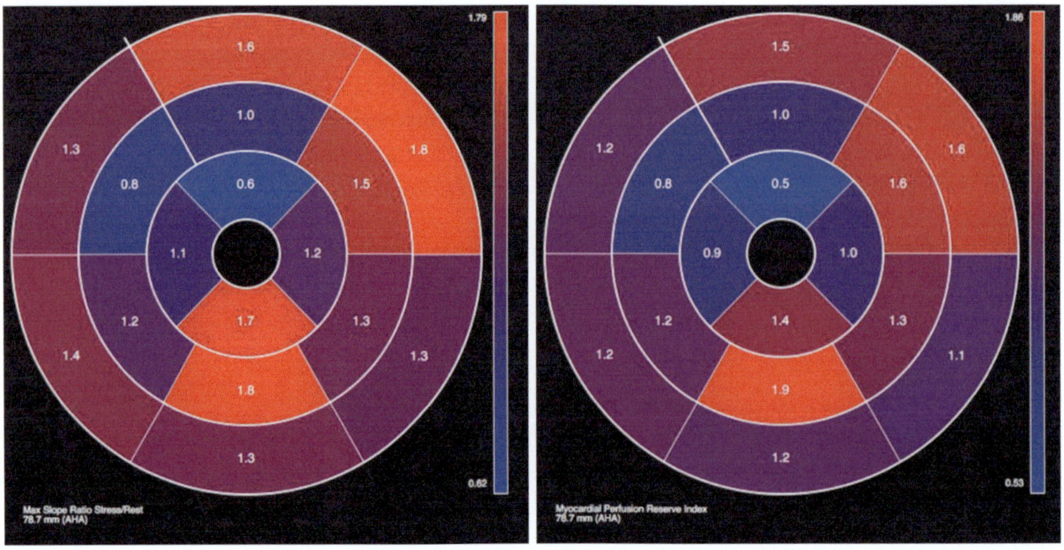

Fig. 6.2 American Heart Association (AHA) 17-segment polar map showing results of maximum upslope stress and rest ratio (left polar map) and myocardial perfusion reserve index (right polar map) using a semiquantitative method

toured. Maximum upslope stress to rest ratio is derived from measuring the initial upslope of the myocardial enhancement at stress and rest but is not corrected by the blood pool. MPR though is corrected by the blood pool. However, it is important to note that the MPR calculated by semiquantitative perfusion is not the same as the MPR calculated by fully quantitative methods since there is signal saturation of the blood pool signal intensity as mentioned earlier which dual bolus and dual sequence help alleviate. Nonetheless, semiquantitative techniques have shown clinically useful prognostic data [26].

Artificial Intelligence-Based Contouring

A major step toward clinical implementation is the use of artificial intelligence (AI) to contour the multitude of perfusion images for the basal, mid-ventricular, and apical slices. The manual contouring and adjustments required for multiple images normally takes ~20 min to perform whilst AI contouring can be accomplished within 1 s [27]. Notably, AI calculated stress MBF and MPR from stress CMR examinations has been shown to be predictive of major adverse cardiovascular events [10].

Diagnostic and Prognostic Value of CMR QP and Its Limitations

Diagnostic Value

Coronary microvascular disease (CMD) and obstructive coronary artery disease (CAD) are two distinct cardiovascular conditions where fully quantitative stress perfusion CMR has a significant role. CMD is attributed to smooth muscle wall thickening, collagen deposition, impaired vasodilation, or increased vasoconstriction. Both CMD and epicardial CAD exhibit similar symptoms such as effort-induced angina pectoris and dyspnea. Moreover, CMD can occur in patients with and without obstructive CAD. Quantitative perfusion measurements can provide additional parameters to help distinguish between these two clinical entities. For example, CMD is typically characterized by diffuse reduction in stress MBF or MPR, whereas obstructive CAD manifests as a regional reduction in MBF or MPR in a coronary territory.

Diagnostic Confidence Utilizing Quantitative Perfusion

A significant benefit of using quantitative perfusion to produce perfusion maps and calculations of stress MBF and MPR is the increase in diagnostic confidence and confirmation of adequate stress achieved with pharmacological agents such as regadenoson, adenosine, dipyridamole, and ATP. In scenarios where a dark rim is present, but the perfusion maps show excellent perfusion, this increases diagnostic certainty that the dark rim is artifactual. Normal appearing myocardial perfusion maps can also increase diagnostic confidence in studies where there is uncertainty with regards to adequate stress.

Clinical Examples

(All images captured are under the copyright of MRI Unit of the Department of Diagnostic Radiology, the University of Hong Kong.)

This part of the review aims at providing real-life clinical examples of application of MRI perfusion imaging. All patients were scanned on a GE 3T SIGNA Premier scanner, undergoing standard multiplanar cine imaging for cardiac function assessment, first pass perfusion imaging for the assessment of rest and stress myocardial perfusion, and late gadolinium enhancement imaging. 0.05 mmol/kg of gadolinium-based contrast agent will be intravenously injected at a peak stress to acquire first-pass stress perfusion (Gadobutrol).

Intravenous adenosine was injected at a rate of 0.14 mg/kg/min for 3 min. If there was inadequate stress response at 2 min, the infusion rate was increased by 50% to 0.21 mg/kg/min for a further 3 min. There was a 10-min interval prior to acquiring rest images, and an additional administration of 0.05 mmol/kg of Gadobutrol was given.

Obstructive CAD

(i) Obstructive CAD patient without revascularization (see Fig. 6.3)
(ii) Patient with previous revascularization (see Fig. 6.4)

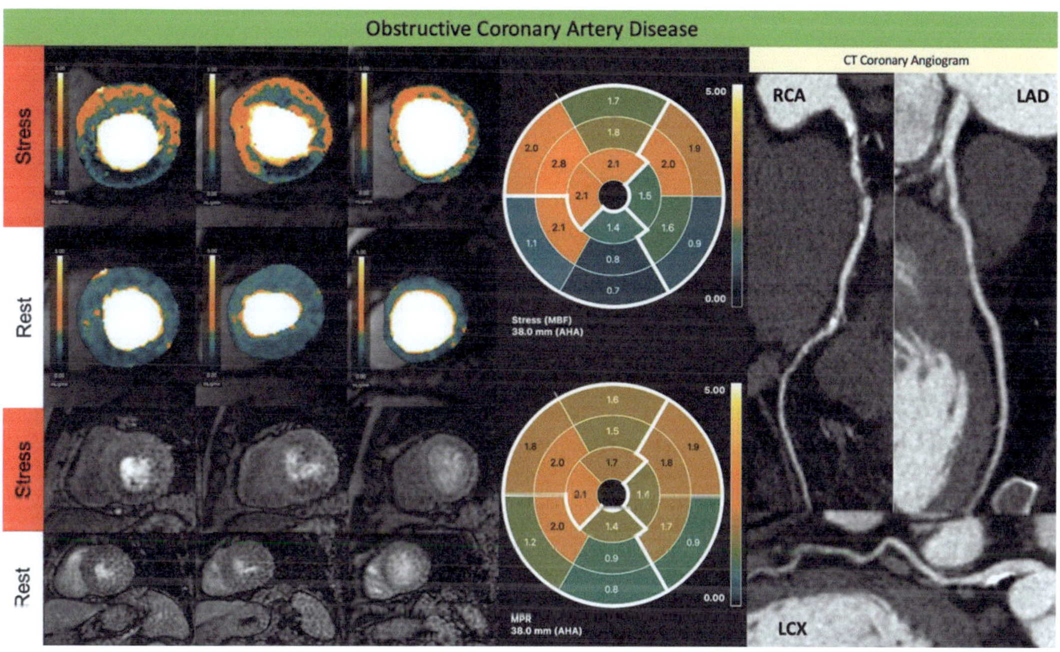

Fig. 6.3 A 70-year-old male with stable angina. There is a stress-induced perfusion defect at the basal inferior, inferoseptal, and mid-ventricular inferior wall which is more clearly demonstrated on the quantitative perfusion images. Global MBF is 1.67 mL/g/min and global MPR is 1.54

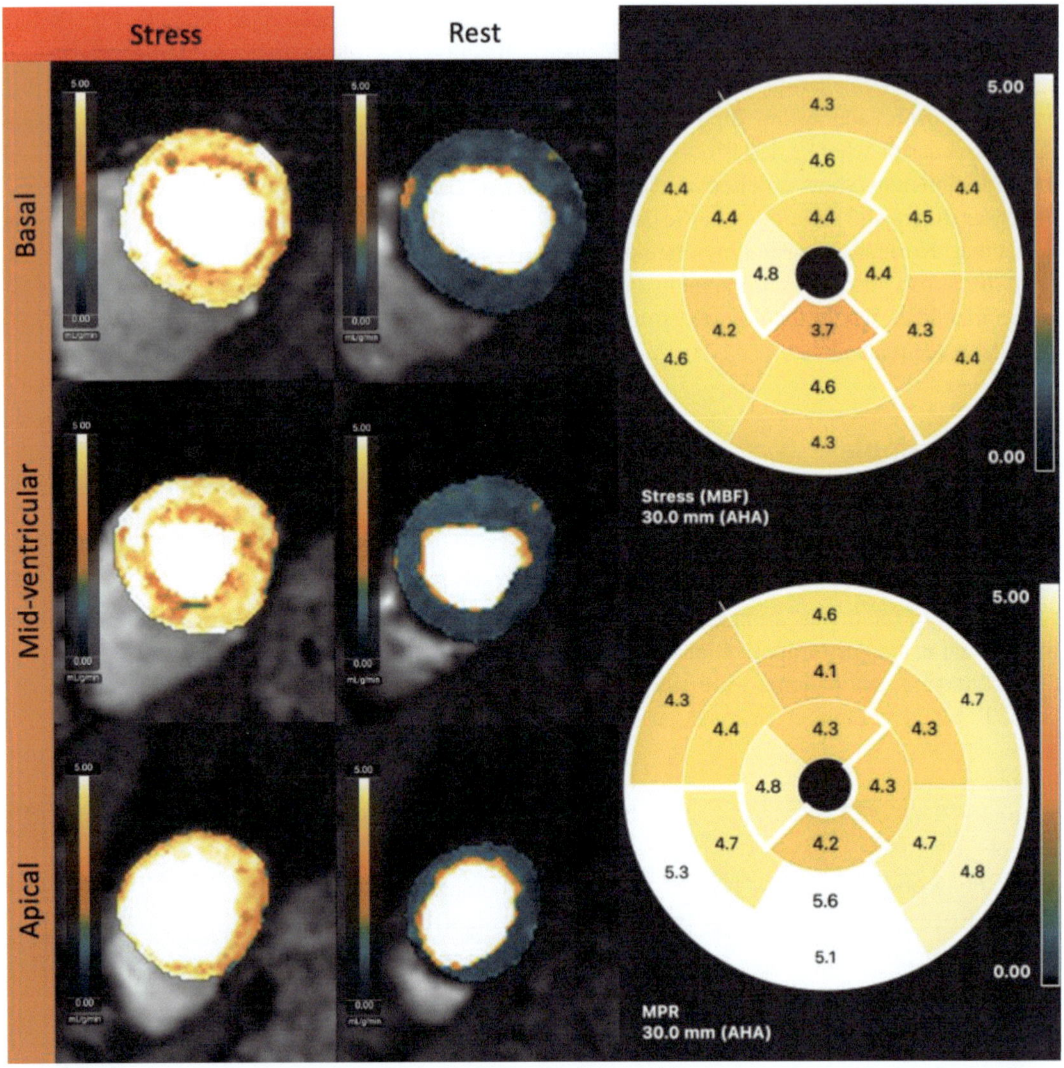

Fig. 6.4 A 72-year-old female with previous percutaneous coronary intervention (PCI). Patient demonstrates normal stress myocardial blood flow and myocardial perfusion reserve can be achieved as shown in the balanced perfusion of overall 17 AHA segments

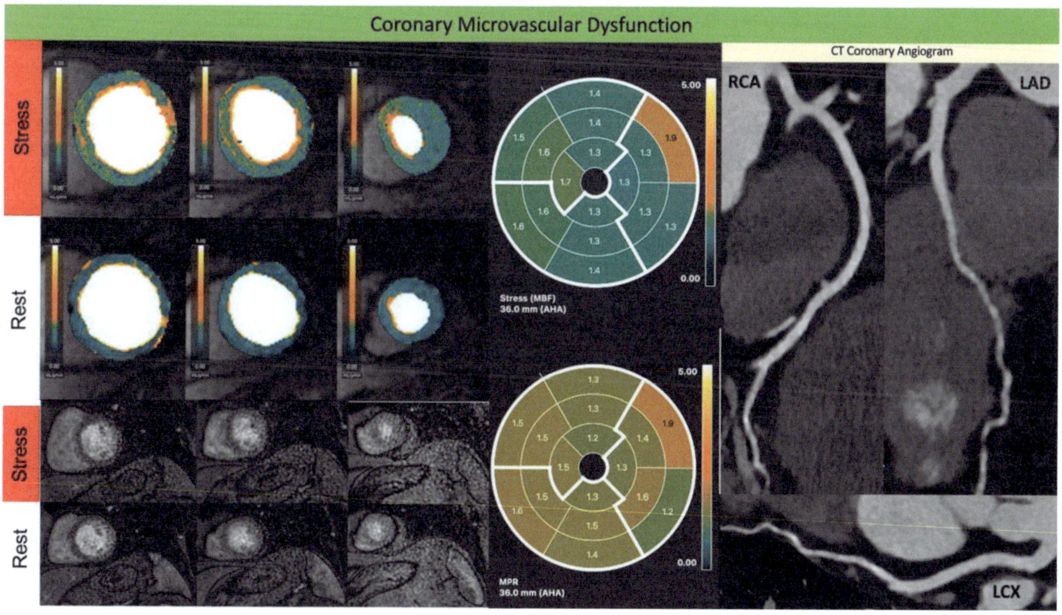

Fig. 6.5 A 62-year-old male with diffuse reduction in perfusion as demonstrated by the turquoise color to the perfusion maps. Together with the CT angiography of no obstructive CAD, the appearances are consistent with coronary microvascular disease (CMD). Quantitative myocardial stress perfusion allows non-invasive detection of CMD

Coronary Microvascular Disease (see Fig. 6.5) Coronary microvascular disease features ischemic ECG changes, stress-induced angina, or more numerically, impaired coronary flow reserve as <2.0–2.5 depending on methodologies. Such criteria can be further validated on stress CMR compared to any other imaging modalities, with its individual clinical context despite the latency and hidden nature of CMD. A previous study has shown that a stress MBF range of 1.82–2.25 ml/g/min is indicative or CMD [5].

Conclusion

Fully quantitative CMR stress perfusion with either dual bolus or dual sequence is a significant development in the assessment of epicardial CAD and CMD. Via advanced mathematical model-dependent or model-independent techniques, stress and rest MBF along with MPR can be calculated accurately. Fully quantitative perfusion holds promise in helping to diagnose CMD and increasing diagnostic confidence.

References

1. Nagel E, et al. Magnetic resonance perfusion measurements for the noninvasive detection of coronary artery disease. Circulation. 2003;108(4):432–7.
2. Kim D, Axel L. Multislice, dual-imaging sequence for increasing the dynamic range of the contrast-enhanced blood signal and CNR of myocardial enhancement at 3T. J Magn Reson Imaging. 2006;23(1):81–6.
3. Elkington AG, et al. Optimization of the arterial input function for myocardial perfusion cardiovascular magnetic resonance. J Magn Reson Imaging. 2005;21(4):354–9.
4. Hsu L-Y, Kellman P, Arai AE. Nonlinear myocardial signal intensity correction improves quantification of contrast-enhanced first-pass MR perfusion in humans. J Magn Reson Imaging. 2008;27(4):793–801.
5. Kotecha T, et al. Automated pixel-wise quantitative myocardial perfusion mapping by CMR to detect obstructive coronary artery disease and coronary microvascular dysfunction: validation against invasive coronary physiology. JACC Cardiovasc Imaging. 2019;12(10):1958–69.
6. Wang S, et al. JACC Imaging 2024; https://www.jacc.org/doi/abs/10.1016/j.jcmg.2024.07.023.
7. Sinha A, Rahman H, Perera D. Coronary microvascular disease: current concepts of pathophysiology, diagnosis and management. Cardiovasc Endocrinol Metab. 2021;10(1):22–30.

8. Taillefer R, et al. Comparison between dipyridamole and adenosine as pharmacologic coronary vasodilators in detection of coronary artery disease with thallium 201 imaging. J Nucl Cardiol. 1996;3(3):204–11.
9. Engblom H, et al. Fully quantitative cardiovascular magnetic resonance myocardial perfusion ready for clinical use: a comparison between cardiovascular magnetic resonance imaging and positron emission tomography. J Cardiovasc Magn Reson. 2017;19(1):78.
10. Knott KD, et al. The prognostic significance of quantitative myocardial perfusion: an artificial intelligence-based approach using perfusion mapping. Circulation. 2020;141(16):1282–91.
11. Drakos S, et al. A cardiovascular magnetic resonance imaging-based pilot study to assess coronary microvascular disease in COVID-19 patients. Sci Rep. 2021;11(1):15667.
12. Sammut EC, et al. Prognostic value of quantitative stress perfusion cardiac magnetic resonance. JACC Cardiovasc Imaging. 2018;11(5):686–94.
13. Vasu S, et al. Regadenoson and adenosine are equivalent vasodilators and are superior than dipyridamole—a study of first pass quantitative perfusion cardiovascular magnetic resonance. J Cardiovasc Magn Reson. 2013;15(1):85.
14. Ng MY, et al. Prognostic value of perfusion cardiovascular magnetic resonance with adenosine triphosphate stress in stable coronary artery disease. J Cardiovasc Magn Reson. 2021;23(1):75.
15. Kramer CM, et al. Standardized cardiovascular magnetic resonance imaging (CMR) protocols: 2020 update. J Cardiovasc Magn Reson. 2020;22(1):17.
16. Hamon M, et al. Meta-analysis of the diagnostic performance of stress perfusion cardiovascular magnetic resonance for detection of coronary artery disease. J Cardiovasc Magn Reson. 2010;12(1):29.
17. Jerosch-Herold M. Quantification of myocardial perfusion by cardiovascular magnetic resonance. J Cardiovasc Magn Reson. 2010;12(1):57.
18. Zierler K. Indicator dilution methods for measuring blood flow, volume, and other properties of biological systems: a brief history and memoir. Ann Biomed Eng. 2000;28(8):836–48.
19. Zierler KL. Theoretical basis of indicator-dilution methods for measuring flow and volume. Circ Res. 1962;10(3):393–407.
20. Hsu LY, et al. Diagnostic performance of fully automated pixel-wise quantitative myocardial perfusion imaging by cardiovascular magnetic resonance. JACC Cardiovasc Imaging. 2018;11(5):697–707.
21. Papanastasiou G, et al. Measurement of myocardial blood flow by cardiovascular magnetic resonance perfusion: comparison of distributed parameter and Fermi models with single and dual bolus. J Cardiovasc Magn Reson. 2015;17(1):17.
22. Chong EYS, et al. JCMR 2024; https://www.journalofcmr.com/article/S1097-6647(24)01112-8/fulltext.
23. Patel AR, et al. Assessment of advanced coronary artery disease: advantages of quantitative cardiac magnetic resonance perfusion analysis. J Am Coll Cardiol. 2010;56(7):561–9.
24. Ishida M, et al. Development of a universal dual-bolus injection scheme for the quantitative assessment of myocardial perfusion cardiovascular magnetic resonance. J Cardiovasc Magn Reson. 2011;13(1):28.
25. KH Leung, et al. EHJ Cardiovascular Imaging 2025; https://academic.oup.com/ehjcimaging/advancearticle/doi/10.1093/ehjci/jeaf339/8364374.
26. Zhou W, et al. Long-term prognosis of patients with coronary microvascular disease using stress perfusion cardiac magnetic resonance. JACC Cardiovasc Imaging. 2021;14(3):602–11.
27. Xue H, et al. Automated inline analysis of myocardial perfusion MRI with deep learning. Radiol Artif Intell. 2020;2(6):e200009.

Quantitative Assessment in Nuclear Cardiology

7

Elisa Franquet, Hui Chong Lau, Thomas S. C. Ng, and Marcelo Fernando Di Carli

Introduction: General Concepts in Nuclear Cardiology and Coronary Artery Disease (CAD)

Nuclear cardiology includes a variety of measurements related to myocardial perfusion, function, contractility, synchrony, metabolism with different substrates, and innervation. It is digital and quantitative at its essence. Decades of work have made possible the development of methods to assess the different aspects of myocardial physiology using different modalities with both established and emerging applications. This chapter will review the role of myocardial perfusion quantification methods in coronary artery disease [1].

Detection and quantification of myocardial ischemia and infarcted myocardium with myocardial perfusion imaging (MPI) is well-established for diagnosing coronary artery disease (CAD) and is a crucial component of CAD management and risk stratification of suspected or known CAD. A main advantage of MPI over other techniques is the availability of standardized and validated quantification methods.

As the epidemiology of disease changes and our understanding of disease pathophysiology increases, the landscape of cardiac imaging and management of coronary artery disease continues to evolve. It is becoming evident that information from MPI using single-photon emission tomography (SPECT), a key component in managing CAD for almost half a century, may be incomplete in certain clinical scenarios. Nowadays, it is common to evaluate patients with a multimodality approach, with coronary CT angiography

E. Franquet (✉)
Division of Nuclear Medicine and Molecular Imaging, Department of Radiology, University of Massachusetts Medical Health, UMass Chan Medical School, Worcester, MA, USA
e-mail: Elisa.franquet-elia@umassmemorial.org

H. C. Lau
Cardiology, Massachusetts General Hospital, Harvard Medical School, Boston, MA, USA

Cardiovascular Imaging Research Center, Massachusetts General Hospital, Harvard Medical School, Boston, MA, USA
e-mail: hclau@mgh.harvard.edu

T. S. C. Ng
Division of Nuclear Medicine and Molecular Imaging, Department of Radiology, Massachusetts General Hospital, Harvard Medical School, Boston, MA, USA

Center for Systems Biology, Massachusetts General Hospital, Harvard Medical School, Boston, MA, USA
e-mail: Sheung.Ng@mgh.harvard.edu

M. F. Di Carli
Division of Nuclear Medicine and Molecular Imaging, Cardiovascular Imaging Department of Radiology, Brigham and Women's Hospital, Harvard Medical School, Boston, MA, USA
e-mail: mdicarli@bwh.harvard.edu

R. Gill, P. Rajiah (eds.), *Quantitative Imaging in the Thorax*,
https://doi.org/10.1007/978-3-032-14103-3_7

becoming the preferred test for patients with low-to-intermediate likelihood of obstructive CAD and MPI now shifting to evaluate patients with higher-risk patients, those with higher cardiometabolic risk factors.

MPI with single-photon emission tomography (SPECT) has been automated for decades with robust imaging analysis algorithms. The concept of myocardial perfusion quantification has been the basis of cardiac nuclear imaging for over half a century. However, as the clinical presentation and epidemiology of CAD are changing, new evaluation methods have been introduced, some of them becoming more relevant than SPECT to answer specific clinical questions that we will discuss later in this chapter.

Methodological Considerations[1]

Myocardial Perfusion Evaluation (MPI)

Coronary artery disease (CAD) continues to be a worldwide leading cause of morbidity and mortality, affecting more than 18.5 million adults in the United States. CAD remains the leading cause of death for men and women, with 605,000 new attacks and 200,000 recurrent attacks based on data from 2005 and 2014 and 9.1 million annual deaths in 2019 [2]. Risk factors are changing with rapidly increasing obesity, diabetes, and other cardiometabolic diseases, and as a consequence, the presentation of CAD is also changing, with an increase in nonobstructive and microvascular disease [3]. Previously, coronary obstructive disease was the most frequent presentation of CAD [4–6]. Single-photon emission computed tomography (SPECT) MPI was able to noninvasively detect the territory of ischemia by a culprit lesion limiting coronary flow, and similarly but more invasively, coronary angiography, which remains the gold standard for detection of obstructive disease. However, the changes in CAD presentation represent diagnostic challenges with the modalities that have been well-established for decades, as CAD presents now with less ischemia on SPECT stress imaging and less obstructive disease in coronary angiography. This new group of disease presentation is called ischemia with nonobstructive coronary artery disease (INOCA). The pathophysiology is still poorly understood, but one of the potential causes of INOCA is thought to be coronarymicrovascular dysfunction (CMD) [7]. One of the diagnostic tools is the assessment of myocardial blood flow (MBF) and myocardial flow reserve (MFR) [3, 4, 8], which requires dynamic acquisition and quantification of the coronary flow. Myocardial perfusion imaging with positron emission tomography (PET) is the most common modality for noninvasive evaluation of MFR. In recent years, the availability and access to other hybrid scanners such as positron emission tomography/computed tomography (PET/CT) and positron emission tracers for perfusion imaging has improved the evaluation and management of coronary artery disease. The changing role of SPECT imaging as CAD presentation evolves and the different methods of myocardial perfusion imaging and quantification will be discussed in this chapter [9].

The coronary arterial system is a continuous network of vessels of decreasing size from the epicardial arteries to the capillaries. Coronary blood flow and myocardial perfusion are regulated by dynamic changes in the resistance of the vessels and arteriolar tone to maintain blood flow and oxygen constant. At rest, oxygen extraction is near maximal, and in situations of higher oxygen demand and depends on coronary blood flow and in situations of higher oxygen demand, demand must be matched by a proportional increase in coronary blood flow to prevent myocardial ischemia [10]. At the epicardial level in CAD, there is a compensatory dilation distal to the areas of stenosis to maintain blood flood at rest. But in situations that require a higher oxygen demand, the compensatory changes cannot accommodate a higher degree of vasodilation and fail to match demand, leading to ischemia, and those areas will receive less blood flow than the remaining of the myocardium [10, 11]. CAD at

[1] Please refer to the Chap. 25 for details of the medical physics considerations of the techniques presented herein.

intramyocardial vessels, arterioles, and capillaries, the so-called microvascular disease, many factors can lead to remodeling and, ultimately attenuation of coronary flow augmentation in response to stress and, if severe enough, can also lead to demand-supply mismatch. This is the basis of stress/rest myocardial perfusion protocols.

Stress imaging can be performed with either exercise or pharmacologic intervention. The choice of radionuclide MPI modality (SPECT or PET) and whether the stress will be exercise or pharmacologic will be tailored to the patient and their context as well as scanner availability. However, any combination of stress and rest imaging is recommended.

Gated myocardial perfusion imaging provides information about reversible (ischemic myocardium) or fixed (infarcted myocardium) perfusion defects, LV function, LV volumes, regional wall motion, and thickening. MPI is indicated in the initial evaluation of patients with stable chest pain or ischemic equivalent and in intermediate to high-risk patients with stable CAD (prior MI, revascularization, arrhythmias, and heart failure). MPI can help decision-making regarding the need for revascularization, provide quantification of ischemia and scarring, and help with risk assessment [12]. Compared to other techniques, the patient's body habitus, presence of pacemaker, arrhythmias, or renal disease do not present limitations. In comparison to other techniques such as MRI or echo, MPI does involve radiation exposure via intravenously administered radiotracers and sometimes low-dose CT, which should always be considered.

The assessment of myocardial perfusion with either SPECT or PET follows the same principle explained above. Regional myocardial perfusion is evaluated at rest and at stress to detect presence of CAD-related perfusion abnormalities or flow-limiting disease by demonstrating differences in perfusion between rest and stress conditions [11]. This means that both rely on detecting regional perfusion differences based on the normalization of tracer uptake to the site of maximum uptake in the left ventricle. This is a known limitation as it can underestimate the presence of multivessel disease or significant left main disease, and while all coronary territories are similarly affected, myocardial perfusion may appear falsely normal or mildly abnormal at stress, the so-called balanced ischemia. In such cases, there are secondary signs that can be helpful in identifying this situation, such as the presence of transient ischemic dilation (TID) or decreased post-stress left ventricular systolic function that would otherwise be normal at rest. Also, in diffuse nonobstructive disease or microvascular disease, myocardial perfusion could also appear relatively normal not revealing the presence of disease in a truly abnormal myocardium.

Differences Between SPECT and PET

While the general principle of myocardial perfusion imaging with SPECT and PET is the same, the modalities have important similarities and technical differences.

SPECT perfusion imaging is the most used stress imaging modality for CAD evaluation, with a sensitivity and specificity ranging from 75% to 85%. It is a widely available technique and less costly than PET. It can be used for both exercise and pharmacologic stress tests. SPECT cardiac imaging technology has markedly improved over the past 15 years. New solid-state cardiac camera systems with cadmium-zinc-telluride (CZT) detectors combined with novel collimator designs, cardiac dedicated collimators, and fan-beam collimation combined with solid-state photodiode detectors and Cs(I) crystal have improved image resolution and increased count sensitivity, allowing reduced injected radiation dose [5]. Limitations such as nonuniform photon attenuation by surrounding soft tissues can be overcome by attenuation correction methods with gadolinium line source, CT, or X-ray. Position-dependent soft tissue attenuation artifacts can be ascertained by observing their presentation when the patient is positioned differently relative to the detectors (from supine to prone or upright depending on the camera). Artifacts from the intense uptake from a nearby bowel in sestamibi studies can be solved by having the patient eat, move, and repeat imaging. However, cameras with NaI crystal detectors are not sensitive enough to quantify myocardial flow as they lack sensitivity and spatial resolution, and therefore microvascular disease, often diffuse, remains undetected on SPECT MPI.

PET scanners provide a higher spatial and temporal resolution compared to SPECT. This translates into better image quality and higher sensitivity for detecting defects sometimes not detected on SPECT but also the possibility of quantifying coronary flow. There are several PET tracers used to evaluate myocardial perfusion. These include ^{13}N-ammonia, ^{82}Rb (rubidium), both FDA-approved, ^{15}O-water (not FDA-approved) [13], and ^{18}F-flurpiridaz (recently FDA approved in 2024) [14–17]. PET imaging is less limited by soft tissue attenuation compared to SPECT, and attenuation correction is performed with a concomitant low-dose CT, similar to SPECT/CT. Some other advantages that PET MPI has are not being limited by nearby intestinal uptake, but there exists some rover from adjacent organs (liver, lung, or stomach) and shorter studies. PET tracers have shorter half-lives than SPECT tracers, and while the protocol length will depend on the tracer of choice, generally the timing between rest and stress studies is shorter, and the overall length of the study decreases considerably. Until the recent approval of flurpiridaz, the main limitation to the broad implementation of PET for evaluation for myocardial perfusion imaging has been the short physical half-life of the previously available isotopes that required an on-site cyclotron or access to a generator. For example, ^{13}N-ammonia has a 10-min half-life and is produced in a cyclotron, ^{15}O has a 2-min half-life and requires cyclotron on site, and ^{82}Rb has a half-life of 75 s, making exercise stress not feasible and also needs an on-site rubidium (^{82}Rb) generator. ^{18}F-Flurpiridaz has a longer half-life (110 min) which is very favorable to those sites without a cyclotron as it can be produced at a regional cyclotron and be distributed, but also, the longer half-life makes an exercise stress possible [18].

Quantification of Myocardial Perfusion

Preparation prior to the studies is crucial to ensure accuracy of the quantification results. For example, caffeine free for at least 12 h is recommended as it is known to interact with the vasodilator effect. In cases where there is high suspicion of vasodilator nonresponder, an alternative would be dobutamine agent.

Quantification methods for regional myocardial perfusion (for both SPECT and PET) have been systemically used because they increase the accuracy of detection of CAD by providing objective and consistent measurements of myocardial perfusion defects, severity, and extent and ultimately helping in prognosis and risk assessment. Commercially available cardiac MPI software packages are available and widely used, and they help standardize the interpretation and analysis of images. They increase readers' confidence and improve intra- and interobserver reproducibility [19]. There are many validated software packages (QPS-QGS, Emory Toolbox, 4D-MSPECT, and Wackers-Liu CQ), and they all follow the same principle.

Perfusion studies should be first evaluated visually in the conventional display of the three sets of tomographic images centered in the left ventricle displayed sequentially in short axis, vertical long axis, and horizontal long axis for qualitative evaluation. Stress and rest images in each axis should be displayed in conjunction for direct comparison. Following that, one should proceed to evaluation of the myocardial quantification.

For quantitative analysis, the first step is the segmentation of the left ventricle from gated and static reconstructed data. MPI software packages automatically select the center of the left ventricle (LV) and the radius defines LV contours. The three-dimensional perfusion distribution is mapped to a standard template to eliminate the variability in LV size and shape between patients [1]. It is crucial to exclude from the segmented LV, radiotracer uptake outside of the heart, such as liver or gastrointestinal tract, so common in technetium-based tracers, as these may result in perfusion defects. To reduce gastrointestinal activity, protocols try to decrease by having patients fast for 2–4 h and give water to drink before the scan. Another source of error can be patient motion during acquisition, which should be screened first by looking at the raw data. MPI software packages also create a three-dimensional display of regional perfusion. This automatic methodology reduces operator interaction at the left ventricular (LV) segmentation stage by performing automatic selection of the processing parameters and producing a reproducible and objective quantitative analysis.

The next step is to extract count densities from each LV short-axis ring through circumferential profiles. The standard 2D graphic display is called a polar map. It is divided following a 17-segment heart model in which each segment is assigned to a coronary artery territory (understanding the variability that exists between coronary anatomy). The highest value in the polar map is assigned 100%, and the rest of the segments are normalized to 100%, providing a relative perfusion map [1, 9, 20]. With the relative perfusion map, one can use thresholds to detect mild, moderate, and severe hypoperfusion and measure regional effects.

On the perfusion distribution, polar map distributions are typically acquired from a population comprising age-matched patients with a low (<5%) pretest likelihood of CAD. However, it is important to note that interpreting studies based on quantitative information alone can lead to higher sensitivity but less specificity. Extracted and normalized relative radiotracer uptake data in reconstructed slices per segment is quantitatively compared against normal data files in healthy patients [9, 19].

Visual identification of the location and extent of the perfusion defect was standardized to the 17-segment model in 2002. The size of the defect is usually estimated semiquantitatively as small (involving one to two segments), medium (involving three to four segments), or large (involving >/= to five segments); or quantitatively with small, medium, and large defects involving <10%, 10%–20%, and ≥20% of the LV, respectively [20].

The severity of hypoperfusion is expressed qualitatively as mild, moderate, or severe, or quantitatively based on the number of standard deviations (SD) below the lower limit of normal for any given myocardial location. Polar maps can then be plotted with defect severity mapped to a color scale, or as the so-called blackout maps where all pixels below normal limits are blacked out. Segments are assigned computed severity scores according to a five-point scale: 0 = normal; 1 = mildly abnormal; 2 = moderately abnormal; 3 = severely abnormal; and 4 = absent.

Segmental scoring is used for both stress and rest. The segmental summed stress score (SSS) and summed rest score provide significant incremental prognostic value for nuclear cardiology [1, 21]. The summed stress score (SSS), the summed rest score (SRS), and the summed difference score (SDS) are then calculated, and they allow to compute the percentage of left ventricle at risk [1, 20].

Standard tools for both SPECT and PET (but with some differences in the computational analysis methods) are available in all the main software packages available commercially.

Global LV Function

Gated imaging allows the assessment of the left ventricular function and its acquisition during each study is strongly encouraged. Parameters that can be calculated include LV ejection fraction (LVEF), end-diastolic volume (EDV), end-systolic volume (ESV), transient ischemic dilation (TID), myocardial mass, and diastolic function at stress and rest. The most common approach to gating is by delineating epicardial and endocardial surfaces from LV segmentation. A volume curve spanning the cardiac cycle is generated, and from the volume curve data, LV end-diastolic volume (EDV), LV end-systolic volume (ESV), LV ejection fraction (LVEF), cardiac output, myocardial mass, and diastolic function parameters (peak and time to peak filling and ejection rates) can then be calculated [9]. LV function calculation is independent of isotope or protocol used and should be performed at rest and after stress. It is reproducible, and several studies have shown that gated MPI and reference standard measurements of quantitative LVEF and LV volumes are concordant. However, it is important to realize that the normal LVEF values with SPECT technology may vary from other methods. When assessing LVEF with SPECT, it is important to realize that the gated image acquisition is indeed performed 30–45 min after the injection of the tracer either at rest or at stress (and therefore 30–45 min following exercise or vasodilator protocol at stress), and the more accurately term to describe the LVEF at stress is "post-stress LVEF." On the contrary, the LVEF calculated on PET during stress reflects the accurate LVEF during peak stress. PET/CT allows a more accurate evaluation of the LVEF reserve (stress ejection fraction-rest ejection fraction), which worsens with obstructive coronary disease and is a marker of severity. A drop in LVEF reserve is a marker of high-risk CAD. The extent and severity of ischemia is inversely proportional to the measured LVEF reserve [22]. Normal LVEF reserve with PET is defined as ≥5% and offers a 97% negative predictive value for excluding left main or three-vessel CAD. Furthermore, a normal LVEF reserve with mildly abnormal PET is predictive of less extensive CAD and may not warrant coronary angiography [23]. It is important to mention that arrythmias, such as atrial fibrillation or frequent premature ventricular contractions (PVCs) can provide poor gating data and therefore underestimate the LVEF.

Transient ischemic dilation (TID) ratio, determined by the ratio of the stress endocardial volume and the rest endocardial volume in static nongated images, is a marker of severe CAD and adverse outcome. TID ratios have been historically established with SPECT, however not widely evaluated with PET. Some data suggests similar ranges compared to SPECT imaging [24].

Coronary Artery Calcification (CAC)

The characterization of coronary-artery calcification by computed tomography shows equivalence with the total coronary calcified atherosclerosis load and the risk of cardiovascular events [25]. Coronary artery calcium (CAC) score is a risk stratification tool based on the amount of calcified plaque in the coronary arteries. CAC score is generated from gated noncontract chest CT. The determination of the CAC score by computed tomography is based on axial slices with a 3 mm thickness acquired prospectively in synchrony with the electrocardiogram at a predetermined moment in the R-R interval, usually in the mid/late diastole. The effective dose of radiation is low. The main quantification system is the Agatson method, determination of calcium volume score, and relative calcium mass score [25]. Hybrid systems SPECT/CT or PET/CT provide CT for attenuation correction, but also, when ECG-gated CT is performed, then CAC can be provided adding value to the CAD assessment, as the presence of coronary artery calcifications increases the incidence of cardiovascular events and new incidence of CAD [3]. The absence of coronary artery calcium (score of 0) is associated with a very low probability of future cardiovascular events; however, we always have to consider those patients that may have underlaying cardiomyopathy from noncalcified plaque that won't be depicted, misguiding diagnosis, prognosis, and therapy management. Cardiac catheterization can help identify areas of luminal narrowing, and PET MPI can provide an accurate assessment of the myocardial perfusion.

Myocardial Blood Flow (PET)

As mentioned earlier in this chapter, PET provides a higher spatial resolution and improves the diagnosis of multivessel disease sing absolute myocardial blood flow quantification. Absolute myocardial blood flow quantification is difficult to obtain by other modalities, as quantification depends on the rapid dynamic acquisition of the injected tracer. Quantifying the absolute regional myocardial blood flow (MBF) and myocardial flow reserve (MFR) with PET is currently the noninvasive reference standard for these measures. The importance of MBF is that it provides unique information about the state of the coronary artery system, combining microcirculation, diffuse disease, and focal CAD that is otherwise not available from nonquantitative methods or other modalities [3, 22, 26].

The quantification of MBF uses the concentration of the radiotracer in blood as a function of time and the uptake by using a selected kinetic model. The ideal perfusion tracer for MBF quantification would have 100% extraction from blood to tissue and 100% retention (no washout) such that the relationship between the MBF and measured activity would be linear. While none of the currently available tracers have a linear relationship, the closest are ^{15}O and ^{13}N-ammonia, which have a tracer uptake rate (K_1) that is close to the true MBF. ^{82}Rb has substantially lower extraction (of approximately 35% at peak exercise) than ^{15}O and ^{13}N-ammonia, and ^{18}F-flurpiridaz appears to have similar to slightly higher extraction and retention values than ^{15}O and ^{13}N-ammonia [27].

Time-activity curves are generated with the measurement of arterial radiotracer activity over time. These should be corrected by to account for tracer binding to plasma proteins, red blood cell uptake, hematocrit, labeled metabolites, etc. Dynamic acquisition with short time frames is required for 3D systems for accurate sampling and integration of arterial blood activity. These frames vary from 5 to 10 s during the first pass extraction through the heart and from 1 to 5 min during the later phase. Limited postprocessing, smoothing, and filtering are important to not impact MBF quantification [27]. Mathematical models that describe the tracer kinetics are used to estimate MBF from time-activity curves. Regional MBF is calculated by the ratio of stress MBF divided by rest MBF. Global MFR provides a measure of diffuse coronary atherosclerosis and microvascular dysfunction. Preserved global MBF (>2 mL min^{-1} g^{-1}) and global MFR (>2) confidently exclude high-risk angiographic CAD; severely reduced global MFR (<1.5) is associated with an increased likelihood of multivessel obstructive disease and should be considered a high-risk feature on PET MPI, and angiographic evaluation may be necessary; flow-limiting CAD should be considered in patients with normal PET MPI and severely reduced regional hyperemic MBF (<1.5 mL min^{-1} g^{-1}) and/or CFR (<1.5) in a single vascular territory [26, 27].

The accuracy of MPI highly depends on an adequate vasodilatory response. As mentioned earlier in the chapter, consuming caffeine before the scan often leads to false negatives. Splenic switch-off is the visual reduction of splenic radiotracer uptake that happens during the stress phase after vasodilator administration. It may serve as a marker for insufficient vasodilator response.

RPP correction: Elevated resting rate pressure product (RPP: blood pressure x heart rate) is often responsible for higher myocardial blood flow at rest, resulting in lower myocardial flow reserve despite adequate peak myocardial blood flow. RPP-corrected resting myocardial flow is performed when RPP is more than 9000 to normalize for abnormally high resting myocardial blood flow, resulting in higher myocardial flow reserve. However, studies have shown that RPP-corrected myocardial flow reserve can potentially result in inaccurate prognostic value in subjects with normal MPI and low uncorrected myocardial flow reserve [28].

In recent years, new research investigating the feasibility of MFR evaluation with the SPECT system has been published with encouraging results. However, more literature and validation are needed. These methods of dynamic acquisition and flow quantification can only be possible with newer and more sensitive detectors such as cadmium zinc telluride (CZT) semiconductor detectors [5]. The main challenge is the difficulty with dynamic and simultaneous acquisition of all projections during the rapid transit of the radiotracer through the left ventricle and myocardium [29]. And despite improved spatial resolution with solid-state cameras, patient and respiratory motion negatively impacts image quality. Data-driven correction methods for respiratory motion are feasible with list mode data acquisition [30].

Case-Based Applications Using Cardiac PET

Normal Scan

A 68-year-old Caucasian female with a history of hyperlipidemia presents with new intermittent left-sided chest pain, dyspnea on exertion, and palpitations (PSVT). She had no known CAD.

She underwent a pharmacological stress-rest PET with ^{82}Rb. She received 0.4 mg of IV regadenoson with an appropriate heart rate response from 58 bpm and 114/71 mmHg to 79 bpm and 100/61 mmHg, with no ischemic ECG changes during the stress test of the exam (Fig. 7.1).

Relative polar maps in stress (left) and rest (center) show homogeneous myocardial perfusion without defects, as seen in the three-axis images; therefore, there are reversible defects recorded (right polar map). The severity is mapped to a color scale ("blackout maps") and show no perfusion defects. The summed stress score (SSS), the summed rest score (SRS), and the summed difference score (SDS) are all zero (Fig. 7.2).

Time activity curves (stress on top, rest on the bottom): The blood pool time-activity curves (green) must start before the injection to ensure appropriate recording of the bolus. They should show a steep increase in counts followed by a drop. The myocardial count time-activity curve must demonstrate a steady uptake of tracer followed by a plateau of counts.

The polar maps on the right indicate the evaluation of flow at stress (top), rest (middle), and reserve (bottom). The CBF calculation per vascular segment is seen in the second column matching the first. At stress, the CBF is normal in all territories.

This patient's PET/CT MPI is normal and therefore there is no evidence of CAD or CMD to explain patient's symptoms, which are confidently interpreted as noncardiac.

Normal Scan with High Calcium Score

A 75-year-old female with hypertension and hyperlipidemia. She presented with dyspnea on exertion. She underwent a cardiac CTA with CAC and an Agatson score of 1857 (left main 82, LAD 1461, LCx 305, and RCA 9).

She underwent a pharmacological stress-rest PET with ^{82}Rb. She received 0.4 mg of IV regadenoson with an appropriate heart rate response from 81 bpm and 146/85 mmHg to 111 bpm and 150/79 mmHg; she had baseline ST-T abnormality

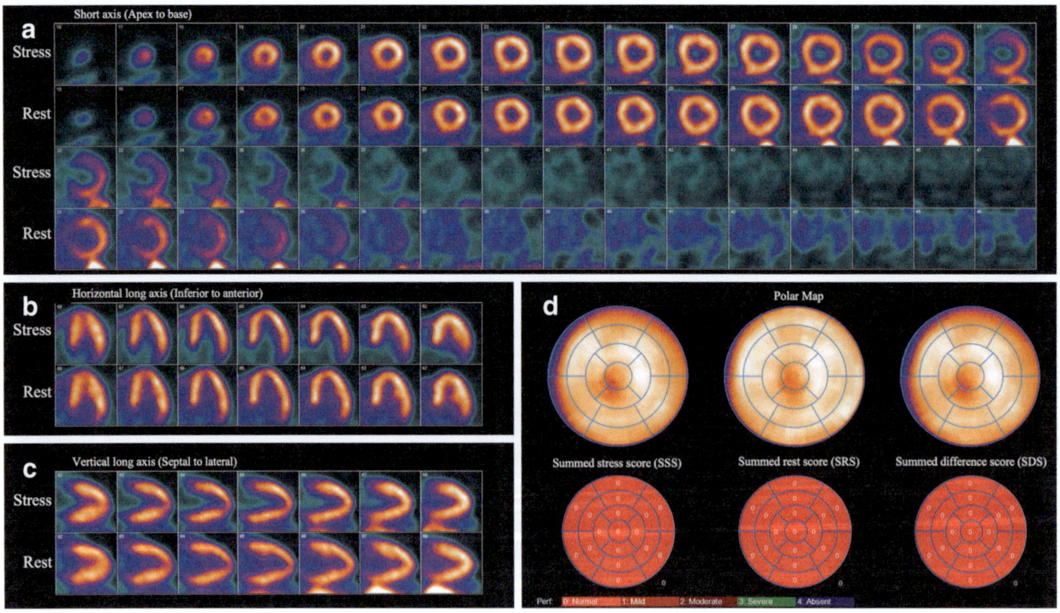

Fig. 7.1 PET perfusion images. The relative myocardial perfusion images are shown (**a–c**). (**a**) Short axis (SA) in stress (first and third rows) and rest (second and fourth rows); (**b**) horizontal long axis (HLA) in stress (first row) and rest (second row); (**c**) vertical long axis (VLA) in stress (first row) and rest (second row); (**d**) the summed rest score (SRS). Images show a homogenous distribution of the tracer both in stress and rest

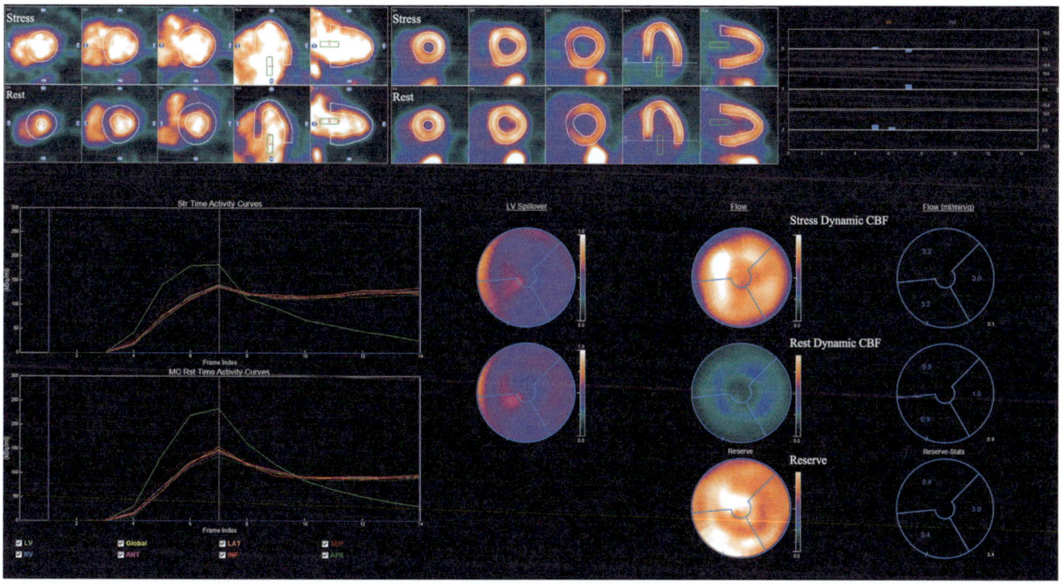

Fig. 7.2 Coronary flow processing. After intravenous injection the tracer and blood pool flow from the right-sided cavities of the heart to the lungs (not shown), and into the left heart (the first set of images on the left at stress-top and rest-bottom), and gradually extracted from the blood pool and retained in the myocardium (second set of images on top at stress-top and rest-bottom). The myocardial ROI (regions of interest) must accurately include the myocardium to accurately calculate the uptake, as demonstrated in the image. The ROI for blood pool sampling (green box) must be reviewed and placed in the same location for rest and stress, without touching the heart's walls to avoid spillover

on EKG. During the stress, she had occasional PAC and non-sustain ventricular tachycardia for six beats and exaggeration of the baseline changes. The EKG was deemed nondiagnostic. No ischemic ECG changes during the stress test of the exam (Fig. 7.3).

The CBF quantification increases normally between rest and stress, and the CFR is normal in all three vascular territories, indicating that, in spite of very high calcium score, there is no obstructive CAD or microvascular disease present. Patient underwent angiographic evaluation due to persistent symptoms, and this revealed non-obstructive CAD with iFR negative at circumflex (0.99). LAD was 30% occluded, circumflex 50%, and RCA 0%. She proceeded with further respiratory workup (Fig. 7.4).

Normal Scan with Low CFR

A 68-year-old female with a history of hyperlipidemia, hypertension, and prediabetes, known CAD with mid LAD occlusion status post PCI in 2021, presents with non-exertional chest pain.

She underwent a pharmacological stress-rest PET with ^{82}Rb. She received 0.4 mg of IV regadenoson with an appropriate heart rate response from 85 bpm and 161/74 mmHg to 103 bpm and 148/79 mmHg. She had baseline NSR, first AV block, and ST-T wave abnormality. During the stress, there were submillimeter ST depression but no EKG ischemic changes. Not shown, calcium burden on the CT portion of the study was severe (Figs. 7.5 and 7.6).

Single Vessel Perfusion Defect with Globally Decreased CFR

A 74-year-old male with history of hypertension and hyperlipidemia who presented with dyspnea on exertion. He also had a history of CABG in 2017 (LIMA to LAD, SVG to OM1, and SVG to RCA).

He underwent a pharmacological stress-rest PET with ^{82}Rb. He received 0.4 mg of IV regadenoson with appropriate heart rate response from 62 bpm and 150/68 mmHg to 85 bpm and

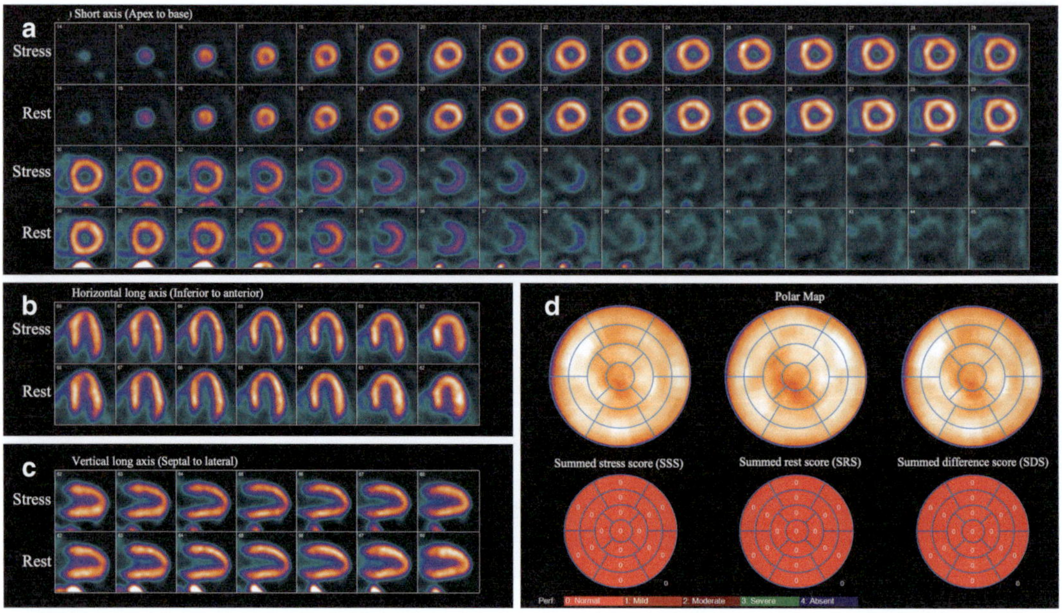

Fig. 7.3 PET perfusion images. The relative myocardial perfusion images are shown (**a**–**c**). (**a**) Short axis (SA) in stress (first and third rows) and rest (second and forth rows); (**b**) horizontal long axis (HLA) in stress (first row) and rest (second row); (**c**) vertical long axis (VLA) in stress (first row) and rest (second row); (**d**) the summed rest score (SRS). Images show homogenous distribution of the tracer both in stress and rest, a normal myocardial perfusion. The relative polar maps at stress (left) and rest (center) shows homogeneous myocardial perfusion without defects. No reversible defects recorded (right polar map). The summed stress score (SSS), the summed rest score (SRS), and the summed difference score (SDS) are all zero

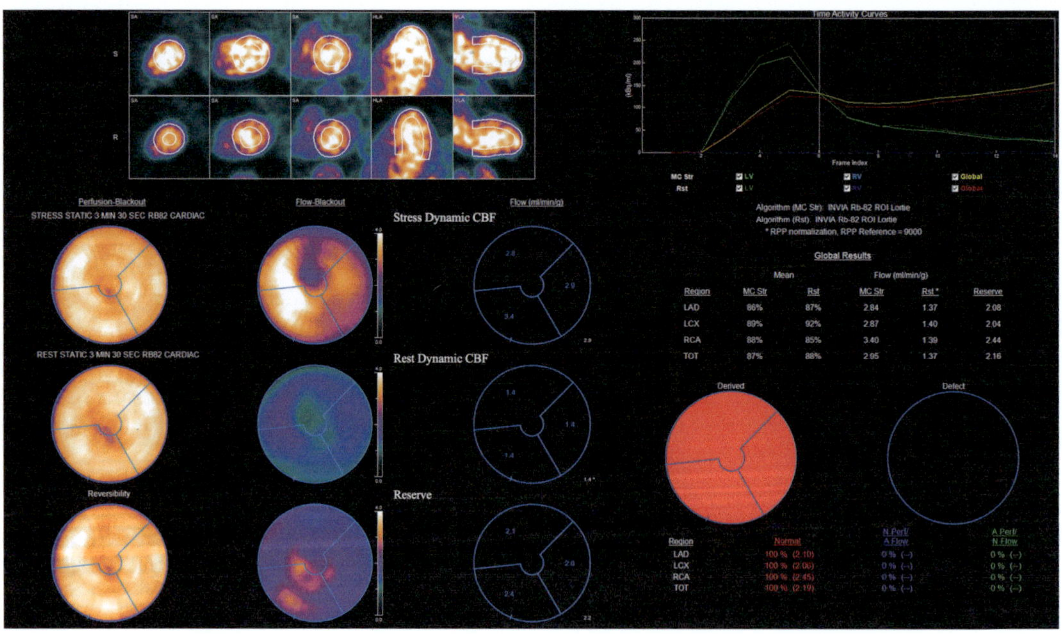

Fig. 7.4 Coronary flow assessment. This case illustrates the presence of blood pool in the ventricles before being retained in the myocardium. Note the blood pool sampling ROI (green box) between the left atrium and ventricle. The blood pool time activity curves are normal (green, stress on top, rest on the bottom). The myocardial count time-activity curves are also normal

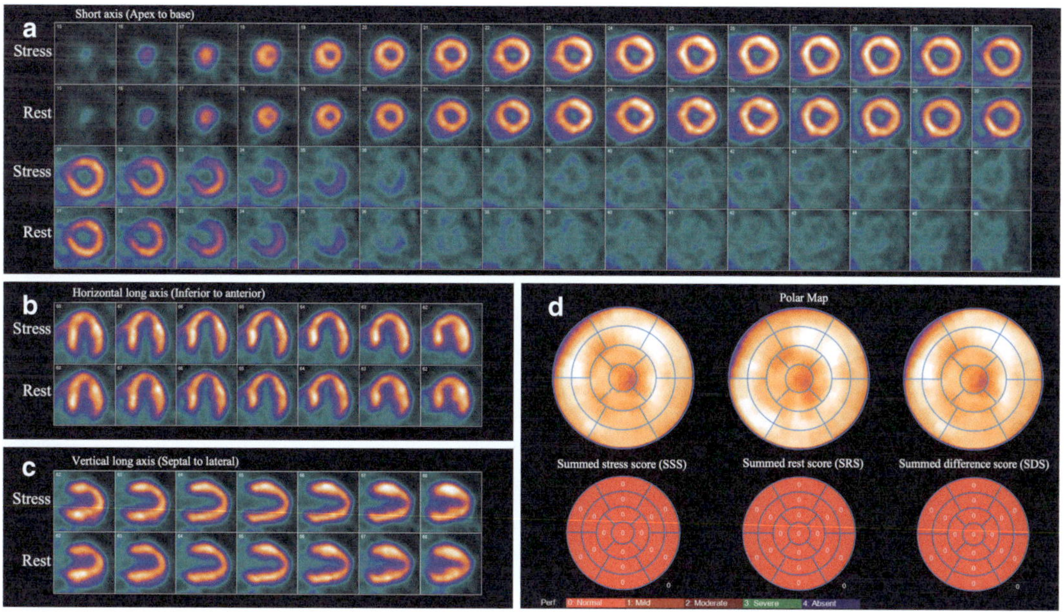

Fig. 7.5 PET perfusion images. The relative myocardial perfusion images are shown (**a–c**) and show homogenous distribution of the tracer both in stress and rest, a normal myocardial perfusion. (**d**) The summed rest score (SRS). The relative polar maps at stress (left) and rest (center) are also normal. The summed stress score (SSS), the summed rest score (SRS), and the summed difference score (SDS) are all zero

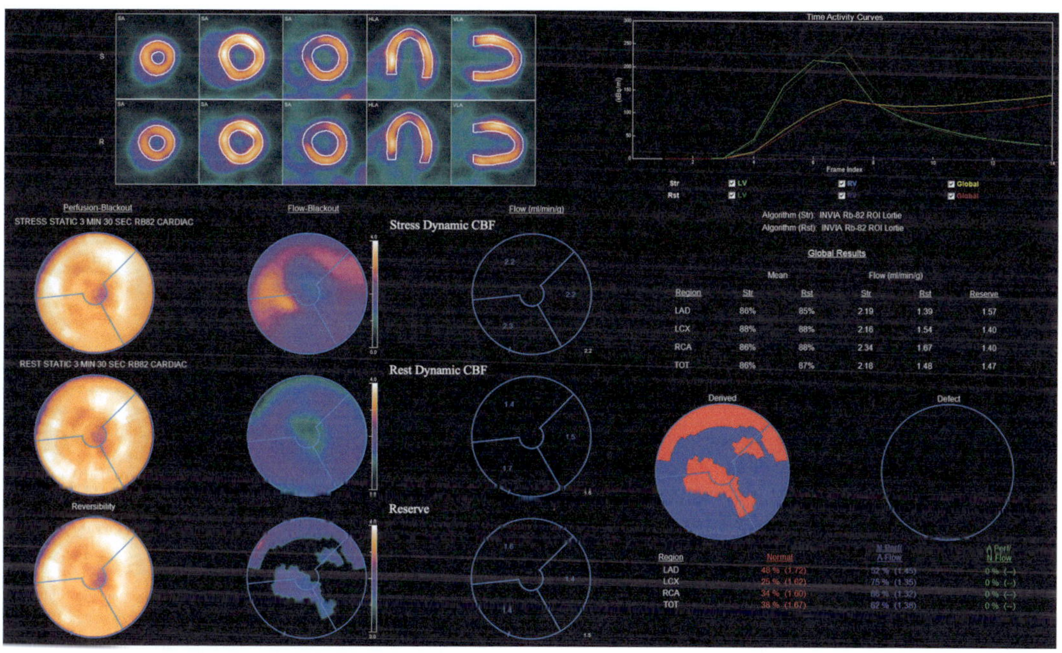

Fig. 7.6 Coronary flow assessment. The quality of the study is good as demonstrated by well-positioned LV ROIs and good blood pool and myocardial time-activity curves. The absolute polar map at stress on the right indicate normal CFR throughout (>2) but only mildly increased from rest yielding a diffusely decreased CFR (<2) (bottom). In this patient, in spite of no evidence of ischemia or infarct, PET demonstrated diffuse poor coronary flow reserve and microvascular disease, for which she underwent medical treatment optimization

116/68 mmHg. He had baseline NSR and no ST changes during stress. Not shown, calcium burden on the CT portion of the study was severe (Figs. 7.7 and 7.8).

Multivessel Disease

A 79-year-old male with history of hypertension and hyperlipidemia. He also had a history of three CABG: LIMA-LAD, SVG-OM, SVG-rPDA more than 30 years ago with known vein graft occlusion, and RCA PCI in 2021.

He underwent a pharmacological stress-rest PET with ^{82}Rb. He received 0.4 mg of IV regadenoson with appropriate heart rate response from 63 bpm and 100/57 mmHg to 85 bpm and 95/51 mmHg. He had baseline NSR and no ST changes during stress on EKG. Not shown, calcium burden on the CT portion of the study was severe (Figs. 7.9 and 7.10).

Perfusion Defect, Normal Coronary Flow

A 62-year-old female with history of hypertension and hyperlipidemia presents with exertional chest pain and dyspnea.

She underwent a pharmacological stress-rest PET with ^{82}Rb. He received 0.4 mg of IV regadenoson with an appropriate heart rate response from 75 bpm and 121/79 mmHg to 100 bpm and 118/75 mmHg. Her EKG showed baseline NSR and first-degree AV block. During the stress test, there were no ischemic changes recorded or symptoms. The calcium burden on the CT portion of the study was mild. During the PET acquisition, patient developed symptoms of prolonged chest pain (Fig. 7.11).

A CTA performed in the emergency room after the PET/CT showed severe stenosis of the LAD (70%–99%), and overall, CAC 153 (left main: 3, LAD: 146, LCx: 2 and RCA: 1). Patient

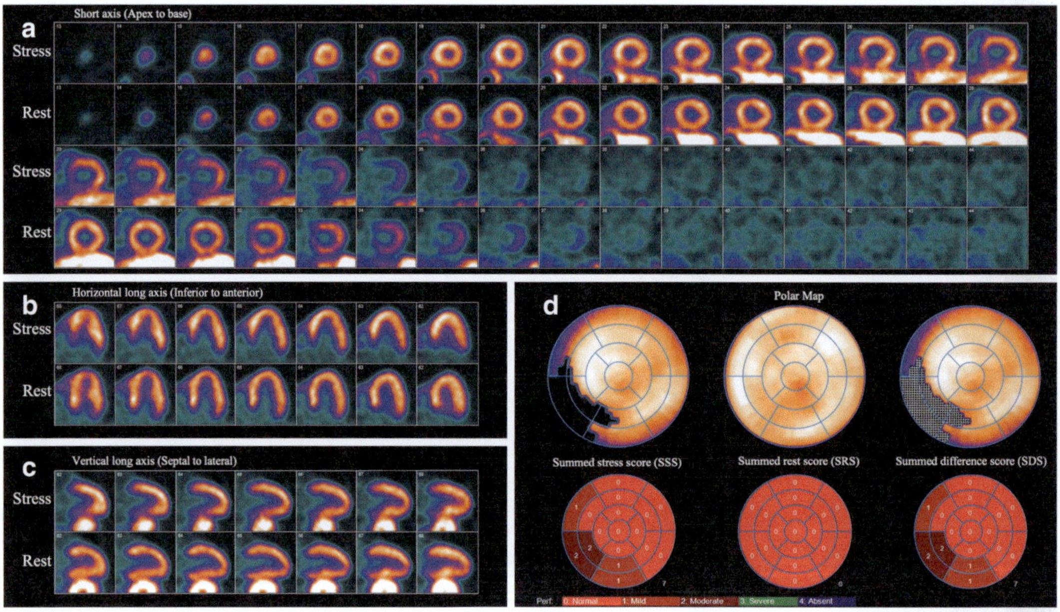

Fig. 7.7 PET perfusion images. The relative myocardial perfusion images show (**a**–**c**) show a small perfusion defect of moderate intensity in the basal and mid inferoseptal segments and complete reversibility at rest. (**d**) The summed rest score (SRS) is 0. The relative polar maps at stress (left) and rest (center) are shown. The summed stress score (SSS) is 7, the summed rest score (SRS) is 0, and the summed difference score (SDS) is 7

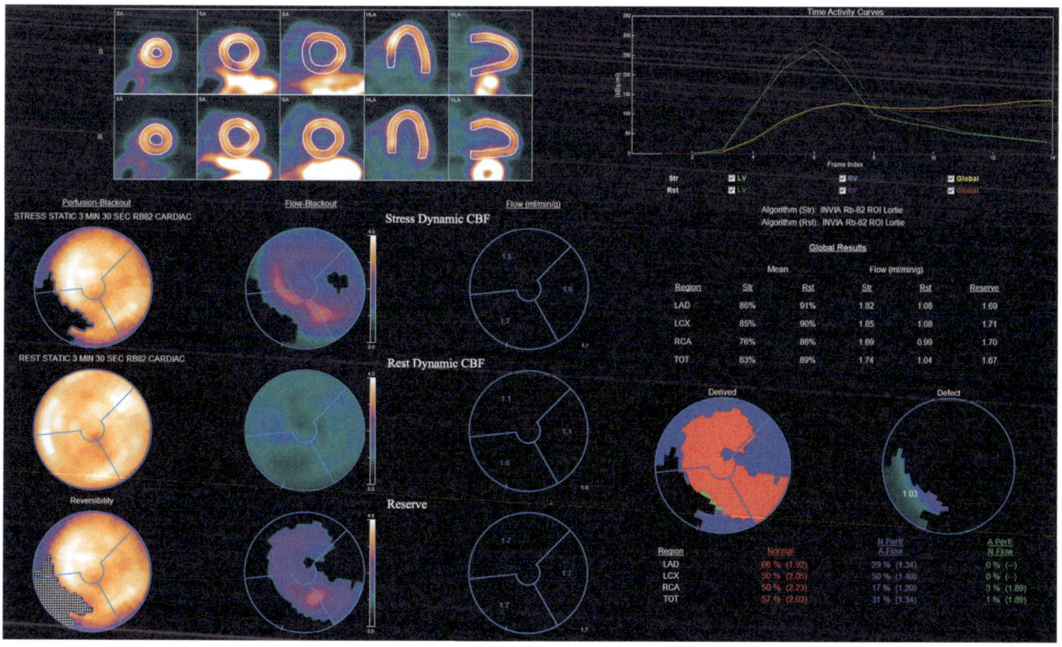

Fig. 7.8 Coronary flow assessment. The quality of the study is good as demonstrated by well-positioned LV ROIs and good blood pool and myocardial time-activity curves. The absolute polar maps on the right indicate diffuse moderate decreased of CBF at stress (top) in all three territories (MBF < 2) and is only mildly increased from rest (middle) yielding a diffusely decreased CFR (bottom). In this patient, while there was evidence of single vessel ischemia, there is also diffuse microvascular disease. This patient is pending intervention and PCI

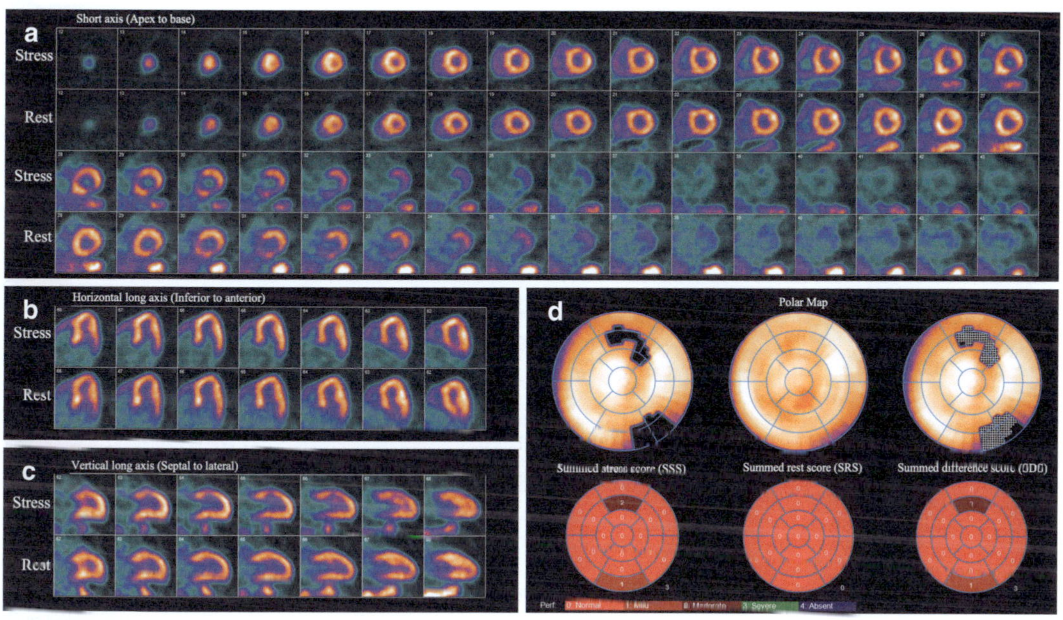

Fig. 7.9 PET perfusion images. The relative myocardial perfusion images show (**a–c**) show a small perfusion defect of mild intensity in the mid anterior wall and basal interolateral wall, both with complete reversibility at rest. (**d**) The summed rest score (SRS)

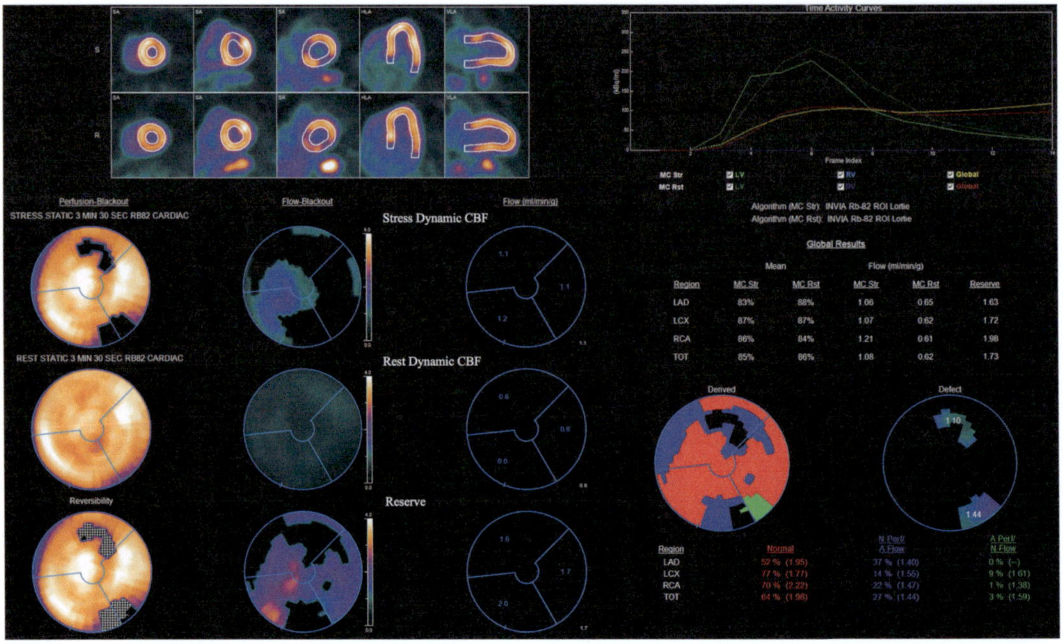

Fig. 7.10 Coronary flow assessment. The quality of the study is good as demonstrated by well-positioned LV ROIs and good blood pool and myocardial time-activity curves. The absolute polar maps on the right indicate diffuse severely decreased CBF at stress (top) in all three territories (MBF < 1.2) and decreased CFR in the territories of ischemia, the LAD and LCx (bottom). In this patient, while there was evidence of single vessel ischemia, there is also diffuse microvascular disease. This patient was managed conservatively with medical treatment optimization

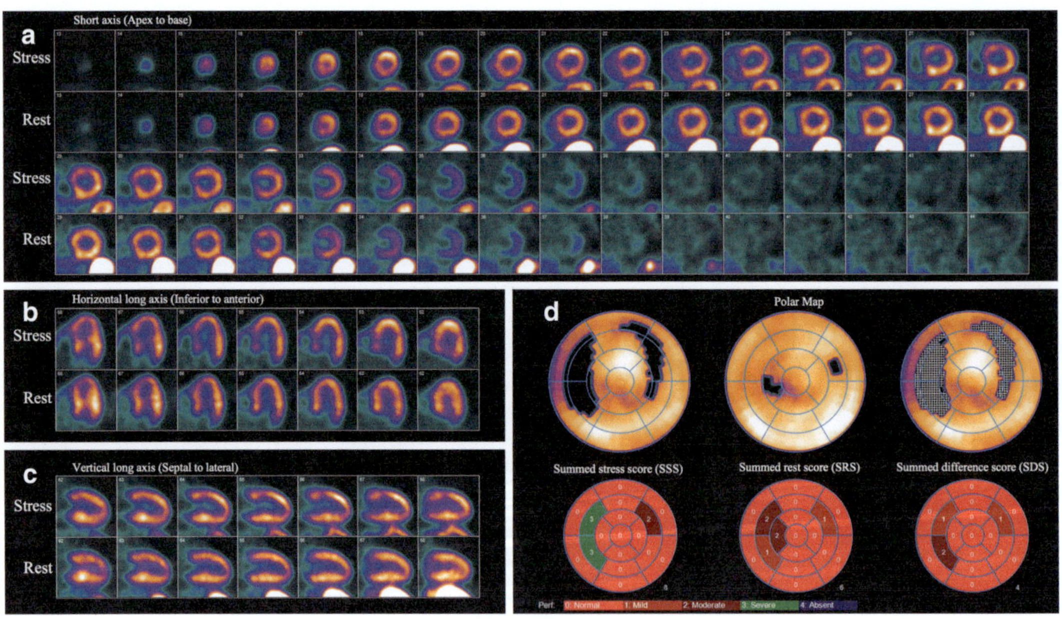

Fig. 7.11 PET perfusion images. The relative myocardial perfusion images show (**a**–**c**) a small perfusion defect of severe intensity in the mid septal wall and a small perfusion defect of mild intensity in the mid anterolateral wall with reversibility. (**d**) The summed rest score (SRS)

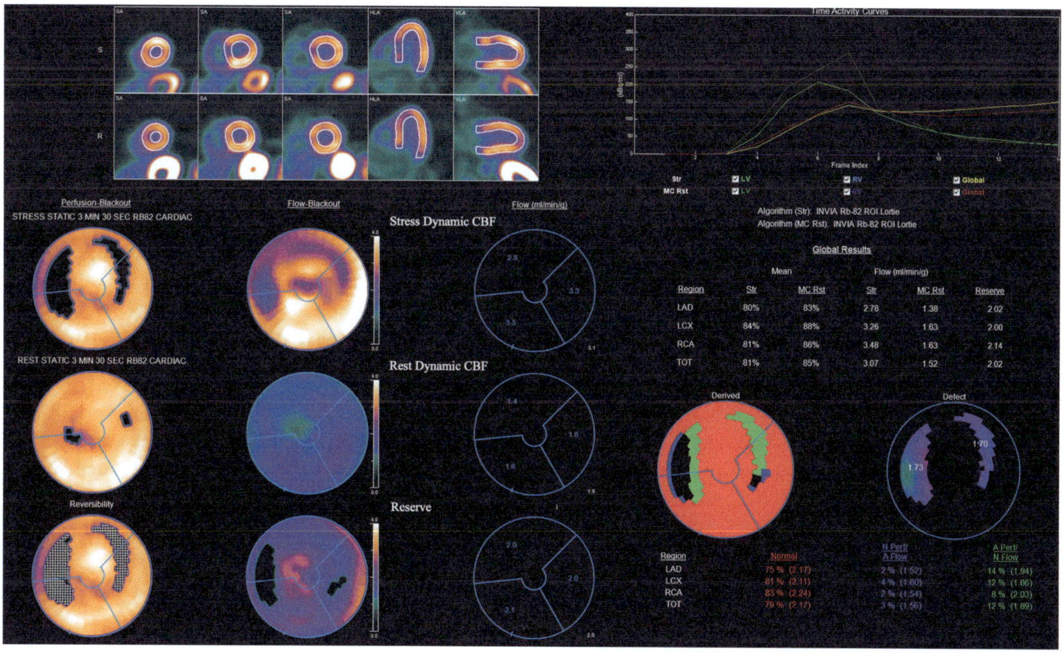

Fig. 7.12 Coronary flow assessment. The quality of the study is good, as demonstrated by well-positioned LV ROIs and good blood pool and myocardial time-activity curves. The absolute polar maps on the indicate normal CBF in all three vascular territories (top) and preserved CFR

underwent angiographic evaluation the next day that showed a patent LM, LAD with proximal to mid-vessel 40% stenosis, small diagonal D1 with 90% ostial stenosis, D2 and D3 small and patent; LCx, OM1 patent, RCA was dominant with 20% mid-vessel disease; PDA and PLV patent. In this case, in spite of absence of flow abnormality, the myocardial perfusion study shows moderate inferoseptal. So, in this patient, in spite of lack of flow abnormalities, the was evidence of ischemia in two territories (LAD and RCA) (Fig. 7.12).

Competing Interests The authors have no conflicts of interest to declare that are relevant to the content of this chapter.

References

1. Garcia EV, Slomka P, Moody JB, Germano G, Ficaro EP. Quantitative clinical nuclear cardiology, part 1: established applications. J Nucl Cardiol. 2020;27(1):189–201.
2. Tsao CW, et al. Heart disease and stroke statistics—2023 update: a report from the American Heart Association. Circulation. 2023;147(8):e93–621.
3. Di Carli MF. Nuclear cardiology and multimodal cardiovascular imaging: a companion to Braunwald's heart disease. 1st ed. Elsevier; 2021. p. 496.
4. Kiso K, Masuda A, Takanami K, Kaneta T, Takase K. Post-ISCHEMIA trial era: reconsideration of the role of nuclear cardiology in patients with chronic coronary artery disease. Ann Nucl Cardiol. 2022;8(1):86–90.
5. Ruddy TD, Kadoya Y, Tavoosi A, Small GR, Wells RG. Advances in single-photon emission computed tomography: hardware, software, and myocardial flow reserve. Cardiol Clin. 2023;41(2):117–27.
6. Di Carli MF. Why will PET be the future of nuclear cardiology? J Nucl Med. 2021;62(9):1189–91.
7. Shah SJ, Lam CSP, Svedlund S, Saraste A, Hage C, Tan RS, et al. Prevalence and correlates of coronary microvascular dysfunction in heart failure with preserved ejection fraction: PROMIS-HFpEF. Eur Heart J. 2018;39(37):3439–50.
8. Lindahl B, Baron T, Albertucci M, Prati F. Myocardial infarction with non-obstructive coronary artery disease. EuroIntervention. 2021;17(11):e875–e87.
9. Motwani M, Berman DS, Germano G, Slomka P. Automated quantitative nuclear cardiology methods. Cardiol Clin. 2016;34(1):47–57.
10. Taqueti VR, Di Carli MF. Coronary microvascular disease pathogenic mechanisms and therapeutic options: JACC state-of-the-art review. J Am Coll Cardiol. 2018;72(21):2625–41.

11. Li DL, Kronenberg MW. Myocardial perfusion and viability imaging in coronary artery disease: clinical value in diagnosis, prognosis, and therapeutic guidance. Am J Med. 2021;134(8):968–75.
12. Dendl K, Koerber SA, Kratochwil C, Cardinale J, Finck R, Dabir M, et al. FAP and FAPI-PET/CT in malignant and non-malignant diseases: a perfect symbiosis? Cancers (Basel). 2021;13(19):4946.
13. Klein R, Celiker-Guler E, Rotstein BH, deKemp RA. PET and SPECT tracers for myocardial perfusion imaging. Semin Nucl Med. 2020;50(3):208–18.
14. Maddahi J, Lazewatsky J, Udelson JE, Berman DS, Beanlands RSB, Heller GV, et al. Phase-III clinical trial of fluorine-18 flurpiridaz positron emission tomography for evaluation of coronary artery disease. J Am Coll Cardiol. 2020;76(4):391–401.
15. Maddahi J, Agostini D, Bateman TM, Bax JJ, Beanlands RSB, Berman DS, et al. Flurpiridaz F-18 PET myocardial perfusion imaging in patients with suspected coronary artery disease. J Am Coll Cardiol. 2023;82(16):1598–610.
16. Packard RR, Huang SC, Dahlbom M, Czernin J, Maddahi J. Absolute quantitation of myocardial blood flow in human subjects with or without myocardial ischemia using dynamic flurpiridaz F 18 PET. J Nucl Med. 2014;55(9):1438–44.
17. Wang J, Mpharm SL, Liu TW, Zhang JM, Chen Y, Li JM, et al. Preliminary and comparative experiment study between (18)F-flurpiridaz and (13) N-NH(3.)H(2)O myocardial perfusion imaging with PET/CT in miniature pigs. Mol Imaging. 2020;19:1536012120947506.
18. Patel KK, Singh A, Bateman TM. The potential of F-18 flurpiridaz PET/CT myocardial perfusion imaging for precision imaging. Curr Cardiol Rep. 2022;24(8):987–94.
19. Acampa W, He W, di Nuzzo C, Cuocolo A. Quantification of SPECT myocardial perfusion imaging. J Nucl Cardiol. 2002;9(3):338–42.
20. Dorbala S, Ananthasubramaniam K, Armstrong IS, Chareonthaitawee P, DePuey EG, Einstein AJ, et al. Single photon emission computed tomography (SPECT) myocardial perfusion imaging guidelines: instrumentation, acquisition, processing, and interpretation. J Nucl Cardiol. 2018;25(5):1784–846.
21. Berman DS, Hachamovitch R, Kiat H, Cohen I, Cabico JA, Wang FP, et al. Incremental value of prognostic testing in patients with known or suspected ischemic heart disease: a basis for optimal utilization of exercise technetium-99m sestamibi myocardial perfusion single-photon emission computed tomography. J Am Coll Cardiol. 1995;26(3):639–47.
22. Hsiao E, Ali B, Blankstein R, Skali H, Ali T, Bruyere J Jr, et al. Detection of obstructive coronary artery disease using regadenoson stress and 82Rb PET/CT myocardial perfusion imaging. J Nucl Med. 2013;54(10):1748–54.
23. Dorbala S, Vangala D, Sampson U, Limaye A, Kwong R, Di Carli MF. Value of vasodilator left ventricular ejection fraction reserve in evaluating the magnitude of myocardium at risk and the extent of angiographic coronary artery disease: a 82Rb PET/CT study. J Nucl Med. 2007;48(3):349–58.
24. Rischpler C, Higuchi T, Fukushima K, Javadi MS, Merrill J, Nekolla SG, et al. Transient ischemic dilation ratio in 82Rb PET myocardial perfusion imaging: normal values and significance as a diagnostic and prognostic marker. J Nucl Med. 2012;53(5):723–30.
25. Neves PO, Andrade J, Moncao H. Coronary artery calcium score: current status. Radiol Bras. 2017;50(3):182–9.
26. Slomka PJ, Moody JB, Miller RJH, Renaud JM, Ficaro EP, Garcia EV. Quantitative clinical nuclear cardiology, part 2: evolving/emerging applications. J Nucl Cardiol. 2021;28(1):115–27.
27. Murthy VL, Bateman TM, Beanlands RS, Berman DS, Borges-Neto S, Chareonthaitawee P, et al. Clinical quantification of myocardial blood flow using PET: joint position paper of the SNMMI cardiovascular council and the ASNC. J Nucl Med. 2018;59(2):273–93.
28. Huck DM, Weber BN, Brown JM, Lopez D, Hainer J, Blankstein R, et al. Prognostic value of myocardial flow reserve vs corrected myocardial flow reserve in patients without obstructive coronary artery disease. J Nucl Cardiol. 2024;37:101854.
29. Zavadovsky KV, Mochula AV, Maltseva AN, Shipulin VV, Sazonova SI, Gulya MO, et al. The current status of CZT SPECT myocardial blood flow and reserve assessment: tips and tricks. J Nucl Cardiol. 2022;29(6):3137–51.
30. Daou D, Sabbah R, Coaguila C, Boulahdour H. Feasibility of data-driven cardiac respiratory motion correction of myocardial perfusion CZT SPECT: a pilot study. J Nucl Cardiol. 2017;24(5):1598–607.

Myocardial Characterization with CT

8

Antonio Esposito, Chiara Gnasso, and Anna Palmisano

Abbreviations

AS	Aortic stenosis
CAD	Coronary artery disease
CMR	Cardiac magnetic resonance
CNR	Contrast-to-noise ratio
CT	Computed tomography
DE	Dual energy
EAM	Electroanatomic map
ECV	Extracellular volume
HCM	Hypertrophic cardiomyopathy
HF	Heart failure
Ht	Hematocrit
HU	Hounsfield unit
ICD	Implantable cardiac defibrillator
LCE	Late contrast enhancement
LGE	Late gadolinium enhancement
LIE	Late iodine enhancement
LVEF	Left ventricle ejection fraction
MINOCA	Myocardial infarction with nonobstructed coronary artery
MVO	Microvascular obstruction
PCD	Photon-counting detector
RFCA	Radiofrequency catheter ablation
ROI	Region of interest
SCD	Sudden cardiac death
SD	Standard deviation
SE	Single energy
TAVR	Transcatheter aortic valve replacement
VMI	Virtual monoenergetic imaging
VT	Ventricular tachycardia

A. Esposito (✉) · C. Gnasso · A. Palmisano
Experimental Imaging Center, IRCCS San Raffaele Scientific Institute, Milan, Italy

School of Medicine, Vita-Salute University, Milan, Italy
e-mail: esposito.antonio@hsr.it; gnasso.chiara@hsr.it; palmisano.anna@hsr.it

Introduction

Pathological Basis of Myocardial Fibrosis

Myocardial fibrosis, the expansion of the cardiac interstitium through the deposition of extracellular matrix proteins, is a common pathophysiologic phenomenon underlying many different myocardial pathological conditions. Three histological types of myocardial fibrosis have been described: replacement, interstitial, and perivascular fibrosis [1].

Replacement fibrosis is usually subsequent to cardiomyocyte necrosis: the loss of cardiomyocyte is replaced by collagen-based scar, with a higher accumulation of collagen type III compared to type I. This type of fibrosis usually leads to systolic dysfunction.

Interstitial and perivascular fibrosis can develop in many cardiomyopathies and in response to hemodynamic changes (such as in

R. Gill, P. Rajiah (eds.), *Quantitative Imaging in the Thorax*,
https://doi.org/10.1007/978-3-032-14103-3_8

severe valvular diseases). In this case, there is a prolonged fibroblastic stimulus leading to a deposition of collagen I fibers surrounding the cardiac muscle bundles (perimysium) or the individual cardiomyocytes (endomysium) or the perivascular space around intramural coronary arterioles [2]. The collagen accumulation shows a topographical variation, increasing from the outer to the inner third of the left ventricular free wall. These types of diffuse fibrosis usually lead to diastolic dysfunction.

Several cell types are implicated in the fibrotic response, either directly producing fibrotic tissue (myofibroblasts) or indirectly secreting profibrotic mediators (lymphocytes, mast cells, vascular cells, macrophages) [3]. Myofibroblasts produce pro-collagen types I and III and secrete other nonstructural extracellular matrix macromolecules, such as the matricellular proteins, that play a pivotal role in the regulation of fibrosis.

Myocardial Fibrosis Assessment: The Role of Imaging

The gold standard for assessing myocardial fibrosis is histology on endomyocardial biopsy; this procedure, however, is invasive and can lead to complications, and it can deliver a false-negative result due to under-sampling.

Cardiac magnetic resonance (CMR) is a noninvasive technique that can assess the presence of both focal and diffuse fibrosis, with good correlation with histology [4]. Focal fibrosis is identified through late gadolinium enhancement (LGE) sequences, whereas diffuse fibrosis can be identified with native and post-contrast T1 mapping and extracellular volume (ECV) calculation. The prognostic advantages of using LGE and ECV have been widely evaluated in a variety of pathological settings and were proven superior to other imaging modalities: CMR is, in fact, the current noninvasive reference standard for myocardial viability assessment [5, 6]. However, CMR is time-consuming, not widely available, may be affected by cardiac devices, and has limited application in patients suffering from claustrophobia. On the contrary, computed tomography (CT) is widely available and offers the advantage of a short acquisition time combined with high spatial resolution. CT imaging of replacement and interstitial fibrosis can be performed using late iodine enhancement (LIE) scan and ECV quantification, respectively.

Iodinated Contrast Media Pharmacokinetics

The rationale behind the possibility of noninvasively assessing myocardial viability is the pharmacokinetics of the contrast materials that both CMR and CT use, which are based on molecules that rapidly and passively diffuse from the vascular space into extracellular tissue but do not enter the intracellular space and that eventually return to the blood pool down the reverse concentration gradient. This "washout phase" occurs over seconds to minutes in healthy myocardium, but when there is an expansion of the extracellular matrix, the pharmacokinetics of these molecules are delayed due to changes in coronary flow rates, capillary permeability, functional capillary density, and the presence of a dense, hydrated collagen matrix [7]. The result is that, in delayed scans, there is a higher concentration of contrast agent in the scar and in areas of expanded extracellular matrix compared to normal myocardium. In CMR, the accumulation of gadolinium-based contrast agents results in a shorter T1 relaxation time, which can be assessed by T1 mapping and visually detected as a hyperintense signal in LGE. Similarly, in CT, in the delayed phase, iodinated contrast medium accumulation in focal scars and diffuse fibrosis areas can be detected as a hyperdense focal area of LIE with an increase in CT attenuation values (in Hounsfield units, HU) [8, 9].

Myocardial ECV_{CT} was first validated in humans by Nacif et al. in 2012 [8]: the authors compared ECV_{CMR} and ECV_{CT} in 24 subjects (both healthy volunteers and those with heart failure) and found a good correlation between the 2 ($r = 0.82$, $p < 0.001$). Bandula et al. validated ECV_{CT} against the gold standard invasive endomyocardial biopsy, as well as ECV_{CMR}

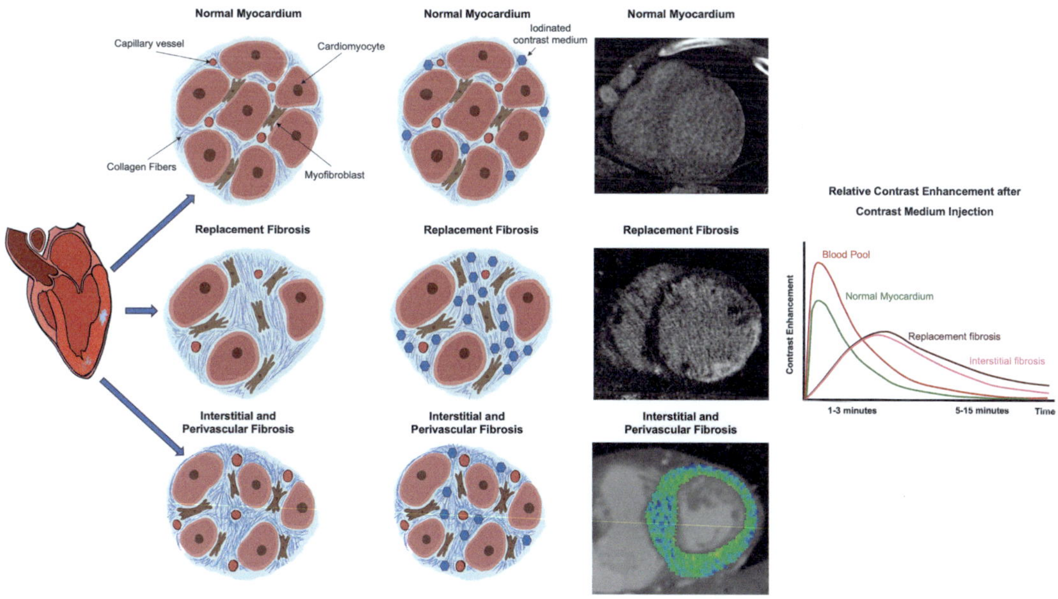

Fig. 8.1 Left: schematic illustration of different types of myocardial fibrosis and iodine distribution after contrast medium administration. Middle: delayed CT in normal myocardium, replacement fibrosis, and interstitial and perivascular fibrosis. Right: representation of relative contrast enhancement of normal and diseased myocardium and blood pool depending on time after the injection

in 23 patients with severe aortic stenosis, and found that ECV_{CT} showed a significant correlation with both histological measures of fibrosis ($r = 0.71, p < 0.001$) and ECV_{CMR} ($r = 0.73$) [10]. The strength of ECV_{CT} quantification relies on its high inter- and intraobserver reproducibility and the ability to visualize coronary anatomy during the same examination [11]. Figure 8.1 depicts a schematic illustration of different types of myocardial fibrosis with iodine accumulation at the equilibrium phased after contrast medium administration.

Focal Fibrosis in CT: Late Iodine Enhancement

Scanning Protocol and Image Reconstruction

LIE_{CT} is obtained from a delayed scan after the injection of contrast medium. Although there is no consensus about the best acquisition time, most studies suggest a delay time range of 3–10 min.

In a reperfused porcine model, Brodoefel et al. compared scans acquired at 3, 5, 10, and 15 min and found that the contrast between viable and scarred myocardium was the greatest at 3 and 5 min [12]. Similarly, Jacquier et al. reported better higher signal-to-noise ratio and better image quality in images obtained at 5 min than in those obtained at 10 min [13]. The lower contrast-to-noise ratio (CNR) of CT compared to CMR and the lack of ability to null the remote myocardium in CT images may hamper the identification of myocardial scars. Previous studies demonstrated a limited sensitivity, despite high specificity, for scar detection, especially at higher tube voltages [14]. Hence, imaging parameters should be optimized to enhance myocardial contrast. At this aim, a low kV scan increases CNR, as demonstrated in a pig model of myocardial infarction submitted to LIE_{CT} using 120, 100, and 80 kV, showing superior contrast and higher agreement with LGE_{CMR} for 80 kV scans [15].

With DE scanners, the image reconstruction has a pivotal role in delayed scans: the use of iodine maps and virtual monoenergetic reconstructions (VMI) can, in fact, facilitate scar detection by enhancing the higher iodine attenuation at virtual monoenergetic lower voltages, due to the proximity of iodine's kedge (33.2 keV). Palmisano et al. demonstrated good agreement in scar detection rates in a clinical setting for both the most and the least experienced readers using 80 kV LIE_{CT} in comparison to CMR, with low radiation exposure [16]. The use of low tube voltages, such as 70 or 80 kV, is effective for delayed scans and permits radiation dose reduction and augmented contrast enhancement [17]. Other studies evaluated the role of VMI reconstructions in the assessment of myocardial scars and demonstrated that 50 keV reconstructions can improve subjective and objective image quality for LIE_{CT} [18, 19]. These studies used dual-layer dual-energy (DE)-CT, allowing for the use of lower tube potential compared to tube-based DE systems, which are bound to a deterioration of spatial and temporal resolution for low-energy reconstructions, which prevents reconstructing images at voltages lower than 70 keV [20]. The recently introduced photon-counting detector (PCD) CT allows for a higher iodine CNR even at lower energy VMI (<60 keV) compared to classic energy-integrating detector CT and VMI at 40–50 keV seems to contribute to better visualization of LIE [21]; studies are needed to identify the best image reconstruction setting in this type of scanner to identify myocardial scars. There is no consensus on whether diastolic or systolic phase acquisition is more appropriate for LIE_{CT} imaging.

CM Injection Protocols

There is no absolute consensus on the contrast dose required for LIE_{CT} imaging; contrast doses used in clinical studies for LIE_{CT} varied from 300 to 700 mgI/kg [22]. Kurobe et al. reported high variability in image quality related to the amount of contrast media per body weight and recommended a dose of 600 mgI/kg (100 mL of 370 mgI/mL contrast agent for a 60 kg patient) for scar assessment on LIE_{CT} [23].

Image Analysis

The interpretation of LIE_{CT} is usually qualitative, based on scar distribution. It can be useful to reformat delayed images to obtain a two-chamber short-axis view and align the images with the angiographic scan, which yields a higher contrast resolution and better distinction of anatomical details. Moreover, it is appropriate to use a narrow window setting [17] and to increase slice thickness (5–10 mm) to emphasize the contrast and reduce noise [24]. Attention should be taken when interpreting the images, in particular to the left ventricular inferior wall, which is susceptible to streak artifacts originating from the diaphragm. Qualitative analysis is particularly useful for identifying the scar pattern and segmental involvement. The correct assessment of scar transmurality is crucial in the diagnostic process for the correct identification of underlying cardiac disease. Despite LIE_{CT}'s ability to depict scars regardless of the transmural involvement, small nonischemic scars could be affected by a limited CNR, resulting in more challenging identification [16]. As regards the quantitative analysis of LIE_{CT}, it has recently become feasible since the introduction of dedicated commercially available software that enables myocardial wall delineation and automatic segmentation of those areas with a higher CT number, superior to a user-defined threshold (e.g., +3 or +5 standard deviation (SD) above the mean for CT number of remote myocardium) [17] resulting able to provide quantitative information about scar mass and percentage.

Diffuse Fibrosis in CT: Extracellular Volume

Scanning Protocol

Currently, no final consensus exists regarding the ideal time point to acquire the delayed scan after contrast injection for ECV quantification: several studies report different time points, usually ranging from 5 to 15 min [25]. Triebel et al. in 2015 compared 5- and 15-min time points post-contrast bolus for equilibrium cardiac CT in 53 patients (26 with systemic amyloidosis and 27 with aortic stenosis) and demonstrated that ECV_{CT} at 5-min post-contrast showed a stronger correlation with ECV_{CMR} than at 15-min post-contrast ($r^2 = 0.85$ compared to 0.74) [26]. Hamdy et al., moreover, evaluated different time points to determine the optimal delay time and found that ECV values were constant at 3, 5, and 7 min, even though there was a trend of lower values at 3 min [27].

Two different scanning protocols should be used to calculate ECV_{CT} based on different scanner systems: the attenuation-based method when using a single-energy (SE) scanner and the spectral method when using a DE or a PCD scanners.

For the attenuation-based protocol, first, a non-enhanced scan is acquired, followed by a delayed acquisition with the same acquisition and reconstruction parameters. ECV_{CT} is then calculated based on the differential attenuation of the myocardium before and after the contrast injection.

When using DE or PCD scanners, ECV_{CT} can be calculated from the iodine map images directly derived from the late enhancement scan; hence, the unenhanced scan is not necessary, and the dose exposure can be reduced.

CM Injection Protocols

There is also no a final consensus regarding the amount of contrast material that should be injected to obtain an adequate ECV_{CT} evaluation. Different injection protocols have been proposed, using a fixed bolus of contrast material, an additional bolus after the angiographic scan, or a body weight-based contrast volume [28]. Takafuji et al. demonstrated no significant differences in ECV_{CT} quantification when using a low-dose injection protocol (346 ± 43 mgI/kg) compared to a higher-dose protocol (571 ± 81 mg/kg) [29]. Therefore, contrast dosing optimized for angio CT scan is considered sufficient for ECV quantification however, ECV quantification and LIE assessment are often combined to adequately answer the clinical question, so the recommended dosage for LIE, around 600 mgI/kg, is used.

Image Analysis

ECV_{CT} quantification differs based on the acquisition protocol. It could be calculated based on the subtraction approach or iodine-specific images. In the subtraction method, ECV_{CT} is calculated based on the differential attenuation of the myocardium and the blood pool before and after the injection of contrast material, corrected by the patient's hematocrit (Ht).

When using a subtraction approach, pre- and post-contrast scans are co-registered, and measurements of HU are obtained by drawing regions of interest (ROIs) in the left ventricular cavity and in the myocardial wall. ECV_{CT} is then calculated based on the formula (Fig. 8.2):

$$ECV_{CT} = (1 - Ht) \times \frac{\Delta HU_{myocardium}}{\Delta HU_{bloodpool}}$$

When using the spectral method, all the quantitative data are automatically extracted from the delayed scan: DE and PCD scanners allow a spectral separation with direct quantification of iodine content. In this case, the ECV_{CT} is obtained from iodine map according to the following formula (Fig. 8.2):

$$ECV_{CT} = (1 - Ht) \times \frac{Iodine_{myocardium}}{Iodine_{bloodpool}}$$

In the case of the spectral method, there is no risk of misalignment between the pre- and post-contrast scan; moreover, this technique is less operator-dependent, which can hamper the ECV_{CT} quantification in the attenuation-based method, where a ROI has to be placed in an unenhanced scan, with poor distinction between myocardium and blood pool, and in a delayed scan, that can be affected by beam-hardening artifacts and image noise [30].

Either with the attenuation-based or the spectral method, the current approach for estimating myocardial ECV requires knowledge of the patient's serum hematocrit, which is not always

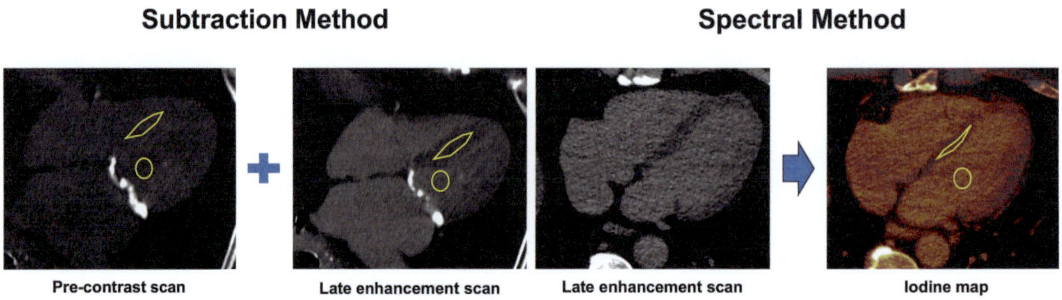

$$ECV_{CT} = (1 - Ht) \times \frac{\Delta HU_{myocardium}}{\Delta HU_{bloodpool}}$$

$$ECV_{CT} = (1 - Ht) \times \frac{Iodine_{myocardium}}{Iodine_{bloodpool}}$$

Fig. 8.2 Schematic illustration of different methods to calculate the ECV. Left: attenuation-based method, based on the acquisition of pre- and post-contrast scan. ROIs are manually drawn in the left ventricular wall and blood pool. Right: Spectral method, suitable for DE scanners or PCD-CT. From the delayed scan, the iodine map is reconstructed, and ROIs are drawn in the left ventricular wall and blood pool to measure iodine concentration. Abbreviations: ECV, extracellular volume; ROI, region of interest; Ht, hematocrit; ΔHUmyo, change in attenuation of the myocardium; ΔHUblood, change in attenuation of the blood pool; (Iodinemyocardium), iodine concentration within the myocardium; (iodine bloodpool), iodine concentration within the blood pool

available. Some authors have proposed the possibility of calculating a synthetic Ht based on the linear association between Ht and blood attenuation on unenhanced or virtual unenhanced scans [31]. However, this linear association and the consequent formula differ based on different scanners and acquisition protocols; hence, a local validation for each center and scanner would be preferable.

Radiation Dose

Radiation dose reduction in LCE_{CT} in the SE approach can be achieved by using prospective electrocardiography-triggered scans without padding (e.g., a fixed 280 ms delay from R-wave can be used). Moreover, low tube potential scans should be used, along with iterative reconstruction algorithms. Delayed scans can be performed at 1–2 mSv [8, 10]. When using a DE system, the same precautions regarding scan triggering should be taken, but it is also possible to reduce the total radiation dose of the examination by eliminating the pre-contrast scan. The ECV can, in fact, be calculated from iodine maps, and there is the possibility of producing virtual non-contrast reconstruction if needed for coronary artery or valvular calcium scoring. Recent studies using PCD-CT for ECV_{CT} quantification report that delayed scans are obtained at 1.2 mSv [32, 33]. Moreover, Aquino et al. reported that the radiation dose for the ECV_{CT} calculation with the spectral method was 40% lower than the attenuation-based method using a PCD-CT (10.1 mGy vs. 16.8 mGy) [33].

LCE_{CT} in the Acute Chest Pain

The management of patients referring to the emergency department (ED) for acute chest pain in the setting of nonspecific signs and symptoms, along with non-characteristic ECG and laboratory test results, is still debated. ROMICAT I and II trials demonstrated that up to 50% of patients with acute chest pain and low-to-intermediate likelihood of acute coronary syndrome have nonobstructive coronary artery disease (CAD), and incorporating CT into a triage strategy can improve the efficacy of clinical decision-making in the emergency department [34, 35]. However, many patients referring to the ED for acute chest pain either do not have a cardiac cause of pain or have a cardiac cause that is not related to coronary arteries, such as myocarditis, myocardial infarction with nonobstructive coronary arteries, or cardiomyopathies. In these patients, CMR sig-

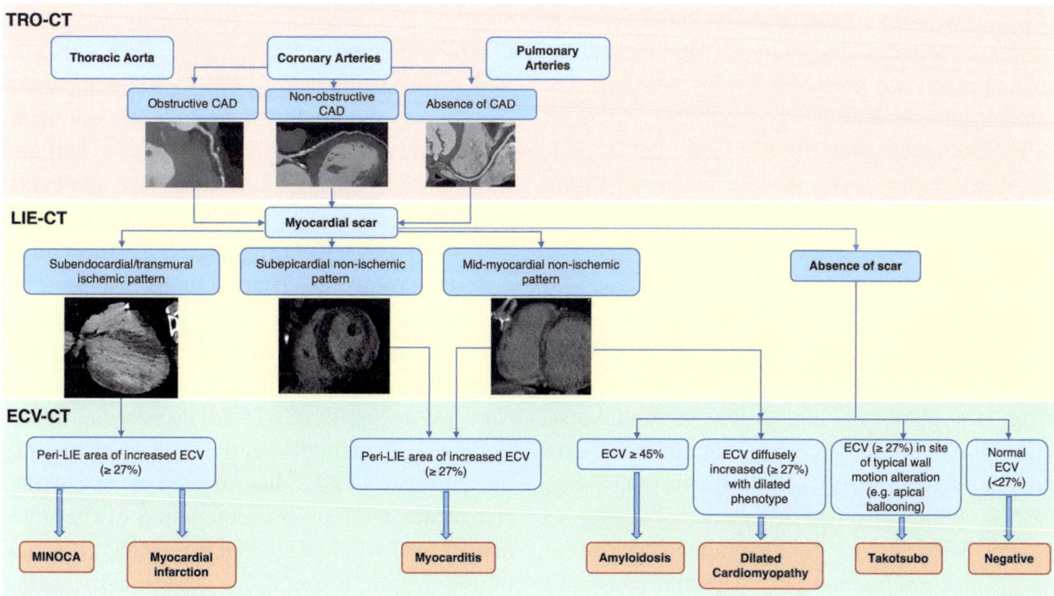

Fig. 8.3 CT-based diagnostic flowchart in patients referring to the emergency room with troponin-positive acute chest pain syndrome, modified from [37]. Triple-rule-out (TRO) CT can be implemented with delayed scans to assess late iodine enhancement (LIE) and extracellular volume (ECV). Based on the presence and pattern of scar, along with ECV alteration, the diagnostic performance of CT significantly increases

nificantly improves the diagnostic rate; however, it has limited availability, especially in the emergency setting, requires long acquisition times and can be affected by cardiac devices. Palmisano et al. proposed a new "multiparametric" CT protocol for patients with acute chest pain and negative findings at triple-rule-out CT, including a 10-min delayed scan to obtain a complete CT-based myocardial characterization. They found that the proposed protocol helped identify the cause of symptoms in 81% of participants, increasing the diagnostic rate of CT from 50% to 90% in the case of angiographic CT implemented with LCE_{CT} [36, 37]. LIE was capable of detecting myocardial scars with ischemic or nonischemic patterns (especially myocarditis), and ECV guided the diagnosis in patients with negative LIE, suggesting the presence of amyloidosis, dilated, or Takotsubo cardiomyopathies. However, the proposed approach was confined to patients with nonobstructive coronary arteries. In a subsequent study, Vignale et al. applied the same multiparametric protocol in patients with obstructive CAD, suggesting a combined evaluation of angiographic CT, wall motion, thickness alteration, and scar on LIE_{CT} [37]. This approach was able to distinguish unstable angina from recent and previous infarction, therefore providing early information useful for patient risk stratification and therapeutic management. Based on this evidences, a multiparametric CT protocol, including the assessment of CAD, function, myocardial remodeling, scar, and ECV_{CT}, could be a valid diagnostic tool in the emergency setting, for patients with acute chest pain and increased troponin levels at low to intermediate risk [38]. Figure 8.3 illustrates the multiparametric CT-based diagnostic flowchart for patients referring to the emergency department for troponin-positive acute chest pain syndrome.

LCE_{CT} in the Dilated Heart

Heart Failure

Heart failure (HF) can be classified into ischemic and nonischemic subtypes based on the underlying cause of dysfunction. The former is characterized by the development of a reparative, focal scar in response to the massive cardiomyocyte necrosis, whereas the latter is supposed to be related to several mechanisms, including microcirculation disorders, leading to the development of reactive, interstitial fibrosis. Scar and interstitial fibrosis play a pivotal role in the structural myocardial remodeling that determines the evolution to diastolic dysfunction and HF [3]. The extent of interstitial fibrosis is, in fact, associated with the prognosis and effectiveness of long-term therapies for heart failure. LIE_{CT} can be added to routine CTA performed to rule out ischemic etiology for distinguishing various cardiomyopathies based on scar pattern identification with good agreement with CMR [39] and to estimate ECV_{CT}, which resulted significantly higher in patients with HF [40, 41] also in the case of preserved ejection fraction [40]. An important cause of nonischemic HF is chemotherapy-induced cardiotoxicity [42]. Tu et al. demonstrated, on a total of 1151 patients with breast cancer treated with anthracyclines, that ECV_{CT} during and after treatment was significantly higher than the baseline and, more importantly, that ECV_{CT} changed significantly earlier than left-ventricle ejection fraction (LVEF) or global longitudinal strain, currently used for early detection of cardiotoxicity: ECV_{CT} changed significantly 3 months after beginning treatment, whereas LVEF did not change until after 6 months [43]. Hence, ECV_{CT} could be used for longitudinal evaluation of cardiotoxicity during chemotherapy treatments.

Ischemic Cardiomyopathy

In patients with suspected or known ischemic cardiomyopathy, a multiparametric CT protocol including LIE_{CT} can be useful for the characterization of different stages of the disease, ranging from the identification of inducible ischemia, of culprit lesion, the severity, and extent of infarction and for prognostication. Indeed, similar to CMR, in patients with CAD candidates to stress CT perfusion, LIE_{CT} must be acquired to discriminate scarred myocardium from inducible perfusion defect [44]. As for LGE_{CMR}, LIE_{CT} is able to identify ischemic scar based on its typical subendocardial or transmural distribution also in a semiquantitative fashion [45], with excellent agreement compared to LGE_{CMR}, showing a sensitivity and specificity of around 98% and 94%, respectively [22]. Larger segmental extent and transmural involvement of LIE_{CT} are associated with worse recovery of LV function at 6-month follow-up and with a higher risk of subsequent hospitalization for heart failure [46–48]. In patients presenting with chest pain, troponin rise, and suspected CAD, LIECT can be combined with routine CT in order to simultaneously rule out obstructive CAD and myocardial infarction [37]. In patients with multivessel disease, the presence of LIE downstream of an obstructive lesion with absent remodeling of the myocardial wall would be useful for the identification of the culprit lesion [37]. Additionally, LIE_{CT} provides excellent contrast resolution for the identification of endoventricular thrombus, and the combined evaluation of CTA showing remodeling of scarred walls suggests previous myocardial infarction [49]. In the case of infarction with a nonobstructed coronary artery (MINOCA), a hypodense rim could be visible on the endocardial border of the scar, indicating the presence of microvascular obstruction (MVO) [37]. MVO is also recognizable in post-PCI patients and has been found to be a known predictor of major adverse cardiac events (MACEs), defined as a composite of cardiac death, congestive heart failure, and myocardial reinfarction (adjusted hazard ratio: 3.74; 95% confidence interval: 2.21–6.34) [50]. Figure 8.4 shows the spectrum of possible findings in postischemic cardiomyopathy on LIE_{CT} images.

Nonischemic Cardiomyopathy

Dilated cardiomyopathy (DCM) is characterized by ventricular dilation and systolic dysfunction, and it represents one of the most common causes of nonischemic heart failure. Many patients present minor structural cardiac abnormalities and express different arrhythmogenic phenotypes before overt heart failure symptoms [51]. In this setting, myocardial characterization plays an

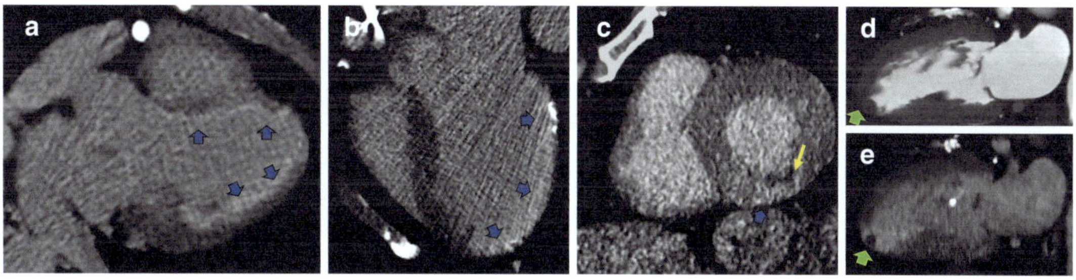

Fig. 8.4 Spectrum of possible findings in ischemic cardiomyopathy on LIE_{CT} images. In (**a**), a large subendocardial scar (blue arrows); in (**b**), a transmural postischemic scar involving the lateral wall from the base to the apex (blue arrows); in (**c**), a focal transmural scar in the inferior mid-ventricular wall with an hypodense subendocardial rim indicating microvascular obstruction (MVO yellow arrow); in (**d**) and (**e**), an apical transmural infarction with a small apical thrombus better visible in the delayed (green arrow in **e**) than in the angiographic scan (green arrow in **d**)

important role in identifying initial structural changes that can allow an early treatment. A recent study investigating the role of ECV_{CT} in predicting MACEs in 70 patients with DCM at long-term follow-up (51 ± 47 months) demonstrated that ECV was the sole independent predictor of MACEs based on a multivariate Cox proportional hazard model including echocardiographic functional assessment [52]. The authors proposed a cutoff of 32.26% based on receiver operating characteristic (ROC) analysis and demonstrated with Kaplan-Meier analysis that patients with a higher ECV_{CT} had significantly higher incidence of MACEs compared to patients with lower values [52].

LCE and ECV in the Hypertrophic Phenotype

In the spectrum of patients presenting with hypertrophic phenotype, the adoption of a CT-based diagnostic workflow, similar to the one commonly used on CMR, including also LIE_{CT} and ECV_{CT}, allows the discrimination of several conditions, including hypertrophic cardiomyopathy (HCM) and amyloidosis, characterized by typical alterations, as well as the assessment of the interstitial myocardial fibrosis that may complicate conditions of pressure overload (e.g., aortic valve stenosis), providing helpful prognostic information.

Hypertrophic Cardiomyopathy

HCM is the most frequent genetic cardiac disease, characterized by a variable clinical course and an increased risk for sudden cardiac death (SCD). Myocardial scar in HCM is typically located in the wall segment with higher thickness, and the percentage of mass involved by a scar at LGE_{CMR} has prognostic implications, being associated with higher arrhythmia. Zhao et al. documented the possibility of characterizing myocardial hypertrophy and scarring with CT in a reliable way, comparing LIE_{CT} and LGE_{CMR} findings in a large cohort of 80 patients with HCM [53]. In particular, LIE_{CT} provided a reliable quantification of scar and of left ventricle wall thickness and had a good correlation with CMR, with a tendency to slightly underestimate the scar burden. These findings were confirmed by Langer et al., who analyzed LCE scans in 30 HCM patients to assess the presence of areas of LIE_{CT} and measured the LIE_{CT} mass through a semiautomatic segmentation, using a threshold of 2SD: they demonstrated a good correlation between LIE mass and LGE mass (7.9 g vs 8.6 g, $r = 0.95$), and a good inter- and intraobserver reliability at qualitative assessment of LIE (0.97 and 0.99) [54]. LIE_{CT} was also found effective in the estimation of scar burden in patients with implantable cardioverter-defibrillator (ICD) and has prognostic implications associated with the recurrence of complex ventricular arrhythmias [55].

Amyloidosis

Systemic amyloidosis is caused by the deposition of misfolded fibrillar protein, which leads to extracellular space expansion and impairment of function. There are two main forms of cardiac amyloidosis, the light chain (AL) and transthyretin (ATTR) amyloidosis, which can be distinguished by the LGE pattern: a global subendocardial scar is more characteristic of an AL amyloidosis, whereas a transmural LGE with a base-to-apex gradient is more common in ATTR amyloidosis [56]. Moreover, especially in cases with absent or nontypical LGE patterns, a marked increase in ECV is pathognomonic for amyloidosis and largely validated. Similarly, LIE_{CT} and ECV_{CT} can provide reliable identification of amyloidosis [57]. Indeed, many authors investigated the role of LCE_{CT} in this clinical setting: Tavoosi et al. demonstrated good reliability by interclass correlation coefficient between ECV_{CT} and ECV_{CMR} in patients with cardiac amyloidosis, both on SE and DE scanners (0.88 and 0.93, respectively) [58]. Gama et al. further evaluated the role of ECV_{CT} on 72 patients with cardiac amyloidosis and enlightened that mean ECV_{CT} values were significantly higher in ATTR forms compared to AL amyloidosis (55.8% ± 10.9% vs 42.7% ± 13.1%, $p < 0.001$). Moreover, over a mean follow-up time of 5.3 ± 2.4 years, the authors demonstrated that global ECV_{CT} had a prognostic role in AL amyloidosis, whereas in ATTR amyloidosis septal ECV_{CT} had a stronger association with all-cause mortality (HR: 1.046, 95% CI 1.003–1.090, $p = 0.037$) [59]. Figure 8.5 illustrates the case of a 78-year-old man with amyloidosis who underwent both CMR and cardiac CT with LCE.

Aortic Stenosis

Aortic valve stenosis (AS) is the most common primary valve disease in developed countries [60]. Chronic pressure overload resulting from progressive valve obstruction induces hypertrophic remodeling in the left ventricle wall, as adaptation contributing to maintain a sufficient cardiac output. The cardiac hypertrophy triggered by pressure

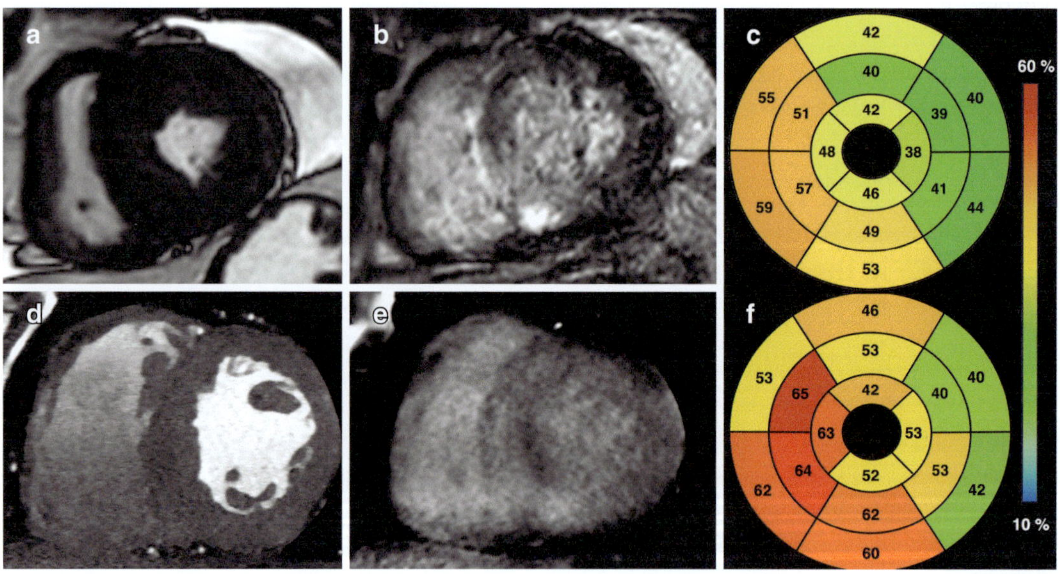

Fig. 8.5 A 78-year-old man diagnosed with ATTR amyloidosis. CMR shows left ventricular hypertrophy (**a**), a transmural area of late gadolinium enhancement involving the whole septum (**b**), along with markedly increased ECV values, especially of the interventricular septum (ECV values between 46% and 59%) (**c**). Cardiac-CT shows the same findings, with left ventricular hypertrophy (**d**), a transmural area of late iodine enhancement involving the whole septum (**e**), and a strong increase in ECV_{CT}, in particular of the interventricular septum, with a segmental distrubution similar to CMR (**f**)

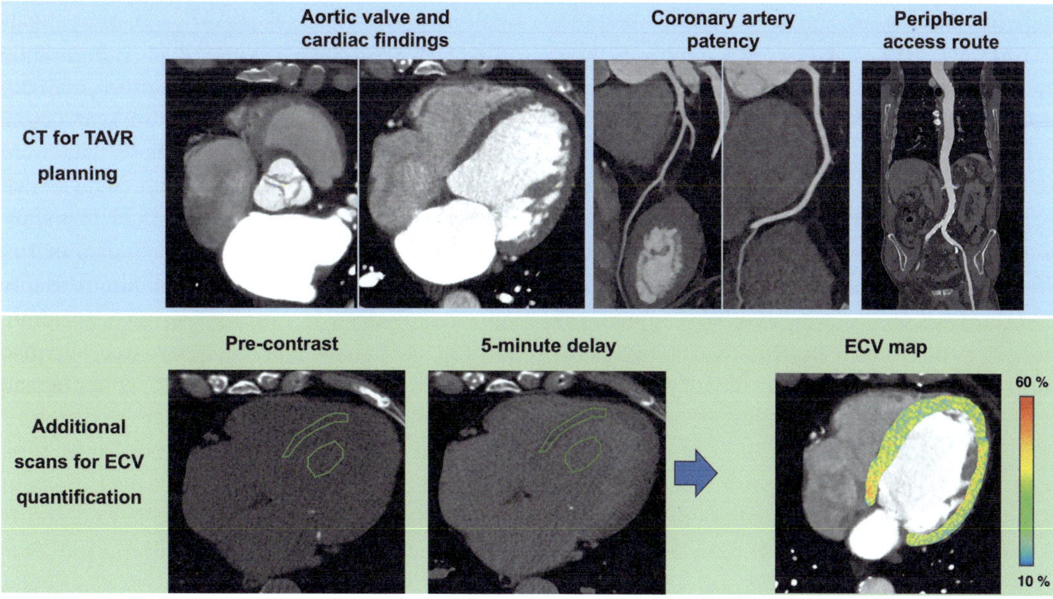

Fig. 8.6 A 84-year-old man diagnosed with severe aortic stenosis with low-flow low-gradient phenotype, candidate to TAVR. The normal CT protocol for TAVR planning was implemented with a delayed scan for ECV quantification. ECV_{CT} was diffusely increased, with global values of 34%. After the procedure, the patient was rehospitalized for heart failure and died 5 months after the treatment for cardiac problems

overload involves both adaptive and maladaptive processes [61], the latter leading to myocyte apoptosis and diffuse interstitial myocardial fibrosis. Azevedo et al. demonstrated that the amount of myocardial fibrosis, by histopathology or LGE, is associated with the degree of left ventricular functional improvement and all-cause mortality after aortic valve replacement in patients with severe AS [62]. Therefore, the estimation of the amount of interstitial fibrosis and myocardial scar in patients with aortic stenosis may improve risk stratification and patient management. Vignale et al. demonstrated, on 159 patients undergoing CT for transcatheter aortic valve replacement (TAVR) planning, that $ECV_{CT} > 31.3\%$ predicts patient mortality and hospitalization for heart failure after TAVR, using a 5-min delayed scan and no additional contrast media injection [53, 63]. Moreover, increased ECV_{CT} was found to be associated with adverse clinical outcomes post-TAVR, also in patients with low-flow, low-gradient AS, which comprise high risk patients [64].

Figure 8.6 shows the case of a patient with severe AS undergoing TAVI who had a high ECV_{CT} burden as assessed at the CT prior to the procedure. Additionally, recent studies have shown a remarkably high prevalence (14%–16%) of ATTR-amyloidosis in the elderly population being considered for TAVR, with a subsequent higher rate of treatment failure. In this setting, ECV_{CT} estimated during routine CT for TAVR planning was found able to detect amyloidosis and to estimate the degree of infiltration with good accuracy compared to bone scintigraphy [59, 64, 65].

LCE in Electrophysiology

Ventricular tachycardia (VT) is a life-threatening condition that can lead to SCD, and radiofrequency catheter ablation (RFCA) is the only potentially curative strategy [47]. Myocardial scar is frequently the substrate for VT, and the identification of scar presence, transmural pattern, and segmental distribution is necessary not only for clarifying the underlying etiology of VT but mostly for guiding RF ablation, suggesting the preferable electroanatomic mapping (EAM) and RFCA approaches (endocardial vs epicardial), and to shorten procedural time and improve procedure success [66]. Despite CMR being the imaging modality of choice for scar characterization, most patients with VT have an ICD that significantly worsens image quality. CT is less affected by ICD artifacts, with less than 2% of myocardial mass nonassessable for shock coils artifacts on posterior mid-basal septum [67, 68]. In patients with ischemic cardiomyopathy, initially, it was proposed to identify areas with wall thickness <5 mm to distinguish scarred from healthy myocardium [49]. However, this approach failed to distinguish subendocardial scars at CMR as well as nonischemic mesocardial scars [69, 70]. LCE_{CT} has been demonstrated to be able to identify myocardial scar substrate for VT independently by the etiology and the transmural involvement with good agreement with scar potetials at EAM and with areas of RFCA, significantly higher than wall thinning [68]. Figure 8.7 shows the comparison between LIE_{CT} images and EAM results for scar detection in two different patients. These data were recently confirmed by Conte et al., showing an agreement between LCE_{CT} and EAM of 94.1% [71]. Moreover, the volumetric CT dataset has the advantage of potentially combining the scar information derived from LCE_{CT} with anatomic information about the coronary tree, cardiac chambers, and epicardial fat and obtaining an integrated 3D model for real-time guidance of EAM and RFCA [68]. The high spatial resolution of the LCE_{CT} dataset further allows the extraction of radiomic parameters that are able to describe fibrosis heterogeneity related to different patterns of myocardial remodeling and risk of ventricular tachycardia recurrence [67]. LCE_{CT} can play a role in the planning of the recently introduced

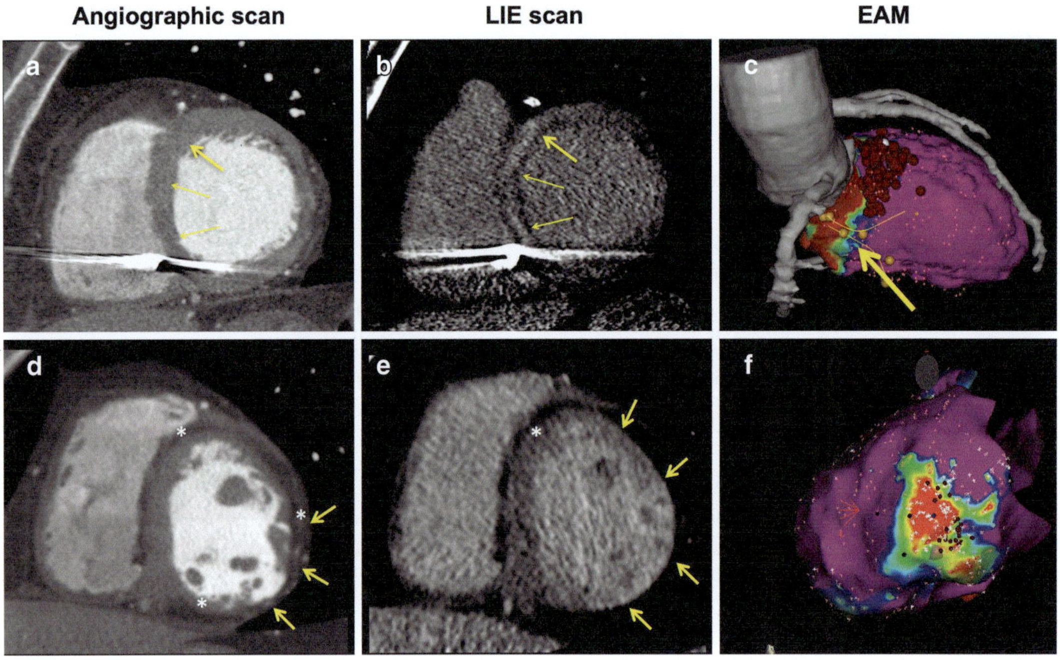

Fig. 8.7 Two exemplifying cases of patients with ventricular tachycardia submitted to CT before EAM and RFCA. At the top is a case of a patient with preserved wall thickness on angiographic scan (**a**) and evidence of a septal mid-wall late enhancement on LIE_{CT} image (**b**). EAM confirmed low voltages in the same area (red areas on **c** indicated by yellow arrow) suggestive for scar; hence, RFCA was performed on the border zone of that region (red dots in **c**). On the bottom, diffuse septal and lateral subepicardial fatty infiltration (white asterisks in **d** and **e**), with wall thinning of lateral wall on CCTA (yellow arrows in **d**) which was characterized by transmural LIE on delayed CT scan (yellow arrows in **e**). These CT findings were suggestive for desmoplakin cardiomyopathy. EAM confirmed altered voltages on lateral mid-basal wall (red area in **f**) and RFCA was performed (red dots in **f**)

stereotactic radio-ablation, which is a potential alternative treatment for high-risk patients [72]. Recently, a hybrid LCE_{CT} FDG-PET approach has been tested in patients with post-myocarditis VT and ICD in order to merge scar information from LCE_{CT} and metabolic information from FDG-PET, suggesting the potentiality of this approach in the identification of active myocarditis from healed myocarditis [73].

References

1. Frangogiannis NG. Cardiac fibrosis. Cardiovasc Res. 2021;117:1450–88.
2. López B, Ravassa S, Moreno MU, José GS, Beaumont J, González A, Díez J. Diffuse myocardial fibrosis: mechanisms, diagnosis and therapeutic approaches. Nat Rev Cardiol. 2021;18:479–98.
3. González A, Schelbert EB, Díez J, Butler J. Myocardial interstitial fibrosis in heart failure: biological and translational perspectives. J Am Coll Cardiol. 2018;71:1696–706.
4. Sibley CT, Noureldin RA, Gai N, et al. T1 mapping in cardiomyopathy at cardiac MR: comparison with endomyocardial biopsy. Radiology. 2012;265:724–32.
5. Haaf P, Garg P, Messroghli DR, Broadbent DA, Greenwood JP, Plein S. Cardiac T1 mapping and extracellular volume (ECV) in clinical practice: a comprehensive review. J Cardiovasc Magn Reson. 2017;18:89.
6. Garcia MJ, Kwong RY, Scherrer-Crosbie M, Taub CC, Blankstein R, Lima J, Bonow RO, Eshtehardi P, Bois JP. State of the art: imaging for myocardial viability: a scientific statement from the American Heart Association. Circ Cardiovasc Imaging. 2020;13:e000053. https://doi.org/10.1161/HCI.0000000000000053.
7. Kim RJ, Albert TSE, Wible JH, Elliott MD, Allen JC, Lee JC, Parker M, Napoli A, Judd RM. Performance of delayed-enhancement magnetic resonance imaging with gadoversetamide contrast for the detection and assessment of myocardial infarction. Circulation. 2008;117:629–37.
8. Nacif MS, Kawel N, Lee JJ, Chen X, Yao J, Zavodni A, Sibley CT, Lima JAC, Liu S, Bluemke DA. Interstitial myocardial fibrosis assessed as extracellular volume fraction with low-radiation-dose cardiac CT. Radiology. 2012;264:876–83.
9. Lardo AC, Cordeiro MAS, Silva C, et al. Contrast-enhanced multidetector computed tomography viability imaging after myocardial infarction. Circulation. 2006;113:394–404.
10. Bandula S, White SK, Flett AS, Lawrence D, Pugliese F, Ashworth MT, Punwani S, Taylor SA, Moon JC. Measurement of myocardial extracellular volume fraction by using equilibrium contrast-enhanced CT: validation against histologic findings. Radiology. 2013;269:396–403.
11. Kurita Y, Kitagawa K, Kurobe Y, Nakamori S, Nakajima H, Dohi K, Ito M, Sakuma H. Estimation of myocardial extracellular volume fraction with cardiac CT in subjects without clinical coronary artery disease: a feasibility study. J Cardiovasc Comput Tomogr. 2016;10:237–41.
12. Brodoefel H, Reimann A, Klumpp B, Fenchel M, Ohmer M, Miller S, Schroeder S, Claussen C, Scheule A, Kopp AF. Assessment of myocardial viability in a Reperfused porcine model. J Comput Assist Tomogr. 2007;31:290–8.
13. Jacquier A, Boussel L, Amabile N, Bartoli JM, Douek P, Moulin G, Paganelli F, Saeed M, Revel D, Croisille P. Multidetector computed tomography in reperfused acute myocardial infarction. Investig Radiol. 2008;43:773–81.
14. Wichmann JL, Bauer RW, Doss M, Stock W, Lehnert T, Bodelle B, Frellesen C, Vogl TJ, Kerl JM. Diagnostic accuracy of late iodine–enhancement dual-energy computed tomography for the detection of chronic myocardial infarction compared with late gadolinium–enhancement 3-T magnetic resonance imaging. Investig Radiol. 2013;48:851–6.
15. Mahnken AH, Bruners P, Mühlenbruch G, Emmerich M, Hohl C, Günther RW, Wildberger JE. Low tube voltage improves computed tomography imaging of delayed myocardial contrast enhancement in an experimental acute myocardial infarction model. Investig Radiol. 2007;42:123–9.
16. Palmisano A, Vignale D, Benedetti G, Del Maschio A, De Cobelli F, Esposito A. Late iodine enhancement cardiac computed tomography for detection of myocardial scars: impact of experience in the clinical practice. Radiol Med. 2020;125:128–36.
17. Oyama-Manabe N, Oda S, Ohta Y, Takagi H, Kitagawa K, Jinzaki M. Myocardial late enhancement and extracellular volume with single-energy, dual-energy, and photon-counting computed tomography. J Cardiovasc Comput Tomogr. 2024;18:3–10. https://doi.org/10.1016/j.jcct.2023.12.006.
18. Liu P, Lin L, Xu C, Han Y, Lin X, Hou Y, Lu X, Vembar M, Jin Z, Wang Y. Quantitative analysis of late iodine enhancement using dual-layer spectral detector computed tomography: comparison with magnetic resonance imaging. Quant Imaging Med Surg. 2022;12:310–20
19. Oda S, Emoto T, Nakaura T, et al. Myocardial late iodine enhancement and extracellular volume quantification with dual-layer spectral detector dual-energy cardiac CT. Radiol Cardiothorac Imaging. 2019;1:e180003.
20. Kalisz K, Rassouli N, Dhanantwari A, Jordan D, Rajiah P. Noise characteristics of virtual monoenergetic images from a novel detector-based spectral CT scanner. Eur J Radiol. 2018;98:118–25.
21. Booij R, van der Werf NR, Dijkshoorn ML, van der Lugt A, van Straten M. Assessment of iodine contrast-

to-noise ratio in virtual monoenergetic images reconstructed from dual-source energy-integrating CT and photon-counting CT data. Diagnostics. 2022;12:1467.
22. Rodriguez-Granillo GA. Delayed enhancement cardiac computed tomography for the assessment of myocardial infarction: from bench to bedside. Cardiovasc Diagn Ther. 2017;7:159–70.
23. Kurobe Y, Kitagawa K, Ito T, et al. Myocardial delayed enhancement with dual-source CT: advantages of targeted spatial frequency filtration and image averaging over half-scan reconstruction. J Cardiovasc Comput Tomogr. 2014;8:289–98.
24. Mendoza DD, Joshi SB, Weissman G, Taylor AJ, Weigold WG. Viability imaging by cardiac computed tomography. J Cardiovasc Comput Tomogr. 2010;4:83–91.
25. Kato S, Misumi Y, Horita N, Yamamoto K, Utsunomiya D. Clinical utility of computed tomography–derived myocardial extracellular volume fraction. JACC Cardiovasc Imaging. 2023;17:516–28. https://doi.org/10.1016/j.jcmg.2023.10.008.
26. Treibel TA, Bandula S, Fontana M, et al. Extracellular volume quantification by dynamic equilibrium cardiac computed tomography in cardiac amyloidosis. J Cardiovasc Comput Tomogr. 2015;9:585–92.
27. Hamdy A, Kitagawa K, Goto Y, Yamada A, Nakamura S, Takafuji M, Nagasawa N, Sakuma H. Comparison of the different imaging time points in delayed phase cardiac CT for myocardial scar assessment and extracellular volume fraction estimation in patients with old myocardial infarction. Int J Cardiovasc Imaging. 2019;35:917–26.
28. Cundari G, Galea N, Mergen V, Alkadhi H, Eberhard M. Myocardial extracellular volume quantification with computed tomography—current status and future outlook. Insights Imaging. 2023;14:156. https://doi.org/10.1186/s13244-023-01506-6.
29. Takafuji M, Kitagawa K, Nakamura S, Hamdy A, Goto Y, Ishida M, Sakuma H. Feasibility of extracellular volume fraction calculation using myocardial CT delayed enhancement with low contrast media administration. J Cardiovasc Comput Tomogr. 2020;14:524–8.
30. Emoto T, Kidoh M, Oda S, et al. Myocardial extracellular volume quantification in cardiac CT: comparison of the effects of two different iterative reconstruction algorithms with MRI as a reference standard. Eur Radiol. 2020;30:691–701.
31. Kim NY, Im DJ, Youn JC, Hong YJ, Choi BW, Kang SM, Lee HJ. Synthetic extracellular volume fraction derived using virtual unenhanced attenuation of blood on contrast-enhanced cardiac dual-energy CT in nonischemic cardiomyopathy. Am J Roentgenol. 2022;218:454–61.
32. Mergen V, Sartoretti T, Klotz E, et al. Extracellular volume quantification with cardiac late enhancement scanning using dual-source photon-counting detector CT. Investig Radiol. 2022;57:406–11.
33. Aquino GJ, O'Doherty J, Schoepf UJ, et al. Myocardial characterization with extracellular volume mapping with a first-generation photon-counting detector CT with MRI reference. Radiology. 2023;307:e222030. https://doi.org/10.1148/radiol.222030.
34. Hoffmann U, Bamberg F, Chae CU, et al. Coronary computed tomography angiography for early triage of patients with acute chest pain. The ROMICAT (Rule Out Myocardial Infarction using Computer Assisted Tomography) trial. J Am Coll Cardiol. 2009;53:1642–50.
35. Chen CL. Coronary CT angiography versus standard evaluation in acute chest pain. N Engl J Med. 2012;367:299–308. https://doi.org/10.1056/nejmoa1201161.
36. Palmisano A, Vignale D, Tadic M, et al. Myocardial late contrast enhancement CT in troponin-positive acute chest pain syndrome. Radiology. 2022;302:545–53.
37. Vignale D, Palmisano A, Colantoni C, Brunetti L, Nicoletti V, Gnasso C, Esposito A. Toward a one-stop shop CT protocol in acute chest pain syndrome. Radiology. 2023;306:E3–4.
38. Carrabba N, Pontone G, Andreini D, et al. Appropriateness criteria for the use of cardiac computed tomography, SIC-SIRM part 2: acute chest pain evaluation; stent and coronary artery bypass graft patency evaluation; planning of coronary revascularization and transcatheter valve procedures; cardiomyopathies, electrophysiological applications, cardiac masses, cardio-oncology and pericardial diseases evaluation. J Cardiovasc Med. 2022;23:290–303.
39. Ohta Y, Kitao S, Yunaga H, Fujii S, Mukai N, Yamamoto K, Ogawa T. Myocardial delayed enhancement CT for the evaluation of heart failure: comparison to MRI. Radiology. 2018;288:682–91.
40. Qi RX, Jiang JS, Shao J, Zhang Q, Zheng KL, Xiao J, Huang S, Gong SC. Measurement of myocardial extracellular volume fraction in patients with heart failure with preserved ejection fraction using dual-energy computed tomography. Eur Radiol. 2022;32:4253–63.
41. Qi RX, Shao J, Jiang JS, Ruan XW, Huang S, Zhang Q, Hu CH. Myocardial extracellular volume fraction quantitation using cardiac dual-energy CT with late iodine enhancement in patients with heart failure without coronary artery disease: a single-center prospective study. Eur J Radiol. 2021;140:109743. https://doi.org/10.1016/j.ejrad.2021.109743.
42. Seidman A, Hudis C, Pierri MK, Shak S, Paton V, Ashby M, Murphy M, Stewart SJ, Keefe D. Cardiac dysfunction in the trastuzumab clinical trials experience. J Clin Oncol. 2002;20:1215–21.
43. Tu C, Shen H, Liu R, et al. Myocardial extracellular volume derived from contrast-enhanced chest computed tomography for longitudinal evaluation of cardiotoxicity in patients with breast cancer treated with anthracyclines. Insights Imaging. 2022;13:85. https://doi.org/10.1186/s13244-022-01224-5.
44. Tanabe Y, Kido T, Kurata A, Kouchi T, Fukuyama N, Yokoi T, Uetani T, Yamashita N, Miyagawa M,

Mochizuki T. Late iodine enhancement computed tomography with image subtraction for assessment of myocardial infarction. Eur Radiol. 2018;28:1285–92.
45. van Assen M, Vonder M, Pelgrim GJ, Von Knebel Doeberitz PL, Vliegenthart R. Computed tomography for myocardial characterization in ischemic heart disease: a state-of-the-art review. Eur Radiol Exp. 2020;4:36.
46. Shapiro MD, Sarwar A, Nieman K, Nasir K, Brady TJ, Cury RC. Cardiac computed tomography for prediction of myocardial viability after reperfused acute myocardial infarction. J Cardiovasc Comput Tomogr. 2010;4:267–73.
47. Sato A, Nozato T, Hikita H, et al. Prognostic value of myocardial contrast delayed enhancement with 64-slice multidetector computed tomography after acute myocardial infarction. J Am Coll Cardiol. 2012;59:730–8.
48. Lessick J, Dragu R, Mutlak D, et al. Is functional improvement after myocardial infarction predicted with myocardial enhancement patterns at multidetector CT? Radiology. 2007;244:736–44.
49. Komatsu Y, Cochet H, Jadidi A, et al. Regional Myocardial Wall thinning at multidetector computed tomography correlates to arrhythmogenic substrate in postinfarction ventricular tachycardia. Circ Arrhythm Electrophysiol. 2013;6:342–50.
50. van Kranenburg M, Magro M, Thiele H, et al. Prognostic value of microvascular obstruction and infarct size, as measured by CMR in STEMI patients. JACC Cardiovasc Imaging. 2014;7:930–9.
51. Ferreira A, Ferreira V, Antunes MM, Lousinha A, Pereira-da-Silva T, Antunes D, Cunha PS, Oliveira M, Ferreira RC, Rosa SA. Dilated cardiomyopathy: a comprehensive approach to diagnosis and risk stratification. Biomedicines. 2023;11:834. https://doi.org/10.3390/biomedicines11030834.
52. Yashima S, Takaoka H, Iwahana T, et al. Evaluation of extracellular volume by computed tomography is useful for prediction of prognosis in dilated cardiomyopathy. Heart Vessel. 2023;38:185–94.
53. Zhao L, Ma X, Feuchtner GM, Zhang C, Fan Z. Quantification of myocardial delayed enhancement and wall thickness in hypertrophic cardiomyopathy: multidetector computed tomography versus magnetic resonance imaging. Eur J Radiol. 2014;83:1778–85.
54. Langer C, Schaefer P, Lutz M, Eden M, Hohnhorst M, Harders H, Faber L, Jansen O, Both M, Frey N. Myocardial fibrosis in hypertrophic cardiomyopathy: volumetric assessment of late enhancement provided by cardiac computed tomography. J Comput Assist Tomogr. 2015;39:797–803.
55. Shiozaki AA, Senra T, Arteaga E, et al. Myocardial fibrosis detected by cardiac CT predicts ventricular fibrillation/ventricular tachycardia events in patients with hypertrophic cardiomyopathy. J Cardiovasc Comput Tomogr. 2013;7:173–81.
56. Dungu JN, Valencia O, Pinney JH, et al. CMR-based differentiation of AL and ATTR cardiac amyloidosis. JACC Cardiovasc Imaging. 2014;7:133–42.
57. Esposito A, Palmisano A, Barbera M, et al. Cardiac computed tomography in troponin-positive chest pain. JACC Cardiovasc Imaging. 2019;12:745–8.
58. Tavoosi A, de Oliveira Brito JB, El Mais H, Small TD, Crean AM, Chow BJW, Small GR. Dual versus single energy cardiac CT to measure extra cellular volume in cardiac amyloidosis: correlations with cardiac MRI. IJC Heart Vasc. 2023;44:101166. https://doi.org/10.1016/j.ijcha.2022.101166.
59. Gama F, Rosmini S, Bandula S, et al. Extracellular volume fraction by computed tomography predicts long-term prognosis among patients with cardiac amyloidosis. JACC Cardiovasc Imaging. 2022;15:2082–94.
60. Osnabrugge RLJ, Mylotte D, Head SJ, Van Mieghem NM, Nkomo VT, LeReun CM, Bogers AJJC, Piazza N, Kappetein AP. Aortic stenosis in the elderly. J Am Coll Cardiol. 2013;62:1002–12.
61. Carabello BA. Is cardiac hypertrophy good or bad? JACC Cardiovasc Imaging. 2014;7:1081–3.
62. Azevedo CF, Nigri M, Higuchi ML, Pomerantzeff PM, Spina GS, Sampaio RO, Tarasoutchi F, Grinberg M, Rochitte CE. Prognostic significance of myocardial fibrosis quantification by histopathology and magnetic resonance imaging in patients with severe aortic valve disease. J Am Coll Cardiol. 2010;56:278–87.
63. Vignale D, Palmisano A, Gnasso C, et al. Extracellular volume fraction (ECV) derived from pre-operative computed tomography predicts prognosis in patients undergoing transcatheter aortic valve implantation (TAVI). Eur Heart J Cardiovasc Imaging. 2023;24:887–96.
64. Tamarappoo B, Han D, Tyler J, et al. Prognostic value of computed tomography–derived extracellular volume in TAVR patients with low-flow low-gradient aortic stenosis. JACC Cardiovasc Imaging. 2020;13:2591–601.
65. Scully PR, Patel KP, Saberwal B, et al. Identifying cardiac amyloid in aortic stenosis. JACC Cardiovasc Imaging. 2020;13:2177–89.
66. Maccabelli G, Tsiachris D, Silberbauer J, et al. Imaging and epicardial substrate ablation of ventricular tachycardia in patients late after myocarditis. Europace. 2014;16:1363–72.
67. Esposito A, Palmisano A, Antunes S, Colantoni C, Rancoita PMV, Vignale D, Baratto F, Della Bella P, Del Maschio A, De Cobelli F. Assessment of remote myocardium heterogeneity in patients with ventricular tachycardia using texture analysis of late iodine enhancement (LIE) cardiac computed tomography (cCT) images. Mol Imaging Biol. 2018;20:816–25.
68. Esposito A, Palmisano A, Antunes S, et al. Cardiac CT with delayed enhancement in the characterization of ventricular tachycardia structural substrate. JACC Cardiovasc Imaging. 2016;9:822–32.
69. Jáuregui B, Soto-Iglesias D, Zucchelli G, et al. Arrhythmogenic substrate detection in chronic ischaemic patients undergoing ventricular tachycardia ablation using multidetector cardiac computed

tomography: compared evaluation with cardiac magnetic resonance. EP Europace. 2021;23:82–90.
70. Yamashita S, Sacher F, Mahida S, et al. Image integration to guide catheter ablation in scar-related ventricular tachycardia. J Cardiovasc Electrophysiol. 2016;27:699–708.
71. Conte E, Carbucicchio C, Catto V, et al. Live integration of comprehensive cardiac CT with electroanatomical mapping in patients with refractory ventricular tachycardia. J Cardiovasc Comput Tomogr. 2022;16:262–5.
72. Conte E, Mushtaq S, Carbucicchio C, et al. State of the art paper: cardiovascular CT for planning ventricular tachycardia ablation procedures. J Cardiovasc Comput Tomogr. 2021;15:394–402.
73. Palmisano A, Vig nale D, Peretto G, et al. Hybrid FDG-PET/MR or FDG-PET/CT to detect disease activity in patients with persisting arrhythmias after myocarditis. JACC Cardiovasc Imaging. 2021;14:288–92.

Myocardial Characterization with MRI

9

Jadranka Stojanovska

Introduction

Cardiac magnetic resonance (CMR) is an emerging imaging modality assessing cardiac morphology, function, flow, and most importantly myocardial tissue integrity. While echocardiography is the first-line imaging modality in patients with cardiovascular diseases, CMR is used to solve clinical conundrums mainly when the question is to identify architectural changes within the myocardial tissue [1]. The advantages of gadolinium administration or different pulse sequences/image contrast techniques enable CMR to evaluate tissue changes and depict tissue edema, fibrosis, scar, deposition of amyloid, sarcoid, or iron with a unique perspective to make the diagnosis, identify findings used for risk stratification and to guide patient's treatment.

However, learning first about myocardial tissue anatomy is paramount before addressing various techniques used for tissue characterization. Therefore, in this chapter, we will cover topics in sequential order from myocardial tissue anatomy, myocardial tissue pathology followed by imaging techniques used for myocardial tissue characterization such as late gadolinium enhancement (LGE), T1 mapping (native and extracellular volume maps), T2-weighted image and T2 mapping, T2* mapping, and fingerprinting.

J. Stojanovska (✉)
Grossman School of Medicine, New York University, New York, NY, USA
e-mail: Jadranka.Stojanovska@nyulangone.org

Myocardial Anatomy

Learning about myocardial tissue anatomy is pivotal to understanding myocardial structure, function, and pathology. Myocardial tissue is composed of parallel aligned cardiomyocytes spaced out with extracelleular space and traversed by the coronary vasculature that brings oxygen to the cardiomyocytes to enable contraction, cardiac lymphatics, and autonomic innervation [2]. Intercalated discs between the cardiomyocytes are responsible for cell-to-cell communication and rapid electrical conduction. In addition, the cardiomyocytes are specialized striated muscle cells responsible for generating synchronized contraction. The extracellular space or the interstitial matrix provides structural support and maintains tissue integrity, supports cardiac pumping, and is being composed of collagen, elastin, and glycans [2]. All of these properties enable proper cardiac function and myocardial perfusion. Furthermore, the heart muscle is composed of three layers. The myocardium is the middle layer of the heart muscle with densely packed myocytes and some amount of extracellular space which varies by sex and age and ranges between 22% and 29% [3], whereas the epicardium is the outer layer, and the subendocardium is the inner layer of the heart muscle (Fig. 9.1a). It is important to note that the subendocardium contracts the most, followed by

R. Gill, P. Rajiah (eds.), *Quantitative Imaging in the Thorax*,
https://doi.org/10.1007/978-3-032-14103-3_9

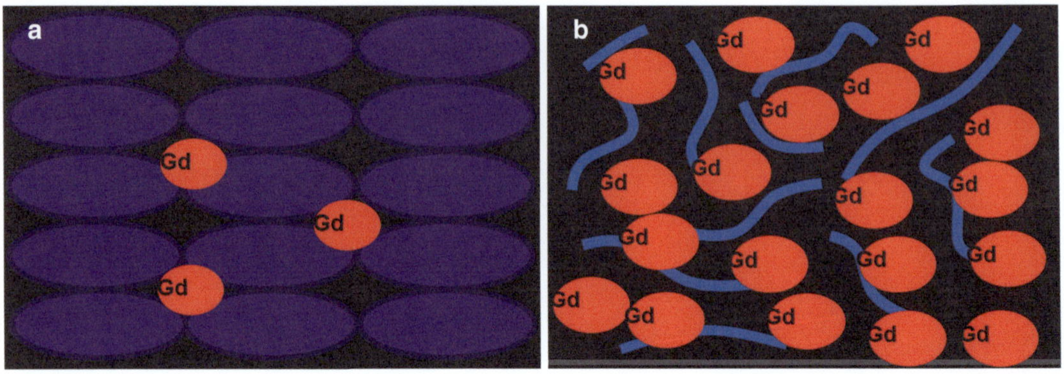

Fig. 9.1 The myocardium is the middle layer of the heart muscle with densely packed myocytes and some amount of extracellular space which varies by sex and age and ranges between 22% and 29% (**a**). The myocardium undergoes pathological changes in the setting of ischemic heart disease, myocarditis, valvular heart disease, and cardiomyopathy that increase the extracellular space (**b**). These changes include inflammation, fibrosis, hypertrophy, and necrosis, leading to ventricular remodeling and impaired function

the mid myocardium; therefore, the oxygen consumption is at the highest level at the subendocardial level [2]. In the setting of ischemia, the subendocardium suffers first from lack of oxygen. The myocardium is found in all four chambers of the heart, being the thickest in the left ventricle followed by the right ventricle and left and right atria.

Pathologic Changes in the Myocardium

The myocardium undergoes pathological changes in the setting of ischemic heart disease, myocarditis, valvular heart disease, cardiomyopathy, etc. These changes include inflammation, fibrosis, hypertrophy, and necrosis, leading to ventricular remodeling and impaired function that confer to different cardiovascular disease processes (Fig. 9.1b). Understanding these pathologic changes is crucial for establishing the diagnosis, risk stratifying patients with cardiovascular diseases, and guide management. The alterations of myocardial anatomical framework can be within the myocytes or the extracellular space which can be further evaluated by CMR.

Cardiac Magnetic Resonance (CMR)

CMR enables noninvasive assessment of tissue changes to facilitate accurate diagnosis, guide decision-making process, monitor treatment response, and risk stratify patients with cardiovascular diseases [4]. CMR has emerged as a powerful tool for myocardial characterization, delving into the insights of the myocardial structure and pathology. While cine (steady state free precession sequence) imaging is an important sequence to elucidate functional abnormality and myocardial remodeling, in this chapter we focus to bring the reader closer to CMR sequences that explore tissue characterization. Furthermore, the following CMR protocol is used for tissue characterization in clinical setting (Fig. 9.2). Of note, the T2-weighted imaging, T2 mapping, native T1 mapping, and T2* mapping are acquired before gadolinium administration. The cine images can be acquired after gadolinium administration to keep the scans efficient, while the late gadolinium enhancement are performed ~10 min after gadolinium injection. Post-gadolinium T1 mapping is acquired at ~15 min post-gadolinium administration.

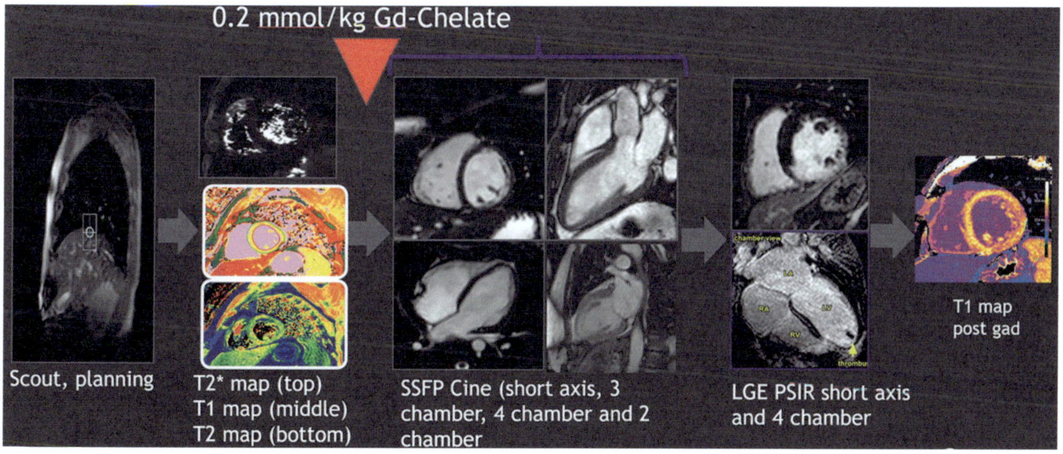

Fig. 9.2 CMR protocol is used for tissue characterization in clinical setting. Of note, the T2-weighted imaging, T2 mapping, native T1 mapping, and T2* mapping are acquired before gadolinium administration. The cine images can be acquired after gadolinium administration to keep the scans efficient, while the late gadolinium enhancement are performed ~10 min after gadolinium injection. Post-gadolinium T1 mapping is acquired at ~15 min post-gadolinium administration

Late Gadolinium Enhancement (LGE)

Late gadolinium enhancement (LGE) imaging is a valuable technique in myocardial tissue characterization that has become the reference standard for noninvasive evaluation of myocardial fibrosis in both ischemic and nonischemic cardiomyopathies [5]. In this paragraph, we will discuss the basic physics principles and clinical applications of LGE imaging in myocardial tissue characterization.

Basic Physics Principles

LGE is an inversion recovery gradient echo sequence that uses 180-degree inversion prepulse to null the myocardium after selecting the appropriate inversion time for each patient so that the scar appears bright and the blood pool gray [5]. This is because the myocardial fibrosis and the normal myocardium have relative different longitudinal recovery (T1) times shortened because of the gadolinium. The LGE acquisition is performed about 10 min postinjection (Fig. 9.3a, b). There are two phases of postinjection of the gadolinium. The first phase is after the injection of the gadolinium when its concentration is present in the first 5 min within the normal myocardium after which the gadolinium washes out. However, in the diseased myocardium where the extracellular volume is expanded, the gadolinium remains in the extracellular space for a longer period of time. Therefore, patients are scanned in approximately 10 min after the gadolinium injection to avoid first pass perfusion within the normal myocardium and identify alterations in the myocardial morphology with retained gadolinium in the extracellular space. The viable myocardium has intact cell membranes, and the myocytes are densely packed between each other with very little extracellular space that allows the gadolinium to go in and wash out within 5 min. Any disease process that expands the extracellular space either by cell death in the setting of myocardial infarction and scar formation with collagen deposition, or deposition of other molecules such as amyloid, sarcoid, or inflammatory cells. This deposition of other cells distorts the myocardial architecture and allows the gadolinium to accumulate in a certain type and pattern that is reflective of the particular disease process. The net result in both scenarios is an increase in extracellular space and changes in washout kinetics.

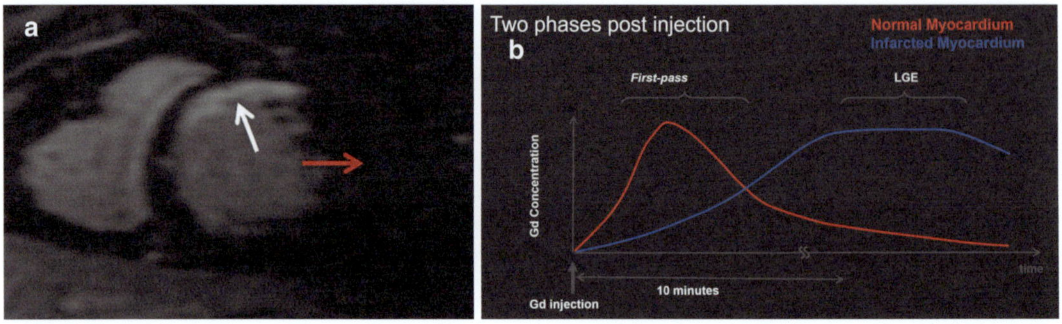

Fig. 9.3 LGE is an inversion recovery gradient echo sequence that uses 180-degree inversion pre-pulse to null the myocardium after selecting the appropriate inversion time for each patient so that the scar appears bright and the blood pool gray (**a**). This is because the myocardial fibrosis and the normal myocardium have relative different longitudinal recovery (T1) times shortened because of the gadolinium. The LGE acquisition is performed about 10 min postinjection (**b**)

Clinical Implications

The normal myocardium demonstrates no late gadolinium enhancement. We diagnose specific type of cardiomyopathy based on the type of accumulation and distribution of late gadolinium enhancement within the myocardium. For example, if LGE is subendocardial or transmural within coronary artery territory, this will indicate nonviable myocardium secondary to prior myocardial infarction (Fig. 9.4a). Patchy LGE is seen in cardiac sarcoid (Fig. 9.4b), whereas subepicardial LGE is seen in patients with sarcoid, myocarditis, Chagas, and Fabry (Fig. 9.4c). Global subendocardial LGE is seen in patients with cardiac amyloid, Loeffler myocarditis, and systemic sclerosis (Fig. 9.4d, e). Patchy nodular septal LGE within hypertrophic myocardium is seen in patients with hypertrophic cardiomyopathy. In addition, enhancement of the pericardium indicates pericarditis. However, LGE as a primary endpoint in CMR is not solely used to diagnose the type of cardiomyopathy based on the pattern and distribution of LGE but to also risk stratify patients which means to identify patients who will experience cardiovascular death or major adverse cardiac event at the earlier time-point compared to patients without LGE. Kim et al. found that 90% of the myocardial segments with near transmural or transmural LGE in patients with ischemic cardiomyopathy did not improve function after revascularization [6]. Furthermore, for patients with nonischemic dilated cardiomyopathy, the pattern and location of LGE is predictive of adverse events. Halliday et al. showed that mid-wall septal LGE is associated with increased mortality in patients with nonischemic dilated cardiomyopathy, while mid-wall septal and lateral wall LGE are associated with greatest sudden cardiac death risk compared to all other types and patterns of LGE [7]. A characteristic pattern of LGE represents a stronger predictor of 1-year mortality in patients with cardiac amyloidosis compared to other non-invasive parameters [8]. A meta-analysis assessed the prognostic value of the extent of LGE in predicting sudden cardiac death in patients with hypertrophic cardiomyopathy using different methods of quantification, thresholds, and clinical profile. The 6 Standard deviation (SD) technique is a highly robust and most utilized reference standard for LGE. The authors identify that LGE 10% is the optimal cut-off to re-stratify intermediate-risk patients using 6SD technique [9].

Conclusion

In summary, the binary outcome of LGE is currently the most important endpoint in the management of cardiovascular diseases. Understanding and recognizing the patterns of LGE allows for accurate diagnosis.

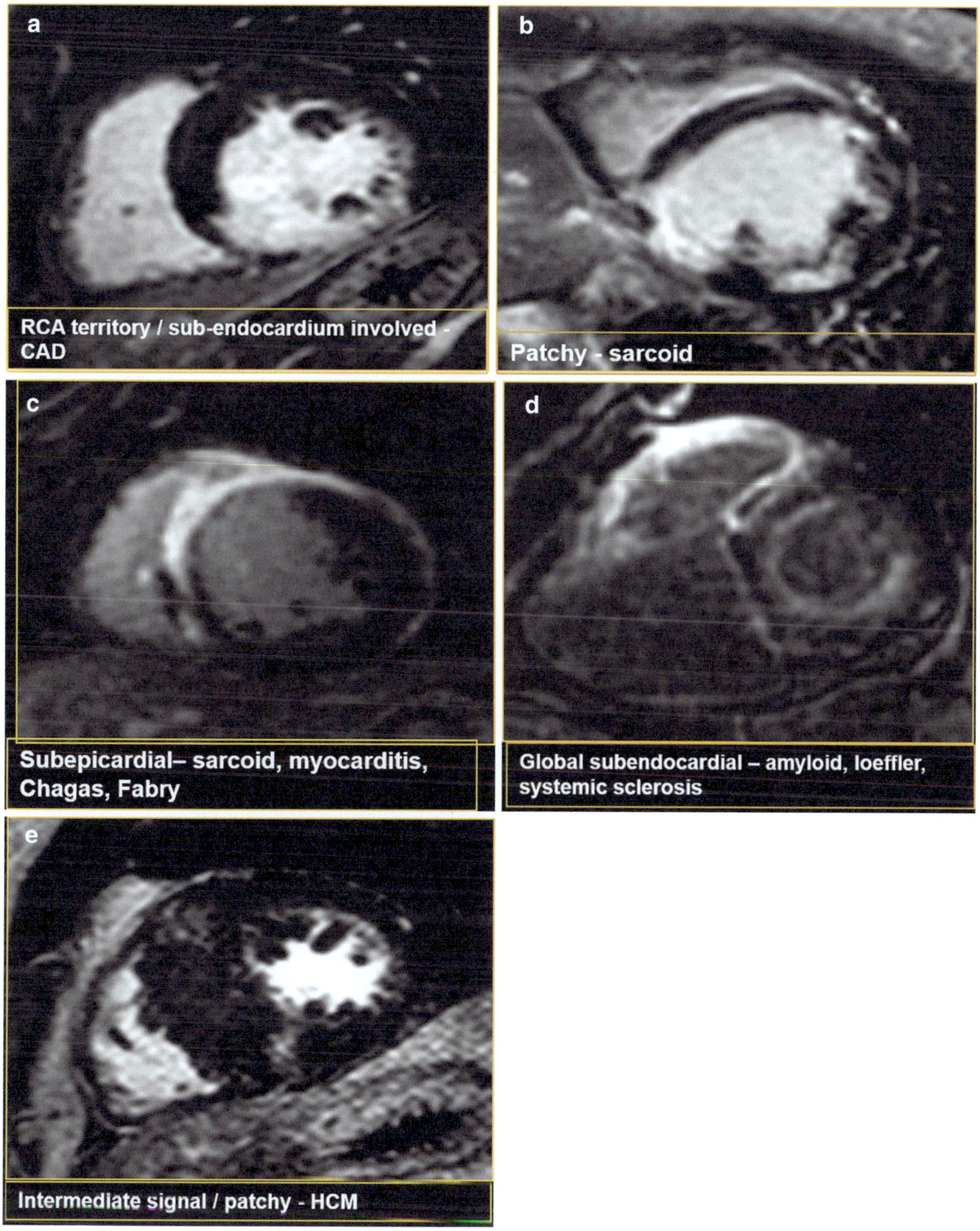

Fig. 9.4 LGE is subendocardial or transmural within coronary artery territory; this will indicate nonviable myocardium secondary to prior myocardial infarction (**a**). Patchy LGE is seen in cardiac sarcoid (**b**), whereas subepicardial LGE is seen in patients with sarcoid, myocarditis, Chagas, and Fabry (**c**). Global subendocardial LGE is seen in patients with cardiac amyloid, Loeffler myocarditis, and systemic sclerosis (**d**). (**e**) Intermediate signal/patchy-HCM

T1 Mapping

While LGE is a gold standard to diagnose patients with different cardiomyopathies, it becomes a challenge for LGE to identify diffuse fibrosis especially when there is a disease in the absence of negative LGE. Therefore, T1 mapping provides quantitative measurements of myocardial relaxation times, allowing for more accurate assessment of tissue properties. Tissue characterization with parametric mapping such as T1 mapping is valuable technique to enable diagnostic, prognostic, and therapeutic decisions in patients with ischemic and nonischemic cardiomyopathy.

Basic Physics

T1 mapping measures the longitudinal time of how rapidly the protons re-equilibrate their spins after being excited by the radiofrequency pulse [10]. The most commonly used sequence is modified look looker inversion recovery sequence acquired in a single breath hold over 17 heart beats which allows the T1 map measurement pre- and post-gadolinium injection. The pre-gadolinium T1 map is called native T1 map and the post-gadolinium T1 map represents ECV map. The signal in the native T1 map represents the myocytes and the interstitial compartment.

Clinical Application

Several tissue properties may change this signal, such as edema, fibrosis, adipose tissue, iron, and amyloid. Edema, fibrosis, and amyloid increase T1 values and adipose tissue and iron decrease T1 times. Furthermore, the native T1 times vary across scanners; therefore, normative range should be established to identify abnormal cases. It is important to note that motion is critical and requires motion correction technique. The signal from ECV map represents extracellular compartment. Fibrosis, inflammation, and amyloidosis are detected with increased extracellular volume. To quantify extracellular volume, the formula takes into account the T1 times of the myocardium and the blood pool pre- and post-gadolinium in addition to the hematocrit (Fig. 9.5a, b). Of note, the percentage of the ECV map obtained from T1 post-gadolinium scans is less variable across the scanners. Parametric mapping has gained a lot of interest and value in the diagnosis of the cardiovascular diseases, prognostication, and monitoring therapy response. The main proven utility of T1 mapping is in the diagnosis of myocarditis, amyloidosis, and check inhibitor cardiotoxicity. T1 mapping is part of the Lake Louise criteria for myocarditis and ECV map has shown a better diagnostic and prognostic utility than LGE and native T1 mapping [11]. In addi-

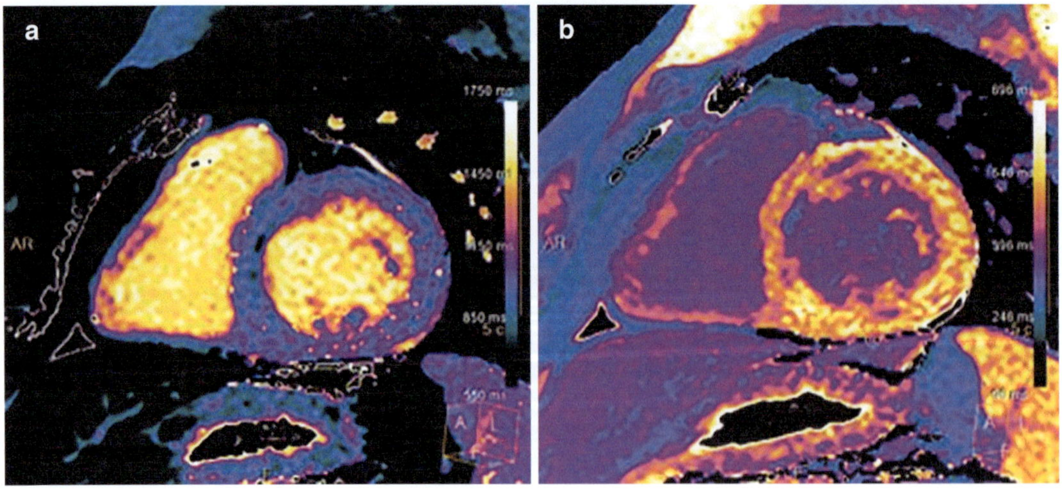

Fig. 9.5 To quantify extracellular volume, the formula takes into account the T1 times of the myocardium (*) and the blood pool (arrowhead) pre- (**a**) and post-gadolinium (**b**) in addition to the hematocrit

tion, T1 mapping is valuable in monitoring disease progression and assessing treatment response in patients with cardiovascular diseases. Changes in T1 relaxation times over time may provide insights in disease status and treatment response in addition to guiding clinical management [12].

Conclusion

In summary, T1 mapping plays a crucial role in myocardial tissue characterization by quantitative assessment of myocardial pathology and myocardial fibrosis as well as monitoring disease progression and evaluating therapeutic efficacy.

T2 Weighted Image and T2 Mapping

Basic Physics Principles

T2-weighted imaging and T2 mapping are CMR imaging techniques that provide valuable information about myocardial edema and inflammation [11]. In this section, we will elucidate the basic physics principles, clinical application, and recent advancement in these two sequences. T2-weighted imaging is double-inversion spin echo sequence with long time to echo and time to repetition relaying on the differences in the T2 relaxation times of the tissue to generate contrast in CMR images and suppressing the signal from the normal myocardium [13]. These images accentuate the regions of altered water content and are sensitive to the presence of myocardial edema and inflammation. It is the best to acquire three short axis images (base, mid cavity, and apical level) in addition to long axis view such as four-chamber view and two-chamber view.

Clinical Application

The main clinical application of T2 weighted imaging is in the diagnosis of myocarditis to evaluate vasogenic edema depicted as high signal intensity predominantly involving the myocardial wall in noncoronary artery distribution. Most commonly, the basal or mid inferolateral wall and/or inferior walls are affected in myocarditis (Fig. 9.5c) [14]. T2-weighted images are also used to differentiate myocarditis from acute infarct in patients with chest pain and increased troponins where patients present with vasogenic edema; however, patients with acute infarct present with cytotoxic edema not visualized on T2 images because of cell swelling. Another indication is to assess acute inflammatory processes in the setting of sarcoid, cardiotoxicity, stress-induced cardiomyopathy, and cardiac transplant rejection. Patients with stress-induced cardiomyopathy usually demonstrate high signal intensity of the mid and apical segments, while the base of the heart is of normal signal [15]. This sequence becomes a routine sequence in the evaluation of nonischemic cardiomyopathy. These images can be evaluated quantitatively and qualitatively. Most common approach is qualitative visualization of regional or diffuse high signal intensity. However, a useful quantitative approach to assess diffuse edema is to measure the signal intensity of the myocardium compared to the adjacent skeletal muscle. If the ratio between the signal intensities of the myocardium and the skeletal muscle is greater than 2 on the T2 weighted CMR in a patient that has not exercised prior to CMR image acquisition then that is indicative of myocardial edema [16].

While this sequence is one of the criterion for the diagnosis of myocarditis based on Lake Louise criteria, there are several challenges associated with this sequence mainly related to image artifact such as motion and variable signal-to-noise ratio [11]. In addition, the interpretation may be subjective; therefore, it is important to correlate the high signal intensity areas with areas of potentially normal myocardium in addition to measure the signal intensity of those regions correlating with the adjacent skeletal muscles.

T2 mapping is a parametric mapping that quantifies T2 relaxation times of myocardial tissue, offers reproducible measurement, and generates parametric color coded maps of T2 relaxation times. This technique provides unique quantitative information of diffuse tissue edema and inflammation. The color coded maps may provide value in visual inspection of abnormal T2 relaxation times to confirm the pathology. The quantitative parametric metrics of tissue properties have revolutionized myocardial tissue characteristics. T2 mapping has found home in the evaluation of infectious/inflammatory myocardial disease such as myocarditis, sarcoidosis, and heart transplant rejection, as well as identifying early changes in the myocardial tissue before the onset of clinical symptoms, facilitating timely intervention and risk stratification. Recent advancements have been focused on good image quality and reproducibility as well as artificial intelligence tool to enable faster and accurate post processing analysis to improve reporting efficiency in the era of increased scanning throughput.

Conclusion

In summary, both T2 weighted and T2 mapping are important tools in CMR to provide unique insights of myocardial edema, inflammation, and tissue composition using qualitative and quantitative assessment. The clinical utility spans a wide range of cardiovascular diseases with essential role in diagnosis, risk stratification, and therapy response providing personalized patient care.

T2* Mapping

Basic Physics Principles

The utility of T2 mapping in clinical setting is very unique and specific in quantification of iron deposition, fibrosis, and different tissue composition within the myocardium. This sequence quantifies the transverse relaxation time (T2*) of tissue, i.e., decay of transverse magnetization in the myocardium following radiofrequency excitation in the presence of parametric substance such as iron [17]. Usually, eight maps are acquired with different echo times in milliseconds (ms) that allow for quantitative post processing by placing a region of interest (ROI) in the interventricular septum. This allows for quantification of T2* values to assess myocardial iron deposition and ascertain the diagnosis and monitor patients with myocardial iron overload cardiomyopathy.

Clinical Application

Clinically, T2* mapping is indicated in patients with hereditary hemochromatosis (Fig. 9.6), thalassemia, and transfusional iron overload.

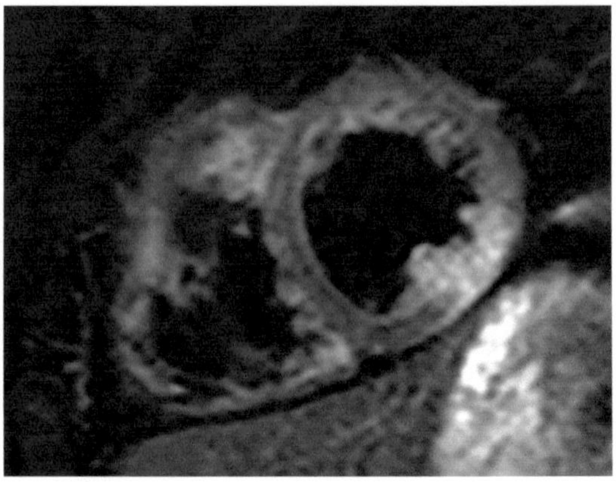

Fig. 9.6 High signal in the mid inferolateral wall and/or inferior walls suggestive of inflammation/edema

Quantifying the presence, extent, and distribution of iron within the myocardium stratifies disease severity based on T2* value. Normal T2* value is 40 ms, mild iron deposition is indicated by T2* value between 20 and 40 ms, and severe form of iron deposition is indicated by T2* value below 20 ms [18]. The T2* value serves as a primary endpoint for patients with the suspicion of iron overload cardiomyopathy to risk stratify these patients for adverse cardiac events such as heart failure and arrhythmias, guide clinical decision-making regarding chelation therapy, and monitor. Recent studies have shown a broader use of T2* mapping in assessing fibrosis, ischemic-reperfusion injury indicating the presence of hemorrhage offering insights into myocardial tissue composition and different disease processes. Several challenges exist related to image acquisition, post-processing, and interpretation that may affect T2* mapping accuracy and reproducibility. Motion artifacts, susceptibility artifacts, and signal-to-noise ratio variation in addition to confounding variables such as edema and inflammation affect the accuracy and interpretation of T2* values underscoring the importance of standardized protocols, post-processing tools, and skilled personnel in acquiring CMR. To optimize T2* mapping acquisition and quantitative accuracy, novel pulse sequences have been developed to address technical challenges. In addition, artificial intelligence and deep learning algorithms have been developed to not only enable automated detection of myocardial iron deposition but also enable sequence acquisition.

Conclusion

In summary, T2* mapping serves as a primary endpoint in patients with suspected iron overload cardiomyopathy facilitating diagnosis, risk stratification, and therapeutic guidance. In addition, T2* mapping has the ability to detect fibrosis and provides useful information in heart failure.

Fingerprinting

Basic Physics Principles

Fingerprinting is the newest and most innovative pulse sequence in CMR realm offering comprehensive quantitative assessment of myocardial tissue properties by using parametric mapping techniques with single co-registered multiparametric scan [19]. This approach streamlines and unifies cardiac MR sequences with one goal to offer a simplified and shortened CMR exams to increase access and efficient patient throughput [20]. Fingerprinting acquires quantitative maps of T1 relaxation time, T2 relaxation time, and proton density fat fraction to generate fingerprints of combined parameters of tissue of interest and enable characterization of myocardial tissue composition and pathology such as edema, fibrosis, and inflammation.

Clinical Application

Clinically, fingerprinting is valuable in patients with ischemic and nonischemic cardiomyopathy as well as assessing treatment response. In patients with ischemic cardiomyopathy, fingerprinting quantifies infarcts myocardium and the salvageable tissue to delineate acute from chronic myocardial infarction using both T1 and T2 mapping techniques, while in patients with myocarditis, quantifies and monitors edema, inflammation, and fibrosis. The role of fingerprinting in patients with nonischemic cardiomyopathies is to provide risk stratification and personalized management strategies by quantifying changes in myocardial architecture such as fibrosis, adipose tissue, and myocardial hypertrophy. However, with every novel imaging sequence, the robustness and repeatability of the technique are crucial in providing accuracy and efficiency of fingerprinting analysis to enable integration with clinical decision. Therefore, recent advancements in fingerprinting have focused on improving spatial resolution and robustness to motion artifacts. Deep machine learning and artificial intelligence have been explored to enhance and speed up the post-processing analysis.

Conclusion

While fingerprinting is not part of the daily clinical practice, it still represents a paradigm shift in myocardial tissue characterization offering quantitative and comprehensive assessment of myocardial tissue to revolutionize myocardial tissue characterization to improve patient outcomes.

References

1. Baldassare L, Ganatra S, Lopez-Mattei J, et al. Advances in multimodality imaging in cardio-oncology: JACC state-of-the-art review. J Am Coll Cardiol. 2022;80(16):1560–78.
2. Chuang ML, Manning WJ, Peshock RM, et al. Normal cardiac anatomy, cardiovascular magnetic resonance. 3rd ed. Philadelphia: Elsevier; 2019. p. 178–191.e2.
3. Roy C, Slimani A, de Meester C, et al. Age and sex corrected normal reference values of T1, T2 T2* and ECV in healthy subjects at 3T CMR. J Cardiovasc Magn Reson. 2017;19:72.
4. Kramer CM, Barkhausen J, Flamm SD, Kim RJ, Nagel E, Society for Cardiovascular Magnetic Resonance Board of Trustees Task Force on Standardized Protocols. Standardized cardiovascular magnetic resonance (CMR) protocols 2013 update. J Cardiovasc Magn Reson. 2013;15:91. https://doi.org/10.1186/1532-429X-15-91.
5. Kellman P, Arai AE. Cardiac imaging techniques for physicians: late enhancement. J Magn Reson Imaging. 2012;36(3):529–42. https://doi.org/10.1002/jmri.23696.
6. Kim RJ, Wu E, Rafael A, et al. The use of contrast-enhanced magnetic resonance imaging to identify reversible myocardial dysfunction. N Engl J Med. 2000;343(20):1445–53.
7. Halliday BP, et al. Outcome in dilated cardiomyopathy related to the extent, location, and pattern of late gadolinium enhancement. JACC Cardiovasc Imaging 2019;12(8 pt 2):1645–55.
8. Austin BA, Tang WHW, Rodriquez ER, et al. Delayed hyper-enhancement magnetic resonance imaging pro-

vides incremental diagnostic and prognostic utility in suspected cardiac amyloidosis. JACC Cardiovasc Imaging. 2009;2(12):1369–77.
9. Kiaos A, Daskalopoulos GN, Kamperidis V, et al. Quantitative late gadolinium enhancement cardiac magnetic resonance and sudden death in hypertrophic cardiomyopathy: a meta-analysis. JACC Cardiovasc Imaging. 2023;16:S1936-878X(23)00346-7.
10. Moon J, Messroghli DR, Kellman P, et al. Myocardial T1 mapping and extracellular volume quantification: a Society for Cardiovascular Magnetic Resonance (SCMR) and CMR Working Group of the European Society of Cardiology consensus statement. J Cardiovasc Magn Reson. 2013;15:92. https://doi.org/10.1186/1532-429X-15-92.
11. Ferreira VM, Schulz-Menger J, Holmvang G, et al. Cardiovascular magnetic resonance in nonischemic myocardial inflammation: expert recommendations. J Am Coll Cardiol. 2018;72(24):3158–76. https://doi.org/10.1016/j.jacc.2018.09.072.
12. Kramer CM, Appelbaum E, Desai MY, et al. Hypertrophic cardiomyopathy registry: the rationale and design of an international, observational study of hypertrophic cardiomyopathy. Am Heart J. 2015;170(2):223–30. https://doi.org/10.1016/j.ahj.2015.05.013.
13. Hundley WG, Bluemke DA, Finn JP, et al. ACCF/ACR/AHA/NASCI/SCMR 2010 expert consensus document on cardiovascular magnetic resonance: a report of the American College of Cardiology Foundation task force on expert consensus documents. J Am Coll Cardiol. 2010;55(23):2614–62. https://doi.org/10.1016/j.jacc.2009.11.011.
14. Friedrich MG, Sechtem U, Schulz-Menger J, et al. Cardiovascular magnetic resonance in myocarditis: a JACC white paper. J Am Coll Cardiol. 2009;53(17):1475–87. https://doi.org/10.1016/j.jacc.2009.02.007.
15. Nandalur KR, Dwamena BA, Choudhri AF, Nandalur MR, Carlos RC. Diagnostic performance of stress cardiac magnetic resonance imaging in the detection of coronary artery disease: a meta-analysis. J Am Coll Cardiol. 2007;50(14):1343–53. https://doi.org/10.1016/j.jacc.2007.06.030.
16. Ferreira VM, Piechnik SK, Dall'Armellina E, et al. Native T1-mapping detects the location, extent and patterns of acute myocarditis without the need for gadolinium contrast agents. J Cardiovasc Magn Reson. 2014;16:36. https://doi.org/10.1186/s12968-014-0036-2.
17. Giri S, Chung YC, Merchant A, et al. T2 quantification for improved detection of myocardial edema. J Cardiovasc Magn Reson. 2009;11:56. https://doi.org/10.1186/1532-429X-11-56.
18. Anderson LJ, Holden S, Davis B, et al. Cardiovascular T2-star (T2*) magnetic resonance for the early diagnosis of myocardial iron overload. Eur Heart J. 2001;22(23):2171–9. https://doi.org/10.1053/euhj.2001.2822.
19. Cruz G, Jaubert O, Botnar RM, Prieto C. Cardiac magnetic resonance fingerprinting: technical developments and initial clinical validation. Curr Cardiol Rep. 2019;21(9):91.
20. Rashid U, Cruz G, Seiberlich N, Hamilton JI. Cardiac MR fingerprinting: overview, technical developments, and applications. J Magn Reson Imaging. 2023;60(5):1753–73.

10 Quantitative MRI of Valvular Heart Disease

Christopher Francois

Introduction

Although severe valvular hear disease (VHD) is relatively uncommon, with a prevalence of 2.5% in the general US, the prevalence increases substantially with age, especially after 75 years. The detection of a murmur on auscultation is the most common indication for imaging of the cardiac valves. This is usually done with transthoracic echocardiography (TTE) and transesophageal echocardiography (TEE). VHD can be an incidental finding on imaging done for other reasons. Cardiac magnetic resonance (CMR) imaging is increasingly used to evaluate acquired and congenital VHD. Although TTE remains the primary imaging modality used in patients with VHD, CMR is indicated when echocardiography quality is insufficient or to obtain complementary information. Advantages of CMR relative to echocardiography include less impact of patient anatomy on image quality, less variability in quantitative parameters related to performer, and the ability to measure flow volumes directly. International guidelines recommend CMR or have indicated that CMR is appropriate for evaluating valvular morphology when incompletely imaged by echocardiography, assessment of pulmonary valve disease, and measurement of transvalvular flow when echocardiography results are uncertain.

This chapter will (A) review the CMR sequences used for evaluating VHD and (B) describe the application of CMR in a variety of congenital and acquired VHD.

C. Francois (✉)
Department of Radiology, Mayo Clinic, Rochester, MN, USA
e-mail: Francois.Christopher@mayo.edu

Sequences

CMR of the cardiac valves is performed with flow sensitive and cineangiography (CINE) sequences. Flow sensitive CMR is performed using phase contrast velocity-encoded techniques (Fig. 10.1). The initial phase contrast sequences developed over 40 years ago have been improved to optimize sensitivity to flow and minimize artifacts. Briefly, in a constant magnetic field, the phases of spinning protons are the same. However, spinning protons exposed to a gradient will precess with different phases, depending on their location within the magnetic field gradient. Moving protons with accumulate a phase shift relative to the stationary protons in adjacent tissues. The difference in phases between moving and adjacent stationary protons is proportional to the velocity of the moving protons.

The most widely used flow CMR sequence is a two-dimensional, one-directional velocity encoded acquisition (2D flow MRI). Two-dimensional flow can be set up to be sensitive to flow through the plane of the acquisition or sensi-

R. Gill, P. Rajiah (eds.), *Quantitative Imaging in the Thorax*,
https://doi.org/10.1007/978-3-032-14103-3_10

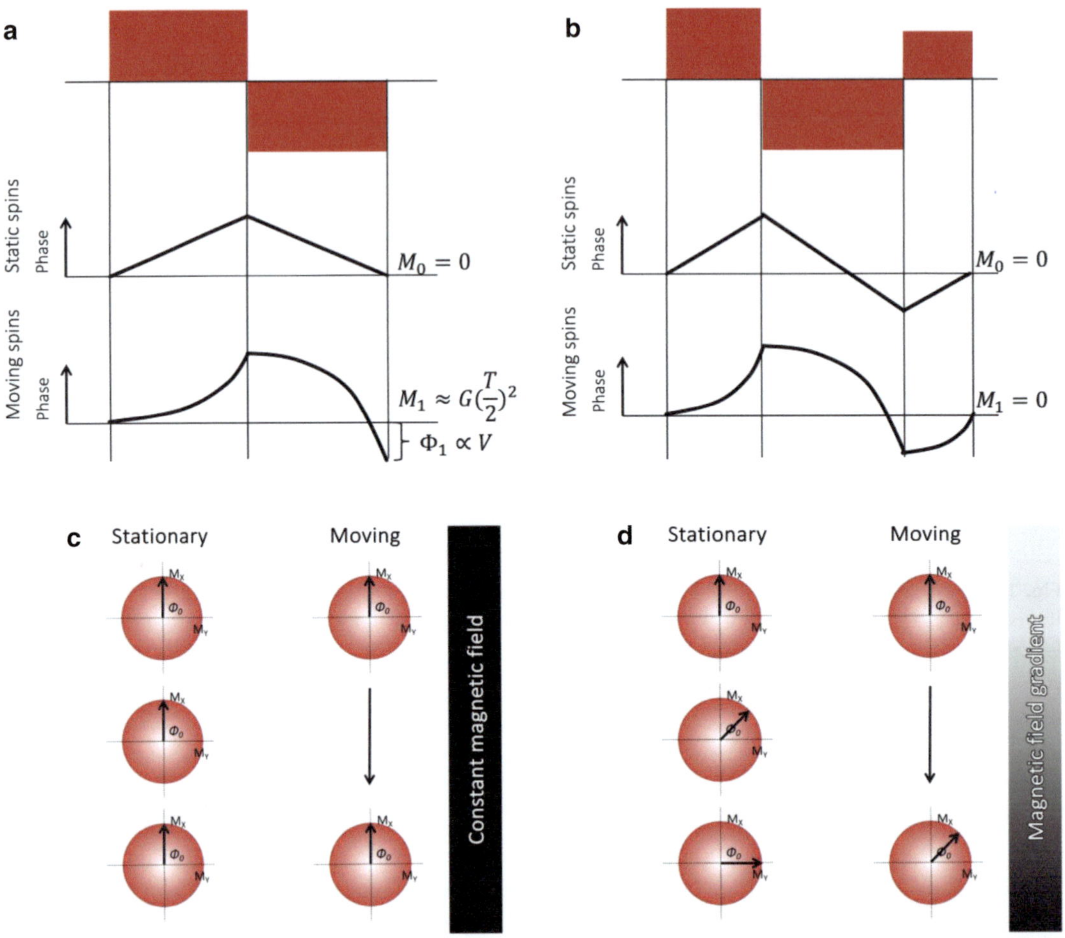

Fig. 10.1 (**a**) Bipolar gradient without flow compensation. The residual phase accumulated after the bipolar gradient by the moving spins is used to calculate the phase difference (Φ). Φ is proportional to the velocity of the moving spins. (**b**) Bipolar gradient with flow compensation. When flow compensation is used, static and moving spins have zero residual phase difference at the end of the bipolar gradient. (**c**) Static and moving tissues all have the same phase, Φ, when in constant magnetic field. (**d**) In a magnetic field gradient, static and moving tissues have different phases, Φ, depending upon their location in the field gradient. The difference in phase between the moving spin and the adjacent stationary spin is proportional to the velocity that the spin is moving

tive to flow within the plane of the acquisition (Fig. 10.2). Within the last 15 years, three-dimensional, three-directional velocity-encoded (4D flow MRI) sequences (Fig. 10.3) have been developed and are now commercially available on all types of MRI scanners. With commercially available software, it is possible to measure flow anywhere within the volume, making measurements orthogonal to the direction of flow (Fig. 10.4). A complete discussion of the sources of error in 2D and 4D flow CMR is beyond the scope of this chapter. However, it is important to be aware of the more common types of error. Errors in flow CMR are frequently related to imperfections in the MR scanner and often referred to as “background errors”—concomitant gradients, eddy currents, and magnetic field non-linearity. These errors can be minimized by optimizing the sequence parameters and at the time of image reconstruction and analysis.

For flow CMR, the velocity encoding should be adjusted to avoid velocity aliasing. The velocity encoding can be determined prior to CMR based on peak velocities detected with echocar-

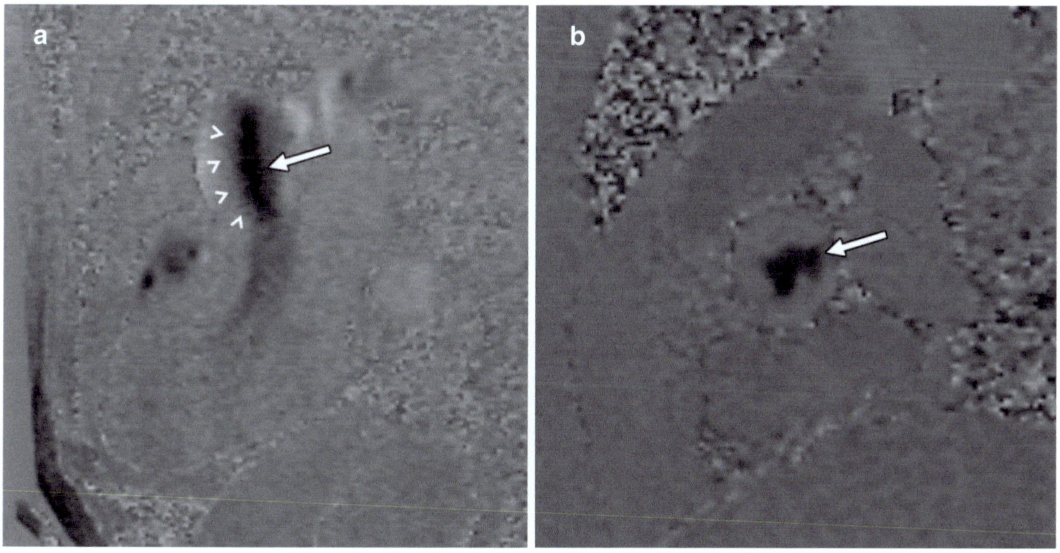

Fig. 10.2 (**a**) Two-dimensional PC CMR with in-plane flow-encoding. In this patient with bicuspid aortic valve, flow-encoding is in the superior-inferior direction such that the aortic valve stenosis jet is clearly visible (arrowheads). Subsequently, the through-plane flow MRI can be set up through the vena contracta (arrow). (**b**) Two-dimensional PC CMR with through-plane flow-encoding. In this flow image acquired perpendicular to the aortic valve (arrow), the signal intensity is proportional to the flow through the imaging plane

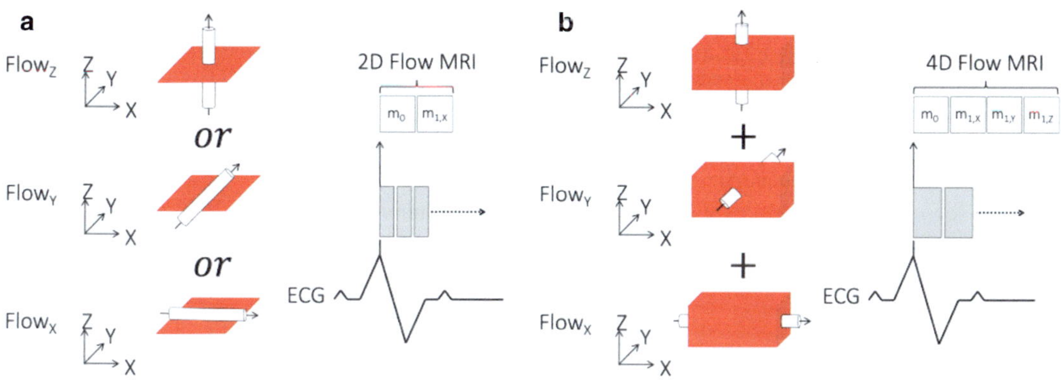

Fig. 10.3 (**a**) Two-dimensional flow MRI is a two-dimensional, cardiac-gated acquisition that is sensitive to flow in one direction and can be in plane or through plane. (**b**) Four-dimensional flow MRI is a three-dimensional, cardiac-gated acquisition that is sensitive to flow in all directions

diography. With 2D flow CMR, if aliasing is detected, the scan should be repeated with higher velocity encoding until the aliasing is no longer present (Fig. 10.5). To measure the peak velocity with flow CMR, the measurements should be done at the vena contracta. With 2D flow CMR, the vena contracta can be determined by quantifying flow velocities on multiple contiguous through-plane 2D flow images or using an in-plane 2D flow acquisition prior to acquiring the through-plane 2D flow. With 4D flow, the vena contracta can be easily identified by adjust the flow color scale to higher velocities until it becomes apparent (Fig. 10.6).

The Society for Cardiovascular Magnetic Resonance (SCMR) recommended sequence parameters for 2D flow MRI are summarized in Table 10.1, and the SCMR recommended sequence parameters for 4D flow MRI are summarized in Table 10.2.

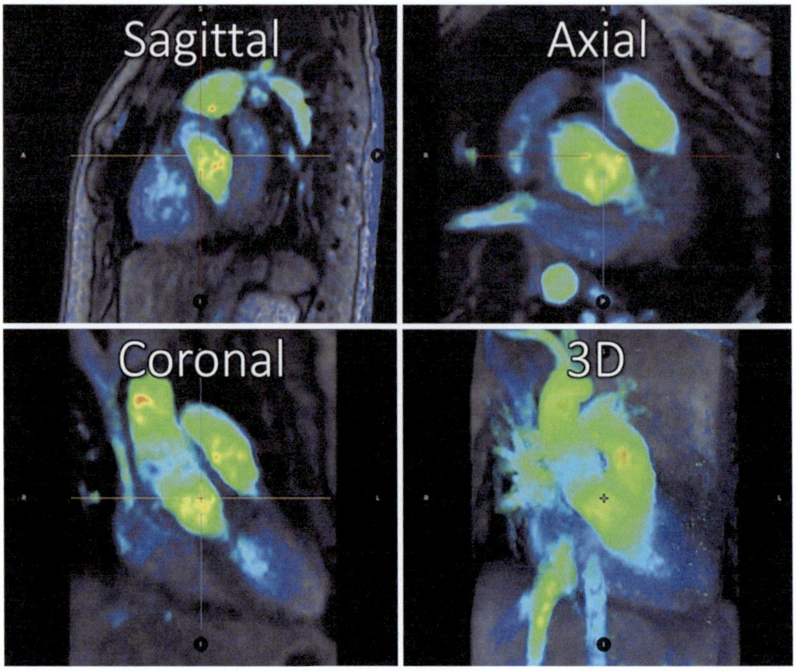

Fig. 10.4 Four-dimensional flow MRI is a three-dimensional, ECG-gated acquisition that is sensitive to flow in all directions. With commercially available software, it is possible to measure flow anywhere within the volume, making measurements orthogonal to the direction of flow

CINE sequences are primarily used to assess the morphology of the valves. CINE sequences are used to measure the size of the valvular annulus. CINE sequences are also used to quantify the severity of valvular stenosis or regurgitation by planimetry, measuring the opening area or the valvular coaptation gap, respectively. A detailed description of the CINE sequences used for VHD have been described in other chapters in this book. CINE-balanced steady-state free precession (bSSFP) is the primary sequence for assessment of valve morphology (Fig. 10.7). CINE-spoiled gradient recalled echo (GRE) can also be used when there is artifact on the CINE bSSFP images (Fig. 10.8). Examples of artifacts on the CINE bSSFP images include spin dephasing from turbulent flow in the setting of severe stenosis or regurgitation and susceptibility artifact from metal from implanted devices.

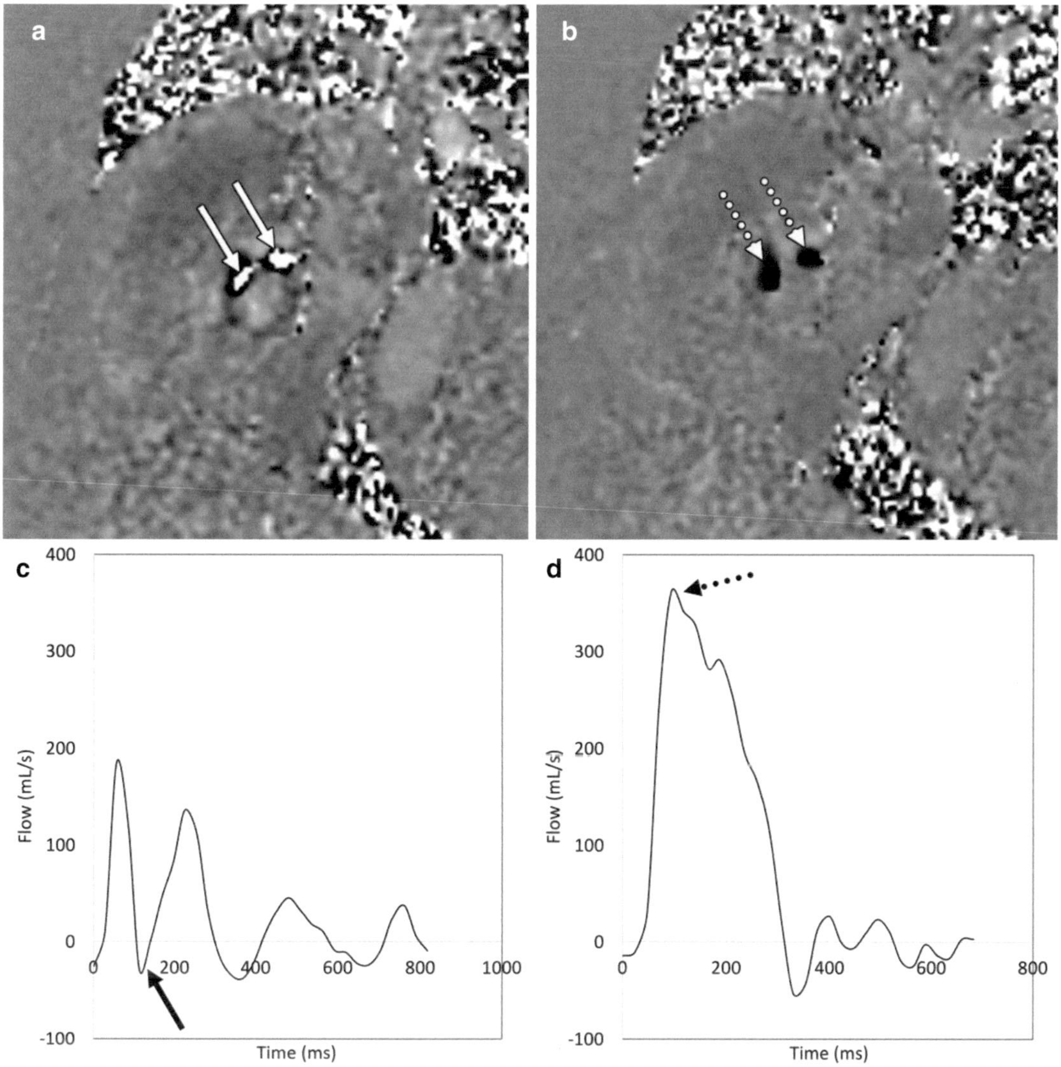

Fig. 10.5 A 52-year-old patient with bicuspid aortic valve and severe aortic valve stenosis. (**a**) Two-dimensional flow MRI acquired with VENC of 300 cm/s reveals substantial aliasing (arrow). (**b**) Two-dimensional flow MRI acquired with VENC of 500 cm/s does not have any aliasing (dotted arrow). (**c**) Flow-time curve for 2D flow MRI acquired with VENC of 300 cm/s has an inverted systolic peak (arrow) due to aliasing. (**d**) Flow-time curve for 2D flow MRI acquired with VENC of 500 cm/s has a normal systolic peak (dotted arrow). The peak systolic velocity was 4.4 m/s, compatible with severe aortic valve stenosis

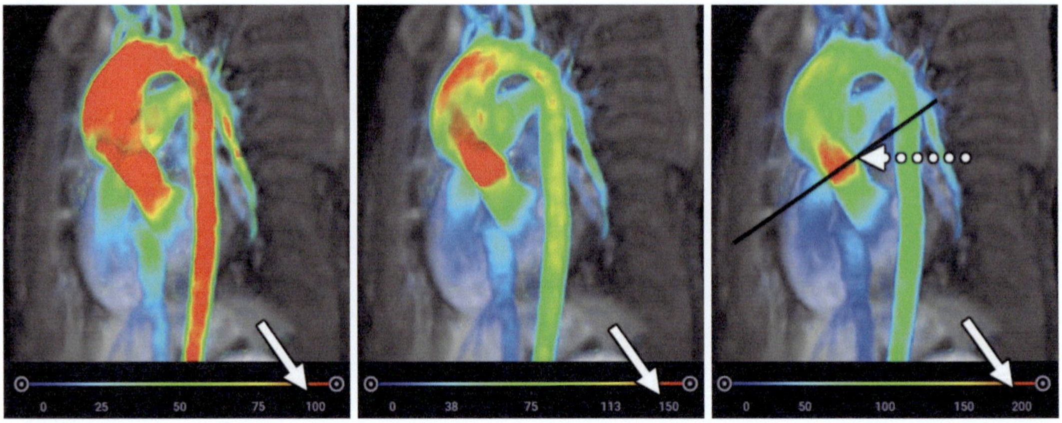

Fig. 10.6 Four-dimensional flow MRI in a patient with bicuspid aortic valve and mild aortic valve stenosis. The color scale is adjusted (arrows) to identify the vena contracta (dotted arrow). Measurement of the peak velocity is performed at the level of the vena contracta (line)

Table 10.1 SCMR recommendations for 2D flow MRI

2D flow MRI parameter	Recommendation(s)	Comment(s)
Field strength	1.5 T or 3.0 T	
In-plane resolution (mm)	1.0–2.0	Adjusted for patient size Should be ≤10% of the diameter of the region of interest
Slice thickness (mm)	5–8	Adjusted for patient size
Reconstructed phases per cardiac cycle	25–30	
Velocity encoding (cm/s)	200	Aortic and pulmonary valves (increase as necessary to avoid aliasing)
	150	Mitral and tricuspid valves
Velocity encoding direction	Through-plane	Flow velocity and volume quantification Orthogonal to the direction of the flow with the valve of interest in the center of the field of view and isocenter of the magnet
	In-plane	Detection of flow direction
Cardiac gating	Retrospective	Prospective can be used if retrospective gating is unavailable
Respiratory motion compensation	Breath-hold	Appropriate for mitral and aortic valves
	Free-breathing, multiple averages	Appropriate tricuspid and pulmonary valves because they are susceptible to respiratory variation due to changes in intrathoracic pressures

Table 10.2 SCMR recommendations for 4D flow MRI

4D flow MRI parameter	Recommendation(s)	Comment(s)
Acquired spatial resolution		
Whole heart (adult)	2.5 mm^3 (≤3.0 mm^3)	Balance between accuracy and scan time
Great vessels (adult)	2.0 mm^3 (≤3.0 mm^3)	
Whole heart (pediatric)	2.0 mm^3 (≤2.5 mm^3)	
Great vessels (adult)	1.5 mm^3 (≤2.0 mm^3)	
Neonates	0.75–1 mm^3 (≤1.5 mm^3)	
Acquired temporal resolution	30 ms (≤50 ms)	Balance between accuracy and scan time
Velocity encoding limit	Maximum expected velocity	10–25% higher than expected maximum velocity

(continued)

Table 10.2 (continued)

4D flow MRI parameter	Recommendation(s)	Comment(s)
Respiratory motion compensation	Optional	
Cardiac motion compensation	Retrospective cardiac gating	Prospective cardiac triggering can be used in patients with arrhythmia
Flip angle (without contrast)	7°	
Flip angle (after contrast)	12–25°	Consider lowering flip angle if acquiring 4D flow MRI late after giving contrast
Contrast administration		Consider in neonates, dissections, or other challenging cases to improve contrast

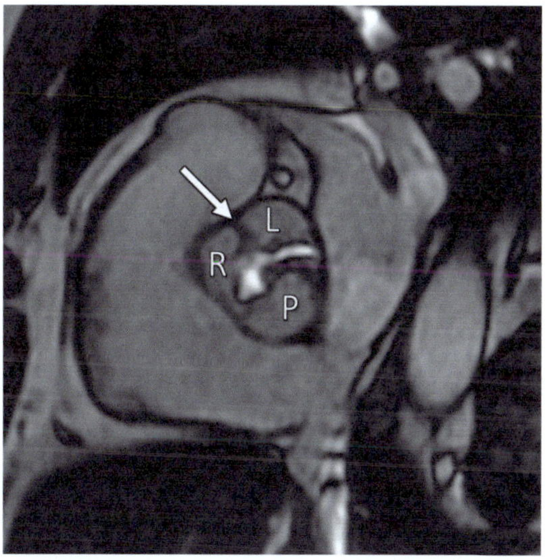

Fig. 10.7 A 42-year-old with bicuspid aortic valve. Balanced steady-state-free precession image shows the morphology of the aortic valve, with fusion of the right (R) and left (L) leaflets and a visible raphe (arrow). P posterior leaflet

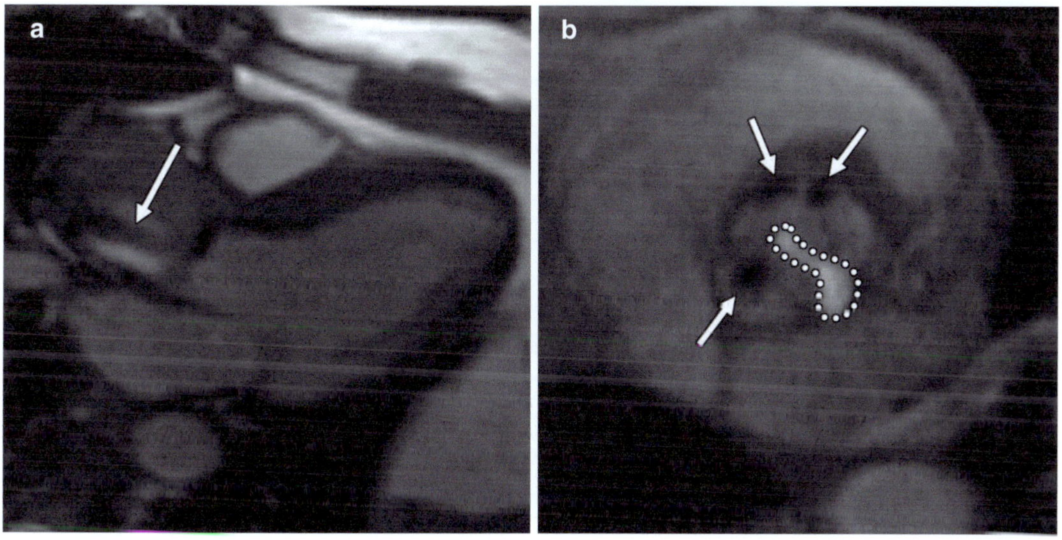

Fig. 10.8 A 71-year-old with severe aortic valve stenosis. (**a**) The spin dephasing jet (arrow) is due to turbulent flow. The severity of stenosis cannot be accurately quantified based on the appearance of the jet on CINE bSSFP images. (**b**) Gradient recalled echo image through the aortic valve shows a small valve opening area (dashed line). The aortic valve leaflet calcifications appear as signal voids on these images (arrows)

Congenital Valve Diseases

Normal and congenital valve morphology is readily assessed by CMR using CINE sequences. When evaluating the cardiac valves, it is essential to assess their thickness and morphology. Congenital abnormalities of the valves can be due to an abnormal number of leaflets or abnormal morphology of the valve leaflets (Fig. 10.9). In extreme cases, the valve can be severely hypoplastic or atretic (Fig. 10.10).

The most common congenital valve abnormality is bicuspid aortic valve (BAV), occurring in approximately 1–2% of the general population. The prevalence of BAV in patients with coarctation of the aorta (50–75%) (Fig. 10.11), Turner syndrome (30%), and William syndrome (30%) is higher than in the general population. BAV can lead to thickening of the aortic valve leaflets, which restricts their mobility and leads to aortic stenosis. BAV is frequently associated with aortic root and ascending aorta enlargement.

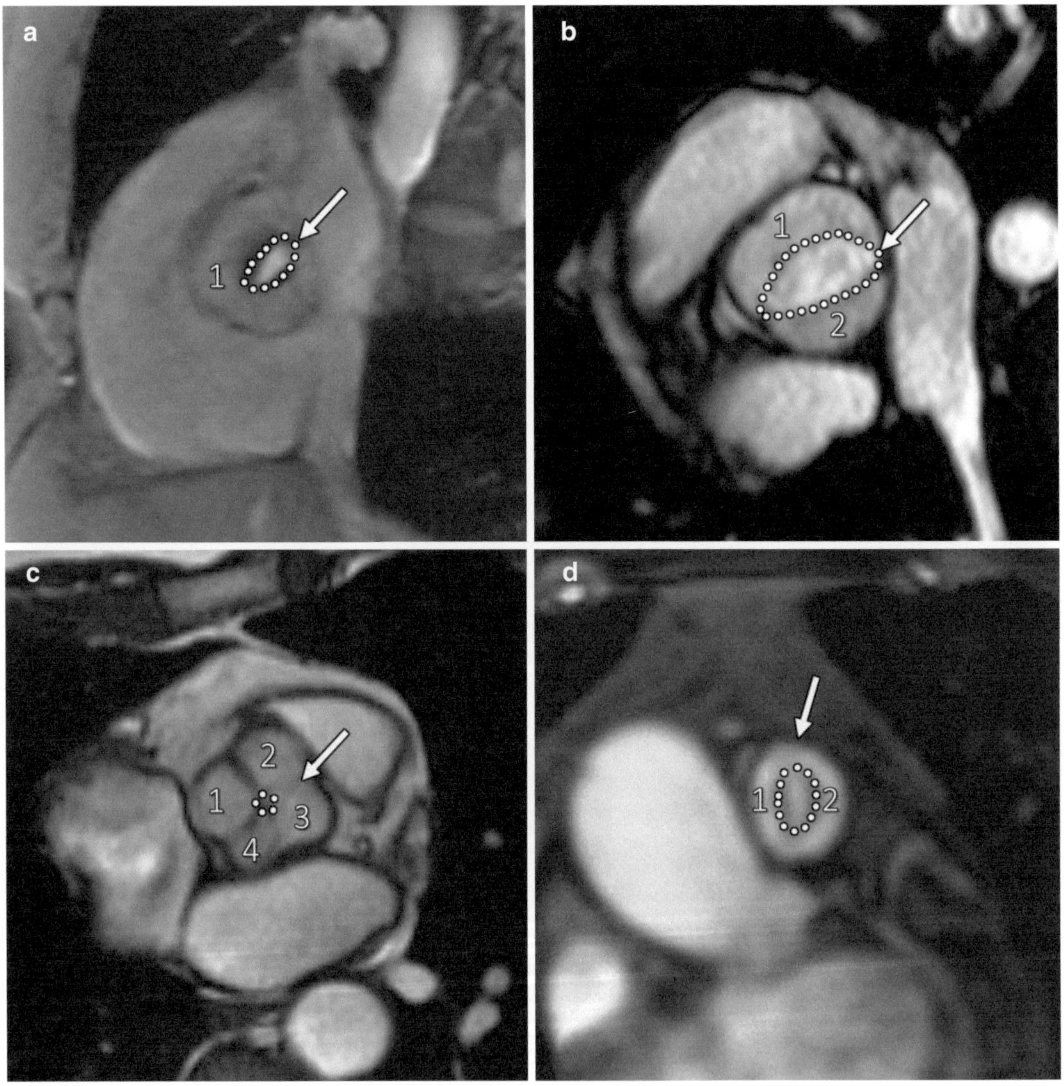

Fig. 10.9 Congenital valve abnormalities due to abnormal number of leaflets. (**a**) Unicuspid aortic valve (arrow) with one leaflet and small opening area (dotted line). (**b**) Bicuspid aortic valve (arrow) with two leaflets and normal opening area (dotted line). (**c**) Quadricuspid aortic valve (arrow) with four leaflets and small coaptation gap (dotted line). (**d**) Bicuspid pulmonary valve (arrow) with two leaflets and small opening area (dotted line)

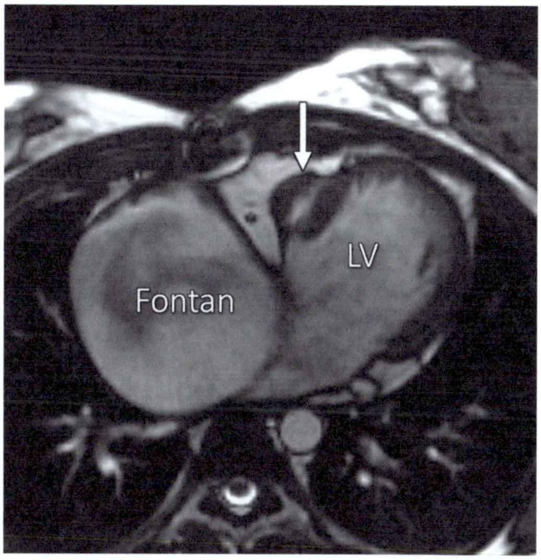

Fig. 10.10 A 34-year-old with tricuspid valve atresia and intra-cardiac Fontan palliation. The right ventricle (arrow) is severely hypoplastic. LV left ventricle

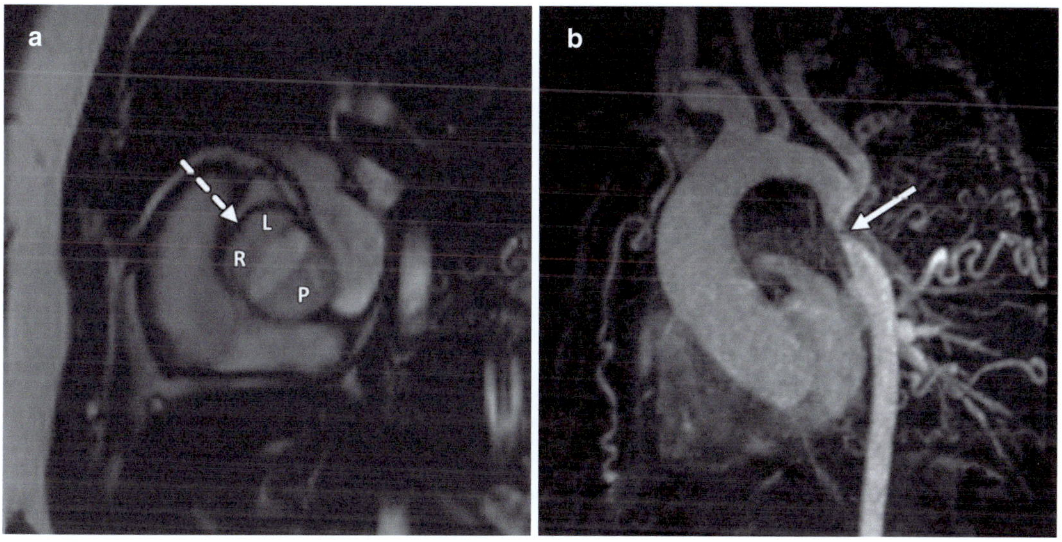

Fig. 10.11 A 22-year-old with bicuspid aortic valve. (**a**) The right and left leaflets are fused and a raphe is visible (dashed arrow). (**b**) The patient also has aortic coarctation (arrow)

As a result, magnetic resonance angiography of the thoracic aorta (Fig. 10.12) should be performed to measure the size of the aortic root and ascending aorta. CINE bSSFP and GRE sequences can be used to evaluate the type of BAV. When evaluating BAV, it is important to determine if there are two or three cusps. In patients with three cusps, the BAV is due to fusion of two of the three leaflets. The fused leaflets may be associated with a raphe.

Congenital abnormalities of the pulmonary, mitral, and tricuspid valves are less common. Ebstein anomaly, due to failure of the septal leaflet of the tricuspid valve to delaminate results in apical displacement of the posterior and septal leaflets of the tricuspid valve (Fig. 10.13). Ebstein anomaly is usually sporadic, and the prevalence is approximately 2–7/100,000 live births. Ebstein anomaly is typically defined as ≥8 mm/m^2 apical displacement of the tricuspid valve relative to the mitral valve. Tricuspid valve regurgitation is present in almost all patients with Ebstein anomaly.

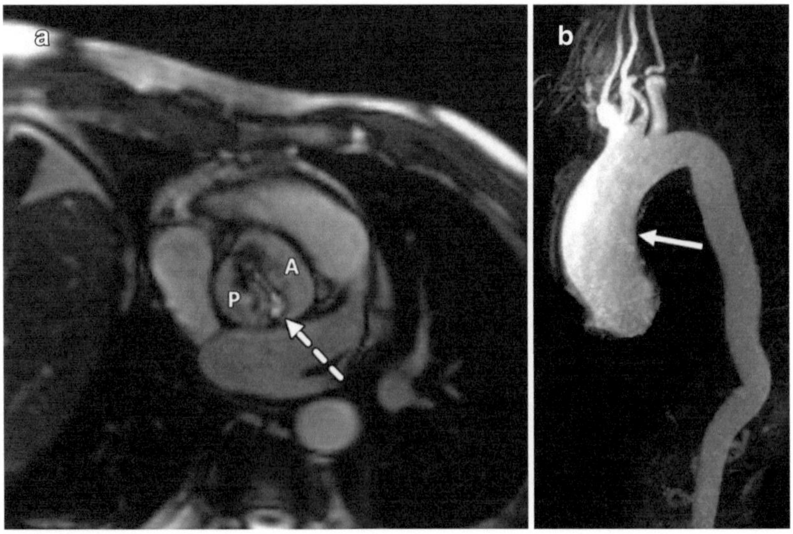

Fig. 10.12 A 42-year-old with bicuspid aortic valve. (**a**) The morphology is of a bicuspid aortic valve with anterior (A) and posterior (P) leaflets. The valve opening area is severely restricted (dashed arrow), compatible with severely aortic valve stenosis. (**b**) Contrast-enhanced magnetic resonance angiography confirmed the presence of an ascending aorta is aneurysm (arrow)

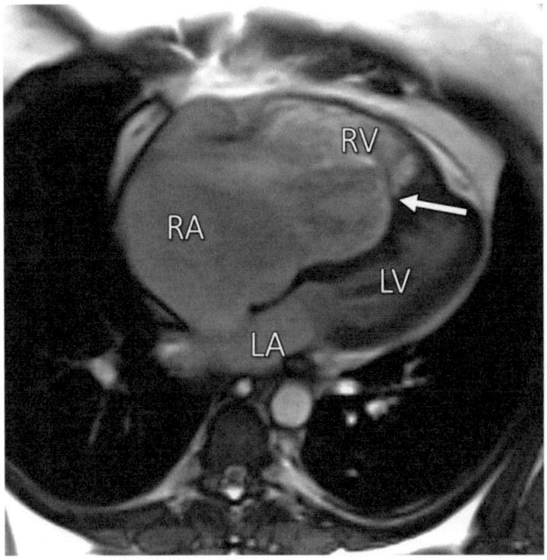

Fig. 10.13 A 30-year-old with Ebstein anomaly. The septal leaflet of the tricuspid valve is apically displaced (arrow) due to incomplete delamination. The right atrium (RA) is severely enlarged. RV right ventricle, LA left atrium, LV left ventricle

Valve Stenosis

Valve stenosis severity can be quantified by measuring the valve opening area by planimetry on CINE images or by measuring the maximum velocity on flow CMR. For planimetry, it is essential to use a thinner slice thickness (≤5 mm) to avoid volume averaging and acquire multiple contiguous CINE slices through the valve of interest to ensure the minimum opening area is included (Fig. 10.14). The valve opening area measured by CMR may differ slightly than the functional area estimated by transthoracic echocardiography using the continuity equation but correlates very well with the area measured by transesophageal echocardiography. In patients with severe valve stenosis, spin dephasing artifact can interfere with the visualization of the valve leaflet tips on CINE bSSFP images. In these cases, CINE GRE should be used.

TTE is routinely performed in patients with aortic valve stenosis (AS) and remains the clinical reference standard for grading AS severity. Limitations of TTE include accuracy in patients with poor acoustic windows, inaccurate aortic annulus diameter measurements, assessment of subvalvular flow acceleration, and inaccuracies in patients with low flow severe aortic valve stenosis. CMR plays an important role in evaluating patients with suboptimal TTE or discordant findings on echocardiography. CMR assessment of AS severity is done with direct planimetry and flow CMR (Fig. 10.15). CMR-based planimetry of the aortic valve area is reproducible with low inter- and intra-reader variability. It is important to keep in mind that with CMR, the aortic valve opening area is measured directly, whereas with echocardiography and invasive catheter angiog-

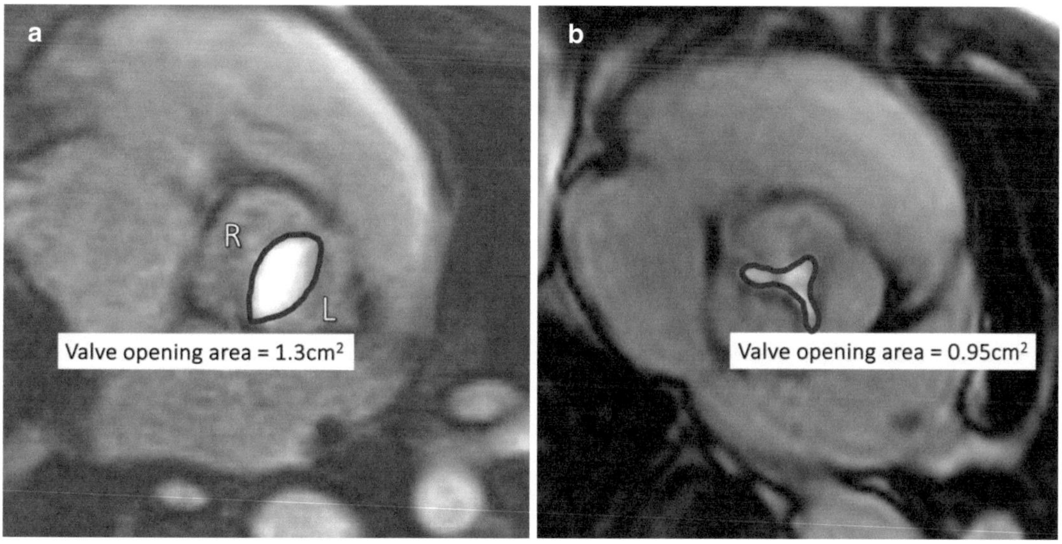

Fig. 10.14 (**a**) A 20-year-old with bicuspid aortic valve with right (R) and left (L) leaflets. The valve opening area (blue line) can be measured by direct planimetry. A valve opening area of 1.3 cm^2 is compatible with moderate aortic valve stenosis. (**b**) A 68-year-old with tricuspid aortic valve and severe aortic valve stenosis based on a valve opening area (blue line) of 0.94 cm^2

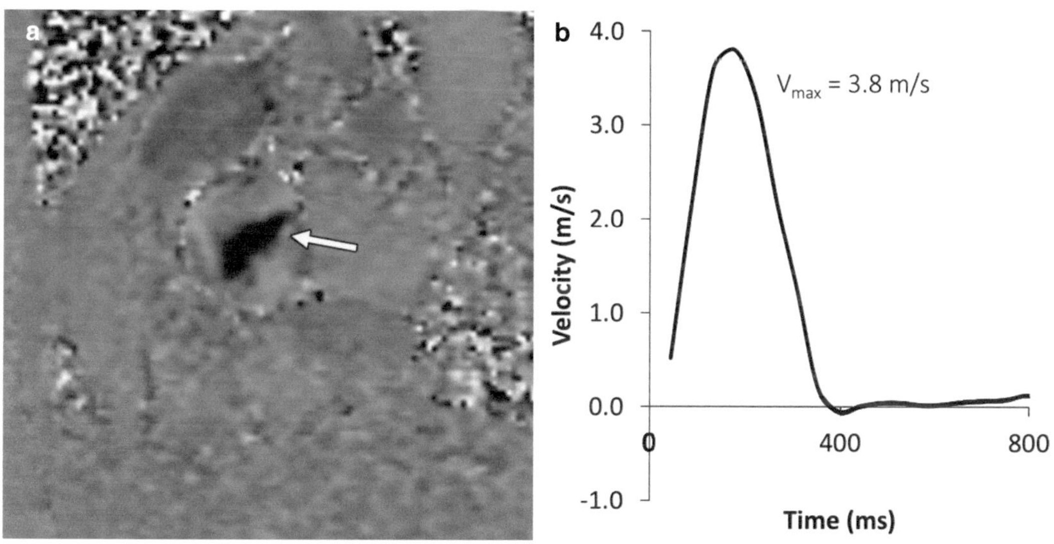

Fig. 10.15 A 24-year-old with bicuspid aortic valve (arrow). Two-dimensional flow MRI through the aortic valve (A) revealed a peak velocity of 3.8 m/s (B), compatible with moderate aortic valve stenosis

raphy, the continuity equation is used to measure the functional orifice area. In general, the aortic valve opening area by direct planimetry is larger than the functional area measured by the continuity equation. Studies have shown that aortic valve area by CMR planimetry <1 cm^2 correlates very well with severe AS by other methods. Similarly, severe AS is highly unlikely to be present when the aortic valve area by CMR planimetry is >1.5 cm^2. Therefore, flow CMR plays an important complementary role in grading AS severity. Two-dimensional flow MRI can be used to estimate the functional aortic valve area by the continuity equation:

$$\text{Functional valve area}\left(\text{FVA}\right)=\text{ventricular ouflow tract}\left(\text{VOT}\right)\text{area}\left(\frac{V_{\text{max,VOT}}}{V_{\text{max,Valve}}}\right)$$

in the same way as echocardiography. In general, the peak velocities by two-dimensional flow MRI are lower than those obtained by echocardiography. CMR is also used in patients with AS to evaluate the impact of AS on the myocardium with tissue characterization sequences. The presence of replacement and diffuse fibrosis can be imaged using late gadolinium enhancement and T1 mapping sequences, respectively. The presence and extent of replacement and diffuse fibrosis in patients with AS have been found to be of significant prognostic value.

Pulmonary valve stenosis (PS) is most often congenital, accounts for approximately 8% of all congenital heart defects, and occurs in approximately 1 in 2000 live births. PS is most often due to a dome-shaped pulmonary valve with decreased opening area. Dysplastic pulmonary valve leaflets are a less common cause of PS. PS is frequently a part of other complex CHD, especially tetralogy of Fallot. Acquired causes of PS include rheumatic and carcinoid valve disease. PS is typically initially evaluated with TTE. However, given the relatively poor acoustic window for imaging the pulmonary valve with echocardiography, CMR is essential for evaluating the etiology and severity of PS. The assessment of PS severity by CMR includes measurement of the opening area by planimetry and the peak velocity from flow CMR (Fig. 10.16). The measurement of right ventricular size and function in patients with PS also is a role for CMR.

Rheumatic heart disease remains a common cause of valvular stenosis worldwide, particularly mitral stenosis (MS). TTE is the most widely used method of evaluating MS through calculation of the mitral valve area by direct planimetry, Doppler pressure halftime, and the continuity equation. If TTE is inadequate, TEE is frequently performed to assess the degree of MS. CMR-based measurements of mitral valve area by planimetry are in strong agreement with those made by TEE with negligible mean differences. An advantage of measuring the mitral valve area by planimetry, rather than using the

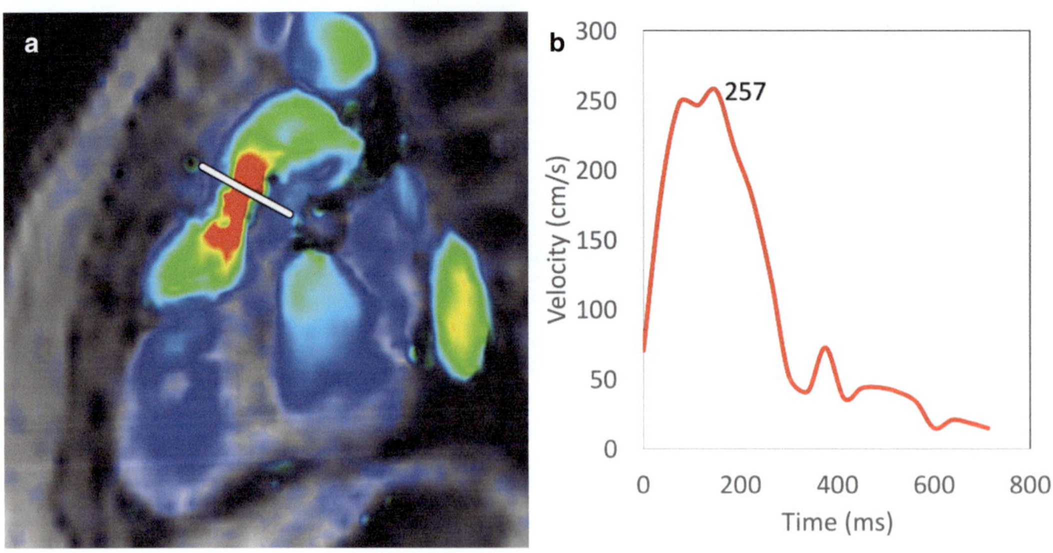

Fig. 10.16 A 10-year-old with congenital pulmonary stenosis. (**a**) Four-dimensional flow MRI revealed flow acceleration through the pulmonary valve. Flow was analyzed at the vena contracta (line). (**b**) Flow velocity-time curve shows a maximum velocity of 257 cm/s, compatible with mild pulmonary valve stenosis

continuity equation, is that it is not affected by heart rate, cardiac output, presence of other valvular heart disease, or other hemodynamic factors. Flow MRI can measure the peak velocity through the mitral valve. Differences between 2D flow MRI and TTE peak velocities are approximately 0.1 m/s. In patients with MS, it is essential to evaluate the effect of MS on the left ventricle and left atrium. In patients with MS, the left ventricle end-systolic volume index and mass index and the left atrial volume index tend to be greater than in healthy controls, and the left ventricle ejection fraction and left atrial emptying fraction are reduced. Abnormal mid-myocardial late gadolinium enhancement can occur in the ventricular septum, in almost 80% of patients at the insertion of the right ventricle.

Tricuspid valve stenosis (TS) is very rare and is usually related to rheumatic heart disease. Other, less common, causes of TS include systemic diseases such as carcinoid syndrome, systemic lupus erythematosus, endomyocardial fibrosis, and antiphospholipid syndrome. In patients with TS, the tricuspid valve leaflets are thickened with restricted mobility. TS is considered severe when the tricuspid valve opening area is <1 cm^2, and the pressure gradient across the tricuspid valve is >5 mmHg. Moderate or severe right atrial enlargement and inferior vena cava dilation are also signs of severe TS.

Suggested CMR criteria for valve stenosis severity are summarized in Table 10.3.

Valve Regurgitation

The degree of aortic (AR) and pulmonary (PR) regurgitation is graded based on the amount of backward flow during diastole is measured relative to the forward flow in systole (Fig. 10.17). This is done with direct measurements of flow through the aortic and pulmonary valves, respectively. When interpreting the degree of pulmonary regurgitation based on the regurgitation fraction, it is important to consider the effects of right ventricular preload on volumes. Therefore, reporting regurgitation volume indexed to body surface area should be considered as well. In patients with AR, the measurement of flow in the descending aorta should also be included because the presence of holodiastolic flow reversal in the descending aorta is another marker of severe AR (Fig. 10.18).

The degree of mitral (MR) and tricuspid (TR) regurgitation is graded based on the amount of backward flow during ventricular systole is measured relative to the forward flow in systole. An advantage of CMR relative to echocardiography in the assessment of MR and TR is that it is not affected by the shape or direction of the regurgitation jet. CMR-derived MR severity has been shown to be a better predictor of left ventricular reverse remodeling than echocardiography derived MR severity. With 2D flow MRI, it is recommended that this be done indirectly by comparing forward flow

Table 10.3 Suggested criteria for grading valve stenosis with CMR

Valve	Stenosis severity	Planimetry area (cm^2)	Flow velocity (m^2)
Aortic	Normal	>2	<2
	Mild	1.5–2	2–3
	Moderate	1–1.5	3–4
	Severe	<1	>4
Pulmonic	Normal	>2	<1–2
	Mild	1.5–2	2–3
	Moderate	1–1.5	3–4
	Severe	<1	>4
Mitral	Normal	>2	
	Mild	1.5–2	
	Moderate	1–1.5	
	Severe	<1	
Tricuspid	Severe	<1	>1.1

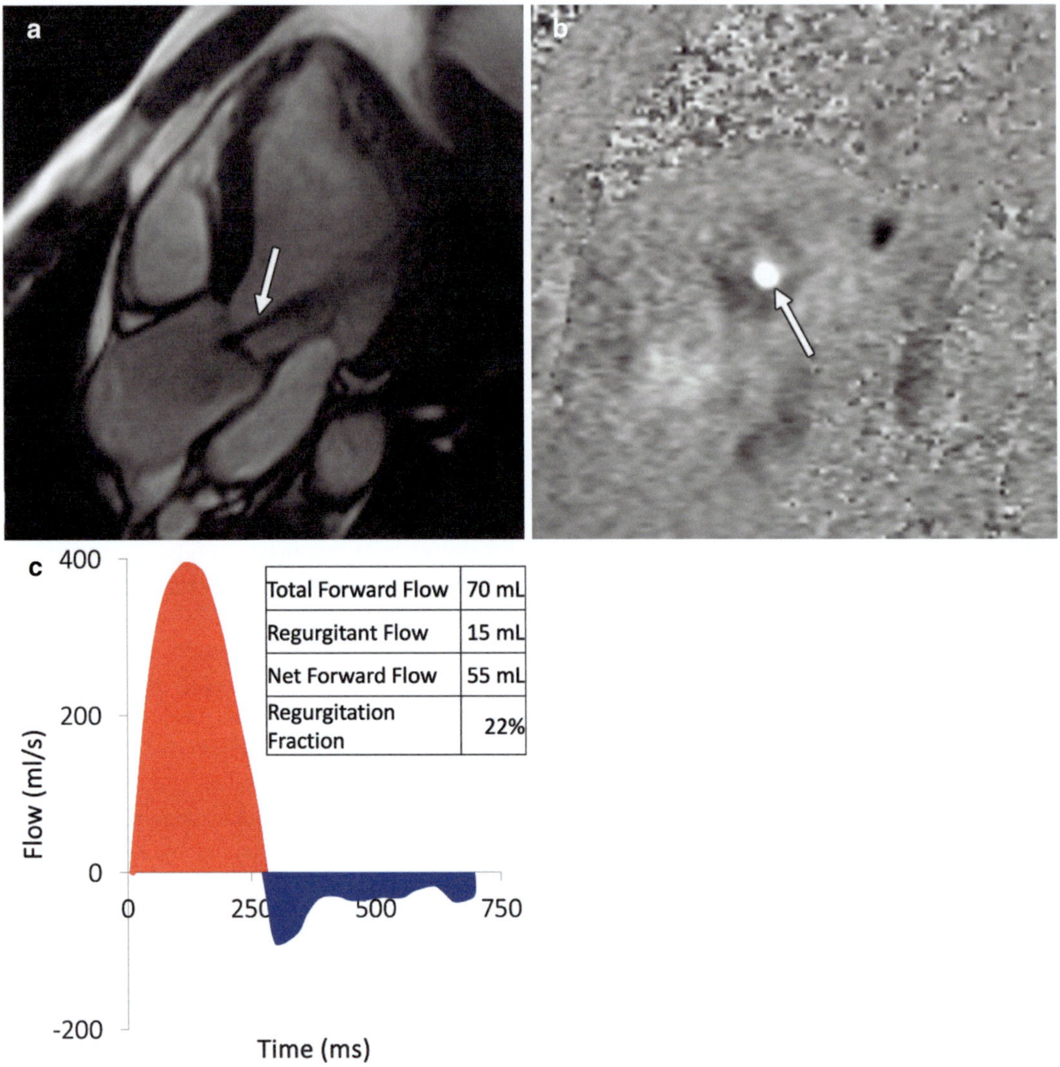

Fig. 10.17 A 43-year-old with aortic valve regurgitation. (**a**) The aortic regurgitation jet (arrow) is apparent on the three-chamber balanced steady-state free precession image. (**b**) Two-dimensional flow MRI acquired below the aortic valve plane, perpendicular to the aortic regurgitation jet is used to quantify the amount of aortic valve regurgitation (arrow). (**c**) The degree of aortic valve regurgitation is calculated from the flow-time curve. The regurgitant flow (red) is divided by the forward flow (blue) to calculate the regurgitation fraction

through the aortic and pulmonary valves to the left and right ventricular stroke volumes by CINE volumetry, respectively (Fig. 10.19). Direct measurements of forward and backward flow through the atrioventricular valves with 2D flow MRI is unreliable due to through-plane motion of the mitral and tricuspid valves. With 4D flow MRI, direct measurements of atrioventricular valve flow can be reliably quantified using valve-tracking software.

In patients with primary MR, multiple thin-slice (≤6 mm) CINE bSSFP acquisitions through the mitral valve should be acquired to assess for mitral valve prolapse and mitral annular disjunction. If mitral annular disjunction is present, the separation of the mitral annulus insertion from the muscular

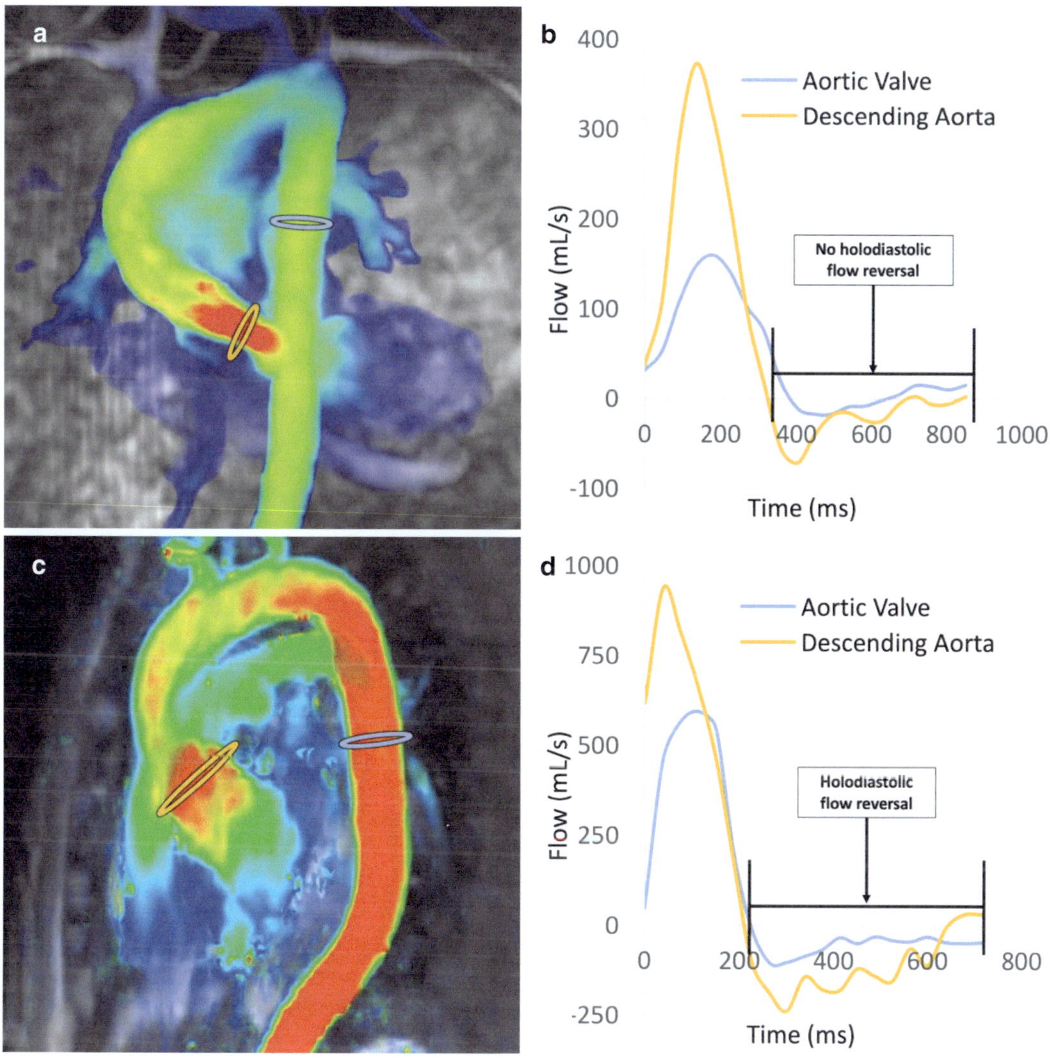

Fig. 10.18 A 24-year-old with bicuspid aortic valve and aortic valve regurgitation. (**a**) Four-dimensional flow MRI was acquired of the aorta and flow analysis at the aortic valve (orange circle) and in the descending aorta (blue circle). (**b**) Flow-time curves for the aortic valve (orange line) and descending aorta (blue line) indicate there is no holodiastolic flow reversal. A 35-year-old with bicuspid aortic valve and aortic valve regurgitation. (**c**) Four-dimensional flow MRI was acquired of the aorta and flow analysis at the aortic valve (orange circle) and in the descending aorta (blue circle). (**d**) Flow-time curves for the aortic valve (orange line) and descending aorta (blue line) indicate there is holodiastolic flow reversal, which is associated with more severe aortic regurgitation

portion of the left ventricle should be measured (Fig. 10.20). The length of the mitral annular disjunction has been shown to be correlated with the amount of late gadolinium enhancement by CMR, a marker of replacement myocardial fibrosis and a risk factor for complex ventricular arrhythmias.

Suggested criteria for valve regurgitation severity are summarized in Table 10.4.

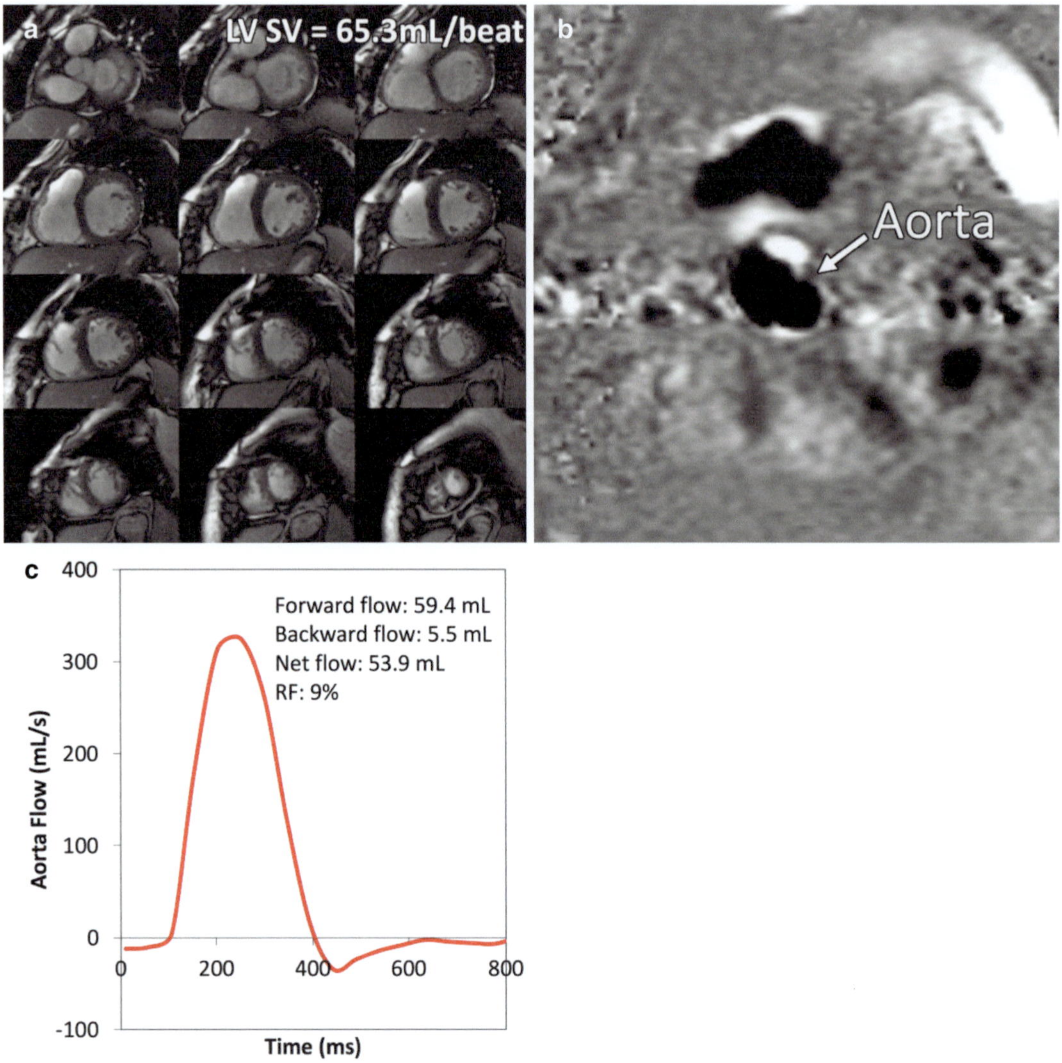

Fig. 10.19 A 56-year-old with mitral valve regurgitation. The degree of mitral valve regurgitation is calculated indirectly from the left ventricular stroke volume derived from the short-axis CINE balanced steady-state free precession images (**a**) and the flow through the aorta (**b**, **c**). In this example, the mitral valve regurgitation volume = 65.3 mL—53.9 mL = 11.4 mL and the mitral valve regurgitation fraction is 11.4/53.9 = 21%

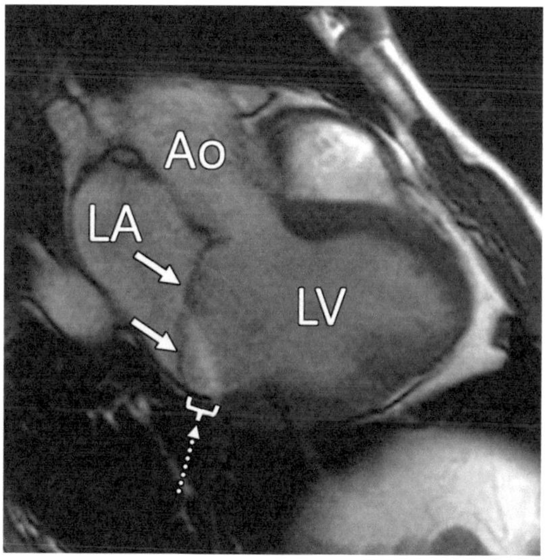

Fig. 10.20 A 40-year-old with bileaflet mitral valve prolapse (solid arrow) and mitral annular disjunction (dotted arrow)

Table 10.4 Suggested criteria for grading valve regurgitation with CMR

Valve	Severity	Regurgitation volume (mL)	Regurgitation fraction (%)
Aortic	Mild		<15
	Moderate		15–35
	Severe		>35
Pulmonic	Mild		<20
	Moderate		20–40
	Severe		>40
Mitral (primary)	Mild		<15–20
	Moderate		20–40
	Severe	≥55	>40
Mitral (secondary)	Mild	<30	
	Moderate	30–60	
	Severe	≥60	
Tricuspid	Mild		≤15
	Moderate		16–48
	Severe		>48

Structural Heart Disease

The use of CMR prior to transcatheter valve replacement is not as well established as cardiac computed tomography (CCT). In fact, CCT is the standard of reference for pre-transcatheter valve replacement assessment. However, CCT requires the use of iodinated contrast agents and exposes patients to ionizing radiation. In patients with contraindications to iodinated contrast agents or in whom minimizing the using of ionizing radiation is desired, CMR is a reasonable alternative. For all transcatheter valve replacement procedures, it is essential to have accurate measurements of the valve annulus dimensions, including diameters, areas, and perimeters. This can be done with contiguous, thin-slice CINE bSSFP and/or 3D bSSFP imaging through the valve of interest.

For transcatheter aortic valve replacement (TAVR), 3D bSSFP imaging, acquired with a non-contrast-enhanced, ECG-triggered, navigator-gated, free-breathing whole heart acquisition has been shown to be noninferior to CCT for aortic annulus sizing.

For transcatheter pulmonary valve replacement (TPVR), CMR can be used to define the shape of the right ventricular outflow tract (RVOT) and measure the size of the pulmonary valve annulus, the distance from the pulmonary valve annulus to the coronary arteries, and the landing zone length. Because the size of the RVOT and pulmonary valve annulus can change by more than 50%, it is important to measure the dimensions in end-systole and end-diastole.

In patients being evaluated prior to transcatheter mitral valve replacement (TMVR) and transcatheter tricuspid valve replacement (TTVR), CMR plays a complementary role to echocardiography and CCT. CMR can play an adjunct role in assessing the morphology and function of the mitral and tricuspid valves. Of note, CMR is inferior to CCT for assessment of the degree of mitral annulus calcification.

Bibliography

1. Nkomo VT, Gardin JM, Skelton TN, Gottdiener JS, Scott CG, Enriquez-Sarano M. Burden of valvular heart diseases: a population–based study. Lancet. 2006;368:1005–11.
2. Chambers JB, et al. Appropriateness criteria for the use of cardiovascular imaging in heart valve disease in adults: a European Association of Cardiovascular Imaging report of literature review and current practice. Eur Heart J. 2017;18:489–98.
3. Myerson SG. Heart valve disease: investigation by cardiovascular magnetic resonance. J Cardiovasc Magn Reson. 2012;14:7.
4. Myerson SG. CMR in evaluating valvular heart disease: diagnosis, severity, and outcomes. JACC Cardiovasc Imaging. 2021;14(10):2020–32.
5. Kramer CM, Barkhausen J, Bucciarelli-Ducci C, et al. Standardized cardiovascular magnetic resonance imaging (CMR) protocols: 2020 update. J Cardiovasc Magn Reson. 2020;22(1):17.
6. Bissel MM, Raimondi F, Ait AL, et al. 4D Flow cardiovascular magnetic resonance consensus statement: 2023 update. J Cardiovasc Magn Reson. 2023;25(1):40.
7. Kupfahl C, Honold M, Meinhardt G, et al. Evaluation of aortic stenosis by cardiovascular magnetic resonance imaging: comparison with established routine clinical techniques. Heart. 2004;90(8):893–901.
8. Mantini C, Di Giammarco G, Pizzicannella J, et al. Grading of aortic stenosis severity: a head-to-head comparison between cardiac magnetic resonance imaging and echocardiography. Radiol Med. 2018;123(9):643–54.
9. Reant P, Lederlin M, Lafitte S, et al. Absolute assessment of aortic valve stenosis by planimetry using cardiovascular magnetic resonance imaging: comparison with transesophageal echocardiography, transthoracic echocardiography, and cardiac catheterisation. Eur J Radiol. 2006;59(2):276–83.
10. Tanaka K, Makaryus AN, Wolff SD. Correlation of aortic valve area obtained by the velocity-encoded phase contrast continuity method to direct planimetry using cardiovascular magnetic resonance. J Cardiovasc Magn Reson. 2007;9(5):799–805.
11. Caruthers SD, Lin SJ, Brown P, et al. Practical value of cardiac magnetic resonance imaging for clinical quantification of aortic valve stenosis: comparison with echocardiography. Circulation. 2003;108(18):2236–43.
12. Adriaans BP, Westenberg JJM, van Cauteren YJM, et al. Clinical assessment of aortic valve stenosis: comparison between 4D flow MRI and transthoracic echocardiography. J Magn Reson Imaging. 2020;51(2):472–80.
13. Uygur B, Celik O, Ustabasioglu FE, et al. Three-dimensional transesophageal echocardiography vs cardiac magnetic resonance in the assessment of planimetric mitral valve area in rheumatic mitral stenosis. Echocardiography. 2018;35:1621–5.
14. Vidula MK, Xu Z, Xu Y, et al. Cardiovascular magnetic resonance characterization of rheumatic mitral stenosis: findings from three worldwide endemic zones. J Cardiovasc Magn Reson. 2022;24:24.
15. Shah S, Jenkins T, Markowitz A, et al. Multimodal imaging of the tricuspid valve: normal appearance and pathological entities. Insights Imaging. 2016;7(5):649–67.
16. Steeds RP, Myerson SG. Imaging assessment of mitral and aortic regurgitation: current state of the art. Heart. 2020;106(22):1769–76.
17. Bolen MA, Popovic ZB, Rajiah P, et al. Cardiac MR assessment of aortic regurgitation: holodiastolic flow reversal in the descending aorta helps stratify severity. Radiology. 2011;260(1):98–104.
18. Kammerlander AA, Wiesinger M, Duca F, et al. Diagnostic and prognostic utility of cardiac magnetic resonance imaging in aortic regurgitation. JACC Cardiovasc Imaging. 2019;12:1474–83.
19. Mercer-Rosa L, Yan W, Kutty S, et al. Quantifying pulmonary regurgitation and right ventricular function in surgically repaired tetralogy of Fallot: a comparative analysis of echocardiography and magnetic resonance imaging. Circ Cardiovasc Imaging. 2012;5:637–43.
20. Puchalski MD, Askovich B, Sower T, et al. Pulmonary regurgitation: determining severity by echocardiography and magnetic resonance imaging. Congenit Heart Dis. 2008;3:168–75.
21. Wald RM, Redington AN, Pereira A, et al. Refining the assessment of pulmonary regurgitation in adults after tetralogy of Fallot repair: should we be measur-

ing regurgitant fraction or regurgitant volume? Eur Heart J. 2009;30:356–61.
22. Garg P, Swift AJ, Zhong L, et al. Assessment of mitral valve regurgitation by cardiovascular magnetic resonance imaging. Nat Rev Cardiol. 2020;17:298–312.
23. Hahn RT, Thomas JD, Khalique OK, et al. Imaging assessment of tricuspid regurgitation severity. JACC Cardiovasc Imaging. 2019;12(3):469–90.
24. Westenberg JJM, Roes SD, Marsan NA, et al. Mitral valve and tricuspid valve blood flow: accurate quantification with 3D velocity-encoded MR imaging with retrospective valve tracking. Radiology. 2008;249(3):792–800.
25. Feneis JF, Kyubwa E, Atianzar K, et al. 4D Flow MRI quantification of mitral and tricuspid regurgitation: reproducibility and consistency relative to conventional MRI. J Magn Reson Imaging. 2018;48(4):1147–58.
26. Reindl M, Lechner I, Holzknecht M, et al. Cardiac magnetic resonance imaging versus computed tomography to guide transcatheter aortic valve replacement: a randomized, open-label, noninferiority trial. Circulation. 2023;148(16):1220–30.
27. Francone M, Budde RPJ, Bremerich J, et al. CT and MR imaging prior to transcatheter aortic valve implantation: standardisation of scanning protocols, measurements and reporting—a consensus document by the European Society of Cardiovascular Radiology (ESCR). Eur Radiol. 2020;30(5):2627–50.
28. Canan A, Ocazionez-Trujillo D, Vargas D, et al. Pre- and postprocedural imaging of transcatheter pulmonary valve implantation. Radiographics. 2022;42(4):991–1011.
29. Naoum C, Blanke P, Cavalcante JL, Leipsic J. Cardiac computed tomography and magnetic resonance imaging in the evaluation of mitral and tricuspid valve disease: implications for transcatheter interventions. Circ Cardiovasc Imaging. 2017;10:e005331.

Quantitative CT and MRI in Planning Transcatheter Interventions for Structural Heart Disease

11

Prabhakar Shantha Rajiah

Introduction

Transcatheter interventions are now increasingly used in the management of structural heart diseases, providing symptomatic relief and improving outcomes without the risks associated with invasive surgical procedures. Imaging plays a key role in the planning of these procedures, including in patient selection and identifying key parameters necessary for transcatheter interventions [1]. Echocardiography is the first-line imaging modality for this pre-procedural assessment, which is widely available in most institutions. Advanced imaging with computed tomography (CT) and magnetic resonance imaging (MRI) provides complementary information to echocardiography. CT has several advantages including rapid acquisition time, high isotropic spatial resolution, good temporal resolution, multiplanar reconstruction capabilities, and large field of view. CT provides key information for patient selection and detection of contraindications for the procedure. CT also provides several quantitative measurements that are important for device selection and sizing. CT is also used as a problem-solving tool following these procedures in characterizing complications that are challenging or indeterminate in echocardiography.

Recent advances in CT have expanded the capabilities of CT for pre-procedural assessment. Photon counting detector (PCD) CT offers ultrahigh-resolution imaging with in-plane spatial resolution of up to 0.1 mm [2]. PCD-CT allows improved visualization of device structure and subtle complications such as small thrombi, hypoattenuated leaflet thickening (HALT), and vegetations [2]. PCD-CT also improves the quantification of stenosis in patients with dense calcified coronary plaques and stents, both of which are limitations in a conventional energy-integrating detector (EID) CT [3]. This can improve the assessment of concomitant coronary artery disease, which is necessary prior to some transcatheter procedures. Using spectral data from PCD-CT or other multi-energy CT (MECT) techniques, calcium can be removed from images, which also improves assessment of luminal stenosis [4]. Conversely, iodine can be removed from images in virtual non-contrast or virtual noniodine images, which can be used to generate calcium score from a contrast-enhanced CTA, thus saving some radiation dose. Low-energy virtual monoenergetic images (VMIs) from MECT techniques enhance the signal of iodinated contrast, which is useful in decreasing the dose of iodinated contrast in patients with severe renal dysfunction and in salvaging suboptimally enhanced CT studies [4]. High-energy VMIs can decrease several artifacts including metallic, beam hardening, and blooming artifacts [4].

P. S. Rajiah (✉)
Department of Radiology, Cardiovascular Radiology Division, Mayo Clinic, Rochester, MN, USA

R. Gill, P. Rajiah (eds.), *Quantitative Imaging in the Thorax*,
https://doi.org/10.1007/978-3-032-14103-3_11

Using iodine maps generated from delayed phase acquisition in MECT or a combination of non-contrast and delayed post-contrast single energy CT, the extracellular volume (ECV) of the myocardium can be quantified. This can be used to identify subclinical cardiac amyloidosis in structural heart disease, which is an adverse prognostic factor [5].

Three-dimensional modeling and printing from CT help with pre-procedural planning and procedural simulation. Using dedicated software, CT data is segmented, and patient-specific 3D models are printed. 3D modeling and printing help the interventional cardiologist in visualizing complex anatomy without the need for knowledge in CT imaging. The interventional procedure can be simulated by using actual devices in the 3D models. Bench testing of various device types and sizes in a 3D-printed model improves correlation with final implanted device and also allows estimation of the risk of paravalvular leak and other complications [6]. Extended reality encompasses virtual, augmented, and mixed reality, which enhance the valuation of complex anatomical information and spatial relationships and improve accuracy of procedural planning [7]. Advances in computational flow modeling offer the potential for hemodynamic information in structural diseases. The use of artificial intelligence (AI) is expected to further enhance the capabilities and workflow of CT, including in patient selection, device sizing, and determination of high-risk features [7].

MRI provides complementary information to echocardiography and CT for select applications [8]. MRI is typically used when there is a contraindication to the use of intravenous iodinated contrast media for CT, such as anaphylactic reaction or severe renal dysfunction. MRI has good spatial and temporal resolutions, multiplanar acquisition capabilities, and large field of view without the need for ionizing radiation. MRI can characterize structural heart disease and quantify ventricular volumes/function, valvular regurgitation/stenosis, and shunts. 2D or 4D phase contrast sequence is used for quantification of valvular heart disease. MRI can also evaluate scar and extracellular volume, especially useful in the assessment of cardiac amyloidosis in patients being considered for transcatheter aortic valve replacement (TAVR). MR angiography with gadolinium is useful in the assessment of access vessels. Non-contrast MRA sequences such as 3D-SSFP and quiescent-interval single-shot (QISS) MRA are useful in the evaluation of access vessels in patients with severe renal dysfunction [9]. The iron-containing ferumoxytol is an off-label alternative to gadolinium in the evaluation of access vessels [10]. Ferumoxytol-MRA and 3D-SSFP sequence are also useful in the assessment of aortic root anatomy for TAVR and right ventricular outflow tract (RVOT) anatomy for transcatheter pulmonary valve replacement (TPVR) [8].

In the following sections, the utility of advanced imaging in the evaluation of commonly performed transcatheter interventions is discussed.

Transcatheter Aortic Valve Replacement

Transcatheter aortic valve replacement (TAVR) is a validated alternative to surgery for patients with severe aortic stenosis. TAVR is well established in severe aortic stenosis with high surgical risk and is also increasingly used in patients with intermediate- to low- surgical risk [11]. Devices used for TAVR are either balloon-expandable (*Sapien*, *Sapien 3*, *Sapien 3 Ultra*, *Sapien XT*), self-expanding, either supra-annular (*Corevalve*, *Evolut R*, *Evolut PRO*, *Allegra*, *ACURATE neo*) or intra-annular (*Portico*, *Navitor*, *Centera*), or mechanically expandable (*LOTUS*). Jenavalve and J-valve are useful in patients with aortic regurgitation [12]. CT provides a comprehensive assessment of the aortic root as well as access vessels and identifies high-risk factors for adverse outcomes (Table 11.1) [13]. MRI is an alternative in patients with severe renal dysfunction [8, 10].

Accurate measurement of the aortic annulus is important for appropriate device and size selection. The aortic annulus is defined within a virtual plane that is aligned to the basal attachment ("hinge") points of the three aortic valve cusps.

Table 11.1 Key CT parameters in pre-procedural assessment of TAVR

Aortic valve	Leaflet anatomy Calcifications—qualitative grading, quantification
Aortic annulus	Diameters (short, long, area-derived, circumference-derived) Perimeter Area
Fluoroscopic angles	Orthogonal view of aortic valve plane, cusp overlap view
Aortic root	Sinus of Valsalva height and width Coronary ostial height from aortic annulus
Sinotubular junction	Diameter Height
Ascending aorta	Diameter, 40 mm above the annulus
Aorta	Kinking, obstruction, thrombi
Iliofemoral arteries	Minimal diameter Calcification Tortuosity

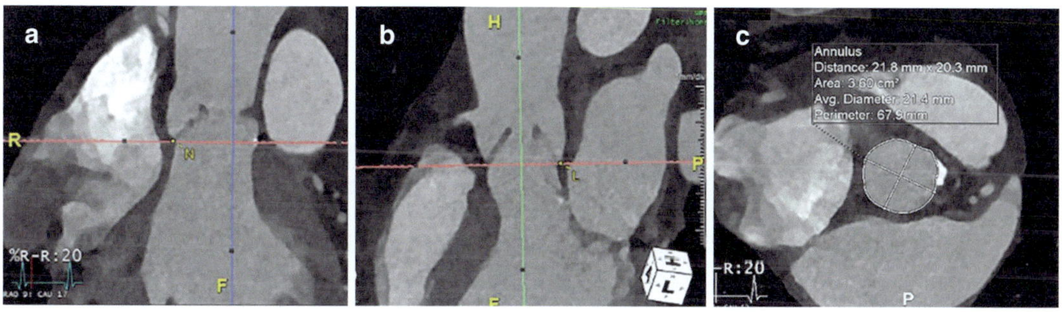

Fig. 11.1 Measurements for TAVR. From coronal (**a**) and sagittal (**b**) multiplanar reconstructions, the hinge points of the aortic annulus are marked, and the annulus is measured in the short-axis plane (**c**)

Due to dynamic changes in the dimensions of the annulus, it is measured from the systolic phase with the largest annular dimension. The annulus can be potentially measured from standard multiplanar reformats in any workstation [13]. However, it is typically measured using dedicated software by either semiautomatic or automatic placement of markers at annulus hinge points. After placement of these markers, various techniques such as cubic spline interpolation, polygon, attenuation-based contour detection, and freehand contour can be used for measurement. Diameters in long and short axis, area, perimeter, and diameters derived from area and perimeter are measured (Fig. 11.1) [13]. Device sizing is based on annular area for balloon-expandable devices and perimeter for self expandable devices. A small amount of device oversizing is used to minimize complications of implantation. It should be noted that the percentage of oversizing is twofold greater based on the area than the perimeter [13].

The aortic valve morphology, i.e., trileaflet, bicuspid, unicuspid, and quadricuspid, is defined. The aortic valve area can be quantified by planimetry, with area < 1.0 cm^2 indicating critical aortic stenosis. Cine imaging shows restricted systolic opening. Valve thickening and calcifications are seen. Calcification in the landing zone (LZ) of the transcatheter aortic valve, i.e., valve cusps, aortic annulus, and left ventricular outflow tract (LVOT), is qualitatively characterized. Single non-protruding focus of calcification is defined as mild. Two or more nodules of calcification or a single nodule with limited protrusion into the annular/subannular lumen indicates moderate calcification. Single or multiple calcified nodules that protrude into the annular lumen or LVOT indicate severe calcification. Extensive calcifications are associated with increased risk of annular rupture and paravalvular regurgitation with expansion of balloon-expandable valves. Higher risk is seen with protruding than flat calcifications, calcifications below the annulus than lower in LVOT, below non-coronary sinus than other sinuses, and with higher percentages of oversizing [13]. There is also increased risk of conduction block from expansion of balloon-expandable valve, especially one that is oversized. A length of membranous ventricular septum of <8 mm is predictive of higher degree of AV block, particularly with deeper implantation. This is measured in the coronal plane at the longest point between the annular level and muscular septum [13].

Coronary artery occlusion is a dreaded complication of TAVR, reported in 0.66% [14]. The risk of coronary occlusion can be predicted based on the sinus of Valsalva (SOV) diameter and the height of the coronary ostium. The coronary ostial height is measured perpendicular to the previously defined annular plane to the lower edge of the left and right coronary ostia (Fig. 11.2). The SOV diameter is measured from cusp to commissure in parallel to the annular plane for the three cusps. The average of the three cusp diameters is used. A coronary ostial height of <12 mm and a SOV diameter of <30 mm indicate high risk for coronary artery occlusion. The diameter and height of the sinotubular junction (STJ) are measured to identify potential risk of injury to the STJ from the valve, particularly with self-expandable valves. The STJ height is measured perpendicular to the annular plane (Fig. 11.2). In low STJ heights, even balloon-expandable valves can reach the STJ and injure it if the diameter is small (Fig. 11.3) [13].

TAVR requires fluoroscopic angulation that provides coplanar view of the aortic annulus without any parallax. CT can identify these angles before the procedure, thus saving fluoroscopic time, radiation dose, and contrast dose. The optimal C-arm angles are reported in LAO or RAO projections and cranial or caudal projections. Typical views are centered on the right coronary cusp or predefined angulations such as LAO 0, LAO 10, and RAO 10 (Fig. 11.4). When the cranial or caudal angulation is >25%, alternative angulations should be provided given the physical restraints of C-arms [13].

Current guidelines require exclusion of significant coronary artery disease (CAD) prior to TAVR [15]. TAVR CT can simultaneously assess coronary arteries, obviating the need for additional coronary angiography for determining CAD. When assessment of coronary arteries is required, beta-blockers may be given to decrease the heart rate. Although nitroglycerine is typically contraindicated in severe aortic stenosis, it can be administered to improved coronary dilatation with appropriate supervision protocol. Recent studies have shown the accuracy of CTA in excluding significant CAD, especially in proximal vessels [15]. There is a high prevalence of dense calcified plaques in these patients with some having coronary stents, which decreases the predictive value and specificity of CTA. Recent studies with ultra-high-resolution mode of PCD CT have shown

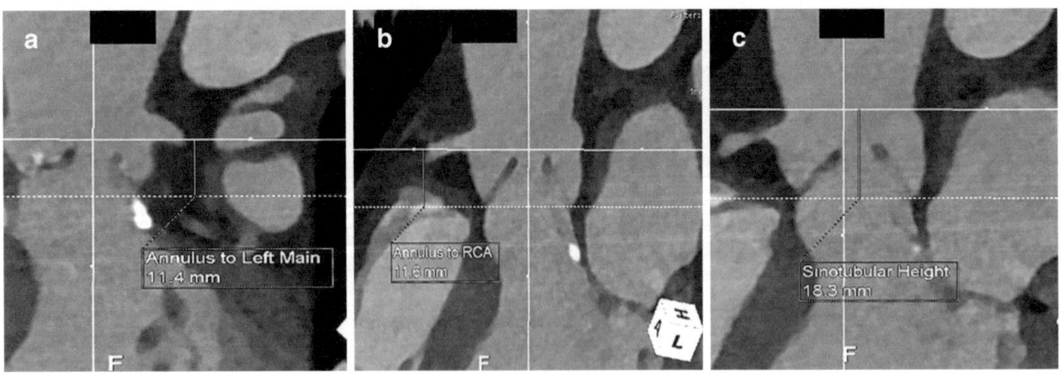

Fig. 11.2 Measurements for TAVR. Distance from the aortic annulus to the left main coronary artery (**a**), right coronary artery (**b**), and sinotubular junction (**c**)

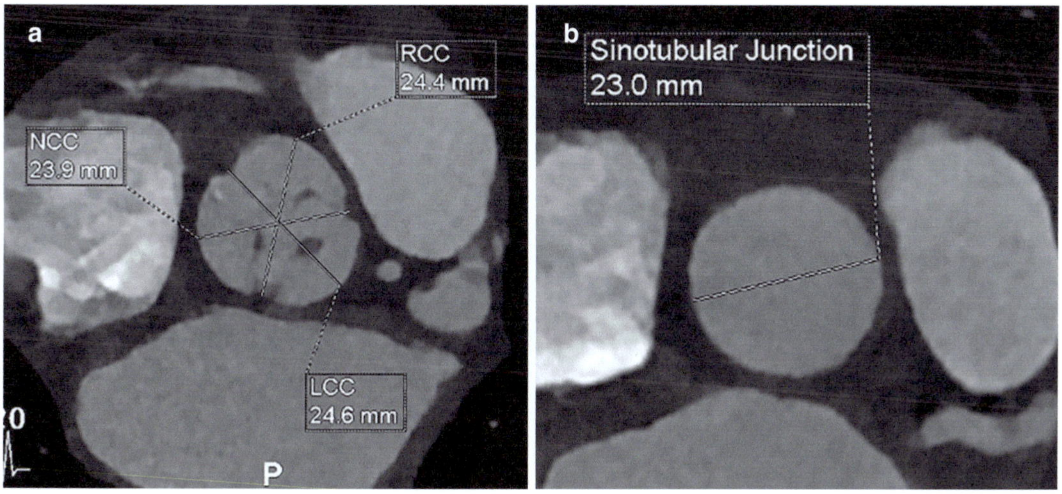

Fig. 11.3 Measurements for TAVR. Measurement of diameters of the aortic root (**a**) and sinotubular junction (**b**)

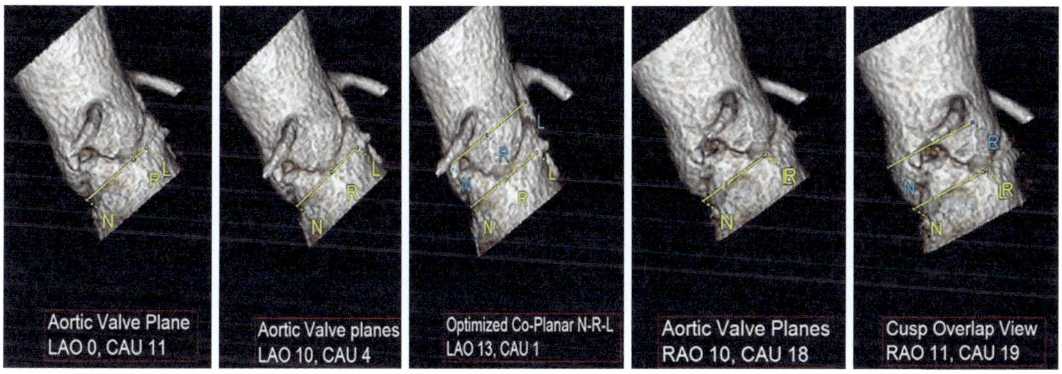

Fig. 11.4 Fluoroscopic angles for TAVR. Simulated fluoroscopic angles needed for the TAVR procedure, including LAO 0, LAO 10, LAO 13, aortic valve plane, and cusp overlap view

improved accuracy with an AUC of 0.92 compared to invasive angiography in the evaluation of these high-risk patients [3]. CT-FFR can improve the diagnostic yield of CT in these patients [16].

Access vessels, commonly iliofemoral arteries, are also evaluated to determine if the large sheaths and delivery systems used in TAVR can be safely introduced without any complications. These are easily measured using CTA performed through the abdomen and pelvis. Key parameters include minimum vessel diameter, calcification, and tortuosity (Fig. 11.5). The minimal luminal diameter is measured using the double-oblique technique, typically using dedicated software that uses centerline placement and curved MPR. The minimal acceptable luminal diameter varies with the device, with >5 mm considered appropriate for most devices. A threshold of sheath: vessel luminal diameter of >1.12 can be used to predict injury [17]. Calcifications can also be qualitatively graded as mild, moderate, and severe. Circumferential calcifications especially at bifurcation or tortuous segments should be mentioned since it can limit expansion of the balloon and can contribute to access failure. Presence of circumferential calcification may require lithotripsy. Calcification in the common femoral artery at access site and high femoral artery bifurcation are noted since they determine the choice of access puncture. Tortuosity of vessels is qualitatively evaluated either on axial or coronal images or volume-rendered reconstruc-

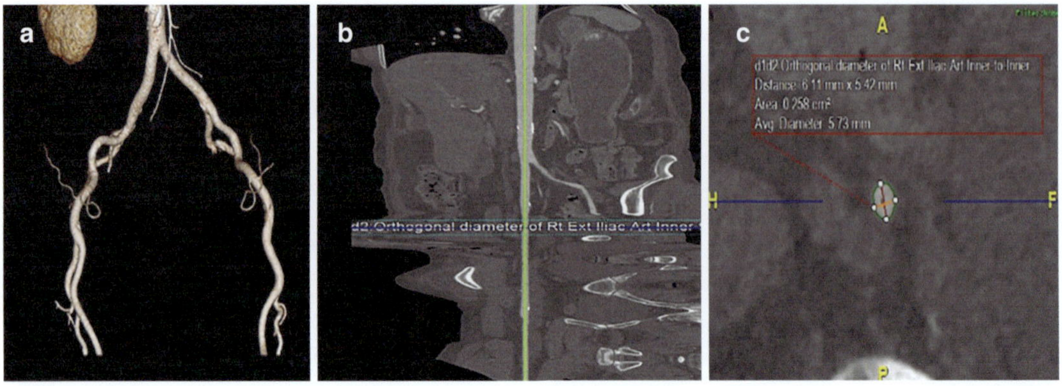

Fig. 11.5 Access vessel evaluation in TAVR. (**a**) 3D volume-rendered view showing mild tortuosity of ilio-femoral arteries. From straightened multiplanar reconstruction of the iliac vessels (**b**) and the minimal diameter of the right external iliac artery is measured (**c**)

Table 11.2 Utility of CT in evaluation of complex TAVR procedures

Indication	Utility of CT
Low-flow, low-gradient aortic stenosis	Aortic valve calcium score to estimate severity of AS
Bicuspid aortic valve	Anatomical classification of bicuspid valve Anatomy of aortic root Definition of annular plane (*third hinge point perpendicular to landing zone*) Supra-annular measurements (*4 mm above annulus*) Calcification burden Aortopathy Aortic angle Coronary anatomy, location, and heights
Aortic regurgitation	Valvular calcifications Annular sizing
Other concomitant valvular diseases	Mitral annular measurements Mitral annular calcifications
Valve-in-valve	Morphology and function of bioprosthetic valve Sizing of the indwelling valve Virtual coronary distance Planning for coronary protective interventions
Difficult femoral access	Subclavian artery—diameter, calcification, tortuosit; Carotid artery- diameter, calcification, tortuosity) Aorta—diameter, calcification IVC—abdominal aorta without calcification; Apical- LV apical aneurysm or thrombus; Distance from LV apex to aortic annulus

tion. Extensive tortuosity is not an absolute contraindication to femoral access, but this may have to be straightened with a sheath.

Complex TAVR

TAVR is also now performed in patients with complex AS, traditionally not considered suitable for TAVR due to complex anatomy and other challenges. CT is a key imaging modality in the pre-procedural evaluation of complex TAVR [18] (Table 11.2).

Valve-in-valve TAVR is performed in patients with failed bioprosthetic aortic valves. CT can demonstrate the structural degeneration in the bioprosthetic valve manifesting as thickening, calcification, and restricted mobility. CT can measure the inner diameter of the surgical valve at the basal ring if surgical details are not available, to determine the appropriate type and size of TAVR valve. Compared to TAVR in native aortic valve, valve-in-valve TAVR is associated with higher risk of coronary artery obstruction of 2.3% due to covering of the coronary ostium by the displaced surgical valve leaflet. CT can predict the risk of coronary occlusion in valve-in-valve TAVR. If the indwelling valve is stentless or if the coronary ostia is above a stented valve, the risk of coronary occlusion is low, and no additional specific measurements are necessary. If the coronary ostia are below the stented valve, a virtual TAVR to coronary (VTC) distance is measured. At the cross-sectional image of the basal ring of the bioprosthetic valve, a virtual cylinder with the same diameter as a fully expanded TAVR is aligned in the middle of the bioprosthetic ring. VTC is calculated between the edge of this cylinder and the coronary artery ostium (Fig. 11.6) [13]. A distance of <4 mm indicates higher risk of coronary occlusion, especially when there is heavy leaflet calcification. In patients with high risk of coronary obstruction, a BASILICA (bioprosthetic or native aortic scallop intentional laceration to prevent iatrogenic coronary obstruction during TAVR) procedure is used to split native or bioprosthetic leaflets. CT coronary eccentricity index can indicate success rate with BASILICA. This is defined as the angle from the center of the coronary ostium to the mid-cusp line in the native valve and midline of each stent post in the bioprosthetic valve. Eccentricity angles of >24.5° for RCA and 19° for LCA are associated with greater risk of coronary occlusion [19].

Low-flow low-gradient severe aortic stenosis can be either classical or paradoxical. Classic LF-LG-AS is associated with low ejection frac-

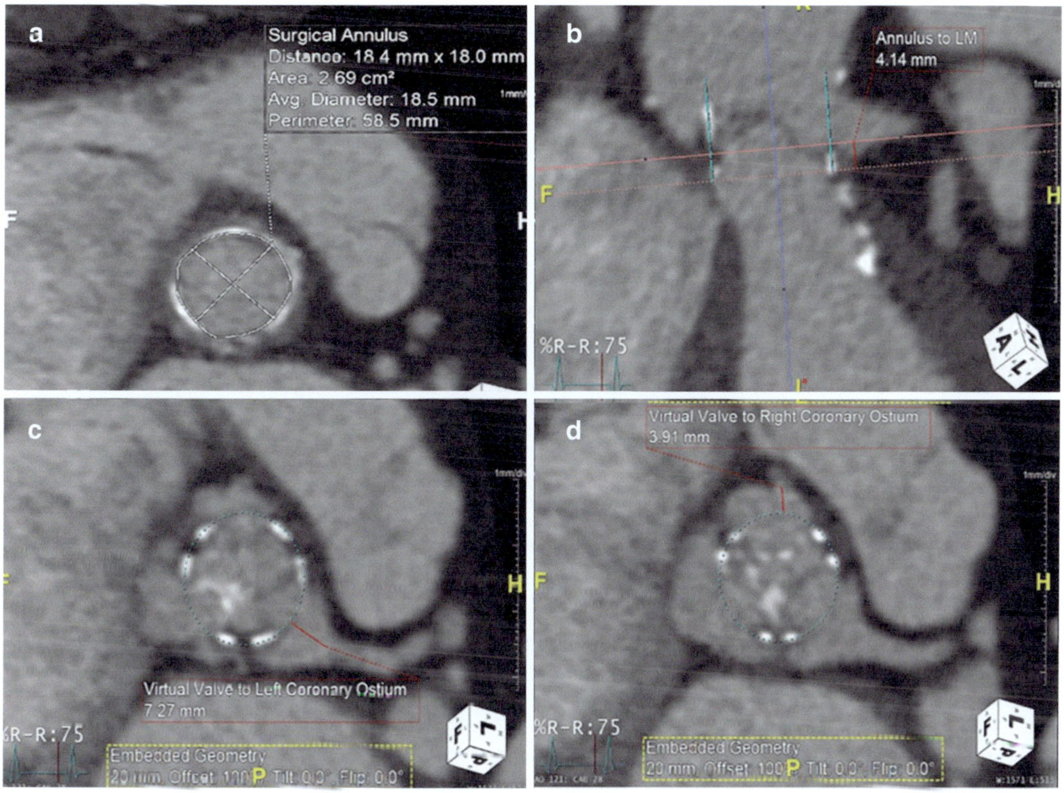

Fig. 11.6 Valve-in-valve TAVR. (**a**) Measurement of the inner diameter of a surgically placed bioprosthetic valve in the aortic position. (**b**) Coronal image shows a virtual cylinder projected from the aortic basal ring to the level of coronary arteries simulating the transcatheter valve. Virtual TAVR to coronary distance for the left coronary artery (**c**) and right coronary artery (**d**)

tion (EF), mean transvalvular gradient, and LV stroke volume (SV), whereas paradoxical LF-LG-AS is associated with normal EF, low mean transvalvular gradient, and low SV. With low flow across a stenosed aortic valve, it is critical to distinguish a true stenosis from a pseudo stenosis caused by severe LV dysfunction or afterload. Low-dose dobutamine stress echocardiography (DSE) is the procedure of choice for this purpose. In DSE, with true LF-LG-AS, normalization of stroke volume leads to increased peak velocity and mean gradient with a persistently decreased effective orifice area (EOA), whereas with pseudo stenosis, the EOA increases without increase in gradient [18]. In patients who cannot have DSE, CT aortic valve calcium scores of ≥2000 in men and ≥ 1200 in women indicates severe AS (Fig. 11.7) [20]. This, however, may not capture the non-calcified valve fibrosis or stenosis from the bicuspid aortic valve (BAV).

bicuspid aortic valve poses challenges for TAVR, including larger dimensions of valve complex, elliptical supra-annular geometry, and flared shape of the aortic valve complex, which predisposes to less circular deployment and larger amount of eccentric leaflet calcifications that compromise optimal expansion. CT or MRI classifies the BAV accurately as fused type (three sinuses, two cusps, two commissures with raphe), two-sinus type (two sinuses and cusps without a raphe), or partial fusion type (three sinuses, cusps, and commissures with a partial fusion of <50% of length) [21]. Delineation of the annular plane for measurement is challenging with BAV of two-sinus type. In addition to the two visualized hinge points, a third hinge point is defined in a plane perpendicular to the landing zone (Fig. 11.8). Regular TAVR measurements can be performed for fusion and partial fusion types. If a supra-annular implantation is considered, measurements are made 4 mm above the annular plane especially with tapered anatomy, which avoids oversizing [18]. Device sizing is based on multiple measurements at multiple levels including area, perimeter, supra-annular or intercommissural distance/area, and linear diameters. The extent and distribution of calcifications provide risk stratification. A horizontal aorta, i.e., an angle of <30° between a plane perpendicular to an aortic annulus and a horizontal reference plane complicates accurate positioning of self-expanding valves. Absence of aortopathy is favorable for TAVR. Coronary anatomy is more variable in BAV, including higher left dominant system and separate ostia for LAD and left circumflex coronary artery (LCX) [18].

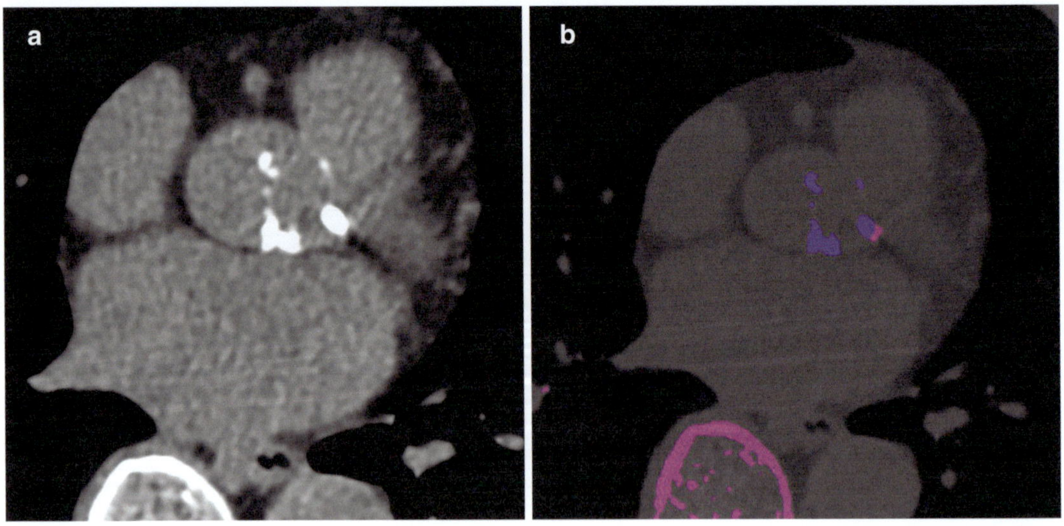

Fig. 11.7 Low-flow low-gradient aortic stenosis. (**a**) non-contrast study shows extensive calcification of the aortic valve leaflets. (**b**) Quantification of the aortic valve calcium resulted in score of 2100, indicating severe aortic stenosis

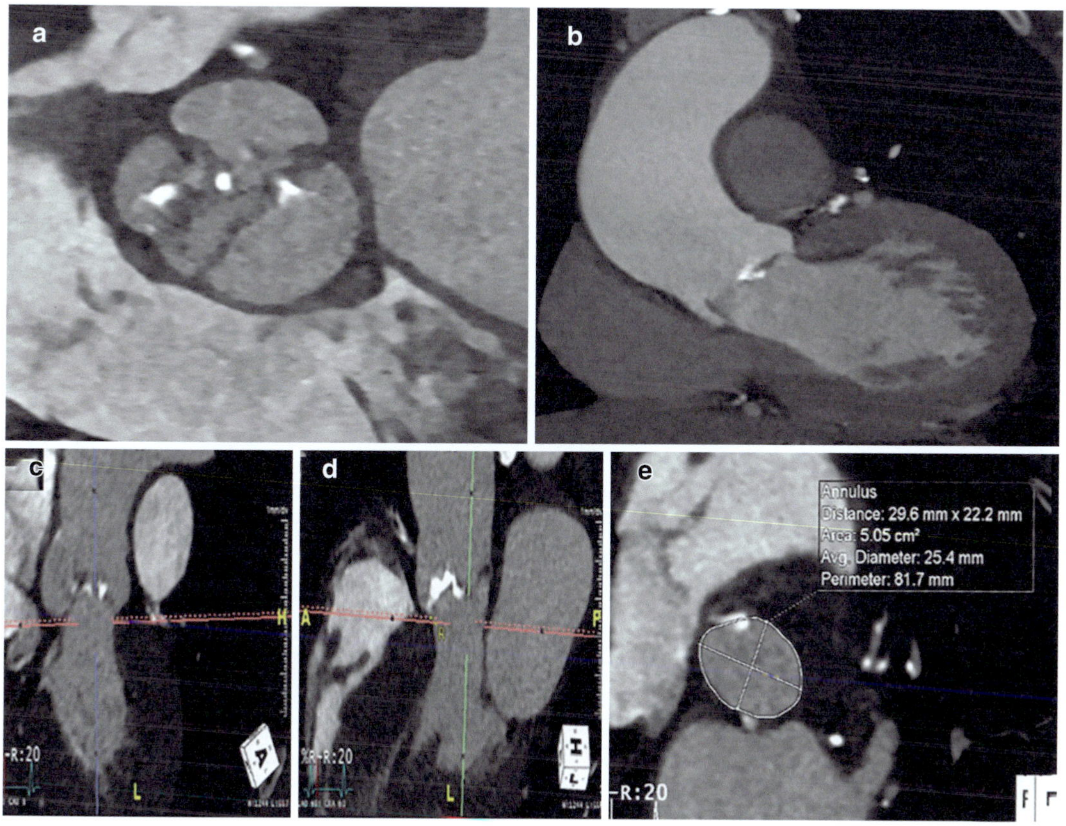

Fig. 11.8 TAVR in bicuspid aortic valve. (**a**) Short-axis view of the aortic valve shows a bicuspid aortic valve with fusion of the right and left leaflets. There is moderate thickening and calcification of the leaflets. (**b**) Coronal CT image shows dilated aortic root and ascending aorta, indicating associated aortopathy. From coronal (**c**) and sagittal (**d**) multiplanar views, markers are placed in hinge points of the aortic annulus. From the short-axis image generated (**e**), the aortic annulus is measured

Aortic valve regurgitation was traditionally not considered for TAVR due to little or no annular calcification and dilated aortic root/ascending aorta that challenges device anchoring and increases risk of device embolization and paravalvular leak. However, AR without significant annular dilatation is favorable for TAVR. Newer second-generation TAVR devices are successful with low complications [22]. Concomitant valvular diseases can also make TAVR challenging. Concomitant mitral regurgitation (MR) is seen in 30% and moderate to severe TR is seen in 24% [23]. A mitral annular diameter of >35.5 mm and mitral annular calcifications are independent predictors of persistent MR following TAVR. Only half of patients with moderate or severe MR or TR associated with AS improve after TAVR [18].

Alternative access vessel is considered for TAVR, if femoral access is not possible. Femoral access is not possible in up to 15% due to unfavorable anatomy, i.e., small vessels, severe calcific atherosclerosis, and extensive tortuosity [24]. Alternative access includes the subclavian artery, common carotid artery, ascending aorta, IVC, or LV apex. CT provides a comprehensive anatomy of these alternative access sites, including the diameter of the vessel and any excessive calcification or tortuosity. For transaortic access, ascending aortic aneurysm and calcification is evaluated. For a transcaval approach, an optimal location in the aorta free of calcification adjacent to the IVC is determined. Any interposed vital structure can also be evlauted. For an apical approach, the distance from the left chest wall to the LV apex and a coaxial aortic valve plane can be determined [13]. Contraindications such as LV apical aneurysm and thrombus can also be evaluated.

Transcatheter Mitral Valve Replacement

Transcatheter mitral valve replacement (TMVR) is an effective option for treating mitral valve disease in patients with high-risk factors for open mitral valve surgery or unfavorable anatomy for minimally invasive mitral valve repair. Multiple devices with various anchoring mechanisms are currently available or being investigated, delivered either by the transeptal or transpical approach. Anchoring mechanisms include radial force (*Intrepid*, *Sapien* 3), apical tether (*Tendyne*), trigone capture and leaflet engagement (*Tiara*), annulus capture and leaflet engagement (*CardiAQ-Edwards*), annular winglets (*NaviGate*), and external anchor (*Caisson*) [25]. TMVR can be performed in the native mitral valve, mitral annular calcification (MAC) (valve-in-MAC), bioprosthetic valve (valve-in-valve), or annuloplasty ring (valve-in-ring). The mitral valve disease itself is evaluated primarily with echocardiography, but CT can also provide complementary information (Table 11.3). In mitral stenosis, the valve leaflets are thickened with restricted diastolic opening. Commissural thickening and calcification are seen in rheumatic heart disease. In mitral regurgitation, incomplete leaflet coaptation is seen in systole. With mitral valve prolapse, the leaflet(s) protrudes >2 mm into the left atrium in systole.

Accurate measurement of the mitral annulus is essential for device sizing. The mitral annulus has a complex three-dimensional saddle-shape, with fibrous anterior one-third and muscular posterior two-thirds. It is possible to measure the mitral annulus in a routine workstation using multiplanar reconstructions and short-axis view of the mitral annulus. However, this task is better performed using a dedicated software that is more robust. Multiple seed points are placed

Table 11.3 Key CT parameters required in pre-procedural assessment for TMVR

Native mitral valve	Morphology of mitral valve apparatus Mitral valve pathology Mitral valve function Mitral annulus dimensions—systole and diastole
Neo-LVOT	Cross-sectional dimensions Aortomitral angle Anterior mitral leaflet length Basal interventricular septal thickness
Virtual prosthesis	Placement angle, offset Fluoroscopic angles
Additional information	Subvalvular apparatus measurements Relationship to left circumflex coronary arteryand coronary sinus Left atrial appendageostium—annulus distance Septal approach—atrial septal anatomy, pathology Transapical approach—best intercostal approach, fluoroscopic angle for coaxial deployment
Valve-in-MAC	Extent of calcifications Thickness Circumference Trigone involvement Leaflet involvement
Valve-in-valve or valve-in-ring	Bioprosthetic valve morphology and function Surgical valve type Inner diameter of surgical valve Leaflet location and height Neo-LVOT

along the 360° circumference of the annulus, from which a cubic spline interpolation of the 3D perimeter of the saddle-shaped annulus is generated. To improve reproducibility, a simplified D-shaped annulus is created by connecting the trigones using a virtual line and eliminating the anterior horn. This D-shaped annulus is then projected onto the short-axis view that represents the 2D D-shaped annulus. From this, the trigone-trigone distance, intercommissural distance, septolateral distance, area, and perimeter are measured (Fig. 11.9). Due to dynamism of the mitral annulus, measurements are made both in end systole and end diastole [25].

Placement of TMVR results in anterior deflection of the anterior mitral leaflet (AML), which narrows the newly created LVOT (neo-LVOT). Neo-LVOT obstruction is the most dreaded complication of TMVR. CT can estimate the size of the anticipated neo LVOT, which allows prediction of neo-LVOT obstruction. A virtual prosthesis, i.e., a 3D model that matches the proposed device, is placed in the annulus at the expected implantation site, typically 80% on the ventricular side and 20% on the atrial side. From a three-chamber end-systolic image, a centerline is created through the LVOT to generate a short-axis curved MPR of neo-LVOT. The smallest neo-LVOT cross-sectional area is measured (Fig. 11.10). Various thresholds of this neo-LVOT area have been proposed, with an area of >170 mm^2 considered to have lower risk of neo-LVOT obstruction [26]. Since the neo-LVOT size is dynamic, recent studies have proposed measuring the size throughout systole. If the patient has small neo-LVOT, this does not exclude TMVR but indicates the need for alternative procedures to mitigate complications. This can be done either by decreasing septal thickness either through

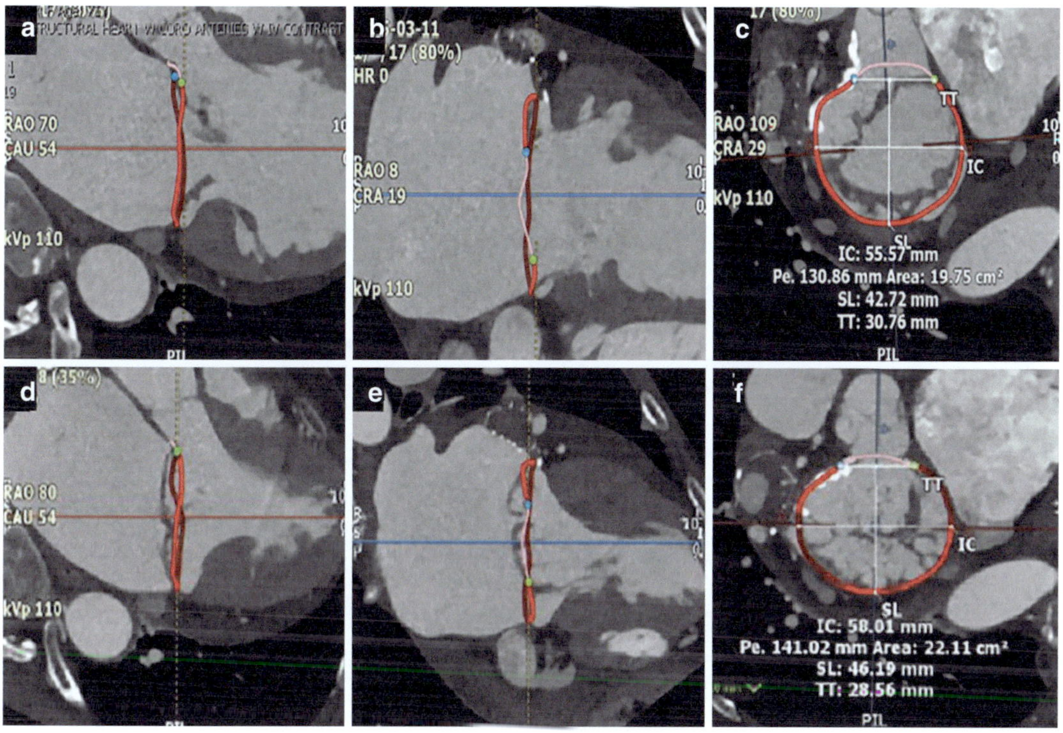

Fig. 11.9 TMVR measurements. The top row shows measurements of the mitral annulus in diastole at 80% R-R interval. From seed points placed in the circumference of the mitral annulus (**a**, **b**), a cubic spline interpolation is obtained. This is then projected on a short-axis image (**c**) to obtain a 2D view from which a D-shaped annulus is generated. Trigone-trigone, septolateral, and intercommissural diameters as well as area and perimeter are measured. Similar measurements are also obtained in systole at 35% R-R interval (**d–f**)

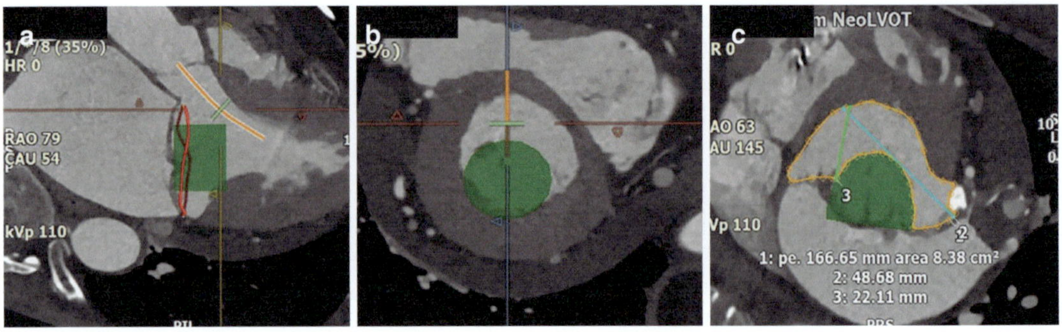

Fig. 11.10 Virtual prosthesis in TMVR. A virtual 29 mm Sapien 3 prosthesis is placed in the mitral annulus with 20% atrial and 80% ventricular offset. A centerline is obtained through the LVOT (yellow) in a three-chamber view (a). The smallest diameter of LVOT is identified in the short-axis image (**b**), from which the area of neo-LVOT is measured. (**c**) In this patient, this area is 838 mm^2, which is considered sufficient

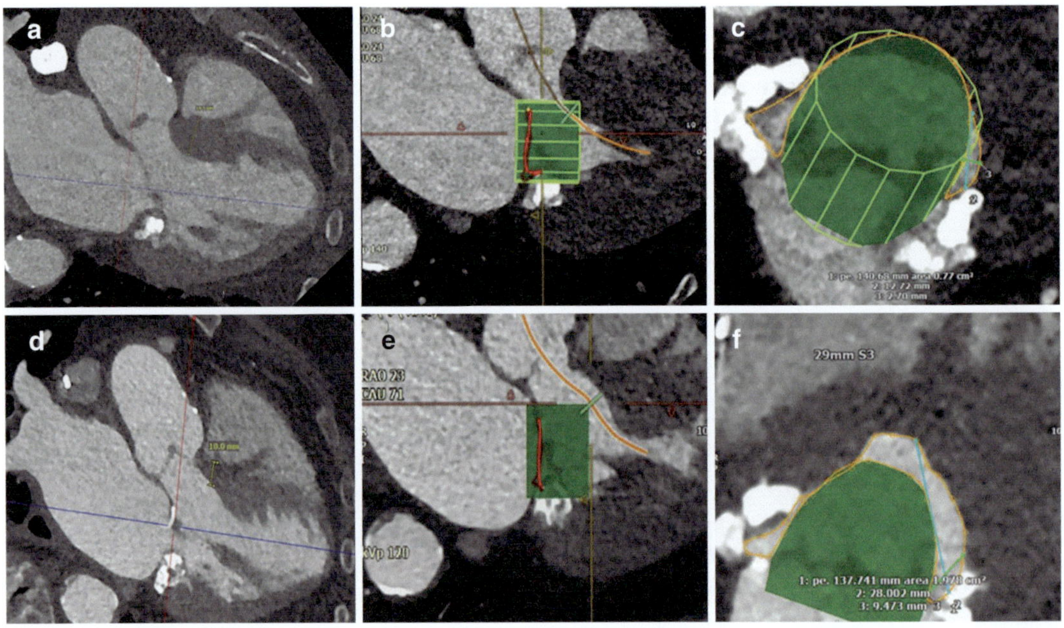

Fig. 11.11 Small neo-LVOT in TMVR. Three-chamber CT reconstruction (**a**) shows severe thickening of the basal anteroseptum, measuring 18.5 mm. Following placement of a 29 mm Sapien 3 virtual prosthesis in the mitral annulus (green), the neo-LVOT is small (**b**), measuring only 77 mm^2 (**c**). Hence, the patient underwent alcohol septal ablation to decrease septal thickness. Follow-up CT performed 2 months later showed decreased thickness of the basal anteroseptum, now measuring 10 mm (**d**). The neo-LVOT is now larger (**e,f**), measuring 198 mm^2, which is now amenable for TMVR (**f**)

alcohol or radiofrequency septal ablation (Fig. 11.11) or transcatheter myotomy (*SESAME- Septal scoring along the midline endocardium*), lacerating the anterior mitral leaflet to create a blood channel to neo-LVOT (LAMPOON (laceration of the anterior mitral leaflet to prevent LVOT obstruction)), or surgically resecting the anterior leaflet [25].

CT can predict fluoroscopic angles that are perpendicular to the mitral annulus for accurate coaxial deployment to decrease fluoroscopic time and contrast doses. A fluoroscopic septolateral view is parallel to the septolateral distance and is

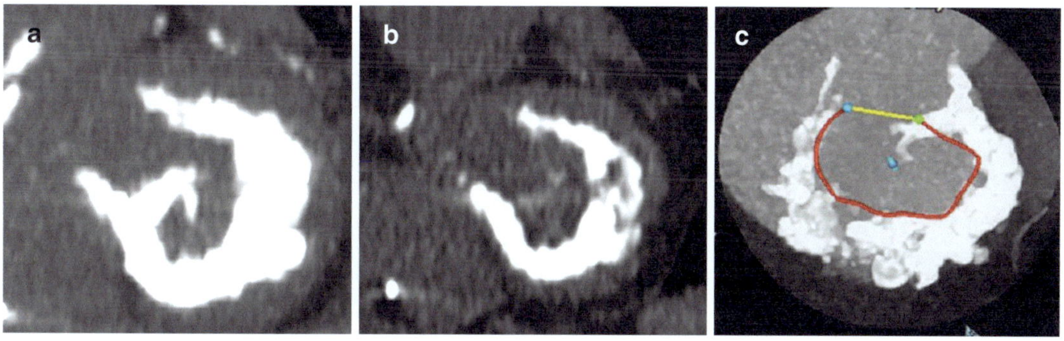

Fig. 11.12 Valve-in-MAC TMVR. Short-axis MIP (**a**) and MPR (**b**) images through the mitral annulus shows extensive mitral annular calcifications that involve more than 270° of circumference with a thickness of 15 mm, involving both leaflets and trigones, with a MAC score of 10. The mitral annulus is measured in (**c**). The extent of calcification allows placement of a TMVR device in the annulus with lower risk of device embolization and paravalvular leaks

the best view to align the device along the mitral annulus. The trigone-trigone view is parallel to the trigone-trigone distance, which however is not possible due to physical C-arm constraints. A compromise view between the SL and trigone-trigone view shows the potential LVOT narrowing. Relationship to the left circumflex coronary artery (LCX) and coronary sinus should be assessed due to potential risk for compression. A virtual guidewire can be placed, and fluoroscopic angle can be simulated [25].

CT provides a comprehensive assessment of the landing zone of the device, i.e., the annulus. In the valve-in-MAC procedure, a prosthetic valve such as Sapien 3 is implanted in the calcium. Adequate calcification is required to anchor the device and prevent device embolization and PVL. A MAC score has been proposed, based on calcium thickness, degree of circumference involved, calcification of one or both trigones, and calcification of one or both leaflets. Out of a maximum score of 10, at least 7 is required for successful valve in MAC (Fig. 11.12) [27]. For devices such as Tiara that are anchored in the basal inferolateral wall, the atrioventricular shelf of the LV myocardium adjacent to the posterior mitral leaflet is evaluated. This shelf is created due to functional mitral regurgitation, and hypertrophy or bulky calcification in this location interferes with anchoring. In mitral annular disjunction, measurements are taken at the landing zone of the device instead of where the posterior mitral leaflet inserts into the left atrium. For apical devices such as Tendyne, subvalvular anatomy, including distance from annulus to papillary muscles, distance between papillary muscles, and distance between papillary muscles and ventricular wall are necessary. LV enlargement may preclude placement of certain devices. For valve-in-valve TMVR, the inner diameter of the surgical prosthesis is useful when there is no surgical history (Fig. 11.13).

For a transapical approach, volumetric CT images help in planning to identify the intercostal space closest to the LV apex and that allows perpendicular deployment of the device to the mitral annulus. Optimal fluoroscopy angle for coaxial deployment can also be obtained. The orthogonal access point is usually anterior or anterolateral to the true apex. For a transseptal approach, CT can characterize interatrial septum, its thickness, and any lesions. The distance from the puncture site to the mitral valve can be estimated [25].

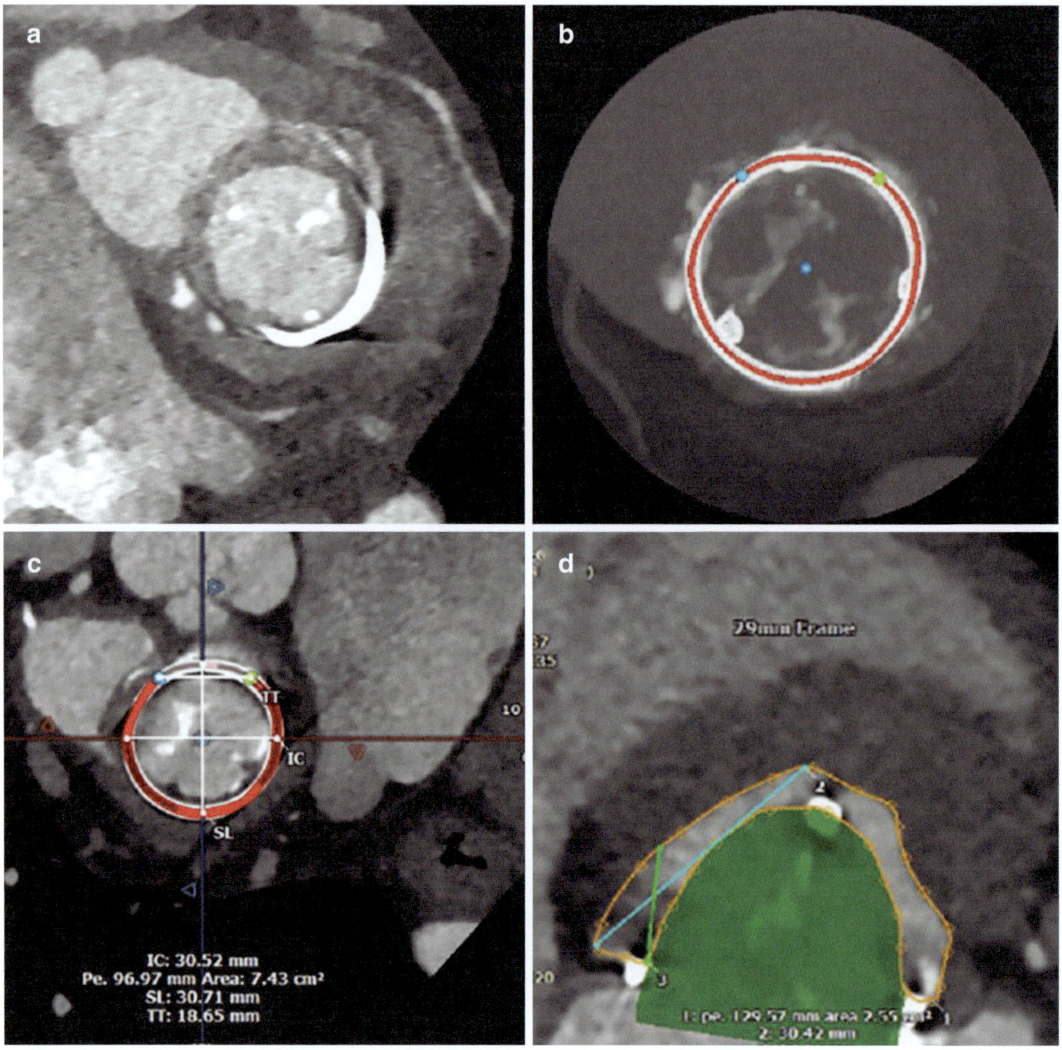

Fig. 11.13 Valve-in-valve TMVR. Short-axis CT image (**a**) shows a degenerated bioprosthetic mitral valve with thickened leaflets. Short-axis MIP image (**b**) shows contouring of the inner portion of the mitral valve prosthesis. From the short-axis image (**c**), various measurements required for device sizing are made. After placement of a virtual 29 mm Sapien prosthesis (**d**), the neo-LVOT is measured, which is 255 mm^2

Transcatheter Tricuspid Valve Intervention

Transcatheter tricuspid valve intervention (TTVI) is an alternative to surgery in the management of patients with severe tricuspid regurgitation (TR) who have high-risk factors for surgery or had previous failed tricuspid valve (TV) surgery. TTVI is challenging due to complex and variable anatomy of the TV apparatus, absence of fibrous support or calcification to anchor the device, and presence of vital structures adjacent to the TV apparatus. The available techniques for TTVI include edge-to-edge plasty, annuloplasty, spacers, valve implantation in preexisting ring/valve or native valve, and heterotopic valve replacement. MRI plays an important role in selecting patients for the procedure, and CT provides comprehensive pre-procedural information [28] (Table 11.4).

Transcatheter edge-to-edge plasty is performed with devices (*Mitraclip*, *Triclip*, *Pascal*) that approximate the TV leaflets to reduce

Table 11.4 Key CT measurements used in the pre-procedural assessment for TTVI

TTVI procedure	Key CT measurements
Edge-to-edge plasty	Coaptation gap Leaflet length Leaflet motion Coplanar angles for grasping Simulation of catheter steering
Annuloplasty	Dimensions of annulus Distance between annulus and right coronary artery Anterior lobe in right atrial appendage; Distance from inferior cavoatrial junction to first hepatic vein
Spacer	Coaptation gap Anatomic regurgitant orifice area Leaflet anatomy, length, motion Dimensions of annulus Dimension of right ventricle Distance between annulus and RV apex Anatomy of RV and anchor site Diameter of left subclavian/axillary vein Distance from left brachiocephalic vein/SVC confluence to RV anchor
Valve replacement in ring/valve	TR mechanism Leaflet morphology and function Dimensions of bioprosthetic valve Fluoroscopy angles
Valve replacement in native valve	Leaflet motion Device lead location, adherence, and redundancy Dimension of annulus Distance between annulus and right coronary artery Papillary muscle location and distance from annulus Fluoroscopy angles IVC to RA offset
Heterotopic valve implantation	TR grade and holosystolic flow reversal (in echo) RV systolic function Dimensions of SVC and IVC Distance between the inferior cavoatrial junction and first hepatic vein Shape of superior cavoatrial junction

TR. Edge-to-edge plasty is performed when there is only up to moderate tethering of TV leaflets, with good leaflet mobility and without leaflet impingement due to devices. Characterization of leaflet anatomy is essential for this technique since clips work only if placed at the medial aspect of leaflets avoiding commissure. There is wide variation in TV leaflet anatomy. The classic three leaflet pattern of anterior, posterior, and septal leaflets is seen in 28–58%, whereas a four-leaflet pattern is seen in 42–52%, two-leaflet configuration is seen in 2–10%, and a five-leaflet configuration is seen in 2–3% [29]. Several measurements are made on the leaflets to help procedural planning. Coaptation gap is the space between the tip of the leaflets, measured on a long-axis view. Tenting measurements including height, area, and angle reflect leaflet tethering, measured on end-systolic four-chamber views. Large coaptation gap of >10 mm, increased tenting height of >10 mm, and increased tenting area of >1.6 cm^2 are not suitable for edge-to-edge repairs. A leaflet length of ≥6 mm or ≥ 9 mm is required for grasping of TV leaflets for the Triclip device [28]. Fluoroscopy angles of coplanar and orthogonal views of the tricuspid annulus (TA) help with catheter steering and coaxial deployment [28].

Annuloplasty reduces TR by decreasing the annular size, which improves leaflet coaptation. Annuloplasty is performed when there is TA dilatation with no more than mild tethering.

Annuloplasty devices can be either directly anchored to the TA (*Cardioband*, *Millipede*, *Trialign*, *Tricinch*) or indirectly placed along the atrioventricular groove (*TRAIPTA*). Dimensions of the TA is important for device sizing in annuloplasty. Similar to the mitral annulus, TA also has an elliptical and saddle-shaped anatomy with two superior and two inferior points. The anterior and posterior portions of TA are muscular, whereas the septal portion is fibrous. With functional TR, annular dilatation occurs at anterior and posterior attachments. Although TA can be measured in a routine workstation using short-axis views of TA from double oblique reconstruction, it is better to measure using dedicated software due to the complex 3D anatomy. Multiple seed points are placed along the circumference of attachment of TV to the myocardium. From a cubic spine interpolation, the 3D perimeter of this annulus is projected on a 2D short-axis image, from which the diameters, perimeter, and area are measured (Fig. 11.14) [28].

The proximity of TA to RCA is also an important parameter required for annuloplasty. The

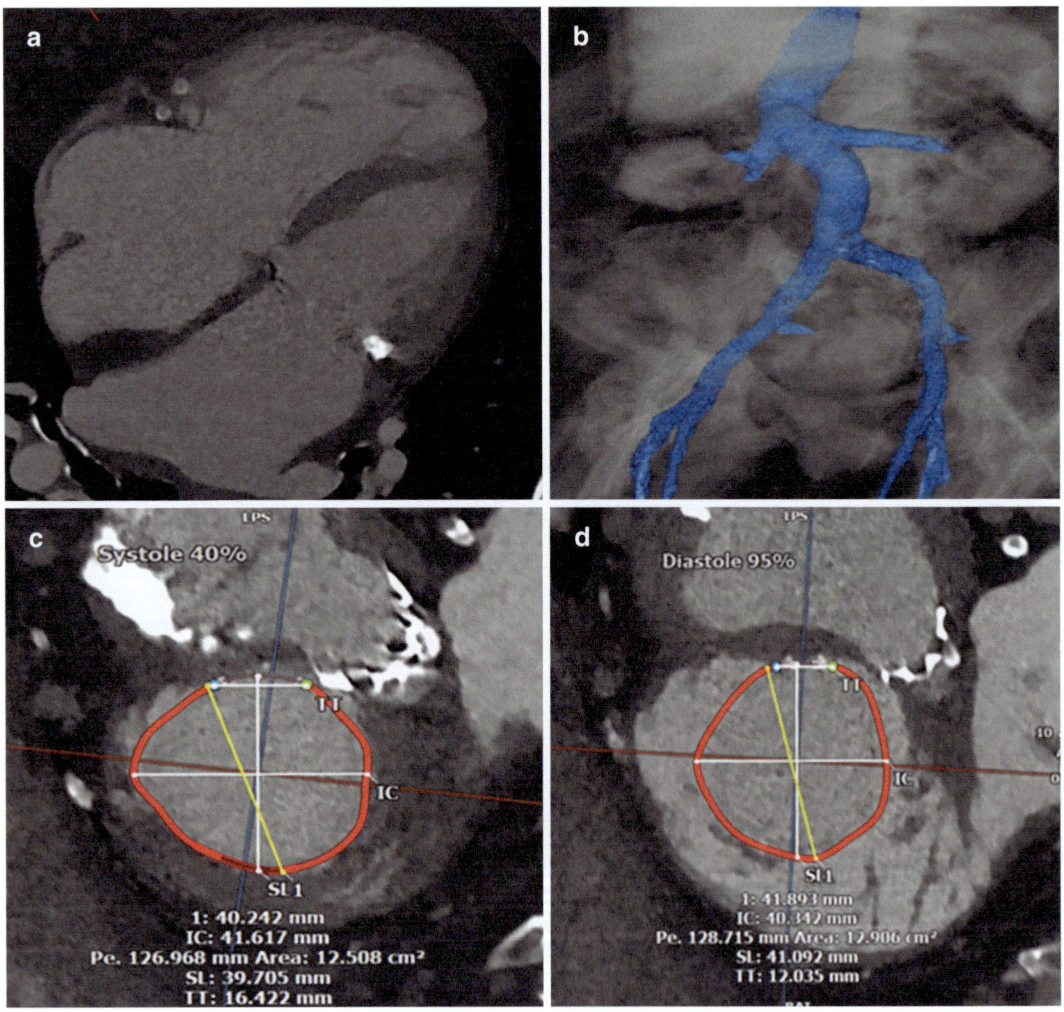

Fig. 11.14 Transcatheter tricuspid valve replacement. Four-chamber reconstructed CT image (**a**) shows wide open tricuspid leaflets and dilated tricuspid annulus, consistent with severe tricuspid regurgitation. There is dilatation of the right ventricle and both atria. (**b**) 3D volume-rendered venographic image shows normal anatomy of the IVC and iliac veins. (**c**, **d**) Measurement of the tricuspid annulus in systole (40 %) and diastole (95 %).

RCA extends in the right atrioventricular groove, seen at the level of the annulus in 65%, crosses the annulus in 25%, and superior to the annulus in 10% [30]. A distance between TA and RCA of >2 mm in CT is considered safe. A TA-RCA distance of <2 mm is seen in 6.6% of patients (van rosendeal). The TriCinch coil also has a stent in IVC to stabilize the system. Hence, the distance between the inferior cavoatrial junction (ICAJ) and the first hepatic vein is measured to estimate the risk of hepatic vein occlusion. The TRAIPTA device is placed in the right AV groove through a puncture in the right atrial appendage. A discrete anteriorly oriented lobe of RAA is important to access the pericardial space [28].

A spacer system (e.g., *Forma*) functions as a surface for leaflet coaptation and reduces TR. Spacer device is useful in patients with severe TR, but without a pacemaker or other devices. Coaptation gap and TA dimension are key pre-procedure measurements necessary for device sizing. The dimension of RV is measured determining device suitability and timing of the procedure. The distance from TA to the RV anchor is measured for estimating the length available for anchoring the device. Papillary muscle anatomy, height, and width are measured to assess any impediments along the anchor pathway. The diameter of the left subclavian and axillary vein is measured to ensure that a large 24F sheath can be accommodated. The distance from the left brachiocephalic vein-SVC confluence to the RV anchor site is measured to evaluate compatibility of the device system. Fluoroscopic angles can also be predicted for planning the procedure [28].

Transcatheter valves (*Sapien 3*, *Melody*) can be placed in patients with failed bioprosthetic valves or rings (valve-in-valve or valve-in-ring procedures). Leaflet morphology and function are important for pre-procedural assessment. In patients without surgical history/notes, CT can provide the inner diameter of the valve size of the prosthetic device. Transcatheter valves (*Evoque*, *Navigate*, *Lux*, *Trisol*, *Cardiovalve*, *Intrepid*) can also be places in patients with native tricuspid valve disease with high-risk factors and unsuitable anatomy for the abovementioned interventions. These unfavorable factors include severe leaflet tethering, large coaptation gap, and device or lead-induced TR. CT can provide information on TA size, distance from RCA, and fluoroscopic angles. CT can also be used to assess leaflet anatomy and mobility, device lead location, papillary muscle location, and IVC to RA offset. Virtual 3D valve implantation can be performed for assessment of the risk of RVOT obstruction, although this is much less common than neo-LVOT obstruction following TMVR. Venous anatomy is assessed due to the larger sheaths and delivery systems used for these procedures from a delayed phase CT of the abdomen and pelvis or lower neck [28].

Heterotopic valve implantation refers to placement of a balloon or self-expandable valve (*Sapien 3*, *Sapien XT*, *Tricvalve*, and *Tricento*) in the IVC, SVC, or both. This reduces the backflow of blood from RV to the cava, which provides symptomatic relief without improving severity of TR. This technique is used in patients who are not eligible for other TTVI procedures. The presence of severe TR with holosystolic flow reversal is essential for the success for this procedure, evaluated using echocardiography. Normal RV systolic function is also important since baseline RV systolic dysfunction can worsen underlying heart failure after heterotopic valve implantation. For device sizing, dimensions of IVC and SVC are measured at various levels. IVC is measured at the ICAJ and at the level of diaphragm. SVC is measured at the superior cavoatrial junction and at the level of the right pulmonary artery. The distance between the ICAJ and the first hepatic vein is measured to assess the risk of hepatic vein occlusion with a distance of <15 mm considered high risk. A funnel-shaped SCAJ also increases the risk of device migration [28].

Transcatheter Pulmonary Valve Replacement

Transcatheter pulmonary valve replacement (TPVR) is used in the treatment of right ventricular outflow tract (RVOT) dysfunction in patients with surgically repaired congenital heart disease who are at high surgical risk. TPVR devices can be placed either in an indwelling RV-PA conduit, native RVOT, or surgical bioprosthetic valves. Balloon-expandable valves (*Melody*, *Sapien 3*, *Sapien XT)* are used when there is a rigid landing zone such as a conduit or bioprosthetic valve with pre-stenting performed for protecting valve housing. Self-expanding valves (*Harmony*, *Pulsta*, *Venus P*, *Alterra*) have been developed for larger native RVOT, which are useful in treatment of pulmonic regurgitation, but cannot expand stenotic segments [31].

CT and MRI provide information required for pre-procedural planning (Table 11.5). The shape of RVOT on CT or MRI helps in determining the complexity of the procedure. Five types have been recognized by Schievano et al. [32]. Type 1 is pyramidal shape that tapers toward pulmonary artery (PA) bifurcation, commonly seen in patch augmentation repair. Type 2 is cylindrical shape with a uniform caliber. Type 3 is inverted pyramidal shape, which is larger toward PA bifurcation. Type 4 is fusiform shape, which is wider centrally with proximal and distal tapering. Type 5 is hourglass shape with central narrowing. Types 2 and 4 are favorable, whereas Types 1, 3, and 5 are unfavorable. For device sizing, the landing zone of the device is measured in double oblique axial reconstructions (Fig. 11.15). Novel devices such as Harmony require multiple measurements including diameters at multiple levels, including sub-valve, mid-valve, supra-valve, mid-trunk, pre-bifurcation, and roof of MPA. In addition, lengths are measured at different levels including sub-valve to supravalvar areas, supra-valve to pre-bifurcation, RVOT to pre-bifurcation, and RVOT to the roof of MPA. Due to the dynamic nature of the RVOT, measurements are made in both systole and diastole (Fig. 11.16). Extensive dynamism is challenging to the TPVR procedure due to difficulty in anchoring the device. For the Harmony device, a fit analysis is performed to determine if there is proximal and distal valve frame interference with PA and RVOT and there is no compression of valve housing. Landing zone can also be measured within a dysfunctional bioprosthesis [31].

Table 11.5 Key CT and MRI measurements used in the evaluation for TPVR

Eligibility for procedure	Quantification of pulmonary regurgitation/stenosis (MRI) Quantification of RV dilatation and RV dysfunction (MRI or CT) Quantification of LV dysfunction
Landing zone/ RVOT/conduit	Shape Diameters Length Dynamism
Need for additional interventions	Branch pulmonary arteries Calcifications Coronary artery location

CT can also identify features that increase the risk of complications and may warrant additional interventional procedures. Circumferential, extensive calcification in the conduit/RVOT indicates a higher risk of rupture with balloon expansion, which is more common in homografts. Extensive calcification indicates the need for pre-stenting (*covered stent or stainless steel*) to provide a rigid landing zone and reduce the risk of rupture with balloon expansion. The location of the coronary artery of <2 mm within RVOT/conduit indicates the risk of coronary artery compression with balloon expansion (Fig. 11.17). This should be assessed in all cardiac phases, with higher risk for anomalous coronary arteries or surgically reimplanted coronary arteries (arterial switch, Ross procedure). The risk is ultimately determined during cardiac catheterization with simultaneous coronary angiography and balloon expansion in RVOT [33]. Anatomy of branch pulmonary arteries is evaluated to determine how high the valve can be implanted. If there is severe stenosis in the proximal PA, this indicates the need for stent placement prior to TPVR [31].

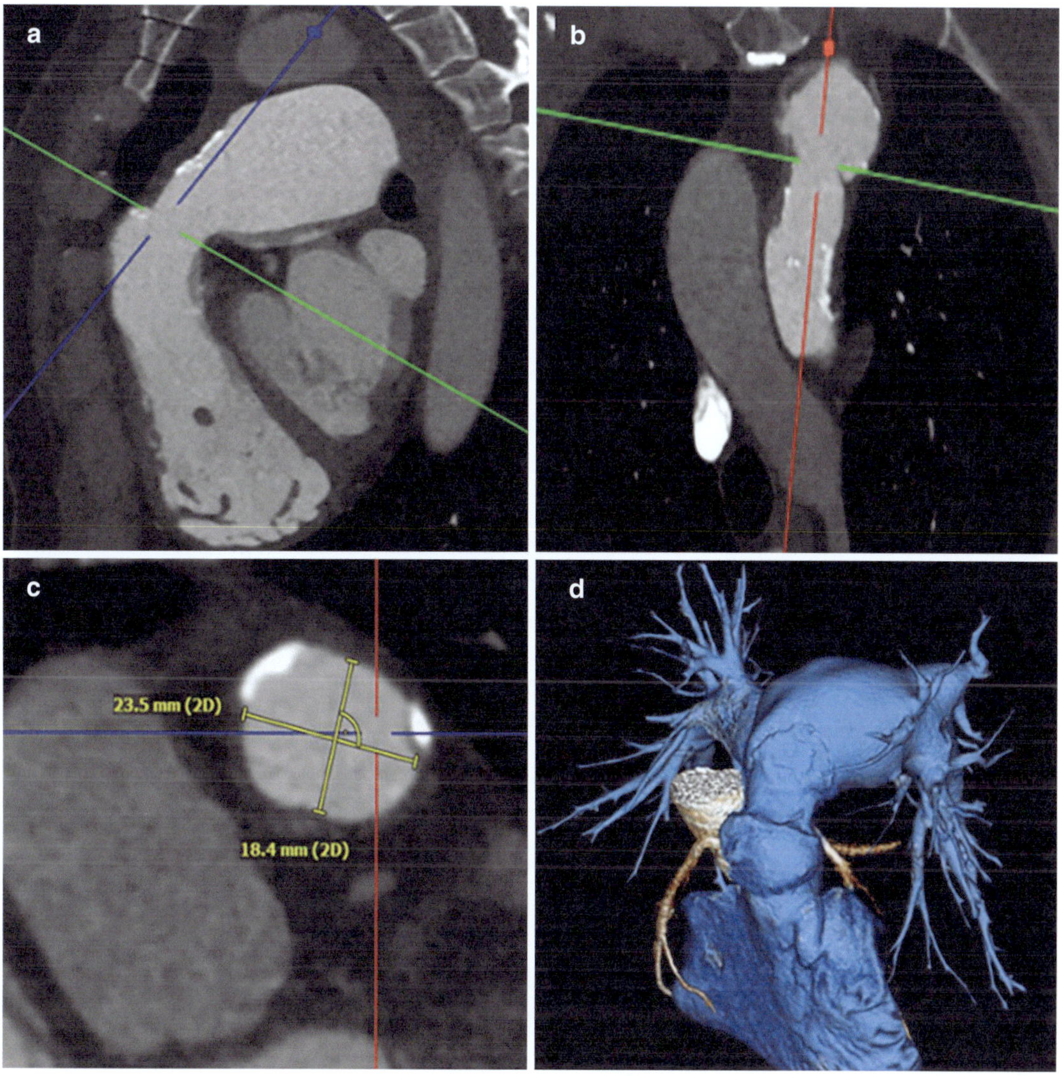

Fig. 11.15 Transcatheter pulmonary valve replacement. A patient with repaired tetralogy of Fallot with a RV-PA conduit was evaluated for TPVR with Melody valve. Sagittal (**a**) and coronal (**b**) CT images show moderate calcification of the homograft due to degeneration. These multiplanar reconstructions are used to generate an orthogonal reconstruction in the short-axis plane (**c**), which is used to measure the landing zone for Melody valve placement. Volume-rendered CT (**d**) image shows the anatomy of the pulmonary homograft and pulmonary arteries

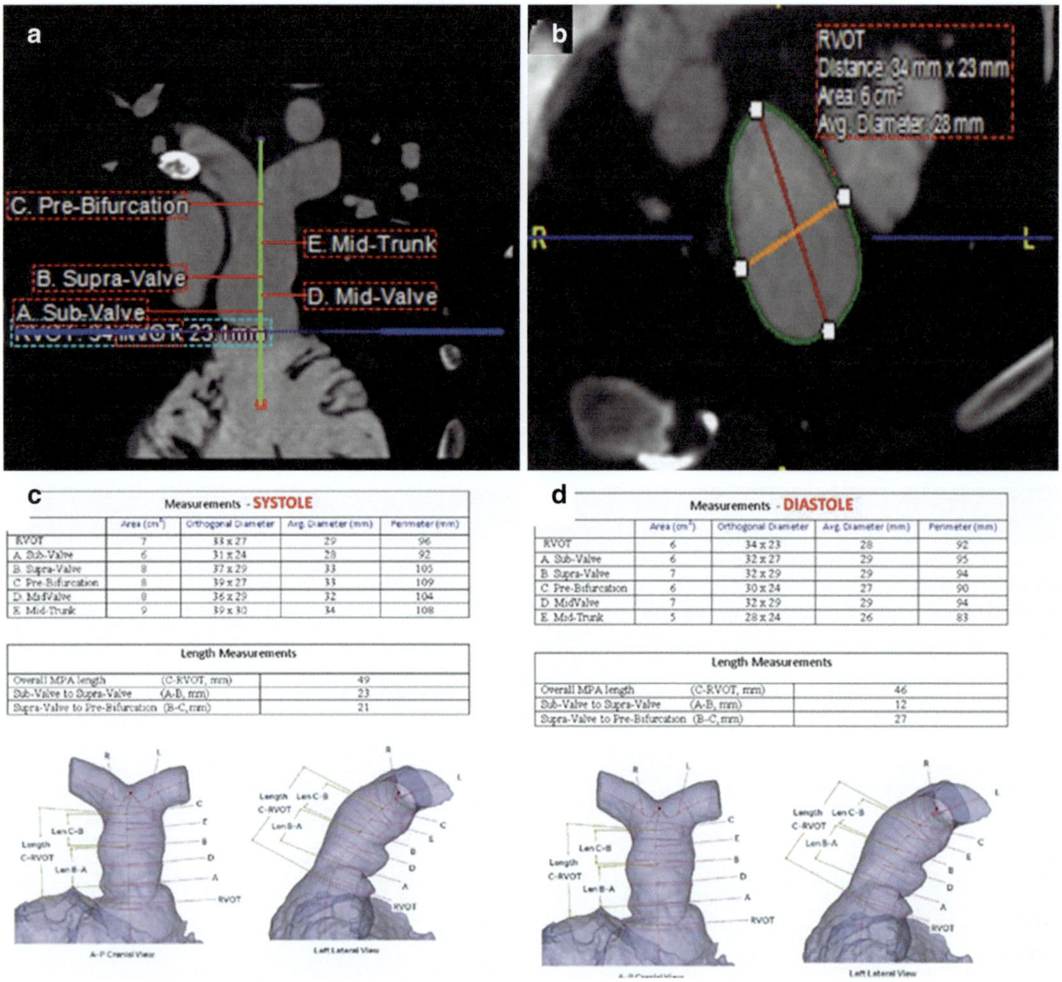

c

Measurements - SYSTOLE	Area (cm²)	Orthogonal Diameter	Avg. Diameter (mm)	Perimeter (mm)
RVOT	7	33 x 27	29	96
A. Sub-Valve	6	31 x 24	28	92
B. Supra-Valve	8	37 x 29	33	105
C. Pre-Bifurcation	8	39 x 27	33	109
D. MidValve	8	36 x 29	32	104
E. Mid-Trunk	9	39 x 30	34	108

Length Measurements	
Overall MPA length (C-RVOT, mm)	49
Sub-Valve to Supra-Valve (A-B, mm)	23
Supra-Valve to Pre-Bifurcation (B-C, mm)	21

d

Measurements - DIASTOLE	Area (cm²)	Orthogonal Diameter	Avg. Diameter (mm)	Perimeter (mm)
RVOT	6	34 x 23	28	92
A. Sub-Valve	6	32 x 27	29	95
B. Supra-Valve	7	32 x 29	29	94
C. Pre-Bifurcation	6	30 x 24	27	90
D. MidValve	7	32 x 29	29	94
E. Mid-Trunk	5	28 x 24	26	83

Length Measurements	
Overall MPA length (C-RVOT, mm)	46
Sub-Valve to Supra-Valve (A-B, mm)	12
Supra-Valve to Pre-Bifurcation (B-C, mm)	27

Fig. 11.16 Pre-procedural assessment for Harmony TPVR. Measurements required for Harmony valve TPVR are measured in long-axis (**a**) and short-axis (**b**) reconstructed images. Several diameters and lengths are measured both in systole (**c**) and diastole (**d**)

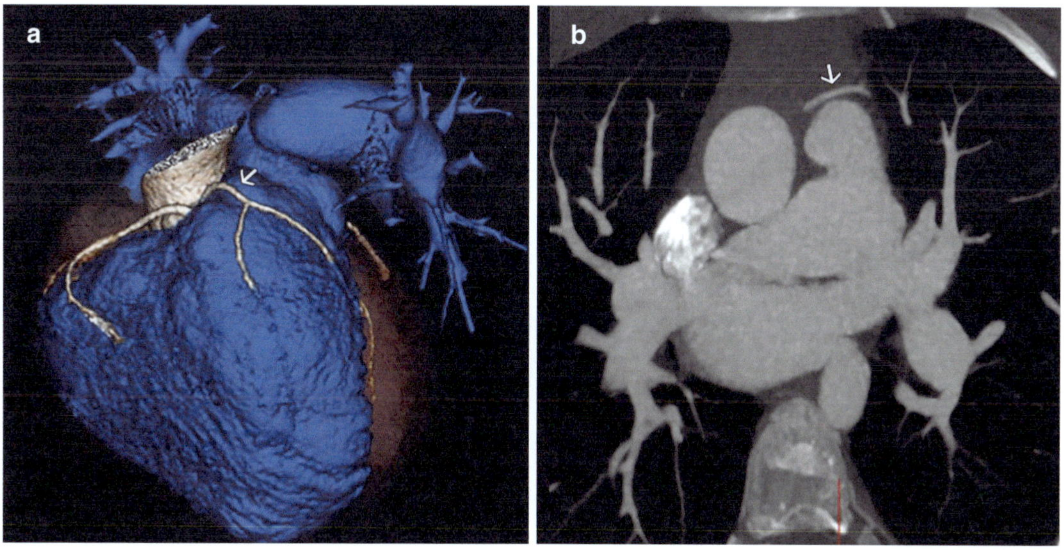

Fig. 11.17 Coronary artery anomaly for TPVR. Volume-rendered 3D (**a**) and axial MIP (**b**) images in a patient being evaluated for TPVR show an anomalous left anterior descending coronary artery originating from the right coronary sinus and coursing (arrow) anterior to the pulmonary homograft. This increases the risk of coronary compression when the balloon-expandable valve is expanded

Transcatheter Left Atrial Appendage Closure

Transcatheter left atrial appendage closure (TLAAC) is an effective treatment strategy with Class IIb recommendation (level of evidence B) for patients with non-valvular atrial fibrillation at increased risk of stroke, especially in patients who need an alternative to oral anticoagulation either due to prior major bleeding event, inability to maintain therapeutic INR, or medical condition/occupation/lifestyle with high risk of trauma [34]. TLAAC devices are placed either through an endocardial approach (*Watchman*, *Watchman FLX*, *Amplatzer cardiac plug*, *Amulet*) or a hybrid endocardial/epicardial (*Lariat*, *Aegis*) approach. The role of pre procedural imaging is to assess contraindications for the device, provide measurements for accurate device sizing, and assess for other anatomical factors. CT provides a comprehensive evaluation of these parameters [35, 36] (Table 11.6).

A thrombus in the LAA is an absolute contraindication to TLAAC due to the risk of thrombus mobilization and stroke. CT with early and delayed phases is as sensitive as trans-esophageal echocardiography (TEE) in the diagnosis of thrombus [37]. A thrombus has low attenuation or < 100 HU in the arterial phase that persists in delayed phases, whereas slow flow is not persistent in the delayed phase. Prone scan, split bolus injection, or dual-energy iodine map can also characterize thrombus. Contraindications for hybrid device include pericardial thickening, calcification and adhesion, large LAA of >4 cm, multilobed LAA with lobes of >4 cm, retro PA LAA, pectus excavatum, and posteriorly rotated heart [35].

Table 11.6 Key parameters required for transcatheter LAAC

Contraindications	LAA thrombus Pericardial abnormalities
LAA characteristics	LAA morphology LAA ostial diameter Device landing zone diameter LAA length
Other parameters	Coumadin ridge thickness Relationship between LAA and left superior pulmonary vein Fluoroscopic angles for largest LAA/landing zone diameter and longest length of LAA Atrial septal anatomy Pulmonary vein anatomy Left atrial size Accessory LAA/LA diverticulum

The LAA has an elliptical orifice in 69% of the population, bounded anterosuperiorly by the coumadin ridge, which separates it from the left superior pulmonary vein (LSPV) and posteroinferiorly by a vestibule, which separates it from the mitral annulus. The shape of the LAA is highly variable, with implications for measurements and treatment [35] (Table 11.7). Accurate measurements of LAA are important to determine the device size accurately. To ensure reproducibility, LAA is measured based on a long-axis view of the LA generated perpendicular to LCX. In this view, the longest view of LAA should be obtained. The LAA is defined as extending from adjacent to the LCX origin to the coumadin ridge. The ostium is measured in cross section. Subsequent measurements differ for devices. For the Watchman device, the landing zone (LZ) is located 10–20 mm distal to the LAA ostium. The LZ diameter is measured from LCx to the leading edge of LZ, and the length is measured from the middle of LZ to the tip of LAA. For Amulet and ACP, the LZ is 12–15 mm distal to the LAA ostium. The LZ diameter is measured perpendicular to the free walls of LAA, and the length is measured from the LAA ostium to the roof of the LAA (Fig. 11.18). Due to dynamism of LAA, measurements are made in the largest dimension in systole. Curved multiplanar reconstructions may help in measuring complex shapes such as chicken wing [35]. CT has been shown to have 100% accuracy in device sizing, with TEE undersizing in 53–62%. Based on TEE, 23% of patients would have been excluded [38]. This potential difference is likely due to volume depletion during fasting for TEE and variations with cardiac cycle. In addition, TEE measures in four different angles and averages measurements.

The thickness of the coumadin ridge estimates the risk of impingement of LSPV by disk and lobe devices like ACP and Amulet. The coumadin ridge is measured either in axial CT or endocardial view, with <5 mm thickness implying a thin ridge [35]. The LAA and LSPV are at the same level in two-thirds of patients, with LAA superior in one-fifth and LSPV superior to LAA in the rest [39]. Close relationship with LSPV may interfere with subsequent ablation of pulmonary vein and venous return. Fluoroscopic angles that mimic the best intraprocedural view of the largest diameter of the ostium and landing zone as well as the longest dimension of LAA without foreshortening can be estimated. Atrial septal thickness and abnormali-

Table 11.7 Shapes of left atrial appendage and implication for TLAAC

Shape	Description	Comments
Windsock	Single lobe, no sharp bend	Easy to measure and implant
Chicken wing	Multiple lobes with a dominant lobe, sharp bend	Most common type Complex procedure Landing zone measurement challenging—curved MPR may help Measure distance from ostium to bend Contraindicated for hybrid approach due to location behind pulmonary artery
Cactus	Multilobulated, each lobe >1 cm Dominant lobe present No sharp bend	Easy to measure and implant
Cauliflower	Multilobulated, short irregular, no dominant lobe or bend	Difficult to identify landing zone Challenging procedure Higher risk of device embolization
Whale tail	Two lobes of similar size	Landing zones measured in each lobe May require two devices
Cone	Rapidly decreasing transverse diameter from ostium to tip	Landing zone diameter changes rapidly, changing device size Higher pressure at the distal aspect—embolization of device

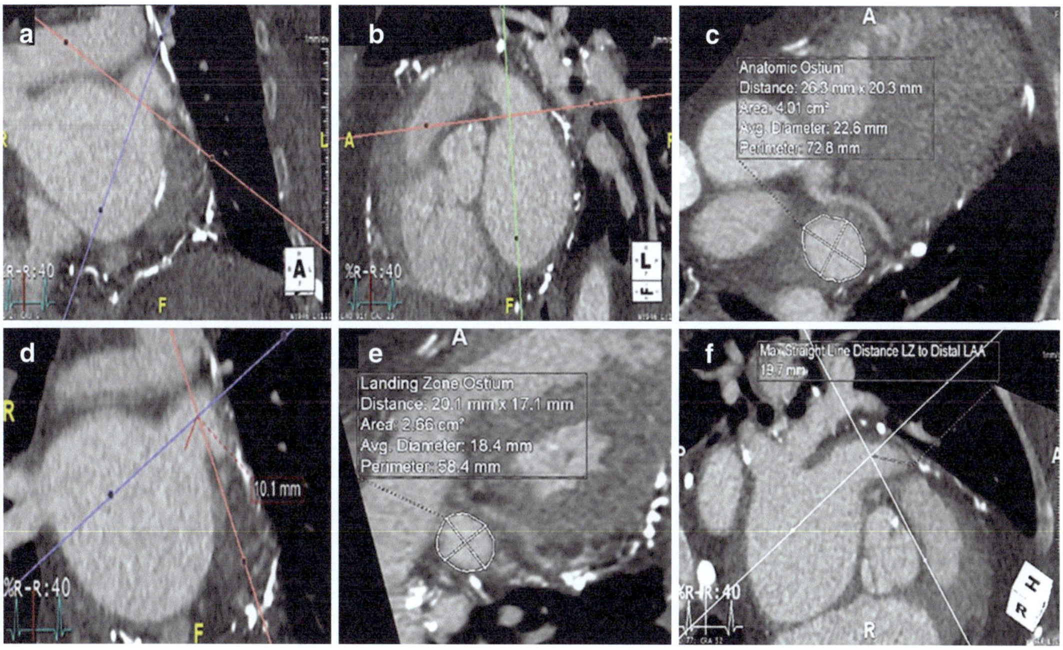

Fig. 11.18 Measurements for transcatheter left atrial appendage closure. From coronal (**a**) and sagittal (**b**) multiplanar reconstructed CT images, a short-axis view of the LAA ostium is generated (**c**), from which the diameters, perimeter, and area of the LAA ostium are measured. For the Watchman device, the landing zone is 10–20 mm distal to the ostium (**d**). The diameter of a proposed landing zone at 10 mm is measured in cross-sectional view (**e**). The length of the LAA is measured from the landing zone to the tip of LAA (**f**)

ties such as lipomatous hypertrophy, patent foramen vale, atrial septal defect, and masses can be evaluated in preparation for atrial septostomy. An optimal site for atrial septal puncture, i.e., postero-inferior location that allows a straight trajectory along the long axis of LAA perpendicular to the ostium, can be identified, and a virtual trajectory and fluoroscopic angle can be calculated [35].

Transcatheter Atrial Septal Defect Closure

Atrial septal defect (ASD) can be closed by a transcatheter approach in those with high surgical risk and favorable anatomy. ASDs can be either secundum (70–80%), primum (10–15%), sinus venosus (5–10%), and coronary sinus defect (1%) [40]. The sinus venosus defect is associated with the partial anomalous pulmonary vein, and the coronary sinus defect is associated with the left-sided SVC. Primum, sinus venosus, and coronary sinus defects as well as those with multiple defects and aneurysmal atrial septum are typically managed with surgery. A secundum defect with suitable anatomy can be treated with transcatheter closure. CT and MRI provide information required for transcatheter closure (Table 11.8).

Table 11.8 Pre-procedural imaging for atrial septal defect closure

Quantification of shunt	2D/4D phase contrast MRI of pulmonic and aortic valves to measure Qp/Qs Direct quantification of shunt
Chamber sizes	Enlarged RA and RV
Pulmonary hypertension	Should be absent
Type of ASD	Secundum and primum are suitable
Size of ASD	10–38 mm
Rim	>5 mm

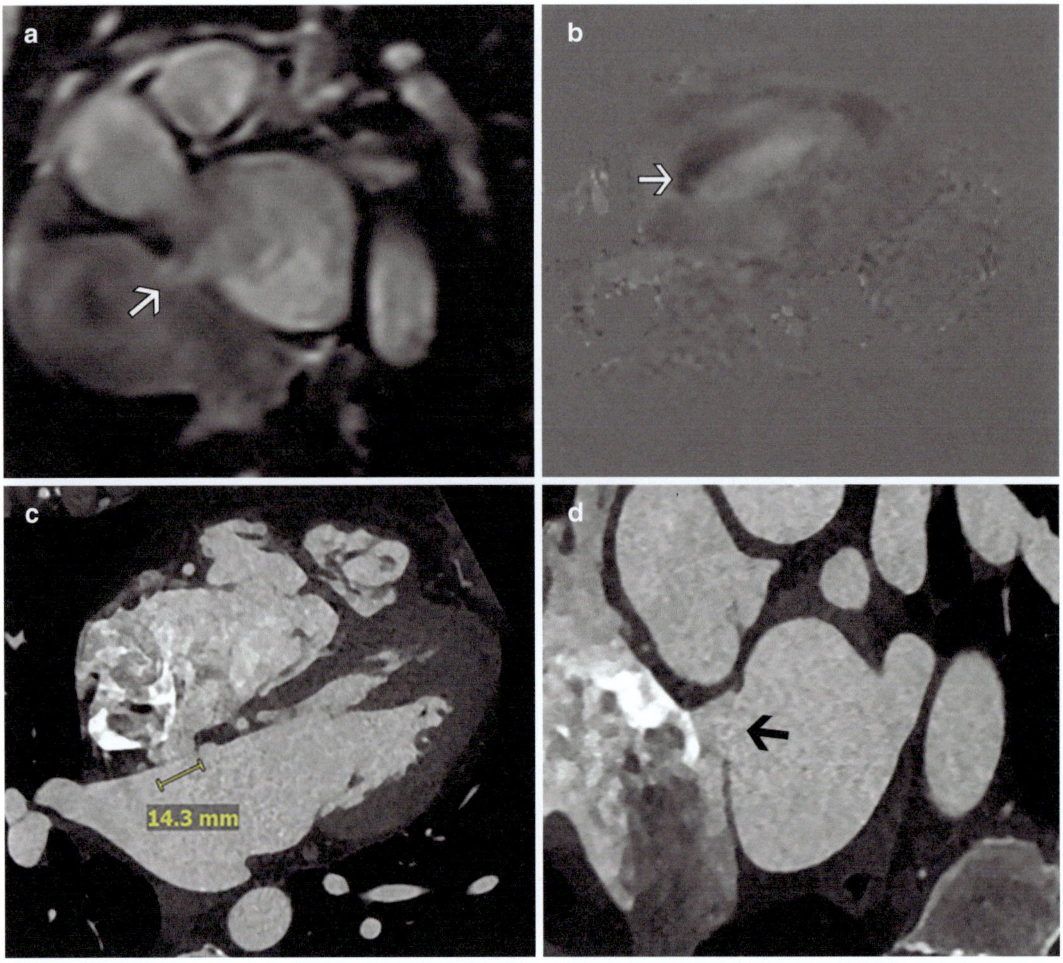

Fig. 11.19 ASD closure. Short-axis cine MR image (**a**) shows a small secundum type of ASD (arrow). (**b**) On a four-chamber phase contrast image, the shunting (arrow) can be shown. The four-chamber reconstructed CT image (**c**) shows the secundum defect measuring 14 mm. There is also enlargement of the RV and RA. (**d**) The short-axis reconstructed CT image (arrow) shows the ASD with deficient superior rim (**d**)

The shunt is quantified using 2D/4D flow MRI with a pulmonary to systemic flow ratio (Qp/Qs) of >1.5, which is considered an indication for closure [41]. RA and RV dilatation without pulmonary hypertension is also an indication. Secundum defect measuring between 10 and 38 mm diameter is suitable for transcatheter closure, with the largest known device measuring 46 mm (Fig. 11.19). A rim of at least 5 mm between the ASD and pulmonary vein, free wall of the atrium, mitral valve and aortic valve (anterosuperior rim), tricuspid valve (anteroinferior rim), coronary sinus, SV (posterosuperior rim), and IVC (posteroinferior rim) is required for anchoring the device. If the rim is insufficient, transcatheter closure is challenging, and hence surgery is preferred. Deficient posteroinferior rim is associated with device embolization toward IVC (Panjwani).

Conclusion

Quantitative imaging plays an important role in pre-procedural assessment for transcatheter interventions for structural heart disease. CT provides comprehensive evaluation that is required for patient selection, device selection, and device sizing. CT also provides parameters that indicate high risk with interventions and predict outcomes. MRI is useful in select cases who cannot have CT due to severe renal dysfunction.

References

1. Rajiah PS. Imaging in transcatheter interventions for structural heart diseases. Semin Roentgenol. 2024;59(1):2.
2. Rajiah PS, Alkhadhi H, Van Mieghem NM, Budde RPJ. Utility of photon counting CT in transcatheter structural heart disease interventions. Semin Roentgenol. 2024;59(1):32–43.
3. Hagar MT, Soschynski M, Saffar R, et al. Accuracy of ultrahigh-resolution photon-counting CT in detecting coronary artery disease in a high-risk population. Radiology. 2023;307(5):e22305.
4. Kalisz K, Halliburton S, Abbara S, et al. Update on cardiovascular applications of multienergy CT. Radiographics. 2017;37(7):1955–74.
5. Scully PR, Patel KP, Saberwal B, et al. Identifying cardiac amyloid in aortic stenosis: ECV quantification by CT in TAVR patients. JACC Cardiovasc Imaging. 2020;13(1):2177–89.
6. El Sabbagh A, Eleid MF, Matsumoto JM, et al. Three-dimensional prototyping for procedural simulation of transcatheter mitral valve replacement in patients with mitral annular calcification. Catheter Cardiovasc Interv. 2018;92(7):E537–49.
7. Androshchuk V, Monttarello N, Lahoti N, et al. Evolving capabilities of computed tomography imaging for transcatheter valvular heart interventions – new opportunities for precision medicine. Int J Cardiovasc Imaging. 2024. https://doi.org/10.1007/s10554-024-03247-z.
8. Proffitt EK, Kaproth-Joslin K, Chaturvedi A, Hobbs SK. Role of magnetic resonance imaging in transcatheter structural heart disease interventions. Semin Roentgenol. 2024;59(1):20–31.
9. Panda A, Francois CJ, Bookwalter CA, et al. Non-contrast magnetic resonance angiography: Techniques, principles and applications. Magn Reson Imaging Clin N Am. 2023;31(3):337–60.
10. Kallianos K, Henry TS, Yeghiazarians Y, et al. Ferumoxytol MRA for transcatheter aortic valve replacement planning with renal insufficiency. Int J Cardiol. 2017;231:255–7.
11. Beerkens FJ, Tang GHL, Kini AS, et al. Transcatheter aortic valve replacement beyond severe aortic stenosis. JACC. 2025;85(9):944–64.
12. Chiarito M, Spirito A, Nicolas J, et al. Evolving devices and materials in transcatheter aortic valve replacement. what to use and for whom. J Clin Med. 2022;11(15):4445.
13. Blanke P, Weir-McCall JR, Achenbach S, et al. Computed tomography imaging in the context of transcatheter aortic valve implantation (TAVI)/transcatheter aortic valve replacement (TAVR): an expert consensus document of the Society of Cardiovascular Computed Tomography. JACC Cardiovasc Imaging. 2019;12(1):1–24.
14. Ribeiro HB, Nombela-Franco L, Urena M, et al. Coronary obstruction following transcatheter aortic valve implantation: a systematic review. JACC Cardiovasc Interv. 2013;6(5):452–61.
15. Renker M, Schoepf UJ, Kim WK. Combined CT coronary artery assessment and TAVI planning. Diagnostics (Basel). 2023;13(7):1327.
16. Peper J, Becker LM, van den Berg H, et al. Diagnostic performance of CCTA and CT-FFR for the detection of CAD in TAVR work-up. J Am Coll Cardiol Interv. 2022;15(11):1140–9.
17. Okuyama K, Jilaihawi H, Kashif M, et al. Transfemoral access assessment for transcatheter aortic valve replacement: evidence-based application of computed tomography over invasive angiography. Circ Cardiovasc Imaging. 2014;8(1):e001995.
18. Kalisz K, Moore A, Chaturvedi A, Rajiah PS. Multimodality imaging in planning of complex TAVR procedures. Semin Roentgenol. 2024;59(1):57–66.
19. Redondo A, Baladron Zorita C, Tchetche D, et al. Commissural versus coronary optimized alignment during transcatheter aortic valve replacement. JACC Cardiovasc Interv. 2022;15(2):135–46.
20. Clavel MA, Burwash IG, Pibarot P. Cardiac imaging for assessing low-gradient severe aortic stenosis. JACC Cardiovasc Imaging. 2017;10(2):185–202.
21. Michelena HI, Della Corte A, Evangelista A, et al. International consensus statement on nomenclature and classification of the congenital bicuspid aortic valve and its aortopathy, for clinical, surgical, interventional and research purposes. Eur J Cardiothorac Surg. 2021;60(3):448–76.
22. Yoon SH, Schmidt T, Bleiziffer S, et al. Transcatheter aortic valve replacement in pure native aortic valve regurgitation. J Am Coll Cardiol. 2017;70(22):2752–63.
23. Holmes DR Jr, Nishimura RA, Grover FL, et al. Annual outcomes with transcatheter valve therapy: from the STS/ACC TVR registry. J Am Coll Cardiol. 2015;66(25):2813–23.
24. Berurtheret S, Karam N, Resseguier N, et al. Femoral versus non femoral peripheral access for transcatheter aortic valve replacement. J Am Coll Cardiol. 2019;74(22):2728–39.
25. Ranganath P, Moore A, Guerrero M, et al. CT for pre- and post-procedural evaluation of transcatheter mitral valve replacement. Radiographics. 2020;40(6):1528–53.
26. Yoon SH, Bleiziffer S, Latib A, et al. Predictors of left ventricular outflow tract obstruction after transcatheter mitral valve replacement. JACC Cardiovasc Interv. 2019;12(2):182–93.
27. Guerrero M, Wang DD, Pursnani A, et al. A cardiac computed tomography-based score to cat-

egorize mitral annular calcification severity and predict valve embolization. JACC Cardiovasc Imaging. 2023;13(9):1945–57.
28. Rajiah PS, Reddy P, Baliyan V, et al. Utility of CT and MRI in tricuspid valve interventions. Radiographics. 2023;43(7):e220153.
29. Hahn RT, Weckbach LT, Noack T, et al. Proposal for a standard echocardiographic tricuspid valve nomenclature. JACC Cardiovasc Imaging. 2021;14(7):1299–305.
30. van Rosendael PJ, Kamperidis V, Kong WKF, et al. Computed tomography for planning transcatheter tricuspid valve therapy. Eur Heart J. 2017;38(9):665–74.
31. Canan A, Ocazionez-Trujillo D, Vargas D, et al. Pre-and post-procedure imaging of transcatheter pulmonary valve implantation. Radiographics. 2022;42(4):991–1011.
32. Schievano S, Coats L, Migliavacca F, et al. Variations in right ventricular outflow tract morphology following repair of congenital heart disease: implications for percutaneous pulmonary valve implantation. J Cardiovasc Magn Reson. 2007;9(4):687–95.
33. Fraisse A, Assaidi A, Mauri L, et al. Coronary artery compression during intention to treat right ventricle outflow with percutaneous pulmonary valve implantation: incidence, diagnosis, and outcome. Catheter Cardiovasc Interv. 2014;83:260–8.
34. January CT, Wann LS, Calkins H, et al. 2019 AHA/ACC/HRS focused update of the 2014 AHA/ACC/HRS guideline for the management of patients with atrial fibrillation: a report of the American College of Cardiology/American Heart Association task force on clinical practice guidelines and the Heart Rhythm Society. J Am Coll Cardiol. 2019;74(1):104–32.
35. Rajiah P, Alkhouli M, Thaden J, et al. Pre-and post-procedural CT of transcatheter left atrial appendage closure devices. Radiographics. 2021;41(3):680–98.
36. Rajiah PS. Imaging evaluation following left atrial appendage closure. Semin Roentgenol. 2024;59(1):121–34.
37. Yu S, Zhang H, Li H. Cardiac computed tomography versus transesophageal echocardiography for the detection of left atrial appendage thrombus: a systematic review and meta-analysis. J Am Heart Assoc. 2021;10(23):e022505.
38. Wang DD, Eng M, Kupsky D, et al. Application of 3-dimensional computed tomographic image guidance to WATCHMAN implantation and impact on early operator learning curve: single-center experience. JACC Cardiovasc Interv. 2016;9(22):2329–40.
39. Syed FF, Noheria A, DeSimone CV, Asirvatham SJ. Left atrial appendage ligation and exclusion technology in the incubator. J Atr Fibrillation. 2015;8(2):1160.
40. Panjwani B, Singh A, Shah A. CT and MR imaging for atrial septal defect repair. Semin Roentgenol. 2024;59(1):103–11.
41. Rajiah P, Kanne JP. Cardiac MRI: part 1, cardiovascular shunts. AJR Am J Roentgenol. 2012;197:W603–20.

Quantitative Imaging in Cardiac Electrophysiology

12

Scott M. Bugenhagen

Introduction

Electrophysiology is a clinical subspecialty of cardiology that seeks to diagnose, manage, and treat a variety of pathological conditions associated with the electrical conduction pathways in the heart. These conditions include ectopic beats such as premature ventricular contractions (PVCs), supraventricular tachycardias such as atrial fibrillation (AF), ventricular arrhythmias such as ventricular tachycardia (VT), and heart blocks that can arise at different positions along the conduction pathways. Arrythmias are common, particularly in older patients, and certain arrythmias may be lethal if left untreated. Treatment options include pharmacologic therapy with antiarrhythmic medications, pacemakers to augment pacing rhythm in the heart, implantable cardioverter defibrillators (ICDs) to provide both pacemaker function and to deliver electrical shocks in the setting of life-threatening arrhythmias such as ventricular fibrillation (VF) and ventricular tachycardia (VT), and ablation procedures to physically alter and eliminate the pathological circuits responsible for triggering and sustaining arrhythmias [1, 2].

Noninvasive imaging plays an important role in evaluating and managing arrhythmias. Quantitative imaging with CT and MRI in particular is increasingly being relied on to provide quantitative information such as size and thickness of anatomical structures, cardiac function, and precise location, pattern, and extent of scar, representing the arrhythmogenic substrate responsible for arrhythmias that is targeted for ablation with invasive procedures. This information can aid the electrophysiologist in diagnosis, pre-procedural treatment planning, and evaluating procedure outcomes. Substrate maps generated with CT or MRI can also provide complimentary information to invasively derived electroanatomic maps (EAMs) that are generated with a variety of invasive mapping techniques and may aid in real-time guidance during ablation procedures [3–6]. In this chapter, we will review clinical applications of CT and MRI in cardiac electrophysiology focusing on established quantitative techniques such as anatomical measurements and scar quantification as well as emerging techniques such as personalized computational modeling of arrhythmias.

Atrial Fibrillation

Atrial fibrillation is a supraventricular tachycardia thought to result from pathological remodeling of cardiac tissues in the atria resulting in scar

S. M. Bugenhagen (✉)
Mallinckrodt Institute of Radiology, Department of Radiology, Washington University School of Medicine, St. Louis, MO, USA
e-mail: sbugenhagen@wustl.edu

R. Gill, P. Rajiah (eds.), *Quantitative Imaging in the Thorax*,
https://doi.org/10.1007/978-3-032-14103-3_12

formation and heterogeneous conduction leading to re-entrant circuits and ectopy originating from myocyte sleeves in the pulmonary veins [7]. It is the most common cardiac arrhythmia encountered in clinical practice, with a prevalence of ~2% [8]. Pulmonary vein isolation, a catheter ablation technique that aims to suppress triggering of AF, is a commonly used second-line therapy after failure of antiarrhythmic medication. It works by generating circumferential scar at the pulmonary vein ostia to electrically isolate and prevent sites of ectopy originating in the pulmonary veins from triggering AF in the atria [9, 10]. Ablation techniques used in pulmonary vein isolation include radiofrequency ablation, cryoablation, and pulsed field electroporation [11].

Pre-procedural Assessment

Noninvasive imaging with CT and MRI is an important component of pre-procedural assessment prior to AF ablation. CT allows for accurate delineation of anatomical structures including measurements such as pulmonary ostia sizes and peri-esophageal fat pad thickness, and MRI allows for localization and quantification of left atrial fibrosis.

Anatomical Assessment

Accurate delineation of anatomical structures is critical for pre-procedural planning prior to AF ablation. CT is the standard modality for anatomical assessment owing to its higher resolution and better definition of fine anatomical structures compared to MRI. CT protocols used for this purpose are generally acquired in the angiographic phase timed for the left atrium and pulmonary veins followed by a delayed phase performed from 60 s to 6 min following injection to evaluate for the presence of thrombus (Fig. 12.1).

Quantification of pulmonary vein anatomy includes assessment of the number and location of pulmonary veins (normally two pulmonary vein ostia are present on both sides), size of each pulmonary vein ostium, and branching distance, defined as the distance from the first branching point to the pulmonary vein ostium. Ostial size measurements are performed on a plane orthogonal to the pulmonary vein ostia, obtained on multiplanar reconstruction (MPR) images on CT (Fig. 12.2). Distance to the first branch point is also performed on MPR images and may require curved MPR for improved accuracy (Fig. 12.2). Ostial size measurements help to inform selection of catheter size and to estimate procedural risk, as smaller ostia (with a minimum diameter of <10 mm) are associated with increased risk of post-procedural stenosis. Branching distance is used to identify the presence of early branching, defined as a branching distance of <10 mm, which is also associated with higher risk for post-procedural stenosis or occlusion of the branching vein [12, 13].

Estimation of the eccentric index, defined as the ratio of the maximum (long axis) diameter to

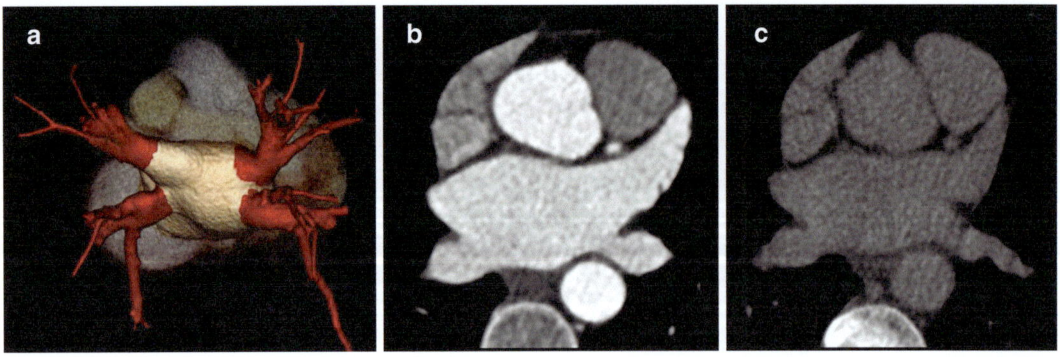

Fig. 12.1 CT pulmonary vein protocol. Contrast-enhanced CT performed for anatomical assessment prior to atrial fibrillation ablation. (**a**) 3D reconstruction of the left atrium and pulmonary veins, with pulmonary veins color-coded in red. (**b**) Contrast-enhanced CT image acquired in the angiographic phase timed for the left atrium and pulmonary veins. (**c**) Delayed phase CT image performed 60 s following image in (**b**)

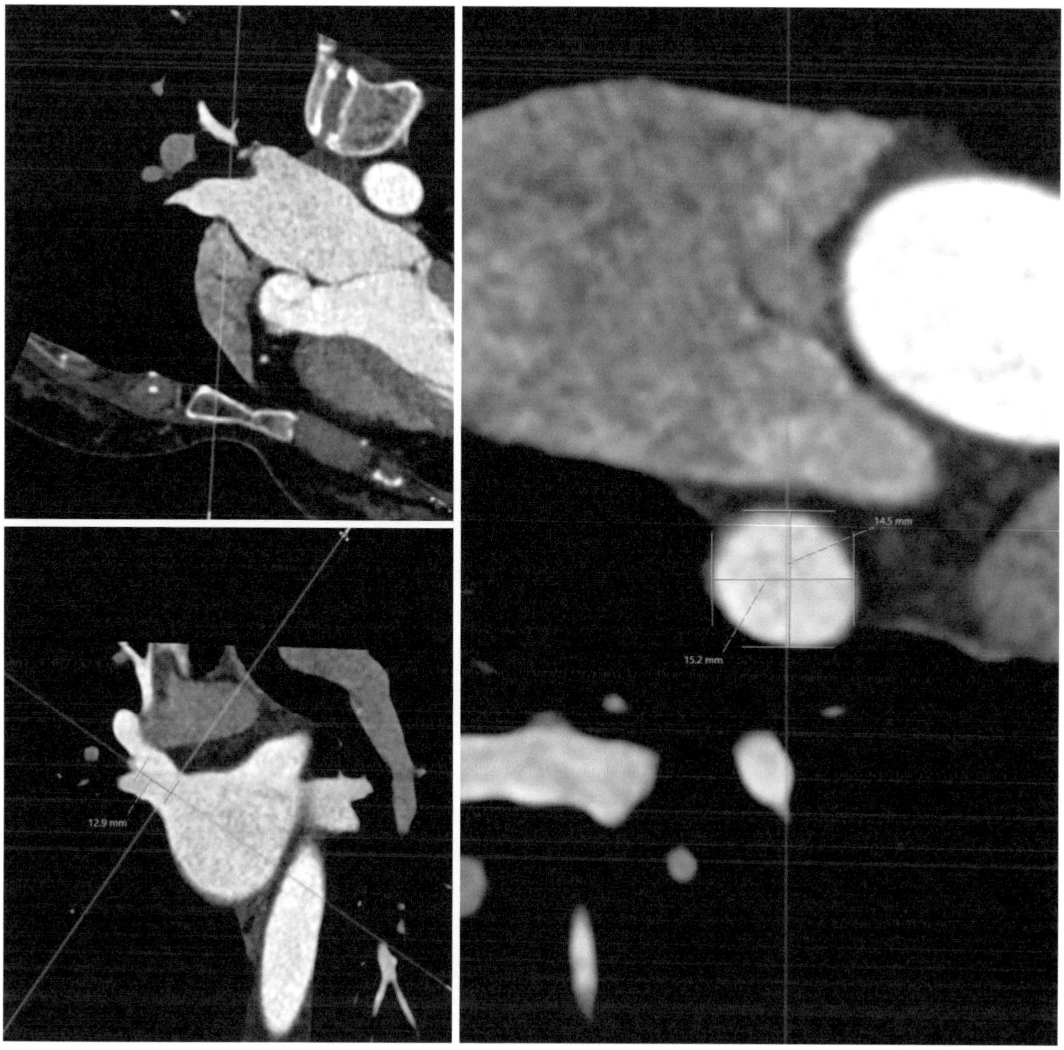

Fig. 12.2 Pulmonary vein ostial size measurement. Pulmonary vein ostial size measurements are performed on a plane orthogonal to the pulmonary vein ostia, obtained on multiplanar reconstruction (MPR) images. In this example, the right superior pulmonary vein ostium is measured which is normal in size

the minimum (short axis) diameter, may also be performed for the left inferior pulmonary vein as a larger eccentric index may complicate isolation in this vein [14] (Fig. 12.3). A narrow angle at the right inferior pulmonary vein and right superior pulmonary vein (less than 40.1° and 79.7°, respectively) has been reported to be associated with incomplete ablation, and the pulmonary vein (PV) angles may occasionally be performed in pre-procedural assessment for this reason. Measurement of PV angle involves identification of a reference line connecting the center of the atrial septum and the midpoint between the left superior and left inferior pulmonary veins. The angle between this reference line and a line perpendicular to a pulmonary vein ostium represents the PV angle (Fig. 12.4) [15].

The location of structures such as the esophagus and phrenic nerve near the pulmonary vein ostia makes them susceptible to damage during pulmonary vein ablation. Pre-procedural evaluation therefore includes localization and measurement of these structures for procedural planning and risk assessment. Regarding the esophagus, its proximity to a specific pulmonary vein ostium or to the posterior wall of the left atrium (if direct

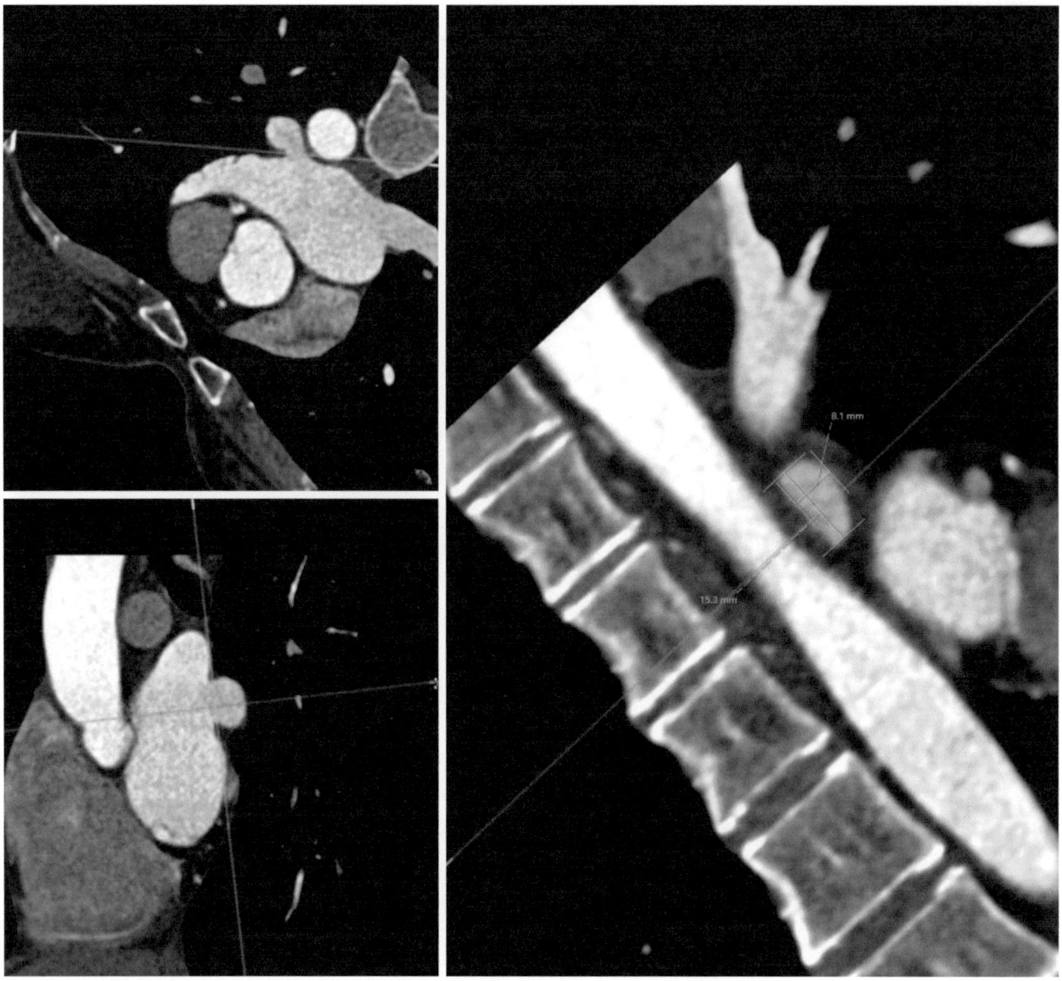

Fig. 12.3 Measurement of pulmonary vein eccentric index. Eccentric index is measured as the ratio of the maximum (long axis) to minimum (short axis) diameter of the pulmonary vein ostium. Measurement is performed on a plane orthogonal to the pulmonary vein ostium. In this example, the left inferior pulmonary vein eccentric index is 15 mm/8 mm ≈ 1.9

LA ablation is planned) is qualitatively reported. If the esophagus is adjacent to a potential ablation site, the thickness of the peri-esophageal fat pad should be reported, which may be used to titrate ablation dose or to plan an alternative ablation approach (Fig. 12.5). Generally, the presence of a fat pad of thickness 0.9 ± 2 mm is considered to be protective [16].

The phrenic nerve is a fine structure that courses along the pericardium often in close proximity to the left atrium. It can occasionally be identified on CT images, but oftentimes it is too small to be confidently identified on imaging. When visible, dedicated software may be used to trace its path, which may be overlayed onto electroanatomic maps to assist in procedural guidance [17]. More often, it is not visible on pre-procedural imaging due to isoattenuation with adjacent structures, in which case its location may be indirectly inferred by identifying the right pericardiophrenic artery (a branch of the internal thoracic artery running parallel to the phrenic nerve) or by identifying phrenic nerve capture while pacing during an ablation procedure (Fig. 12.6). A phrenic nerve location of

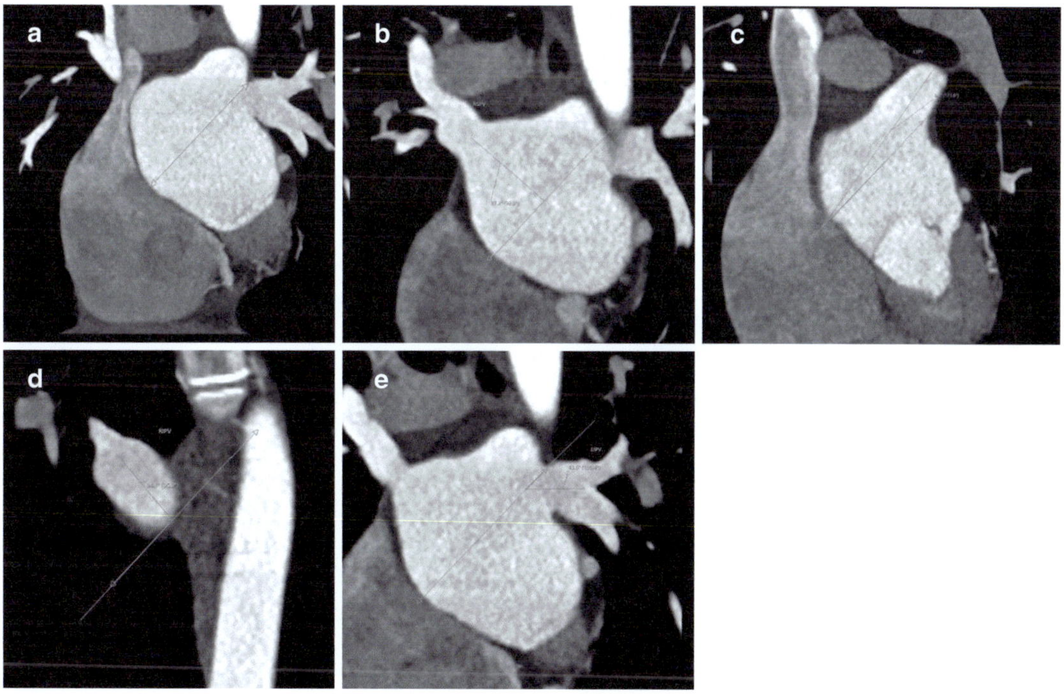

Fig. 12.4 Measurement of pulmonary vein angle. Pulmonary vein angle (PVA) is measured relative to a reference line connecting the center of the atrial septum to the midpoint between the left superior and left inferior pulmonary veins (**a**). The angle is measured between this reference line and a line perpendicular to a pulmonary vein ostium. In this example, the right superior PVA is 87° (**b**), the left superior PVA is 8° (**c**), the right inferior PVA is 84° (**d**), and the left inferior PVA is 44° (**e**)

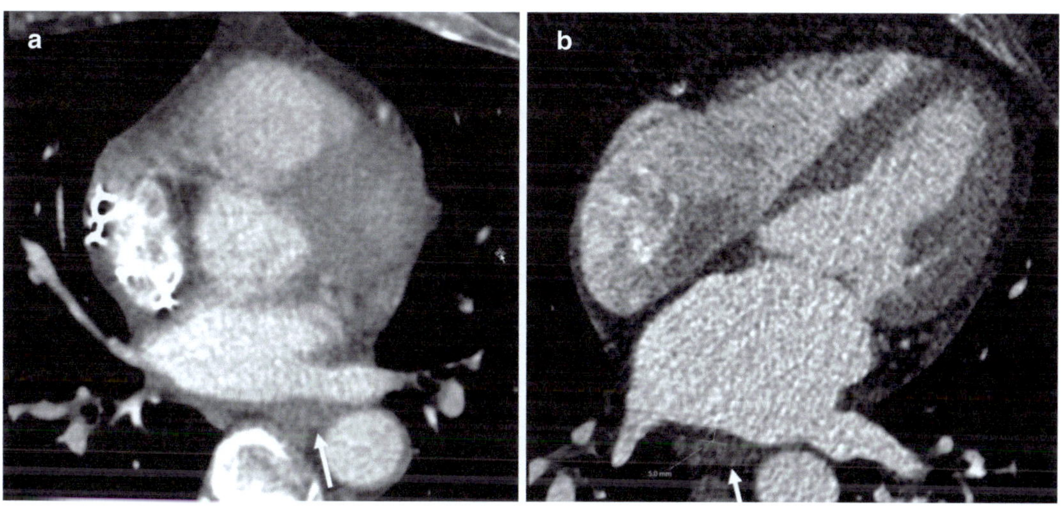

Fig. 12.5 Location esophagus and thickness of fat pad. (**a**) In this patient, the esophagus (arrow) is located immediately adjacent to the left inferior pulmonary vein with essentially no intervening peri-esophageal fat which increases risk for esophageal perforation. (**b**) In this patient, the esophagus (arrow) is located midline with a significant amount (5 mm) of protective peri-esophageal fat, suggesting much less risk for perforation in this patient compared to the patient in (**a**)

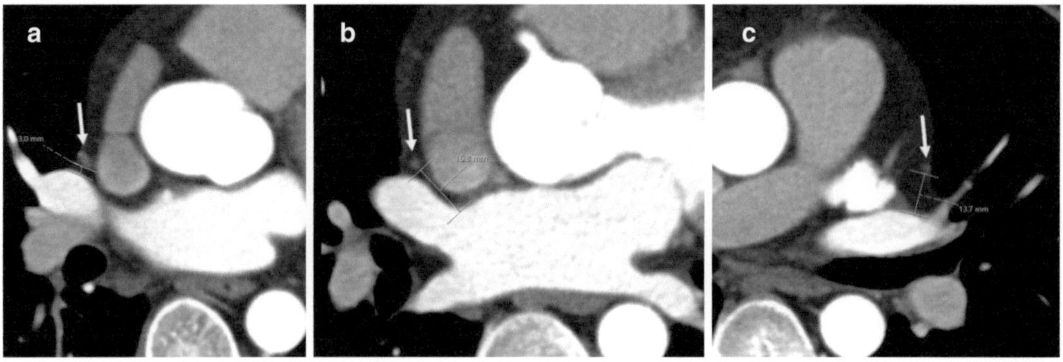

Fig. 12.6 Identifying location of phrenic nerve. (**a**) The right pericardiophrenic neurovascular bundle is directly visualized on CT (arrow) and is located 3 mm from the adjacent right superior pulmonary vein. (**b**) However, this distance is 17 mm from the right superior pulmonary vein ostium, which is a sufficient distance that risk is not significantly elevated for this patient. (**c**) The left pericardiophrenic neurovascular bundle (arrow) is located 14 mm from the left superior pulmonary vein, and an even larger distance from the left superior pulmonary vein ostium (not visualized on this image)

<10 mm of the right superior pulmonary vein is at higher risk for injury [18].

In addition to identifying anatomical structures, pre-procedural imaging with CT is used to identify left atrial thrombus, which is an absolute contraindication to AF ablation due to a high risk of thrombus embolization associated with the ablation procedure. Distinguishing thrombus from slow-filling artifact can be difficult on the angiographic phase, and a delayed phase is usually built into pre-ablation scan protocols for this reason. A well-defined filling defect that persists on delayed phase images is consistent with left atrial thrombus (Fig. 12.7). Generally, specificity for identifying thrombus increases with a longer delay, reaching 100% at 6 min delay [19]. Quantitative approaches have been developed that may be used to identify thrombus on a single angiographic phase on CT. In one algorithmic approach, the ratio of Hounsfield units (HUs) measured at the proximal and distal aspect of the atrial appendage and standard deviation (SD) at the distal aspect are measured, which are used in the decision tree of the algorithm [20]. Other approaches using radiomics have also demonstrated mixed degrees of success [21]. Generally, inclusion of a delayed phase offers superior specificity to these single-phase approaches. As an alternative to CT, MRI may be used to identify LA thrombus; the sensitivity and specificity of detection approach 100% and 99.2% using a late gadolinium enhancement (LGE) sequence with an inversion time of 600 ms [22].

Substrate Identification

Atrial fibrillation (AF) results from pathological remodeling in the left atrium that leads to LA fibrosis representing the substrate responsible for developing arrhythmias [7]. AF itself leads to progressive structural changes resulting in development of additional fibrosis and progressive worsening of severity of atrial arrhythmias [23]. These arrhythmias may be treated by PV isolation as described above as well as homogenization, which aims to eliminate electrical activity in an area of atrial substrate, and de-channeling, which aims to ablate channels/gaps remaining in an ablation scar from prior ablation treatments [24]. The critical component to success in these approaches is the accurate identification of substrate targets.

While preprocedural imaging for LA substrate identification is not routinely performed at all centers, some centers apply MRI for this purpose. MRI allows sensitive detection of fibrosis using 3D high-resolution late gadolinium enhancement (LGE) sequences with fat saturation using a respiratory and cardiac cycle gated technique (navigator sequence) 15–30 min following contrast administration. The LA wall may be segmented by subtracting an epicardial segmentation from a

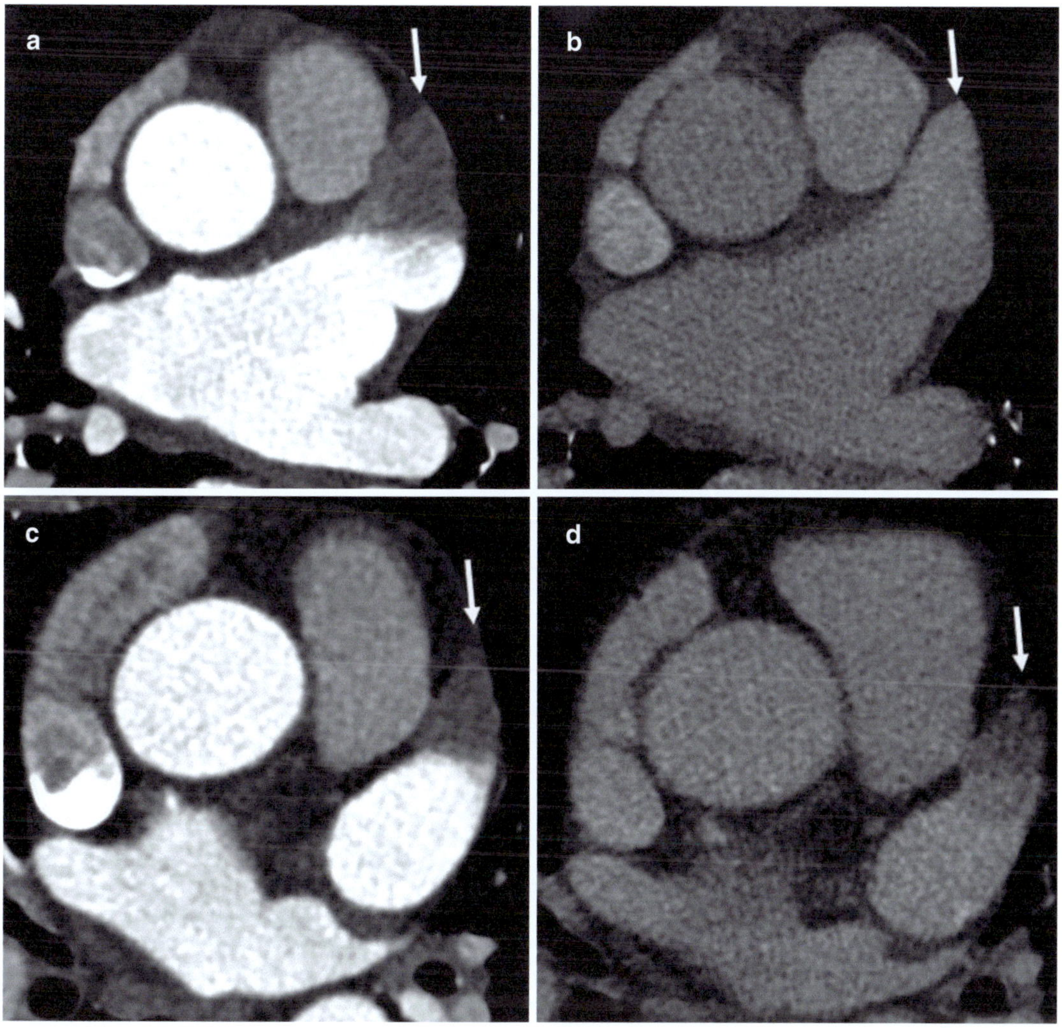

Fig. 12.7 Evaluating for left atrial appendage thrombus on delayed phase images. (**a**) CT image in the angiographic phase demonstrated a filling defect in the left atrial appendage. (**b**) However, the delayed phase image performed 60 s following (**a**) demonstrates fill-in, compatible with slow filling artifact. (**c**) CT image on another patient shows a similar filling defect on the angiographic phase. (**d**) However, in this patient the filling defect persists on the delayed phase image consistent with a left atrial appendage thrombus

separate endocardial segmentation. Areas of fibrosis may then be identified within the segmented atrial wall using either standard deviation (SD)-based (using a cutoff of 2–4 SD) or full-width-at-half-maximum (FWHM)-based thresholding methods (Fig. 12.8) [25]. Alternatively, rather than simple binary thresholding, an image intensity ratio (IIR) representing the ratio of image intensity between the LA wall and blood pool may be assigned to each voxel of the LA wall, where an IIR of 1.2 is used to define areas of scar. IIR values have been shown to correlate well with electrogram voltages measured during invasive electroanatomic voltage mapping [26].

Segmentation of scar within the LA wall using any of the above methods may then be used to quantify the volume percentage of LA fibrosis. This percentage may be used to classify the extent of LGE into one of four Utah grades, defined as I (0–10%), II (10–20%), III (20–30%), and IV (>30%). The Utah grade can assist in pre-procedural planning, where lower grades (I, II,

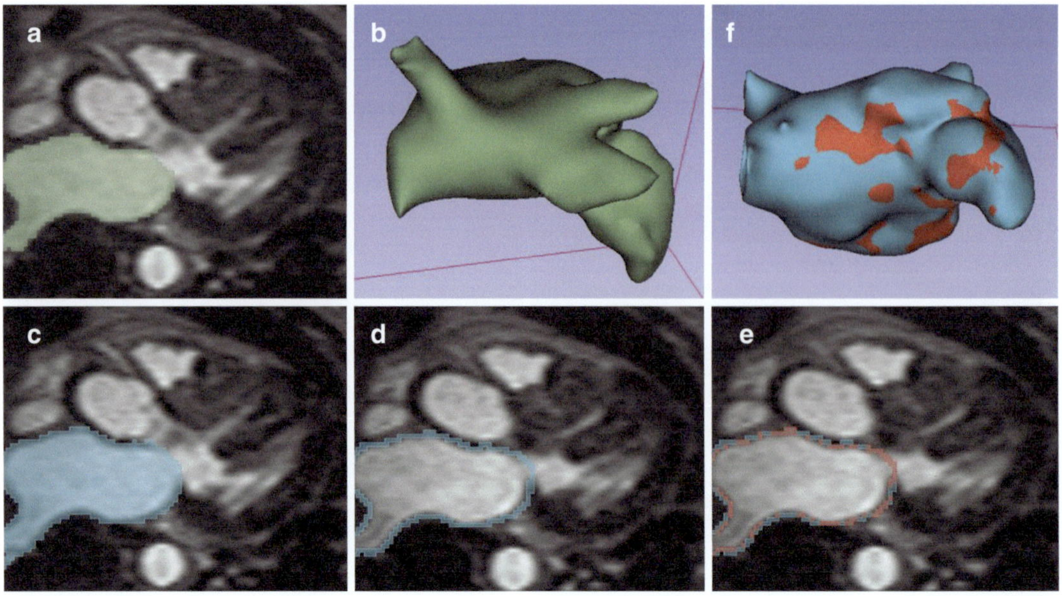

Fig. 12.8 Quantifying left atrial fibrosis on MRI. Left atrial (LA) fibrosis may be quantified on a 3D high-resolution whole heart late gadolinium enhancement navigator (cardiac and respiratory gated) sequence performed 15–30 min following contrast administration. Steps to quantify fibrosis include (**a**) segmentation of the LA blood pool, with 3D segmentation of the LA blood pool shown in (**b**). (**c**) This segmentation is then expanded by 2.5 mm to create a larger segmentation from which the blood pool segmentation is subtracted, producing a 3D shell representing the LA wall (**d**). Thresholding is performed on this shell using a cutoff of 2–4 standard deviations above normal myocardium. (**e**) This produces a new segmentation representing LA scar (red) which is superimposed on the segmentation of normal LA wall (blue). (**f**) 3D representation of the LA wall (blue) with superimposed areas of scar (red)

and localized III) may be amenable to PV isolation with or without homogenization, whereas higher grades (III and IV) are associated with a lower likelihood of ablation success suggesting that a non-ablative approach may be more suitable in these patients [25].

CT may also be used for substrate identification using similar SD- or FWHM-based thresholding techniques as MRI or using a CT image attenuation ratio (IAR, representing the ratio of image attenuation in Hounsfield units between the LA wall and blood pool) to segment areas of LA scar. Similar to IIR, IAR has been shown to have good correlation to invasively recorded bipolar voltages. However, while spatial resolution is higher in CT compared to MRI, the contrast to noise ratio is lower in CT, which may reduce sensitivity for detection [27]. A novel alternative CT-based method for substrate identification that takes better advantage of the higher resolution of CT compared to MRI uses quantification of LA wall thickness rather than contrast enhancement (Fig. 12.9). A LA wall thickness map is derived by solving the Laplace equation over a finite element mesh derived from the LA wall segmentation [28]. Areas of thin LA wall (<1.9 mm) have been shown to correlate well with areas of low voltage (<0.5 mV) corresponding to sites of scar on EAM [29]. Thicker areas have been shown to be associated with a higher rate of AF recurrence suggesting that higher ablation dose may be required in these areas [30].

In addition to LA thickness, higher left atrial epicardial adipose tissue (EAT) volume and attenuation have also been shown to correlate with areas of lower voltage on EAM and to be associated with recurrent AF [31, 32]. EAT surrounding the LA may be segmented by applying a thresholding mask with attenuation values ranging between −200 to −190 (lower limit) and −50 to −30 (upper limit) HU [32, 33] (Fig. 12.10). Novel approaches using radiomics and machine

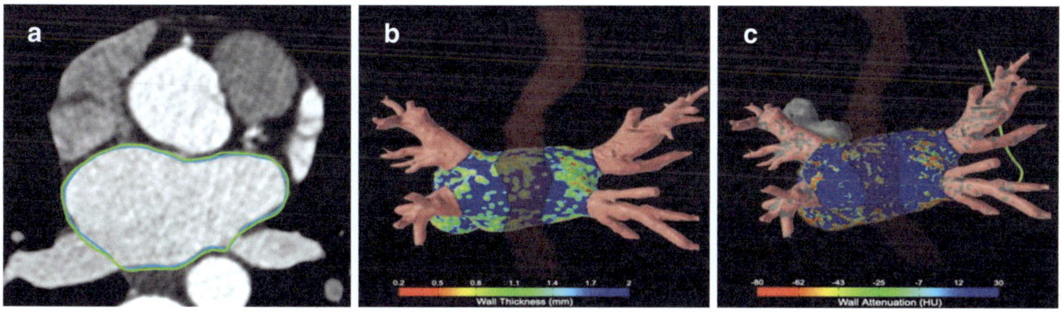

Fig. 12.9 Quantifying left atrial fibrosis on CT. Left atrial (LA) fibrosis may be quantified on CT using either a thickness map or a wall attenuation map. (**a**) To construct the LA thickness map, the outer (green) and inner (blue) surfaces of the left atrium are segmented. (**b**) This segmentation is used to produce a finite element mesh from which the Laplace equation may be solved to obtain a map of LA wall thickness. (**c**) Alternatively, a wall attenuation map may be produced by quantifying the ratio of Hounsfield units between the LA wall and blood pool on a delayed enhancement phase of imaging obtained 15–30 min following contrast administration. (Panels **b** and **c** are reproduced with permission from *Radiographics* from Ref. [79])

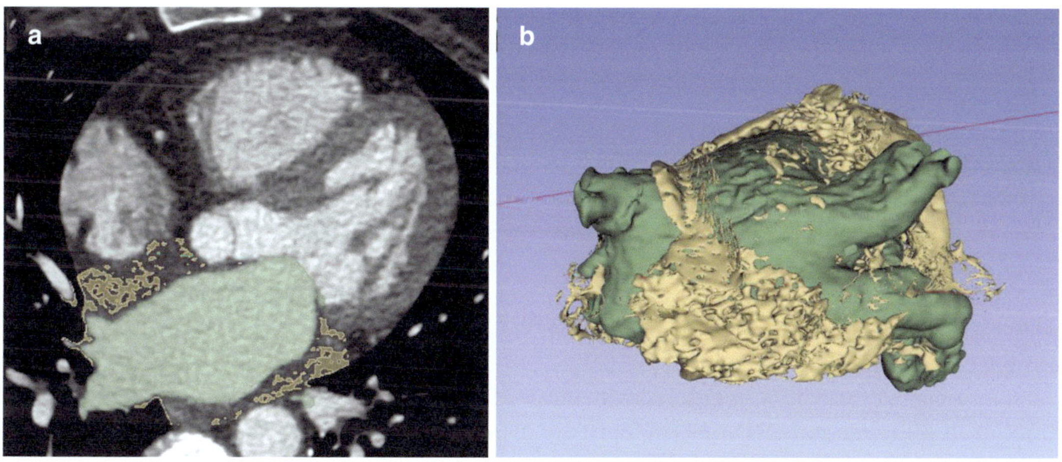

Fig. 12.10 Quantifying left atrial epicardial adipose tissue on CT. (**a**) Left atrial (LA) epicardial adipose tissue (EAT) may be quantified by segmenting the peri-atrial fat using a thresholding mask, in this case between −190 and −30 Hounsfield units. (**b**) 3D reconstruction of the segmented LA blood pool (green) and LA EAT (yellow)

learning have also been applied to EAT analysis to predict risk of AF recurrence with variable results [33, 34].

Procedural Guidance

AF ablation is guided by invasively derived electroanatomic mapping (EAM) systems to generate an anatomical 3D shell of the endocardial surface of the left atrium. These systems localize the position of catheters in contact with the endocardial surface using either a low-intensity magnetic field generated by inductors at the tip of the catheter or an electric field induced by electrodes at the tip of the catheter [35]. As position recordings are obtained only at select points where the catheters are in contact with the endocardial surface, the 3D shells generated by EAM are limited by under-sampling resulting in incomplete geometry [35]. However, the preprocedural imaging techniques described above allow for co-registration of anatomical data derived from CT or MRI with the cloud map of position points derived from EAM so that generation of a complete anatomical map may be

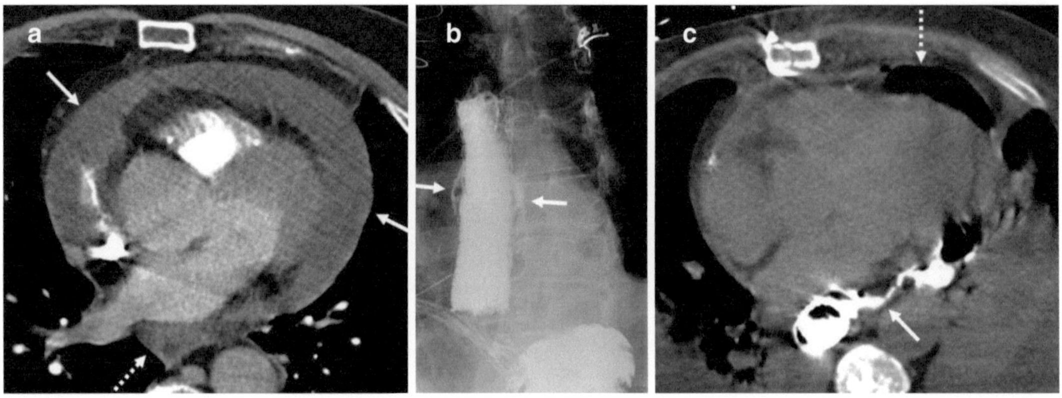

Fig. 12.11 Post-procedural complications of LA ablation. This patient received a LA ablation for management of refractor atrial fibrillation. (**a**) Large pericardial effusion (arrows) is seen on CT performed 1 week following ablation, in addition to thickening of the adjacent esophagus with peri-esophageal fat stranding (dotted arrow) concerning for pericardio-esophageal fistula. (**b**) The fistula was managed with placement of an esophageal stent; however, fluoroscopy demonstrated extraluminal contrast (arrows) concerning for persistent fistula. (**c**) CT performed following fluoroscopy confirms presence of a large residual pericardio-esophageal fistula with contrast (arrow) and gas (dotted arrow) emanating from the esophagus into the pericardium

performed with fewer EAM-derived position points. This co-registration may also incorporate substrate maps derived from pre-procedural imaging from CT or MRI as described above, which is especially useful for ablation strategies aiming to target or enclose areas of atrial scar in addition to standard PV isolation. Additional anatomical structures identified on pre-procedural imaging may also be co-registered with the EAM map allowing the electrophysiologist to view the position of these structures in relation to ablation targets in real time, for example, to avoid or reduce ablation energy at regions close to the esophagus in posterior wall or PV ostium ablation or regions close to the sinoatrial coronary artery during LA roof ablation [36]. As mentioned above, the phrenic nerve may be too small to confidently identify on pre-procedural imaging in which case its position may be inferred intra-procedurally via pacing-induced phrenic nerve capture.

Post-procedural Evaluation

While not routinely performed, CT or MRI may be obtained following a LA ablation procedure to evaluate for complications when suspected or to evaluate the success of ablation especially in cases of refractory AF. Potential complications include PV stenosis, PV thrombosis (often with associated pulmonary infarct), and atrioesophageal fistula formation, which may manifest as gas in the cardiac chambers or pericardial effusion (Fig. 12.11). Indirect signs of atrioesophageal fistula include left atrial wall thickening with adjacent fat stranding in the mediastinum [37]. Complications are usually better assessed by CT owing to its higher sensitivity for detecting these findings.

In evaluating the success of ablation, MRI with LGE is usually preferred owing to its higher sensitivity for evaluating fibrosis. In general, scaring due to ablation has higher IIR with lower wall thickness compared to fibrosis caused directly by AF [25]. Success of ablation may be quantified by generating a difference map between post- and pre-treatment fibrosis. Successful ablation results in lower overall post-procedural fibrosis burden, whereas residual or progressive fibrosis burden is often seen with AF recurrence. Repeat ablation may be useful in some cases, namely, for homogenization of incompletely ablated existing scar or ablation gap connection in the setting of gaps in linear atrial or PV ablation scars [38, 39].

Ventricular Tachycardia

Ventricular tachycardia (VT) is a wide complex tachyarrhythmia arising from the ventricle that may be fatal when left untreated. It is classified as sustained or non-sustained based on duration lasting more than or less than 30 s. The morphology may be monomorphic or polymorphic and can degenerate into ventricular fibrillation and ultimately result in cardiac arrest [40]. Catheter ablation is a commonly used second-line therapy for VT ablation after failure of antiarrhythmic medications [41].

Pre-procedural Assessment

CT and MR play an important role in peri-procedural management of VT, particularly in the pre-ablation phase of management where it can aid in diagnosis and ablation planning. Specific applications of pre-procedural imaging include evaluating ICD candidacy, diagnosing the etiology of VT, anatomical assessment, and substrate identification. Electrocardiographic imaging (ECGi), a novel quantitative imaging technology that uses computational modeling techniques applied to anatomical geometry of the epicardial heart surface and torso from CT, is also used routinely as a complementary tool for substrate identification in centers with access to the technology [42].

ICD Candidacy

In general, CT or MR imaging is indicated in any patient undergoing evaluation prior to VT ablation. At a minimum, cross-sectional imaging provides a means for accurate documentation of ejection fraction, which is required by guidelines for determining ICD candidacy. Specifically, guidelines recommend ICD in patients with symptomatic HF (NYHA class II–III) and LVEF of ≤35% after ≥3 months of optimal medical therapy in patients expected to survive ≥1 year [43]. Of the available imaging modalities for quantifying ejection fraction, cardiac MR is considered the gold standard and the preferred modality for documenting LVEF for the purpose of ICD candidacy determination [44].

Quantification of ejection fraction on MRI usually relies on manual or semiautomated segmentation of ventricle cavity volumes during the best systolic and best diastolic cardiac phases (Fig. 12.12). This is usually done on the two-chamber short-axis series, but other views are used simultaneously to ensure that the volumes included are contained within the valve planes defining the ventricular volume. Specialized software may be used to semiautomate the contouring process by identifying the valve planes and interpolating between segmented slices. Some software allows fully automated segmentation using AI techniques [45]. However, these often rely on the radiologist to evaluate the accuracy of the segmentations and correct for any errors.

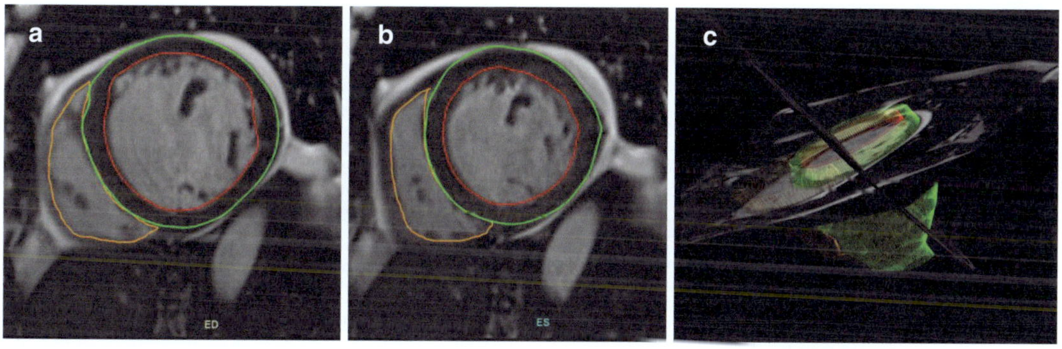

Fig. 12.12 Evaluating ICD candidacy using MRI to quantify ejection fraction. Patient with dilated cardiomyopathy undergoing MRI to determine ICD candidacy. (**a**, **b**) LVEF is quantified on MRI by segmenting the endocardial (red) surface of the left ventricle at both end-diastole (**a**) and end-systole (**b**). RVEF may similarly be obtained by segmenting the RV endocardial surface (orange). LV epicardial segmentation (green) may also be performed if LV wall mass is required. (**c**) Dedicated software uses the above segmentation to create 3D volumes that may be used to calculate ejection fraction

Once segmentations are generated on each slice, ventricular volumes are then calculated by generating a full 3D geometry using geometric interpolation between the slices. Ejection fraction is calculated as $(LVEDV - LVESV)/LVEDV$.

Etiology of VT

Oftentimes, the etiology of cardiomyopathy responsible for VT and whether there is associated structural heart disease and/or scar is unknown at the time of presentation. Having a specific diagnosis is important in guiding further workup and formulating a management plan, including the decision of whether or not to ablate. Deciding whether to ablate and the best approach for ablation depends heavily on specific features of structural disease and scar and on the specific type of cardiomyopathy. For evaluating etiology and determining presence of structural heart disease and scar, cardiac MR is considered the gold standard [46]. Ideally, cardiac MR should be performed in any patient with newly diagnosed ventricular tachycardia prior to ICD implantation. However, if an ICD is already present, a wideband GRE sequence can be performed at a CIED capable center to reduce off-resonance artifact [47]. Alternatively, contrast-enhanced MDCT can be performed instead if MRI is not an option.

A useful starting point in establishing etiology is in classifying cardiomyopathy as ischemic or nonischemic. The hallmark of ischemic cardiomyopathy is the presence of subendocardial infarct/scar following a vascular distribution, often with associated aneurysmal dilation and wall thinning in the area of scar [48]. On MRI, scar is characterized by an area of subendocardial LGE in the region of infarct. On CT, scar is characterized by wall thinning and hypoperfusion on the angiographic phase and delayed contrast enhancement on the delayed (~10 min) phase. An important feature to report is the degree of transmurality of the scar, with >50% wall thickness involvement indicative of nonviable scar (Fig. 12.13). Typically, ablations for subendocardial scars of ischemic cardiomyopathy are targeted using a subendocardial ablation approach, although full-thickness scars may benefit from an epicardial or combined approach.

Nonischemic cardiomyopathy is a broad category encompassing all forms of cardiomyopathy

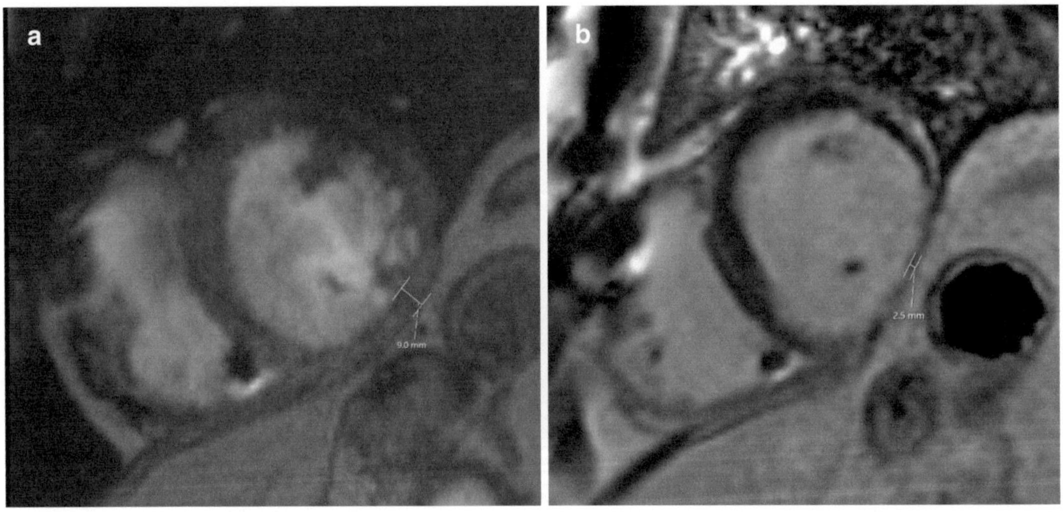

Fig. 12.13 Assessing viability in ischemic cardiomyopathy. Viability may be determined on MRI by the degree of transmurality of an infarct, where infarct thickness of >50% of the wall thickness is considered nonviable (**a**). The wall thickness may be measured in diastole on short-axis cine images, in this case measuring 9 mm in the region of infarct (**b**). It can be difficult to distinguish enhancing wall from adjacent blood pool. Therefore, the thickness of remaining viable nonenhancing wall may be measured instead, and this may be subtracted from wall thickness obtained from (**a**) to obtain thickness of scar. In this case, the scar involves 72% thickness of the inferolateral wall, consistent with a nonviable circumflex distribution infarct

not associated with coronary ischemic disease. The specific etiology can often be determined based on specific patterns of LGE on cardiac MR [49], although sometimes the pattern is nonspecific, and a specific diagnosis requires correlating with additional clinical information. Acute myocarditis can be diagnosed on imaging according to the Lake Louise criteria, where diagnosis requires fulfilling the two main criteria of T1 and T2 abnormalities [50]. Abnormal T1 signal is defined by either presence of LGE or elevated T1 relaxation times or extracellular volume. T1 mapping allows computation of voxel-wise T1 relaxation times using special balanced SSFP acquisition sequences such as MOLLI. Specific cutoffs for normal and abnormal relaxation times are generally scanner specific. Likewise, abnormal T2 signal is defined by increased T2 relaxation times on T2-mapping sequences or based on global or regional elevated signal on standard T2 images (where ratio of myocardial to skeletal muscle signal of ≥2 is considered abnormal) (Fig. 12.14). VT can result from scarring as a sequela of myocarditis, characterized by a subepicardial scar classically affecting the lateral wall (Fig. 12.14D).

Hypertrophic cardiomyopathy (HCM) can also be diagnosed based on imaging by demonstration of maximum LV wall thickness of >15 mm in the absence of another cause of LV

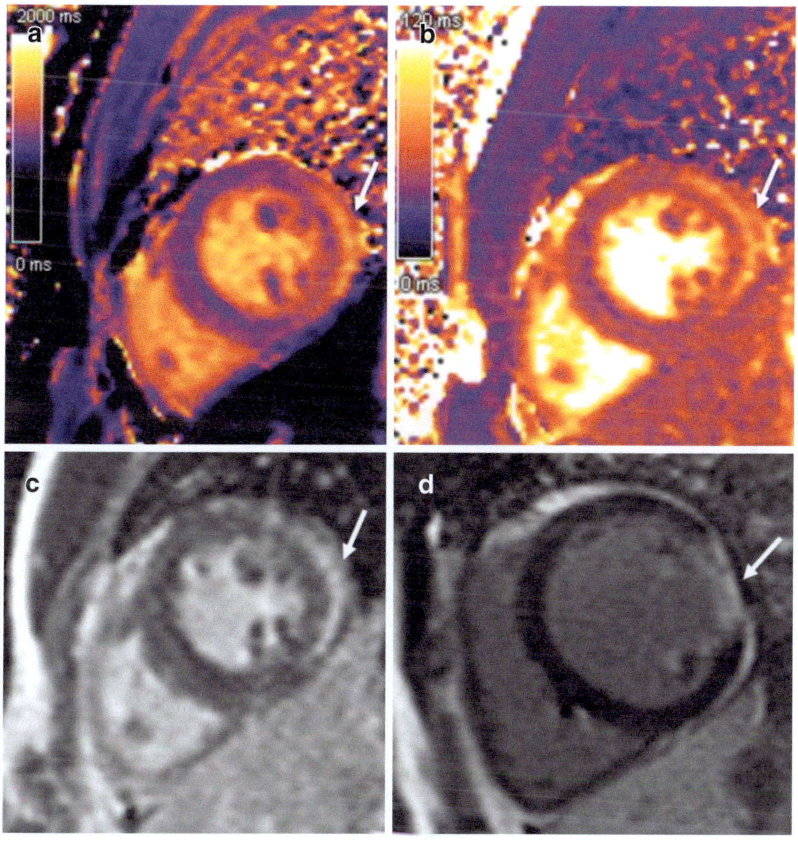

Fig. 12.14 Myocarditis. A 21-year-old patient presenting with acute chest pain and PVCs. (**a**, **b**) Elevated signal is seen on both T1 maps (**a**) with relaxation times above 1050 ms (arrow) and on T2 maps (**b**) with relaxation times above 55 ms (arrow) at the mid subepicardial lateral wall. (**c**) There is corresponding LGE (arrow) in the regions of T1 and T2 signal elevation. Together, these findings are diagnostic of acute myocarditis. (**d**) A 27-year-old patient (different patient from above) with history of myocarditis with frequent PVCs and sustained monomorphic VT, with MRI showing full thickness scar (arrow) at the mid lateral wall. Patient subsequently underwent ablation of this scar with improvement in symptoms

hypertrophy. VT is a potential complication of HCM with twofold increased risk of sudden cardiac death when LGE exceeds 15% as determined by manual planimetry or semiautomated thresholding methods (discussed further below) [51]. Scar associated with HCM is often patchy and mesocardial in distribution (Fig. 12.15). Arrhythmogenic right ventricle cardiomyopathy (ARVC) is another nonischemic cardiomyopathy with imaging-based diagnosis, with major criteria involving RV wall akinesia or dyssynchrony and either of RV dilation (ratio of RV end-diastolic volume to body surface area of 110 mL/m^2 in male patients of 100 mL/m^2 in female patients) or decreased RV ejection fraction (RVEF <40%) [52]. In general, identification of scar in the RV wall is limited on imaging, but recognizing the diagnosis of ARVC may help direct electroanatomic mapping to the right ventricle (Fig. 12.16).

Sarcoidosis is another nonischemic cardiomyopathy that often demonstrates a nonspecific pattern of scar. Most often, sarcoidosis is characterized by subepicardial or mesocardial distribution often with a patchy/nodular pattern of enhancement that can affect any wall of the myocardium but with a relatively higher propensity for the inferior basal wall. Current guidelines recommend ICD placement in patients with cardiac sarcoidosis with LVEF ≤35% (class I recommendation) or in patients with LVEF >35% and percent LGE > 5.7% (class IIa recommendation) [53]. In determining candidacy for ablation, the electrophysiologist will want to know whether the inflammation of sarcoidosis is acute or chronic, as management of acute inflammation may include treatment with steroids prior to considering ablation. In the acute setting, findings on cardiac MR include elevated T2 signal indicating edema (which may be defined using parameters as above) with myocardial thickening in the affected regions, whereas in the chronic setting, there is absence of elevated T2 signal often with thinning in the affected regions [49]. FDG-PET is particularly helpful in distinguishing acute from chronic sarcoidosis, with areas of active inflammation demonstrating elevated FDG uptake in the affected areas (Fig. 12.17).

Substrate Identification

In both ischemic and nonischemic cardiomyopathy, the distribution of arrhythmogenic scar (sub-

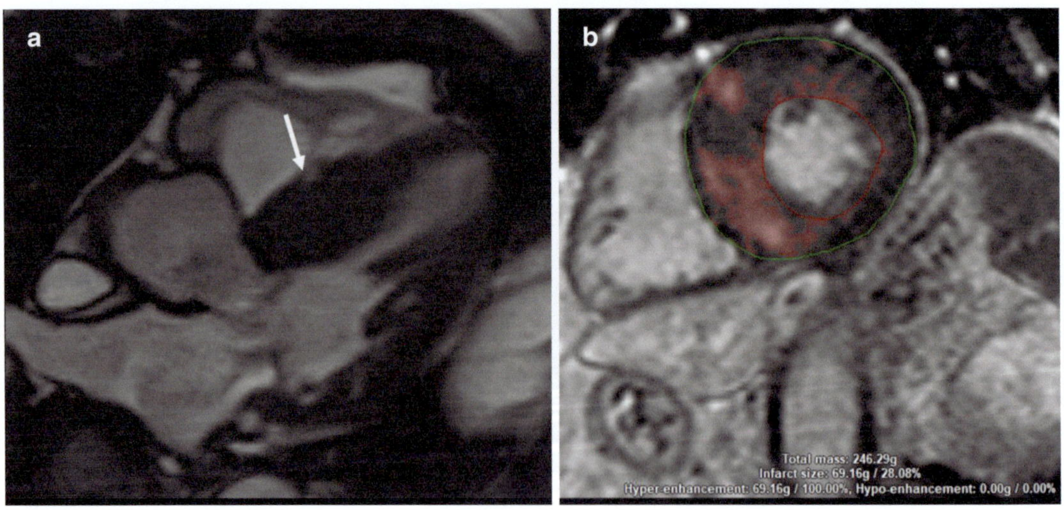

Fig. 12.15 Evaluating ICD candidacy in hypertrophic cardiomyopathy. A 62-year-old patient with hypertrophic cardiomyopathy. (**a**) MRI four-chamber long-axis cine images show marked thickening of the basal to mid septal wall (arrow) compatible with asymmetric septal variant hypertrophic cardiomyopathy. (**b**) Late gadolinium enhancement (LGE) images demonstrate extensive patchy LGE comprising 28% of the LV wall (highlighted in red), which qualifies this patient for ICD placement

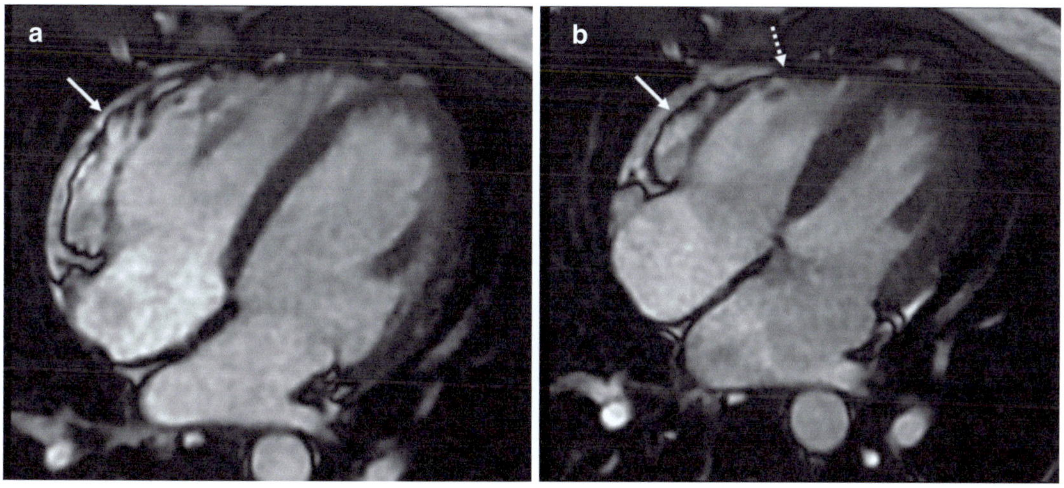

Fig. 12.16 Arrhythmogenic right ventricle cardiomyopathy (ARVC). A 31-year-old patient with new onset VT requiring cardioversion. MRI shows dilated RV (arrow) with reduced right ventricle ejection fraction (quantified as 36%). In comparing diastolic (**a**) and systolic (**b**) four-chamber long-axis cine images, there is apparent focal dyskinesis with focal bulging (arrow) and "crinkling" (dotted arrow) of the RV free-wall compatible with the "accordion sign" of ARVC

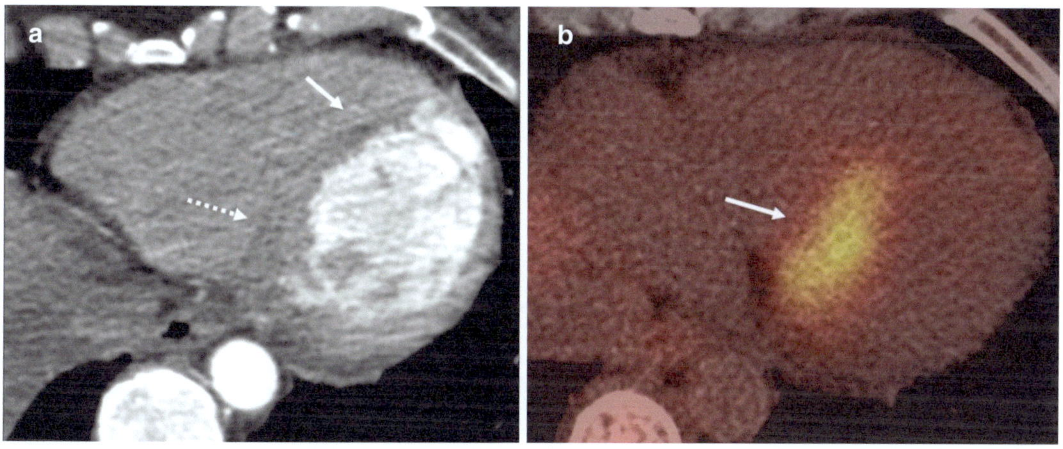

Fig. 12.17 Acute on chronic cardiac sarcoidosis. A 57-year-old patient with cardiac sarcoidosis with recurrent VT refractory to sotalol. (**a**) CT demonstrates areas of focal thinning corresponding to fibrous scar at the apical septum (solid arrow) and focal thickening corresponding to active area of inflammation at the basal septum (dotted arrow). (**b**) PET demonstrates FDG uptake at the area of thickening confirming the presence of active inflammation in this region. Given the active inflammation, the patient was treated with a different immunomodulating agent which led to resolution of active disease on a follow-up scan and no recurrence of VT

strate) provides the electrophysiologist with valuable information regarding the most suitable approach for ablation (endocardial vs. epicardial or combined approach for midmyocardial or transmural scar) along with the specific areas of the myocardium on which to focus effort during electroanatomic mapping studies. As discussed above, this substrate mapping is ideally performed with LGE imaging on MRI but can also be performed on CT using delayed phase images in patients with contraindications to MRI. MRI-derived substrate maps have been shown to correlate with both abnormal voltages and VT isthmus sites identified on electroanatomic maps, and in one study were even shown to identify isthmus sites in scar areas not identified by voltage mapping [44]. CT-derived substrate maps have been shown to allow prediction of abnormal voltages (<1.5 mV) in 81.7% of analyzed segments, and 84% of abnormal voltages were mapped a maximum of 10 mm from CT-segmented scar [54, 55]. Dual energy technique has also been used, in which iodine mapping and virtual monoenergetic images can be used to improve the contrast-to-noise ratio of scar.

Generally, scar is subdivided into two zones, core and gray zone, based on the relative values of signal intensity (SI) on MRI (or signal attenuation in terms of Hounsfield units on CT) (Fig. 12.18). The presence and distribution of border zone are known to affect the risk of sudden cardiac death and the need for ICD [56]. While there are no consensus definitions for quantifying scar, several heuristic thresholding methods have been published, the most common of which include the full-width-at-half-maximum (FWHM) thresholding method, and the standard deviation (SD)-based method. While exact definitions may vary, one such definition of the FWHM-based method categorizes the scar core as regions with SI ≥ 50% of maximal SI of infarct and gray zone as regions with SI ≥ maximum SI of myocardium but <50% of maximum SI of the infarct. A definition of the SD-based method categorizes scar core as regions with SI > 3 SD of the SI of the total myocardium and gray zone as regions with 2 SD ≤ SI < 3 SD; however, cutoffs ranging from 2 SD to 6 SD have been used [57, 58]. Typically, these thresholding techniques are supplemented with manual planimetry to remove areas with artifactually elevated signal such as regional interfaces of the myocardium with adjacent structures, as volume averaging and other artifacts in these regions tend to overestimate scar burden [59].

Anatomical Assessment

Apart from distribution of scar, the feasibility and risk of a specific ablation approach may also be determined by other anatomical features such as the proximity of scar to vital structures such as the coronary arteries and phrenic nerve, the presence of thrombus, and the presence of unstable features such as ventricle wall pseudoaneurysms. For an epicardial approach specifically, the presence of pericardial adhesions or calcifications and the thickness of the epicardial fat pad are important features in determining the suitability of an epicardial approach (Fig. 12.19). Although not an absolute contraindication, a fat pad of ≤10 mm is desired, and epicardial ablations in the presence of excessive fat (>10 mm) have been shown to be ineffective [60]. For an endocardial approach, excessive trabeculations can cause poor contact with catheter electrodes, which may lead to low amplitude signal that

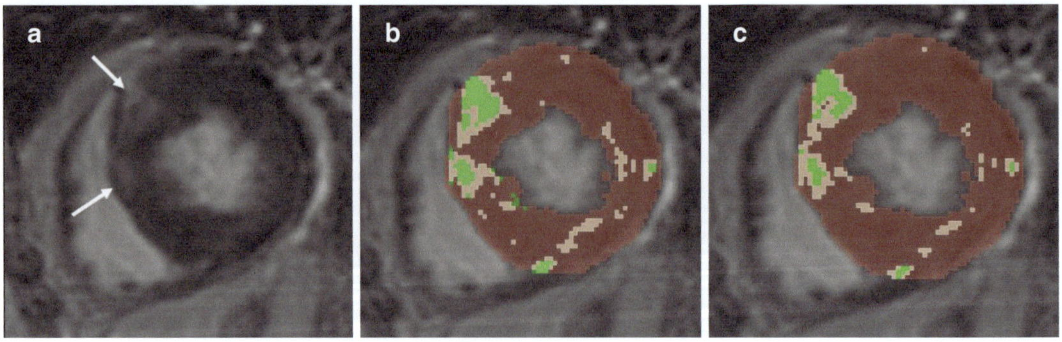

Fig. 12.18 Substrate mapping of scar core and grey zone. Patient with hypertrophic cardiomyopathy showing multifocal patchy LGE on MRI (**a**, arrows). Scare core and gray zone may be quantified using several different semiautomated thresholding techniques. In (**b**), scar core (green) is segmented using FWHM technique with threshold of 45% and gray zone (tan) using FWHM threshold of 30%. In (**c**), scar core is segmented using standard deviation (SD) technique with threshold of 6 standard deviations and grey zone using SD threshold of 3 SD. Both options produce qualitatively similar segmentation of scar

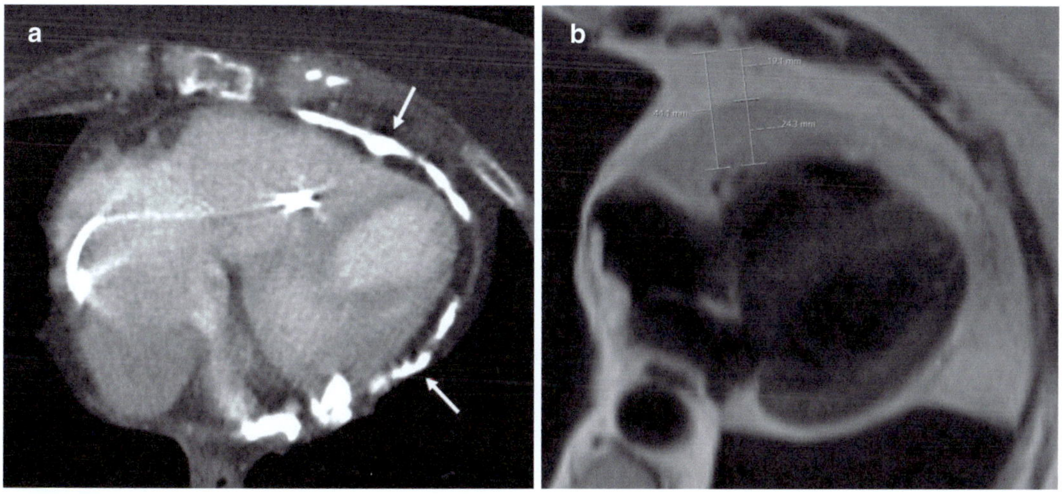

Fig. 12.19 Anatomical assessment prior to VT ablation. The presence of pericardial calcifications (**a**, arrows) and excessively thick (>10 mm) epicardial fat (**b**) are relative contraindications for an epicardial ablation approach. In **b**, there is exuberant epicardial fat measuring 24 mm in thickness with an additional thick layer of mediastinal fat measuring 19 mm anteriorly. Neither of these patients would be good candidates for epicardial ablation

may mimic a scar. Issues with access may also be problematic, for example, in the setting of occluded or anatomically prohibitive veins, for example, with interrupted inferior vena cava. For substrate in the peri-mitral region, ablation may be performed through the coronary sinus, and patency or other anomalies of the coronary sinus should be evaluated.

Electrocardiographic Imaging (ECGi)

ECGi is a novel quantitative imaging technique that allows noninvasive reconstruction of epicardial voltage maps and activation maps using a large number (~250) of body surface potential recordings obtained from electrodes placed on a vest worn on the torso along with three-dimensional anatomical heart-torso imaging using gated CT obtained with axial resolution between 0.6 and 1 mm (Fig. 12.20). The technique relies on assumptions regarding the bioelectric field induced by the heart including the following [42]:

1. Capacitive effects of the conducting medium are negligible.
2. Inductive effects of the conducting medium are negligible.
3. Boundary conditions can be reduced to static electric fields.
4. Torso volume is a homogeneous passive conductor (no current sources).

These assumptions allow Maxwell's equations to be reduced to the electrostatic field equations governed by the Laplace equation:

$$\Delta V = 0 \tag{12.1}$$

Using the boundary element method applied to the torso and epicardial surface mesh obtained from segmenting the heart and torso on CT, the Laplace equation is discretized to the following form:

$$V_{\mathrm{T}} = AV_{\mathrm{E}} \tag{12.2}$$

where V_{T} corresponds to the body surface potential map obtained from the electrode vest and V_{E} is the predicted epicardial voltage map obtained from inverting Eq. (12.2) [61].

Much like substrate mapping with MRI or CT, ECGi is useful in preoperative planning by providing a priori prediction of the location of arrhythmogenic substrate through predicted voltage maps and also offers prediction of the location of potential VT isthmus sites or focal activation sites through predicted activation maps (discussed further below in the next section). Studies have shown a moderate correlation between ECGi and epicardial electroanatomic

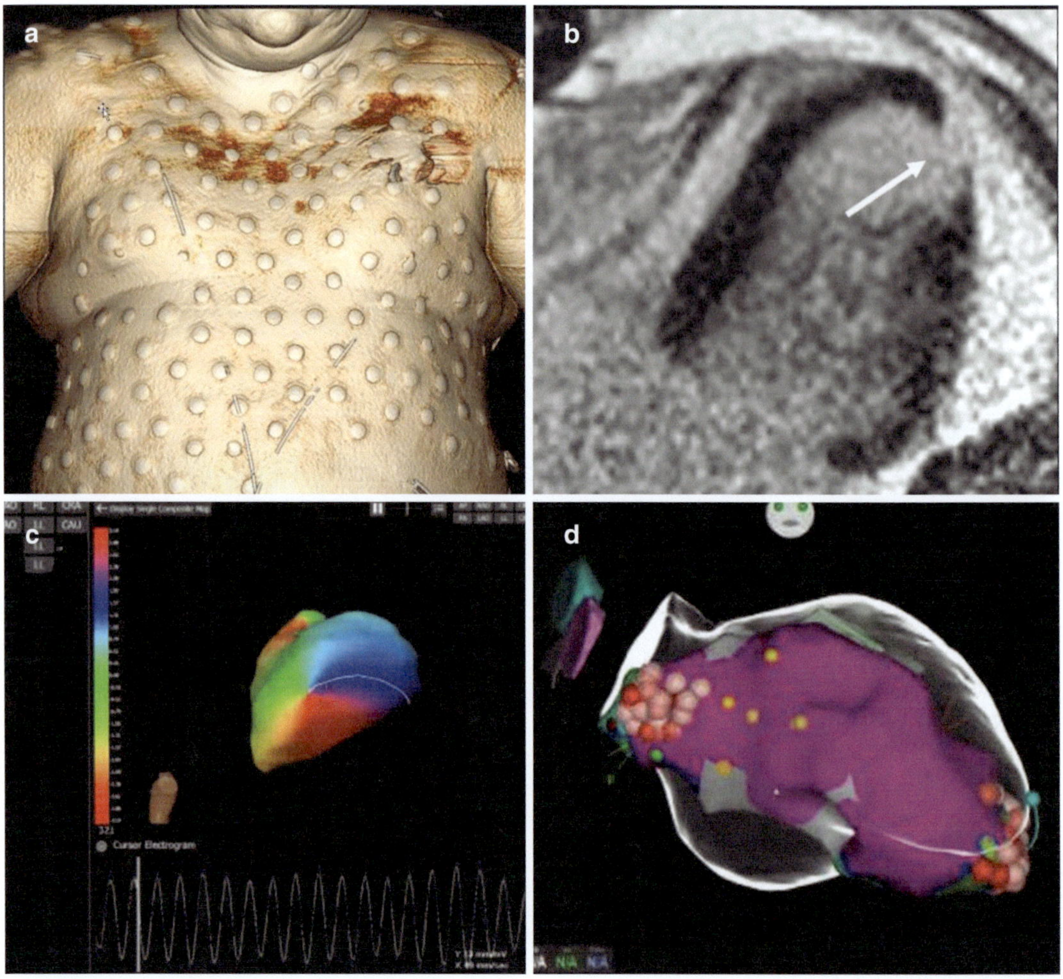

Fig. 12.20 Electrocardiographic imaging (ECGi). This novel technique uses a vest with a large number (~250) electrodes, seen as radiopaque studs on topogram (**a**). This patient had a focal full thickness infarct at the inferolateral apex (**b**, arrow). (**c**) ECGi was performed which mapped VT exit site to the basal LV septum. EAM showed focal low voltage both at the region of infarct and at the septal LVOT, and pacemapping and entrainment mapping both confirmed critical isthmus at the septal LVOT. (**d**) Ablation was performed at both sites with resolution of VT (small spheres correspond to ablation lesions). (Panel **c** is reproduced with permission from *Radiographics* from Ref. [79])

voltage maps obtained during catheter ablation of VT, localizing sites of epicardial focal activation to a resolution of 13.2 mm [62]. A powerful feature of ECGi is its ability to generate a complete voltage or activation map using data from just a single heart beat in a pre-procedural setting, which is especially useful in patients with hemodynamically unstable VT who cannot tolerate the long periods of VT required in EAM mapping on the procedure table.

ECGi is particularly useful in stereotactic ablative radiotherapy (SBRT), which is a beam-focused radiation therapy allowing high dose per fraction (25–40 Gy) to targeted volumes of tissue that is used as an alternative noninvasive ablation technique in high-risk or treatment-refractory VT [63]. Pre-procedure planning prior to SBRT entails substrate imaging much like in standard EAM-guided catheter ablation (Fig. 12.21), and due to the high risk in these cases, invasive electroanatomic mapping is usually not performed in SBRT. Results of ECGi imaging may be used to develop a customized treatment plan prescribing beam intensity and positioning.

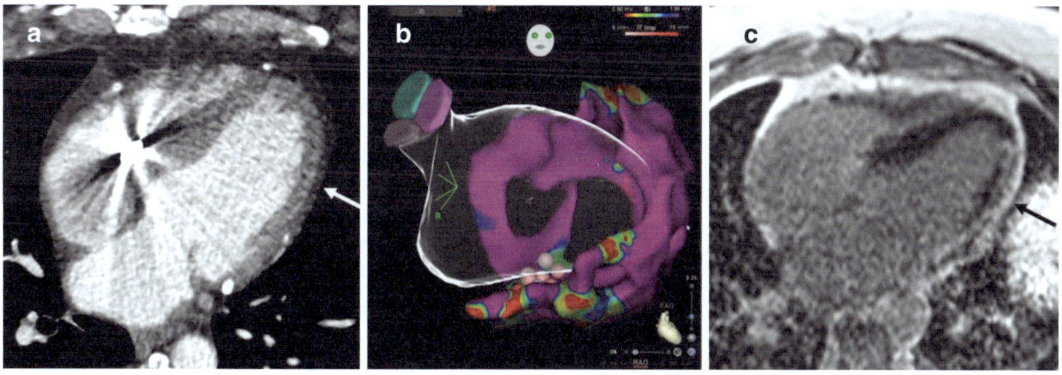

Fig. 12.21 Evaluation prior to stereotactic beam radiation therapy (SBRT) in high-risk VT. Patient with ischemic cardiomyopathy with extremely refractory VT. (**a**) CT shows wall thinning at the lateral wall (arrow). (**b**) Electroanatomic maps obtained with subepicardial approach showed sites of abnormal voltage at the region of wall thinning (red areas correspond to areas of low voltage). (**c**) Patient continued having frequent VT following ablation, despite MRI showing full-thickness ablation at the inferior wall (arrow). Therefore, the patient was subsequently referred for SBRT

Intra-procedural Imaging

Ultimately, the goal of VT ablation is to eliminate the arrhythmogenic substrate responsible for initiating and propagating ventricular tachycardia. For reentry-type arrhythmias, this involves ablating the critical isthmus responsible for reentry, whereas for focal-type arrhythmias (PVCs), this involves ablating the focal activation site(s). For catheter-based ablation, these sites are identified through detailed invasive electroanatomic mapping studies performed in the electrophysiology lab. The basic toolset of EAM mapping includes (1) activation mapping, (2) entrainment mapping, (3) pace mapping, and (4) substrate mapping [41]. Activation mapping is used to obtain the sequence of myocardial activation during ventricular tachycardia and is used to identify a site of origin of a focal VT or critical isthmus site for reentrant VT. Entrainment mapping is a technique used for mapping critical components of a reentry circuit and is used to confirm that a suspected isthmus site identified on activation mapping corresponds to a true critical VT isthmus site. Pace mapping is an alternative mapping technique that, unlike activation and entrainment mapping which require induction of VT, can be performed in sinus rhythm. This is useful in cases where initiating ventricular tachycardia is difficult or in hemodynamically unstable ventricular tachycardia that cannot be tolerated for more than brief periods of time. In general, pace mapping is used most often for confirming sites of activation in focal VT and has limited utility in reentrant VT.

Electroanatomical substrate mapping, much like substrate mapping obtained from imaging, seeks to map regions of scar tissue to identify ablation targets. In electroanatomical substrate mapping, areas of abnormal substrate are identified based on properties of electrograms such as low voltage (<0.5 mV is considered abnormal, whereas >1.5 mV is considered normal) in areas of dense scar or as slow or delayed conduction (late potentials) and fractionated electrograms in areas of gray zone. Its precision for identifying critical sites of origin is much less compared to the above EAM techniques, but it is useful in cases of non-inducible or poorly tolerated VT or in cases of unmappable VT where a site of origin cannot be confidently identified using the other mapping techniques [41].

A powerful technique in the intra-procedural setting is in combining pre-procedural imaging with electroanatomic mapping. In this technique, 3D maps of substrate obtained from MRI and/or CT can be imported into the EAM software for interactive visualization that can help direct electroanatomic mapping in real time. Other features of imaging can also be imported, including the location of vital structures such as the coronary arteries obtained from CTA, which can help direct ablation away from areas that may result in injury to these structures [64]. Activation and substrate maps from ECGi may similarly be imported and visualized in real time [62]. The advantage of displaying this information during EAM is that mapping effort may be focused on areas of suspected VT origin predicted from pre-procedure imaging, which may substantially reduce ablation and fluoroscopic times.

Post-procedural Imaging

While not routinely performed, imaging in the post-procedural setting may be considered if there are suspected complications such as

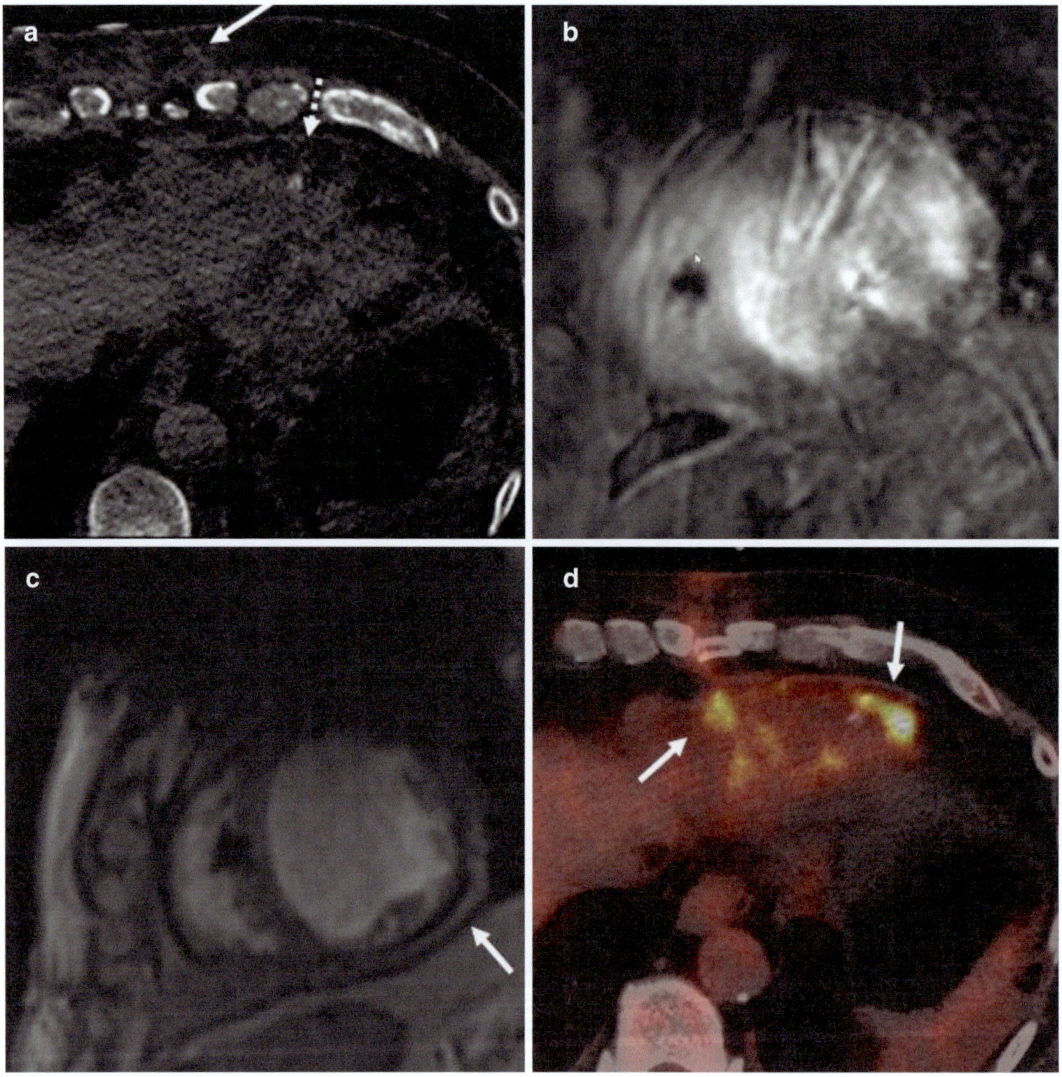

Fig. 12.22 Post-procedural imaging following VT ablation. Patient with nonischemic cardiomyopathy with refractory VT despite multiple prior ablations, who underwent recent epicardial ablation complicated by RV perforation during pericardial access requiring open repair. (**a**) CT images show sternotomy changes (arrow) with post-surgical changes of RV wall repair (dotted arrow). (**b**, **c**) MR images show large area of thinning in the inferior and lateral walls (**c**, arrow), but otherwise limited evaluation for LGE in setting of CIED despite wideband GRE sequence (**b**). (**d**) PET shows foci of inflammation limited to the RV repair and sternotomy sites (arrows) consistent with post-operative inflammation. Patient continued having VT and was subsequently referred for SBRT

steam-pop, pericardial effusion, or suspected injury to vital structures resulting in complications such as myocardial perforation or diaphragmatic elevation in phrenic nerve injury. Post-procedural imaging is also occasionally performed to characterize features of the ablation scar such as location and transmurality. For example, this may be performed in the setting of VT recurrence to determine whether complete ablation of the sites of targeted myocardium was achieved, or whether there are areas of incomplete ablation or other sites of substrate that may benefit from additional ablation (Fig. 12.22).

Cardiac Resynchronization Therapy

Ventricular dyssynchrony is caused by dyssynchronous timing of mechanical contractions either in segments of the LV (intraventricular desynchrony) or between the right and left ventricles (interventricular desynchrony). This can be caused by conduction abnormalities such as bundle branch block, intraventricular conduction delay, and scar. Cardiac resynchronization therapy (CRT, also referred to as biventricular pacing) is a treatment strategy that can improve synchrony by strategic placement of pacing leads in the right atrium, in the right ventricle, and in a coronary vein branch, with the goal of achieving optimal shortening of QRS, a marker of dyssynchrony (with longer QRS indicating a worse degree of dyssynchrony).

It is important to identify whether a patient might respond to CRT a priori, as it is an expensive and invasive procedure with approximately 20–30% of patients showing no improvement after CRT [65]. Quantitative imaging, particularly with MRI but also possible with gated CT, is particularly helpful in this regard. Strain imaging techniques can be used to estimate time to peak contraction in the different myocardial segments, and LGE imaging can identify sites of scar. Using this information, the lead may be placed at the site of latest contraction in a region absent of scar [66]. Alternatively, the lead may be placed at the site of latest electrical activation, which may be determined noninvasively using ECGi or 12-lead ECG [67–69].

Imaging-Based Computational Modeling

Computational modeling approaches have emerged as a promising tool for predicting and understanding treatment responses for a variety of arrhythmias. While not yet approved for clinical use, they have gained significant traction in this direction in applications such as evaluating ICD candidacy, planning ablation procedures, and optimizing lead placement for CRT. Generally, these approaches seek to develop patient-specific models ("digital twin") or population representative models ("virtual cohorts") of cardiac electrophysiology at the cell, tissue, and whole organ level to simulate and predict treatment responses to therapies or ablation procedures. The models are personalized using anatomical segmentations of the heart and distribution of infarct and border zone, which are typically obtained from MRI as described above [70–72].

For determining ICD candidacy, the personalized models allow determination of a Virtual-heart Arrhythmia Risk Predictor (VARP), which offers a more predictive metric for arrhythmia risk than the currently used clinical metrics LVEF and percent LGE. The predictor is considered positive when an arrhythmia is induced by virtual pacing at any of several uniformly distributed pacing sites in the left and right ventricles [73, 74]. For pre-ablation planning, ablation targets are identified from simulated AF or VT, and virtual ablation lesions may then be generated in the model as nonconductive lesions at the targeted sites [75, 76]. For VT, the model can determine whether the lesions result in VT non-inducibility to evaluate the effectiveness of the planned ablation lesion. If VT is inducible, either due to additional VT circuits or new VT circuits resulting from the ablation, additional targets may be identified and simulated until VT is no longer inducible [77]. In CRT, resolving the electrical dyssynchrony does not necessarily improve mechanical dyssynchrony and vice versa. Multiscale computational models accounting for patient-specific electrophysiology, electromechanics, and hemodynamics offer the potential to better optimize lead location and device settings, though the complexity of the models currently limits their use clinically [78].

Conclusion

Quantitative imaging using CT and MRI plays a critical role in many clinical electrophysiology applications. Modern quantitative imaging techniques allow for accurate anatomical assessment and precise localization and quantification of arrhythmogenic substrate that may assist the electrophysiologist in planning and executing ablation procedures and evaluating procedure outcomes. Quantitative imaging also plays an important role in evaluating ICD candidacy and in optimizing lead placement in CRT. Novel quantitative techniques such as ECGi and patient-specific computational modeling also rely heavily on information provided by CT and MRI, such as anatomical features and scar distribution, and may supplement information obtained from imaging alone and electroanatomic mapping to better guide management decisions.

References

1. Tse G. Mechanisms of cardiac arrhythmias. J Arrhythm. 2016;32(2):75–81. https://doi.org/10.1016/j.joa.2015.11.003. Epub 2015 Dec 17.
2. Costantini O. Basic principles of cardiac electrophysiology. Med Clin North Am. 2019;103(5):767–74.
3. Knackstedt C, Schauerte P, Kirchhof P. Electro-anatomic mapping systems in arrhythmias. Europace. 2008;10 Suppl 3:iii28–34.
4. Koutalas E, Rolf S, Dinov B, Richter S, Arya A, Bollmann A, Hindricks G, Sommer P. Contemporary mapping techniques of complex cardiac arrhythmias – identifying and modifying the arrhythmogenic substrate. Arrhythm Electrophysiol Rev. 2015;4(1):19–27.
5. Sy RW, Thiagalingam A, Stiles MK. Modern electrophysiology mapping techniques. Heart Lung Circ. 2012;21(6–7):364–75.
6. Gimelli A, Ernst S, Liga R. Multi-modality imaging for the identification of arrhythmogenic substrates prior to electrophysiology studies. Front Cardiovasc Med. 2021;8:640087.
7. Staerk L, Sherer JA, Ko D, Benjamin EJ, Helm RH. Atrial fibrillation: epidemiology, pathophysiology, and clinical outcomes. Circ Res. 2017;120(9):1501–17.
8. Kornej J, Börschel CS, Benjamin EJ, Schnabel RB. Epidemiology of atrial fibrillation in the 21st century: novel methods and new insights. Circ Res. 2020;127(1):4–20.
9. Haïssaguerre M, Jaïs P, Shah DC, Takahashi A, Hocini M, Quiniou G, Garrigue S, Le Mouroux A, Le Métayer P, Clémenty J. Spontaneous initiation of atrial fibrillation by ectopic beats originating in the pulmonary veins. N Engl J Med. 1998;339(10):659–66.
10. Oral H, Knight BP, Tada H, Ozaydin M, Chugh A, Hassan S, Scharf C, Lai SW, Greenstein R, Pelosi F Jr, Strickberger SA, Morady F. Pulmonary vein isolation for paroxysmal and persistent atrial fibrillation. Circulation. 2002;105(9):1077–81.
11. Parameswaran R, Al-Kaisey AM, Kalman JM. Catheter ablation for atrial fibrillation: current indications and evolving technologies. Nat Rev Cardiol. 2021;18(3):210–25.
12. Wittkampf FH, Vonken EJ, Derksen R, Loh P, Velthuis B, Wever EF, Boersma LV, Rensing BJ, Cramer MJ. Pulmonary vein ostium geometry: analysis by magnetic resonance angiography. Circulation. 2003;107(1):21–3.
13. Rajiah P, Kanne JP. Computed tomography of pulmonary venous variants and anomalies. J Cardiovasc Comput Tomogr. 2010;4(3):155–63.
14. Ang R, Hunter RJ, Baker V, et al. Pulmonary vein measurements on pre-procedural CT/MR imaging can predict difficult pulmonary vein isolation and phrenic nerve injury during cryoballoon ablation for paroxysmal atrial fibrillation. Int J Cardiol. 2015;195:253–8.
15. Matsumoto Y, Muraoka Y, Funama Y, Mito S, Masuda T, Sato T, Akita T, Awai K. Analysis of the anatomical features of pulmonary veins on pre-procedural cardiac CT images resulting in incomplete cryoballoon ablation for atrial fibrillation. J Cardiovasc Comput Tomogr. 2019;13(2):118–27.
16. Lemola K, Sneider M, Desjardins B, Case I, Han J, Good E, Tamirisa K, Tsemo A, Chugh A, Bogun F, Pelosi F Jr, Kazerooni E, Morady F, Oral H. Computed tomographic analysis of the anatomy of the left atrium and the esophagus: implications for left atrial catheter ablation. Circulation. 2004;110(24):3655–60.
17. Squara F, Desjardins B, Marchlinski FE, Supple GE. Prospective 3-dimensional computed tomography segmentation of the pericardiac right phrenic nerve in the setting of atrial fibrillation ablation. Circ Arrhythm Electrophysiol. 2014;7(3):561–2.
18. Horton R, Di Biase L, Reddy V, Neuzil P, Mohanty P, Sanchez J, Nguyen T, Mohanty S, Gallinghouse GJ, Bailey SM, Zagrodzky JD, Burkhardt JD, Natale A. Locating the right phrenic nerve by imaging the right pericardiophrenic artery with computerized

tomographic angiography: implications for balloon-based procedures. Heart Rhythm. 2010;7(7):937–41.

19. Spagnolo P, Giglio M, Di Marco D, Cannaò PM, Agricola E, Della Bella PE, Monti CB, Sardanelli F. Diagnosis of left atrial appendage thrombus in patients with atrial fibrillation: delayed contrast-enhanced cardiac CT. Eur Radiol. 2021;31(3):1236–44.
20. Tanaka M, Yasuoka R, Nagano T, et al. A novel method to demonstrate thrombus formation of the left atrial appendage in patients with persistent atrial fibrillation by cardiac computed tomography. Int J Cardiol Heart Vasc. 2021;36:100866.
21. Ebrahimian S, Digumarthy SR, Homayounieh F, et al. Use of radiomics to differentiate left atrial appendage thrombi and mixing artifacts on single-phase CT angiography. Int J Cardiovasc Imaging. 2021;37(6):2071–8.
22. Kitkungvan D, Nabi F, Ghosn MG, et al. Detection of LA and LAA thrombus by CMR in patients referred for pulmonary vein isolation. JACC Cardiovasc Imaging. 2016;9(7):809–18.
23. Wijffels MC, Kirchhof CJ, Dorland R, Allessie MA. Atrial fibrillation begets atrial fibrillation. A study in awake chronically instrumented goats. Circulation. 1995;92(7):1954–68.
24. Fochler F, Yamaguchi T, Kheirkahan M, Kholmovski EG, Morris AK, Marrouche NF. Late gadolinium enhancement magnetic resonance imaging guided treatment of post-atrial fibrillation ablation recurrent arrhythmia. Circ Arrhythm Electrophysiol. 2019;12(8):e007174.
25. Siebermair J, Kholmovski EG, Marrouche N. Assessment of left atrial fibrosis by late gadolinium enhancement magnetic resonance imaging: methodology and clinical implications. JACC Clin Electrophysiol. 2017;3(8):791–802.
26. Khurram IM, Beinart R, Zipunnikov V, Dewire J, Yarmohammadi H, Sasaki T, Spragg DD, Marine JE, Berger RD, Halperin HR, Calkins H, Zimmerman SL, Nazarian S. Magnetic resonance image intensity ratio, a normalized measure to enable interpatient comparability of left atrial fibrosis. Heart Rhythm. 2014;11(1):85–92.
27. Ling Z, McManigle J, Zipunnikov V, Pashakhanloo F, Khurram IM, Zimmerman SL, Philips B, Marine JE, Spragg DD, Ashikaga H, Calkins H, Nazarian S. The association of left atrial low voltage regions on electroanatomic mapping with low attenuation regions on cardiac computed tomography perfusion imaging in patients with atrial fibrillation. Heart Rhythm. 2015;12(5):857–64.
28. Bishop M, Rajani R, Plank G, Gaddum N, Carr-White G, Wright M, O'Neill M, Niederer S. Three-dimensional atrial wall thickness maps to inform catheter ablation procedures for atrial fibrillation. Europace. 2016;18(3):376–83.
29. Nakatani Y, Sakamoto T, Yamaguchi Y, Tsujino Y, Kataoka N, Kinugawa K. Left atrial wall thickness is associated with the low-voltage area in patients with paroxysmal atrial fibrillation. J Interv Card Electrophysiol. 2020;58(3):315–21.
30. Zuo K, Li K, Liu M, Li J, Liu X, Liu X, Zhong J, Yang X. Correlation of left atrial wall thickness and atrial remodeling in atrial fibrillation: study based on low-dose-ibutilide-facilitated catheter ablation. Medicine (Baltimore). 2019;98(15):e15170.
31. Wong CX, Ganesan AN, Selvanayagam JB. Epicardial fat and atrial fibrillation: current evidence, potential mechanisms, clinical implications, and future directions. Eur Heart J. 2017;38(17):1294–302.
32. Shao Y, Chen L, Chen W, Sang C, Xu C, Zhang C. Left atrial epicardial adipose tissue is associated with low voltage zones in the left atrium in patients with non-valvular atrial fibrillation. Front Cardiovasc Med. 2022;9:924646.
33. Bodagh N, Williams MC, Vickneson K, Gharaviri A, Niederer S, Williams SE. State of the art paper: cardiac computed tomography of the left atrium in atrial fibrillation. J Cardiovasc Comput Tomogr. 2023;17(3):166–76.
34. Yang M, Cao Q, Xu Z, Ge Y, Li S, Yan F, Yang W. Development and validation of a machine learning-based radiomics model on cardiac computed tomography of epicardial adipose tissue in predicting characteristics and recurrence of atrial fibrillation. Front Cardiovasc Med. 2022;9:813085.
35. Rolf S, Hindricks G, Sommer P, Richter S, Arya A, Bollmann A, Kosiuk J, Koutalas E. Electroanatomical mapping of atrial fibrillation: review of the current techniques and advances. J Atr Fibrillation. 2014;7(4):1140.
36. Tops LF, Schalij MJ, den Uijl DW, Abraham TP, Calkins H, Bax JJ. Image integration in catheter ablation of atrial fibrillation. Europace. 2008;10 Suppl 3:iii48–56.
37. Gupta A, Perera T, Ganesan A, Sullivan T, Lau DH, Roberts-Thomson KC, Brooks AG, Sanders P. Complications of catheter ablation of atrial fibrillation: a systematic review. Circ Arrhythm Electrophysiol. 2013;6(6):1082–8.
38. Mont L, Roca-Luque I, Althoff TF. Ablation lesion assessment with MRI. Arrhythm Electrophysiol Rev. 2022;11:e02.
39. Parmar BR, Jarrett TR, Kholmovski EG, Hu N, Parker D, MacLeod RS, Marrouche NF, Ranjan R. Poor scar formation after ablation is associated with atrial fibrillation recurrence. J Interv Card Electrophysiol. 2015 Dec;44(3):247–56.
40. Baldzizhar A, Manuylova E, Marchenko R, Kryvalap Y, Carey MG. Ventricular tachycardias: characteristics and management. Crit Care Nurs Clin North Am. 2016;28(3):317–29.
41. Guandalini GS, Liang JJ, Marchlinski FE. Ventricular tachycardia ablation: past, present, and future perspectives. JACC Clin Electrophysiol. 2019;5(12):1363–83.
42. Rudy Y. Noninvasive electrocardiographic imaging of arrhythmogenic substrates in humans. Circ Res. 2013;112(5):863–74.

43. Zipes DP, Camm AJ, Borggrefe M, et al. ACC/AHA/ESC 2006 guidelines for management of patients with ventricular arrhythmias and the prevention of sudden cardiac death—executive summary: a report of the American College of Cardiology/American Heart Association Task Force and the European Society of Cardiology Committee for Practice Guidelines (Writing Committee to Develop Guidelines for Management of Patients with Ventricular Arrhythmias and the Prevention of Sudden Cardiac Death) Developed in collaboration with the European Heart Rhythm Association and the Heart Rhythm Society. Eur Heart J. 2006;27(17):2099–140. https://doi.org/10.1093/eurheartj/ehl199.
44. Wijnmaalen AP, van der Geest RJ, van Huls van Taxis CF, et al. Head-to-head comparison of contrast-enhanced magnetic resonance imaging and electroanatomical voltage mapping to assess post-infarct scar characteristics in patients with ventricular tachycardias: real-time image integration and reversed registration. Eur Heart J. 2011;32(1):104–14.
45. Avendi MR, Kheradvar A, Jafarkhani H. Fully automatic segmentation of heart chambers in cardiac MRI using deep learning. J Cardiovasc Magn Reson. 2016;18(Suppl 1):P351.
46. Salerno M, Sharif B, Arheden H, et al. Recent advances in cardiovascular magnetic resonance: techniques and applications. Circ Cardiovasc Imaging. 2017;10(6):e003951. https://doi.org/10.1161/CIRCIMAGING.116.003951.
47. Jenista ER, Wendell DC, Azevedo CF, Klem I, Judd RM, Kim RJ, Kim HW. Revisiting how we perform late gadolinium enhancement CMR: insights gleaned over 25 years of clinical practice. J Cardiovasc Magn Reson. 2023;25(1):18.
48. Sirajuddin A, Mirmomen SM, Kligerman SJ, et al. Ischemic heart disease: noninvasive imaging techniques and findings. Radiographics. 2021;41(4):990–1021. https://doi.org/10.1148/rg.2021200125.
49. Cummings KW, Bhalla S, Javidan-Nejad C, Bierhals AJ, Gutierrez FR, Woodard PK. A pattern-based approach to assessment of delayed enhancement in nonischemic cardiomyopathy at MR imaging. Radiographics. 2009;29(1):89–103. https://doi.org/10.1148/rg.291085052.
50. Ferreira VM, Schulz-Menger J, Holmvang G, et al. Cardiovascular magnetic resonance in nonischemic myocardial inflammation: expert recommendations. J Am Coll Cardiol. 2018;72(24):3158–76.
51. Chan RH, Maron BJ, Olivotto I, et al. Prognostic value of quantitative contrast-enhanced cardiovascular magnetic resonance for the evaluation of sudden death risk in patients with hypertrophic cardiomyopathy. Circulation. 2014;130(6):484–95.
52. Marcus FI, McKenna WJ, Sherrill D, et al. Diagnosis of arrhythmogenic right ventricular cardiomyopathy/dysplasia: proposed modification of the task force criteria. Circulation. 2010;121(13):1533–41.
53. Kazmirczak F, Chen KA, Adabag S, et al. Assessment of the 2017 AHA/ACC/HRS guideline recommendations for implantable cardioverter-defibrillator implantation in cardiac sarcoidosis. Circ Arrhythm Electrophysiol. 2019;12(9):e007488.
54. Tian J, Jeudy J, Smith MF, et al. Three-dimensional contrast-enhanced multidetector CT for anatomic, dynamic, and perfusion characterization of abnormal myocardium to guide ventricular tachycardia ablations. Circ Arrhythm Electrophysiol. 2010;3(5):496–504. https://doi.org/10.1161/CIRCEP.109.889311.
55. Esposito A, Palmisano A, Antunes S, et al. Cardiac CT with delayed enhancement in the characterization of ventricular tachycardia structural substrate: relationship between CT-segmented scar and electro-anatomic mapping. JACC Cardiovasc Imaging. 2016;9(7):822–32.
56. Acosta J, Fernández-Armenta J, Borràs R, et al. Scar characterization to predict life-threatening arrhythmic events and sudden cardiac death in patients with cardiac resynchronization therapy: the GAUDI-CRT study. JACC Cardiovasc Imaging. 2018;11(4):561–72.
57. Aljaroudi WA, Flamm SD, Saliba W, Wilkoff BL, Kwon D. Role of CMR imaging in risk stratification for sudden cardiac death. JACC Cardiovasc Imaging. 2013;6(3):392–406.
58. Zhang L, Huttin O, Marie PY, Felblinger J, Beaumont M, Chillou C, Girerd N, Mandry D. Myocardial infarct sizing by late gadolinium-enhanced MRI: comparison of manual, full-width at half-maximum, and n-standard deviation methods. J Magn Reson Imaging. 2016;44(5):1206–17.
59. Schulz-Menger J, Bluemke DA, Bremerich J, Flamm SD, Fogel MA, Friedrich MG, Kim RJ, von Knobelsdorff-Brenkenhoff F, Kramer CM, Pennell DJ, Plein S, Nagel E. Standardized image interpretation and post-processing in cardiovascular magnetic resonance – 2020 update: Society for Cardiovascular Magnetic Resonance (SCMR): Board of Trustees Task Force on Standardized Post-Processing. J Cardiovasc Magn Reson. 2020;22(1):19.
60. Desjardins B, Morady F, Bogun F. Effect of epicardial fat on electroanatomical mapping and epicardial catheter ablation. J Am Coll Cardiol. 2010;56(16):1320–7.
61. Salinet J, Molero R, Schlindwein FS, et al. Electrocardiographic imaging for atrial fibrillation: a perspective from computer models and animal experiments to clinical value. Front Physiol. 2021;12:653013.
62. Graham AJ, Orini M, Zacur E, et al. Simultaneous comparison of electrocardiographic imaging and epicardial contact mapping in structural heart disease. Circ Arrhythm Electrophysiol. 2019;12(4):e007120.
63. Robinson CG, Samson PP, Moore KMS, et al. Phase I/II trial of electrophysiology-guided noninvasive cardiac radioablation for ventricular tachycardia. Circulation. 2019;139(3):313–21.
64. Cochet H, Komatsu Y, Sacher F, et al. Integration of merged delayed-enhanced magnetic resonance imaging and multidetector computed tomography for the guidance of ventricular tachycardia abla-

tion: a pilot study. J Cardiovasc Electrophysiol. 2013;24(4):419–26.
65. Sieniewicz BJ, Gould J, Porter B, Sidhu BS, Teall T, Webb J, Carr-White G, Rinaldi CA. Understanding non-response to cardiac resynchronisation therapy: common problems and potential solutions. Heart Fail Rev. 2019;24(1):41–54.
66. Rajiah PS, Kalisz K, Broncano J, et al. Myocardial strain evaluation with cardiovascular MRI: physics, principles and clinical applications. Radiographics. 2022;42(4):968–90.
67. Parreira L, Tsyganov A, Artyukhina E, et al. Non-invasive three-dimensional electrical activation mapping to predict cardiac resynchronization therapy response: site of latest left ventricular activation relative to pacing site. Europace. 2023;25(4):1458–66.
68. Jia P, Ramanathan C, Ghanem RN, Ryu K, Varma N, Rudy Y. Electrocardiographic imaging of cardiac resynchronization therapy in heart failure: observation of variable electrophysiologic responses. Heart Rhythm. 2006;3(3):296–310.
69. Melgaard J, van Dam PM, Sommer A, et al. Non-invasive estimation of QLV from the standard 12-lead ECG in patients with left bundle branch block. Front Physiol. 2022;13:939240.
70. Trayanova NA, Lyon A, Shade J, Heijman J. Computational modeling of cardiac electrophysiology and arrhythmogenesis. Physiol Rev. 2024;104:1265–333.
71. Lopez-Perez A, Sebastian R, Izquierdo M, Ruiz R, Bishop M, Ferrero JM. Personalized cardiac computational models: from clinical data to simulation of infarct-related ventricular tachycardia. Front Physiol. 2019;10:580.
72. Cluitmans M, Walton R, Plank G. Editorial: computational methods in cardiac electrophysiology. Front Physiol. 2023;14:1231342.
73. Arevalo HJ, Vadakkumpadan F, Guallar E, Jebb A, Malamas P, Wu KC, Trayanova NA. Arrhythmia risk stratification of patients after myocardial infarction using personalized heart models. Nat Commun. 2016;7:11437.
74. Deng D, Arevalo HJ, Prakosa A, Callans DJ, Trayanova NA. A feasibility study of arrhythmia risk prediction in patients with myocardial infarction and preserved ejection fraction. Europace. 2016;18(suppl 4):iv60–6.
75. Ashikaga H, Arevalo H, Vadakkumpadan F, Blake RC, Bayer JD, Nazarian S, Muz Zviman M, Tandri H, Berger RD, Calkins H, Herzka DA, Trayanova NA, Halperin HR. Feasibility of image-based simulation to estimate ablation target in human ventricular arrhythmia. Heart Rhythm. 2013;10:1109–16.
76. Zahid S, Whyte KN, Schwarz EL, Blake RC III, Boyle PM, Chrispin J, Prakosa A, Ipek EG, Pashakhanloo F, Halperin HR, Calkins H, Berger RD, Nazarian S, Trayanova NA. Feasibility of using patient-specific models and the "minimum cut" algorithm to predict optimal ablation targets for left atrial flutter. Heart Rhythm. 2016;13:1687–98.
77. Trayanova NA, Pashakhanloo F, Wu KC, Halperin HR. Imaging based simulations for predicting sudden death and guiding ventricular tachycardia ablation. Circ Arrhythm Electrophysiol. 2017;10(7):e004743.
78. Lee AWC, Costa CM, Strocchi M, Rinaldi CA, Niederer SA. Computational modeling for cardiac resynchronization therapy. J Cardiovasc Transl Res. 2018;11(2):92–108.
79. Bugenhagen S, Kolluri N, Tan N, Morris M, Rajiah PS. Utility of CT and MRI in cardiac electrophysiology. Radiographics. 2024;44(9):e230222.

13 Cardiology Perspective: Approaches to Multimodality Quantitative Imaging in Cardio-Oncology Patients

Sonia F. Epstein and Ming Hui Chen

Introduction: A Case Study

A 64-year-old woman is referred to oncology for treatment of early stage, left-sided, human epidermal growth factor receptor 2-positive (HER2+) breast cancer. Her treatment plan includes lumpectomy, doxorubicin (240 mg/ml^2), cyclophosphamide, paclitaxel, trastuzumab, hormonal therapy, and radiotherapy (45 Gy).

In patients with left-sided breast cancer, the heart lies in close proximity to the left breast—and even in the radiation field. As part of the computed tomography (CT) planning protocol and during her radiotherapy treatment, the radiation oncologist and radiology technologists coach the patient in deep inspiration breath hold (DIBH) maneuvers. With each deep breath, this simple and widely utilized radiation technique developed by Chen et al. displaces the patient's heart caudally and posteriorly away from the left breast radiation field [1] (Fig. 13.1). In doing so, the radiation dose to the patient's heart and left anterior descending artery (LAD), the major coronary artery that supplies the left ventricle (LV) in most individuals, decreases by 67% and 73% percent, respectively [2]. Quantitative CT imaging has made the implementation of this technique possible. It is only with 3D localization of the breast cancer and the precise coordinates of the CT scan that it is possible to deliver radiation to the tumor at precisely the correct moment during DIBH when the heart and the breast are farthest apart and also to cut off the radiation beam precisely as the breast moves out of the prescribed radiation field as the chest deflates with expiration [3]. Quantitative CT imaging has been critical to detecting adverse cardiopulmonary issues in cancer patients, but also has helped minimize radiation to the coronaries without compromising treatment to the tumor—thereby improving cancer outcomes overall.

Cardiovascular disease (CVD) is a central concern for cancer patients and survivors and their physicians, in part because therapies, like radiation, also damage the heart muscle, valves, coronary and carotid arteries, and vasculature, potentially leading to heart failure (HF), cardiomyopathy, coronary artery disease (CAD), and/or stroke [4]. DIBH, a cardioprotective strategy, is just one example of how the field of radiology intersects with the rapidly evolving cardio-oncology subspeciality, which addresses the unique cardiovascular needs of the 18.1 million cancer survivors in the United States today [5, 6]. With improvements in cancer screening and treatment, a record number of individuals are

S. F. Epstein
Boston Children's Hospital, Boston, MA, USA

M. H. Chen (✉)
Boston Children's Hospital, Boston, MA, USA

Harvard Medical School, Boston, MA, USA

Dana-Farber Cancer Institute, Boston, MA, USA
e-mail: MingHui.Chen@childrens.harvard.edu

R. Gill, P. Rajiah (eds.), *Quantitative Imaging in the Thorax*,
https://doi.org/10.1007/978-3-032-14103-3_13

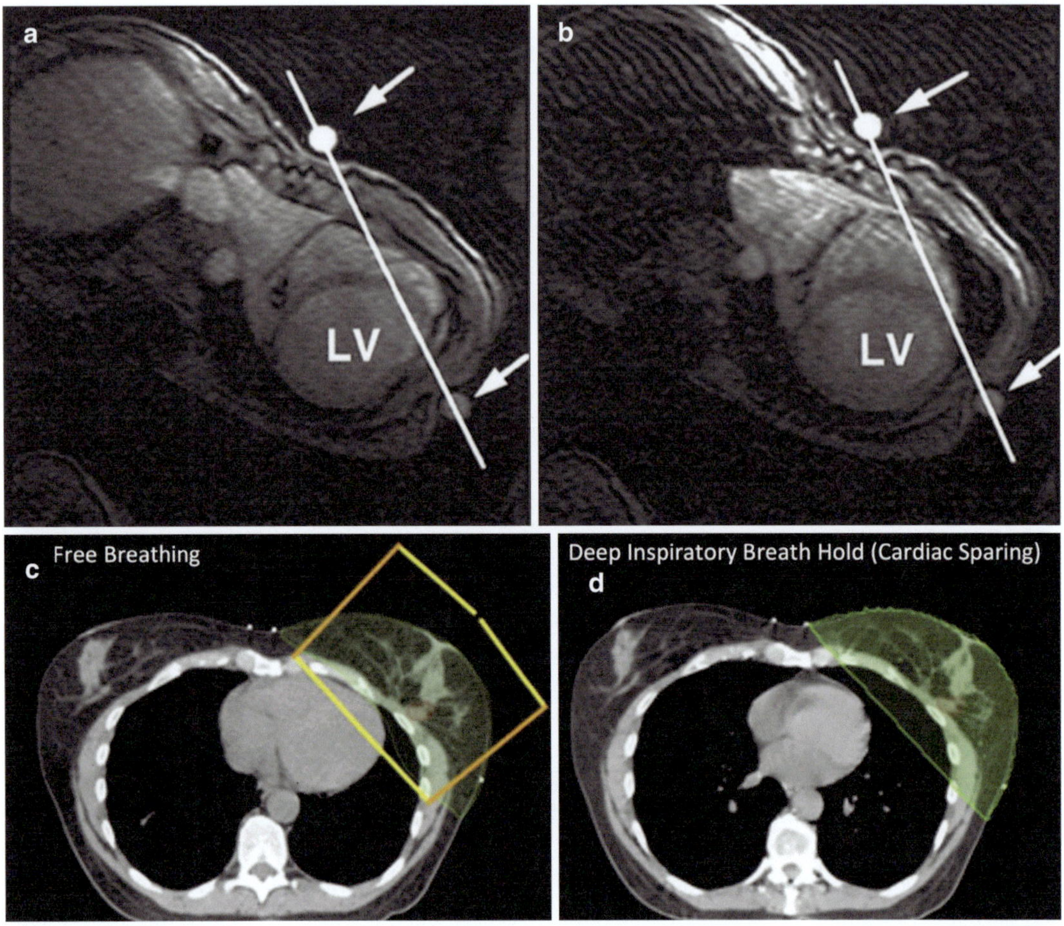

Fig. 13.1 Impact of Breath Hold on Decreasing Cardiac Radiation. Radiation planning for patients with left-sided breast cancer shows proximity of the left heart and ventricle (LV) to the breast cancer radiation portal with (**a, c**) free breathing, and then (**b, d**) the displacement of the heart outside the radiation portals with deep inspiratory breath hold (DIBH). DIBH during radiation planning is a technique piloted by Chen et al. (top panels, magnetic resonance images) [1]. This technique is now routinely used during radiation therapy for breast cancer (bottom panels, cardiac computed tomography images, adapted from Tanguturi et al. [3])

surviving cancer, with nearly half of all survivors being alive ten or more years post-diagnosis [5]. These triumphs for cancer survivorship have been and will continue to be achieved with robust monitoring of cardiovascular health before, during, and beyond cancer treatment.

In this chapter, we describe the utility of multimodality quantitative cardiothoracic imaging in cardio-oncology from a cardiology and lifespan perspective. This allows radiologists and radiation oncologists to gain perspective on what cardiac providers caring for these patients seek when they refer the patients for chest and cardiac imaging and the role that imaging plays throughout patients' oncological treatment and survivorship journey (Fig. 13.2).

Multimodality cardiothoracic imaging plays a critical role in cardiovascular risk assessment prior to cancer treatment, cardiotoxicity assessment during treatment, and surveillance for cardiotoxicity and atherosclerotic CVD (ASCVD) post-treatment and among long-term survivors. Furthermore, advanced imaging techniques are integral to clinical research, where high precision and quantitation are important for serial imaging [7, 8].

The chapter begins with an overview of the multiple manifestations of cardiotoxicity and subsequently provides detail of the uses of rele-

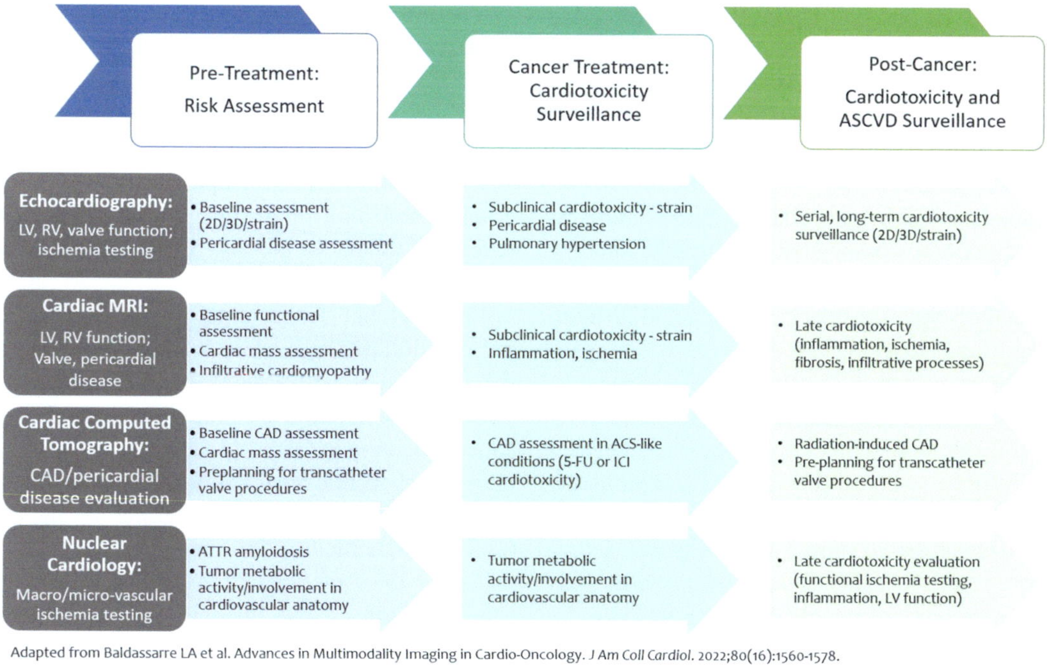

Fig. 13.2 Chest and quantitative cardiac imaging play essential roles pre-, during, and post-cancer treatment [7]. Echocardiography, cardiac MRI, cardiac computed tomography, and nuclear imaging are used in surveillance, evaluation, and diagnosis of a range of cardiovascular conditions that may occur during oncological treatment and across the survivorship continuum

vant thoracic imaging modalities in the detection and treatment of cardiotoxicity. Echocardiography is the first-line imaging modality for cardio-oncology patients, but cardiac magnetic resonance imaging (CMR), cardiac computed tomography (CCT), positron emission therapy (PET), and cardiac single-photon emission computerized tomography (SPECT) also provide key diagnostic, quantitative and/or prognostic information. The chapter concludes with special consideration of common imaging issues, namely, those associated with cardiac imaging in female patients who comprise the majority of long-term cancer survivors, in childhood cancer patients and survivors, and in under-resourced settings.

Defining Cardiotoxicity

Historically, cardiotoxicity has been associated with HF induced by anthracycline chemotherapy agents (including doxorubicin, daunorubicin, idarubicin, etc.), which are a mainstay of treatment for many important cancers including breast cancer, lymphoma, and sarcomas. This phenomenon was recognized not long after the introduction of this drug class in the 1960s [9]. Trastuzumab, introduced in the late 1990s in the United States for the treatment of HER2+ metastatic breast cancer, was transformative in the care of breast cancer patients and also recognized early on to be associated with HF and/or declines in left ventricular ejection fraction (LVEF), especially when used in conjunction with anthracycline therapy [10].

There are, however, many other well-recognized forms of cardiotoxicity, such as the late effects of radiation therapy (RT), which include CAD, valvular heart disease, myocardial fibrosis, conduction system disorders, pericardial disease, and autonomic dysfunction, in addition to HF and cardiomyopathy. Radiation-induced cardiotoxicity may present up to decades post-treatment and is especially prevalent in long-term survivors of Hodgkin lymphoma (HL), treated in the 1960–1990s with high-dose mediastinal or mantle radiation (a field that involves the neck to the mid-thoracic region or the neck to the abdomen). Over the past two decades, with the advancement of targeted cancer therapies, myriad other cardiovascular toxicities associated with cancer therapy have been highlighted, such as myocarditis, pericardial disease, vascular toxicities, and arrhythmias (Table 13.1) [11].

The term "cancer therapy-related cardiac dysfunction" (CTRCD) has emerged to specifically refer to the continuum of asymptomatic decreases in LVEF to symptomatic HF, a spectrum that is commonly seen with anthracycline- and trastuzumab-based protocols. The term CTRCD is used here to indicate this effect, while other toxicities such as myocarditis are referred to by name explicitly, in line with other reports [7].

Though the exact definition of asymptomatic CTRCD varies across the field of oncology and cardiology, many cite an absolute decrease in LVEF of ≥10 EF units to less than approximately 50–55%; declines in LVEF are further classified clinically as symptomatic or asymptomatic and also by severity (mild/moderate/severe CTRCD). In the last 5–10 years, newer imaging biomarkers have been introduced, such as peak global longitudinal strain (GLS), a deformation parameter that provides a quantitative measure of cardiac muscle contractile function [12]. Clinical cardiology societies have added a decline in GLS and elevation of cardiac biomarkers to diagnostic definitions of asymptomatic CTRCD [11, 13]. A definition of CTRCD, specifically for imagers, was introduced by the American College of Cardiology Cardio-Oncology and Imaging Council and is provided in Table 13.2 [7, 11].

Table 13.1 Utility of cardiothoracic imaging modalities in cardio-oncology

Imaging modality	Utility	Common cancer therapies for referred patients	Examples	Advantages and disadvantages
Echocardiography	LV/RV structure and function Assessment for CTRCD or subclinical cardiotoxicity Valvular disease Pericardial disease Functional ischemia assessment Pulmonary hypertension	Anthracyclines HER2-targeted therapies ICIs Radiation HSCT VEGF inhibitors BTK inhibitors Proteasome inhibitors Fluoropyrimidines CAR-T-cell therapies	LVEF assessment with 3D echocardiography and GLS before anthracycline/HER2-targeted treatment and for serial monitoring/surveillance during/after treatment Stress echocardiography for evaluation of radiation-induced coronary artery disease in patient with ambiguous CCTA	Pros: Frontline imaging technique for cardiotoxicity Versatile and widely accessible Can be used at bedside Cons: Variability with operator/observer experience (especially strain) Poor echocardiographic windows challenge image interpretation (more common with mastectomy, breast implants, lung disease, and obesity)
Cardiac magnetic imaging	LV/RV structure and function Assessment for CTRCD or subclinical cardiotoxicity Myocarditis Valvular function Pericardial disease Ischemia assessment (stress CMR) Vascular toxicity Other inflammation; fibrosis; infiltrative processes	Anthracyclines HER2-targeted therapies ICIs Radiation HSCT VEGF inhibitors BTK inhibitors Proteasome inhibitors Fluoropyrimidines CAR-T-cell therapies	Assessment for myocarditis (with T1/T2 mapping and LGE sequences) in patients treated with ICIs presenting with arrhythmia/hemodynamic instability or other CV symptoms Evaluation of constrictive pericarditis (with real-time cine and phase contrast sequences) in patients with history of radiation with CV symptoms	Pros: High image quality and resolution Cross-sectional imaging Tissue characterization Cons: Higher cost; reduced accessibility Contraindications for gadolinium (i.e., in pregnant patients) or for patients with metal devices Prolonged scan time and breath holds

(continued)

Table 13.1 (continued)

Imaging modality	Utility	Common cancer therapies for referred patients	Examples	Advantages and disadvantages
Cardiac computed tomography	CAD/radiation-induced CAD assessment ASCVD assessment Pericardial disease Transcatheter valve repair/TAVR preplanning	ICIs Proteasome inhibitors Radiation HSCT Fluoropyrimidines	Evaluate for CAD in acute coronary syndrome-like response to 5-FU or ICI CCTA for assessment of suspected ischemia in patient on HF-associated treatments/with HF symptoms	Pros: Widely available Rapid test time Noninvasive and definitive CAD evaluation with CCTA; subclinical CAD evaluation CAC scoring and plaque characterization and FFR assessment for hemodynamic significance Cons: Radiation exposure Contraindications for iodinated contrast Prolonged breath holds Calcification in those with history radiation may influence assessment of coronary lesions
Nuclear imaging (SPECT; PET)	Macro- or microvascular ischemia LV functional assessment Transthyretin amyloidosis	ICIs Proteasome inhibitors Radiation HSCT Fluoropyrimidines	Evaluation of CAD prior to initiation of therapy associated with ischemia or thrombosis Quantification of myocardial blood flow and myocardial flow reserve with PET in patients with CAD	Pros: SPECT widely available for ischemia assessment Superior accuracy of PET for quantitative ischemia assessment and identifying nonobstructive CAD Cons: Radiation exposure SPECT susceptible to attenuation artifacts PET largely limited to academic medical centers

5-FU 5-fluorouracil, *ASCVD* atherosclerotic cardiovascular disease, *BTK* Bruton's tyrosine kinase inhibitors, *CAC* coronary artery calcium, *CAD* coronary artery disease, *CAR-T* chimeric T-cell antigen therapy, *CCTA* cardiac computed tomography angiography, *CMR* cardiac magnetic resonance imaging, *CTRCD* cancer therapy-related cardiac dysfunction, *GLS* global longitudinal strain, *HER2* human epidermal growth factor receptor 2, *HSCT* hematopoietic stem cell transplantation, *ICI* immune checkpoint inhibitor, *LGE* late gadolinium enhancement, *LV* left ventricle, *LVEF* LV ejection fraction, *PET* positron emission therapy, *RV* right ventricle, *SPECT* single-photon emission computerized tomography, *TAVR* transcatheter aortic valve replacement, *VEGF* vascular endothelial growth factor. Refer to citations for further information regarding the summary above [7, 8, 26]

Table 13.2 ACC Cardio-Oncology and Imaging Council 2022 definition of CTRCD for imagers[a]

Definite CTRCD: LVEF reduction of ≥10% to value <50% Possible CTRCD: LVEF reduction ≥10% to value 50–55% LVEF reduction <10% to value <50% Reduction in GLS of ≥15% without significant LVEF reduction	Imaging modality: 3D volumetric echocardiography primarily recommended for LVEF assessment CMR preferred to 2D assessment of LVEF

[a]This definition for imagers complements the International Cardio-Oncology Society's clinical categories of cardiotoxicity [7, 11]

Imaging Modalities Relevant to Cardio-Oncology

Echocardiography

Echocardiography is the first-line modality for evaluating CTRCD and other cardiotoxicities due to its accessibility, portability, cost-effectiveness, and lack of associated radiation (Table 13.1) [13–16]. LVEF measured on echocardiography helps identify the risk of CTRCD; therefore, baseline echocardiographic assessment before the commencement of treatment with a potentially cardiotoxic therapy is essential. Baseline echocardiography allows for (a) risk assessment for HF, (b) assessment of the need for medical management of cardiac function during treatment, (c) adjustment of antineoplastic regimens to the patient's cardiac function if necessary, and (d) establishment of a baseline for long-term surveillance [16, 17]. During and after cancer treatment, echocardiography continues to be critical to monitoring cardiovascular health.

Echocardiographic evaluation of LVEF in cancer patients is ideally performed with the use of 3D imaging, which minimizes geometric assumptions in the determination of overall LV systolic function. Integration of GLS measurement from three views can also be obtained and quantitated [8, 13]. 3D imaging is preferred to 2D imaging due to its lack of geometric assumptions and its better reproducibility and greater accuracy in detecting an abnormal LVEF, but cost and limited availability of trained operators still limit its widespread use. For 2D LVEF assessment, the modified Simpson's biplane method should be used. Ultrasound-enhancing contrast agents should be used to improve image quality if two or more LV segments are difficult to visualize. CMR (discussed below) can also be used to evaluate LVEF if 3D echo imaging is not feasible or readily available or there are poor acoustic windows or data discrepancies between noninvasive studies. Multi-gated acquisition nuclear imaging (MUGA) is considered as a third-line modality, but its use is not preferred secondary to the associated radiation exposure [13].

In addition to LVEF, baseline echocardiography can be used to evaluate wall motion score index, right ventricular (RV) function, LV diastolic function, valve disease, and pericardial disease, which may be compromised due to treatment with cardiotoxic therapies [7, 13]. Stress echocardiography can also be used to evaluate patients at risk of CAD from treatment, including those treated with anticancer drugs such as fluorouracil (antimetabolite), bevacizumab (a monoclonal antibody), or sorafenib and sunitinib (multi-targeted tyrosine kinase inhibitors), to name a few. Patients who have received chest radiation are also at high risk for coronary artery disease, which may occur decades after radiation exposure. Stress echocardiography in addition to detecting ischemia can unmask subclinical LV dysfunction and decreased contractile reserve [16].

During cancer therapy, echocardiology is recommended to monitor for CTRCD or other forms of cardiotoxicity, though frequency of screening varies based on the patient, cardiotoxic agent being used, and existing guidelines. For anthracyclines, repeat echocardiography at administration of cardiotoxic doses (250 mg/ml^2 doxorubicin equivalent) is recommended (AHA) [8], with suggested repetition for every 50 mg/ml^2 administered thereafter (ACC) [7]. Guidelines also differ regarding the appropriate frequency of echocardiographic screening for trastuzumab-induced toxicity, with a range from every 3 months (per US Food and Drug Administration recommendations) to more patient-tailored but less specific recommendations [4, 13]. Other cardiotoxic therapies for which echocardiographic screening before, during, and after cancer treatment is suggested are outlined in Table 13.1.

LVEF is a reliable but imperfect indicator of cardiotoxicity [18]. In addition to being subject to vendor and operator variability, it is dependent on LV end-diastolic and end-systolic volumes, which can be impacted by volume depletion or afterload. GLS (myocardial deformation) may be a more sensitive predictor of cardiotoxicity and help distinguish patients with borderline-abnormal LVEF who may be at elevated risk of adverse cardiac outcomes with treatment with cardiotoxic therapies [18, 19]. There is evidence in breast cancer patients that LV strain measurements decline prior to subsequent decreases in LVEF [20]. Strain may be measured with Doppler tissue imaging or 2D speckle-tracking echocardiography (STE), with 2D STE preferred because of the lack of angle dependency [16]. The use of the same vendor and (ideally) the same observer for serial strain imaging is highly recommended due to inter-vendor and inter-observer variability [21].

For cancer survivors, echocardiographic screening is a cornerstone of cardiac surveillance. The same parameters as described above are relevant to serial testing, with the frequency of testing dependent on the risk level, cardiotoxic agents used during treatment, and symptoms of the patient [16]. For serial LVEF and especially GLS testing, the use of the same software is recommended due to inter-vendor variability [18]. For GLS analysis, a decrease of >15% from baseline has been suggested as abnormal, but research is ongoing [8, 13, 16]. The SUCCOUR trial, an international randomized controlled trial designed to assess differences between GLS- and LVEF-guided therapies in patients being monitored for anthracycline cardiotoxicity, did not find added benefit of utilizing GLS-guided interventions [22]; however, the study's clinical endpoint (change in LVEF) may not represent the longer-term impact of GLS-guided therapy as explicitly as rarer but more significant endpoints, such as incident HF [23, 24]. Furthermore, it is possible that the association between early reductions in GLS and subsequent CTRCD is also impacted by compensatory changes in global circumferential strain, wall thickness, or LV diameter [25, 26].

Cardiac Magnetic Resonance Imaging

Since its early use in the 1980s, magnetic resonance imaging for the cardiovascular system has been an important tool for examining LV and RV anatomy and function, as well as for identifying myocardial ischemia with nuclear imaging [16]. More recently, CMR has been integrated into cardio-oncology research and practice, especially in cases where results of echocardiographic study are inconclusive or require further investigation. There is, however, still limited availability and a higher cost of CMR compared to echocardiography. CMR is now best used to perform quantitative assessment of LVEF and considered the gold standard for noninvasive LVEF assessment. Thus, CMR can complement echocardiography in its surveillance roles before, during, and after treatment. It may be especially important in serial follow-up of new anticancer agents, where repeated measures of LV or RV chamber dimensions is needed to determine small incremental changes, or for assessment of myocarditis.

Complementary Functions to Echocardiography

The advantages of CMR for anatomical study include its ability to visualize and delineate a wide range of cardiovascular tissue and functional characteristics, which may refine baseline cardiovascular risk assessment and cardiotoxicity surveillance during and after treatment. CMR offers superior definition between endocardial and epicardial borders, a wide variability in scanning views, high spatial resolution, and reliance on fewer geometric assumptions than those required for echocardiographic calculation of chamber volumes. Moreover, like echocardiography, CMR is noninvasive and requires no radiation exposure. However, the modality is not widely accessible, requires a high level of technical expertise, is of much higher cost, and requires longer scanning time for the patient, which has contributed to its limited use [27].

CMR, however, is the reference standard for the determination of LV volumes and LVEF through steady-state free precession (SSFP) cine sequences due to its high resolution, accuracy, and reproducibility. CMR has been shown to identify LVEF below 50% with more accuracy than both 3D and 2D echocardiography, which may make it a preferred technique for LVEF measurement in patients with confirmed or suspected CTRCD. This may be useful at any point of the treatment timeline, but especially in the context of determining whether to discontinue anthracycline or other cancer therapies [16, 28, 29]. Furthermore, for research studies of new agents that require repeated measures of LVEF, CMR provides less variability of the LVEF measurement that may be key in determining effects of new agents utilizing a smaller sample size. CMR complements echocardiography in other applications as well, such as evaluation of diastolic dysfunction (discussed in the next section).

Lastly, radiation-induced cardiac injury can cause calcification of valve leaflets and/or structure, with CMR studies of individuals over 20 years post-radiotherapy (median dose 40 Cy) finding valve disease in 42% of patients [30]. Though valve function is best analyzed on echocardiography, CMR provides additional details that may be clinically useful especially prior to surgery or percutaneous intervention. CMR helps quantify the severity of valvular disease by providing information on valve size and area, transvalvular gradients, and regurgitant volumes/fractions.

Tissue Characterization: Restrictive Cardiomyopathy and Myocarditis

Tissue characterization with CMR is especially important in the care of patients treated with ionizing radiation. Ionizing thoracic radiation is predominantly associated with restrictive cardiomyopathy with diastolic dysfunction, often due to myocardial stiffening from fibrotic tissue. Radiation-induced fibrosis may increase the risk of CAD, cardiomyopathy, valvular heart disease, arrhythmias, and pericardial disease up to decades post-treatment [31]. Gadolinium typically accumulates in areas of fibrosis and appears brightly on T1-weighted sequences, making CMR imaging with late gadolinium enhancement (LGE) useful in the assessment of patients with a history of radiation [29]. Newer tissue characterization methods, including T1 mapping and extracellular volume (ECV) fraction estimation, can be used as surrogate markers of myocardial fibrosis and have been linked to HF risk, though applications to clinical care have remained limited.

During and after cancer treatment, CMR allows for noninvasive distinction between causes of restrictive cardiomyopathy, such as amyloidosis or radiation-induced myocardial replacement fibrosis [29]. Pericardial disease in some form (including asymptomatic pericardial calcifications, effusions, and acute or chronic constrictive pericarditis leading to progressive HF) is prevalent years after radiation and can also occur as a side effect of chemotherapy or with graft-versus-host disease post-stem cell transplantation [32]. Tissue characterization can help determine the extent of inflammation and degree of abnormal pericardial thickening, and functional assessments of ventricular filling can help clarify the hemodynamic impact of pericardial disease.

A growing application of CMR tissue characterization techniques in the cardio-oncology setting is for the diagnosis of myocarditis, which can occur acutely during cancer treatment. Immune checkpoint inhibitors (ICIs), a novel class of anticancer agents, trigger immunological responses that have been shown to be highly effective in targeting a wide and ever-expanding range of aggressive cancers (including metastatic skin, lung, and gastrointestinal cancers, lymphomas, and others) [33, 34]. However, ICIs can also result in an undesired attack on the myocardium, usually within 1–3 months of initiating the therapy [35]. ICI myocarditis is rare (~1% incidence) and can have diverse clinical manifestation, from subclinical myocarditis with no, mild, or nonspecific symptoms, such as fatigue, to fulminant HF with cardiogenic shock, which carries significant associated mortality [33]. Risk factors are still being studied but may involve an underlying autoimmune disease [36].

Because of the wide variability in associated symptoms, ICI-myocarditis can be difficult to diagnose. Normal ECG/serum troponin levels do not exclude ICI-myocarditis, nor do abnormal findings exclude other diagnoses such as coronary ischemia. In patients suspected of myocarditis, CMR is the gold-standard noninvasive diagnostic test. LGE with CMR has been found in up to ~75% of ICI-myocarditis patients, despite most patients in some case series having normal or borderline LVEF [29, 35]. The 2018 Louis Lake criteria for CMR-based diagnosis recommend the use of at least one T1-based criterion (increased myocardial T1 relaxation times, ECV, or LGE) with at least one T2-based criterion (increased myocardial T2 relaxation times, visible myocardial edema, or increased T2 signal intensity ratio) [37].

Finally, CMR can quantitate the extent of myocardial infarction and related results of vascular obstruction (discussed in the next section). Stress perfusion aids in the assessment of CAD, where perfusion defects are observed in ischemic myocardium. While CMR can aid in CAD assessment, cardiac computed tomography and coronary angiography can provide a more rapid, targeted assessment of coronary artery stenosis.

Cardiac Computed Tomography

Cardiac computed tomography (CCT), discussed in the introduction to this chapter, plays an essential role in radiation therapy planning: it helps distinguish between different tissue types, improves targeted radiation, and helps spare healthy tissue and organs (i.e., heart and lungs) from radiation exposure through techniques such as DIBH. This section discusses the role of CCT in cardio-oncology from a diagnostic and risk assessment perspective across the timeline of cancer treatment. In particular, we describe the utility of CCT in evaluating coronary artery disease, delineating coronary arteries and representing chamber volumes and cardiovascular anatomy, and in providing functional data, all of which may be important before, during, and after cancer treatment.

Coronary Artery Disease in Cancer Patients

Radiation-induced CAD (RICAD) is highly prevalent among long-term cancer survivors treated with radiation to the chest. It has been shown to be the most common cardiovascular effect in HL survivors 40 years after treatment, with a 3.2-fold increase in standardized incidence ratio of CAD compared to the general population. CAD as a first event was found to have a cumulative incidence of one in five among patients 60 years or older who were treated for HL before age 25 [38]. Furthermore, breast cancer survivors treated with radiation have been shown to have a 7.4% increase in major coronary events (myocardial infarction, coronary revascularization, or death from ischemic heart disease) per gray, beginning 5 years post-radiation and into the third decade beyond, with no apparent plateau [39]. The 10-year cumulative incidence of hospitalization for CAD among breast cancer survivors was over 3% [40]. Diagnostic work-up for CAD may also be required for patients receiving tyrosine kinase inhibitors such as nilotinib and ponatinib, 5-fluorouracil, or other agents promoting atherosclerosis, vasospasm, or vascular toxicities that may present with angina.

CCT is essential to the quantification of coronary calcification and noninvasive assessment of CAD, as well as determination of hemodynamic significance of coronary lesions. Automated quantitative coronary artery calcium scoring (CAC) with CCT imaging is a quick, noninvasive, and cost-effective technique for quantifying CVD risk in patients, especially prior to cancer treatment. Higher pretreatment CAC scores have been associated with increased rates of adverse cardiac outcomes in patients with breast and lung cancer, diffuse large B-cell lymphoma, and others [41, 42]. Since non-electrocardiographic-gated chest CT imaging is routinely used for cancer staging, treatment planning, and surveillance, baseline CAC assessment is possible for many cancers and is suggested for all cancer patients prior to treatment by a 2022 expert consensus document from the Society of Cardiovascular Computed Tomography [43]. Serial monitoring for subclinical ASCVD may be indicated (both non-ECG-gated and ECG-gated scores can be used, as they provide similar results) [44].

CAC scores can inform clinical decision-making (i.e., statin therapy with lifestyle modification in those with CAC > 100) or perhaps factor in the choice of antineoplastic agents in high-risk patients with high CAC scores, with the understanding that all cardiac therapies support the primary goal of optimally tolerated treatment directed at the cancer [45]. The association of CAC scoring and CV outcomes has been demonstrated in breast cancer survivors, but the prognostic power and ideal screening frequency for CAC remain undetermined [45, 46].

CCT Angiography

CCT angiography (CCTA) provides noninvasive anatomical information on coronary stenosis and obstruction. It is a widely accessible, noninvasive alternative to coronary angiography, especially in patients with a high risk of bleeding and in cardio-oncology in general, where certain subsets of patients are at high risk for CAD. CCTA offers excellent negative predictive value (NPV) in the exclusion of obstructive CAD and can be used as a screening test for high-risk cancer survivors who have many other comorbidities. The results of CCTA spare many patients from the need for invasive cardiac catheterization. It should be noted that the positive predictive value (PPV) of CCTA, or sensitivity of diagnosing coronary lesions, is lower: 48% PPV vs. 99% NPV for ≥70% stenosis in the prospective, multicenter ACCURACY trial [47]. Therefore, if there is a strong clinical suspicion of CAD, either before or after the CCTA, cardiac catheterization may need to be performed not only for diagnosis but also for management (i.e., stent placement).

In recent years, CCTA-derived fractional flow reserve (FFR_{CT}) has emerged as an important tool for noninvasively investigating the functional impact of coronary lesions, thereby helping inform recommendations for either percutaneous or surgical revascularization. FFR_{CT} may help reduce the number of unnecessary revascularization procedures by providing additional information on the hemodynamic significance of observed anatomical stenoses (FFR_{CT} > ~0.80 considered "normal" and ≤0.75 or 0.80 indicating a high likelihood of hemodynamic significance) [48]. Symptomatic patients with intermediate anatomic stenosis (30–70%) with FFR_{CT} values >0.80 have been shown to have comparable prognoses to those with lesions <30% when invasive angiography is deferred.

Other CCT Applications in Patients with Radiation History

Many long-term HL survivors treated with mediastinal radiation develop valvular stenosis involving the left-sided valves (either the mitral valve or more commonly the aortic valve). Patients with significant aortic stenosis may eventually require either percutaneous or surgical valve replacement (TAVR or SAVR). CCT can quantify the valve area, valve leaflet dimensions, and 3D valvular structure/substructure and is used as an important part of pre-planning and device sizing prior to percutaneous or surgical valve interventions, such as TAVR or SAVR. Cardiac CT planning has improved the outcomes of these procedures [49].

CCT is also the modality of choice to assess the pericardium for thickness and calcification in patients with constrictive pericarditis, which can result from prior chest radiation.

PET/SPECT

Nuclear imaging techniques, which include SPECT and PET, have well-established roles in cardiology. In cancer patients and survivors, SPECT- and PET-based myocardial perfusion imaging (MPI) allows for the noninvasive diagnosis and evaluation of myocardial ischemia and myocardial infarction through LV tracer uptake; however, these techniques require radiation exposure.

SPECT-based perfusion imaging has been observed to be predictive of major adverse cardiac events when combined with anatomic imaging [50]. SPECT techniques that reduce radiation exposure, such as high-resolution cadmium-zinc telluride detectors and stress-first protocols, may be especially relevant for cardio-oncology patients [8]. SPECT imaging with 99m-technetium-pyrophosphate has also improved diagnosis and initiation of treatment for cardiac transthyretin amyloidosis.

While SPECT is historically the most widely used technique in cardiac nuclear imaging, due to the availability of SPECT cameras and relatively lower cost, quantitative myocardial perfusion with PET is becoming more prevalent. Advantages of PET include its higher diagnostic accuracy, bolstered by accurate attenuation correction, lower associated radiation dose than for SPECT, and shorter exam time for CAD assessment [51]. PET imaging allows for quantification of myocardial blood flow (MBF) and myocardial flow reserve (MFR), a ratio of MBF at maximum stress to rest, which has been shown to predict adverse outcomes. (Ongoing research is exploring the feasibility of estimating MBF and MRF from standard SPECT MPI scans.) [52] These parameters can aid in risk stratification of patients with CAD and guide decisions regarding performance and timing of revascularization. Importantly, these quantitative indices also play a role in diagnosing microvascular disease in the absence of obstructive epicardiac CAD, which can be particularly relevant to cardio-oncology patients [53, 54].

Microvascular damage and vascular toxicity is increasingly appreciated as a mechanism of cardiotoxicity related to treatment with antimetabolites, anti-microtubule agents, alkylating agents, and radiation and especially newer targeted therapies such as vascular endothelial growth factor (VEGF) inhibitors and tyrosine kinase inhibitors [55]. Targeting VEGF, an essential growth and survival factor for endothelial cells, is well documented to cause hypertension and may lead to adverse vascular events including aortic dissection, stroke, and arterial and venous thrombosis. The risk of HF in patients on VEGF inhibitors has been shown to be highest among those with preexisting CAD. Thus, perfusion imaging techniques may play an important role in evaluating at-risk patients before, during, and after treatment [56].

Finally, there are promising applications of quantitative radiology techniques in developing new biomarkers for cardiotoxicity. Fluorodeoxyglucose labeled with fluorine-18 PET associated with CT (^{18}F-FDG PET/CT) is a widely used technique in oncology to diagnose, stage, and monitor tumors in cancer patients because the ^{18}F-FDG tracer reflects levels of cellular metabolism. Notably, cardiomyocytes exposed to anthracyclines may also increase metabolic activity in the context of the proinflammatory, oxidative environment induced by anthracyclines, thereby justifying uptake of ^{18}F-FDG as an early biomarker of anthracycline-induced cardiotoxicity [57, 58]. A study of HL patients found correlations between increased ^{18}F-FDG uptake in the LV and decreased LVEF post-chemotherapy, even though differences between pre- and post-chemotherapy LVEF were not significant [59]. Similarly, in breast cancer patients, both LV and RV uptake of ^{18}F-FDG were found to correlate with cardiotoxicity development [60].

ICI treatment has also been associated with increased ^{18}F-FDG uptake, but its utility in risk stratification and quantification of atherosclerotic inflammatory activity remains unconfirmed. Somatosensin receptors are highly expressed in inflammatory cells, and primitive findings suggest that somatosensin receptor-based PET/CT (^{68}Ga-DOTATOC PET/CT) could aid in diagnosis of ICI-induced myocarditis in patients who do not have evident myocardial damage on CMR [61]. Dozens of other tracers associated with inflammation, sympathetic innervation, metabolism, and fibrosis have been proposed to have diagnostic or prognostic utility in cardio-oncology [62]. Though these findings cannot yet be clinically applied, the finding that metabolic biomarkers of cardiotoxicity change prior to physiological alterations represents an exciting area for further research and highlights the integral role that radiopharmaceutical and radiological techniques may play in cardiotoxicity assessment as the cardio-oncology field continues to evolve.

Imaging in Special Populations

Female Cancer Patients

Cardiotoxicity is highly salient to the care of female cancer patients and survivors. Risk of anthracycline-induced cardiotoxicity is higher in female cancer patients compared to males, and many breast cancer treatments are also cardiotoxic. Recently, the need for a sex- and gender-informed approach to cardio-oncology has been described [63, 64]. Biological changes at critical life stages, including menarche, pregnancy, and menopause, put female cancer patients and survivors at a unique risk of cardiovascular disease, necessitating a lifespan-based approach to cardio-oncology care [63]. Here, we discuss relevant imaging considerations in female survivors of breast cancer and in pregnant patients with a history or current diagnosis of cancer.

Breast Cancer

One in eight women will be diagnosed with breast cancer in her lifetime, making it the most common cancer among women and in the general population. The opening to this chapter described how the deep inspiration breath hold technique can be used in CT planning scans and during radiotherapy to reduce radiation dose to the left heart. Of note, left-sided breast cancer is more prevalent than right-sided cancer, putting women at additional risk of receiving left heart radiation [65]. Direct associations between radiation dose and risk of major coronary events in breast cancer survivors have been elucidated. Here, we describe opportunities to improve CVD surveillance and prevention in breast cancer survivors.

Reconstructive surgery is common after breast cancer treated with full or partial mastectomy. With laws mandating insurance coverage of mastectomy-related procedures, the prevalence of breast reconstruction is growing [66]. However, tissue expanders and breast implants can compromise cardiothoracic image quality. In a small retrospective study of women with silicone expanders and implants, one half of the study group was deemed to have had studies with inadequate echocardiographic image quality [67]. This often occurs due to poor acoustic windows, shadows, and artifacts obstructing views of the chambers and valves. Image quality enhancement is a key tool in mitigating these challenges, but optimal strategies have yet to be determined [68]. Subcostal view-based longitudinal strain may be a reliable alternative to apical view-based longitudinal strain in patients who have undergone post-reconstructive surgery, though this approach requires further study.

Beyond difficulties in echocardiographic imaging, attenuation artifacts can challenge SPECT imaging in women with silicone- or saline-containing implants [69]. Furthermore, CMR may not be indicated for patients with soft tissue expanders due to their associated magnetic ports [68].

A cross-disciplinary effort between radiologists, cardiologists, oncologists, reconstructive surgeons, and biomedical engineers is needed to identify the shortcomings of typical imaging strategies for breast cancer patients who have had reconstructive surgery [66]. Failure to perform adequate cardiac imaging in this population can lead to under- or misdiagnosis and poor cardiac outcomes. Thus, radiology modalities that offer better attenuation correction, such as PET, or those that are unaffected by the presence of implants, such as CCTA or CAC assessment, are integral to assessment of cardiovascular and cardiothoracic disease.

Ongoing studies are exploring a demonstrated correlation between CAC and breast arterial calcification (BAC) seen on mammography, which suggest that mammography could aid in cardiovascular risk stratification [70]. Finally, evaluation of CMR in this population is warranted [66]. The CareBest study (Cardiac Magnetic Resonance for Early Detection of Cardiotoxicity in Breast Cancer) is examining the prognostic value of adding a 3-minute cardiac imaging protocol to breast MRI examinations for breast cancer survivors, with the aim of determining whether LV volume and EF, LV strain, native T1, ECV, and T2 values acquired in the mid-LV are prognostic for major cardiac events [71]. Going forward, the utility of CMR for detection of pericardial diseases (common after radiation) or myocarditis (associated with immunotherapies approved for breast cancer treatments) will also improve the cardio-oncology care of breast cancer survivors.

Pregnancy

Cardio-oncological management in pregnant cancer patients and survivors presents unique challenges due to increased risks involved for both parent and fetus. During pregnancy, the heart is subjected to increased hemodynamic stress with increased output and blood redirection to the uterus and placenta; this, combined with generalized vascular dilatation, can increase or unmask cardiovascular dysfunction [72]. While pregnant patients without a cancer history may present with chest pain and shortness of breath during pregnancy, cancer survivors with prior cardiotoxicity related to cancer therapeutics have a high (28%) weighted incidence of LV dysfunction or HF during pregnancy and therefore require especially close cardiovascular surveillance [73].

As in nonpregnant individuals, echocardiography is the first-line cardiovascular imaging modality. In contrast, CMR protocols utilizing gadolinium-based contrast agents should not be performed due to their potential to cross the placenta and the unknown effects on the fetus [74]. During pregnancy, LVEF, RVEF, and pulmonary artery systolic pressures are expected to remain the same, but LA diameter, LV end-diastolic diameter, and LV mass are expected to increase [74].

Exercise or dobutamine stress echocardiography can provide useful evaluations of cardiac reserve, which is especially important to evaluate prior to pregnancy, labor, and delivery [7]. Imaging techniques that include ionizing radiation (i.e., PET/SPECT) are typically avoided due to possible fetal exposure to ionization. However, radiation fields that include the pelvic area are rarely needed in the assessment of cardiovascular conditions, and thus risks of fetal exposure are low for cardiovascular radiography, fluoroscopy, and CT [74, 75]. The American College of Obstetricians and Gynecologists has published guidelines on the use of diagnostic imaging during pregnancy and categorizes chest radiography as a "very low-dose" examination (fetal radiation dose of 0.0005–0.01 mGy) [76].

Childhood Cancer Patients and Survivors

As of 2020, nearly 496,000 cancer survivors in the United States were first diagnosed when they were under the age of 20 years [77]. As in adults, there have been encouraging increases in survival of childhood cancers, necessitating increased attention to the long-term care of this population. Minimizing radiation exposure is a core consideration in this population, given cardiotoxicity's association with younger age at radiation and time elapsed since exposure. Thus, fast acquisition CCTA and PET protocols may be considered for survivors of childhood cancer [8].

Furthermore, techniques that detect subclinical cardiac changes may be useful for long-term surveillance of survivors of childhood cancers. The large St. Jude's cohort of childhood cancer survivors has shown that although only 5.8% of participants have abnormal 3D LVEF (<50%) a median of 23 years post-diagnosis, nearly a third of those with normal 3D LVEF had cardiac dysfunction by GLS (28%) [26, 78]. It has been demonstrated that abnormal GLS is associated with future cardiomyopathy in patients treated with anthracyclines who have normal 3D LVEF [79]. CMR also has utility in pediatric cancer survivors with normal LVEF, with increased ECV, a marker of diffuse fibrosis, associated with anthracycline exposure, markers of adverse ventricular remodeling, and lower VO_2 max. However, the role of CMR in cardiac surveillance for childhood cancer survivors remains relatively unexplored [80].

Early detection of cardiovascular disease in survivors of childhood cancer can improve outcomes, justifying consistent echocardiographic surveillance, in accordance with guideline recommendations [81]. Unfortunately, screening in accordance with these guidelines has been shown to be low, but some outreach interventions have been shown to increase participation [82]. Future research may elucidate optimal strategies for long-term screening in this population.

Under-Resourced Populations in the United States

Modern imaging techniques have revolutionized the quality of cardiovascular care, especially for vulnerable populations such as cancer patients and survivors. However, there remain barriers to accessible and affordable cardio-oncology care and associated imaging components. While cardio-oncology clinics are becoming more widespread, they remain predominantly located in major academic centers in urban areas [7]. More expensive imaging modalities, such as CMR and PET/CT, and diagnostic-quality scanners that produce high-quality images may not be available at under-resourced hospitals, which disproportionately serve vulnerable minority and low-income communities [83]. Furthermore, CMR for early detection of cardiac effects of cancer-related therapies is a non-reimbursed service that can pose a substantial financial burden [84].

Motion artifacts from lower-quality scanners can challenge diagnostic efforts, leading to later or missed diagnoses that directly impact health outcomes. The utility of many of the quantitative measurements discussed previously depends on high-quality imaging: for example, poor echocardiographic imaging can distort strain values, and poor lumen delineation can compromise FFR_{CT} measurement on CCTA. Further, if institutions lack skilled technologists, as may be the case in under-resourced settings, there is also an increased risk of worse health outcomes [85]. In a study of breast cancer mammography, technologist-associated image quality indicators, including positioning, compression, and sharpness, were worse in low-income populations and correlated with later stage at breast cancer diagnosis [86]. The same issues may apply to cardiovascular imaging.

Notably, artificial intelligence (AI) may play a role in augmenting clinician expertise and decreasing health disparities: while many studies of AI in radiology have focused on improving diagnosis, which may be useful in some under-resourced settings, others have proposed using AI to improve equity by translating instructions for patients during imaging examinations, which can improve image quality and therefore patient outcomes [87].

Despite the challenges of integrating multimodality imaging in under-resourced settings, there have been multiple encouraging case studies in recent years. One community hospital, which began its cardio-oncology program through the collaboration of two cardiologists, a nurse practitioner, an oncologist, and a clinical pharmacist, expanded its capacity over time by networking with a larger medical center and optimizing productivity through the work of advanced practice clinicians [88]. Another program, which incorporated elements of both community-based and academic-based programs, received support from professional societies in its growth. It prioritized significant use of multimodality imaging (mostly echocardiography-based) and referral for invasive testing/imaging. Notably, CMR was used in only 4.6% of the cardio-oncology patients at the new clinic, secondary to challenges related to insurance [84].

Ultimately, to increase access to quality cardio-oncology care, buttressed by advanced quantitative cardiovascular imaging, there must be robust collaboration between cardiologists, oncologists, radiologists, and others at the local, state, and national level, especially through engagement with established professional organizations. In turn, these organizations can engage with stakeholders, including governmental representatives, insurers, regulators, and philanthropies, to improve the equity and availability of advanced imaging as part of cardio-oncology care [89]

References

1. Chen MH, Chuang ML, Bornstein BA, Gelman R, Harris JR, Manning WJ. Impact of respiratory maneuvers on cardiac volume within left breast radiation portals. Circulation. 1997;96:3269–72.
2. Bergom C, Currey A, Desai N, Tai A, Strauss JB. Deep inspiration breath hold: techniques and advantages for cardiac sparing during breast cancer irradiation. Front Oncol. 2018;8:87. Published 2018 Apr 4. https://doi.org/10.3389/fonc.2018.00087.
3. Tanguturi SK, Lyatskaya Y, Chen Y, Catalano PJ, Chen MH, Yeo WP, et al. Prospective assessment of deep inspiration breath-hold using 3-dimensional surface tracking for irradiation of left-sided breast cancer. Pract Radiat Oncol. 2015;5(6):358–65. https://doi.org/10.1016/j.prro.2015.06.002.
4. Sturgeon KM, Deng L, Bluethmann SM, Zhou S, Trifiletti DM, Jiang C, et al. A population-based study of cardiovascular disease mortality risk in US cancer patients. Eur Heart J. 2019;40(48):3889–97. https://doi.org/10.1093/eurheartj/ehz766.
5. American Cancer Society. Cancer treatment & survivorship facts & figures 2022–2024. Atlanta: American Cancer Society; 2022.
6. Miller KD, Nogueira L, Devasia T, Mariotto AB, Yabroff KR, Jemal A, Kramer J, Siegel RL. Cancer treatment and survivorship statistics, 2022. CA Cancer J Clin. 2022;72(5):409–36. https://doi.org/10.3322/caac.21731.
7. Baldassarre LA, Ganatra S, Lopez-Mattei J, et al. Advances in multimodality imaging in cardio-oncology: JACC state-of-the-art review. J Am Coll Cardiol. 2022;80(16):1560–78. https://doi.org/10.1016/j.jacc.2022.08.743.
8. Addison D, Neilan TG, Barac A, et al. Cardiovascular imaging in contemporary cardio-oncology: a scientific statement from the American Heart Association. Circulation. 2023;148(16):1271–86. https://doi.org/10.1161/CIR.0000000000001174.
9. Ritchie JL, Singer JW, Thorning D, Sorensen SG, Hamilton GW. Anthracycline cardiotoxicity: clinical and pathologic outcomes assessed by radionuclide ejection fraction. Cancer. 1980;46:1109–16.
10. Seidman A, Hudis C, Pierri MK, Shak S, Paton V, Ashby M, Murphy M, Stewart SJ, Keefe D. Cardiac dysfunction in the trastuzumab clinical trials experience. J Clin Oncol. 2002;20(5):1215–21. https://doi.org/10.1200/JCO.2002.20.5.1215. PMID: 11870163.
11. Herrmann J, Lenihan D, Armenian S, et al. Defining cardiovascular toxicities of cancer therapies: an International Cardio-Oncology Society (IC-OS) consensus statement. Eur Heart J. 2022;43(4):280–99. https://doi.org/10.1093/eurheartj/ehab674.
12. Liu JE, Barac A, Thavendiranathan P, Scherrer-Crosbie M. Strain imaging in cardio-oncology. JACC CardioOncol. 2020;2(5):677–89. https://doi.org/10.1016/j.jaccao.2020.10.011.
13. Lyon AR, López-Fernández T, Couch LS, Asteggiano R, Aznar MC, Bergler-Klein J, Boriani G, Cardinale D, Cordoba R, Cosyns B, Cutter DJ, de Azambuja E, de Boer RA, Dent SF, Farmakis D, Gevaert SA, Gorog DA, Herrmann J, Lenihan D, Moslehi J, Moura B, Salinger SS, Stephens R, Suter TM, Szmit S, Tamargo J, Thavendiranathan P, Tocchetti CG, van der Meer P, van der Pal HJH, ESC Scientific Document Group. 2022 ESC guidelines on cardio-oncology developed in collaboration with the European Hematology Association (EHA), the European Society for Therapeutic Radiology and Oncology (ESTRO) and the International Cardio-Oncology Society (IC-OS). Eur Heart J. 2022;43(41):4229–361. https://doi.org/10.1093/eurheartj/ehac244. Erratum in: Eur Heart J. 2023 May 7;44(18):1621.
14. Armenian SH, Lacchetti C, Barac A, Carver J, Constine LS, Denduluri N, Dent S, Douglas PS, Durand JB, Ewer M, Fabian C, Hudson M, Jessup M, Jones LW, Ky B, Mayer EL, Moslehi J, Oeffinger K, Ray K, Ruddy K, Lenihan D. Prevention and monitoring of cardiac dysfunction in survivors of adult cancers: American Society of Clinical Oncology clinical practice guideline. J Clin Oncol. 2017;35(8):893–911. https://doi.org/10.1200/JCO.2016.70.5400.
15. Dobson R, Ghosh AK, Ky B, Marwick T, Stout M, Harkness A, Steeds R, Robinson S, Oxborough D, Adlam D, Stanway S, Rana B, Ingram T, Ring L, Rosen S, Plummer C, Manisty C, Harbinson M, Sharma V, Pearce K, Lyon AR, Augustine DX, British Society of Echocardiography (BSE) and the British Society of Cardio-Oncology (BCOS). BSE and BCOS guideline for transthoracic echocardiographic assessment of adult cancer patients receiving anthracyclines and/or trastuzumab. JACC CardioOncol. 2021;3(1):1–16. https://doi.org/10.1016/j.jaccao.2021.01.011.
16. Plana JC, Galderisi M, Barac A, Ewer MS, Ky B, Scherrer-Crosbie M, Ganame J, Sebag IA, Agler DA, Badano LP, Banchs J, Cardinale D, Carver J, Cerqueira M, DeCara JM, Edvardsen T, Flamm SD, Force T, Griffin BP, Jerusalem G, Liu JE, Magalhães A, Marwick T, Sanchez LY, Sicari R, Villarraga HR, Lancellotti P. Expert consensus for multimodality imaging evaluation of adult patients during and after cancer therapy: a report from the American Society of Echocardiography and the European Association of Cardiovascular Imaging. J Am Soc Echocardiogr. 2014;27(9):911–39. https://doi.org/10.1016/j.echo.2014.07.012.
17. Curigliano G, Lenihan D, Fradley M, Ganatra S, Barac A, Blaes A, Herrmann J, Porter C, Lyon AR, Lancellotti P, Patel A, DeCara J, Mitchell J, Harrison E, Moslehi J, Witteles R, Calabro MG, Orecchia R, de Azambuja E, Zamorano JL, Krone R, Iakobishvili Z, Carver J, Armenian S, Ky B, Cardinale D, Cipolla CM, Dent S, Jordan K, ESMO Guidelines Committee. Management of cardiac disease in cancer patients throughout oncological treatment: ESMO consensus recommendations. Ann Oncol. 2020;31(2):171–90. https://doi.org/10.1016/j.annonc.2019.10.023.

18. Lorenzini C, Lamberti C, Aquilina M, Rocca A, Cortesi P, Corsi C. Reliability of left ventricular ejection fraction from three-dimensional echocardiography for cardiotoxicity onset detection in patients with breast cancer. J Am Soc Echocardiogr. 2017;30(11):1103–10. https://doi.org/10.1016/j.echo.2017.06.025. Epub 2017 Aug 16. PMID: 28822666.
19. Mousavi N, Tan TC, Ali M, Halpern EF, Wang L, Scherrer-Crosbie M. Echocardiographic parameters of left ventricular size and function as predictors of symptomatic heart failure in patients with a left ventricular ejection fraction of 50–59% treated with anthracyclines. Eur Heart J Cardiovasc Imaging. 2015;16(9):977–84. https://doi.org/10.1093/ehjci/jev113. Epub 2015 Apr 29. PMID: 25925220.
20. Sawaya H, Sebag IA, Plana JC, et al. Assessment of echocardiography and biomarkers for the extended prediction of cardiotoxicity in patients treated with anthracyclines, taxanes, and trastuzumab. Circ Cardiovasc Imaging. 2012;5(5):596–603. https://doi.org/10.1161/CIRCIMAGING.112.973321.
21. Galderisi M, Cosyns B, Edvardsen T, Cardim N, Delgado V, Di Salvo G, et al. Standardization of adult transthoracic echocardiography reporting in agreement with recent chamber quantification, diastolic function, and heart valve disease recommendations: an expert consensus document of the European Association of Cardiovascular Imaging. Eur Heart J Cardiovasc Imaging. 2017;18:1301–10.
22. Negishi T, Thavendiranathan P, Penicka M, Lemieux J, Murbraech K, Miyazaki S, Shirazi M, Santoro C, Cho GY, Popescu BA, Kosmala W, Costello B, la Gerche A, Mottram P, Thomas L, Seldrum S, Hristova K, Bansal M, Kurosawa K, Fukuda N, Yamada H, Izumo M, Tajiri K, Sinski M, Vinereanu D, Shkolnik E, Banchs J, Kutty S, Negishi K, Marwick TH. Cardioprotection using strain-guided management of potentially cardiotoxic cancer therapy: 3-year results of the SUCCOUR trial. JACC Cardiovasc Imaging. 2023;16(3):269–78. https://doi.org/10.1016/j.jcmg.2022.10.010. Epub 2022 Nov 16. PMID: 36435732.
23. Negishi T, Thavendiranathan P, Negishi K, Marwick TH, SUCCOUR Investigators. Rationale and design of the strain surveillance of chemotherapy for improving cardiovascular outcomes: the SUCCOUR trial. JACC Cardiovasc Imaging. 2018;11(8):1098–105. https://doi.org/10.1016/j.jcmg.2018.03.019. Epub 2018 Jun 13. PMID: 29909105.
24. Lopez-Mattei JC, Hassan S. The SUCCOUR trial: a cardiovascular imager's perspective. American College of Cardiology; 2021. https://www.acc.org/Latest-in-Cardiology/Articles/2021/04/16/13/09/The-SUCCOUR-Trial. Accessed 23 Jan 2024.
25. Narayan HK, French B, Khan AM, Plappert T, Hyman D, Bajulaiye A, et al. Noninvasive measures of ventricular–arterial coupling and circumferential strain predict cancer therapeutics–related cardiac dysfunction. JACC Cardiovasc Imaging. 2016;9:1131–41.
26. Plana JC, Thavendiranathan P, Bucciarelli-Ducci C, Lancellotti P. Multi-modality imaging in the assessment of cardiovascular toxicity in the cancer patient. JACC Cardiovasc Imaging. 2018;11(8):1173–86. https://doi.org/10.1016/j.jcmg.2018.06.003. Erratum in: JACC Cardiovasc Imaging 2019 Jan;12(1):224. PMID: 30092972.
27. Christodoulou AG, Cruz G, Arami A, Weingärtner S, Artico J, Peters D, Seiberlich N. The future of CMR: all-in-one vs. real-time CMR (part 1). J Cardiovasc Magn Reson. 2024;26(1):100997. https://doi.org/10.1016/j.jocmr.2024.100997.
28. Armstrong AC, Gidding S, Gjesdal O, Wu C, Bluemke DA, Lima JA. LV mass assessed by echocardiography and CMR, cardiovascular outcomes, and medical practice. JACC Cardiovasc Imaging. 2012;5:837–48.
29. Harries I, Liang K, Williams M, Berlot B, Biglino G, Lancellotti P, Plana JC, Bucciarelli-Ducci C. Magnetic resonance imaging to detect cardiovascular effects of cancer therapy: *JACC CardioOncology* state-of-the-art review. JACC CardioOncol. 2020;2(2):270–92. https://doi.org/10.1016/j.jaccao.2020.04.011.
30. Machann W, Beer M, Breunig M, et al. Cardiac magnetic resonance findings in 20-year survivors of mediastinal radiotherapy for Hodgkin's disease. Int J Radiat Oncol Biol Phys. 2011;79:1117–23.
31. Mrotzek SM, Rassaf T, Totzeck M. Cardiovascular damage associated with chest irradiation. Front Cardiovasc Med. 2020;7:41. Published 2020 Mar 20. https://doi.org/10.3389/fcvm.2020.00041.
32. Belzile-Dugas E, Eisenberg MJ. Radiation-induced cardiovascular disease: review of an underrecognized pathology. J Am Heart Assoc. 2021;10(18):e021686. https://doi.org/10.1161/JAHA.121.021686. Epub 2021 Sep 6. Erratum in: J Am Heart Assoc. 2023 May 16;12(10):e027687.
33. Tan S, Day D, Nicholls SJ, Segelov E. Immune checkpoint inhibitor therapy in oncology: current uses and future directions: *JACC: CardioOncology* state-of-the-art review. JACC CardioOncol. 2022;4(5):579–97. Published 2022 Dec 20. https://doi.org/10.1016/j.jaccao.2022.09.004.
34. Arcari L, Tini G, Camastra G, et al. Cardiac magnetic resonance imaging in immune check-point inhibitor myocarditis: a systematic review. J Imaging. 2022;8(4):99. Published 2022 Apr 5. https://doi.org/10.3390/jimaging8040099.
35. Mahmood SS, Fradley MG, Cohen JV, et al. Myocarditis in patients treated with immune checkpoint inhibitors. J Am Coll Cardiol. 2018;71(16):1755–64. https://doi.org/10.1016/j.jacc.2018.02.037.
36. Ganatra S, Neilan TG. Immune checkpoint inhibitor-associated myocarditis. Oncologist. 2018;23(8):879–86. https://doi.org/10.1634/theoncologist.2018-0130.
37. Ferreira VM, Schulz-Menger J, Holmvang G, et al. Cardiovascular magnetic resonance in nonischemic myocardial inflammation: expert recommendations. J Am Coll Cardiol. 2018;72(24):3158–76.

38. van Nimwegen FA, Schaapveld M, Janus CP, Krol AD, Petersen EJ, Raemaekers JM, Kok WE, Aleman BM, van Leeuwen FE. Cardiovascular disease after Hodgkin lymphoma treatment: 40-year disease risk. JAMA Intern Med. 2015;175(6):1007–17. https://doi.org/10.1001/jamainternmed.2015.1180. PMID: 25915855.
39. Darby SC, Ewertz M, McGale P, Bennet AM, Blom-Goldman U, Brønnum D, Correa C, Cutter D, Gagliardi G, Gigante B, Jensen MB, Nisbet A, Peto R, Rahimi K, Taylor C, Hall P. Risk of ischemic heart disease in women after radiotherapy for breast cancer. N Engl J Med. 2013;368(11):987–98. https://doi.org/10.1056/NEJMoa1209825. PMID: 23484825.
40. Abdel-Qadir H, Tai F, Croxford R, et al. Characteristics and outcomes of women developing heart failure after early stage breast cancer chemotherapy: a population-based matched cohort study. Circ Heart Fail. 2021;14(7):e008110. https://doi.org/10.1161/CIRCHEARTFAILURE.120.008110.
41. Gal R, van Velzen SGM, Hooning MJ, et al. Identification of risk of cardiovascular disease by automatic quantification of coronary artery calcifications on radiotherapy planning CT scans in patients with breast cancer. JAMA Oncol. 2021;7(7):1024–32. https://doi.org/10.1001/jamaoncol.2021.1144.
42. Shen H, Lian Y, Yin J, Zhu M, Yang C, Tu C, Peng Y, Li X, Zhang J. Cardiovascular risk stratification by automatic coronary artery calcium scoring on pretreatment chest computed tomography in diffuse large B-cell lymphoma receiving anthracycline-based chemotherapy: a multicenter study. Circ Cardiovasc Imaging. 2023;16(2):e014829. https://doi.org/10.1161/CIRCIMAGING.122.014829. Epub 2023 Feb 7. PMID: 36748459.
43. Lopez-Mattei J, Yang EH, Baldassarre LA, Agha A, Blankstein R, Choi AD, Chen MY, Meyersohn N, Daly R, Slim A, Rochitte C, Blaha M, Whelton S, Dzaye O, Dent S, Milgrom S, Ky B, Iliescu C, Mamas MA, Ferencik M. Cardiac computed tomographic imaging in cardio-oncology: an expert consensus document of the Society of Cardiovascular Computed Tomography (SCCT). Endorsed by the International Cardio-Oncology Society (ICOS). J Cardiovasc Comput Tomogr. 2023;17(1):66–83. https://doi.org/10.1016/j.jcct.2022.09.002. Epub 2022 Sep 15. PMID: 36216699.
44. Marrero N, Blumenthal RS, Patel J, Whelton SP, American College of Cardiology. Integrating CAC scores into risk stratification of patients undergoing cancer treatment. 2023. Available from: https://www.acc.org/Latest-in-Cardiology/Articles/2023/09/12/10/38/Integrating-CAC-Scores-Into-Risk-Stratification-of-Patients-Undergoing-Cancer-Treatment.
45. Velusamy R, Nolan M, Murphy A, Thavendiranathan P, Marwick TH. Screening for coronary artery disease in cancer survivors. JACC CardioOncol. 2023;5(1):22–38. Available from: https://doi.org/10.1016/j.jaccao.2022.12.007.
46. Puckett LL, Saba SG, Henry S, Rosen S, Rooney E, Filosa SL, Gilbo P, Pappas K, Laxer A, Eacobacci K, Kapyur AN, Robeny J, Musial S, Chaudhry A, Chaudhry R, Lesser ML, Riegel A, Ramoutarpersaud S, Rahmani N, Shah A, Papas V, Dawodu T, Charlton J, Knisely JPS, Lee L. Cardiotoxicity screening of long-term, breast cancer survivors-The CAROLE (Cardiac-Related Oncologic Late Effects) Study. Cancer Med. 2021;10(15):5051–61. https://doi.org/10.1002/cam4.4037. Epub 2021 Jul 10. PMID: 34245128; PMCID: PMC8335805.
47. Budoff MJ, Dowe D, Jollis JG, et al. Diagnostic performance of 64-multidetector row coronary computed tomographic angiography for evaluation of coronary artery stenosis in individuals without known coronary artery disease: results from the prospective multicenter ACCURACY (Assessment by Coronary Computed Tomographic Angiography of Individuals Undergoing Invasive Coronary Angiography) trial. J Am Coll Cardiol. 2008;52:1724–32. https://doi.org/10.1016/j.jacc.2008.07.031.
48. Nørgaard BL, Fairbairn TA, Safian RD, Rabbat MG, Ko B, Jensen JM, Nieman K, Chinnaiyan KM, Sand NP, Matsuo H, Leipsic J, Raff G. Coronary CT angiography-derived fractional flow reserve testing in patients with stable coronary artery disease: recommendations on interpretation and reporting. Radiol Cardiothorac Imaging. 2019;1(5):e190050. https://doi.org/10.1148/ryct.2019190050.
49. Blanke P, Weir-McCall JR, Achenbach S, Delgado V, Hausleiter J, Jilaihawi H, Marwan M, Nørgaard BL, Piazza N, Schoenhagen P, Leipsic JA. Computed tomography imaging in the context of transcatheter aortic valve implantation (TAVI)/transcatheter aortic valve replacement (TAVR): an expert consensus document of the Society of Cardiovascular Computed Tomography. JACC Cardiovasc Imaging. 2019;12(1):1–24. https://doi.org/10.1016/j.jcmg.2018.12.003. PMID: 30621986.
50. Pazhenkottil AP, Benz DC, Gräni C, Madsen MA, Mikulicic F, von Felten E, Fuchs TA, Moch BH, Stehli J, Lüscher TF, Gaemperli O, Buechel RR, Kaufmann PA. Hybrid SPECT perfusion imaging and coronary CT angiography: long-term prognostic value for cardiovascular outcomes. Radiology. 2018;288(3):694–702. https://doi.org/10.1148/radiol.2018171303.
51. Danad I, Raijmakers PG, Driessen RS, et al. Comparison of coronary CT angiography, SPECT, PET, and hybrid imaging for diagnosis of ischemic heart disease determined by fractional flow reserve. JAMA Cardiol. 2017;2(10):1100–7. https://doi.org/10.1001/jamacardio.2017.2471.
52. Wells RG, Bengel FM, Camoni L, Cerudelli E, Cuddy-Walsh SG, Diekmann J, Han L, Kadoya Y, Kawaguchi N, Keng YJF, Miyagawa M, Ratner H, Teng XF, Ruddy TD. Multicenter evaluation of the feasibility of clinical implementation of SPECT myocardial blood flow measurement: intersite variability and imaging time. Circ Cardiovasc Imaging.

2023;16(10):e015009. https://doi.org/10.1161/CIRCIMAGING.122.015009.

53. Nayfeh M, Ahmed AI, Saad JM, Alahdab F, Al-Mallah M. The role of cardiac PET in diagnosis and prognosis of ischemic heart disease: optimal modality across different patient populations. Curr Atheroscler Rep. 2023;25(7):351–7. https://doi.org/10.1007/s11883-023-01107-0.
54. Geltman EM, Henes CG, Senneff MJ, Sobel BE, Bergmann SR. Increased myocardial perfusion at rest and diminished perfusion reserve in patients with angina and angiographically normal coronary arteries. J Am Coll Cardiol. 1990;16(3):586–95. https://doi.org/10.1016/0735-1097(90)90347-r. PMID: 2387931.
55. Campia U, Moslehi JJ, Amiri-Kordestani L, Barac A, Beckman JA, Chism DD, Cohen P, Groarke JD, Herrmann J, Reilly CM, Weintraub NL. Cardio-oncology: vascular and metabolic perspectives: a scientific statement from the American Heart Association. Circulation. 2019;139(13):e579–602. https://doi.org/10.1161/CIR.0000000000000641. Erratum in: Circulation 2019 Apr 9;139(15):e838-e839. PMID: 30786722; PMCID: PMC6530491.
56. Touyz RM, Herrmann J. Cardiotoxicity with vascular endothelial growth factor inhibitor therapy. NPJ Precis Oncologia. 2018;2:13. Published 2018 May 8. https://doi.org/10.1038/s41698-018-0056-z.
57. Becker MMC, Arruda GFA, Berenguer DRF, Buril RO, Cardinale D, Brandão SCS. Anthracycline cardiotoxicity: current methods of diagnosis and possible role of 18F-FDG PET/CT as a new biomarker. Cardiooncology. 2023;9(1):17. https://doi.org/10.1186/s40959-023-00161-6. PMID: 36973762; PMCID: PMC10041777.
58. Bauckneht M, Ferrarazzo G, Fiz F, Morbelli S, Sarocchi M, Pastorino F, Ghidella A, Pomposelli E, Miglino M, Ameri P, Emionite L, Ticconi F, Arboscello E, Buschiazzo A, Massimelli EA, Fiordoro S, Borra A, Cossu V, Bozzano A, Ibatici A, Ponzoni M, Spallarossa P, Gallamini A, Bruzzi P, Sambuceti G, Marini C. Doxorubicin effect on myocardial metabolism as a prerequisite for subsequent development of cardiac toxicity: a translational 18F-FDG PET/CT observation. J Nucl Med. 2017;58(10):1638–45. https://doi.org/10.2967/jnumed.117.191122. Epub 2017 Jun 23. PMID: 28646013.
59. Sarocchi M, Bauckneht M, Arboscello E, et al. An increase in myocardial 18 fluorodeoxyglucose uptake is associated with left ventricular ejection fraction decline in Hodgkin lymphoma patients treated with anthracycline. J Transl Med. 2018;16(1):1–8. https://doi.org/10.1186/s12967-018-1670-9.
60. Kim J, Cho S-G, Kang S-R, et al. Association between FDG uptake in the right ventricular myocardium and cancer therapy-induced cardiotoxicity. J Nucl Cardiol. 2020;27(6):2154–63. https://doi.org/10.1007/s12350-019-01617-y.
61. Boughdad S, Latifyan S, Fenwick C, et al. 68Ga-DOTATOC PET/CT to detect immune checkpoint inhibitor-related myocarditis [published correction appears in J Immunother Cancer. 2022 May;10(5):e003594corr1]. J Immunother Cancer. 2021;9(10):e003594. https://doi.org/10.1136/jitc-2021-003594.
62. Kelly JM, Babich JW. PET tracers for imaging cardiac function in cardio-oncology. Curr Cardiol Rep. 2022;24(3):247–60. https://doi.org/10.1007/s11886-022-01641-4.
63. Chen MH, Epstein SF. Tailored to a woman's heart: gender cardio-oncology across the lifespan. Curr Cardiol Rep. 2023;25(11):1461–74. https://doi.org/10.1007/s11886-023-01967-7. Epub 2023 Oct 11. PMID: 37819431.
64. Canale ML, Bisceglia I, Gallucci G, Russo G, Camerini A, Di Fusco SA, Paccone A, Camilli M, Fiscella D, Lestuzzi C, Turazza FM, Gulizia MM, Pavan D, Maurea N, Gabrielli D, Oliva F, Colivicchi F. Women at heart: introducing gender cardio-oncology. Front Cardiovasc Med. 2022;9:974123. https://doi.org/10.3389/fcvm.2022.974123. PMID: 36505385; PMCID: PMC9726754.
65. Amer MH. Genetic factors and breast cancer laterality. Cancer Manag Res. 2014;16(6):191–203. https://doi.org/10.2147/CMAR.S60006.
66. Oren O, Blankstein R, Bhatt DL. Addressing imaging pitfalls to reduce cardiovascular disease misdiagnosis in patients with breast cancer following reconstruction. JAMA Cardiol. 2022;7(2):123–5. https://doi.org/10.1001/jamacardio.2021.4564. PMID: 34730778.
67. Pignatti M, Mantovani F, Bertelli L, Barbieri A, Pacchioni L, Loschi P, De Santis G. Effects of silicone expanders and implants on echocardiographic image quality after breast reconstruction. Plast Reconstr Surg. 2013;132(2):271–8. https://doi.org/10.1097/PRS.0b013e31829e7bec. PMID: 23897326.
68. Ositelu K, Trevino A, Tong A, Chen MH, Akhter N. Challenges in cardiovascular imaging in women with breast cancer. Curr Cardiol Rep. 2023;25(10):1247–55. https://doi.org/10.1007/s11886-023-01941-3. Epub 2023 Aug 29. PMID: 37642930.
69. Stinis CT, Lizotte PE, Movahed MR. Impaired myocardial SPECT imaging secondary to silicon- and saline-containing breast implants. Int J Cardiovasc Imaging. 2006;22(3-4):449–55. https://doi.org/10.1007/s10554-005-9068-1. Epub 2006 Mar 15. PMID: 16538430.
70. Yoon YE, Kim KM, Han JS, Kang SH, Chun EJ, Ahn S, Kim SM, Choi SI, Yun B, Suh JW. Prediction of subclinical coronary artery disease with breast arterial calcification and low bone mass in asymptomatic women: registry for the women health cohort for the BBC study. JACC Cardiovasc Imaging. 2019;12(7 Pt 1):1202–11. https://doi.org/10.1016/j.jcmg.2018.07.004. Epub 2018 Aug 15. PMID: 30121271.
71. Hong YJ, Kim GM, Han K, Kim PK, Lee SA, An E, Lee JY, Lee HJ, Hur J, Kim YJ, Kim MJ, Choi BW. Cardiotoxicity evaluation using magnetic reso-

nance imaging in breast cancer patients (CareBest): study protocol for a prospective trial. BMC Cardiovasc Disord. 2020;20(1):264. https://doi.org/10.1186/s12872-020-01497-y. PMID: 32493217; PMCID: PMC7268598.
72. Honigberg MC, Sarma AA. Pregnancy among survivors of childhood cancer: cardiovascular considerations. Curr Treat Options Cardiovasc Med. 2018;20(7):54. https://doi.org/10.1007/s11936-018-0650-y. PMID: 29923132.
73. Nolan M, Oikonomou EK, Silversides CK, et al. Impact of cancer therapy-related cardiac dysfunction on risk of heart failure in pregnancy. JACC CardioOncol. 2020;2(2):153–62. Published 2020 Jun 16. https://doi.org/10.1016/j.jaccao.2020.04.007.
74. Bello NA, Bairey Merz CN, Brown H, Davis MB, Dickert NW, El Hajj SC, Giullian C, Quesada O, Park K, Sanghani RM, Shaw L, Volgman AS, Wenger NK, Williams D, Pepine CJ, Lindley KJ, American College of Cardiology Cardiovascular Disease in Women Committee and the Cardio-Obstetrics Work Group. Diagnostic Cardiovascular Imaging and Therapeutic Strategies in Pregnancy: JACC Focus Seminar 4/5. J Am Coll Cardiol. 2021;77(14):1813–22. https://doi.org/10.1016/j.jacc.2021.01.056. PMID: 33832607; PMCID: PMC8221542.
75. Colletti PM, Lee KH, Elkayam U. Cardiovascular imaging of the pregnant patient. AJR Am J Roentgenol. 2013;200(3):515–21. https://doi.org/10.2214/AJR.12.9864. PMID: 23436839.
76. ACOG. ACOG Committee Opinion: Number 723: guidelines for diagnostic imaging during pregnancy and lactation. Obstet Gynecol. 2017;130:e210–6.
77. NCCR. NCCR*Explorer: an interactive website for NCCR cancer statistics [Internet]. National Cancer Institute; 2023 Sept 7. [updated 2023 Sept 8; cited 2024 Feb 19]. Available from: https://nccrexplorer.ccdi.cancer.gov.
78. Armstrong GT, Joshi VM, Ness KK, Marwick TH, Zhang N, Srivastava D, Griffin BP, Grimm RA, Thomas J, Phelan D, Collier P, Krull KR, Mulrooney DA, Green DM, Hudson MM, Robison LL, Plana JC. Comprehensive echocardiographic detection of treatment-related cardiac dysfunction in adult survivors of childhood cancer: results from the St. Jude lifetime cohort study. J Am Coll Cardiol. 2015;65(23):2511–22. https://doi.org/10.1016/j.jacc.2015.04.013. PMID: 26065990; PMCID: PMC4539123.
79. Ehrhardt MJ, Liu Q, Mulrooney DA, Rhea IB, Dixon SB, Lucas JT Jr, Sapkota Y, Shelton K, Ness KK, Srivastava DK, McDonald A, Robison LL, Hudson MM, Yasui Y, Armstrong GT. Improved cardiomyopathy risk prediction using global longitudinal strain and N-terminal-pro-B-type natriuretic peptide in survivors of childhood cancer exposed to cardiotoxic therapy. J Clin Oncol. 2024;42:JCO2301796. https://doi.org/10.1200/JCO.23.01796.
80. Leerink JM, de Baat EC, Feijen EAM, et al. Cardiac disease in childhood cancer survivors: risk prediction, prevention, and surveillance: *JACC CardioOncology* state-of-the-art review. JACC CardioOncol. 2020;2(3):363–78. Published 2020 Sep 15. https://doi.org/10.1016/j.jaccao.2020.08.006.
81. Children's Oncology Group. Long-term follow-up guidelines for survivors of childhood, adolescent, and young adult cancers, version 6.0. Children's Oncology Group; 2023.
82. Zabih V, Kahane A, O'Neill NE, Ivers N, Nathan PC. Interventions to improve adherence to surveillance guidelines in survivors of childhood cancer: a systematic review. J Cancer Surviv. 2019;13:713–29. https://doi.org/10.1007/s11764-019-00790-w.
83. Morgan RL, Karam SD, Bradley CJ. Ethnic disparities in imaging utilization at diagnosis of non-small cell lung cancer. J Natl Cancer Inst. 2020;112(12):1204–12.
84. Sadler D, Chaulagain C, Alvarado B, et al. Practical and cost-effective model to build and sustain a cardio-oncology program. Cardiooncology. 2020;6:9. Published 2020 Jul 16. https://doi.org/10.1186/s40959-020-00063-x.
85. Waite S, Scott J, Colombo D. Narrowing the gap: imaging disparities in radiology. Radiology. 2021;299(1):27–35. https://doi.org/10.1148/radiol.2021203742. Epub 2021 Feb 9. PMID: 33560191.
86. Rauscher GH, Conant EF, Khan JA, Berbaum ML. Mammogram image quality as a potential contributor to disparities in breast cancer stage at diagnosis: an observational study. BMC Cancer. 2013;13(1):208.
87. Davis MA, Lim N, Jordan J, Yee J, Gichoya JW, Lee R. Imaging artificial intelligence: a framework for radiologists to address health equity, from the *AJR* special series on DEI. AJR Am J Roentgenol. 2023;221(3):302–8. https://doi.org/10.2214/AJR.22.28802. Epub 2023 Feb 22. PMID: 37095660.
88. Sundlöf DW, Patel BD, Schadler KC, et al. Development of a cardio-oncology program in a community hospital. JACC CardioOncol. 2019;1(2):310–3. Published 2019 Dec 17. https://doi.org/10.1016/j.jaccao.2019.09.004.
89. Sadler D, Arnold A, Herrmann J, Daniele A, Silva CMPDC, Ghosh AK, Szmit S, Khan RI, Raez L, Blaes A, Brown SA. Reaching across the Aisle: cardio-oncology advocacy and program building. Curr Oncol Rep. 2021;23(6):64. https://doi.org/10.1007/s11912-021-01059-1. PMID: 33855620; PMCID: PMC8045572.

14 Quantitative Imaging of Pericardial and Epicardial Fat

Michail C. Mavrogiannis
and Charalambos Antoniades

Introduction

The pericardium (originating from the Greek περί, "around," and κάρδιον, "heart") is a dual-layered sac that envelops the heart and the roots of the great blood vessels and lies in the anterior mediastinum. Its main functions are to secure the heart within the mediastinum, provide lubrication, and offer protection against infections. In the clinical setting, pericardial diseases can manifest either in isolation or as part of systemic disorders [1, 2]. Assessment of the pericardium and pericardial spaces is of great importance for diagnosing and managing conditions such as acute pericarditis, pericardial effusion, cardiac tamponade, and constrictive pericarditis. In addition, the study of adipose tissue depots adjacent to the pericardium using modern imaging techniques provides unique insights into cardiometabolic disease and metabolically unhealthy obesity [1, 3].

M. C. Mavrogiannis
Radcliffe Department of Medicine, Division of Cardiovascular Medicine, University of Oxford, Oxford, UK
e-mail: Michail.mavrogiannis@wolfson.ox.ac.uk

C. Antoniades (✉)
Acute Multidisciplinary Imaging and Interventional Centre, Radcliffe Department of Medicine, Division of Cardiovascular Medicine, University of Oxford, Oxford, UK
e-mail: Charalambos.antoniades@cardiov.ox.ac.uk

The pericardial sac comprises two main layers: an outer fibrous layer, the parietal pericardium, and an inner double-layered serous sac. The parietal pericardium is attached to the sternum via the superior and inferior sternopericardial ligaments. Inferiorly, it is connected to the central tendon of the diaphragm, while superiorly, it is attached to the tunica adventitia of the great vessels and the pre-tracheal fascia [4]. The fibrous pericardium offers protection against infections as it acts as an anatomical barrier, while also securing the heart within the mediastinum with its pericardial attachments. The inner serous double-layered sac comprises a parietal layer, which is firmly attached to the parietal pericardium and a visceral layer (visceral pericardium), a mesothelial cell layer covering the heart and great vessels. The part of the visceral pericardium that interfaces with the myocardium is also known as the epicardium. Beneath the visceral layer lies a thin layer of dense fibrous connective tissue, often with varying amounts of fatty tissue. Within the two layers of the serosal pericardium lies the pericardial space. Under normal conditions, it contains up to 50 mL of pericardial fluid, which is a plasma ultrafiltrate [5]. The pericardial fluid lubricates the heart's surfaces, minimizing friction during mechanical function. At the heart's base, the reflections of the pericardial sac create extensions of the pericardial cavity called pericardial sinuses, including the transverse sinus located behind the ascending

R. Gill, P. Rajiah (eds.), *Quantitative Imaging in the Thorax*,
https://doi.org/10.1007/978-3-032-14103-3_14

aorta and the oblique sinus situated behind the left atrium (LA), effectively separating the posterior LA wall from the pericardial space.

Adjacent to the pericardium lie two thoracic visceral fat depots, the epicardial adipose tissue (EAT) and the pericardial adipose tissue (PAT). Anatomically, EAT is enclosed between the cardiac surface and the visceral pericardium, while PAT sits externally to the pericardium and surrounding the cardiac silhouette [6, 7] (Fig. 14.1). Within EAT, the perivascular adipose tissue (PVAT) surrounding the coronary arteries is also present. PVAT is defined as the layer of the adipose tissue located in a radial distance from the vascular wall equal to one luminal diameter of the adjacent vessel. This definition applies to the PVAT surrounding vessels up to a luminal diameter of 2 cm. For vessels with a luminal diameter of >2 cm, by convention, PVAT is defined as the adipose tissue within a distance of 2 cm from the outer vessel wall [7]. As visceral fat depots, both EAT and PAT are metabolically active and secrete a number of adipokines, exerting both protective and deleterious effects on the cardiovascular system [3]. In addition, their secretome correlates with systemic metabolic status and insulin resistance with EAT potentially acting as a key regulator of metabolically unhealthy obesity and metabolic syndrome. Indeed, EAT volume correlates with different cardiovascular entities such as coronary artery disease (CAD) and atrial fibrillation (AF) [8]. The biological properties of PVAT are different compared to the rest of the EAT. However, there is a gradual transition between PVAT and non-PVAT within EAT.

The utilization of multiple imaging techniques for the comprehensive diagnostic evaluation of pericardial diseases and the quantification of PAT and EAT as well as the PVAT surrounding the coronary arteries has emerged as an essential approach for contemporary clinical practice and the study of cardiometabolic disorders and metabolically unhealthy obesity [1, 3].

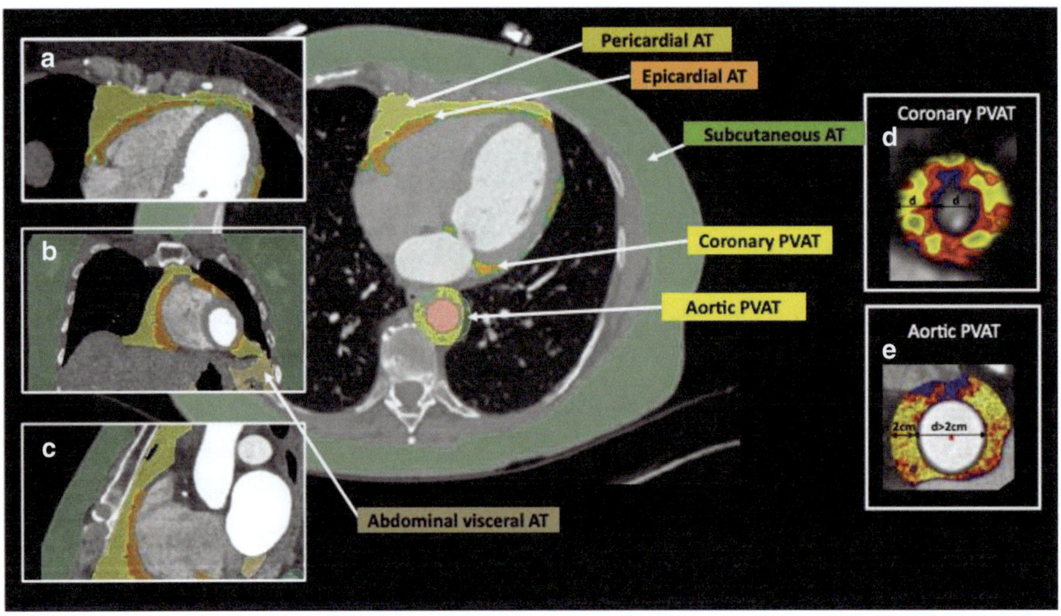

Fig. 14.1 Imaging of human adipose tissue depots by computed tomography. Axial (**a**), coronal (**b**), and sagittal (**c**) views of the chest showing subcutaneous, visceral abdominal, and thoracic (including the pericardial and epicardial) adipose tissues. Reconstruction of the perivascular adipose tissue (PVAT) around an epicardial coronary artery (**d**) and thoracic aorta (**e**). PVAT is defined as the adipose tissue lying within a radial distance from the outer vessel wall equal to the vessel diameter (or at a maximum distance of 2 cm in the case of large vessels with a diameter of >2 cm, like the aorta). (With permissions from Antoniades et al. [7])

Imaging of the Pericardial Space

CMR

Cardiac magnetic resonance (CMR) can only depict the parietal layer of the normal pericardium as the inner visceral layer is not thick enough to be visualized. The appearance of the normal pericardium is that of a thin curvilinear structure aligning with the myocardial contours surrounded by varying amounts of the adipose tissue. It is best visualized along the right ventricular free wall and the cardiac base due to the sparse presence of fat in those areas. Identifying the pericardium along the inferolateral wall is often challenging due to the existence of pulmonary parenchyma.

Measuring the normal pericardium is most effectively done using high-resolution single-slice dark blood T1-weighted spin echo imaging. In these images, the pericardium appears as a thin, low-intensity layer, typically encircled by areas of high-signal fatty tissue in the majority of regions [9, 10]. Cine steady-state free precession (SSFP) imaging sequence generates images with high spatial and temporal resolution. On cine SSFP imaging, the pericardium appears hypointense, while pericardial fluid and fat appear bright with the former slightly more intense than the latter. In addition, pericardial thickness can typically measure up to 3 mm on cine SSFP imaging as opposed to 0.5–1 mm measured on autopsy studies. This discrepancy is attributed to partial volume effects, cardiac motion, inclusion of pericardial fluid, and the presence of chemical shift artifact [11] (Fig. 14.2). CMR also allows the evaluation of structures like the transverse pericardial sinus and the pre-aortic and retro-aortic pericardial recesses. A small quantity of pericardial fluid is typically present in the pericardial space and can be visualized in black blood and cine images. On cine images, it is normal to observe unrestricted movement of the myocardium against the pericardium.

CMR serves as a valuable supplementary diagnostic tool for various pericardial conditions, particularly when echocardiography results are inconclusive, there is suspicion of localized disease, and echocardiographic image quality is less than optimal or when additional underlying issues are suspected [12]. CMR offers insights into the extent of pericardial disease and abnormalities in adjacent structures and enables precise measurements of pericardial and related structures. Moreover, it excels in tissue characterization, providing an assessment of potential inflammation. The examination of pericardial conditions with CMR encompasses morphological imaging to evaluate pericardial structure and conduct tissue characterization, as well as functional imaging to assess ventricular function and intracardiac flows.

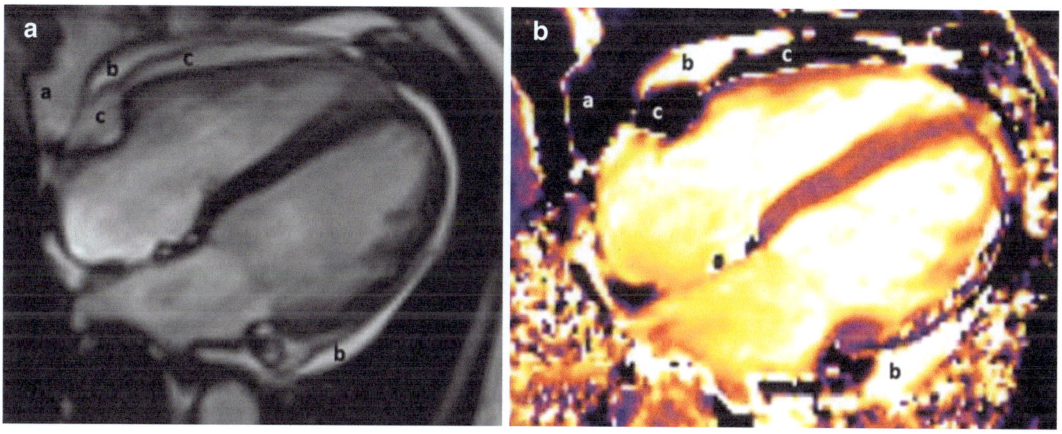

Fig. 14.2 The contribution of native T1 mapping techniques to separate the fat from fluid. Four-chamber view, balanced steady-state free precession (b-SSFP) imaging (**a**) and native T1 mapping technique (**b**). Pericardial fat (**a**), pericardial fluid (**b**), and epicardial fat (**c**). (From Vidalakis et al. [12], licensed under CC-BY 4.0)

The major advantages of CMR include the detailed anatomic description of pericardial space providing useful morphologic and functional information and the evaluation of associated extracardiac disease, safety, and repeatability. In addition, the lack of ionizing radiation is a major strength of CMR. On the other hand, limitations of CMR include overestimation of pericardial thickness resulting from the movement of pericardial layers, insufficient spatial resolution, and chemical artifacts occurring at the adipose tissue-fluid interface on cine CMR. CMR is also time consuming, costs more than most imaging modalities, cannot visualize calcifications, and cannot be used as a bedside examination for critically ill patients. CMR, finally, can be only used in hemodynamically stable patients. Table 14.1 summarizes the strengths and limitations of CMR and computed tomography (CT) for the assessment of pericardial diseases.

CT

Computed tomography (CT) is a widely accessible technique with a rapid acquisition time of just a few seconds. Modern CT scanners offer excellent spatial resolution, typically less than 1.0 mm. They also provide high temporal resolution and specialized imaging methods that synchronize image capture with the patient's electrocardiogram (ECG gated CT) or retrospectively select X-ray data from suitable cardiac cycle segments for image reconstruction, reducing the impact of motion artifacts [14].

While cardiac CT is primarily used to visualize coronary arteries, it also offers detailed imaging of all cardiac structures, including the pericardium. The pericardium can be seen in both non-contrast and contrast-enhanced CT scans. After the administration of intravenous contrast, it is possible to detect enhanced thickening of the pericardium in cases of suspected pericarditis or tumor infiltration [15–17]. However, the CT appearance of the pericardium is similar to that of the myocardium, and, as a result, it is most clearly visible when it is surrounded by fat and not immediately adjacent to the myocardium (Fig. 14.3). It typically appears as a thin line, most prominently on the front surface of the heart. The absence of visualizing the pericardium on CT, especially on the posterior heart surface, does not necessarily indicate a complete absence of the pericardium. Moreover, CT scans exhibit a high sensitivity for detecting pericardial calcification.

When evaluating pericardial thickness, it is essential to ensure that measurements are taken in planes providing a perfectly orthogonal view of the pericardium. On high-resolution CT scans, the typical pericardial thickness falls within the range of 1–2 mm. The upper limit of normal for the thinnest part of the pericardium is 0.7 mm in thin-slice CT and 1.2 mm in thick-slice CT [18]. In high-resolution CT, the upper limit of normal for the thickest section is 2 mm [15, 17]. However, it is worth noting that thicknesses of up to 4 mm have also been reported as within the normal range [19]. The most challenging aspect of assessing pericardial thickening lies in the fact that, due to overlapping CT attenuation values, it can be difficult to differentiate a slightly thickened pericardium from small accumulations of pericardial fluid.

Table 14.1 Strengths and limitations of CMR and CCTA for the assessment of pericardial diseases and conditions

	CMR	CCTA
Pericardial thickness	+++	+++
Constriction	+++	++
Effusion	+++	+++
Inflammation	+++	+/–
Tissue/fluid characterization	+++	++
Calcification	n/a	+++

Adopted from Antonopoulos et al. [13]

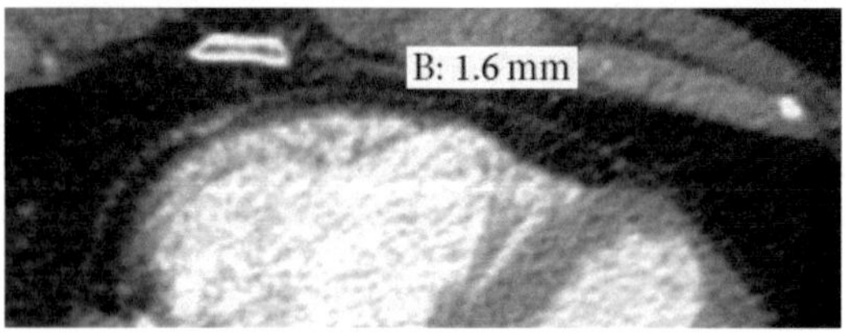

Fig. 14.3 Normal pericardium on a gated contrast-enhanced axial CT. (From Czum et al. [20], licensed under CC-BY 3.0)

The advantages of CT include the ability to provide detailed anatomic description of the pericardial space with excellent spatial and temporal resolution. In addition, CT can provide useful information in the evaluation of extracardiac disease and can reproducibly depict areas of the pericardium. Image acquisition time is faster than CMR, while CT can also detect pericardial calcification. The major limitation of the modality is the exposure to ionizing radiation. CT, also, cannot be used as a bedside examination for critically ill patients and is addressed only to hemodynamically stable patients.

Evaluating the Pericardial Cavity

Pericardial effusion includes a diverse range of pathologies. Processes that cause pericardial inflammation can increase pericardial fluid production. Such conditions include exudative fluid accumulation due to hemopericardium, purulent effusions, and malignancy. Alternatively, transudative fluid accumulation can occur as a result of reduced reabsorption and an elevation in systemic venous pressure, as seen in congestive heart failure or pulmonary hypertension. Non-inflammatory effusions are often transudative except for chylopericardium, which can present as one of the few exudative non-inflammatory effusions, posing diagnostic challenges. It is important to highlight that in around 50% of cases, no specific cause is found, and the pericardial effusion is categorized as idiopathic [21]. Additionally, pericardial effusions can be classified based on the acuity of presentation (acute, subacute, and chronic), size (mild, moderate, or large), and their impact on hemodynamics (absence of any hemodynamic effects, cardiac tamponade, and effusive-constrictive) [22].

CMR Assessment of Pericardial Effusions

Transthoracic echocardiography (TTE) is considered the first-line test for the initial assessment of a pericardial effusion. CMR, however, can provide detailed anatomical display and accurate three-dimensional quantitative assessment of the pericardial cavity. In addition, CMR is useful in assessing pericardial thickness, identifying concomitant inflammation, and recognizing potential complications, such as cardiac tamponade. With its broader thoracic coverage, CMR can also identify the underlying cause of pericardial effusions and associated conditions of adjacent structures.

According to the size classification of pericardial effusions, they can be categorized as trivial (only seen in systole), small (<1 cm), moderate (1–2 cm), and large (>2 cm) when evaluated using CMR [1]. SSFP cine imaging and contrast-enhanced phase-sensitive inversion recovery (PSIR) can be utilized to assess the size and location of pericardial effusion. SSFP cine imaging can also identify potential hemodynamic complications. Furthermore, signal characteristics obtained through CMR can assist in the qualitative assessment of pericardial effusions, distinguishing between transudates and exudates. The majority of effusions show high T2-weighted and SSFP signals. Transudates typically exhibit low signal on T1-weighted images and high signal on gradient-echo cine images, while blood products and protein-rich exudates (e.g., due to infection and malignancy) show low T2- and high T1-weighted signals with heterogeneous appearance [23].

The signal characteristics of hemorrhagic effusions (hemopericardium) depend on the duration of the pathology. In general, hemopericardium exhibits high-signal intensity in both T1 and T2 images due the high concentration of protein within the fluid [24]. However, on gradient-echo SSFP images, hemopericardium in the acute phase exhibits low signal intensity, while in the chronic state, this low signal intensity exhibits inhomogeneities consistent with calcifications, fibrosis, or hemosiderin deposition.

CMR can serve as a valuable complementary or confirmatory test for ruling out localized cardiac tamponade where the assessment of hemodynamics with echocardiography yields atypical results and the presence of tamponade remains uncertain. However, its use in the majority of cardiac tamponade cases, which are medical emergencies, is limited. Cine SSFP imaging and real-time free-breathing cine imaging can demonstrate diastolic compression of the right ventricular free wall, early systolic collapse of the right atrium, and potential displacement of the interventricular septum to the left side during early inspiration [25].

CT Assessment of Pericardial Effusions

Small amounts of fluid in the pericardial space and recesses, particularly around the posterior and inferior aspects of the heart and the left atrial appendage, can be detected using cardiac CT in healthy individuals (incidental finding) [26]. Additionally, in cases of pericardial effusion, CT is effective at clearly outlining the anatomical distribution of pericardial fluid. The CT attenuation values can provide indications about the type and origin of the effusion. Densities higher than that of water (above 10 HU) suggest a high protein content. Hemorrhagic effusions typically exhibit a density of over 30 HU. However, in cases of chronic hemopericardium, the density tends to decrease over time. To distinguish acute hemorrhagic effusions from nonhemorrhagic ones, a CT attenuation value exceeding 30 HU demonstrated a sensitivity of 100% and specificity of 70% [17]. CT, like CMR, does not play a role in managing acute, life-threatening cardiac tamponade. However, it can be beneficial in assessing the feasibility of percutaneous pericardiocentesis, especially in cases involving loculated or complex effusions [27].

Evaluating the Pericardium

Pericarditis

Pericardial inflammation (pericarditis) is a relatively common clinical entity accounting for ~3.0% of admissions to cardiology departments. It can present as acute, subacute, or recurrent pericarditis with the latter occurring in around 15–30% of patients who have experienced an episode of acute pericarditis. Recurrent pericarditis is associated with poor prognosis. In the majority of cases, pericarditis is considered idiopathic. Other causes include infectious diseases, malignancies, autoimmune disorders, uremia, invasive cardiothoracic procedures, and trauma of the chest [20]. Chest irradiation and myocardial infarction can also cause pericarditis. Pericarditis can be accompanied by pericardial effusion, while it can also lead to cardiac tamponade or constriction, with distinct morphological and functional imaging features. The diagnostic approach of pericarditis does not pose significant challenges. Echocardiography is the first-line imaging modality. However, CMR and CT can offer additional diagnostic and prognostic information.

Using CMR in Acute, Subacute, and Recurrent Pericarditis

On CMR, the presentation of acute pericarditis includes different degrees of pericardial thickening (normal to mildly thickened), edema, and late gadolinium enhancement (LGE) (Fig. 14.4). On black blood T1-weighted spin-echo images, the pericardium appears hypointense, while a thickness of ≥3 mm is highly suggestive of pericarditis [28]. In cases where pericardial effusion allows the distinction of the two pericardial layers, inflammation of the visceral pericardium can become visible. Increased signal intensity on T2-short tau inversion recovery (STIR) images is compatible with acute pericarditis with edema, while the presence of pericardial LGE with normal pericardial T2-STIR signal is highly suggestive of a subacute process. CMR can be also used to assess the extension of inflammation to adjacent tissues such as the epicardial fat and myocardium.

CMR can help guide diagnosis and risk stratification in cases of recurrent pericarditis. Inflammation can be quantified as a volumetric parameter using pericardial LGE [29]. As CMR has a good negative predictive value in assessing pericardial thickness and inflammation, it can be used to monitor diseases and guide care. Semiquantitative or quantitative assessment of

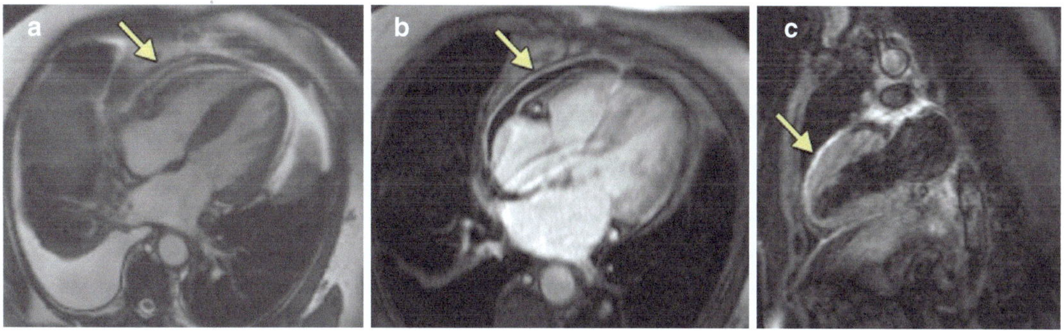

Fig. 14.4 CMR imaging of acute pericarditis. (**a**) Demonstrates thickening of both visceral and parietal layers (arrow) with a small pericardial effusion and large right pleural effusion on balanced steady-state free precession (b-SSFP). (**b**) Early gadolinium enhancement where both pericardial layers enhance, suggesting pericardial inflammation (arrow). (**c**) The pericardium appears as bright signal on T2-weighted short tau inversion recovery (T2-W STIR) (arrow), suggesting an edematous, inflammatory process. (From Dawson et al. [30], licensed under CC-BY 4.0)

pericardial LGE is useful in identifying individuals at risk for recurrence or with unfavorable prognosis.

Systemic inflammatory disorders such as rheumatoid arthritis can cause both acute and recurrent pericarditis, which can be either symptomatic (inflammation and pericardial effusion) or asymptomatic (pericardial effusion). On CMR, the subepicardial or mid-wall myocardial LGE pattern correlates with the activity of the disease and can facilitate initial investigation. In addition, pericarditis findings can be prominent in post-myocardial infarction (post-MI) patients, usually in close proximity to the infarction area [31]. CMR findings can be indicative of inflammation providing clinically valuable information for patients with nontypical post-MI chest pain with atypical ECG and/or laboratory results.

Using CT in Acute, Subacute, and Recurrent Pericarditis

In acute pericarditis, CT can identify small pericardial effusion and minimal pericardial thickening that might not be captured by echocardiography. Characterization of pericardial fluid is also possible to identify underlying causes. For example, attenuation greater than that of water is highly indicative of an exudate with potential causes including malignancy, infection, or hemopericardium [32]. In complicated acute pericarditis with moderate-to-large effusion but without tamponade, CT can be used when transthoracic echocardiography (TTE) is not diagnostic. In cases with a potential traumatic cause, especially when associated injuries to adjacent structures are suspected (e.g., penetrating injury or gastric/esophageal perforation), it is reasonable to consider CT.

Pericardial Constriction

Constrictive pericarditis (CP) is characterized by the presence of a thick, noncompliant, inflamed, and/or calcified pericardium. This restricts the heart's ability to fill properly by preventing the transmission of changes in intrathoracic pressure during respiration. In developed countries, constrictive pericarditis is primarily associated with factors such as previous cardiac surgery, pericarditis, and radiation therapy to the mediastinum [33], while in developing countries, causes include immunosuppressive conditions and tuberculosis [34]. In cases of chronic constriction, pericardial effusion is typically absent.

Using CMR in Constrictive Pericarditis

CMR can reliably identify signs of constrictive physiology even when increased pericardial thickness is not present [35]. Signs of constriction include abrupt cessation of diastolic filling, septal bounce, or respiro-phasic variation in septal excursion on real-time free-breathing cine sequences. In addition, CMR can identify atrial enlargement. However, CMR cannot readily differentiate pericardial calcification from pericardial thickening as it appears as low signal on all sequences [21]. Overall, the diagnostic accuracy of CMR for constrictive pericarditis, which is mainly based on the assessment of pericardial thickness and relative interventricular septal excursion, is excellent. CMR assessment of pericardial LGE and inflammatory biomarkers can potentially predict the reversibility of constrictive pericarditis with anti-inflammatory regiments [36]. Finally, in a small number of constrictive pericarditis cases, increased pericardial thickness or hemodynamic features of constriction might be absent posing significant diagnostic challenges and stressing the need for a multimodality imaging approach.

Using CT in Constrictive Pericarditis

In CT, the presence of thickened pericardium does not confirm constriction. Increased pericardial thickness can be observed during the postoperative period, in conditions like uremia, rheumatic heart disease, sarcoidosis, or as a consequence of radiation therapy. About 20% of cases with constriction may not display pericardial thickening on CT [37]. Furthermore, CT cannot assess the hemodynamic significance of a thickened pericardium. Therefore, while the appearance of "pericardial thickening" on CT can provide support in cases of suspected constriction, it is not definitive of the condition. Similarly, a normal pericardial thickness cannot rule out constriction [38]. CT can effectively identify the presence and exact extent of pericardial calcification compared to CMR. In cases where constriction is suspected, the discovery of pericardial calcification should be considered a significant finding [39]. However, calcification alone does not enable a diagnosis of constrictive pericarditis and a multimodality approach should be considered.

Evaluating Epicardial Fat

Using CT

Modern Approaches in Quantifying EAT

The development of novel imaging techniques and the integration of computational systems in the analysis and interpretation of medical images have opened up new possibilities for measuring the volume of the adipose tissue or, potentially, assessing its "quality" using complex image post-processing techniques. Different imaging modalities provide varying amounts and types of information, but CT is widely regarded as the gold standard for visualizing and characterizing the epicardial adipose tissue. This is due to its exceptional spatial resolution, full coverage of the heart's volume, and the distinctive attenuation signals of the adipose tissue, which typically fall within the range of −30 to −190 HU [7]. However, manual quantification of the adipose tissue is a labor-intensive, time-consuming process and is not typically included in the routine interpretation of coronary CT angiography (CCTA). Deep learning models can bridge this efficiency gap and contribute to the development of automated EAT segmentation algorithms [40]. Using a single network, West et al. have developed a deep-learning technique for the automated segmentation and quantification of EAT from CCTA images using, for the first time, a large cohort of patient scans. Their automated segmentation algorithm was trained and validated in approximately 4000 scans, including technically challenging populations, sourced from an international multicenter prospective cohort study [41]. Overall, this novel deep-learning network (DLN) reduces the average quantification time from 18 min to 12 s indicating that such approaches could potentially become part of standard of care [42] (Fig. 14.5).

Prognostic Value of EAT Volume

EAT volume, clinically measured on contrast or non-contrast CT, is associated with cardiovascular disease (CVD) markers and outcomes includ-

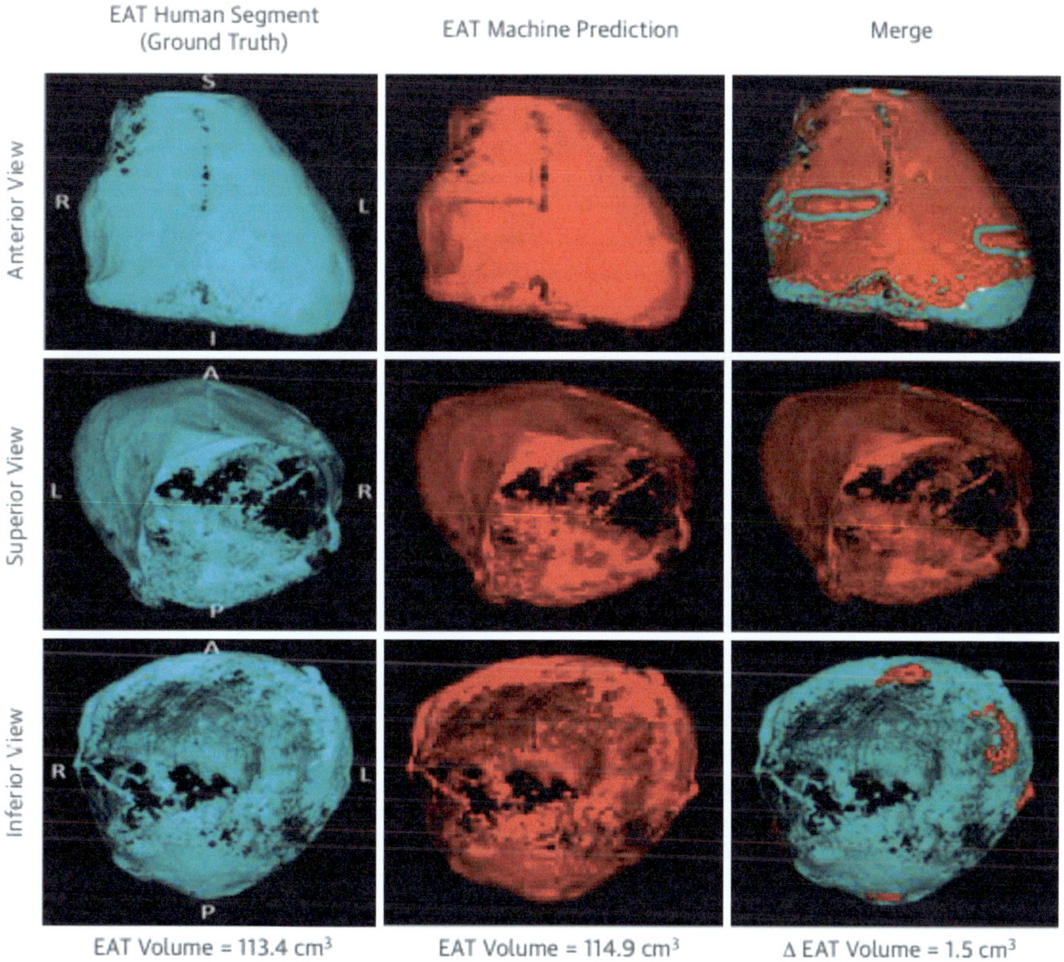

Fig. 14.5 A single CCTA demonstrating human expert segmentation as ground truth, automated machine segmentation, and a merge. A anterior, I inferior, L left, P posterior, R right, S superior. (Reproduced from West et al. [42])

ing the presence of atherosclerosis and coronary artery disease (CAD) and the progression of coronary calcification, atrial fibrillation, and heart failure. A number of studies have focused on the prognostic value of EAT volume in regard to all-cause mortality and cardiovascular events highlighting its role in predicting and stratifying cardiovascular risk (Table 14.2). In addition, it has been shown that EAT volume can predict nonfatal myocardial infarction (MI) and stroke, independent of body mass index (BMI) and after adjusting for relevant risk factors [12]. EAT volume has been also associated with metabolically unhealthy visceral obesity and diabetes. EAT releases adipokines that can influence cardiovascular physiology in an endocrine manner by entering the systemic circulation. EAT, a visceral adipose tissue depot, is highly vascular and releases its secretome into the bloodstream, primarily exerting deleterious effects on the cardiovascular system in an endocrine manner [3]. In addition to its endocrine effects on the cardiovascular system, the adipose tissue can also directly influence the heart and the vascular wall. This influence occurs through paracrine mechanisms (i.e., by molecules diffusing to nearby cells) or vasocrine processes (i.e., mediated by the local micro-circulation). The bidirectional communication between the EAT and cardiovascular system and any discordance between the two can be

Table 14.2 Studies highlighting the prognostic value of EAT volume

Outcome	Studies
Coronary artery disease	Alexopoulos et al. [43], Nakanishi et al. [44], Goeller et al. [45], Ito et al. [46]
Coronary calcification	Yerramasu et al. [47], Goeller et al. [45], Nakanishi et al. [48]
Heart failure	Fontes-Carvalho et al. [49], Khawaja [50]
Major adverse cardiovascular events	Mahabadi et al. [51], Goeller et al. [45], West et al. [42]
Atrial fibrillation	Nagashima et al. [52], Nalliah et al. [8], West et al. [42]
Visceral obesity and diabetes	Wang et al. [53], Versteylen et al. [54], Chun et al. [55], Milanese et al. [56]
Mortality	Kwon et al. [57], Christensen et al. [58], D'Marco et al. [59], West et al. [42]

a cause of detrimental effects on the vasculature and related tissues.

Assessing Pericardial AT (PAT) Volume

PAT volume has been associated with insulin resistance and subsequent diabetes while pro-inflammatory mediators, cytokines, and chemokines secreted by visceral fat depots are involved in systemic inflammation and insulin resistance, which precedes diabetes development [60]. PAT, as defined in a 2023 European Society of Cardiology (ESC) Clinical Consensus Statement, sits externally to the pericardium and surrounding the cardiac silhouette [7]. Different quantification methods have been used to assess PAT volume with DL-based body composition analysis being used the most among studies [61, 62]. While PAT volume correlates with insulin resistance, it is not strongly associated with high-risk plaque features or coronary artery disease compared to EAT [63]. As such, due to its anatomical distance from coronary arteries and the heart, PAT is considered a more "systemic" visceral fat depot.

Assessing EAT Quality

In general, "healthy" EAT, along with relevant visceral adipose tissue depots such as PAT, exhibit smaller adipocytes, which are increased in number compared to the subcutaneous adipose tissue [64]. Obesity and insulin resistance are characterized by hyperbolic lipid accumulation. Lipid accumulation and downregulation of preadipocyte factors that inhibit adipogenesis results in adipocytes undergoing hypertrophy (increase in size). On CT, the adipose tissue appears with lower attenuations as attenuation metrics reflect adipocyte size [45]. In addition, a metabolically dysfunctional adipose tissue correlates with systemic inflammation. Dysfunctional EAT presents a number of specific characteristics that differentiate it from a healthy fat tissue, driven by abnormal adipogenesis, development of fibrotic tissue, angiogenesis, and other molecular characteristics [65]. As these changes lead to striking alterations in adipose tissue texture, they can be captured through specific changes in the radiomic profile of the adipose tissue in CT imaging. Such alterations in EAT readings have been associated with serum levels of lipids, plaque inflammatory markers, and major adverse cardiovascular events [45].

Assessing Perivascular Adipose Tissue (PVAT) Around Coronary Arteries

The role of PVAT goes beyond offering structural support as a physical barrier of the blood vessels. In the last decades, a number of studies have highlighted the contribution of PVAT in the vessels' function via the secretion of vasoactive factors (adipokines) with paracrine (outside-in) effects on the vascular wall. In addition, PVAT has the capacity to sense signals released from the vessel wall (inside-out) that alter its biological behavior. This bidirectional interplay between PVAT and the vascular wall represents a crosstalk mechanism between the two tissues [66]. Paracrine signals originating from vascular cells lead to phenotypic alterations of PVAT adipocytes, which in response adjust the content of their secretome. The modified secretome exerts paracrine effects back on to the vascular wall. This crosstalk between PVAT and the vessel wall can take various forms in healthy and diseased states.

The high spatial resolution and the ability to detect distinct attenuation signals of fat render

CT the gold standard for capturing and characterizing PVAT. PVAT can "sense" signals from the inflamed vascular wall and change its composition. More specifically, PVAT alters its lipid/water composition from a greater lipophilic to a greater relative aqueous component due to inflammation-induced lipolysis and suppressed adipogenesis. This shift from a lipophilic to an aqueous phase correlates with a shift in attenuation on computed tomography (CT) toward more positive HU values. Mean pericoronary adipose tissue attenuation (PCAT) changes as the balance between the lipid and the aqueous phase of the perivascular adipose tissue changes around inflamed arteries. However, this measure is affected by several technical, biological, and anatomical factors, which need to be considered when using this metric to estimate coronary inflammation. The perivascular fat attenuation index (pFAI) is a metric developed to quantify the 3D attenuation gradients in CCTA imaging of PVAT, and it is corrected for technical scan parameters [64] (Fig. 14.6). The pFAI technology has been validated, both from biological and clinical perspectives. Currently, it is considered the principal CCTA biomarker of coronary inflammation.

While the analysis of FAI around the proximal segments of epicardial coronary arteries can be used as a surrogate of the overall coronary inflammatory burden, FAI can also provide lesion-specific analysis. However, this additional tool has not been yet validated and is not recommended for clinical use. Its use is mainly targeted in the provision of valuable insights for research and experimental purposes. FAI tends to increase

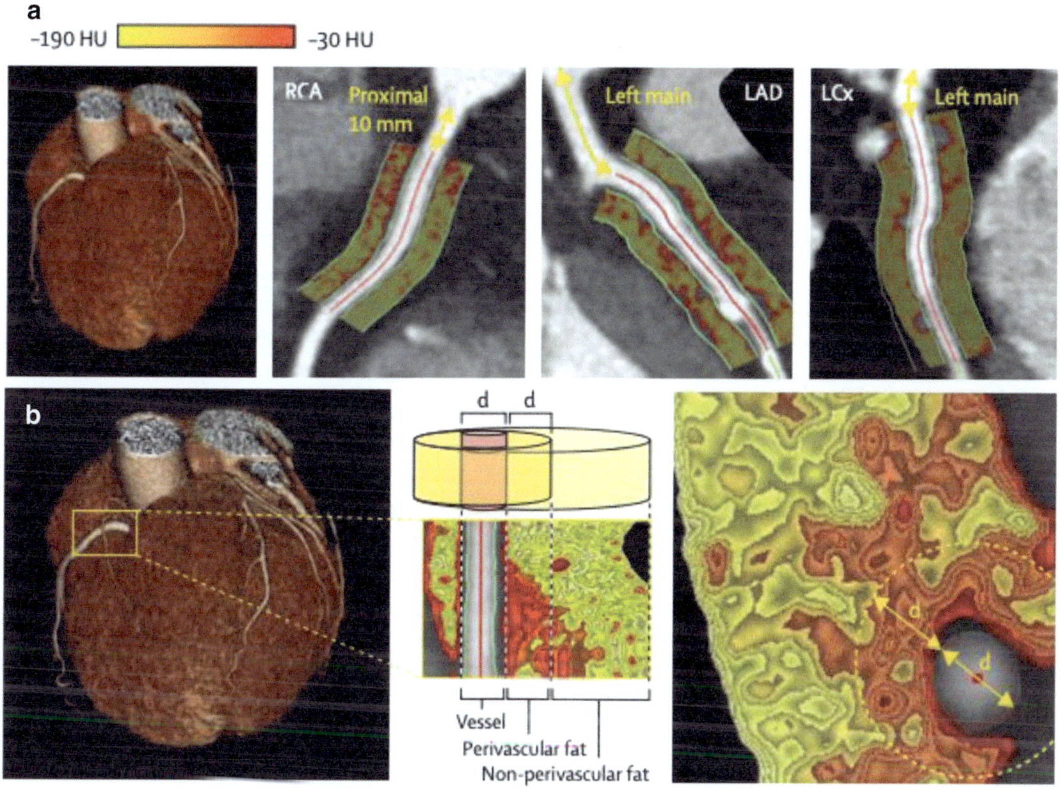

Fig. 14.6 Perivascular FAI analysis around epicardial coronary vessels. (**a**) Perivascular FAI phenotyping of the proximal segments of all three major epicardial coronary vessels, with corresponding FAI color maps. (**b**) Example of perivascular FAI phenotyping around the proximal RCA. Perivascular fat was defined as fat within a radial distance equal to the diameter (*d*) of the vessel. FAI fat attenuation index, HU Hounsfield unit, LAD left anterior descending artery, LCx left circumflex artery, RCA right coronary artery. (From Oikonomou et al. [69], licensed under CC-BY 4.0)

incrementally around ruptured plaques or plaques that exhibit the so-called vulnerable phenotype in individuals with ST-elevation myocardial infarction (STEMI), non-ST-elevation myocardial infarction (NSTEMI), and unstable angina [64]. Moreover, in patients with acute coronary syndromes (ACS), FAI is higher around atherosclerotic coronary segments, while it can predict progression of non-calcified plaque [67]. The FAI technology has been validated against the imaging "gold standard" for the detection of adipose tissue inflammation, the uptake of 18F-deoxyglucose (FDG) using positron emission tomography (PET) and has shown to provide excellent sensitivity and specificity to detect adipose tissue inflammation [68].

Pericoronary FAI is a crude method to estimate inflammation of coronary arteries [69]. It is measured by applying post-processing techniques on standard CCTA images, and, as a result, FAI measurement suffers from technical limitations such as motion artifacts and heart rhythm abnormalities. In research studies, FAI performs adequately well. However, translating this technology into a clinically applicable tool is challenging as attenuation values on CCTA are influenced by numerous technical, biological, and anatomical factors [70]. FAI score addresses these limitations as it adjusts FAI values for age, sex, further scan technical parameters, and biological and anatomical factors, providing a standardized, vessel-specific (separately for all three epicardial coronary arteries) metric of coronary inflammation [71]. FAI score is currently the only regulatory cleared metric of coronary inflammation derived from CCTA in Europe. The clinical interpretation of FAI score should be based on age- and sex-specific nomograms. An FAI score above the 75th percentile for the patient's age and sex in the LAD or RCA, or above the 95th percentile in the LCx, indicates that the individual is exposed to high inflammatory risk, while an FAI score above the 90th percentile in either the LAD or the RCA is considered as very high risk.

FAI score was integrated in a prognostic AI algorithm along with clinical risk factors such as diabetes, smoking, hyperlipidemia, and hypertension, as well as atherosclerotic plaque burden and characteristics of vulnerable plaque as detected on CCTA to generate the 8-year % risk of the individual patient for a fatal cardiac event (AI-Risk algorithm) [71]. Compared to a baseline risk model including traditional risk factors only, the AI-Risk algorithm significantly improved risk discrimination and classification. In addition, the model's incremental prognostic value was maintained even after incorporating the modified Duke CAD index in the baseline model. The prognostic AI model was developed on US population and validated on European population before being incorporated into a medical device for clinical use. The use of the AI-Risk algorithm has been proposed in a recent ESC Clinical Consensus Statement as an addition to classic risk calculators, to provide a more comprehensive risk prediction when a CCTA is available [7] (Fig. 14.7).

The extraction of radiomic features from PVAT and the use of ML techniques can generate novel sophisticated biomarkers that could enhance the detailed characterization of PVAT [73]. Different forms of inflammation can result in a diversity of imaging texture changes in PVAT, influenced by varying degrees of perivascular lipolysis, adipogenesis, edema, fibrosis, and angiogenesis [3]. Utilizing "ground truth" data extracted from tissue biopsies to train radiomic signatures of PVAT from CCTA had led to the development of "radiotranscriptomic" signatures of vascular inflammation. Indeed, through the utilization of AT biopsies of individuals undergoing heart surgery along with matching CCTA images, ML signatures were developed to capture inflammation, fibrosis, and vascularity from the radiomic phenotype of the adipose tissue and to generate the fat radiomic profile (FRP). In a cohort of 5487 participants from the SCOT-HEART [74] and CRISP-CT [69], it was shown that such signatures have the power to independently predict adverse cardiovascular outcomes beyond traditional risk factors [73]. Similar radiotranscriptomic approaches have been also used to develop noninvasive imaging biomarkers to support clinical decision-making. Kotanidis et al. have developed a platform that can quantify cytokine-driven vascular inflammation from routine CT scans in patients

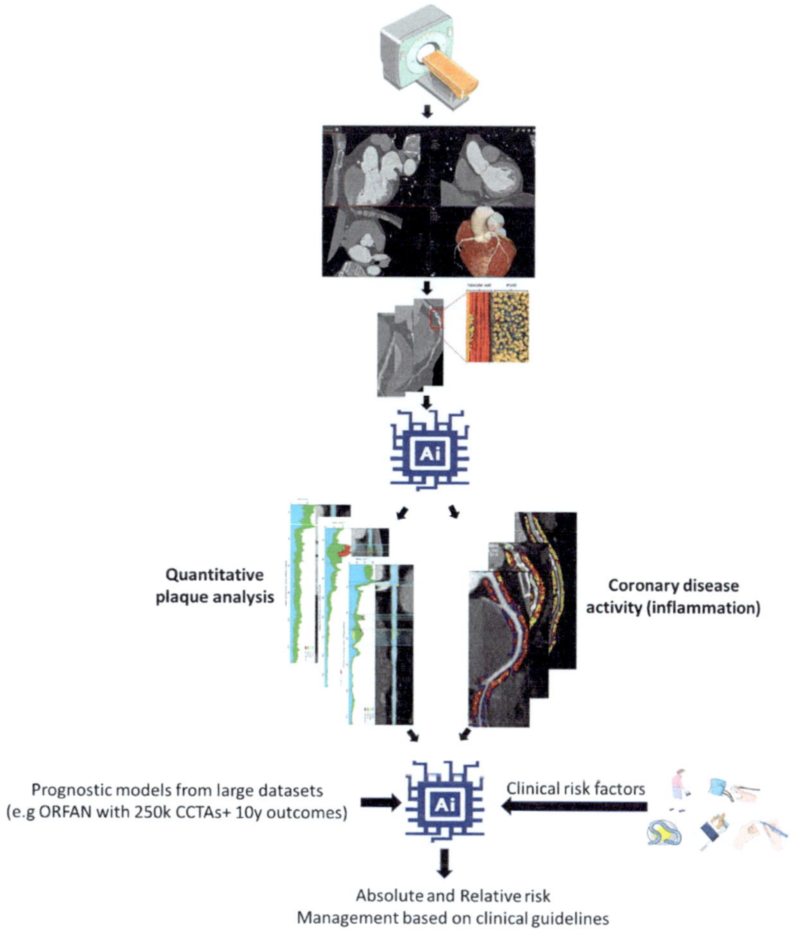

Fig. 14.7 Artificial intelligence-assisted image interpretation for the assessment of coronary artery disease, prediction of patient's risk, and deployment of personalized medical management. (Reproduced with permission by Antoniades et al. [72])

with COVID-19. This novel radiotranscriptomic signature has the potential to predict thrombosis and the likelihood of death in COVID-19 patients while also enabling the identification of patients who are likely to respond well to treatment (i.e., dexamethasone) [75].

Using CMR

CMR can only depict the parietal layer of the normal pericardium as the inner visceral layer is not thick enough to be visualized, and, as a result, the pericardial area assessment always includes both the epicardial and pericardial fat compartments. Therefore, epicardial and pericardial fat can be quantified en bloc but not separately, which poses significant limitations. Adipose tissue volumes can be quantified using CMR by combining T1-weighted images without and with fat saturation preparation. Another notable limitation, however, is the need for standardized image quality to facilitate the assessment of adipose tissue quality, which is essential for making valid between-patient comparisons.

While basic measurements of the total epicardial and pericardial adipose tissue volumes using MRI can provide useful insights about the predictive value of visceral obesity in the general population [76], this tends to be significantly lower in comparison to volumetric quantification of EAT using CT [42]. Same as in CCTA, manual quantification of the adipose tissue is inefficient. Automated EAT and PAT segmentation techniques have been developed showing promising results for large-scale, fast scan analysis (Fig. 14.8). Automatically quantified

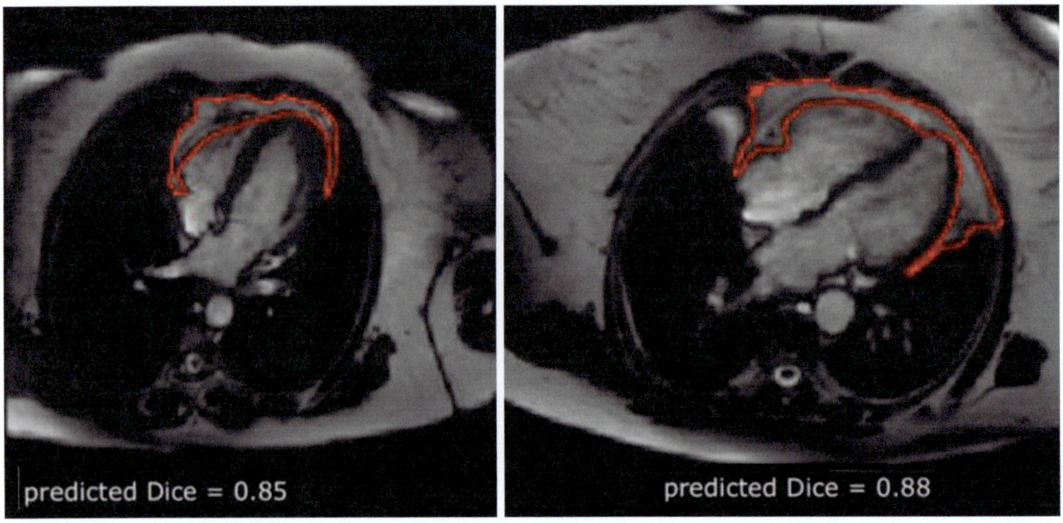

Fig. 14.8 Automated en bloc EAT and PAT segmentation and its predicted segmentation quality. The Dice score provides a quality-control measure with scores <0.7 indicating poor segmentation quality. (From Bard et al. [77], licensed under CC-BY 4.0) [76]

volumes of the combined EAT and PAT area using CMR have been associated with unhealthy cardiovascular structure and function, regardless of baseline comorbidities, vascular risk factors, inflammatory markers, and various noninvasive and imaging measures of obesity. However, a more in-depth qualitative assessment of visceral fat depots and radiomic analysis of images is not yet available using CMR techniques.

Conflict of Interest MCM is a consultant at WHO. C.A. declares several patents (US10,695,023B2, PCT/GB2017/053262, GB2018/1818049.7, GR20180100490, GR20180100510) licensed to Caristo Diagnostics. C.A. is the immediate past Chair of the British Atherosclerosis Society. C.A., is Founder, shareholder, director and consultant of Caristo Diagnostics, a University of Oxford Spinout company. C.A. declares honoraria from Amarin, Silence Therapeutics, Abcentra, Amgen, Nodthera, Novartis, UCB and Caristo Diagnostics. R.A.K. declares honoraria from Abbott and Amarin.

References

1. Adler Y, Charron P, Imazio M, Badano L, Barón-Esquivias G, Bogaert J, et al. 2015 ESC guidelines for the diagnosis and management of pericardial diseases: the task force for the diagnosis and management of pericardial diseases of the European Society of Cardiology (ESC) endorsed by: the European Association for Cardio-Thoracic Surgery (EACTS). Eur Heart J. 2015;36(42):2921–64.
2. Imazio M, Gaita F. Diagnosis and treatment of pericarditis. Heart. 2015;101(14):1159–68.
3. Oikonomou EK, Antoniades C. The role of adipose tissue in cardiovascular health and disease. Nat Rev Cardiol. 2019;16(2):83–99.
4. Hoit BD. Anatomy and physiology of the pericardium. Cardiol Clin. 2017;35(4):481–90.
5. Tabaksblat MY, Halpern DG, Argulian E, Herzog E. Anatomy and physiology of the pericardium. Management of pericardial disease. Springer International Publishing; 2014. p. 3–10.
6. Antonopoulos AS, Antoniades C. The role of epicardial adipose tissue in cardiac biology: classic concepts and emerging roles. J Physiol. 2017;595(12):3907–17.
7. Antoniades C, Tousoulis D, Vavlukis M, Fleming I, Duncker DJ, Eringa E, et al. Perivascular adipose tissue as a source of therapeutic targets and clinical biomarkers. Eur Heart J. 2023;44(38):3827–44.
8. Nalliah CJ, Bell JR, Raaijmakers AJA, Waddell HM, Wells SP, Bernasochi GB, et al. Epicardial adipose tissue accumulation confers atrial conduction abnormality. J Am Coll Cardiol. 2020;76(10):1197–211.
9. Sechtem U, Tscholakoff D, Higgins CB. MRI of the normal pericardium. AJR Am J Roentgenol. 1986;147(2):239–44.
10. Stark DD, Higgins CB, Lanzer P, Lipton MJ, Schiller N, Crooks LE, et al. Magnetic resonance imaging of the pericardium: normal and pathologic findings. Radiology. 1984;150(2):469–74.
11. Spodick DH. Pericardial disease. JAMA. 1997;278(9):704.

12. Vidalakis E, Kolentinis M, Gawor M, Vasquez M, Nagel E. CMR in pericardial diseases – an update. Curr Cardiovasc Imaging Rep. 2020;13(4):14.
13. Antonopoulos AS, Vrettos A, Androulakis E, Kamperou C, Vlachopoulos C, Tsioufis K, et al. Cardiac magnetic resonance imaging of pericardial diseases: a comprehensive guide. Eur Heart J Cardiovasc Imaging. 2023;24(8):983–98.
14. Halliburton SS. Recent technologic advances in multi-detector row cardiac CT. Cardiol Clin. 2009;27(4):655–64.
15. Wang ZJ, Reddy GP, Gotway MB, Yeh BM, Hetts SW, Higgins CB. CT and MR imaging of pericardial disease. Radiographics. 2003;23 Spec No:S167–80.
16. Verhaert D, Gabriel RS, Johnston D, Lytle BW, Desai MY, Klein AL. The role of multimodality imaging in the management of pericardial disease. Circ Cardiovasc Imaging. 2010;3(3):333–43.
17. O'Leary SM, Williams PL, Williams MP, Edwards AJ, Roobottom CA, Morgan-Hughes GJ, et al. Imaging the pericardium: appearances on ECG-gated 64-detector row cardiac computed tomography. Br J Radiol. 2010;83(987):194–205.
18. Bull RK, Edwards PD, Dixon AK. CT dimensions of the normal pericardium. Br J Radiol. 1998;71(849):923–5.
19. Breen JF. Imaging of the pericardium. J Thorac Imaging. 2001;16(1):47–54.
20. Czum JM, Silas AM, Althoen MC. Evaluation of the pericardium with CT and MR. ISRN Cardiol. 2014;2014:174908.
21. Imazio M. Pericardial involvement in systemic inflammatory diseases. Heart. 2011;97(22):1882–92.
22. Permanyer-Miralda G. Acute pericardial disease: approach to the aetiologic diagnosis. Heart. 2004;90(3):252–4.
23. Al-Mallah MH, Almasoudi F, Ebid M, Ahmed AM, Jamiel A. Multimodality imaging of pericardial diseases. Curr Treat Options Cardiovasc Med. 2017;19(12):89.
24. Lazaros G, Antonopoulos AS, Lazarou E, Vlachopoulos C, Foukarakis E, Androulakis A, et al. Long-term outcome of pericardial drainage in cases of chronic, large, hemodynamically insignificant, C-reactive protein negative, idiopathic pericardial effusions. Am J Cardiol. 2020;126:89–93.
25. Aldweib N, Farah V, Biederman RWW. Clinical utility of cardiac magnetic resonance imaging in pericardial diseases. Curr Cardiol Rev. 2018;14(3):200–12.
26. Bogaert J, Centonze M, Vanneste R, Francone M. Cardiac and pericardial abnormalities on chest computed tomography: what can we see? Radiol Med. 2010;115(2):175–90.
27. Friedrich MG, Sechtem U, Schulz-Menger J, Holmvang G, Alakija P, Cooper LT, et al. Cardiovascular magnetic resonance in myocarditis: a JACC white paper. J Am Coll Cardiol. 2009;53(17):1475–87.
28. Rajiah P. Cardiac MRI: part 2, pericardial diseases. AJR Am J Roentgenol. 2011;197(4):W621–34.
29. Kumar A, Sato K, Verma BR, Ala CK, Betancor J, Yzeiraj E, et al. Quantitative assessment of pericardial delayed hyperenhancement helps identify patients with ongoing recurrences of pericarditis. Open Heart. 2018;5(2):e000944.
30. Dawson D, Rubens M, Mohiaddin R. Contemporary imaging of the pericardium. JACC Cardiovasc Imaging. 2011;4(6):680–4.
31. Caforio ALP, Adler Y, Agostini C, Allanore Y, Anastasakis A, Arad M, et al. Diagnosis and management of myocardial involvement in systemic immune-mediated diseases: a position statement of the European Society of Cardiology Working Group on myocardial and pericardial disease. Eur Heart J. 2017;38(35):2649–62.
32. Yared K, Baggish AL, Picard MH, Hoffmann U, Hung J. Multimodality imaging of pericardial diseases. JACC Cardiovasc Imaging. 2010;3(6):650–60.
33. Ling LH, Oh JK, Schaff HV, Danielson GK, Mahoney DW, Seward JB, et al. Constrictive pericarditis in the modern era: evolving clinical spectrum and impact on outcome after pericardiectomy. Circulation. 1999;100(13):1380–6.
34. Mayosi BM. Contemporary trends in the epidemiology and management of cardiomyopathy and pericarditis in sub-Saharan Africa. Heart. 2007;93(10):1176–83.
35. Chetrit M, Natalie Szpakowski N, Desai MY. Multimodality imaging for the diagnosis and treatment of constrictive pericarditis. Expert Rev Cardiovasc Ther. 2019;17(9):663–72.
36. Cremer PC, Tariq MU, Karwa A, Alraies MC, Benatti R, Schuster A, et al. Quantitative assessment of pericardial delayed hyperenhancement predicts clinical improvement in patients with constrictive pericarditis treated with anti-inflammatory therapy. Circ Cardiovasc Imaging. 2015;8(5):e003125.
37. Sohal S, Mathai SV, Lipat K, Kaur A, Visveswaran G, Cohen M, et al. Multimodality imaging of constrictive pericarditis: pathophysiology and new concepts. Curr Cardiol Rep. 2022;24(10):1439–53.
38. Talreja DR, Edwards WD, Danielson GK, Schaff HV, Tajik AJ, Tazelaar HD, et al. Constrictive pericarditis in 26 patients with histologically normal pericardial thickness. Circulation. 2003;108(15):1852–7.
39. Xu B, Kwon DH, Klein AL. Imaging of the pericardium: a multimodality cardiovascular imaging update. Cardiol Clin. 2017;35(4):491–503.
40. Commandeur F, Goeller M, Razipour A, Cadet S, Hell MM, Kwiecinski J, et al. Fully automated CT quantification of epicardial adipose tissue by deep learning: a Multicenter study. Radiol Artif Intell. 2019;1(6):e190045.
41. Oxford Heart, Vessels, and Fat Cohort. The ORFAN study. 2019. [Internet]. https://www.oxhvf.com/the-orfan-study/.
42. West HW, Siddique M, Williams MC, Volpe L, Desai R, Lyasheva M, et al. Deep-learning for epicardial adipose tissue assessment with computed tomography: implications for cardiovascular risk prediction. JACC Cardiovasc Imaging. 2023;16(6):800–16.

43. Alexopoulos N, McLean DS, Janik M, Arepalli CD, Stillman AE, Raggi P. Epicardial adipose tissue and coronary artery plaque characteristics. Atherosclerosis. 2010;210(1):150–4.
44. Nakanishi K, Fukuda S, Tanaka A, Otsuka K, Jissho S, Taguchi H, et al. Persistent epicardial adipose tissue accumulation is associated with coronary plaque vulnerability and future acute coronary syndrome in non-obese subjects with coronary artery disease. Atherosclerosis. 2014;237(1):353–60.
45. Goeller M, Achenbach S, Marwan M, Doris MK, Cadet S, Commandeur F, et al. Epicardial adipose tissue density and volume are related to subclinical atherosclerosis, inflammation and major adverse cardiac events in asymptomatic subjects. J Cardiovasc Comput Tomogr. 2018;12(1):67–73.
46. Ito T, Suzuki Y, Ehara M, Matsuo H, Teramoto T, Terashima M, et al. Impact of epicardial fat volume on coronary artery disease in symptomatic patients with a zero calcium score. Int J Cardiol. 2013;167(6):2852–8.
47. Yerramasu A, Dey D, Venuraju S, Anand DV, Atwal S, Corder R, et al. Increased volume of epicardial fat is an independent risk factor for accelerated progression of sub-clinical coronary atherosclerosis. Atherosclerosis. 2012;220(1):223–30.
48. Nakanishi R, Rajani R, Cheng VY, Gransar H, Nakazato R, Shmilovich H, et al. Increase in epicardial fat volume is associated with greater coronary artery calcification progression in subjects at intermediate risk by coronary calcium score: a serial study using non-contrast cardiac CT. Atherosclerosis. 2011;218(2):363–8.
49. Fontes-Carvalho R, Fontes-Oliveira M, Sampaio F, Mancio J, Bettencourt N, Teixeira M, et al. Influence of epicardial and visceral fat on left ventricular diastolic and systolic functions in patients after myocardial infarction. Am J Cardiol. 2014;114(11):1663–9.
50. Khawaja T, Greer C, Chokshi A, Chavarria N, Thadani S, Jones M, et al. Epicardial fat volume in patients with left ventricular systolic dysfunction. Am J Cardiol. 2011;108(3):397–401.
51. Mahabadi AA, Berg MH, Lehmann N, Kälsch H, Bauer M, Kara K, et al. Association of epicardial fat with cardiovascular risk factors and incident myocardial infarction in the general population: the Heinz Nixdorf Recall Study. J Am Coll Cardiol. 2013;61(13):1388–95.
52. Nagashima K, Okumura Y, Watanabe I, Nakai T, Ohkubo K, Kofune T, et al. Association between epicardial adipose tissue volumes on 3-dimensional reconstructed CT images and recurrence of atrial fibrillation after catheter ablation. Circ J. 2011;75(11):2559–65.
53. Wang CP, Hsu HL, Hung WC, Yu TH, Chen YH, Chiu CA, et al. Increased epicardial adipose tissue (EAT) volume in type 2 diabetes mellitus and association with metabolic syndrome and severity of coronary atherosclerosis. Clin Endocrinol. 2009;70(6):876–82.
54. Versteylen MO, Takx RAP, Joosen IAPG, Nelemans PJ, Das M, Crijns HJGM, et al. Epicardial adipose tissue volume as a predictor for coronary artery disease in diabetic, impaired fasting glucose, and non-diabetic patients presenting with chest pain. Eur Heart J Cardiovasc Imaging. 2012;13(6):517–23.
55. Chun H, Suh E, Byun AR, Park HR, Shim KW. Epicardial fat thickness is associated to type 2 diabetes mellitus in Korean men: a cross-sectional study. Cardiovasc Diabetol. 2015;14:46.
56. Milanese G, Silva M, Bruno L, Goldoni M, Benedetti G, Rossi E, et al. Quantification of epicardial fat with cardiac CT angiography and association with cardiovascular risk factors in symptomatic patients: from the ALTER-BIO (alternative cardiovascular BIO-imaging markers) registry. Diagn Interv Radiol. 2019;25(1):35–41.
57. Kwon SS, Choi K, Da Nam B, Lee H, Cho NJ, Park BW, et al. Epicardial adipose tissue radiodensity is associated with all-cause mortality in patients undergoing hemodialysis. Sci Rep. 2021;11(1):23090.
58. Christensen RH, von Scholten BJ, Hansen CS, Jensen MT, Vilsbøll T, Rossing P, et al. Epicardial adipose tissue predicts incident cardiovascular disease and mortality in patients with type 2 diabetes. Cardiovasc Diabetol. 2019;18(1):114.
59. D'Marco LG, Bellasi A, Kim S, Chen Z, Block GA, Raggi P. Epicardial adipose tissue predicts mortality in incident hemodialysis patients: a substudy of the Renagel in new dialysis trial. Nephrol Dial Transplant. 2013;28(10):2586–95.
60. Liu J, Fox CS, Hickson D, Sarpong D, Ekunwe L, May WD, et al. Pericardial adipose tissue, atherosclerosis, and cardiovascular disease risk factors: the Jackson heart study. Diabetes Care. 2010;33(7):1635–9.
61. Koitka S, Kroll L, Malamutmann E, Oezcelik A, Nensa F. Fully automated body composition analysis in routine CT imaging using 3D semantic segmentation convolutional neural networks. Eur Radiol. 2021;31(4):1795–804.
62. Kroll L, Nassenstein K, Jochims M, Koitka S, Nensa F. Assessing the role of pericardial fat as a biomarker connected to coronary calcification-a deep learning based approach using fully automated body composition analysis. J Clin Med. 2021;10(2):356.
63. Lu MT, Park J, Ghemigian K, Mayrhofer T, Puchner SB, Liu T, et al. Epicardial and paracardial adipose tissue volume and attenuation – association with high-risk coronary plaque on computed tomographic angiography in the ROMICAT II trial. Atherosclerosis. 2016;251:47–54.
64. Antonopoulos AS, Sanna F, Sabharwal N, Thomas S, Oikonomou EK, Herdman L, et al. Detecting human coronary inflammation by imaging perivascular fat. Sci Transl Med. 2017;9(398):eaal2658.

65. Antonopoulos AS, Tousoulis D. The molecular mechanisms of obesity paradox. Cardiovasc Res. 2017;113(9):1074–86.
66. Mancio J, Oikonomou EK, Antoniades C. Perivascular adipose tissue and coronary atherosclerosis. Heart. 2018;104(20):1654–62.
67. Marwan M, Hell M, Schuhbäck A, Gauss S, Bittner D, Pflederer T, et al. CT attenuation of Pericoronary adipose tissue in normal versus atherosclerotic coronary segments as defined by intravascular ultrasound. J Comput Assist Tomogr. 2017;41(5):762–7.
68. Kwiecinski J, Dey D, Cadet S, Lee SE, Otaki Y, Huynh PT, et al. Peri-coronary adipose tissue density is associated with 18F-sodium fluoride coronary uptake in stable patients with high-risk plaques. JACC Cardiovasc Imaging. 2019;12(10):2000–10.
69. Oikonomou EK, Marwan M, Desai MY, Mancio J, Alashi A, Hutt Centeno E, et al. Non-invasive detection of coronary inflammation using computed tomography and prediction of residual cardiovascular risk (the CRISP CT study): a post-hoc analysis of prospective outcome data. Lancet. 2018;392(10151):929–39.
70. Boussoussou M, Vattay B, Szilveszter B, Simon J, Lin A, Vecsey-Nagy M, et al. The effect of patient and imaging characteristics on coronary CT angiography assessed pericoronary adipose tissue attenuation and gradient. J Cardiovasc Comput Tomogr. 2023;17(1):34–42.
71. Oikonomou EK, Antonopoulos AS, Schottlander D, Marwan M, Mathers C, Tomlins P, et al. Standardized measurement of coronary inflammation using cardiovascular computed tomography: integration in clinical care as a prognostic medical device. Cardiovasc Res. 2021;117(13):2677–90.
72. Antoniades C, Patel P, Antonopoulos AS. Using artificial intelligence to study atherosclerosis, predict risk and guide treatments in clinical practice. Eur Heart J. 2023;44(6):437–9.
73. Oikonomou EK, Williams MC, Kotanidis CP, Desai MY, Marwan M, Antonopoulos AS, et al. A novel machine learning-derived radiotranscriptomic signature of perivascular fat improves cardiac risk prediction using coronary CT angiography. Eur Heart J. 2019;40(43):3529–43.
74. SCOT-HEART Investigators, Newby DE, Adamson PD, Berry C, Boon NA, Dweck MR, et al. Coronary CT angiography and 5-year risk of myocardial infarction. N Engl J Med. 2018;379(10):924–33.
75. Kotanidis CP, Xie C, Alexander D, Rodrigues JCL, Burnham K, Mentzer A, et al. Constructing custom-made radiotranscriptomic signatures of vascular inflammation from routine CT angiograms: a prospective outcomes validation study in COVID-19. Lancet Digit Health. 2022;4(10):e705–16.
76. Ardissino M, McCracken C, Bard A, Antoniades C, Neubauer S, Harvey NC, et al. Pericardial adiposity is independently linked to adverse cardiovascular phenotypes: a CMR study of 42 598 UK biobank participants. Eur Heart J Cardiovasc Imaging. 2022;23(11):1471–81.
77. Bard A, Raisi-Estabragh Z, Ardissino M, Lee AM, Pugliese F, Dey D, et al. Automated quality-controlled cardiovascular magnetic resonance pericardial fat quantification using a convolutional neural network in the UK biobank. Front Cardiovasc Med. 2021;8:1–11.

Quantitative Imaging of the Aorta 15

Meghavi Mashar, Ritu R. Gill,
and Jonathan M Goldstein

Introduction

Quantitively imaging of the aorta is vital in a variety of pathology for surgical intervention, whether it is for perioperative planning or for assessing severity. These may be static to assess aortic size at various points or dynamic to assess other characteristics such as pressure gradients or flow. Currently, there is extensive use of cross-sectional imaging with computed tomography (CT) and magnetic resonance (MR) angiography with 3D datasets. Most imaging modalities to monitor aneurysms are CT angiography and MR angiography with 3D dataset. Consistency of measurement is essential to allow accurate assessment, but published guidance is unfortunately highly variable across modalities, timing during the cardiac cycle (end systole vs. end diastole), reporting cross-sectional values (inner luminal diameter, outer luminal diameter) or leading edge to leading edge (i.e. the outer wall of the aorta to the inner). Moreover, it is unclear whether these measurements should be normalised to age, sex and body surface area. However, note should be made that a single measurement of any 2D view cannot fully capture any asymmetry and thus two orthogonal measurements are recommended.

For static measurements, there are key sites where measurements need to be taken: aortic annulus, aortic sinuses, sinotubular junction, mid-ascending aorta, high ascending aorta below the origin of the brachiocephalic trunk, aortic arch and descending aorta [1]. In echocardiography, these are from the parasternal long-axis view and typically using the leading edge to leading edge method (Fig. 15.1).

Historically aortic valve annulus measurements were not felt to be needed for open repair, given that the surgeon can easily assess this during open repair. However, given the trend towards transcatheter and transapical-implanted valves, assessing annular size and the iliofemoral vessels is needed for appropriate prosthesis selection. Traditionally, this has been assessed through echocardiography, but gated multidetector CT can provide both long- and short-axis measurements, which is useful given that the annulus is more ovoid than round [2]. Evaluation on CT involves creating a 3D reconstruction paralleling the parasternal long axis seen on echocardiography. Ideally, double oblique transverse measurements should be taken perpendicular to the long

M. Mashar · R. R. Gill (✉) · J. M. Goldstein
Department of Radiology, Columbia University
Medical Center, New York, NY, USA
e-mail: mmashar@bidmc.harvard.edu;
RG3675@CUMC.COLUMBIA.EDU;
jmg2362@cumc.columbia.edu

R. Gill, P. Rajiah (eds.), *Quantitative Imaging in the Thorax*,
https://doi.org/10.1007/978-3-032-14103-3_15

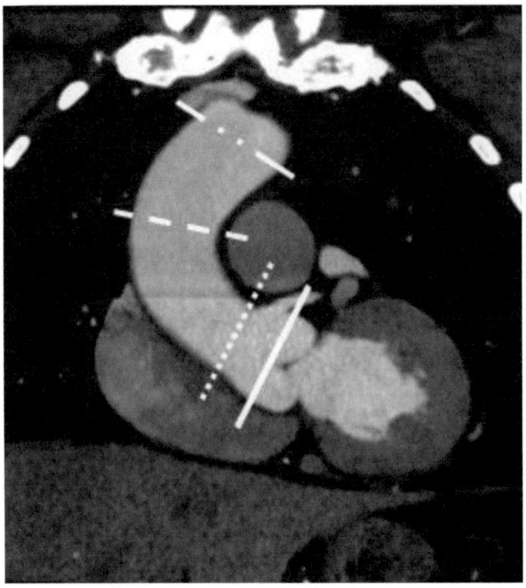

Fig. 15.1 Coronal oblique CT of the chest of a 66-year-old ascending aortic anatomic landmarks typically measured. Aortic annulus (long dashed lunch), aortic sinuses of Valsalva (solid white line), sinotubular junction (dotted white line), mid-ascending aorta (dashed white line), and high ascending aorta (dashed and dotted line)

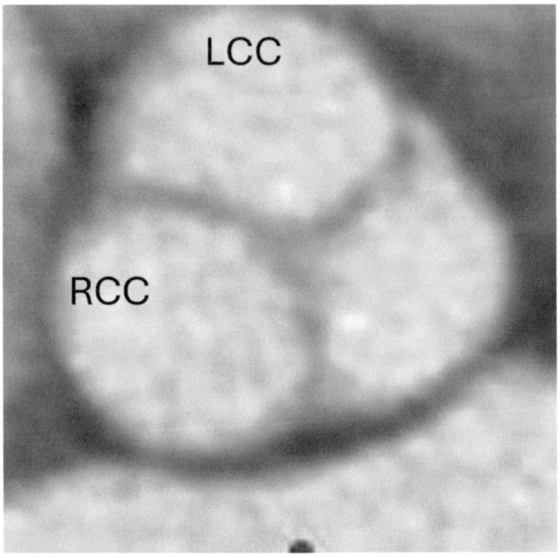

Fig. 15.2 Computerised tomography measurements of the sinus of Valsalva diameters in a short-axis view. LCC left coronary cusp, NCC noncoronary cusp, RCC right coronary cusp. Dotted line, cusp-commissure measurement; solid line, cusp-to-cusp measurement

axis of the aorta, with the maximal and minimal diameters of the basal ring just below the hinge points (where the aortic valve cusps attach to the aortic annulus) in the systolic phase where maximal valve opening is present. Whilst there are notable differences in valve measurements between MDCT and echocardiography [3], it is unclear whether this has an impact on procedural success.

The next site of measurement is the aortic sinus, of which there are three, right, left and non-coronary. This is also the site of the origin of the coronary arteries (Fig. 15.2). Two different types of measurements are common here: cusp-cusp and cusp-commissure. A study found that end-diastolic cusp-commissure measurements, whilst being 2–3 mm smaller than cusp-cusp measures, were closer [4] to the original reference echocardiography measurements from the Framingham Heart Study [5]. However another study of Marfan's patients showed that cusp-to-cusp diameters were closer to TTE measurements for patients with TAAs with cusp- commissure measurements underestimating the true diameters [6].

Gated MR angiography clearly has advantages for longer-term follow-up compared to MDCT. In addition to the absence of radiation exposure, in a younger population such as those with connective tissue disease, respiratory motion artefact also poses less of an issue. There are many non-contrast MR sequences that are available for aortic assessment with good contrast and signal-to-noise ratio. These are mainly balanced steady-state free precession (SSFP) sequences: fast imaging employing steady-state acquisition (FIESTA), true fast imaging with steady-state precession (FISP) and balanced fast field echo (FFE) sequences [7].

Since the 1980s, 2D phase-contrast MRI with CINE sequences has been used for anatomical and quantitative evaluation of blood flow. ECG-gated 2D balanced SSFP sequences perpendicular to the aortic root in two planes can be used to assess the aortic valve and root, with contrast-enhanced MRA to assess the remainder of the aorta. 3D balanced SSFP sequences with prospective ECG triggering and respiratory navigation may avoid the need for contrast, though this is susceptible to 'dark band artefact'.

4D flow MRI has the added ability to measure flow velocity in three directions over time through velocity-encoded cine sequences. Whilst 2D CINE phase-contrast MRI allows evaluation of haemodynamic parameters in a single 2D slice, 4D flow MRI can provide a more holistic perspective with added information of the temporal and spatial blood flow over the entire segments [8]. This allows selection of any location in the 3D volume of data and calculation of multiple haemodynamic parameters including total flow, peak pressure gradient and peak and mean velocities, which have also demonstrated good concordance with similar metrics derived from echocardiography [9, 10]. This has also allowed research on a plethora of potentially useful haemodynamic biomarkers, which have been studied in a variety of conditions.

The main techniques in the aorta that have been studied have been ^{18}F-fluoride PET/CT and ^{18}F-fluorodeoxyglucose (^{18}F-FDG), detecting calcification and inflammation, respectively. ^{18}F-Fluoride binds to a hydroxyapatite crystal and preferentially binds to areas of newly developing microcalcification but does not bind to areas of macrocalcification given that the hydroxyapatite is internalised and not available for binding [11]. ^{18}F-FDG PET uses labelled glucose, which accumulates with metabolically active cells, and inflammation is considered a key driver of many aortic pathologies. As such, it can be very sensitive though variably specific. Reported parameters are maximum tissue-to-background ratios (TBR_{max}) and maximum standard uptake values (SUV_{max}).

Aortic Valve Disease

Aortic Stenosis

Aortic valvular disease affects 0.9% of the general population [12]. Aortic stenosis is the most common valvular disease affecting 12.4% of the population and 3.4% of severe AS in those 75 and older [13]. The aetiology was once considered to be degenerative in nature secondary to ageing, but recent work has demonstrated there may be similarities to atherosclerosis with an inflammatory infiltrate and progressive calcium deposition [14]. Intervention is undertaken in symptomatic patients with severe disease and asymptomatic patients with severe disease and associated left ventricular impairment based on size and systolic function. Haemodynamic parameters that are assessed to grade severity include peak velocity (≥4 m/s), mean pressure gradient (≥40 mmHg) and aortic valve area (≤1.0 cm^2) [15].

Transthoracic echocardiography with Doppler has been the mainstay of aortic stenosis assessment and allows characterisation of aortic valve anatomy, function and haemodynamic and information regarding left ventricular mass and function. However, it does have limitations due to patient factors such as being unable to align exactly with the direction of maximal blood flow velocity and assessing left ventricular outflow tract diameter due to calcification and its oblong shape. 4D flow MRI may be of value to provide functional information regarding aortic stenosis. A study has compared TTE and 4D PC-MR to 2D PC-MR [16] and found 4D PC-MR to improve concordance of different aortic stenosis parameters including peak jet velocity, mean transvalvular pressure gradient and aortic valve area compared to echocardiography.

Echocardiography also continues to miss one third of people with left ventricular dysfunction as they have normal ejection fraction, a relatively insensitive echocardiography-derived quantitative marker [17]. 2D cardiac MR is the gold standard to assess LV volumes and patterns of ventricular remodelling (can still be of use with more accurate information on left ventricular characteristics [18, 19]). Importantly, it can provide an assessment of myocardial fibrosis, which results in heart failure and death secondary to aortic stenosis [20].

The earliest derived technique is late gadolinium enhancement (LGE) where post-contrast T1 sequences demonstrate areas of high T1 signal in areas of LGE demonstrates mid-wall replacement fibrosis and correlates with histological fibrosis [21] and high-sensitivity troponin I levels [22]. LGE is known to be an independent predictor of all-cause mortality with an eightfold risk of increased death [19, 23, 24]. It also has an added advantage of discovering other deposition patterns revealing other concomitant pathologies common in those with aortic stenosis such as myocardial infarction, which shows a subendocardial/transmural pattern [25].

Diffuse fibrosis is harder to detect by LGE due to the lack of normal adjacent myocardium to generate visual contrast. Other measures have been derived to allow T1 mapping where the signal from each voxel is calculated and can then be displayed as a colour map. These include native T1 relaxation time, post-contrast T1, partition coefficient (λ, ratio of T2 signal change (pre- and post-contrast) in the myocardium and blood pool, extracellular volume fraction (ECV, $\lambda \times (1 -$ haematocrit)) and fibrosis volume (ECV × end-diastolic volume) [26].

Extracellular volume fraction demonstrates good reproducibility and closely correlates with collagen volume fraction on histology [27–30]. However, given that ECV is relative to the mass of the left ventricle, balanced increase in both fibrosis and left ventricle mass, balanced increases cannot be detected. A review thus proposes that fibrosis volume may be a more accurate measure of absolute fibrosis [23] though this has yet to be investigated. Clinically, native T1 relaxation time and extracellular volume fraction have been extensively studied, but inhomogenously, and have yielded variable results with regard to prognosticating aortic stenosis patients.

There are subgroups of patient where routine markers of severity derived from echocardiography underestimate the degree of a disease. Certain subgroups of aortic stenosis will show low flow (stroke volume < 35 ml/m^2), discordant with low aortic valve area. Subtypes include the classic low flow-low gradient type where there is left ventricle systolic dysfunction and paradoxical low flow-low gradient where the ejection fraction is preserved. Low-dose dobutamine stress echocardiography can differentiate the classic low flow-low gradient aortic stenosis from a primarily ventricular pathology causing reduced contractility and is recommended in guidelines [12]. On induced stress, severe aortic stenosis causes an increased mean valve gradient with stable low cross-sectional area of the valve.

CT calcium scoring, namely, the Agatston score, is derived from gated non-contrast CT and may also aid differentiation in some of these subgroups. The Agatston score accounts for both weight and density and correlates well with the weight of calcium in specimens of explanted aortic valves [31]. Moreover, it closely correlates with echocardiogram-derived haemodynamic measures of aortic stenosis severity [14, 32, 33] with recent data indicating a role in prognostication.

Thresholds to stratify moderate and severe aortic stenosis have recently been proposed by a study of 451 patients, which were later applied to a larger cohort of 794 patients where they demonstrated strong positive predictive value with all-cause mortality. Moreover, the correlation increased with worsening ejection fraction and stenosis severity as detected by echocardiogram. These varied between men (≥2065 AU) and women (≥1274 AU) even accounting for different aortic valve areas (≥476 AU/cm^2) and (≥292 AU/cm^2) for both, respectively [34]. For paradoxical low flow-low gradient aortic stenosis, aortic valve CT calcium scoring, discussed below, may be beneficial to aid differentiation of this subgroup [35]. These patients may be higher risk and benefit from valve replacement [36] though more data is needed [37].

Functional imaging may also be useful for assessing calcification. In aortic stenosis, ^{18}F-fluoride acts as a marker of calcification activity with histological correlates to alkaline phosphatase and osteocalcin [38] and can predict where new areas of calcium will form. Uptake demonstrates a positive correlation with advanced aortic stenosis [39] and disease progression at 1–2 years [22, 40]. This may also be of value in better understanding the pathogenenesis of the condition. In aortic stenosis, higher levels of ^{18}F-FDG have been seen in patients compared to controls with a moderate correlation with disease severity. However, there is a caveat as myocardial uptake may contaminate the signal from the aortic valve [23].

Cardiac MR has also showed promise in a study of ex vivo explanted aortic valves where it demonstrated high sensitivity and specificity for identification of both calcification and fibrosis. Unfortunately, in vivo imaging of the valve using CMR is not possible due to leaflet motion [41]. In addition to determining severity, quantitative imaging derived from CT angiography or MR angiography may be of value for preoperative planning particularly for minimally invasive procedures as mentioned above. Recent data has shown that artificial intelligence algorithms may allow semiautomatic segmentation of characteristics such as the aortic valve area on CT angiography, with greater concordance with echocardiography measurements compared to manual segmentation [42]. Practically, most guidelines and thresholds are still centred completely around echocardiography. Thus, it does not appear that cross-sectional imaging will replace echocardiography in the near future.

Aortic Regurgitation

Transthoracic echocardiography is the gold standard [8] to assess valve morphology, aetiology, severity and left ventricular remodelling. However, the assessment is more complex. Macroscopic features, such as leaflet prolapse, poor leaflet closure (non-coaptation) and length and width of regurgitant death, contribute to assessment of severity [43]. These are used in conjunction with more quantitative measures of severity such as the ratio of regurgitant jet to the left ventricular outflow tract width (>65%) [44], rate of deceleration of aortic regurgitation Doppler jet (<200 ms) [43], diastolic flow reversal in the aorta with high end-diastolic velocity (>20 cm/s) [45] and regurgitant fraction (>50%) [46]. 2D cardiac MR may provide more accurate calculation of regurgitation volume and fraction with greater reproducibility than echocardiography but also demonstrates good concordance with echocardiography values. However, one study shows that a regurgitation fraction of greater than 33% predicted the need for surgery within 3 years.

Left ventricular end-systolic diameter of greater than 5.0 cm is associated with a 20% risk of progression or mortality [47]. Systolic impairment is a poor prognostic feature, and surgical intervention is recommended in asymptomatic disease with the presence of left ventricular dilatation [13]. 2D cardiac MR once again has a role in assessing left ventricular volumes and ejection fraction though its expense renders it a less widely utilised technique than echocardiography. However, left ventricular end-diastolic volumes of >246 ml have been associated with a high likelihood of future symptoms and surgery [48].

Aortic Aneurysm

Aortic aneurysm is a focal dilatation of the aorta involving all three layers of the aortic wall, intima, media and adventitia. Thoracic aneurysms most commonly occur in the sixth and seventh decades of life, more commonly affecting men two four times more than women. The clinically silent nature of this condition makes it challenging to truly estimate its prevalence and incidence. Clinical presentation is largely secondary to complications such as rupture or dissection, and many such cases are attributed to other causes, particularly when a postmortem examination is not carried out. Small studies have estimated the incidence as 10.4 cases per 100,000 patient-years [49]. These are most commonly degenerative in aetiology and can be associated with an abdominal aortic aneurysm in approximately 25% of cases. Risk factors are the same as those for atherosclerotic disease, namely, smoking, hypertension and hypercholesterolaemia [50].

The mean rate of aneurysm growth substantially varies but is reported as up to 0.4 cm per year [51]. Factors influencing the rate of growth include initial size or localisation but also concomitant presence of valve disease and connective tissue disease. Aneurysms are occult and thus may have a high morbidity. Symptoms do not develop until the aneurysm has expanded sufficiently to exert mass effect on other structures, erode into bone or until there are complications such as dissection or rupture. The risk of rupture and thoracic aneurysm size are closely linked, greater than 5 cm is 20%, greater than 6 cm is 40% and greater than 7 cm is over 50% [52]. Abdominal aortic aneurysms are similar in behaviour. Rupture has an incidence of 1–5% [53, 54] with a mortality rate of 81% [55]. Rupture is associated with enlargement and weakening of the aortic wall. Many have described pathological processes involving increased inflammatory infiltrate, extracellular matrix breakdown, changes in smooth muscle cell type in the aortic wall, oxidative stress and neovascularisation [56].

Elective surgical intervention for a patient without another underlying cardiovascular abnormality or connective tissue is at 5.0–5.5 cm [57–59]. The Yale Centre of Thoracic Aortic Disease recommends intervention at a growth rate of 1 cm or more per year or rapid aneurysm enlargement to that size. However, those with a bicuspid aortic valve, family history of early dissection coarctation, small adult body size (ratio of aortic area to body height > 10 cm^2/m) or a concomitant need for other cardiac surgery may undergo intervention at much smaller aortic diameters [58]. Intervention involves aortic stent graft implantation or open repair. Extensive research has gone into finding non-invasive predictors of expansion.

The role of CT in aneurysm evaluation is largely for assessment of aneurysm growth, which is usually undertaken by systematic measurements as outlined above. Determining maximum aorta dimension is vital, and this should include both true and false lumens. A cross-sectional image is generated perpendicular to the aortic centreline, as assessed in double-oblique multiplanar reformats. Moreover, CT provides a useful tool for operative planning for endovascular graft insertion.

A plethora of quantitative markers derived from MRI have been studied, which can be categorised as haemodynamic, molecular and wall biomarkers to attempt to predict the risk of progression. Unfortunately, the majority of studies have either been in animal models or small retrospective cohort studies and are beyond the scope of this review with limited prospective studies assessing meaningful clinical endpoints including growth, rupture or repair. Most studies have used 4D flow MRI to assess haemodynamic biomarkers whilst dynamic contrast-enhanced (DCE) MRI has been used to assess molecular and wall biomarkers. Another key technique used for wall biomarkers is MR elastography. However, none of these studies demonstrate a quantitative threshold for any of these biomarkers, which limits their use in clinical practice.

Laminar flow with consistent and high flow velocity is a necessity for normal arterial wall function. In contrast, vortex flow represents orthogonal flow deviation around a centreline through the aorta [1]. Small studies with MRI data have demonstrated a correlation between vortex flow and supra-physiological helix flow in those with a dilated ascending aorta, but also an association between the strength of both and aortic arch and descending aortic diameter [1, 60]. Marfan's syndrome patients have been shown to have an increased degree of vortex flow in the descending aorta, whilst high strength non-physiological helical flow was seen at the aortic root [61]. However, these studies have heavily relied on visual assessment or semi-quantitative assessment of flow in the aorta instead of using a standardised grading scale limiting reproducibility.

Arterial endothelial cells function as mechanoreceptors [62] and detect a specific amount of wall shear stress (WSS), which stimulate atheroprotective pathways. Wall shear stress is the force per unit cross-sectional area exerted by a boundary by a moving fluid and vice versa [63]. Low wall shear stress can result in dysfunctional regulation of endothelial cells, which can cause wall remodelling and dilatation. This is mostly estimated by near-wall-blood flow velocity gradient. One study looked at rupture stretch, the pressure required to rupture surgically resected aneurysmal tissue from ascending aortic aneurysm patients in vitro and found it to be correlated with time-averaged wall shear stress [64]. Low time-averaged wall shear stress thus is likely to be linked to decreased aneurysm wall strength. Similarly, lower peak systolic wall shear stress has been seen in patients with a dilated ascending aorta and also showed an inverse correlation with ascending aortic diameter [1]. Specifically, other studies have demonstrated lower peak systolic wall shear stress in patients with abdominal aortic aneurysms and in dilated segments of the aorta compared to non-dilated segments.

Limited prospective studies exist, though in a small cohort of 30, decreased wall shear stress was associated with a growth rate of 2 mm in six patients [65]. Oscillatory shear index (OSI) represents beat-to-beat variation in WSS, and when this parameter is high, it induces an inflammatory response and the generation of reactive oxygen species. High oscillatory shear index and low wall shear stress have been linked to atherogenesis, a key element of the pathogenesis of aneurysm formation [66].This may be through the upregulation of NADPH oxidase, production of reactive oxygen species and modification of low-density lipoprotein, a known precursor [67].

A correlation has been demonstrated between oscillatory shear index and ascending aorta [1] dilatation, whilst another study demonstrated higher OSI in infra-renal abdominal aortic aneurysms compared to adjacent non-dilated segments of the aorta [68]. Though another study found no difference comparing those with infra-renal aortic aneurysms and controls, both of a similar age and younger patients [69].

Flow stasis allows platelet adhesion and thrombus formation. This may have some potential as a quantitative marker, though correlation with abdominal aortic aneurysm progression has not truly been demonstrated. One study investigated the feasibility of three methods of analysing 4D flow MRI data: conventional volumetric residence time (VRT), mean velocity analysis (MVA) and particle travel distance (TDA) and found the latter had good agreement with flow visualisation [70].

Flow displacement is the distance from the centreline of the aorta in the proximal and tubular planes. This has been demonstrated to be higher in dilated aortic aneurysms versus non-dilated aortic aneurysms [71], and another prospective clinical study has shown that flow displacement rates of >5% were associated with diameter growth [66]. These studies have mainly centred around abdominal aortic aneurysms (AAAs), and the biomarkers studied include wall stiffness, wall microvasculature and late gadolinium enhancement. Wall stiffness is an indication of wall strength and distinct from wall shear stress. This is best evaluated by MR elastography, through the use of wave propagation, and allows assessment of aortic stiffness [72]. Peak stress and burst pressure are two metrics that are inversely proportional to aortic stiffness as calculated by MRE, which has been replicated in both human [73] and animal studies [74]. Aortic aneurysm development has been strongly associated with wall extracellular matrix degradation through matrix metalloproteinases, chronic inflammatory infiltrate and extensive neovascularisation [73].

Dynamic contrast-enhanced MRI (DCE-MRI) can be used to demonstrate contrast uptake and to calculate quantitative parameters such as the volume transfer constant of gadolinium into the extracellular space (K^{trans}). K^{trans} incorporates the permeability, microvascular flow and surface area of the microvasculature and shows a moderate correlation to the maximal AAA diameter [75]. Other DCE-MRI-derived parameters including the area under the curve for the initial enhancement slope and the gradient of the slope may be associated with growth rate, independent of the maximal diameter as demonstrated in one retrospective study [76].

Late gadolinium enhancement may act as a surrogate marker for inflammation and may indicate a greater risk of progression and rupture. PET-MRI was used to demonstrate that the presence of concomitant late gadolinium enhancement and FDG enhancement was related to aneurysm expansion rate [77].

Molecular Biomarkers

Inflammatory infiltrate has been demonstrated in end-stage abdominal aortic aneurysms, and symptoms appear to be more common in inflammatory abdominal aortic aneurysms [78]. The majority of work on molecular biomarkers has been in animal studies except a single study in humans on ultrasmall superparamagnetic particles of iron oxide.

USPIO are small particles between 10 and 30 nm in MRI contrast agents, which can persist in the blood stream and can be taken up by tissue macrophages [79]. The latter are key in the inflammatory process of AAAs. USPIO uptake has been demonstrated on T2* images, and histology demonstrated correlation with macrophage infiltration, which seemed to correlate with the rate of growth of AAAs [80]. A large prospective study replicated these results and also demonstrated correlation with rupture and death, but this was not independent of other clinical actors such as baseline AAA diameter [81].

Other newer contrast agents can also detect other important molecular markers linked to AAA progression [82] such as matrix metalloproteinases (MMP 2 [83], MMP9 [84], ADAMTS4 [85]) and key components of the cell wall such as elastin, specifically tropoelastin, which is produced by a dysfunctional matrix [86], and adventitial collagen [87]. Thus far, these have only been studied in animal models.

Predominantly similar radiotracers have been used with different cross-sectional imaging modalities in a handful of studies. However, there has been insufficient clinical data to try and establish true quantitative thresholds. ^{18}F-FDG PET/CT was the most common, whilst in one study, ^{18}F-NaF PET/CT and ^{18}F-FDG PET/MRI have been used [88]. The relationship between different radiotracers and clinical prognosis of AAA have had inconsistent results. For ^{18}F-FDG PET/CT, the majority of small cohort studies have demonstrated more negative than positive correlations, though it may be useful in predicting AAA growth rate in specific subgroups [89]. Unfortunately, ^{18}F-FDG PET is not specific, given that it accumulates in any cells metabolising glucose, including other processes, such as atherosclerosis [89]. ^{18}F-FDG PET/MRI has also been investigated by a single study. FDG hot spots (though not SUV_{max} or TBR_{max}) were correlated with recent AAA growth, whilst late gadolinium enhancement in the aneurysm wall was also correlated with an increased median growth rate [90]. A single study investigating ^{18}F-sodium fluoride PET/CT found a significant correlation between TBR_{max} and AAA expansion adjusted by known risk factors as well as clinical outcomes of repair and rupture [91]. Whilst it shows promise, more investigation is needed.

Repair and Complications

Endovascular aneurysm repair is the treatment of choice for aneurysmal disease given its better mortality compared to open surgical repair [92–94]. Type II endoleak is the most common type of endoleak [95] postoperatively, which is a retrograde filling of the sac following graft placement. Dynamic CT and MR imaging may show higher sensitivity for endoleak detection [96].

4D flow MRI shows promise to provide quantitative metrics that may aid in the diagnosis and management of type II endoleaks. One study demonstrated higher initial peak flow velocity and amplitude of dynamics of blood flow in the persistent vessels supplying those with unresolved type II endoleaks at 1 year [97] (Fig. 15.3).

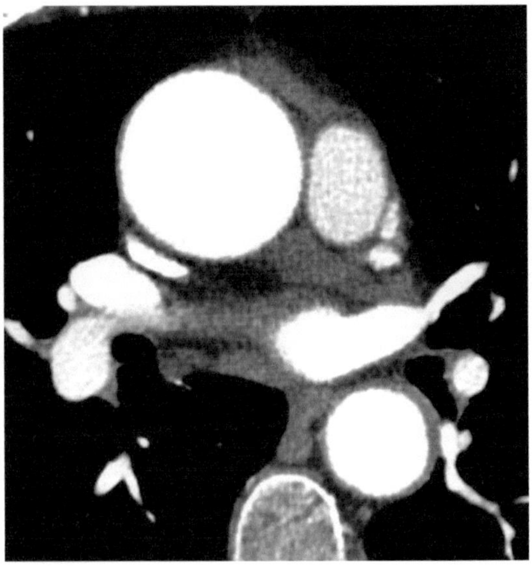

Fig. 15.3 Contrast-enhanced CT of the chest. Ascending aortic aneurysm

Acute Aortic Syndromes

Aortic Dissection

Aortic dissection occurs due to a tear in the intima creating a false passage. Acute Type A dissection is life threatening and necessitates imminent repair; thus, quantitative imaging unfortunately has a limited role to play (Figs. 15.4 and 15.5).

Type B aortic dissection involves the aorta distal to the origin of the brachiocephalic trunk. This can be defined as complicated, depending on the presence of aortic rupture, refractory pain, rapid aortic expansion, uncontrollable hypertension or malperfusion of vessels arising from the aorta or uncomplicated. Complicated Type B dissection has a significantly higher mortality of 16.1% versus 2.6% for uncomplicated [98]. This may impede blood to branches arising from the false lumen with subsequent solid organ ischaemia/infarction. The other possible complication is progressive enlargement of the pseudoaneurysm and rupture.

Treatment involves covering the primary tear with a stent graft to allow collapse of the false lumen and positive aortic remodelling. Imaging may occasionally reveal a more distal tear in addition to the one supplying the false lumen, and failure to cover this may require subsequent intervention.

Maximal aortic diameter is the main quantitative measure, which is associated with aortic complications, demonstrated in multiple studies [99]. An initial analysis supported a cut-off of 41 mm with a larger baseline aortic diameter being predictive of aortic enlargement [100]. Another metric with a strong evidence basis is the patency of the false lumen. Full thrombosis of the false lumen prevents blood entry, thereby reducing pressurisation and exerting a protective effect. In contrast, full patency allows ongoing pressurisation with remodelling and weakening of the outer wall of the false lumen [101]. Partial thrombosis may be the most high-risk state with a higher rate of aortic complications and patient mortality [102], though it is unclear when it may represent favourable adaptation. Measurements of the false lumen have been studied to gauge the development of aneurysmal growth; however, the majority of these lack substantial clinical evidence. Some studies have tried to generate quantitative metrics of high-risk false lumen characteristics, summarised in Table 15.1.

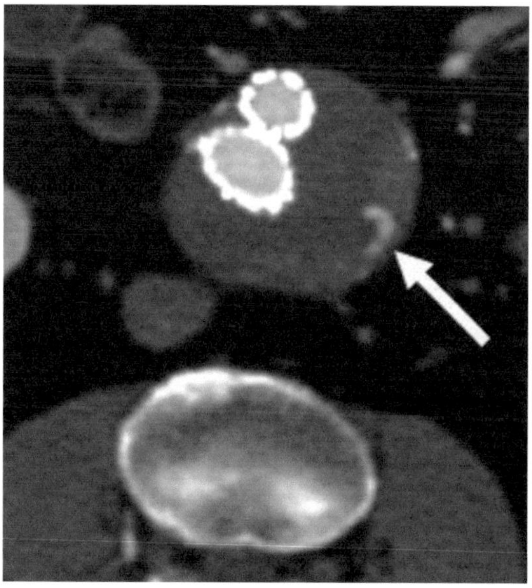

Fig. 15.4 Contrast-enhanced CT of the abdomen. Patient status post-endovascular aneurysm repair. White arrow shows filling of the aneurysm sac, secondary to a Type 2 endoleak

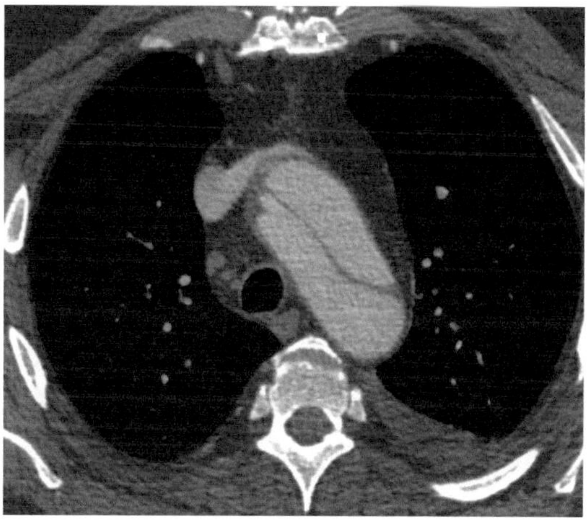

Fig. 15.5 Aortic dissection flap seen in the arch of the aorta on contrast-enhanced CT the chest

Primary entry tear location and size have been shown to inconsistently predict dissection-

Table 15.1 Quantitative measures predictive of progression of aortic aneurysm progression

Quantitative measure	Threshold	Implication
False aneurysm area [103]	≥922 m^2	Increased risk of complications: Limb ischaemia Dissection progression Rupture
True lumen compression [104] (TL/TL + FL)	<25%	Increase rate of dissection-related events but not mortality
TL volume/FL volume [105]	<0.8	Predictive of aortic intervention
FL structure and location [106]	Location: inner aortic curvature Shape: elliptical TL and saccular FL	Increased aortic growth rate
FL circumferential extent: angular distance in degrees between two FL insertion points on the intimal flap [107][a]	>249°	Predicts adverse events: Aortic rupture Rapid growth Aneurysm formation

TL true lumen, *FL* false lumen
[a]This parameter is unaffected by the variable position of the dissection flap

related adverse events and mortality. A value of 10 mm was described from a small cohort study with 85% sensitivity and 87% specificity. A more proximal location of tear was also associated with dissection-related adverse events [75]. However, another retrospective study showed no correlation between entry-tear distance from the left subclavian artery and the aortic growth rate, though single-entry tears were more commonly associated with high rates of aortic diameter [108].

More complex imaging techniques, namely, 3D reconstructed dynamic CT and MRI, are of limited use in clinical practice due to a small number of studies limited by heterogeneity of data and small sample sizes. Specific haemodynamic parameters and other metrics have been investigated by reconstructed CT images making 3D models of the aorta with computational models superimposed to simulate aortic flow in the true and false lumens. These can be used to calculate parameters from computational fluid dynamics. A few of the parameters and their key findings have been summarised in Table 15.2.

4D flow MRI has been able to characterise flow in the true and false lumens, fenestrations and entry tears and post-treatment assessment [90]. Larger primary entry tears have been positively correlated with overall flow, peak flow and flow velocities in the false lumen and are negatively correlated with true lumen flow velocity [118], paralleling CT findings. 4D flow MR has been shown to detect fenestrations more effectively than combined 2D MR and MRA [119]. Moreover, a small study found that higher net flow in the false lumen was associated with increased rate of aortic expansion. One study characterised the false lumen ejection fraction, a measure of retrograde flow at the dominant entry tear. In a small retrospective study, false lumen ejection fraction was increased in those with false lumen enlargement [120], with a subsequent follow-up study correlating this with aortic growth rate [121]. Another small study correlated false lumen ejection fraction and absolute pressure difference between the false lumen and ejection fraction as independent factors of aortic growth (≥3 mm/year) [122]. A complete discussion of all the studies and findings of quantitative metrics in animal models and in vitro models is beyond the scope of this chapter but has been reported elsewhere.

The SVS and STS have introduced updated reporting standards for Type B aortic dissection (TBAD), including a new classification system that standardises descriptions of aortic dissection [123]. The chronicity classification has been extended to over 90 days, replacing the previous range of 14–90 days. Additionally, a "high risk" category has been added to the acuity classification to better differentiate patient conditions.

Table 15.2 Summary of Parameters and associations

Parameter	Finding
Size of primary entry tear (mm)	Larger primary entry tear increases false lumen flow rate [109]
Number of re-entry tears	Decreased number of re-entry treats increases flow rate in the false lumen [110]
False lumen flow (%)	Elevated percentage total aortic flow passing through the false lumen is associated with increased risk of aneurysm formation and expansion [111]
Wall shear stress (WSS) (dyn/cm^2)	Increased WSS associated with aortic growth and risk of retrograde Type A aortic dissection [86, 112] Decreased WSS associated with increased FL thrombus formation [113]
Transluminal pressure gradient (cm^2/dyn)	Increased gradient corresponds to false lumen dilatation, tear propagation and increased risk of malperfusion [84, 114–116]

Adapted from Zilber et al. [117]

False lumen reporting has been refined, with "entry flow" now replacing "endoleak" to more accurately describe flow sources. The definition of aortic remodelling has also been clarified, with clearer criteria for positive and negative remodelling based on lumen size and aortic diameter. Aortic remodelling has been redefined for clarity, emphasizing that it should describe changes in the entire aorta, not just the stent graft area. Positive aortic remodelling is characterised by false lumen reduction without total aortic growth, true lumen expansion without total aortic growth or a reduction in total aortic diameter with variable changes in lumen size. Conversely, negative aortic remodelling is defined by the opposite changes or a failure to meet the criteria for positive remodelling. Overall, these updates aim to improve consistency in research and enhance clinical communication.

The TEM classification effectively addresses several limitations of prior systems by identifying "non-A, non-B" as a distinct category, thereby eliminating uncertainty and facilitating rapid decision-making in the emergency department. A comprehensive diagnostic evaluation is essential when applying the TEM system, as it supports the surgical team in providing the most appropriate management. The system highlights high-risk anatomical variants, such as Type A dissections with an entry point in the aortic arch, enabling clinicians to better assess risks and optimise survival outcomes. Additionally, it incorporates malperfusion status, allowing for accurate predictions of in-hospital mortality and promoting consideration of more aggressive treatment when indicated (Figs. 15.6 and 15.7, Table 15.3).

Intramural Haematoma and Penetrating Atherosclerotic Ulcer

Intramural haematoma occurs due to rupture of the vaso-vasorum, causing accumulation of blood in the intimal/medial layer without a tear. In contrast, penetrating atherosclerotic ulcer occurs secondary to atherosclerotic plaque erosion and inflammation, with resultant focal outpouching in the intimal layer to the internal elastic lamina. Whilst cross-sectional imaging has the potential to evaluate feeding vessels and blood pool, unfortunately ongoing research is still required (Fig. 15.8).

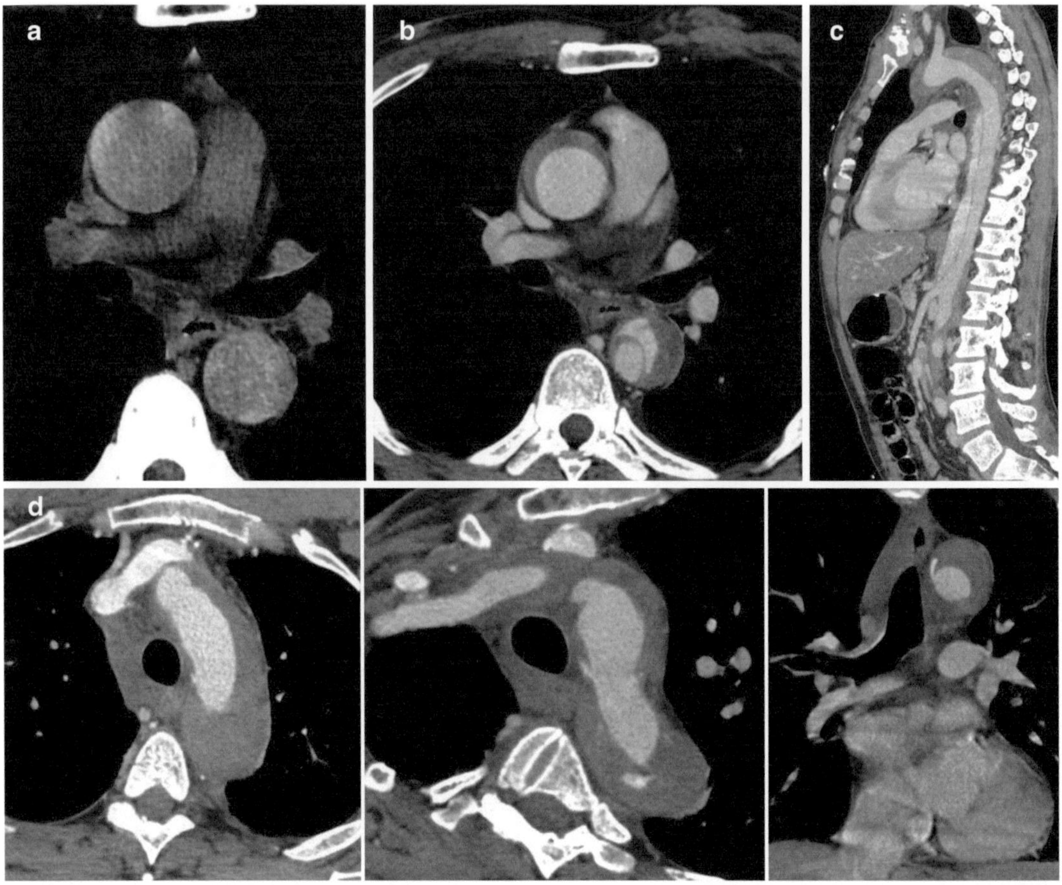

Fig. 15.6 (**a**) Showing IMH in the ascending and likely some IMH in descending. (**b**) Post contrast again showing IMH in the ascending with partially thrombosed dissection in descending. (**c**) Just showing extent of dissection

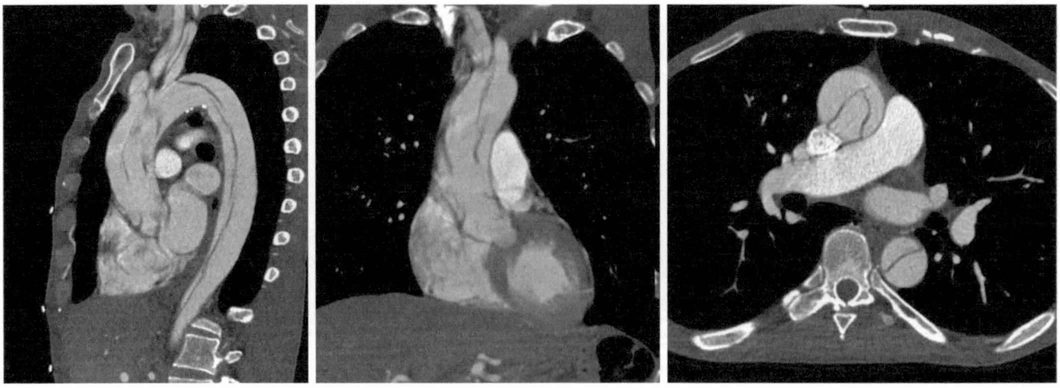

Fig. 15.7 D-upon close inspection, we see the actual tear of the dissection in the aortic arch on these axial, oblique sagittal, and oblique coronal images showing that this is really a type B dissection with retrograde extension rather than a type A sagittal, coronal, and axial images of a classic type A dissection with entry tear in the ascending aorta

Table 15.3 Combined TEM classification table for acute aortic dissection (AAD)

Category	Description
Type (T)	Defines if the dissection involves the *ascending aorta (A), descending aorta (B), or non-A, non-B*
Entry tear location (E)	*E0*: No visible tear
	E1: Ascending aorta
	E2: Aortic arch
	E3: Descending aorta
Malperfusion (M)	*M0*: No malperfusion
	M1: Coronary malperfusion (heart involvement)—*High mortality, requires emergency surgery for Type A E1 M1*
	M2: Supra-aortic malperfusion (brain involvement)
	M3: Visceral/renal/iliac malperfusion—*Non-A, non-B dissections often require the highest rate of aortic re-intervention*
Clinical implications	*Survival rates are lowest* in Type A dissections, especially with *entry tears in the arch (E2)*
	Total arch replacement is commonly required for *E2 and E3 cases*
	The *TEM system incorporates modern imaging and endovascular treatments*, improving diagnosis and outcome prediction

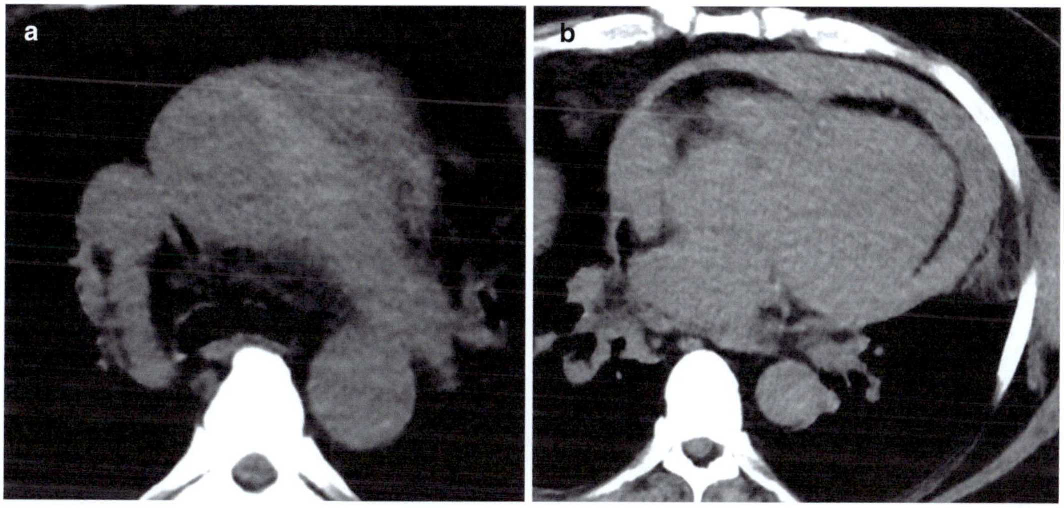

Fig. 15.8 (**a**) Showing IMH in the ascending/arch. (**b**) Non-contrast showing hemopericardium, concerning for signs of rupture

Coarctation of Aorta

Aortic coarctation is a congenital condition where there is a narrowing of the aorta, either before, at the level of or after the ligamentum arteriosum. This has implications for the risk of future aortic pathologies. The pressure gradient through the stenosis and post-stenotic loss of pressure guides treatment [124], generally when the systolic pressure gradient is >20 mmHg [125]. 4D flow MRI offers a non-invasive alternative to measure flow at variable points, whilst other conventionally used methods such as catheterisation and echocardiography are invasive and allow limited 3D visualisation, respectively. A study has shown good concordance in pressure measurements at five locations in the aorta between catheter angiography and 4D flow MRI [125]. Moreover, 4D flow MRI allows anatomical mapping of collaterals [123]. Overall, this technique holds promise for peri-operative assessment and management of aortic coarctation.

References

1. Freeman LA, Young PM, Foley TA, Williamson EE, Bruce CJ, Greason KL. CT and MRI assessment of the aortic root and ascending aorta. AJR Am J Roentgenol. 2013;200(6):W581–92. https://doi.org/10.2214/AJR.12.9531. PMID: 23701088.
2. Delgado V, Ng AC, van de Veire NR, van der Kley F, Schuijf JD, Tops LF, de Weger A, Tavilla G, de Roos A, Kroft LJ, Schalij MJ, Bax JJ. Transcatheter aortic valve implantation: role of multi-detector row computed tomography to evaluate prosthesis positioning and deployment in relation to valve function. Eur Heart J. 2010;31(9):1114–23. https://doi.org/10.1093/eurheartj/ehq018. Epub 2010 Feb 19. PMID: 20173197.
3. Messika-Zeitoun D, Serfaty JM, Brochet E, Ducrocq G, Lepage L, Detaint D, Hyafil F, Himbert D, Pasi N, Laissy JP, Iung B, Vahanian A. Multimodal assessment of the aortic annulus diameter: implications for transcatheter aortic valve implantation. J Am Coll Cardiol. 2010;55(3):186–94. https://doi.org/10.1016/j.jacc.2009.06.063. PMID: 20117398.
4. Burman ED, Keegan J, Kilner PJ. Aortic root measurement by cardiovascular magnetic resonance: specification of planes and lines of measurement and corresponding normal values. Circ Cardiovasc Imaging. 2008;1(2):104–13. https://doi.org/10.1161/CIRCIMAGING.108.768911. Epub 2008 Jul 30. PMID: 19808527.
5. Vasan RS, Larson MG, Benjamin EJ, Levy D. Echocardiographic reference values for aortic root size: the Framingham Heart Study. J Am Soc Echocardiogr. 1995;8(6):793–800. https://doi.org/10.1016/s0894-7317(05)80003-3. PMID: 8611279.
6. Amsallem M, Milleron DO, Jondeau G, Ou P. Comparative assessment of thoracic aortic aneurysms by trans-thoracic echocardiography versus computerized tomography. In: ESCR 2014 EPOS. 2014. https://epos.myesr.org/poster/escr/escr2014/416. Accessed 30 Aug 2024.
7. Nayak KS, Hargreaves BA, Hu BS, Nishimura DG, Pauly JM, Meyer CH. Spiral balanced steady-state free precession cardiac imaging. Magn Reson Med. 2005;53(6):1468–73. https://doi.org/10.1002/mrm.20489. PMID: 15906302.
8. Stankovic Z, Allen BD, Garcia J, Jarvis KB, Markl M. 4D flow imaging with MRI. Cardiovasc Diagn Ther. 2014;4(2):173–92. https://doi.org/10.3978/j.issn.2223-3652.2014.01.02. PMID: 24834414; PMCID: PMC3996243.
9. Bock J, Frydrychowicz A, Lorenz R, Hirtler D, Barker AJ, Johnson KM, Arnold R, Burkhardt H, Hennig J, Markl M. In vivo noninvasive 4D pressure difference mapping in the human aorta: phantom comparison and application in healthy volunteers and patients. Magn Reson Med. 2011;66(4):1079–88. https://doi.org/10.1002/mrm.22907. Epub 2011 Mar 24. Erratum in: Magn Reson Med. 2014 Aug;72(2):601. PMID: 21437978.
10. Stalder AF, Russe MF, Frydrychowicz A, Bock J, Hennig J, Markl M. Quantitative 2D and 3D phase contrast MRI: optimized analysis of blood flow and vessel wall parameters. Magn Reson Med. 2008;60(5):1218–31. https://doi.org/10.1002/mrm.21778. PMID: 18956416.
11. Irkle A, Vesey AT, Lewis DY, Skepper JN, Bird JL, Dweck MR, Joshi FR, Gallagher FA, Warburton EA, Bennett MR, Brindle KM, Newby DE, Rudd JH, Davenport AP. Identifying active vascular microcalcification by (18)F-sodium fluoride positron emission tomography. Nat Commun. 2015;6:7495. https://doi.org/10.1038/ncomms8495. PMID: 26151378; PMCID: PMC4506997.
12. Nkomo VT, Gardin JM, Skelton TN, Gottdiener JS, Scott CG, Enriquez-Sarano M. Burden of valvular heart diseases: a population-based study. Lancet. 2006;368(9540):1005–11. https://doi.org/10.1016/S0140-6736(06)69208-8. PMID: 16980116.
13. Vavilis G, Bäck M, Bárány P, Szummer K. Epidemiology of aortic stenosis/aortic valve replacement (from the Nationwide Swedish Renal Registry). Am J Cardiol. 2022;163:58–64. https://doi.org/10.1016/j.amjcard.2021.09.046. Epub 2021 Nov 16. PMID: 34799087.
14. Sverdlov AL, Ngo DT, Chapman MJ, Ali OA, Chirkov YY, Horowitz JD. Pathogenesis of aortic stenosis: not just a matter of wear and tear. Am J Cardiovasc Dis. 2011;1(2):185–99. Epub 2011 Jul 28. PMID: 22254198; PMCID: PMC3253493.
15. Otto CM, Nishimura RA, Bonow RO, Carabello BA, Erwin JP 3rd, Gentile F, Jneid H, Krieger EV, Mack M, McLeod C, O'Gara PT, Rigolin VH, Sundt TM 3rd, Thompson A, Toly C. 2020 ACC/AHA guideline for the management of patients with valvular heart disease: executive summary: a report of the American College of Cardiology/American Heart Association Joint Committee on clinical practice guidelines. Circulation. 2021;143(5):e35–71. https://doi.org/10.1161/CIR.0000000000000932. Epub 2020 Dec 17. Erratum in: Circulation. 2021 Feb 2;143(5):e228. doi: 10.1161/CIR.0000000000000960. Erratum in: Circulation. 2021 Mar 9;143(10):e784. doi: 10.1161/CIR.0000000000000966. PMID: 33332149.
16. Adriaans BP, Westenberg JJM, van Cauteren YJM, Gerretsen S, Elbaz MSM, Bekkers SCAM, Veenstra LF, Crijns HJGM, Wildberger JE, Schalla S. Clinical assessment of aortic valve stenosis: comparison between 4D flow MRI and transthoracic echocardiography. J Magn Reson Imaging. 2020;51(2):472–80. https://doi.org/10.1002/jmri.26847. Epub 2019 Jun 30. PMID: 31257647; PMCID: PMC7004028.
17. Cramariuc D, Cioffi G, Rieck AE, Devereux RB, Staal EM, Ray S, Wachtell K, Gerdts E. Low-flow aortic stenosis in asymptomatic patients: valvular-arterial impedance and systolic function from the SEAS substudy. JACC Cardiovasc Imaging.

2009;2(4):390–9. https://doi.org/10.1016/j.jcmg.2008.12.021. PMID: 19580719.
18. Armstrong AC, Gidding S, Gjesdal O, Wu C, Bluemke DA, Lima JA. LV mass assessed by echocardiography and CMR, cardiovascular outcomes, and medical practice. JACC Cardiovasc Imaging. 2012;5(8):837–48. https://doi.org/10.1016/j.jcmg.2012.06.003. PMID: 22897998; PMCID: PMC3501209.
19. Bellenger NG, Burgess MI, Ray SG, Lahiri A, Coats AJ, Cleland JG, Pennell DJ. Comparison of left ventricular ejection fraction and volumes in heart failure by echocardiography, radionuclide ventriculography and cardiovascular magnetic resonance; are they interchangeable? Eur Heart J. 2000;21(16):1387–96. https://doi.org/10.1053/euhj.2000.2011. PMID: 10952828.
20. Hein S, Arnon E, Kostin S, Schönburg M, Elsässer A, Polyakova V, Bauer EP, Klövekorn WP, Schaper J. Progression from compensated hypertrophy to failure in the pressure-overloaded human heart: structural deterioration and compensatory mechanisms. Circulation. 2003;107(7):984–91. https://doi.org/10.1161/01.cir.0000051865.66123.b7. PMID: 12600911.
21. Azevedo CF, Nigri M, Higuchi ML, Pomerantzeff PM, Spina GS, Sampaio RO, Tarasoutchi F, Grinberg M, Rochitte CE. Prognostic significance of myocardial fibrosis quantification by histopathology and magnetic resonance imaging in patients with severe aortic valve disease. J Am Coll Cardiol. 2010;56(4):278–87. https://doi.org/10.1016/j.jacc.2009.12.074. PMID: 20633819.
22. Chin CW, Shah AS, McAllister DA, Joanna Cowell S, Alam S, Langrish JP, Strachan FE, Hunter AL, Maria Choy A, Lang CC, Walker S, Boon NA, Newby DE, Mills NL, Dweck MR. High-sensitivity troponin I concentrations are a marker of an advanced hypertrophic response and adverse outcomes in patients with aortic stenosis. Eur Heart J. 2014;35(34):2312–21. https://doi.org/10.1093/eurheartj/ehu189. Epub 2014 May 14. PMID: 24829362; PMCID: PMC4156973.
23. Dweck MR, Joshi S, Murigu T, Alpendurada F, Jabbour A, Melina G, Banya W, Gulati A, Roussin I, Raza S, Prasad NA, Wage R, Quarto C, Angeloni E, Refice S, Sheppard M, Cook SA, Kilner PJ, Pennell DJ, Newby DE, Mohiaddin RH, Pepper J, Prasad SK. Midwall fibrosis is an independent predictor of mortality in patients with aortic stenosis. J Am Coll Cardiol. 2011;58(12):1271–9. https://doi.org/10.1016/j.jacc.2011.03.064. PMID: 21903062.
24. Barone-Rochette G, Piérard S, Meester D, de Ravenstein C, Seldrum S, Melchior J, Maes F, Pouleur AC, Vancraeynest D, Pasquet A, Vanoverschelde JL, Gerber BL. Prognostic significance of LGE by CMR in aortic stenosis patients undergoing valve replacement. J Am Coll Cardiol. 2014;64(2):144–54. https://doi.org/10.1016/j.jacc.2014.02.612. PMID: 25011718.
25. Everett RJ, Newby DE, Jabbour A, Fayad ZA, Dweck MR. The role of imaging in aortic valve disease. Curr Cardiovasc Imaging Rep. 2016;9:21. https://doi.org/10.1007/s12410-016-9383-z. Epub 2016 Jun 7. PMID: 27375833; PMCID: PMC4896976.
26. Higgins DM, Moon JC. Review of T1 mapping methods: comparative effectiveness including reproducibility issues. Curr Cardiovasc Imaging Rep. Springer US. 2014;7:1–10.
27. Flett AS, Hayward MP, Ashworth MT, Hansen MS, Taylor AM, Elliott PM, McGregor C, Moon JC. Equilibrium contrast cardiovascular magnetic resonance for the measurement of diffuse myocardial fibrosis: preliminary validation in humans. Circulation. 2010;122(2):138–44. https://doi.org/10.1161/CIRCULATIONAHA.109.930636. Epub 2010 Jun 28. PMID: 20585010.
28. Kammerlander AA, Marzluf BA, Zotter-Tufaro C, Aschauer S, Duca F, Bachmann A, Knechtelsdorfer K, Wiesinger M, Pfaffenberger S, Greiser A, Lang IM, Bonderman D, Mascherbauer J. T1 mapping by CMR imaging: from histological validation to clinical implication. JACC Cardiovasc Imaging. 2016;9(1):14–23. https://doi.org/10.1016/j.jcmg.2015.11.002. Epub 2015 Dec 9. PMID: 26684970.
29. Fontana M, White SK, Banypersad SM, Sado DM, Maestrini V, Flett AS, Piechnik SK, Neubauer S, Roberts N, Moon JC. Comparison of T1 mapping techniques for ECV quantification. Histological validation and reproducibility of ShMOLLI versus multibreath-hold T1 quantification equilibrium contrast CMR. J Cardiovasc Magn Reson. 2012;14(1):88. https://doi.org/10.1186/1532-429X-14-88. PMID: 23272651; PMCID: PMC3552758.
30. White SK, Sado DM, Fontana M, Banypersad SM, Maestrini V, Flett AS, Piechnik SK, Robson MD, Hausenloy DJ, Sheikh AM, Hawkins PN, Moon JC. T1 mapping for myocardial extracellular volume measurement by CMR: bolus only versus primed infusion technique. JACC Cardiovasc Imaging. 2013;6(9):955–62. https://doi.org/10.1016/j.jcmg.2013.01.011. Epub 2013 Apr 10. PMID: 23582361.
31. Messika-Zeitoun D, Aubry MC, Detaint D, Bielak LF, Peyser PA, Sheedy PF, Turner ST, Breen JF, Scott C, Tajik AJ, Enriquez-Sarano M. Evaluation and clinical implications of aortic valve calcification measured by electron beam computed tomography. Circulation. 2004;110(3):356–62. https://doi.org/10.1161/01.CIR.0000135469.82545.D0. Epub 2004 Jul 12. PMID: 15249504.
32. Cowell SJ, Newby DE, Burton J, White A, Northridge DB, Boon NA, Reid J. Aortic valve calcification on computed tomography predicts the severity of aortic stenosis. Clin Radiol. 2003;58(9):712–6. https://doi.org/10.1016/s0009-9260(03)00184-3. PMID: 12943644.
33. Cueff C, Serfaty J-M, Cimadevilla C, Laissy J-P, Himbert D, Tubach F, et al. Measurement of aor-

tic valve calcification using multislice computed tomography: correlation with haemodynamic severity of aortic stenosis and clinical implication for patients with low ejection fraction. Heart. BMJ Publishing Group Ltd and British Cardiovascular Society. 2011;97:721–6.

34. Clavel MA, Pibarot P, Messika-Zeitoun D, Capoulade R, Malouf J, Aggarval S, Araoz PA, Michelena HI, Cueff C, Larose E, Miller JD, Vahanian A, Enriquez-Sarano M. Impact of aortic valve calcification, as measured by MDCT, on survival in patients with aortic stenosis: results of an international registry study. J Am Coll Cardiol. 2014;64(12):1202–13. https://doi.org/10.1016/j.jacc.2014.05.066. PMID: 25236511; PMCID: PMC4391203.
35. Clavel MA, Messika-Zeitoun D, Pibarot P, Aggarwal SR, Malouf J, Araoz PA, Michelena HI, Cueff C, Larose E, Capoulade R, Vahanian A, Enriquez-Sarano M. The complex nature of discordant severe calcified aortic valve disease grading: new insights from combined Doppler echocardiographic and computed tomographic study. J Am Coll Cardiol. 2013;62(24):2329–38. https://doi.org/10.1016/j.jacc.2013.08.1621. Epub 2013 Sep 24. PMID: 24076528.
36. Dayan V, Vignolo G, Magne J, Clavel MA, Mohty D, Pibarot P. Outcome and impact of aortic valve replacement in patients with preserved LVEF and low-gradient aortic stenosis. J Am Coll Cardiol. 2015;66(23):2594–603. https://doi.org/10.1016/j.jacc.2015.09.076. PMID: 26670058.
37. Mehrotra P, Jansen K, Flynn AW, Tan TC, Elmariah S, Picard MH, Hung J. Differential left ventricular remodelling, and longitudinal function distinguishes low flow from normal-flow preserved ejection fraction low-gradient severe aortic stenosis. Eur Heart J. 2013;34(25):1906–14. https://doi.org/10.1093/eurheartj/eht094. Epub 2013 Mar 26. PMID: 23533186; PMCID: PMC3858103.
38. Dweck MR, Jenkins WS, Vesey AT, Pringle MA, Chin CW, Malley TS, Cowie WJ, Tsampasian V, Richardson H, Fletcher A, Wallace WA, Pessotto R, van Beek EJ, Boon NA, Rudd JH, Newby DE. 18F-sodium fluoride uptake is a marker of active calcification and disease progression in patients with aortic stenosis. Circ Cardiovasc Imaging. 2014;7(2):371–8. https://doi.org/10.1161/CIRCIMAGING.113.001508. Epub 2014 Feb 7. PMID: 24508669.
39. Dweck MR, Jones C, Joshi NV, Fletcher AM, Richardson H, White A, Marsden M, Pessotto R, Clark JC, Wallace WA, Salter DM, McKillop G, van Beek EJ, Boon NA, Rudd JH, Newby DE. Assessment of valvular calcification and inflammation by positron emission tomography in patients with aortic stenosis. Circulation. 2012;125(1):76–86. https://doi.org/10.1161/CIRCULATIONAHA.111.051052. Epub 2011 Nov 16. PMID: 22090163.
40. Jenkins WS, Vesey AT, Shah AS, Pawade TA, Chin CW, White AC, Fletcher A, Cartlidge TR, Mitchell AJ, Pringle MA, Brown OS, Pessotto R, McKillop G, Van Beek EJ, Boon NA, Rudd JH, Newby DE, Dweck MR. Valvular (18)F-fluoride and (18) F-fluorodeoxyglucose uptake predict disease progression and clinical outcome in patients with aortic stenosis. J Am Coll Cardiol. 2015;66(10):1200–1. https://doi.org/10.1016/j.jacc.2015.06.1325. PMID: 26338001.
41. Le Ven F, Tizón-Marcos H, Fuchs C, Mathieu P, Pibarot P, Larose E. Valve tissue characterization by magnetic resonance imaging in calcific aortic valve disease. Can J Cardiol. 2014;30(12):1676–83. https://doi.org/10.1016/j.cjca.2014.09.036. Epub 2014 Oct 7. PMID: 25475469.
42. Tuncay V, Prakken N, van Ooijen PM, Budde RP, Leiner T, Oudkerk M. Semiautomatic, quantitative measurement of aortic valve area using CTA: validation and comparison with transthoracic echocardiography. Biomed Res Int. 2015;2015:648283. https://doi.org/10.1155/2015/648283. Epub 2015 Jun 29. PMID: 26221603; PMCID: PMC4499628.
43. Lancellotti P, Tribouilloy C, Hagendorff A, Popescu BA, Edvardsen T, Pierard LA, Badano L, Zamorano JL, Scientific Document Committee of the European Association of Cardiovascular Imaging. Recommendations for the echocardiographic assessment of native valvular regurgitation: an executive summary from the European Association of Cardiovascular Imaging. Eur Heart J Cardiovasc Imaging. 2013;14(7):611–44. https://doi.org/10.1093/ehjci/jet105. Epub 2013 Jun 3. PMID: 23733442.
44. Perry GJ, Helmcke F, Nanda NC, Byard C, Soto B. Evaluation of aortic insufficiency by Doppler color flow mapping. J Am Coll Cardiol. 1987;9(4):952–9. https://doi.org/10.1016/s0735-1097(87)80254-1. PMID: 3558992.
45. Tribouilloy C, Avinée P, Shen WF, Rey JL, Slama M, Lesbre JP. End diastolic flow velocity just beneath the aortic isthmus assessed by pulsed Doppler echocardiography: a new predictor of the aortic regurgitant fraction. Br Heart J. 1991;65(1):37–40. https://doi.org/10.1136/hrt.65.1.37. PMID: 1993128; PMCID: PMC1024460.
46. Siani A, Perone F, Costantini P, Rodolfi S, Muscogiuri G, Sironi S, Carriero S, Pavon AG, van der Bilt I, van Rosendael P, Broekhuizen L, Teske A, Cramer MJ, Guglielmo M. Aortic regurgitation: a multimodality approach. J Clin Ultrasound. 2022;50(8):1041–50. https://doi.org/10.1002/jcu.23299. PMID: 36218214; PMCID: PMC9828136.
47. Bonow RO, Lakatos E, Maron BJ, Epstein SE. Serial long-term assessment of the natural history of asymptomatic patients with chronic aortic regurgitation and normal left ventricular systolic function. Circulation. 1991;84(4):1625–35. https://doi.org/10.1161/01.cir.84.4.1625. PMID: 1914102.
48. Myerson SG, d'Arcy J, Mohiaddin R, Greenwood JP, Karamitsos TD, Francis JM, Banning AP,

Christiansen JP, Neubauer S. Aortic regurgitation quantification using cardiovascular magnetic resonance: association with clinical outcome. Circulation. 2012;126(12):1452–60. https://doi.org/10.1161/CIRCULATIONAHA.111.083600. Epub 2012 Aug 9. PMID: 22879371.

49. Clouse WD, Hallett JW Jr, Schaff HV, Gayari MM, Ilstrup DM, Melton LJ 3rd. Improved prognosis of thoracic aortic aneurysms: a population-based study. JAMA. 1998;280(22):1926–9. https://doi.org/10.1001/jama.280.22.1926. PMID: 9851478.

50. Reed D, Reed C, Stemmermann G, Hayashi T. Are aortic aneurysms caused by atherosclerosis? Circulation. 1992;85(1):205–11. https://doi.org/10.1161/01.cir.85.1.205. PMID: 1728451.

51. Thompson SG, Brown LC, Sweeting MJ, the RESCAN Collaborators, et al. Systematic review and meta-analysis of the growth and rupture rates of small abdominal aortic aneurysms: implications for surveillance intervals and their cost-effectiveness. Health Technol Assess. 2013;17:1–118. Available from: https://www.ncbi.nlm.nih.gov/books/NBK261038/, https://doi.org/10.3310/hta17410.

52. De Backer J, Muiño-Mosquera L, Campens L. How to measure the aorta in the setting of genetic aortic disease. European Society of Cardiology. https://www.escardio.org/Councils/Council-on-Cardiovascular-Genomics/Cardiovascular-Genomics-Insight/Volume-3/how-to-measure-the-aorta-in-the-setting-of-genetic-aortic-disease.

53. Parkinson F, Ferguson S, Lewis P, Williams IM, Twine CP. South East Wales vascular network. Rupture rates of untreated large abdominal aortic aneurysms in patients unfit for elective repair. J Vasc Surg. 2015;61(6):1606–12. https://doi.org/10.1016/j.jvs.2014.10.023. Epub 2015 Feb 7. PMID: 25661721.

54. Powell JT, Sweeting MJ, Brown LC, Gotensparre SM, Fowkes FG, Thompson SG. Systematic review and meta-analysis of growth rates of small abdominal aortic aneurysms. Br J Surg. 2011;98(5):609–18. https://doi.org/10.1002/bjs.7465. Epub 2011 Mar 17. PMID: 21412998.

55. Reimerink JJ, van der Laan MJ, Koelemay MJ, Balm R, Legemate DA. Systematic review and meta analysis of population based mortality from ruptured abdominal aortic aneurysm. Br J Surg. 2013;100(11):1405–13. https://doi.org/10.1002/bjs.9235. PMID: 24037558.

56. Cho MJ, Lee MR, Park JG. Aortic aneurysms: current pathogenesis and therapeutic targets. Exp Mol Med. 2023;55(12):2519–30. https://doi.org/10.1038/s12276-023-01130-w. Epub 2023 Dec 1. PMID: 38036736, PMCID: PMC10766996.

57. Elefteriades JA. Indications for aortic replacement. J Thorac Cardiovasc Surg. 2010;140(6 Suppl):S5–9; discussion S45–51. https://doi.org/10.1016/j.jtcvs.2010.10.001. PMID: 21092797.

58. David TE. Surgical treatment of ascending aorta and aortic root aneurysms. Prog Cardiovasc Dis. 2010;52(5):438–44. https://doi.org/10.1016/j.pcad.2009.12.005. PMID: 20226961.

59. Coady MA, Rizzo JA, Hammond GL, Kopf GS, Elefteriades JA. Surgical intervention criteria for thoracic aortic aneurysms: a study of growth rates and complications. Ann Thorac Surg. 1999;67(6):1922–6; discussion 1953–8. https://doi.org/10.1016/s0003-4975(99)00431-2. PMID: 10391339.

60. Von Knobelsdorff-Brenkenhoff F, Trauzeddel RF, Barker AJ, et al. Blood flow characteristics in the ascending aorta after aortic valve replacement—a pilot study using 4D-flow MRI. Int J Cardiol. 2014;170(3):426–33.

61. Guala A, Teixido-Tura G, Dux-Santoy L, et al. Decreased rotational flow and circumferential wall shear stress as early markers of descending aorta dilation in Marfan syndrome: a 4D flow CMR study. J Cardiovasc Magn Reson. 2019;21(1):63.

62. Ando J, Yamamoto K. Vascular mechanobiology: endothelial cell responses to fluid shear stress. Circ J. 2009;73(11):1983–92. https://doi.org/10.1253/circj.cj-09-0583. Epub 2009 Oct 5. PMID: 19801852.

63. Katritsis D, Kaiktsis L, Chaniotis A, Pantos J, Efstathopoulos EP, Marmarelis V. Wall shear stress: theoretical considerations and methods of measurement. Prog Cardiovasc Dis. 2007;49(5):307–29. https://doi.org/10.1016/j.pcad.2006.11.001. PMID: 17329179.

64. Condemi F, Campisi S, Viallon M, et al. Relationship between ascending thoracic aortic aneurysms hemodynamics and biomechanical properties. IEEE Trans Biomed Eng. 2020;67(4):949–56.

65. Korpela T, Kauhanen SP, Kariniemi E, et al. Flow displacement and decreased wall shear stress might be associated with the growth rate of an ascending aortic dilatation. Eur J Cardiothorac Surg. 2022;61(2):395–402.

66. Takehara Y, Isoda H, Takahashi M, Unno N, Shiiya N, Ushio T, Goshima S, Naganawa S, Alley M, Wakayama T, Nozaki A. Abnormal flow dynamics result in low wall shear stress and high oscillatory shear index in abdominal aortic dilatation: initial in vivo assessment with 4D-flow MRI. Magn Reson Med Sci. 2020;19(3):235–46. https://doi.org/10.2463/mrms.mp.2019-0188. Epub 2020 Jul 13. PMID: 32655086; PMCID: PMC7553816.

67. Hwang J, Ing MH, Salazar A, Lassègue B, Griendling K, Navab M, Sevanian A, Hsiai TK. Pulsatile versus oscillatory shear stress regulates NADPH oxidase subunit expression: implication for native LDL oxidation. Circ Res. 2003;93(12):1225–32. https://doi.org/10.1161/01.RES.0000104087.29395.66. Epub 2003 Oct 30. PMID: 14593003; PMCID. PMC4433384.

68. Takehara Y, Isoda H, Takahashi M, et al. Abnormal flow dynamics result in low wall shear stress and high oscillatory shear index in abdominal aortic

dilatation: initial in vivo assessment with 4D-flow MRI. Magn Reson Med Sci. 2020;19(3):235–46.
69. Trenti C, Ziegler M, Bjarnegård N, et al. Wall shear stress and relative residence time as potential risk factors for abdominal aortic aneurysms in males: a 4D flow cardiovascular magnetic resonance case–control study. J Cardiovasc Magn Reson. 2022;24(1):18.
70. Ziegler M, Welander M, Lantz J, et al. Visualizing and quantifying flow stasis in abdominal aortic aneurysms in men using 4D flow MRI. Magn Reson Imaging. 2019;57:103–10.
71. Kauhanen SP, Hedman M, Kariniemi E, et al. Aortic dilatation associates with flow displacement and increased circumferential wall shear stress in patients without aortic stenosis: a prospective clinical study. J Magn Reson Imaging. 2019;50(1):136–45.
72. Kolipaka A, Illapani VS, Kenyhercz W, et al. Quantification of abdominal aortic aneurysm stiffness using magnetic resonance elastography and its comparison to aneurysm diameter. J Vasc Surg. 2016;64(4):966–74.
73. Reeps C, Pelisek J, Seidl S, Schuster T, Zimmermann A, Kuehnl A, Eckstein HH. Inflammatory infiltrates and neovessels are relevant sources of MMPs in abdominal aortic aneurysm wall. Pathobiology. 2009;76(5):243–52. https://doi.org/10.1159/000228900. Epub 2009 Oct 2. PMID: 19816084.
74. Dong H, Russell DS, Litsky AS, et al. In vivo aortic magnetic resonance elastography in abdominal aortic aneurysm: a validation in an animal model. Investig Radiol. 2020;55(7):463–72.
75. Nguyen VL, Backes WH, Kooi ME, et al. Quantification of abdominal aortic aneurysm wall enhancement with dynamic contrast-enhanced MRI: feasibility, reproducibility, and initial experience. J Magn Reson Imaging. 2014;39(6):1449–56.
76. Zhou A, Leach JR, Zhu C, et al. Dynamic contrast-enhanced MRI in abdominal aortic aneurysms as a potential marker for disease progression. J Magn Reson Imaging. 2023;58:1258–67.
77. Kuzniar M, Tegler G, Wanhainen A, et al. Feasibility of assessing inflammation in asymptomatic abdominal aortic aneurysms with integrated 18F-fluorodeoxyglucose positron emission tomography/magnetic resonance imaging. Eur J Vasc Endovasc Surg. 2020;59(3):464–71.
78. Choke E, Thompson MM, Dawson J, et al. Abdominal aortic aneurysm rupture is associated with increased medial neovascularization and overexpression of proangiogenic cytokines. Arterioscler Thromb Vasc Biol. 2006;26(9):2077–82.
79. Trivedi RA, Mallawarachi C, U-King-Im JM, et al. Identifying inflamed carotid plaques using in vivo USPIO-enhanced MR imaging to label plaque macrophages. Arterioscler Thromb Vasc Biol. 2006;26(7):1601–6.
80. Richards JM, Semple SI, MacGillivray TJ, et al. Abdominal aortic aneurysm growth predicted by uptake of ultrasmall superparamagnetic particles of iron oxide: a pilot study. Circ Cardiovasc Imaging. 2011;4(3):274–81.
81. The MA3RS Study Investigators. Aortic wall inflammation predicts abdominal aortic aneurysm expansion, rupture, and need for surgical repair. Circulation. 2017;136(9):787–97.
82. Rabkin SW. The role matrix metalloproteinases in the production of aortic aneurysm. Prog Mol Biol Transl Sci. 2017;147:239–65.
83. Chew DK, Orshal JM, Khalil RA. Elastase-induced suppression of endothelin-mediated ca2+ entry mechanisms of vascular contraction. Hypertension. 2003;42(4):818–24.
84. Chew DK, Conte MS, Khalil RA. Matrix metalloproteinase-specific inhibition of ca2+ entry mechanisms of vascular contraction. J Vasc Surg. 2004;40(5):1001–10.
85. Kaufmann JO, Brangsch J, Kader A, et al. ADAMTS4-specific MR probe to assess aortic aneurysms in vivo using synthetic peptide libraries. Nat Commun. 2022;13(1):2867.
86. Lavin B, Lacerda S, Andia ME, et al. Tropoelastin: an in vivo imaging marker of dysfunctional matrix turnover during abdominal aortic dilation. Cardiovasc Res. 2020;116(5):995–1005.
87. Adams LC, Brangsch J, Reimann C, et al. Simultaneous molecular MRI of extracellular matrix collagen and inflammatory activity to predict abdominal aortic aneurysm rupture. Sci Rep. 2020;10(1):15206.
88. Baolei G, Can C, Peng L, Yan S, Cheng Y, Hui T, Minzhi L, Daqiao G, Weiguo F. Molecular imaging of abdominal aortic aneurysms with positron emission tomography: a systematic review. Eur J Vasc Endovasc Surg. 2021;62(6):969–80. https://doi.org/10.1016/j.ejvs.2021.08.010. Epub 2021 Oct 22. PMID: 34696984.
89. Tarkin JM, Joshi FR, Rudd JH. PET imaging of inflammation in atherosclerosis. Nat Rev Cardiol. 2014;11(8):443–57. https://doi.org/10.1038/nrcardio.2014.80. Epub 2014 Jun 10. PMID: 24913061.
90. Kuzniar M, Tegler G, Wanhainen A, Ahlström H, Mani K, Hansen T. Feasibility of assessing inflammation in asymptomatic abdominal aortic aneurysms with integrated 18F-fluorodeoxyglucose positron emission tomography/magnetic resonance imaging. Eur J Vasc Endovasc Surg. 2020;59(3):464–71. https://doi.org/10.1016/j.ejvs.2019.04.004. Epub 2019 Nov 8. PMID: 31708339.
91. Forsythe RO, Dweck MR, McBride OMB, Vesey AT, Semple SI, Shah ASV, Adamson PD, Wallace WA, Kaczynski J, Ho W, van Beek EJR, Gray CD, Fletcher A, Lucatelli C, Marin A, Burns P, Tambyraja A, Chalmers RTA, Weir G, Mitchard N, Tavares A, Robson JMJ, Newby DE. 18F-sodium fluoride uptake in abdominal aortic aneurysms: the SoFIA3 study. J Am Coll Cardiol. 2018;71(5):513–23. https://doi.org/10.1016/j.jacc.2017.11.053. PMID: 29406857; PMCID: PMC5800891.

92. United Kingdom EVAR Trial Investigators, Greenhalgh RM, Brown LC, Powell JT, Thompson SG, Epstein D, Sculpher MJ. Endovascular versus open repair of abdominal aortic aneurysm. N Engl J Med. 2010;362(20):1863–71. https://doi.org/10.1056/NEJMoa0909305. Epub 2010 Apr 11. PMID: 20382983.
93. Prinssen M, Verhoeven EL, Buth J, Cuypers PW, van Sambeek MR, Balm R, Buskens E, Grobbee DE, Blankensteijn JD, Dutch Randomized Endovascular Aneurysm Management (DREAM) Trial Group. A randomized trial comparing conventional and endovascular repair of abdominal aortic aneurysms. N Engl J Med. 2004;351(16):1607–18. https://doi.org/10.1056/NEJMoa042002. PMID: 15483279.
94. Lederle FA, Kyriakides TC, Stroupe KT, Freischlag JA, Padberg FT Jr, Matsumura JS, Huo Z, Johnson GR, OVER Veterans Affairs Cooperative Study Group. Open versus endovascular repair of abdominal aortic aneurysm. N Engl J Med. 2019;380(22):2126–35. https://doi.org/10.1056/NEJMoa1715955. PMID: 31141634.
95. Marchiori A, von Ristow A, Guimaraes M, Schönholz C, Uflacker R. Predictive factors for the development of type II endoleaks. J Endovasc Ther. 2011;18(3):299–305. https://doi.org/10.1583/10-3116.1. PMID: 21679064.
96. Sakata M, Takehara Y, Katahashi K, Sano M, Inuzuka K, Yamamoto N, Sugiyama M, Sakahara H, Wakayama T, Alley MT, Konno H, Unno N. Hemodynamic analysis of Endoleaks after endovascular abdominal aortic aneurysm repair by using 4-dimensional flow-sensitive magnetic resonance imaging. Circ J. 2016;80(8):1715–25. https://doi.org/10.1253/circj.CJ-16-0297. Epub 2016 Jun 29. PMID: 27357219.
97. Katahashi K, Sano M, Takehara Y, Inuzuka K, Sugiyama M, Alley MT, Takeuchi H, Unno N. Flow dynamics of type II endoleaks can determine sac expansion after endovascular aneurysm repair using four-dimensional flow-sensitive magnetic resonance imaging analysis. J Vasc Surg. 2019;70(1):107–116.e1. https://doi.org/10.1016/j.jvs.2018.09.048. Epub 2019 Feb 18. PMID: 30792053.
98. Afifi RO, Sandhu HK, Leake SS, Boutrous ML, Kumar V 3rd, Azizzadeh A, Charlton-Ouw KM, Saqib NU, Nguyen TC, Miller CC 3rd, Safi HJ, Estrera AL. Outcomes of patients with acute type B (DeBakey III) aortic dissection: a 13-year, single-center experience. Circulation. 2015;132(8):748–54. https://doi.org/10.1161/CIRCULATIONAHA.115.015302. PMID: 26304666; PMCID: PMC4548541.
99. Spinelli D, Benedetto F, Donato R, et al. Current evidence in predictors of aortic growth and events in acute type B aortic dissection. J Vasc Surg. 2018;68(6):1925–1935.e8.
100. Kato M, Bai H, Sato K, et al. Determining surgical indications for acute type B dissection based on enlargement of aortic diameter during the chronic phase. Circulation. 1995;92(9 Suppl):II107–12.
101. Kunishige H, Myojin K, Ishibashi Y, Ishii K, Kawasaki M, Oka J. Predictors of surgical indications for acute type B aortic dissection based on enlargement of aortic diameter during the chronic phase. Jpn J Thorac Cardiovasc Surg. 2006;54(11):477–82.
102. Tsai TT, Evangelista A, Nienaber CA, et al. Partial thrombosis of the false lumen in patients with acute type B aortic dissection. N Engl J Med. 2007;357(4):349–59.
103. Chang CP, Liu JC, Liou YM, Chang SS, Chen JY. The role of false lumen size in prediction of in-hospital complications after acute type B aortic dissection. J Am Coll Cardiol. 2008;52(14):1170–6.
104. Evangelista A, Salas A, Ribera A, et al. Long-term outcome of aortic dissection with patent false lumen: predictive role of entry tear size and location. Circulation. 2012;125(25):3133–41.
105. Lavingia KS, Larion S, Ahanchi SS, et al. Volumetric analysis of the initial index computed tomography scan can predict the natural history of acute uncomplicated type B dissections. J Vasc Surg. 2015;62(4):893–89. [Published correction appears in J Vasc Surg 2016;63(4):1133.].
106. Tolenaar JL, van Keulen JW, Jonker FH, et al. Morphologic predictors of aortic dilatation in type B aortic dissection. J Vasc Surg. 2013;58(5):1220–5.
107. Sailer AM, van Kuijk SM, Nelemans PJ, et al. Computed tomography imaging features in acute uncomplicated Stanford type-B aortic dissection predict late adverse events. Circ Cardiovasc Imaging. 2017;10(4):e005709.
108. Tolenaar JL, van Keulen JW, Trimarchi S, et al. Number of entry tears is associated with aortic growth in type B dissections. Ann Thorac Surg. 2013;96(1):39–42.
109. Cheng Z, Wood NB, Gibbs RG, Xu XY. Geometric and flow features of type B aortic dissection: initial findings and comparison of medically treated and stented cases. Ann Biomed Eng. 2015;43(1):177–89.
110. Ben Ahmed S, Dillon-Murphy D, Figueroa CA. Computational study of anatomical risk factors in idealized models of type B aortic dissection. Eur J Vasc Endovasc Surg. 2016;52(6):736–45.
111. Shang EK, Nathan DP, Fairman RM, et al. Use of computational fluid dynamics studies in predicting aneurysmal degeneration of acute type B aortic dissections. J Vasc Surg. 2015;62(2):279–84.
112. Osswald A, Karmonik C, Anderson JR, et al. Elevated wall shear stress in aortic type B dissection may relate to retrograde aortic type A dissection: a computational fluid dynamics pilot study. Eur J Vasc Endovasc Surg. 2017;54(3):324–30.
113. Menichini C, Xu XY. Mathematical modeling of thrombus formation in idealized models of aortic dissection: initial findings and potential applications. J Math Biol. 2016;73(5):1205–26.
114. Munshi B, Parker LP, Norman PE, Doyle BJ. The application of computational modeling for risk

prediction in type B aortic dissection. J Vasc Surg. 2020;71(5):1789–1801.e3.
115. Zhang Y, Lu Q, Feng J, et al. A pilot study exploring the mechanisms involved in the longitudinal propagation of acute aortic dissection through computational fluid dynamic analysis. Cardiology. 2014;128(2):220–5.
116. Tse KM, Chiu P, Lee HP, Ho P. Investigation of hemodynamics in the development of dissecting aneurysm within patient-specific dissecting aneurismal aortas using computational fluid dynamics (CFD) simulations. J Biomech. 2011;44(5):827–36.
117. Zilber ZA, Boddu A, Malaisrie SC, Hoel AW, Mehta CK, Vassallo P, Burris NS, Roldán-Alzate A, Collins JD, François CJ, Allen BD. Noninvasive morphologic and hemodynamic evaluation of type B aortic dissection: state of the art and future perspectives. Radiol Cardiothorac Imaging. 2021;3(3):e200456. https://doi.org/10.1148/ryct.2021200456. PMID: 34235440; PMCID: PMC8250421.
118. Liu D, Fan Z, Li Y, et al. Quantitative study of abdominal blood flow patterns in patients with aortic dissection by 4-dimensional flow MRI. Sci Rep. 2018;8(1):9111.
119. Allen BD, Aouad PJ, Burris NS, et al. Detection and hemodynamic evaluation of flap fenestrations in type B aortic dissection with 4D flow MRI: comparison with conventional MRI and CT angiography. Radiol Cardiothorac Imaging. 2019;1(1):e180009.
120. Burris NS, Nordsletten DA, Sotelo JA, et al. False lumen ejection fraction predicts growth in type B aortic dissection: preliminary results. Eur J Cardiothorac Surg. 2020;57(5):896–903.
121. Burris NS, Patel HJ, Hope MD. Retrograde flow in the false lumen: marker of a false lumen under stress? J Thorac Cardiovasc Surg. 2019;157(2):488–91.
122. Marlevi D, Sotelo JA, Grogan-Kaylor R, Ahmed Y, Uribe S, Patel HJ, Edelman ER, Nordsletten DA, Burris NS. False lumen pressure estimation in type B aortic dissection using 4D flow cardiovascular magnetic resonance: comparisons with aortic growth. J Cardiovasc Magn Reson. 2021;23(1):51. https://doi.org/10.1186/s12968-021-00741-4. PMID: 33980249; PMCID: PMC8117268.
123. Lombardi JV, Hughes GC, Appoo JJ, Bavaria JE, Beck AW, Cambria RP, Charlton-Ouw K, Eslami MH, Kim KM, Leshnower BG, Maldonado T, Reece TB, Wang GJ. Society for Vascular Surgery (SVS) and Society of Thoracic Surgeons (STS) reporting standards for type B aortic dissections. J Vasc Surg. 2020;71(3):723–47. https://doi.org/10.1016/j.jvs.2019.11.013. Epub 2020 Jan 27. PMID: 32001058.
124. Riesenkampff E, Fernandes JF, Meier S, et al. Pressure fields by flow-sensitive, 4D, velocity-encoded CMR in patients with aortic coarctation. JACC Cardiovasc Imaging. 2014;7(9):920–6. https://doi.org/10.1016/j.jcmg.2014.03.017.
125. Burris NS, Hope MD. 4D flow MRI applications for aortic disease. Magn Reson Imaging Clin N Am. 2015;23(1):15–23. https://doi.org/10.1016/j.mric.2014.08.006.

Pulmonary Hypertension

16

Julia Niemierko, Katarzyna Sienkiewicz, Wojciech Cytawa, and Jadwiga Fijałkowska

Pathophysiology of Pulmonary Hypertension

Pulmonary hypertension is a complex and progressive disorder characterized by increased pressure in pulmonary circulation, leading to right heart dysfunction and potentially fatal complications. It is defined by a mean pulmonary arterial pressure (mPAP) greater than 20 mmHg at rest during right heart catheterization. The European Society of Cardiology (ESC) has classified pulmonary hypertension into five groups based on similar pathophysiological mechanisms, clinical presentation, hemodynamic characteristics, and therapeutic management [23].

These groups are as follows:

- Group 1: Pulmonary arterial hypertension (PAH)—primarily affects the small pulmonary arteries and is characterized by increased vascular resistance. It includes idiopathic PAH, hereditary PAH, and PAH associated with various conditions such as connective tissue disorders, congenital heart diseases, HIV infection, and drug/toxin exposure.
- Group 2: PH due to left heart disease—occurs as a result of left-sided heart conditions, such as heart failure with reduced ejection fraction, valvular heart diseases, or left ventricular diastolic dysfunction. Increased left atrial pressure is transmitted to the pulmonary circulation, leading to PH.
- Group 3: PH due to lung diseases and/or hypoxia—includes PH associated with chronic obstructive pulmonary disease (COPD), interstitial lung diseases, sleep-disordered breathing, and other lung disorders. Hypoxia, inflammation, and remodeling of the pulmonary vasculature contribute to the development of PH.
- Group 4: Chronic thromboembolic pulmonary hypertension (CTEPH)—is a unique form of PH caused by chronic thromboembolic occlusion of pulmonary arteries. It is a consequence of unresolved or recurrent pulmonary embolism. Surgical or interventional treatment may be necessary to alleviate the obstruction and improve pulmonary hemodynamics.
- Group 5: PH with unclear and/or multifactorial mechanisms—encompasses PH conditions that do not fit into the previous categories or have overlapping features. It includes PH associated with blood, systemic, and metabolic disorders.

J. Niemierko (✉) · K. Sienkiewicz
Department of Radiology, Medical University Hospital of Gdańsk, Gdańsk, Poland

W. Cytawa
Department of Nuclear Medicine, Medical University of Gdańsk, Gdańsk, Poland

J. Fijałkowska
2nd Department of Radiology, Medical University of Gdańsk, Gdańsk, Poland

R. Gill, P. Rajiah (eds.), *Quantitative Imaging in the Thorax*,
https://doi.org/10.1007/978-3-032-14103-3_16

Cardiopulmonary Interactions

In its natural state, arterial pulmonary circulation is low-resistance low-pressure system. Pulmonary arteries larger than 1 mm are predominantly composed of parallel elastic laminae, which results in small resistance. Their high compliance allows them to accommodate cardiac output with very little blood pressure fluctuation, and it maximizes distribution of blood to the peripheral alveoli. These features ultimately allow for proper gas exchange. In arteries smaller than 1 mm, the wall gradually includes more smooth muscles; capillary and precapillary arteries contribute significantly to the pulmonary vascular resistance (PVR) and are the site of the greatest pressure drop within the pulmonary circulation.

Pulmonary hypertension (PH) leads to a wide range of anatomical changes in the pulmonary vasculature and interdependent structures. Persistent elevation in pulmonary arterial pressure triggers structural remodeling of the pulmonary vessels. These changes collectively result in the narrowing and occlusion of the small pulmonary arteries, contributing to increased vascular resistance and impaired blood flow [22]. Vascular remodeling leads to increased PA stiffness and decreased compliance. As a result, pressure and resistance in the pulmonary circulation rises. In consequence, the pulmonary arteries get dilated to compensate for the changes in the pulmonary flow. Initially, there is no change in right ventricular geometry and function (asymptomatic compensated state). With time, increased pulmonary arterial pressure and vascular resistance impose a significant afterload on the right ventricle. The right ventricle initially undergoes adaptive changes, such as hypertrophy and remodeling, to maintain cardiac output against the increased pulmonary vascular resistance. However, chronic pressure overload and remodeling eventually lead to right ventricular dilation, impaired contractility, and right heart failure. This maladaptive response contributes to disease progression and poor clinical outcome in PH patients [60].

Cardiopulmonary interactions in PH involve various mechanisms, including ventricular interdependence, altered left ventricular filling, and abnormal cardiac output distribution. Ventricular interdependence refers to the close anatomical and functional relationship between the right and left ventricles. In PH, increased right ventricular pressure and volume overload can impede left ventricular diastolic filling, leading to reduced left ventricular stroke volume and cardiac output. This impaired left ventricular function can further exacerbate right ventricular dysfunction [13].

Abnormal gas exchange is another crucial aspect of cardiopulmonary interactions in PH. The disease process leads to ventilation-perfusion mismatch, reduced pulmonary capillary bed, and impaired oxygen diffusion in the lungs [22]. These abnormalities result in decreased oxygenation and exercise intolerance, further compromising cardiac function and overall exercise capacity in PH patients.

Additionally, pulmonary vascular remodeling and endothelial dysfunction in PH can lead to altered production and release of vasoactive substances. These substances, such as endothelin-1 and nitric oxide, play critical roles in regulating vascular tone and systemic hemodynamics. Imbalances in their production contribute to pulmonary vasoconstriction, pulmonary arterial remodeling, and impaired vasodilation, further exacerbating the cardiopulmonary interactions in PH [21].

Imaging Algorithm

PH is a complex disease with diverse etiologies and a wide range of radiological manifestations. Initial suspicion of PH often arises from observations on chest radiography, where notable findings include enlarged right heart and pulmonary arteries, as well as an elevated cardiac apex. Furthermore, radiographic features related to underlying causes, such as interstitial lung disease, may be apparent.

When proximal pulmonary and cardiac enlargement is evident on chest radiography, patients are frequently referred for echocardiography, a noninvasive imaging modality capable of identifying cardiac causes of PH. If echocardiography reveals the presence of cardiac shunts, further evaluation through MRI is warranted.

In cases where underlying lung disease is suspected, patients are typically directed toward high-resolution computed tomography (HRCT) or CT pulmonary angiography (CTPA) for a comprehensive assessment. These imaging techniques provide detailed information about lung parenchyma and pulmonary vasculature, assisting in the identification and characterization of lung-related causes of PH.

However, in situations where CTPA findings present with ambiguity, ventilation-perfusion (V/Q) scintigraphy is a valuable diagnostic tool, particularly for the evaluation of chronic thromboembolic pulmonary hypertension (CTEPH). V/Q scintigraphy offers functional insights by assessing pulmonary ventilation and perfusion, aiding in the detection of perfusion abnormalities associated with CTEPH.

Pulmonary angiography has historically been regarded as the established standard for evaluating pulmonary vascular anatomy. However, alternative imaging methods like CT and MR angiography have gained recognition as noninvasive diagnostic options. One notable advantage of pulmonary angiography is the possibility to perform right heart catheterization (RHC) simultaneously. While several tests may indicate a diagnosis of pulmonary hypertension, RHC remains the standard of reference for diagnosis of PH [2].

Echocardiography

Echocardiography is an essential tool in raising suspicion of pulmonary hypertension. However, it is not sufficient to make a definitive diagnosis and cannot firmly differentiate between different types of PH, with the exception of group 2, i.e., PH secondary to left heart disease where it provides accurate data on either valvular or left ventricular function. The complex anatomy of the RV is a challenge for echocardiographic assessment. RV enlargement can be suspected if it is larger than LV in the four-chamber view, but estimation of RV volumes and ejection fraction requires 3D imaging. The evaluation of echocardiographic findings in PH requires a comprehensive approach, as there is no single parameter specific to the diagnosis.

One of the primary echocardiographic measures to suspect PH is the peak velocity of the tricuspid regurgitant flow. If it is greater than 2.8 m/s, it must be correlated with other echocardiographic features to determine the likelihood of PH and the need for further diagnostic testing [23].

Computed Tomography

The primary CT signs suggesting the presence of PH include an enlarged main pulmonary artery (MPA) diameter, an elevated MPA-to-aorta ratio (Fig. 16.1), and enlarged right heart chambers. Numerous studies [29, 32, 36, 47, 49] have shown a direct correlation between the diameter of the MPA and mPAP as measured with right heart catheterization. Based on the Framingham Study, the sex-specific normative cutoff values for the MPA diameter on non-contrast, ECG-gated cardiac multidetector CT are 29 mm for men and 27 mm for women. The same study established the cutoff for the MPA-to-aorta ratio as 0.9 for both sexes [58].

In the setting of parenchymal lung disease, the specificity of a dilated MPA in predicting PH is

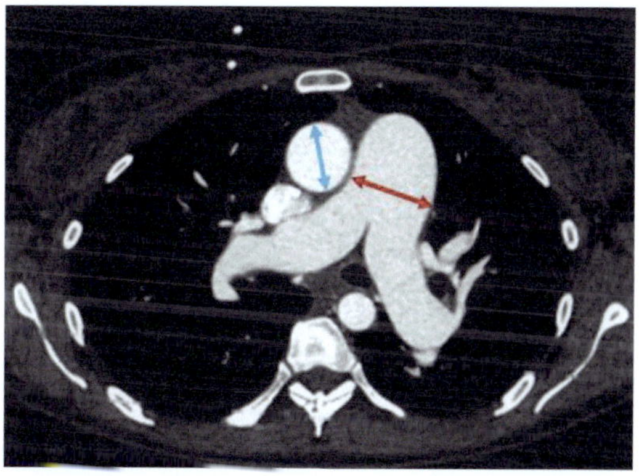

Fig. 16.1 Axial, contrast-enhanced image through the chest shows the measurements of pulmonary artery (red arrow) and aortic (blue arrow) diameters

even higher when additionally the segmental artery-to-bronchus ratio is increased in multiple pulmonary lobes [56].

A dilated MPA poses a risk of higher morbidity and mortality, particularly due to compression of neighboring structures [18]. A MPA diameter >4 cm and a MPA-to-aorta ratio >1.21 pose a higher risk of left main coronary artery compression and subsequent left ventricular (LV) ischemia [37].

The ratio of RV to LV in computed tomography pulmonary angiography (CTPA) >1 is a surrogate marker for RV dysfunction because it correlates with the increase in RV afterload. Diagnostic CT models have shown that the combination of three parameters (MPA diameter ≥30 mm, RV outflow tract (RVOT) wall thickness ≥6 mm, and septal deviation ≥140° [or RV/LV ratio ≥ 1]) is highly predictive of PH [52] (Fig. 16.2).

Right pulmonary artery (RPA) distensibility measured by ECG-gated CTPA has proven to be a sensitive and specific marker for pulmonary hypertension. The cross-sectional area of the RPA is obtained midway between the origin and its first anterior branch at every 10% of the cardiac cycle to assess maximal and minimal diameter. RPA distensibility is significantly lower in patients with pulmonary hypertension compared to healthy controls. The upper cutoff value for identifying patients with pulmonary hypertension is 16.5% [44].

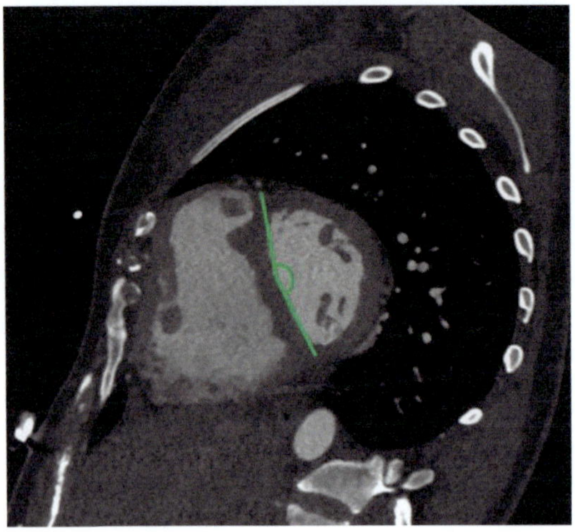

Fig. 16.2 Short-axis CTPA image through the heart demonstrates the measurement of the septal deviation

Several studies have provided evidence supporting the role of coronary sinus (CS) dilatation as a predictive factor for PH [25, 39, 62]. Unlike other measurements that can be influenced by changes in the cardiac cycle, heart diseases, or contractile motion artifacts, the CS exhibits a greater degree of stability. This makes it a reliable indicator for assessing PH. When the width of the CS exceeds 11 mm, it raises suspicion regarding the presence of PH and suggests the need for further evaluation [25]. This threshold value serves as a practical guide for radiologists to identify individuals who may be at risk for PH and require additional diagnostic testing.

As an exponent of RV failure, the reflux of contrast into the inferior vena cava (IVC) can be observed in patients PH. The severity of reflux can be assessed semi-quantitatively using Groves' six-point scale, which provides a grading system for evaluating the extent of reflux into the IVC [19]. Grade 1 indicates no reflux into the IVC, while grade 6 signifies reflux into the IVC with opacification of distal hepatic veins. In the context of PH, contrast reflux is typically significant, with grades 4 to 6 being commonly associated with the condition [4].

Pulmonary hypertension associated with left heart disease (Group 2) is defined as mPAP exceeding 20 mmHg and a pulmonary capillary wedge pressure (PCWP) of more than 15 mmHg. The CT-derived enlarged left atrial area is an independent and strong predictor of increased PCWP in patients with suspected PH and can help distinguish patients with PH due to left heart disease from patients with other types of PH [10].

Dual-Energy Computed Tomography

Dual-energy computed tomography (DECT) of the chest offers a comprehensive approach for the quantitative assessment of pulmonary hypertension patients. This imaging technique enables the measurement of traditional parameters while simultaneously allowing functional analysis of the lung and perfusion analysis via iodine maps [3]. DECT closely resembles standard, ungated CTPA, but it incorporates a saline flush to minimize artifacts associated with the superior vena cava. Various DECT acquisition technologies are available from different vendors, broadly classified as prospective techniques (occurring before patient scanning) and retrospective techniques (occurring after patient scanning).

Regardless of the technique used, DECT capitalizes on the distinct absorption properties of iodinated contrast media at low and high kilovoltage. The acquisition involves simultaneous data acquisition at both 140 kVp and 80 kVp, which is then employed to generate an iodine perfusion map of the lung parenchyma using a subtraction technique. The quantification of perfused blood volume (PBV) images is achieved by calculating the iodine content in a single voxel. Additionally, the utilization of iodine presence or absence within a voxel enables the creation of a lung vessel map (Fig. 16.3).

Although DECT images measure iodine at a single time point and are not strictly perfusion images, studies have confirmed their effectiveness as surrogate markers of lung perfusion [16, 34]. Perfusion defects observed in DECT exhibit a strong correlation with planar V/Q and single-photon emission computed tomography (SPECT) V/Q images [28]. The size of these detected perfusion defects can be quantified absolutely or in relation to the total lung volume, and both parameters demonstrate a correlation with right heart strain [6]. In the context of chronic thromboembolic pulmonary hypertension (CTEPH), quantitative lung PBV outperforms qualitative PBV in terms of its correlation with the cardiac index [50].

Cardiac Magnetic Resonance

Cardiac magnetic resonance (CMR) is considered the gold standard imaging modality for assessing cardiac volumes and function also providing data on flow, myocardial deformation, and tissue characterization. It provides unique insights into cardiac remodeling and progressive heart dysfunction that occurs during chronic pressure overload in PH. The prognosis and long-term outcome of PH patients primarily correlate with RV function, and therefore, CMR parameters hold prognostic value and can be used to monitor treatment response [23].

Morphology

Magnetic resonance imaging provides accurate and reproducible measurements of the heart chambers obtained from a stack of steady-state free procession (SSFP) cine images by endo- and epicardial border segmentation.

The initial RV response to increased afterload in PH is hypertrophy, followed by RV dilatation and dysfunction. As a result of impaired diastolic RV function, together with an enlarged tricuspid annulus and subsequent tricuspid regurgitation, the right atrium eventually also dilates. In all types

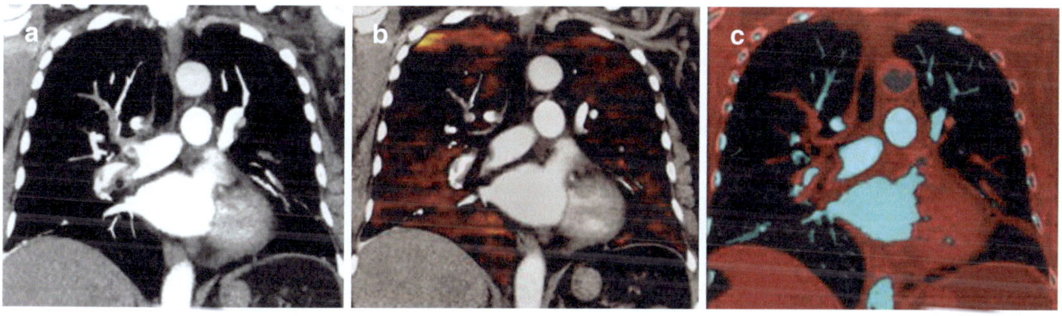

Fig. 16.3 Computed tomography angiography (**a**), fused perfused blood volume (**b**), and fused lung vessel map images (**c**) of a patient with acute pulmonary embolism. On the CTA image (**a**), multiple filling defects are observed bilaterally within the pulmonary arteries, corresponding to the presence of the embolic material. The fused PBV image (**b**) reveals perfusion defects within the lung parenchyma supplied by the obstructed pulmonary arteries. On the fused lung vessel map image (**c**), vessels containing iodine are color-coded blue, while those without iodine are color-coded red, making the identification of the embolism easier

of PH, the right chambers undergo similar adaptive changes in response to increased pulmonary resistance (Fig. 16.4). However, the appearance of the left side of the heart depends on the type of PH:

1. In advanced precapillary PH with concomitant RV dysfunction, both left chambers may become smaller due to chronic underfilling. This promotes apoptosis, eventually resulting in reduced LV mass [8, 51].
2. In isolated postcapillary PH (group 2 in the PH classification), left ventricle (LV) and/or valve impairment lead to subsequent PH development. In this type of PH, the left atrium (LA) is enlarged (usually larger than the right atrium), but the appearance of the LV depends on the primary disease [23].

Each type of PH can lead to alterations in LV geometry, resulting in a change in its shape to resemble the letter "D". It is a result of increased pressure in the RV, which leads to a shift of the intraventricular septum toward the LV. The LV eccentricity index (LVEI) can be assessed in short-axis planes (SAX) by calculating the ratio of LV cross-sectional diameters at the mid-segment level. Normally, the LVEI in systolic phase should not be greater than 1.2, and in the

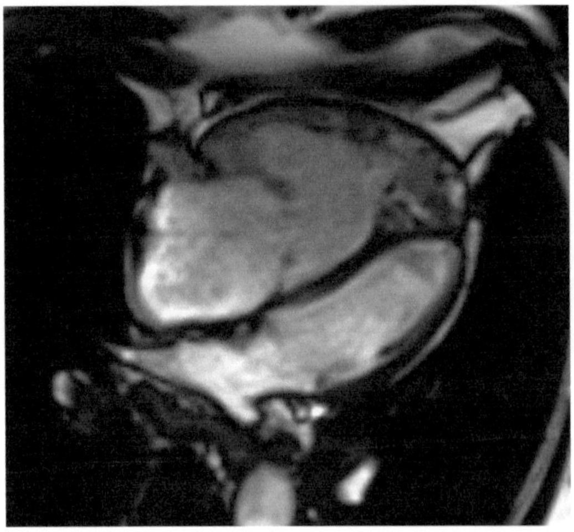

Fig. 16.4 CMR, 4-chamber cine diastolic stillframe. Typical cardiac morphology in a patient with PH (all types except type 2). Significant enlargement of both right chambers with relatively small left heart chambers

presence of PH, it tends to increase [53] (Fig. 16.5).

Another parameter, the ventricular mass index (VMI), is obtained by dividing the total RV mass by the LV mass and can be used as a marker of PH with high sensitivity and specificity if it is greater than 0.4 [53].

Volumes

Volumes are measured from a stack of SSFP SAX cine images (RV may also be assessed from transaxial planes) by per-slice segmentation of endocardium borders in maximum diastole and systole. When RV is enlarged, it can extend beyond the atrioventricular groove in basal SAX slices and resemble a "shoulder" around the right atrium that is usually visible only in diastolic phase. This complex anatomy must be taken into consideration to correctly evaluate RV volumes (Fig. 16.6).

Volumetric parameters play a significant role in the comprehensive assessment of 1-year mortality risk according to the ESC guidelines for PH [23]. A multiparametric approach, including clinical, invasive, laboratory, and imaging tests, is used to describe the risk, which is divided into three categories: low, intermediate, and high. The CMR values utilized in this classification include: right ventricle ejection fraction (RVEF), stroke volume index (SVI), and right ventricle end-systolic volume index (RVESVI) (Table 16.1).

Chronic right-sided pressure overload leads to RV failure and a decrease in RV stroke volume (RVSV). Together with altered LV geometry, this contributes to a reduction in LV preload and volumes. In precapillary PH, left ventricular ejection fraction (LVEF) is usually preserved, but LV underfilling leads to a decrease in left ventricular stroke volume (LVSV) and cardiac output [51].

Repeated volumetric assessments during PH treatment provide insights into long-term prognosis and help adjust medical strategies to improve patients' outcomes [23]. Risk of mortality in PAH is higher if a decrease in LVEDVI, LVESVI, RVEF and/or increase in RVEDVI or RVESVI is observed in serial CMR examinations [1].

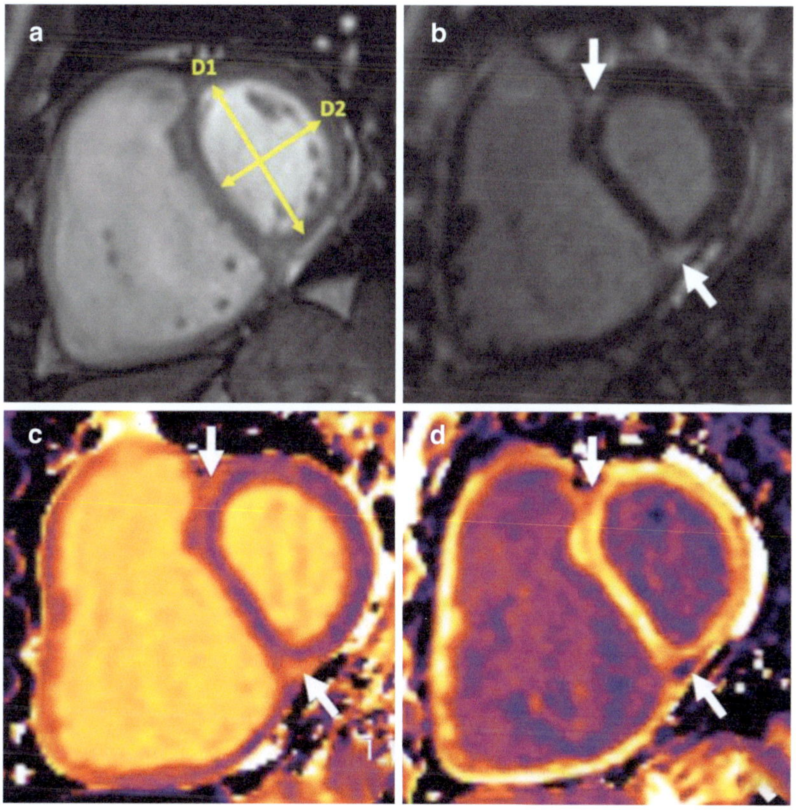

Fig. 16.5 Short axis images of a patient with PH: (**a**) Steady-state free procession (SSFP) cine image in diastole. Intraventricular septum shift altered LV geometry. The left ventricle eccentricity index (LVEI) is calculated by measuring the ratio of the anterior-inferior (D2) and septal-posterolateral (D1) cavity dimensions at the mid-ventricular level; (**b**–**d**) white arrows indicate fibrosis in both insert points in LGE image (**b**), native T1 Mapping (**c**), and ECV Map (**d**)

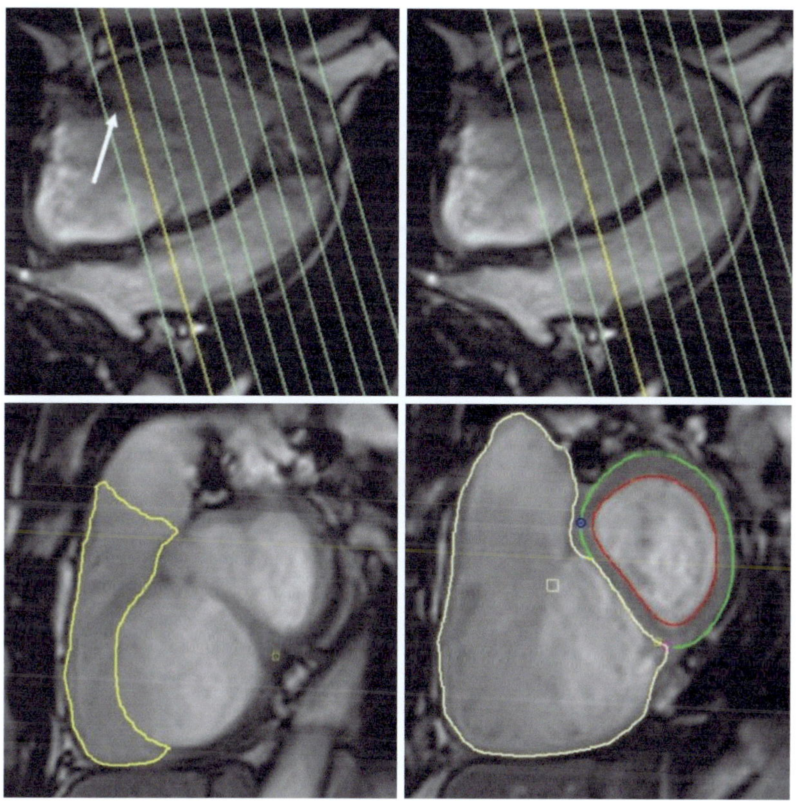

Fig. 16.6 Enlarged RV extend beyond the atrioventricular groove (white arrow). In the most basal short-axis (SAX) slice, the RV may resemble a "shoulder" around the right atrium. RV's complex anatomical features should be considered to obtain accurate measurements. SAX SSFP cine images with ventricular segmentation (bottom images) and their cross-sections on the long axis 4-chamber view (top images)

Table 16.1 Measurements in the imaging of PH

	Parameter	Value/change in PH	Significance/comment
Morphology/ volumes (CMR and CT)	RV size and volume[a]	Enlarged in pre- and postcapillary PH	Result of progressive right ventricle dysfunction
	RV mass in pre- and postcapillary PH[a]	Enlarged CMR: 1. Papillary muscles included in RV mass: Females >71 g / males >95 g 2. Papillary muscles included in blood pool: Females >48 g / males >54 g CT: RVOT thickness ≥6 mm	Adaptation to increased afterload
	Right atrium (RA)[a]	Enlarged	Secondary to right ventricle diastolic dysfunction and increased afterload, can be exacerbated by concomitant tricuspid regurgitation
	LV size and volumes[a]	1. Precapillary PH: normal or decreased 2. Postcapillary PH Enlarged: e.g., dilated cardiomyopathy, ischemic injury, mitral regurgitation Normal or decreased: e.g., restrictive cardiomyopathy, mitral stenosis	1. Result of chronic underfilling 2. Primary due to left ventricle or left valvular diseases which cause subsequent PH development
	LV mass in precapillary PH[a]	Normal or reduced	Chronic underfilling promotes apoptosis
	LA[a]	1. Precapillary PH: Normal or smaller 2. Postcapillary PH: Enlarged (usually LA > RA)	1. Result of chronic underfilling 2. Result of left ventricle diastolic dysfunction or increased left ventricle pre- or afterload
	LVEI (CMR and CT)	In systole: LVEI ≥1,2 In diastole: LVEI ≥1,17	Change in left ventricle geometry secondary to increased pressure in right ventricle
	Intraventricular septum deviation (CT)	≥140 degrees	
	VMI = total RV mass/ total LV mass (CMR)	VMI > 0,4	PH may be suspected with high sensitivity and specificity

(continued)

Table 16.1 (continued)

	Parameter	Value/change in PH	Significance/comment
	RV/LV ratio in 4CH view (CT)	≥1	Correlates with the increase in RV afterload
	RPA distensibility = (RPA area max- RPA area min) / RPA area max ×100% (CT)	<16,5%	Requires multiphase CT imaging
	MPA (MR and CT)	Enlarged: 1. MR: Females:>31 mm (systolic diameter) Males: >33 mm (systolic diameter) 2. CT Females: 27 mm Males: 29 mm	
	MPA-to-aorta ratio (CT)	>0.9	
	Segmental artery-to-bronchus ratio (CT, only for group 3 of PH)	>1:1	Measured in the setting of dilated MPA, obtained in 3–4 pulmonary lobes on axial CT images.
	Groves' scale of the IVC reflux severity	Grade 1: no contrast reflux into the IVC Grade 2: trace contrast reflux into the IVC Grade 3: contrast reflux limited to the IVC Grade 4: contrast reflux into the IVC and hepatic veins near confluence Grade 5: contrast in the IVC, reaching mid-part of hepatic veins Grade 6: contrast in the IVC reaching hepatic veins in the peripheral hepatic parenchyma	Semi-quantitative assessment
	Volumetric parameters in 1-year mortality risk stratification according to ESC guidelines	1. Low <5%: RVEF >54% SVI >40 ml/m^2 RVESVI <42 ml/m^2 2. Intermediate 5–20% RVEF 37–54% SVI 26-40 ml/m^2 RVESVI 42–54 ml/m^2 3. High >20% RVEF <37% SVI < 26 ml/m^2 RVESVI >54 ml/m^2	Part of multiparametric approach that also includes clinical, invasive, and laboratory tests
	Repeated volumetric assessment—Prognosis in PAH	1. Increased mortality: RVEF decrease RVEDVI/ RVESVI increase LVEDVI decrease LVSVI decrease 2. Risk of clinical worsening: RVEF decrease RVEDVI/ RVESVI increase	Repeated CMR assessment may improve treatment results

(continued)

Table 16.1 (continued)

	Parameter	Value/change in PH	Significance/comment
STRAIN (CMR)	RV longitudinal, circumferential, and radial strain	Decreased	No exact cut-off values
	LV circumferential strain	Decreased	Typically in the interventricular septum in mid-segments level
FLOW (CMR)	Pulmonary flow velocities	Mean MPA velocity <11.7 cm/s suggests mean pulmonary pressure >25 mmHg	All velocities in the MPA are decreased in PH
	RAC of MPA (MPA systolic area- MPA diastolic area)/ MPA diastolic area x100%	RAC <40%	Prognostic value
	Shunts analysis: Qp:Qs = forward flow in MPA: forward flow in ascending aorta	1. Normal: Qp:Qs = 1:1 2. Significant left to right shunt Qp:Qs >1.5:1 3. Eisenmenger syndrome, shunt flow from right to left Qp < Qs	Eisenmenger syndrome is associated with advanced PH
	WSS (4D flow)	Decreased	Reduced vasodilation
Pulmonary Transit Time (CMR)	PTT = maximum LV enhancement time – maximum RV enhancement time	>6.5 seconds	Higher risk of adverse outcome in PAH Measured from first-pass perfusion scans
Tissue Characterisation (CMR)	LGE	In both insert points	Macroscopic fibrosis
	T1 mapping	Increased in both insert points	Reflects diffuse fibrosis
Perfusion (CMR)	Right and left ventricle perfusion	Decreased	Contribute to ischemic RV injury in PH
Lung V/Q Scan	Lung ventilation/ perfusion	≥1 segmental or ≥2 subsegmental perfusion defects with preserved ventilation suggest PE	Normal V/Q scan practically excludes CTEPH
	Lung counts vs. total-body counts on a perfusion scan	$\frac{\text{Totalbodycounts} - \text{Lungcounts}}{\text{Totalbodycounts}} \times 100\% > 6\%$ suggests right-to-left shunt	Detects and quantifies right-to-left shunt
First-Pass RNA	Qp:Qs	Qp:Qs >1.2 suggests left-to-right shunt	Detects and quantifies left-to-right shunt
MYOCARDIAL PERFUSION SCAN	RV/LV uptake ratio	RV/LV >0.35 suggestive for PH	Non–attenuation-corrected SPECT images; sensitivity of 72% and specificity of 70% for detection of PH

CMR cardiac magnetic resonance, *CT* computed tomography, *RV* right ventricle, *PH* pulmonary hypertension, *RVOT* right ventricular outflow tract, *RA* right atrium, *LV* left ventricle, *LA* left atrium, *LVEI* left ventricle eccentricity index, *VMI* ventricular mass index, *4CH view* four-chamber view, *RPA* right pulmonary artery, *MPA* main pulmonary artery, *IVC* inferior vena cava, *RVEF* right ventricular ejection fraction, *SVI* stroke volume index, *RVESVI* right ventricular end-systolic volume index, *PAH* pulmonary arterial hypertension, *RAC* relative area change, *WSS* wall shear stress, *PTT* pulmonary transit time, *LGE* late gadolinium enhancement, *V/Q* ventilation/perfusion, *PE* pulmonary embolism, CTEPH chronic thromboembolic pulmonary hypertension, *RNA* radionuclide angiography

[a]Reference CMR values are available in "Reference ranges ("normal values") for cardiovascular magnetic resonance (CMR) in adults and children: 2020 update" [26]

Strain

Myocardial deformation or strain, measured using CMR, can be obtained by different techniques, most commonly by myocardial feature tracking (MFT) method, which follows myocardial displacement and velocity using block matching techniques from SSFP cine images. It measures a change in myocardial length during cardiac cycle and can be assessed in three directions: longitudinal, circumferential, and radial.

Strain abnormalities in PH patients can be detected before other features of ventricular dysfunction develop, thus playing a role in the early identification of subclinical myocardial impairment [11, 61]. RV analysis is more complicated due to its thinner wall; however, RV longitudinal, circumferential, and radial strain may be reliably obtained and all of them tend to decrease in PH. Left ventricular circumferential strain, particularly in mid-wall segments, may also be reduced [57].

Strain curves also provide information on the RV mechanical dyssynchrony (Fig. 16.7). Increased RV wall tension is caused by combina-

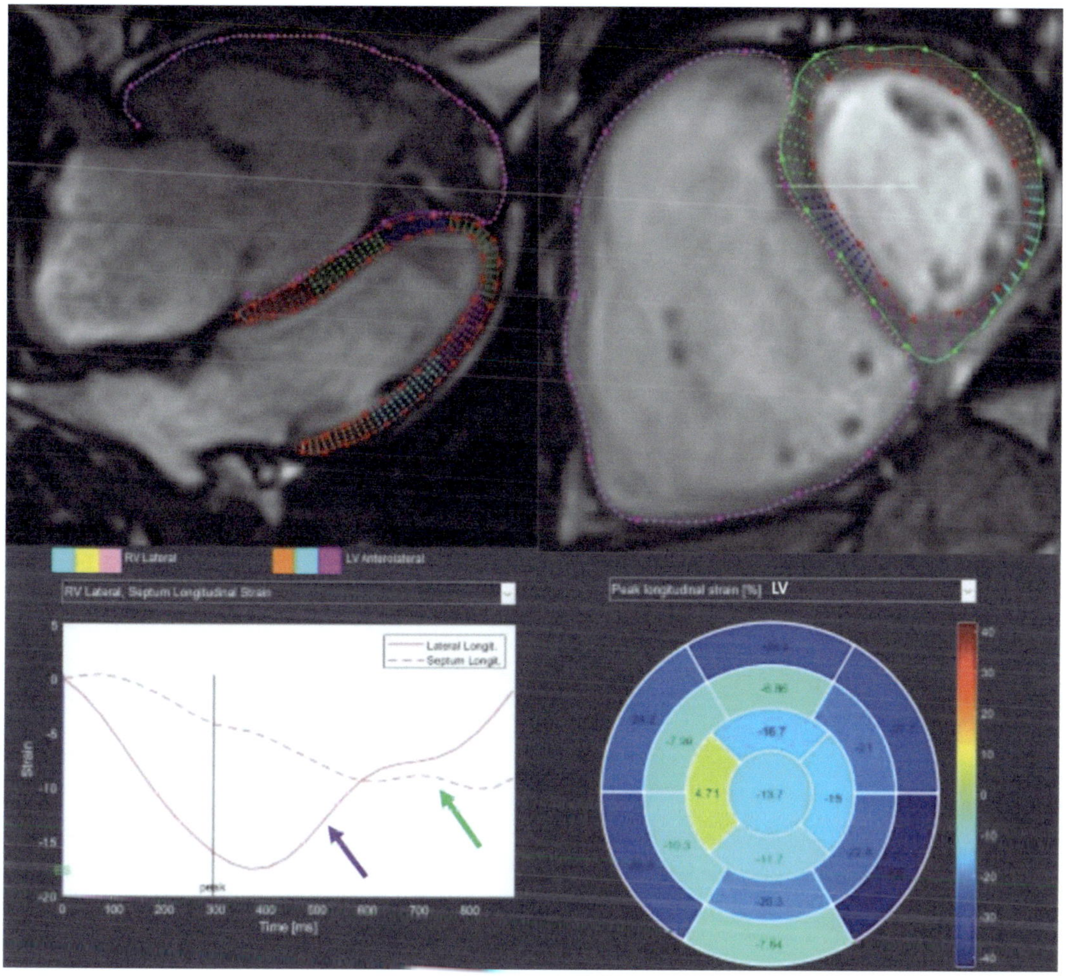

Fig. 16.7 Myocardial feature tracking (MFT) strain analysis in long- and short-axis planes. The graph shows RV longitudinal strain with mechanical dyssynchrony between intraventricular septum (green arrow) and RV free wall (purple arrow). Global longitudinal strain for RV: −11.3. In the left lower corner, a bull-eye presentation of left ventricle longitudinal strain for 17 segments according to AHA segmentation, LV global longitudinal strain: −16.5

tion of pressure overload, resulting from elevated pulmonary vascular resistance and volume overload induced by tricuspid regurgitation. This results in prolongation of RV contraction time compared to the LV. Postsystolic shortening, where the RV myocardium continues to contract after pulmonary valve closure, may also be observed [33].

Flow

Two-dimensional phase-contrast imaging is an established method for assessing flow parameters in large blood vessels. Patients with PH typically have lower pulmonary blood flow velocities [12]. The MPA flow curve in PH may show a shortening of the acceleration time (from the beginning of systole to peak velocity) and a characteristic notch (deceleration) in the mid-systolic phase [42] (Fig. 16.8). In PH, flow in the MPA can be helical and may form characteristic retrograde flow, typically in the dorsal part of the MPA, in the mid- and end-systolic phases [12, 42] (Fig. 16.9).

Patients with congenital heart disease and significant left-to-right shunts are at risk of developing PH. The ratio of total pulmonary blood flow to the total systemic blood flow (Qp:Qs) is obtained by comparing forward flow in the MPA and ascending aorta. Left-to-right shunt is considered hemodynamically significant when Qp:Qs ratio is greater than 1.5:1 (Fig. 16.10). In patients with a coexisting shunt and advanced PH, a gradual decrease in Qp:Qs may be observed until flow reversal through the congenital defect occurs from right-to-left; this condition is known as Eisenmenger syndrome [7].

An increase in pulmonary vascular resistance results in MPA stiffness. Cross-sectional magnitude 2D phase-contrast images of the MPA throughout the cardiac cycle allow the assessment of pulmonary compliance. The change in area of the MPA between diastole and systole, expressed as a percentage, provides a parameter known as the relative area change (RAC). RAC of less than 40% is highly sensitive in detecting

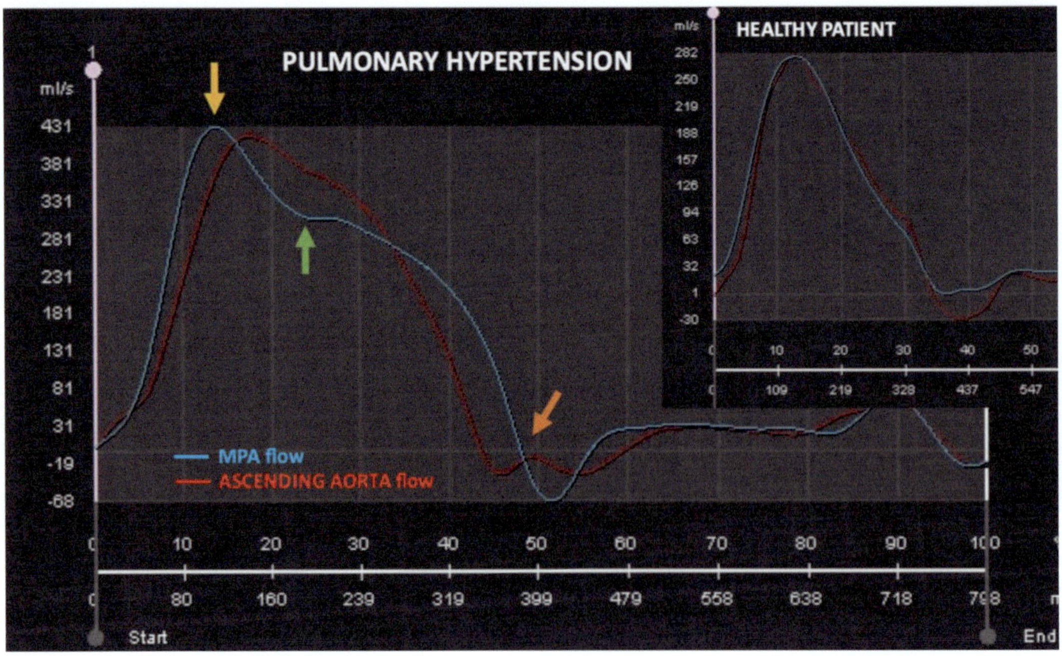

Fig. 16.8 2D phase contrast (2D PC) imaging. The main pulmonary artery (MPA) flow pattern (blue curve): yellow arrow—short acceleration time (from the beginning of forward flow to its peak); green arrow—mid-systolic notch (deceleration) of flow; orange arrow—prolongation of pulmonary flow versus aortic flow (red curve) that reflects mechanical dyssynchrony and is a result of prolonged RV contraction time. In the right upper corner: 2D PC flow curves in a healthy patient

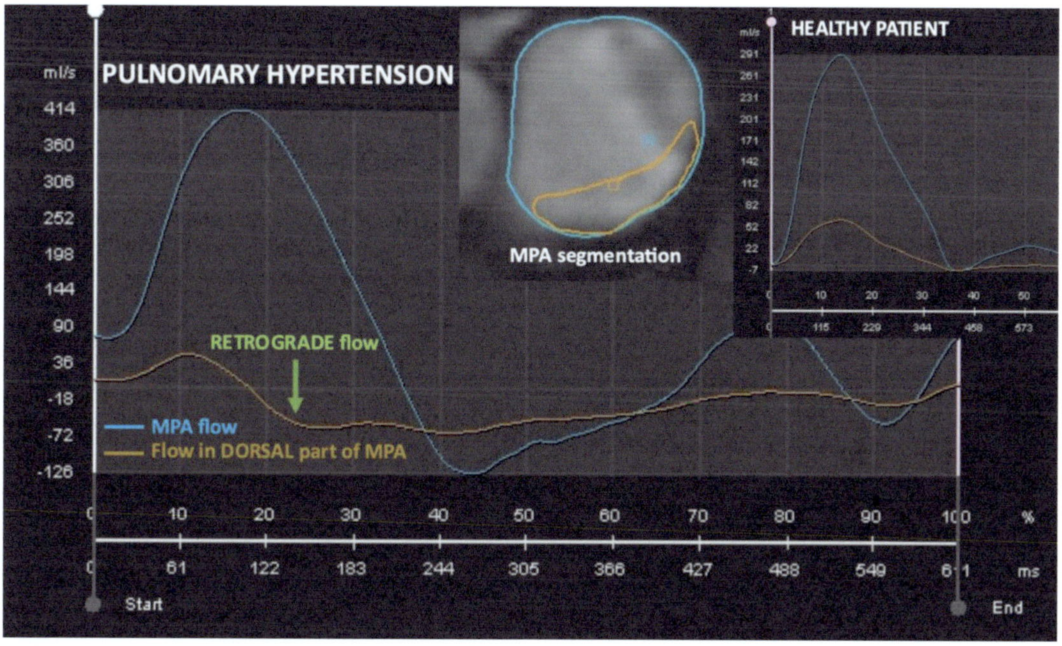

Fig. 16.9 2D phase contrast (2D PC) imaging. Flow in the main pulmonary artery (MPA, blue curve). In mid- and end-systole, flow in the dorsal part of the MPA is retrograde (orange curve, green arrow) as a result of helical flow trajectory, which is typical for pulmonary hypertension. Upper middle section: MPA magnitude image with segmentation used to obtain the curves in PH patient. Upper right corner: 2D PC flow curves in a healthy patient

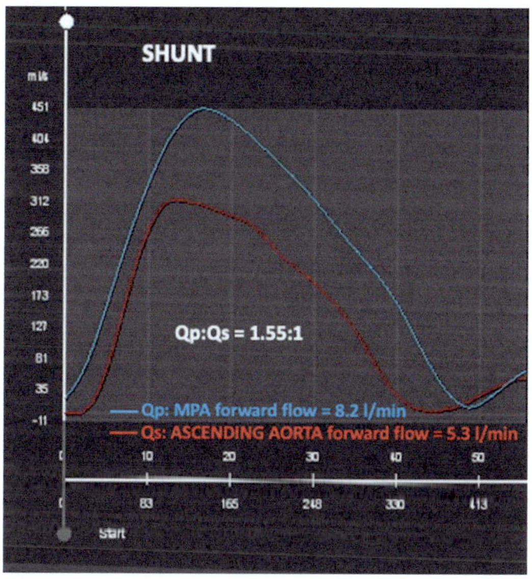

Fig. 16.10 A patient with left-to-right shunt resulting from the right upper pulmonary vein draining into the vena cava superior. 2D phase contrast flow curves show significant left to right shunt with Qp:Qs =1.55:1. Blue curve: MPA flow = 8.2 l/min of forward flow. Red curve: ascending aorta flow = 5.3 l/min of forward flow

elevated mPAP [8, 45] (Fig. 16.11). A relatively new technique, four-dimensional flow, provides temporal and three-dimensional flow data along the entire heart and great vessels. It introduces novel parameters like wall shear stress (WSS), which reflect the shear force of the flow near the vessel wall. In PH, reduced WSS fails to stimulate endothelial cells to release nitric oxide and promote vasodilation, thus contributing to adverse vascular remodeling [12].

Pulmonary Transit Time

In PH, due to high vascular resistance and RV failure, it takes more time for blood to pass through the pulmonary circulation, resulting in prolonged pulmonary transit time (PTT) (Fig. 16.12). PTT is measured from first-pass contrast perfusion scans by subtracting the RV maximum enhancement time from the LV maximum enhancement time. If PTT exceeds 6.5 seconds, there is a higher risk of adverse outcome in PAH [54].

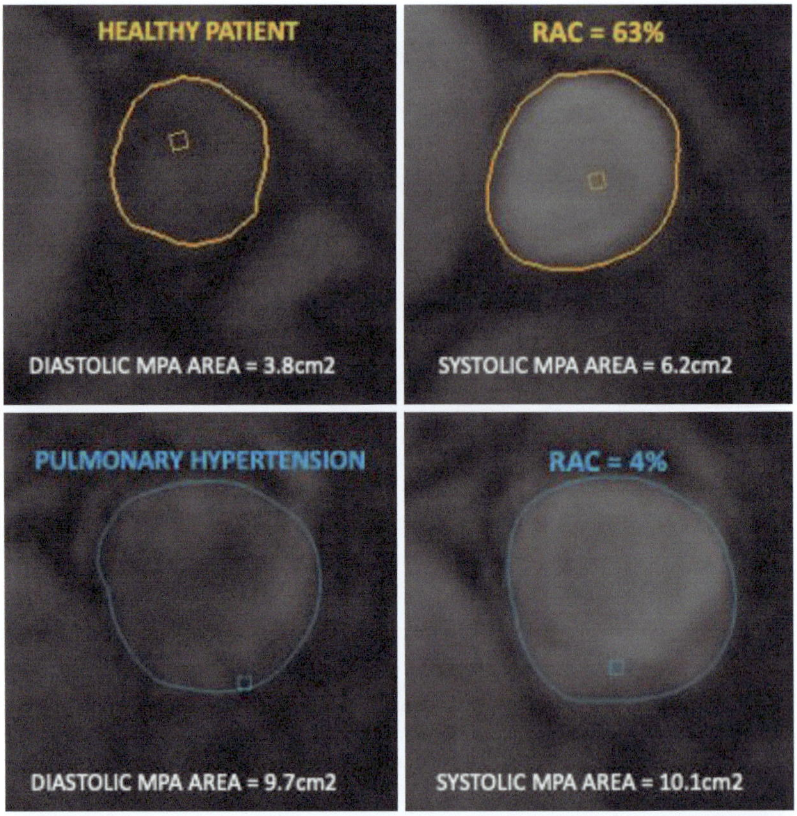

Fig. 16.11 Magnitude 2D phase contrast imaging. Relative area change (RAC) of pulmonary artery in a healthy patient (orange segmentation) and a patient with PH (blue segmentation). RAC = (MPA systolic area- MPA diastolic area/MPA diastolic area) ×100%

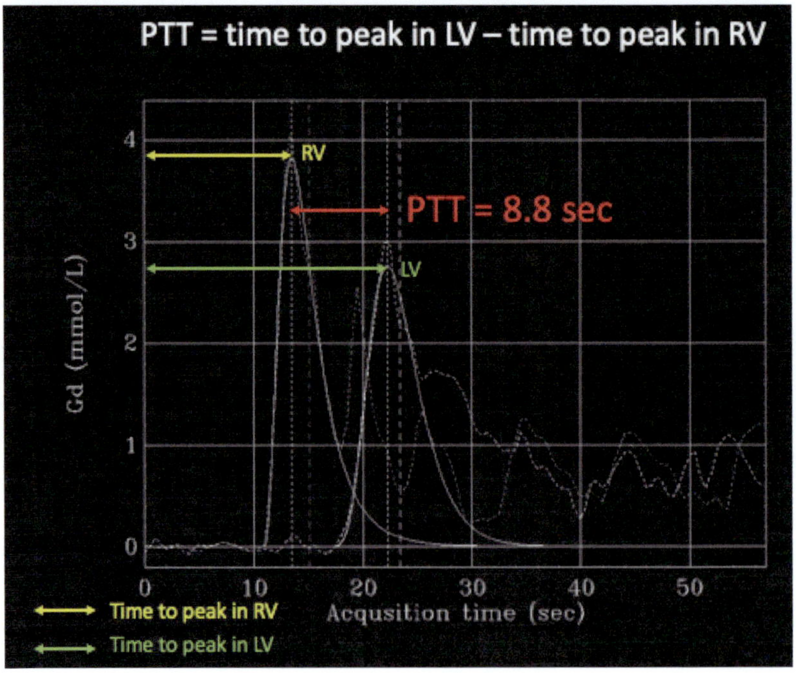

Fig. 16.12 First-pass contrast perfusion scan in a patient with PH. The graph depicts curves representing the enhancement in each of the ventricles over time. The PTT is calculated by subtracting the peak enhancement time of the RV from the peak enhancement time of the LV. In this patient, the PTT is prolonged, measuring 8.8 seconds

Tissue Characterization

PH patients typically present areas of late gadolinium enhancement (LGE) along both septal RV insertion points. These correlate with increased pulmonary artery pressure, RV remodeling, reduced RV contractility, and worse outcomes [12]. In the absence of macroscopic LGE, diffuse fibrosis at the insertion sites can be detected by increased native T1 mapping [46] (Fig. 16.5).

Perfusion

Perfusion abnormalities are observed in PH. RV hypertrophy without corresponding expansion of the coronary tree, together with reduced stroke volume and low systemic blood pressure, can adversely affect coronary flow. Myocardial perfusion may be evaluated in stress CMR studies using a vasodilator, either regadenoson or adenosine. In PH, myocardial perfusion reserve indices of both ventricles tend to be decreased. Reduced perfusion leads to ischemia and further exacerbation of RV dysfunction [12, 59].

Radionuclide Scans

Quantitative Nature of Radionuclide Imaging

Imaging in nuclear medicine is achieved by registration of photons emitted by the patient's body after administration of a radiopharmaceutical. The numbers of photons detected by a scintillation camera at a position corresponding to a pixel in the image are termed "counts." The number of counts in a certain area defined as a region of interest (ROI) for planar imaging or a volume of interest (VOI) for tomographic scans is related to the signal intensity of photons and is assumed to be a proportional measure of the radiotracer uptake. Counts ratios for various ROIs or VOIs may be used to detect differences in activity uptakes and therefore can be used as a quantitative measure of clinically relevant factors. An example of a relative quantification is the calculation of the split function of paired organs, e.g., kidneys in a dynamic renal scintigraphy. The change in activity uptake over time can be important in assessing the biokinetics of a particular organ or tissue. One can assume that a normal tissue follows a certain time-activity curve and that a change in the shape of the curve may reveal significant changes in the functional behavior of the organ [24].

Lung Ventilation/Perfusion (V/Q) Scan

Lung V/Q scan is a combination of ventilation and perfusion scans performed successively, commonly indicated in patients with suspicion of pulmonary embolism (PE). Ventilation scan requires inhalation of radioactive gas, e.g., kryptonium-81 m, Technegas® (a gaseous suspension of graphite nanoparticles labeled with technetium-99 m) or an aerosol of ^{99m}Tc-DTPA (diethylenetriaminepentaacetic acid). On the other hand, perfusion scan is performed after intravenous injection of a suspension of macroaggregated albumin (MAA) labeled with technetium-99 m, which become temporarily implanted in the lung capillaries. The number of ^{99m}Tc-MAA particles varies between 200,000 and 400,000 and results in temporal occlusion of approximately 1/1000 of pulmonary capillaries. In cases of perfusion defects in at least one segmental or two subsegmental regions with preserved ventilation (so called V/Q mismatch), pulmonary embolism (PE) is usually diagnosed. According to the ESC/ERS guidelines for the diagnosis and treatment of PH, V/Q lung scintigraphy may be used as a screening method in the diagnosis of CTEPH (Fig. 16.13). The sensitivity and specificity of planar V/Q scintigraphy in diagnosing CTEPH is

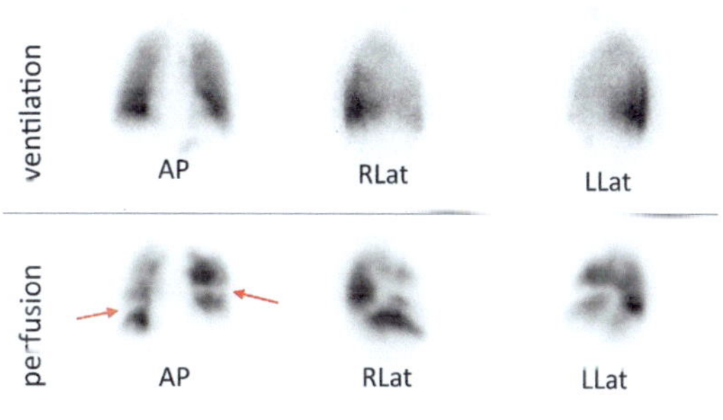

Fig. 16.13 Lung V/Q scan of a patient with pulmonary embolism. Red arrows depict segmental perfusion defects with preserved ventilation. (Courtesy of dr med. Stanisław Piszczek from Nuclear Medicine Department, Military Institute of Medicine, Warsaw, Poland)

96–97% and 90–95%, respectively [27], while a normal V/Q scan practically excludes CTEPH [5]. Tomographic or SPECT V/Q scan also performed in a hybrid manner as SPECT/CT (scintigraphic and anatomical imaging acquired by a hybrid gamma camera equipped with a CT scanner) has a higher sensitivity than planar imaging and generates fewer indeterminate results [20, 40, 41]. The main limitation of V/Q scan in the differential diagnosis of PH is that it cannot help to discriminate pulmonary veno-occlusive disease (PVOD) from idiopathic PAH [48]. PVOD is a rare (~10%) cause of idiopathic PAH, and the results of lung scintigraphy in this clinical entity may present equivocally, as patchy perfusion defects or even as defects resembling subsegmental emboli [17, 55].

Of note, when ^{99m}Tc-MAA is detected in liver, kidneys, or brain, it suggests the presence of right-to-left cardiac shunt. Intracardiac shunts are an important cause of PAH. In normal conditions, ^{99m}Tc-MAA after intravenous injection is almost entirely captured in the lung capillary system, while in the case of right-to-left shunts, some particles bypass the lung circulation, enter systemic blood stream, and localize in the capillaries of other organs [43]. The magnitude of the shunt can be estimated in a whole-body scan performed after injection of ^{99m}Tc-MAA, by measuring the lungs counts and total body counts and inserting them in the following formula:

$$\%\text{Shunt} = \frac{\text{Totalbodycounts} - \text{Lungcounts}}{\text{Totalbodycounts}} \times 100\%$$

In healthy individuals, only 4–6% of the injected ^{99m}Tc-MAA bypass the lungs. A shunt of >6% is characteristic for the right-to-left shunt [38].

Extra-lung ^{99m}Tc-MAA accumulation can also be seen in hepatic failure with macroscopic intrapulmonary shunts (hepatopulmonary syndrome), in congenital pulmonary arteriovenous malformations (Osler-Weber-Rendu disease), and in patients who have undergone cavopulmonary anastomotic surgery [43].

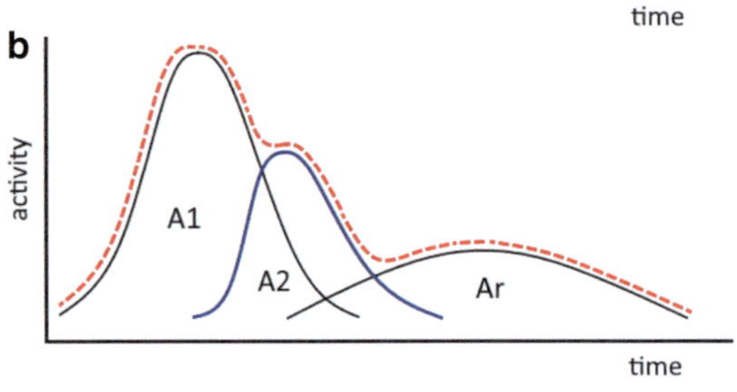

Fig. 16.14 Time-activity curve acquired from a pulmonary ROI in a healthy individual (**a**). A1 corresponds to initial pass of activity through the lungs; Ar shows recirculated activity through lungs after circulating in the body. A2 shows early recirculation through lungs shortly after first pass in left-to-right shunt (**b**). (Adapted from MacDonald and Burrell [31])

Quantifying the Heterogeneity of Lung Perfusion

The lung perfusion scans can be used for quantitative assessment of the uniformity of lung perfusion by means of perfusion index (P index) based on calculation of perfused area rate (PAR) at various percentage thresholds of maximal pixel radioactivity. Using the P index, one can quantify the uniformity of lung perfusion which tends to be lower in severe PH, with the appearance of various degrees of diffuse patchy defects. The P index correlates significantly with the mPAP measured invasively in patients with primary PH. Therefore, the quantitative analysis of lung perfusion scans may provide a noninvasive indicator of pulmonary hypertension severity. Moreover, in patients receiving long-term vasodilator therapy (PGI_2), performing the follow-up studies and comparing the P indexes may help to depict the improvement in the remodeling effect on the pulmonary vasculature. Hence, the quantitative analysis of irregular distribution of radiotracer on lung perfusion scans can provide useful information about the severity of disease and the effect of therapy [15].

First-Pass Radionuclide Angiocardiography (FP-RNA)

FP-RNA is a diagnostic nuclear procedure based on dynamic imaging of the first pass of an intravenously injected radiopharmaceutical through the heart, lungs, and blood vessels. Sequential analysis of scintigrams and plotting time-activity curve (TAC) over heart chambers or lungs allows to diagnose various cardiac or vascular abnormalities and quantification of intracardiac shunts. Technically, the procedure can be performed after bolus injection of ^{99m}Tc-pertechnetate, ^{99m}Tc-labeled albumin or red blood cells. By plotting TAC from a pulmonary ROI, normally a two-phase curve is obtained, where the left peak (higher and thinner) corresponds to the first pass of radiotracer through the lungs, and the right peak (lower and wider) shows recirculation in the systemic blood pool (Fig. 16.14a). In the left-to-right shunt, one can observe early recirculation of the radiopharmaceutical through the lungs marked as the additional peak on the descending slope of the left peak, which represents the shunt component (Fig. 16.14b). The shunt ratio Qp:Qs is then calculated as (A1 + A2)/A1, where A1 is the area under the primary fitted curve and A2 is the area under the secondary (shunt) fitted curve [14]. The ratio of Qp:Qs > 1.2 suggests left-to-right shunt.

Left and Right Ventricular Ejection Fraction

It should be emphasized that in patients with contraindications to CMR or with inappropriate acoustic window making interpretation of echocardiography difficult, FP-RNA can also be used to estimate the left and right ventricular ejection fraction. Moreover, at equilibrium, after the entire bloodpool is uniformly labeled with ^{99m}Tc, *multigated acquisition* (MUGA), also known as equilibrium radionuclide angiography (ERNA) can be performed, which is a reliable and reproducible method of measuring the right ventricular ejection fraction, provided that the study is performed as SPECT [9].

Myocardial Perfusion Scintigraphy (MPS)

MPS is commonly used for the assessment of myocardial perfusion abnormalities in patients with ischemic heart disease. Due to limited spatial resolution, it is almost exclusively used to assess left ventricular perfusion; however, in PH resulting in pressure overload and hypertrophy of the right ventricle, it can be used to quantify its wall thickness. The right and left ventricular free walls (RV/LV) uptake ratio measured in ^{99m}Tc-tetrofosmin myocardial SPECT correlates significantly with both pulmonary artery systolic pressure and RV wall thickness. The RV/LV ratio of 0.35 on non-attenuation-corrected SPECT images has a sensitivity of 72% and a specificity of 70% for the detection of significant elevation of pulmonary artery pressure. Hence, the RV/LV uptake ratio measured on MPS images can be used to identify patients with high pulmonary artery pressure or RV hypertrophy [35].

Also, a target to background (T/B) ratio obtained by placing the target ROI within the right ventricular wall and the background ROI over the adjacent lung tissue in MPS can serve as a semi-quantitative measure of the severity of PAH. The T/B ratio has a high potential to discriminate moderate/severe from mild PAH, with the cutoff value of 1.855 allowing to diagnose moderate/severe PAH with sensitivity of 86.7% and specificity of 100% [30].

Key Points

- Pulmonary hypertension is defined by a mean pulmonary arterial pressure greater than 20 mmHg at rest during right heart catheterization.
- Clinically PH is divided into: PAH (group 1), PH due to left heart disease (group 2), PH due to lung diseases and/or hypoxia (group 3), CTEPH (group 4), PH with unclear and/or multifactorial mechanisms (group 5).
- Quantitative imaging parameters can be evaluated in echocardiography, computed tomography, cardiac magnetic resonance, and

radionuclide scans. These measurements may help in identifying the etiology of PH.
- While several tests may facilitate early detection of PH and be used to monitor the progress of the disease, the right heart catheterization remains the standard of reference for establishing diagnosis of PH.

Acknowledgements We are grateful to prof. Edyta Szurowska, Head of the second Department of Radiology, Medical University of Gdańsk, Poland for her support, prof. Marcin Fijałkowski from the first Department of Cardiology, Medical University of Gdańsk and dr Karolina Dorniak from the Division of Cardiac Diagnostics, Medical University of Gdańsk for their critical appraisal of the manuscript and to dr Jacek Teodorczyk from the Department of Nuclear Medicine, Medical University of Gdańsk, for reviewing sections of this chapter. We would like to express our special gratitude to Luke Rothman for the detailed proofreading the manuscript.

References

1. Alabed S, Shahin Y, Garg P, et al. Cardiac-MRI predicts clinical worsening and mortality in pulmonary arterial hypertension. JACC Cardiovasc Imaging. 2021;14:931–42. https://doi.org/10.1016/j.jcmg.2020.08.013.
2. Aluja Jaramillo F, Gutierrez FR, Díaz Telli FG, et al. Approach to pulmonary hypertension: from CT to clinical diagnosis. Radiographics. 2018;38:357–73. https://doi.org/10.1148/rg.2018170046.
3. Ameli-Renani S, Rahman F, Nair A, et al. Dual-energy CT for imaging of pulmonary hypertension: challenges and opportunities. Radiographics. 2014;34:1769–90. https://doi.org/10.1148/rg.347130085.
4. Aviram G, Cohen D, Steinvil A, et al. Significance of reflux of contrast medium into the inferior vena cava on computerized tomographic pulmonary angiogram. Am J Cardiol. 2012;109:432–7. https://doi.org/10.1016/j.amjcard.2011.09.033.
5. Bajc M, Schümichen C, Grüning T, et al. EANM guideline for ventilation/perfusion single-photon emission computed tomography (SPECT) for diagnosis of pulmonary embolism and beyond. Eur J Nucl Med Mol Imaging. 2019;46:2429–51. https://doi.org/10.1007/s00259-019-04450-0.
6. Bauer RW, Frellesen C, Renker M, et al. Dual energy CT pulmonary blood volume assessment in acute pulmonary embolism—correlation with D-dimer level, right heart strain and clinical outcome. Eur Radiol. 2011;21:1914–21. https://doi.org/10.1007/s00330-011-2135-1.
7. Baumgartner H, De Backer J, Babu-Narayan SV, et al. 2020 ESC guidelines for the management of adult congenital heart disease. Eur Heart J. 2021;42:563–645. https://doi.org/10.1093/eurheartj/ehaa554.
8. Bradlow WM, Gibbs JSR, Mohiaddin RH. Cardiovascular magnetic resonance in pulmonary hypertension. J Cardiovasc Magn Reson. 2012;14:6. https://doi.org/10.1186/1532-429X-14-6.
9. Corbett JR, Akinboboye OO, Bacharach SL, et al. ASNC announcement. J Nucl Cardiol. 2009;16:164. https://doi.org/10.1007/s12350-008-9027-z.
10. Currie BJ, Johns C, Chin M, et al. CT derived left atrial size identifies left heart disease in suspected pulmonary hypertension: derivation and validation of predictive thresholds. Int J Cardiol. 2018;260:172–7. https://doi.org/10.1016/j.ijcard.2018.02.114.
11. De Siqueira MEM, Pozo E, Fernandes VR, et al. Characterization and clinical significance of right ventricular mechanics in pulmonary hypertension evaluated with cardiovascular magnetic resonance feature tracking. J Cardiovasc Magn Reson. 2016;18:39. https://doi.org/10.1186/s12968-016-0258-x.
12. Freed BH, Collins JD, François CJ, et al. MR and CT imaging for the evaluation of pulmonary hypertension. JACC Cardiovasc Imaging. 2016;9:715–32. https://doi.org/10.1016/j.jcmg.2015.12.015.
13. Friedberg MK, Redington AN. Right versus left ventricular failure: differences, similarities, and interactions. Circulation. 2014;129:1033–44. https://doi.org/10.1161/CIRCULATIONAHA.113.001375.
14. Friedman JD, Berman DS, Borges-Neto S, et al. ASNC announcement. J Nucl Cardiol. 2009;16:330. https://doi.org/10.1007/s12350-009-9061-5.
15. Fukuchi K, Hayashida K, Nakanishi N, et al. Quantitative analysis of lung perfusion in patients with primary pulmonary hypertension. J Nucl Med. 2002;43:757.
16. Fuld MK, Halaweish AF, Haynes SE, et al. Pulmonary perfused blood volume with dual-energy CT as surrogate for pulmonary perfusion assessed with dynamic multidetector CT. Radiology. 2013;267:747–56. https://doi.org/10.1148/radiol.12112789.
17. Galiè N, Humbert M, Vachiery J-L, et al. 2015 ESC/ERS guidelines for the diagnosis and treatment of pulmonary hypertension. Kardiologia Polska (Polish Heart J). 2015;73:1127–206. https://doi.org/10.5603/KP.2015.0242.
18. Galiè N, Saia F, Palazzini M, et al. Left main coronary artery compression in patients with pulmonary arterial hypertension and angina. J Am Coll Cardiol. 2017;69:2808–17. https://doi.org/10.1016/j.jacc.2017.03.597.
19. Groves AM, Win T, Charman SC, et al. Semi-quantitative assessment of tricuspid regurgitation on contrast-enhanced multidetector CT. Clin Radiol. 2004;59:715–9. https://doi.org/10.1016/j.crad.2004.02.007.
20. Grüning T, Drake BE, Farrell SL, Nokes T. Three-year clinical experience with VQ SPECT for diagnosing pulmonary embolism: diagnostic performance. Clin Imaging. 2014;38:831–5. https://doi.org/10.1016/j.clinimag.2014.04.003.

21. Hassoun PM, Mouthon L, Barberà JA, et al. Inflammation, growth factors, and pulmonary vascular remodeling. J Am Coll Cardiol. 2009;54:S10–9. https://doi.org/10.1016/j.jacc.2009.04.006.
22. Hopkins N, McLoughlin P. The structural basis of pulmonary hypertension in chronic lung disease: remodelling, rarefaction or angiogenesis? J Anat. 2002;201:335–48. https://doi.org/10.1046/j.1469-7580.2002.00096.x.
23. Humbert M, Kovacs G, Hoeper MM, et al. 2022 ESC/ERS guidelines for the diagnosis and treatment of pulmonary hypertension. Eur Heart J. 2022;43:3618–731. https://doi.org/10.1093/eurheartj/ehac237.
24. IAEA. Quantitative nuclear medicine imaging: concepts, requirements and methods. Vienna: International Atomic Energy Agency; 2014.
25. Isaacs D, Hazany S, Gamst A, et al. Evaluation of the coronary sinus on chest computed tomography in patients with and without pulmonary artery hypertension. J Comput Assist Tomogr. 2009;33:513–6. https://doi.org/10.1097/RCT.0b013e3181949b19.
26. Kawel-Boehm N, Hetzel SJ, Ambale-Venkatesh B, et al. Reference ranges ("normal values") for cardiovascular magnetic resonance (CMR) in adults and children: 2020 update. J Cardiovasc Magn Reson. 2020;22:87. https://doi.org/10.1186/s12968-020-00683-3.
27. Konstantinides SV, Meyer G, Becattini C, et al. 2019 ESC guidelines for the diagnosis and management of acute pulmonary embolism developed in collaboration with the European Respiratory Society (ERS): the task force for the diagnosis and management of acute pulmonary embolism of the European Society of Cardiology (ESC). Eur Respir J. 2019;54:1901647. https://doi.org/10.1183/13993003.01647-2019.
28. Kreitner K-F. Noninvasive imaging of pulmonary hypertension. Semin Respir Crit Care Med. 2014;35:099–111. https://doi.org/10.1055/s-0033-1363456.
29. Lange TJ, Bornia C, Stiefel J, et al. Increased pulmonary artery diameter on chest computed tomography can predict borderline pulmonary hypertension. Pulm circ. 2013;3:363–8. https://doi.org/10.4103/2045-8932.113175.
30. Liu M, Qin C, Xia X, et al. Semi-quantitative assessment of pulmonary arterial hypertension associated with congenital heart disease through myocardial perfusion imaging. Hell J Nucl Med. 2017;20:204–10. https://doi.org/10.1967/s002449910600.
31. MacDonald A, Burrell S. Infrequently performed studies in nuclear medicine: part 1. J Nucl Med Technol. 2008;36:132. https://doi.org/10.2967/jnmt.108.051383.
32. Mahammedi A, Oshmyansky A, Hassoun PM, et al. Pulmonary artery measurements in pulmonary hypertension: the role of computed tomography. J Thorac Imaging. 2013;28:96–103. https://doi.org/10.1097/RTI.0b013e318271c2eb.
33. Marcus JT, Gan CT-J, Zwanenburg JJM, et al. Interventricular mechanical asynchrony in pulmonary arterial hypertension. J Am Coll Cardiol. 2008;51:750–7. https://doi.org/10.1016/j.jacc.2007.10.041.
34. Masy M, Giordano J, Petyt G, et al. Dual-energy CT (DECT) lung perfusion in pulmonary hypertension: concordance rate with V/Q scintigraphy in diagnosing chronic thromboembolic pulmonary hypertension (CTEPH). Eur Radiol. 2018;28:5100–10. https://doi.org/10.1007/s00330-018-5467-2.
35. Mazraeshahi RM, Striet J, Oeltgen RC, Gerson MC. Myocardial SPECT images for diagnosis of pulmonary hypertension and right ventricular hypertrophy. J Nucl Med Technol. 2010;38:175. https://doi.org/10.2967/jnmt.110.080200.
36. McCall RK, Ravenel JG, Nietert PJ, et al. Relationship of Main pulmonary artery diameter to pulmonary arterial pressure in scleroderma patients with and without interstitial fibrosis. J Comput Assist Tomogr. 2014;38:163–8. https://doi.org/10.1097/RCT.0b013e3182aa7fc5.
37. Mesquita SMF, Castro CRP, Ikari NM, et al. Likelihood of left main coronary artery compression based on pulmonary trunk diameter in patients with pulmonary hypertension. Am J Med. 2004;116:369–74. https://doi.org/10.1016/j.amjmed.2003.11.015.
38. Mettler FA, Guiberteau MJ. Essentials of nuclear medicine imaging: expert consult – online and print. London: Elsevier Health Sciences; 2012.
39. Młynarski R, Młynarska A. Coronary sinus diameter as a potential marker of right ventricle impairment. IJERPH. 2022;19:2217. https://doi.org/10.3390/ijerph19042217.
40. Reinartz P, Wildberger JE, Schaefer W, et al. Tomographic imaging in the diagnosis of pulmonary embolism: a comparison between V/Q lung scintigraphy in SPECT technique and multislice spiral CT. J Nucl Med. 2004;45:1501.
41. Roach PJ, Schembri GP, Bailey DL. V/Q scanning using SPECT and SPECT/CT. J Nucl Med. 2013;54:1588. https://doi.org/10.2967/jnumed.113.124602.
42. Reiter U, Reiter G, Fuchsjäger M. MR phase-contrast imaging in pulmonary hypertension. BJR. 2016;89:20150995. https://doi.org/10.1259/bjr.20150995.
43. Remy-Jardin M, Ryerson CJ, Schiebler ML, et al. Imaging of pulmonary hypertension in adults: a position paper from the Fleischner Society. Radiology. 2021;298:531–49. https://doi.org/10.1148/radiol.2020203108.
44. Revel M-P, Faivre J-B, Remy-Jardin M, et al. Pulmonary hypertension: ECG-gated 64-section CT angiographic evaluation of new functional parameters as diagnostic criteria. Radiology. 2009;250:558–66. https://doi.org/10.1148/radiol.2502080315.
45. Sanz J, Kariisa M, Dellegrottaglie S, et al. Evaluation of pulmonary artery stiffness in pulmonary hypertension with cardiac magnetic resonance. JACC Cardiovasc Imaging. 2009;2:286–95. https://doi.org/10.1016/j.jcmg.2008.08.007.

46. Saunders LC, Johns CS, Stewart NJ, et al. Diagnostic and prognostic significance of cardiovascular magnetic resonance native myocardial T1 mapping in patients with pulmonary hypertension. J Cardiovasc Magn Reson. 2018;20:78. https://doi.org/10.1186/s12968-018-0501-8.
47. Scelsi CL, Bates WB, Melenevsky YV, et al. Egg-and-Banana sign: a novel diagnostic CT marker for pulmonary hypertension. Am J Roentgenol. 2018;210:1235–9. https://doi.org/10.2214/AJR.17.19208.
48. Seferian A, Helal B, Jaïs X, et al. Ventilation/perfusion lung scan in pulmonary veno-occlusive disease. Eur Respir J. 2012;40:75–83. https://doi.org/10.1183/09031936.00097911.
49. Shimizu K, Tsujino I, Sato T, et al. Performance of computed tomography-derived pulmonary vasculature metrics in the diagnosis and haemodynamic assessment of pulmonary arterial hypertension. Eur J Radiol. 2017;96:31–8. https://doi.org/10.1016/j.ejrad.2017.09.010.
50. Si-Mohamed SA, Zumbihl L, Turquier S, et al. Lung dual-energy CT perfusion blood volume as a marker of severity in chronic thromboembolic pulmonary hypertension. Diagnostics. 2023;13:769. https://doi.org/10.3390/diagnostics13040769.
51. Sjögren H, Kjellström B, Bredfelt A, et al. Underfilling decreases left ventricular function in pulmonary arterial hypertension. Int J Cardiovasc Imaging. 2021;37:1745–55. https://doi.org/10.1007/s10554-020-02143-6.
52. Swift AJ, Dwivedi K, Johns C, et al. Diagnostic accuracy of CT pulmonary angiography in suspected pulmonary hypertension. Eur Radiol. 2020;30:4918–29. https://doi.org/10.1007/s00330-020-06846-1.
53. Swift AJ, Rajaram S, Condliffe R, et al. Diagnostic accuracy of cardiovascular magnetic resonance imaging of right ventricular morphology and function in the assessment of suspected pulmonary hypertension results from the ASPIRE registry. J Cardiovasc Magn Reson. 2012;14:40. https://doi.org/10.1186/1532-429X-14-40.
54. Swift AJ, Telfer A, Rajaram S, et al. Dynamic contrast–enhanced magnetic resonance imaging in patients with pulmonary arterial hypertension. Pulm Circ. 2014;4:61–70. https://doi.org/10.1086/674882.
55. Szturmowicz M, Kacprzak A, Szołkowska M, et al. Pulmonary veno-occlusive disease: pathogenesis, risk factors, clinical features and diagnostic algorithm — state of the art. Adv Respir Med. 2018;86:131–41. https://doi.org/10.5603/ARM.2018.0021.
56. Tan RT, Kuzo R, Goodman LR, et al. Utility of CT scan evaluation for predicting pulmonary hypertension in patients with parenchymal lung disease. Chest. 1998;113:1250–6. https://doi.org/10.1378/chest.113.5.1250.
57. Tello K, Dalmer A, Vanderpool R, et al. Cardiac magnetic resonance imaging-based right ventricular strain analysis for assessment of coupling and diastolic function in pulmonary hypertension. JACC Cardiovasc Imaging. 2019;12:2155–64. https://doi.org/10.1016/j.jcmg.2018.12.032.
58. Truong QA, Massaro JM, Rogers IS, et al. Reference values for normal pulmonary artery dimensions by noncontrast cardiac computed tomography: the Framingham Heart Study. Circ Cardiovasc Imaging. 2012;5:147–54. https://doi.org/10.1161/CIRCIMAGING.111.968610.
59. Vogel-Claussen J, Skrok J, Shehata ML, et al. Right and left ventricular myocardial perfusion reserves correlate with right ventricular function and pulmonary hemodynamics in patients with pulmonary arterial hypertension. Radiology. 2011;258:119–27. https://doi.org/10.1148/radiol.10100725.
60. Vonk Noordegraaf A, Chin KM, Haddad F, et al. Pathophysiology of the right ventricle and of the pulmonary circulation in pulmonary hypertension: an update. Eur Respir J. 2019;53:1801900. https://doi.org/10.1183/13993003.01900-2018.
61. Xu J, Yang W, Zhao S, Lu M. State-of-the-art myocardial strain by CMR feature tracking: clinical applications and future perspectives. Eur Radiol. 2022;32:5424–35. https://doi.org/10.1007/s00330-022-08629-2.
62. Zhang C, Xin Q, Xu H, et al. Value of coronary sinus during computed tomography pulmonary angiography for predicting pulmonary hypertension in patients with acute pulmonary embolism. Cardiol Discov. 2023;3:78–84. https://doi.org/10.1097/CD9.0000000000000090.

Quantitative Evaluation of Pulmonary Embolism

17

Deepa Gopalan

Introduction

Pulmonary embolism (PE) is the life-threatening manifestation of venous thromboembolism (VTE) and is the third most common cause of cardiovascular death after myocardial infarction and stroke. The natural history of PE is to resolve over time, but a gamut of long-term sequelae has been described in survivors. The "post-PE syndrome" may be associated with one or more of the following: functional limitation, impaired gas exchange, abnormal pulmonary artery flow dynamics, and cardiac dysfunction [1]. The extreme manifestation of post-PE syndrome is chronic thromboembolic pulmonary disease (CTEPD) where there are perfusion defects without pulmonary hypertension followed by the more serious phenomenon of chronic thromboembolic pulmonary hypertension (CTEPH). Imaging is integral to the diagnosis and risk stratification of both acute and chronic pulmonary thromboembolism.

D. Gopalan (✉)
Department of Radiology, Hammersmith Hospital, Imperial College Healthcare NHS Trust, London, UK
e-mail: d.gopalan@nhs.net

Morphological Abnormalities of Pulmonary Thromboembolism on CT Pulmonary Angiography (CTPA)

A structured systematic approach is required to comprehend the broad spectrum of abnormalities that can be seen on CT in acute and chronic thromboembolism.

A. *Angiographic Features*

The most common direct finding of acute PE is a central intraluminal filling defect surrounded by rim of contrast material yielding a "polo mint" and "railway track" appearances when observed in the plane perpendicular and parallel to the vessel long axis respectively. Large clots that are draped over the pulmonary trunk bifurcation is referred to as "saddle embolus." The clots form an acute angle with the vessel wall and are often located at bifurcations. Complete occlusion is characterised by homogenous lack of contrast opacification and the vessel with acute clot is often distended. It is important to carefully review the right sided cardiac chambers and the inferior vena cava for the presence of a mobile clot-in-transit; this has an estimated incidence of 2–6% and possibly even higher in patients with severe PE and is associated with increased 30-day mortality [2].

Chronic thromboembolism is characterized by wall adherent eccentric thrombus that may or may not be calcified. The clot forms obtuse

R. Gill, P. Rajiah (eds.), *Quantitative Imaging in the Thorax*,
https://doi.org/10.1007/978-3-032-14103-3_17

angles and concave surfaces with the vessel wall. Instead of the smooth proximal to distal vessel gradation, there may be abrupt truncations in the vessel calibre. Vessels that are occluded shortly after origin may have blind ending pouch defects. Chronically tapered vessels are of overall small calibre or completely cut-off. Incomplete recanalization results in intravascular slits, bands, and webs of fibrous tissue and stenosis with or without post-stenotic dilatation. The webs are typically <1 mm in thickness and located at bifurcations and are generally better visualised on multiplanar reformats. Systemic collaterals often from bronchial circulation or also from intercostals and inferior phrenic arteries are frequently seen in chronic PE. Anastomoses can be present between bronchial arteries and precapillary pulmonary arterioles as well as postcapillary venules and small veins [3]. These anastomoses are important for maintaining the viability of ischemic pulmonary parenchyma downstream of proximal pulmonary artery obstructions. The delineation of bronchial circulation would require a slightly delayed phase CT, and hence, their presence may be missed if the CTPA has been optimised just for the pulmonary circulation.

Absent or heterogenous flow in the pulmonary veins, termed "pulmonary vein sign" can be present in both acute and chronic thromboembolism. It is thought to be the consequence of diminished venous return into an underfilled left atrium and is an ancillary feature that can be readily visualised on CTPA [4]. PVS is more frequent in chronic thromboembolism and shows resolution following successful pulmonary endarterectomy [5].

B. *Pulmonary Parenchyma*

Acute PE can be complicated by pulmonary infarcts that manifest on CT as wedge-shaped subpleural ground glass opacities with or without a rim of consolidation (reverse halo sign). A characteristic finding of chronic PE is mosaic attenuation with geographic pattern of lung attenuation (gray areas being normally perfused lung and black areas with reduced perfusion and lower vessel count). Multifocal atelectatic subpleural band-like opacites are the consequence of prior pulmonary infarcts. Occasionally, the infarcts may cavitate and may be further complicated with concomitant infection.

CT can also demonstrate features of cor pulmonale such as contrast medium reflux in to dilated IVC and hepatic veins, pleural and pericardial effusions, ascites, and subcutaneous oedema.

C. *Cardiac Chambers*

The cardiac chamber abnormalities are outlined under the section on quantification.

Acute Pulmonary Embolism

The management strategy of patients with acute PE requires accurate and rapid risk assessment involving three components: (1) clinical evaluation, (2) laboratory measures reflecting myocardial injury, and (3) estimation of the right ventricular size and/or function by CT and/or echocardiography.

Conventional CTPA: Quantification of Cardiovascular Signs

Right Ventricular Dysfunction

The traditional view that life-threatening acute PE equated with anatomically massive clot burden has been challenged by numerous studies highlighting the importance of the underlying cardiopulmonary function in determining the clinical outcome. Acute PE causes elevation of pulmonary vascular resistance leading to right ventricular dysfunction (RVD). which has been proven to be a major determinant of short-term mortality [6]. To reconcile clinical outcomes with cardiopulmonary function and embolus burden, the terms low-risk, submassive (or intermediate-risk), and massive (or high-risk) are used with the latter two categories defined by the presence of right heart strain and hemodynamic instability (systolic blood pressure < 90 mmHg), respectively [7]. This differentiation is crucial as it defines the threshold at which patients are deemed to be at sufficient risk to justify aggressive treatments such as systemic thrombolysis and advanced clot removal techniques such as catheter-directed thrombolysis, catheter-based thrombectomy, and surgical thrombectomy [8, 9].

The right ventricle (RV) to left ventricle (LV) diameter ratio, an established sign of RV dilatation on echocardiography, is also the main surrogate criterion for RVD on CT as it correlates with the increase in afterload induced by the acute clot on ventricular function [8, 10, 11]. In a meta-analysis, increased RV/LV diameter ratio on CT had a fivefold higher risk for PE-related mortality, conferring the strongest risk association [12]. There is conflicting evidence showing lack of correlation between CT-derived ventricular ratio and PE prognosis, particularly in normotensive patients [13, 14]. The apparent contradictions underscore the heterogeneity of PE-related data, reflecting the variations in study design, mortality rates, and endpoints. A comprehensive meta-analysis of 49 studies looking at clinical outcomes in patients with acute PE confirmed that across all end points, ventricular diameter ratio on CT had the strongest predictive value and most robust evidence base for adverse clinical outcomes [15].

The right and left ventricular diameters are calculated by measuring the maximum diameter of the RV and LV in the short axis in the axial plane, from the innermost aspect of the interventricular septum to the free wall of the ventricles, perpendicular to the long axis of the heart [16, 17] (Fig. 17.1). There are a few controversies regarding the best method for deriving the RV/LV ratio. Firstly, given the complex three-dimensional geometry of the right heart, reconstructed four-chamber views derived from multiplanar reformats have been advocated as the more precise and hence superior approach when compared to transaxial measurements for quantification of the ventricular ratio [18, 19]. But manual reconstructions can be cumbersome and time-consuming, requiring the use of dedicated software, whereas axial measurements are simple, do not necessitate too much additional effort, and are reproducible [20]. Crucially, the axial measurements have been shown to yield comparative results to the four-chamber reconstructions [21, 22]. Automated artificial intelligence algorithms based post-processing tools are now available to compute the RV/LV diameter ratio to provide an objective metric of RVD and have high accuracy and low failure rates [23–25].

Interestingly, the majority of the CT studies evaluating the use of RV/LV ratio for acute PE

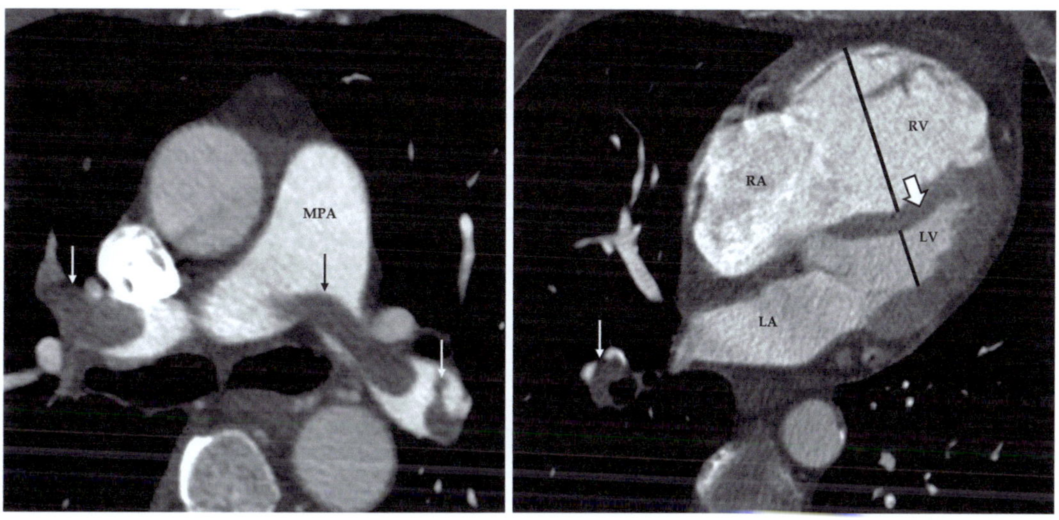

Fig. 17.1 Axial CTPA images of a 48-year-old with acute onset severe dyspnea, syncope and positive biomarkers demonstrates acute pulmonary embolism associated with right heart strain. Left panel: Saddle embolus draping across the main pulmonary artery (MPA) in to right and left pulmonary arteries (arrows). Right panel: Markedly dilated right ventricle (RV) with right to left ventricular (LV) ratio of 3.0*, leftward bowing of interventricular septum (block arrow), enlargement of right atrium (RA) and small left atrium (LA) *Ventricular diameter is maximal distance between ventricular endocardium and interven tricular septum perpendicular to long axis of heart. The RV:LV ratio is calculated by measuring the maximum diameters (thick black lines) of right and left ventricles.

risk stratification have not used EKG-gated protocols. In a small cohort of 62 patients, Scheffel et al. [26] demonstrated that not only did the ventricular ratios derived from four-chamber views on ECG-gated CT have less intra- and interobserver variability compared to non-EKG-gated CTs but they were also better predictors of short-term outcome with fewer patients being falsely classified as being at high risk. But CTPAs in routine clinical practice are not EKG-gated and although inferior for cardiac chamber assessment, the RV/LV ratio measured on non-EKG-gated CTPA has been shown to be reliable in most real-world cases of acute PE with good reproducibility.

While it is broadly accepted that increased ventricular diameter ratios on CT are associated with worse prognosis, the optimal CT cutoff value to predict RVD is the subject of ongoing discussion. A ratio of ≥ 0.9 is frequently but not always associated with worse prognosis and hence a higher threshold value is necessary for better risk assessment. Some studies have proposed a ratio of >1.0 [27, 28], while a higher threshold of >1.5 has been used by others [17, 29, 30]. The current European Society of Cardiology/European Respiratory guidelines on acute PE state that a ratio of 1.2 or higher is associated with an increased all-cause mortality [8].

Biomarkers of cardiac injury can also be used for PE risk stratification. Troponin, a marker of myocardial injury, is elevated in patients with acute PE who are at high risk of short-term death and adverse outcome events [114]. An elegant study by Granot et al. [31] demonstrated that RV/LV ratio >3 had a 95% likelihood of elevated troponin levels compared to 22% when RV/LV ratio was <2.0 and with 30-day mortality rate of 18% compared to 6%, respectively.

Another feature of RVD, adapted from echocardiography, is the straightening and bowing of the interventricular septum (IVS) in PE patients, first described on CT by Oliver et al. [32]. The progressively dysfunctional RV displaces the septum toward the left ventricle which in turn impairs the LV preload. The association between IVS bowing on CT and PE severity is not consistent in the existing literature. Some authors found no correlation between IVS position and PE-related mortality [33–36], while others have found it to be a more frequent finding in severe PE [17, 19, 37, 38] with significant relation to adverse outcomes. In a robust meta-analysis by Meinel et al. [15], abnormal septal curvature was significantly associated with all-cause mortality as well as PE-related mortality, a finding that suggests that IVS bowing has high specificity for RVD on CT. This is further supported by a recent publication that showed the presence of IVS bowing was able to predict thrombolytic usage [39]. A three-point scale can be used on CT to assess the position of the IVS. A septum that is convex toward the RV is classified as normal, while abnormal positions will include either a flattened septum or one that is convex toward the LV. Simple as it may sound, the observance of septal bowing on CT is affected by high interobserver variability [13, 37, 40].

Although it is not possible to perform direct evaluation of RV function on a non-EKG-gated CT, the prolongation of the transit time during the test bolus of intravenous contrast medium can provide an important clue to underlying RVD. Li et al. [41] showed that a delay in the bolus curve upslope time >6 s had a predictive value nearly equal to that of the CT anatomy-based measures, even when adjusted using multivariate analysis in patients with acute PE. The presence of concomitant conditions such as diffuse lung disease or pulmonary hypertension can also increase the length of test bolus curve and caution must be exercised before attributing this feature to acute PE alone.

Other Vascular Signs

Contrast medium refluxing into the inferior vena cava and hepatic veins may be an indirect sign of tricuspid valve insufficiency that may develop secondary to RV dilatation and reduced cardiac output. The reflux may serve as a dynamic feature of acute right heart failure as it has been shown to correlate with PE-related mortality [33]. Groves et al. [42] proposed a six-point scale for gradation of the reflux (1 = no IVC reflux;

2 = trace of reflux into IVC only; 3 = reflux into IVC but not hepatic veins; 4 = reflux into IVC and proximal hepatic veins; 5 = reflux into IVC and mid-hepatic veins; and 6 = reflux into IVC and opacifying distal hepatic veins). Reflux grades ≥4 have been shown to be associated with increased 30-day mortality in patients with acute PE [43]. The presence of IVC reflux has also been shown to be significantly associated with the need for mechanical ventilation and increased duration of intensive care unit treatment [35] and attributable mortality [39]. But the sign must be interpreted with caution as its specificity for RV dysfunction is diminished at high rates of contrast medium injection.

Several other vascular CT parameters have been proposed for real-time risk stratification of PE such as main pulmonary artery diameter >29 mm, increased ratio of pulmonary artery to ascending aorta, distension of the superior vena cava and azygos vein, dilated coronary sinus >9 mm [44], and the presence of concomitant coronary artery calcification [45–47], but these metrics are less important compared with the direct measurement of ventricular size as their predictive value is not consistent.

Pulmonary artery distensibility is a measure of vascular remodeling and vessel wall stiffness. In a normally compliant vessel, the distensibility ranges between 20% and 25% of the minimal diameter [48]. On EKG-gated CT, it is possible to calculate pulmonary artery distensibility by looking at the percentage change in the cross-sectional area of the PA in diastole and systole (maximum systolic diameter minus minimum diastolic diameter divided by the minimal diastolic diameter). Measurements are made perpendicular to the longitudinal axis of the PA on axial and coronal views. In a small study investigating the PA distensibility on CT in normal cohorts versus thromboembolism, the control group had a normative value of 25.9 ± 5.7% with a decrease in distensibility in acute severe PE [49]. PA distensibility is reduced in severe acute PE [50, 51].

Pulmonary infarction, seen in one third of patients with acute PE, has also been investigated as a potential prognostic marker [35, 52]. In a recent study with the large cohort of acute PE patients with pulmonary infarction, there was no correlation between infarction and poorer outcomes; furthermore, there was no difference in the rate of reperfusion therapies required by patients with and without infarction [53].

Pulmonary Arterial Obstruction

Cardiac status is a more accurate indicator of the magnitude of PE rather than the severity of angiographic obstruction. However, the pulmonary artery obstruction index (PAOI), a semiquantitative measure of clot burden, can be useful for risk stratification and monitoring of patients requiring an objective repetitive assessment, e.g., the effects of thrombolytic therapy. In the late 1990s, Bankier et al. [54] adapted the original angiographic indices of Miller et al. [55] and Walsh et al. [56] to helical CT. Subsequently, newer scoring systems designed specifically for CTPA have evolved; of these, the Qanadli et al. [57] and Mastora et al. [58] scores have gained the most application.

The Qanadli score considers both complete and partial vascular obstruction and integrates it with the residual lung perfusion [57]. Ten segmental arteries (three upper lobes, two middle lobe/lingula, three lower lobes) are assigned to each lung. One point is given to each segmental artery with a clot. If the thrombus is in a more proximal branch, the score would equal the number of the segmental branches that arose distal to the proximal artery. The unit score per artery is multiplied by a weighting factor for the residual perfusion distal to the clot (0 = no thrombus; 1 = partial occlusion, 2 = total occlusion) to give a maximum total score of 40 per patient. The obstruction index is simple and reproducible even in cases of anatomical variations. The Mastora scoring [58] uses a five-point scale (1, <25%; 2, 25–49%; 3, 50–74%; 4, 75–99%; 5, 100%) based on the percentage of obstruction to determine the central, peripheral, and global CT severity scores. Aside from its complexity, the accuracy of this score has not been validated.

The value of PAOI for prediction of PE severity, RV failure, and short-term clinical outcome is contentious. Some studies have shown an association between PAOI and mortality after acute PE [17, 36, 57, 59, 60], while others have challenged the assertion that obstructive indices correlate with mortality [13, 33, 61, 62]. The inconsistencies could potentially reflect the heterogeneity of study population as the CT obstruction scoring does not take into account preexisting comorbidities that may affect the cardiovascular reserve. Moreover, the discrepancy between the hemodynamic severity and mechanical obstruction could be due to pulmonary vasoconstriction mediated by vasoactive amines and systemic arterial hypoxemia [63].

Based on the PAOI, Qanadli et al. [57] divided the patients with PE in a high-risk (PAOI ≥20) and low-risk (PAOI <20) groups. A CT obstruction index of 40% or greater could identify 90% of patients with RV dilatation. Van der Meer et al. [36] reported a 11.2-fold increased risk of PE-specific 3-month mortality with a PAOI of 40% or higher despite anticoagulation, while Sen et al. had a 5.7-times increased mortality with PAOI higher than 36.5% as well as a higher rate of intensive care requirement [59]. Wong et al. proposed a novel "tipping point" between increasing thrombus load and RV decompensation as they found a strong correlation between PAOI and RV/LV diameter only after the obstruction index reached a defined threshold [11]. Despite the controversy regarding PAOI and PE mortality, there seems to be a strong correlation between PAOI and RV/LV ratio. Several studies have shown that PAOI can differentiate between patients with and without RVD [64–66]. Patients with PAOI >40% and RV/LV ratio >1.0 have significantly worse outcome [36].

Recently, a composite score called the combined Qanadli index (Qanadli score, RV/LV ratio, and pulmonary infarction) was shown to improve the odds ratio from 13 to 16 for predicting changes in cardiovascular parameters and short-term mortality in patients with pulmonary embolism [67].

It is also possible to do semiautomated estimates of clot volume burden using segmentation and region growing algorithms that have been shown to be accurate and reproducible [68]. There is good correlation between the automated quantification of clot volume and manual PAOI scoring [69]. In addition to improving measurement reliability, the computer-assisted techniques could reduce the time taken for quantification.

Atrial Size in Acute PE

Another pathophysiological consequence of massive PE with severe RVD is a decrease in right heart output and subsequent underfilling of left heart chambers. In conjunction with the IVS bowing and attendant diminished LV preload, there is a reduction in the cardiac output resulting in hypotensive shock. Few CT studies have described a decrease in left atrial (LA) size and reduced diameter of pulmonary veins, a consequence of diminished venous return [70, 71]. Furthermore, there is a significant negative correlation between the left atrial size and the embolic burden. A high PAOI is associated with small left and larger right atrial cavity size on CT [72, 73]. Using an automated software for volumetric analysis, Aviram et al. [74] showed that acute PE patients with LA volume ≤ 62 mL had significantly higher mortality rate of 19.6% compared to 8.9% in those with LA volume > 62 mL. A systematic review [75, 76] of 6 studies with 990 patients showed significant correlation between the longest left to right and anteroposterior diameters of the left atrium and the PAOI. Patients who died within 30 days of the acute event had significantly small LA volume compared to survivors. Despite the ease with which LA size can be measured on CT, current prediction models do not include LA size as large volume validation is lacking.

Chronic Thromboembolism

The imaging strategy for chronic thromboembolism involves a multimodality approach, tailored to confirm the diagnosis, evaluate the disease distribution, and assess the severity of pulmonary hypertension, followed by a multidisciplinary team discussion to determine the optimal therapeutic intervention.

Unlike acute PE, chronic thromboembolism is characterized by a gradual but progressive increase in RV afterload and pulmonary vascular resistance caused by mechanical obstruction and secondary remodeling of small arteries. Although the pulmonary arterial abnormalities demonstrated on imaging are integral to decision-making, the major determinant of long-term prognosis is RV dysfunction leading to irreversible RV failure [76]. Hence, estimation of cardiac function and PH severity is a core precept in the evaluation of chronic thromboembolism. *Cardiac MRI is the standard of care for assessment of RV function and will be dealt with in the pulmonary hypertension chapter.*

Dual-Energy CT (DECT) for Pulmonary Thromboembolism

DECT involves acquisition of two simultaneous or near-simultaneous datasets at different x-ray energy levels and can be performed using technologies that operate at the source level (dual-source, rapid voltage switching, dual-spin, split-beam) and/or at the detector level (dual-layer, photon counting CT). As each method has its own foibles, it is important that users get acquainted with the system that is at their disposal. The DE datasets can be used to distinguish specific materials with large atomic numbers such as iodine and xenon, based on their unique X-ray absorption characteristics with the differing X-ray energy spectra, thereby extending the CT capabilities beyond the standard densitometric assessment [77]. Optimal energy level will vary according to the scan technology. The material of interest is user-defined to create a two- or three-material decomposition technique depending on the available hardware (e.g., iodine-enhanced images generated by subtracting water from contrast-enhanced DECT images). It is pivotal to understand that images should only be evaluated for the material pairs to which they correspond. For example, water images look different depending on the material pair used for reconstruction (e.g., water [calcium] vs. water [iodine] images) [78]. The effective patient dose depends strongly on the dual-energy technology that is employed. Higher-end scanners are typically radiation-dose neutral with appropriate protocols [79]. Unlike conventional CTPA where it is preferable to have optimized opacification within pulmonary arteries, the homogeneity of the iodine map is determined by adequate attenuation of the downstream pulmonary capillary system. Hence, higher iodine concentration (>300 mg I/mL) and a slightly longer acquisition of up to 7 s may be necessary [80].

The data from the two energy spectra are used to calculate the distribution of iodine in the lung parenchyma after intravenous contrast material administration. Post-processing software is used to produce a visual panorama of the iodine distribution called pulmonary perfused blood volume (PBV) maps. The PBV maps are color coded (typically a 16-bit color scale) and can be superimposed as a color-fused overlay over the conventional anatomic CT data to produce CTPA DE perfusion maps. 3D reconstructions are not only useful to get a visual overview of reduced perfusion but also for quantification as the extent of the defects may be underestimated with uniplanar assessment. It is important to remember that DE perfusion reflects enhancement of the lung parenchyma at a single time point that indirectly displays blood volume as opposed to time-resolved dynamic CT perfusion and hence is only a surrogate marker of perfusion.

Virtual monoenergetic images (VMI) derived from DECT can prospectively facilitate reduction in the total amount of required contrast material needed for CTPA by up to 50% at photon energy of 50 keV as shown by Yuan et al. [81] without affecting image quality. The second most common cause of suboptimal CTPA after motion artifacts is substandard contrast enhancement. Up to 10% of CTPA studies are nondiagnostic, with 40% of these relating to poor contrast enhancement [82]. As VMI at low energy levels have higher image contrast and thus can increase vascular attenuation, it can be used retrospectively for salvaging studies with suboptimal vascular opacification [83, 84]. High-energy VMI images are useful to reduce metallic artifacts.

Using similar principles of material decomposition, inhaled xenon-enhanced DECT can be used to visualize the ventilatory component and delineate ventilation-perfusion mismatch analogous to VQ scintigraphy [85–88]. While early reports have established technical feasibility, the application has not undergone robust validation as there are many practical challenges such as the need for specific equipment, high cost, additional radiation dose, and side effects associated with Xenon gas. But the principle reinforces the growing importance of modern CT techniques in the diagnosis of thromboembolic disease.

DECT technique has matured since its introduction in 2006, and it is now possible to perform visual analysis of perfusion abnormalities as well as objective quantification.

Patterns of DECT Perfusion Abnormalities

A perfusion defect is characterized by a focal area of lung parenchyma with reduction in iodine concentration below the stated threshold [89]. The classical defect in acute and chronic PE is a peripheral wedge-shaped or triangular focus of hypoattenuation in lobar, segmental, or subsegmental distribution. This is different to the patchy defects seen in pulmonary arterial hypertension and hence can be used to differentiate between PAH and thromboembolic disease [90]. The combined use of standard CPTA for pulmonary arterial morphology and DECT iodine maps has been shown to have a sensitivity and specificity of 100% for CTEPH diagnosis of CTEPH [91]. DECT can also distinguish perfusion defects due to vascular causes from those secondary to airways disease. Chronic thromboembolism is characterized by perfusion defects that are concordant with the hypoattenuated (dark) areas of mosaic attenuation. Moreover, higher iodine concentration in the hyperattenuated (bright) areas of mosaic attenuation is indicative of a vascular rather than airway abnormality [92].

Pitfalls in DECT Interpretation

Not all perfusion defects are attributable to thromboembolism. Beam hardening artifacts from dense contrast material in the vena cava, innominate veins, and cardiac chambers can cause pseudo-perfusion defects. Lesser artifacts can be caused by pulsatile cardiac motion (mainly right middle lobe and lingula) and respiratory diaphragmatic movement (predominantly in the lung bases). There is also a gravity-dependent variation in regional blood flow. In supine posture, the volume of blood is higher in the dorsal part of the lung [93, 94]. Disease entities such as emphysema, pneumonia, atelectasis, fibrosis, and pleural effusion can cause perfusion heterogeneity mimicking thromboembolism [89, 95–97]. Therefore, it is necessary to analyze the iodine maps in conjunction with the morphological images. This combination approach is also useful to identify pulmonary infarction which is characterized by a perfusion defect that is larger than the accompanying corresponding lung parenchymal abnormality [89]. The PBV values are affected by a variety of parameters. These include factors that can influence vascular enhancement such as injection technique, arm position, the timing and shape of the contrast bolus, the age of the patient [98], and underlying cardiopulmonary status (e.g., prolongation of the transit times with heart failure).

Effects of Collateral Circulation

Following PA occlusion, blood flow via the systemic collateral circulation can increase by as much as 30% relative to the original flow [99]. This phenomenon is more frequently observed with chronic PE and can contribute to different patterns of perfusion abnormalities in chronic thromboembolism. The injected iodinated contrast medium can pass into the lung via the pulmonary as well as systemic collateral circulation and hence it is possible to gain additional insights into the physiological effects of PE using DECT. Not only are the systemic collaterals more common in chronic PE compared to acute PE, but they are also noted to be significantly frequent ipsilateral to the lungs with perfusion defects compared to lungs without perfusion defects [100]. A dual-phase (early and late) DECT protocol has been used to explore the differences in the regional perfusion patterns in patients with acute and chronic PE. In a small study of 42 patients (24 acute and 18 chronic PE), Hong et al. [101] showed greater enhancement of lung segments in the delayed phase in chronic PE due to infilling of the initial PBV defects by the systemic collaterals. Koike et al. [102] also demonstrated PBV differences between acute and chronic PE phase, emphasizing the enhanced role of systemic collaterals in chronic PE. More recently, prolonged transit time due to increase in PVR has also been proposed as a cause for the delayed increased lung enhancement [103].

DECT Quantification

There is a lack of standardization for the analytical methods that can be used for DECT assessment of lung perfusion defects. A perfusion scoring system was first proposed in 2010 by Chae et al. [104]. Each lung is divided into 10 segments (three in both upper lobes, two in the middle lobe and lingula, and five in both lower lobes). The perfusion defect is graded on a three-point scale: 0 = normal perfusion, 1 = moderately reduced perfusion, 2 = profoundly reduced or absent perfusion. Thieme et al. [105] used a lobar perfusion method based on an incremental percentage of the volume of each lobe with perfusion defects (Grade 0 = 0% [i.e., no defect], Grade 1 = 1–25%, Grade 2 = 26–50%, Grade 3 = 51–75%, Grade 4 = 76–99%, Grade 5 = 100%, i.e., complete defect) with a weighting factor given to number of involved segments to derive a perfusion defect score (P-score). A simplified approach was taken by Takagi et al. [106] by using a three-point scale (0 = no defect, 1 = defect in <50% of a segment, 2 = ≥50% of a segment).

Manual perfusion scores are user-dependent and cumbersome and hence not useful in routine clinical practice. However, DECT has benefited from a decade of technological advances; the introduction of automated quantification of global and regional pulmonary perfusion has facilitated significant reduction of post-processing steps. But quantification cannot be performed in picture archiving and communications system platform and requires the use of proprietary vendor software.

The 3D measurements of the defects can be improved by doing volumetric quantification, whereby the volume of perfusion defects relative to the total lung volume is calculated [107, 108] (Fig. 17.2). PBV can be expressed as a relative

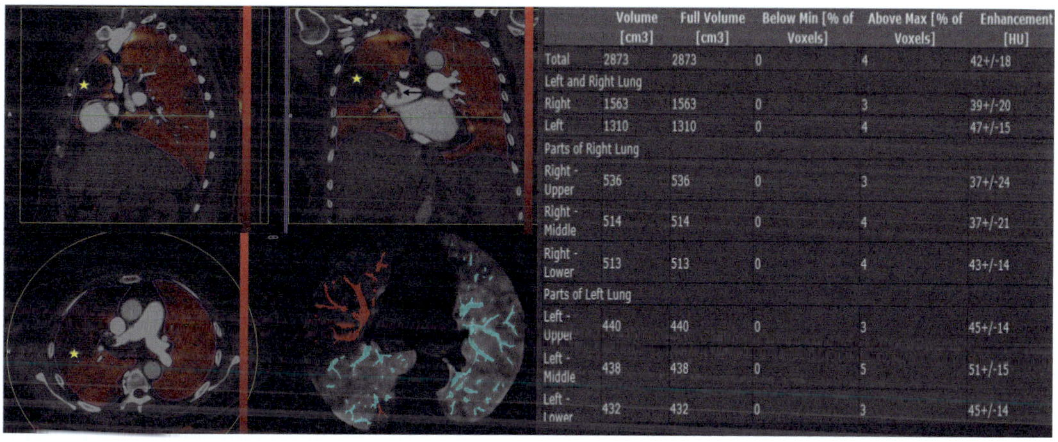

	Volume [cm3]	Full Volume [cm3]	Below Min [% of Voxels]	Above Max [% of Voxels]	Enhancement [HU]
Total	2873	2873	0	4	42+/-18
Left and Right Lung					
Right	1563	1563	0	3	39+/-20
Left	1310	1310	0	4	47+/-15
Parts of Right Lung					
Right - Upper	536	536	0	3	37+/-24
Right - Middle	514	514	0	4	37+/-21
Right - Lower	513	513	0	4	43+/-14
Parts of Left Lung					
Left - Upper	440	440	0	3	45+/-14
Left - Middle	438	438	0	5	51+/-15
Left - Lower	432	432	0	3	45+/-14

Fig. 17.2 Acute pulmonary embolism in a 34-year-old female with antiphospholipid syndrome. Dual-energy computed tomography (DECT) lung perfusion quantification generates iodine distribution maps (or lung iodine perfused blood volume (iPBV) maps) that highlight regional blood flow within the pulmonary parenchyma. Left panel: The dedicated software shows pulmonary embolism (arrows) and perfusion defects (star) in the right lung. Right panel: DECT map obtained with volume analysis software shows perfusion defect volume. Hounsfield units (HU) (iodine enhancement level) as lung iPBV values are calculated automatically in several patterns (whole lung, left and right lungs, and the upper, middle and lower lungs). The results are typically reported as the absolute volume or the percentage of the total lung volume affected by the perfusion defect.

value per unit volume or as per unit mass when normalized by lung density [109]. Alterations in breathing and the resultant extent of lung inflation will have significant effect on the perfusion per unit volume [110] for the perfusion per unit mass as the lung tissue mass does not vary much with the respiratory cycle [111].

An important limitation of DECT is that it only provides a relative PBV measurement, comparing iodine intensity across different lobes to identify focal perfusion defects. Hence, most of the DECT-based studies rarely report the physical units of the perfusion maps. Using a rapid kVp switching scanner, Wu et al. demonstrated the iodine density for normal lung to be 1.89 mg/mL (0.85–3.29 mg/mL) with significant differences between normal lung parenchyma, nonocclusive perfusion defects, and occlusive perfusion defects [112]. More recently, using a dual-source DECT protocol, chronic thromboembolic patients were shown to have decreased lung HU (median 27 vs. 39), lower PBV values (median 39 vs. 62), and higher PA peak/lung HU ratio (median 17 vs. 11) when compared with acute PE, findings that were attributed to alterations in the structural integrity of the vascular bed with progressive vascular remodeling and small vessel disease in chronic PE [113]. PBV quantification by DECT has been shown to have excellent intra- and interobserver reliability [114]. Recently, a proof-of-concept study in four patients showed that effective atomic number-based quantitative PBV maps (PBV Z_{eff}) were superior to the standard (PBV_{iodine}) DECT iodine maps for PBV quantification, but this work would need further validation in larger human cohort.

Applications of DECT in Thromboembolic Disease

The complementary advantages between standard CTPA and DECT in pulmonary thromboembolism could be applied to clinical practice in numerous ways.

Enhanced Visualization of Clots

The clinical importance of DECT is underscored by a recent meta-analysis of seven studies which demonstrated a high pooled positive likelihood ratio for PE detection. Hence, DECT could potentially be useful as a prevalence independent, rule-in test [115]. The detection of peripheral clots is also improved with DECT [116] but it is important to acknowledge that the management of subsegmental emboli is contentious [117]. In a retrospective analysis of 1144 DECT examinations, a small incremental benefit was demonstrated as an additional 1% had a new diagnosis of acute PE with the use of iodine maps [118]. Perfusion defects usually correspond to the area of an occluded vessel but can also be seen in the absence of a demonstrable intravascular clot [119] or a visible pulmonary parenchymal abnormality. These could be the consequence of microcirculatory obstruction or persistent hypoperfusion secondary to vasoconstrictive mediators. Conversely, perfusion may be preserved when the clot is either nonocclusive or partially occlusive [120, 121]. Only 6–9% of nonocclusive clots are associated with perfusion defects compared to 82–95% of occlusive thrombus [122]. It is therefore important to interrogate PBV maps in conjunction with the standard morphological CTPA images.

Risk Stratification

Multiple studies have explored the correlation between pulmonary perfused blood volumes and other traditional CT markers of PE severity [66, 104, 105, 107, 108, 123–128]. Both manual and automatic PBV quantification have been shown to have moderate to high negative correlation with PA obstruction score and axial RV/LV diameter ratio [66, 104, 128], serum troponin [105], and D-dimer [108]. Higher perfusion defect score is associated with lower survival and worse clinical outcomes [124]. In a retrospective analysis of 53 patients with acute PE, Bauer et al. [108] demonstrated that the relative hazard ratio for death increased by a factor of up to 10 in patients with perfusion defects >5% relative to lung volume. A global PBV value of <60% is associated with higher occurrence of ICU admission [123]. Despite a lack of correlation between perfusion defect volume and pulmonary artery obstruction score, Apfaltrer et al. [107] found that patients with low perfusion defect volume were low-risk cases who did not require intensive monitoring and treatment. In a very recent study, the perfusion defect volume was shown to have the potential to be an independent prognostic marker as it was able to predict adverse outcomes independent of clinical pretest scoring as well as visual assessment of PE severity [129]. Conversely, in a propensity-matched study of 480 patients with acute PE undergoing standard CTPA or DECT, PBV quantification offered no added benefit over CT ventricular diameter ratio for predicting all-cause death within 30 days [130]. The discrepancy could relate to the heterogenous population, outcome variations, as well as methodological differences in DECT quantification between different studies.

Different DECT-based functional parameters have been used in the evaluation of chronic PE and CTEPH. DECT perfusion imaging allows for improved detection of segmental and peripheral chronic thromboembolism [131, 132]. DECT can also provide insights into alterations in the vascular bed in CTED compared to CTEPH. In a small study involving 28 matched CTED and CTEPH patients, Saeedan et al. [133] demonstrated higher perfusion defect score in CTEPH and more unilateral disease in CTED, but after propensity score matching, there were no statistically significant differences in any of the functional DECT parameters between the two groups. Several studies have explored the correlation between reduced PBV and hemodynamic markers of severity in CTEPH [100, 106, 134–136]. A significant correlation was seen with some studies [106, 134, 135], while only a weak to moderate association was seen with others [136, 137]. This discrepancy could be due to the heterogeneity in the CTEPH samples that were studied. In a recent retrospective review of 78 CTEPH cases, Abozeed et al. showed that perfusion defect score, clot burden score, and a combined score had positive correlation with mPAP and PVR but the magnitude of correlation was weak [138]. Using standard-phase DECT, increased central and reciprocal reduction in peripheral parenchymal enhancement expressed as the ratio PAenh/WLenh (pulmonary artery enhancement and volumetric enhancement of whole lung) has been shown to correlate well with PVR [139]. More recently, this ratio was demonstrated to be the single best dual-phase DECT metric for PVR correlation [103].

Recently, deep learning automated lung segmentation technique was used to define hypoperfusion on a per-pixel basis and calculate the global and lobar hypoperfused lung volume (HLV), a measure of the spatial extent of impairment compared to PBV which is an average of parenchymal iodine concentration. In 51 CTEPH patients, Bird et al. [140] demonstrated that global HLV correctly distinguished CTEPH patients from controls (AUV 0.84), had higher specificity relative to global PBV (64% vs. 51%), and had strong correlation with preoperative PVR ($\rho = 0.81$) and a moderate correlation with the change in PVR after pulmonary endarterectomy ($\rho = -0.70$) in patients with surgically defined segmental disease. However, this is a single institution observational and retrospective study in a small patient cohort and hence required broader validation.

Follow-Up for Assessment of Disease Progression

DECT could be used to evaluate the extent of revascularization following acute PE. Wu et al. [112] demonstrated a significant difference in iodine densities before and after treatment with anticoagulation. Persistence of perfusion defect on DECT could be due to incomplete clot resolution or fragmentation [139]. But the VQ literature has shown that about 40% of survivors of acute PE have persistent perfusion defects although only a small proportion go on to develop chronic thromboembolism [141].

Serial Monitoring for Evaluation of Response to Treatment

Serial quantification of perfusion can be useful to monitor response to therapeutic intervention. In a small study of 16 BPAs in 8 patients, PBV maps before and after balloon pulmonary angioplasty for CTEPH correlated with hemodynamic metrics such as pulmonary artery pressure and pulmonary vascular resistance [142]. The same authors showed that in 17 patients with 57 BPA sessions, DECT was also shown to be more reliable than SPECT imaging in the assessment of improvement after BPA [143]. More recently, the efficacy of BPA as assessed by improvement in the lung perfusion heterogeneity on PBV showed positive correlation with hemodynamic parameters as well as exercise capacity [144]. Similarly, an improvement in perfusion blood volume corresponding to the successful removal of chronic thromboembolic material has also been demonstrated following pulmonary endarterectomy [145]. While these are promising, it must be emphasized that these studies involved small patient cohorts from single centers and hence require validation on a larger scale.

Tissue Characterization

DECT data are useful for the detection and tissue characterization of intravascular thrombotic material using the material decomposition method. In addition to analyzing iodine distribution in the lung parenchyma, using a dedicated software algorithm, it is also possible to evaluate the iodine content of pulmonary vessels. This is useful to differentiate true clots from flow artifacts and partial volume effects [146]. DECT parameters have also been used for differentiating pulmonary artery sarcoma from thrombus. In a small study of 25 patients, Chang et al. [147] showed that while there was no significant difference in standard HU between the two entities, the iodine HU (27.9 vs. 10.6 HU) and iodine concentration values (1.49 vs. 0.61) were significantly higher in the sarcoma group.

Intermodality Correlation Between DECT, MR Perfusion, and VQ Scintigraphy

There are intrinsic methodological as well as physiological differences between DECT and other perfusion imaging modalities. As previously emphasized, DECT iodine maps are only a surrogate marker of perfusion as the iodine distribution is studied at a single time point. This contrasts with true perfusion measurements accorded by dynamic contrast-enhanced MRI (DCE-MR) where serial time point measurements are made following intravenous administration of contrast material. DCE-MR perfusion is a radiation-free noninvasive technique that has been shown to be useful in the screening and monitoring of CTEPH following therapeutic intervention [148–152]. Although CT is disadvantaged by radiation constraints, it has higher spatial resolution and is more practical than MRI with shorter examination times and wider availability. DECT has been shown to be a non-inferior alternative to MRI in estimating CTEPH severity and post-therapy follow-up [153]. In a small group of 20 CTEPH patients, there was comparable quantification of lung perfusion defects between MR and DECT with good spatial agreement and a similar significant reduction in the perfusion defects following pulmonary endarterectomy. Perfusion scintigraphy using ^{99m}Tc-macroaggregated albumin (MAA) is the first pass technique reflecting the distribution of the radiotracer solely in the pulmonary circulation as the MAA particles are trapped in the pulmonary capillary bed. Using first-generation scanners, Thieme et al. [154] first compared DECT with VQ scintigraphy and demonstrated good agreement between the two modalities with sensitivities and specificities of 75 and 80% on a per-patient basis and 83 and 99% on a per-segment basis, respectively, for acute PE. In the follow-up of acute PE patients, DECT was shown to perform as well as SPECT for the detection of chronic thromboembolic disease [155]. There is an excellent patient-level agreement between PBV maps on DECT and V/Q scintigraphy for CTEPH diagnosis [156, 157]. Recently, a similarly high level of agreement was found for the quantitative correlation of the severity of perfusion defects between DECT and SPECT VQ [158]. However, there is only a modest to moderate agreement at the segmental level between the two modalities, primarily due to the fundamental intermodality differences in the depiction of the distal pulmonary circulation [159].

Functional Respiratory Imaging

Functional respiratory imaging (FRI) is a quantitative post-processing technique based on multidetector CT and computational fluid dynamics

(CFD) that can provide objective information on the pulmonary intravascular volumes and geometry. Automated lung vessel segmentation, 3D reconstruction of the intraparenchymal vasculature, and vascular volume quantitation are performed using proprietary software.

In a small cohort of 18 CTEPH patients and 15 controls, Rahaghi et al. [160] used this approach to elegantly demonstrate the effects of pulmonary vascular remodeling. The blood volume is expressed as a function of cross-sectional area of the vessel (e.g., BV5 and BV > 10 = blood volume of vessels with a cross-sectional area of ≤5 and >10 mm^2, respectively, in a region of interest). CTEPH patients showed engorgement of proximal vessels, reduction in the small-vessel volume (objective evidence of vascular pruning), and asymmetry in the arterial and venous vascular beds with increased arterial tortuosity. The loss of distal vasculature had significant correlation to increased PVR.

Quantitative evaluation of the morphologic alterations in the small pulmonary vessels has also been evaluated in acute PE and may have a role in phenotyping and prognostication [161, 162]. Analysis of CT scans of 17 patients involved in the SEATTLE II study (acute massive or submassive PE with evidence of right heart strain treated with catheter-directed fibrinolysis) [163] showed that decreased distal venous volume and increased distal arterial-venous difference were associated with baseline RV dilation; the latter metric was also predictive of the degree of RV decompression after therapy [164]. In a single institution retrospective study of 703 patients identified as having intermediate-risk PE, a decrease in the small arterial vessel fraction and dilated main pulmonary artery on the baseline diagnostic CT were both predictors of chronic oxygen requirement on discharge [162].

Conclusion

The imaging diagnosis of pulmonary thromboembolism has undergone significant change and development in the past 25 years. Unprecedented advances in CT technology have allowed imaging to evolve from simple visual perception of morphological abnormalities to a more objective approach with the capability of deriving various physiological parameters that can enhance the ability to improve diagnosis, prognostication, and therapy monitoring. Dual-energy imaging offers new additional insights into pulmonary vascular physiology in patients with acute and chronic thromboembolism. An exponential body of scientific evidence has accumulated in parallel to the technical innovations and increased availability of DECT systems. However, the lack of single uniform methodology for PBV measurements independent of the scanner type poses a pertinent challenge contributing to the underutilization of DECT in routine clinical practice. There is an unmet need for standardizing DECT quantification and establishing platform-specific normative values. Simpler and standardized algorithms are needed to make perfusion quantification feasible in the emergent setting.

References

1. Sista AK, Klok FA. Late outcomes of pulmonary embolism: the post-PE syndrome. Thromb Res. 2018;164:157–62.
2. Barrios D, Rosa-Salazar V, Morillo R, Nieto R, Fernández S, Zamorano JL, et al. Prognostic Significance of Right Heart Thrombi in Patients With Acute Symptomatic Pulmonary Embolism: Systematic Review and Metaanalysis. Chest. 2017;151[2]:409–16.
3. Dorfmüller P, Günther S, Ghigna MR, Thomas de Montpréville V, Boulate D, Paul JF, et al. Microvascular disease in chronic thromboembolic pulmonary hypertension: a role for pulmonary veins and systemic vasculature. Eur Respir J. 2014;44[5]:1275–88.
4. Gopalan D, Nordgren-Rogberg A, Le EPV, Pavey H, Tarkin J, Nyrén S, et al. Abnormal Pulmonary Venous Filling: An Adjunct Feature in the Computed Tomography Pulmonary Angiogram Assessment of Chronic Thromboembolic Pulmonary Hypertension. JAHA. 2020;9[21]:e018075.
5. Gopalan D, Riley JYJ, Leong K, Guo HH, Zamanian RT, Hsi A, et al. Pulmonary Vein Sign on Computed Tomography Pulmonary Angiography in Proximal and Distal Chronic Thromboembolic Pulmonary Hypertension With Hemodynamic Correlation. J Thorac Imaging. 2023 May 1;38[3]:159–64.
6. Grifoni S, Olivotto I, Cecchini P, Pieralli F, Camaiti A, Santoro G, et al. Short-term clinical outcome of patients with acute pulmonary embolism, normal

blood pressure, and echocardiographic right ventricular dysfunction. Circulation. 2000;101:2817–22.
7. Jaff MR, McMurtry MS, Archer SL, Cushman M, Goldenberg N, Goldhaber SZ, et al. Management of massive and submassive pulmonary embolism, iliofemoral deep vein thrombosis, and chronic thromboembolic pulmonary hypertension: a scientific statement from the American Heart Association. Circulation. 2011;123:1788–830.
8. Konstantinides SV, Meyer G, Becattini C, Bueno H, Geersing GJ, Harjola VP, et al. 2019 ESC guidelines for the diagnosis and management of acute pulmonary embolism developed in collaboration with the European Respiratory Society [ERS]. Eur Heart J. 2020;41:543–603.
9. Stevens SM, Woller SC, Baumann Kreuziger L, Bounameaux H, Doerschug K, Geersing GJ, et al. Executive summary: antithrombotic therapy for VTE disease: second update of the CHEST guideline and expert panel report. Chest. 2021;160:2247–59.
10. Henzler T, Roeger S, Meyer M, Schoepf UJ, Nance JW, Haghi D, et al. Pulmonary embolism: CT signs and cardiac biomarkers for predicting right ventricular dysfunction. Eur Respir J. 2012;39:919–26.
11. Wong LF, Akram AR, McGurk S, Van Beek EJR, Reid JH, Murchison JT. Thrombus load and acute right ventricular failure in pulmonary embolism: correlation and demonstration of a 'tipping point' on CT pulmonary angiography. Br J Radiol. 2012;85:1471–6.
12. Vedovati MC, Germini F, Agnelli G, Becattini C. Prognostic role of embolic burden assessed at computed tomography angiography in patients with acute pulmonary embolism: systematic review and meta-analysis. J Thromb Haemost. 2013;11:2092–102.
13. Araoz PA, Gotway MB, Harrington JR, Harmsen WS, Mandrekar JN. Pulmonary embolism: prognostic CT findings. Radiology. 2007;242:889–97.
14. Jiménez D, Lobo JL, Monreal M, Moores L, Oribe M, Barrón M, et al. Prognostic significance of multidetector CT in normotensive patients with pulmonary embolism: results of the protect study. Thorax. 2014;69:109–15.
15. Meinel FG, Nance JW, Schoepf UJ, Hoffmann VS, Thierfelder KM, Costello P, et al. Predictive value of computed tomography in acute pulmonary embolism: systematic review and meta-analysis. Am J Med. 2015;128:747–759.e2.
16. Schoepf UJ, Kucher N, Kipfmueller F, Quiroz R, Costello P, Goldhaber SZ. Right ventricular enlargement on chest computed tomography: a predictor of early death in acute pulmonary embolism. Circulation. 2004;110:3276–80.
17. Collomb D, Paramelle PJ, Calaque O, Bosson JL, Vanzetto G, Barnoud D, et al. Severity assessment of acute pulmonary embolism: evaluation using helical CT. Eur Radiol. 2003;13:1508–14.
18. Quiroz R, Kucher N, Schoepf UJ, Kipfmueller F, Solomon SD, Costello P, et al. Right ventricular enlargement on chest computed tomography: prognostic role in acute pulmonary embolism. Circulation. 2004;109:2401–4.
19. Kang DK, Thilo C, Schoepf UJ, Barraza JM, Nance JW, Bastarrika G, et al. CT signs of right ventricular dysfunction: prognostic role in acute pulmonary embolism. JACC Cardiovasc Imaging. 2011;4:841–9.
20. Ende-Verhaar YM, Kroft LJM, Mos ICM, Huisman MV, Klok FA. Accuracy and reproducibility of CT right-to-left ventricular diameter measurement in patients with acute pulmonary embolism. PLoS One. 2017;12:e0188862.
21. Kamel EM, Schmidt S, Doenz F, Adler-Etechami G, Schnyder P, Qanadli SD. Computed tomographic angiography in acute pulmonary embolism: do we need multiplanar reconstructions to evaluate the right ventricular dysfunction? J Comput Assist Tomogr. 2008;32:438–43.
22. Stein PD, Matta F, Yaekoub AY, Goodman LR, Sostman HD, Weg JG, et al. Reconstructed 4-chamber views compared with axial imaging for assessment of right ventricular enlargement on CT pulmonary angiograms. J Thromb Thrombolysis. 2009;28:342–7.
23. Sharkey MJ, Taylor JC, Alabed S, Dwivedi K, Karunasaagarar K, Johns CS, et al. Fully automatic cardiac four chamber and great vessel segmentation on CT pulmonary angiography using deep learning. Front Cardiovasc Med. 2022;9:983859.
24. González G, Jiménez-Carretero D, Rodríguez-López S, Kumamaru KK, George E, San José Estépar R, et al. Automated axial right ventricle to left ventricle diameter ratio computation in computed tomography pulmonary angiography. Fraidenraich D, editor. PLoS One. 2015;10:e0127797.
25. Foley RW, Glenn-Cox S, Rossdale J, Mynott G, Burnett TA, Brown WJH, et al. Automated calculation of the right ventricle to left ventricle ratio on CT for the risk stratification of patients with acute pulmonary embolism. Eur Radiol. 2021;31:6013–20.
26. Scheffel H, Stolzmann P, Leschka S, Desbiolles L, Seifert B, Marincek B, et al. Ventricular short-axis measurements in patients with pulmonary embolism: effect of ECG-gating on variability, accuracy, and risk prediction. Eur J Radiol. 2012;81:2195–202.
27. Contractor S, Maldjian PD, Sharma VK, Gor DM. Role of helical CT in detecting right ventricular dysfunction secondary to acute pulmonary embolism. J Comput Assist Tomogr. 2002;26:587–91.
28. Lim KE, Chan CY, Chu PH, Hsu YY, Hsu WC. Right ventricular dysfunction secondary to acute massive pulmonary embolism detected by helical computed tomography pulmonary angiography. Clin Imaging. 2005;29:16–21.
29. Lerchbaumer MH, Ebner M, Ritter CO, Steimke L, Rogge NIJ, Sentler C, et al. Prognostic value of right atrial dilation in patients with pulmonary embolism. ERJ Open Res. 2021;7:00414–2020.

30. Reid JH, Murchison JT. Acute right ventricular dilatation: a new helical CT sign of massive pulmonary embolism. Clin Radiol. 1998;53:694–8.
31. Granot Y, Rozenbaum Z, Ziv-Baran T, Fares R, Milwidsky A, Berliner S, et al. Correlation between CT-derived cardiac chamber volume, myocardial injury and mortality in acute pulmonary embolism. Thromb Res. 2021;205:63–9.
32. Oliver TB, Reid JH, Murchison JT. Interventricular septal shift due to massive pulmonary embolism shown by CT pulmonary angiography: an old sign revisited. Thorax. 1998;53:1092–4; discussion 1088–9.
33. Ghaye B, Ghuysen A, Willems V, Lambermont B, Gerard P, D'Orio V, et al. Severe pulmonary embolism: pulmonary artery clot load scores and cardiovascular parameters as predictors of mortality. Radiology. 2006;239:884–91.
34. Moroni AL, Bosson JL, Hohn N, Carpentier F, Pernod G, Ferretti GR. Non-severe pulmonary embolism: prognostic CT findings. Eur J Radiol. 2011;79:452–8.
35. Heyer CM, Lemburg SP, Knoop H, Holland-Letz T, Nicolas V, Roggenland D. Multidetector-CT angiography in pulmonary embolism-can image parameters predict clinical outcome? Eur Radiol. 2011;21:1928–37.
36. van der Meer RW, Pattynama PMT, van Strijen MJL, van den Berg-Huijsmans AA, Hartmann IJC, Putter H, et al. Right ventricular dysfunction and pulmonary obstruction index at helical CT: prediction of clinical outcome during 3-month follow-up in patients with acute pulmonary embolism. Radiology. 2005;235:798–803.
37. Kang DK, Ramos-Duran L, Schoepf UJ, Armstrong AM, Abro JA, Ravenel JG, et al. Reproducibility of CT signs of right ventricular dysfunction in acute pulmonary embolism. AJR Am J Roentgenol. 2010;194:1500–6.
38. Shayganfar A, Hajiahmadi S, Astaraki M, Ebrahimian S. The assessment of acute pulmonary embolism severity using CT angiography features. Int J Emerg Med. 2020;13:15.
39. Karri J, Truong T, Hasapes J, Trujillo DO, Chua S, Shiralkar K, et al. Correlating computed tomography pulmonary angiography signs of right ventricular strain in pulmonary embolisms to clinical outcomes. Ann Thorac Med. 2020;15:64–9.
40. Samaranayake CB, Craigie M, Kempny A, Bell PT, McCann A, Wahi S, et al. Right heart strain assessment on CTPA following acute pulmonary embolism: interobserver variability between expert radiologists and physicians. Respir Med. 2022;200:106928.
41. Li C, Lin CT, Kligerman SJ, Hong SN, White CS. Enhancement characteristics of the computed tomography pulmonary angiography test bolus curve and its use in predicting right ventricular dysfunction and mortality in patients with acute pulmonary embolism. J Thorac Imaging. 2015;30:274–81.
42. Groves AM, Win T, Charman SC, Wisbey C, Pepke-Zaba J, Coulden RA. Semi-quantitative assessment of tricuspid regurgitation on contrast-enhanced multidetector CT. Clin Radiol. 2004;59:715–9.
43. Aviram G, Rogowski O, Gotler Y, Bendler A, Steinvil A, Goldin Y, et al. Real-time risk stratification of patients with acute pulmonary embolism by grading the reflux of contrast into the inferior vena cava on computerized tomographic pulmonary angiography. J Thromb Haemost. 2008;6:1488–93.
44. Cozzi D, Moroni C, Cavigli E, Bindi A, Caviglioli C, Nazerian P, et al. Prognostic value of CT pulmonary angiography parameters in acute pulmonary embolism. Radiol Med. 2021;126:1030–6.
45. Ng ACC, Chung T, Yong ASC, Wong HSP, Chow V, Celermajer DS, et al. Long-term cardiovascular and noncardiovascular mortality of 1023 patients with confirmed acute pulmonary embolism. Circ Cardiovasc Qual Outcomes. 2011;4:122–8.
46. Heidinger BH, DaBreo D, Kirkbride RR, Santos M, Carroll BJ, Feldman SA, et al. Risk assessment of acute pulmonary embolism utilizing coronary artery calcifications in patients that have undergone CT pulmonary angiography and transthoracic echocardiography. Eur Radiol. 2021;31:2809–18.
47. Williams MC, Morley NCD, Muir KC, Reid JH, van Beek EJR, Murchison JT. Coronary artery calcification is associated with mortality independent of pulmonary embolism severity: a retrospective cohort study. Clin Radiol. 2019;74:973.e7–973.e14.
48. Botney MD. Role of hemodynamics in pulmonary vascular remodeling: implications for primary pulmonary hypertension. Am J Respir Crit Care Med. 1999;159:361–4.
49. Wu DK, Hsiao SH, Lin SK, Lee CY, Yang SH, Chang SM, et al. Main pulmonary arterial distensibility: different presentation between chronic pulmonary hypertension and acute pulmonary embolism. Circ J. 2008;72:1454–9.
50. Wang D, Yang F, Zhu X, Cui S, Dong S, Zhang Z, et al. CTPA pulmonary artery distensibility in assessment of severity of acute pulmonary embolism and right ventricular function. Medicine (Baltimore). 2021;100:e24356.
51. Yang F, Wang D, Cui S, Zhu Y, Liu L, Ji M, et al. Decreased pulmonary artery distensibility as a marker for severity in acute pulmonary embolism patients undergoing ECG-gated CTPA. J Thromb Thrombolysis. 2021;51:748–56.
52. Revel MP, Triki R, Chatellier G, Couchon S, Haddad N, Hernigou A, et al. Is it possible to recognize pulmonary infarction on multisection CT images? Radiology. 2007;244:875–82.
53. Lio KU, O'Corragain O, Bashir R, Brosnahan S, Cohen G, Lakhter V, et al. Clinical outcomes and factors associated with pulmonary infarction following acute pulmonary embolism: a retrospective observational study at a US academic Centre. BMJ Open. 2022;12:e067579.
54. Bankier AA, Janata K, Fleischmann D, Kreuzer S, Mallek R, Frossard M, et al. Severity assessment of acute pulmonary embolism with spiral CT:

evaluation of two modified angiographic scores and comparison with clinical data. J Thorac Imaging. 1997;12:150–8.
55. Miller GA, Sutton GC, Kerr IH, Gibson RV, Honey M. Comparison of streptokinase and heparin in treatment of isolated acute massive pulmonary embolism. Br Med J. 1971;2:681–4.
56. Walsh P, Greenspan R, Simon M, Hyers T, Woosley P, Cole C. An angiographic severity index for pulmonary embolism. Circulation. 1973;47:101–8.
57. Qanadli SD, El Hajjam M, Vieillard-Baron A, Joseph T, Mesurolle B, Oliva VL, et al. New CT index to quantify arterial obstruction in pulmonary embolism: comparison with angiographic index and echocardiography. AJR Am J Roentgenol. 2001;176:1415–20.
58. Mastora I, Remy-Jardin M, Masson P, Galland E, Delannoy V, Bauchart JJ, et al. Severity of acute pulmonary embolism: evaluation of a new spiral CT angiographic score in correlation with echocardiographic data. Eur Radiol. 2003;13:29–35.
59. Sen HS, Abakay Ö, Cetincakmak MG, Sezgi C, Yilmaz S, Demir M, et al. A single imaging modality in the diagnosis, severity, and prognosis of pulmonary embolism. Biomed Res Int. 2014;2014:470295.
60. Abdelwahab HW, Arafa S, Bondok K, Batouty N, Bakeer M. Relationship between clot burden in pulmonary computed tomography angiography and different parameters of right cardiac dysfunction in acute pulmonary embolism. Cardiovasc J Afr. 2020;31:21–4.
61. Ghuysen A, Ghaye B, Willems V, Lambermont B, Gerard P, Dondelinger RF, et al. Computed tomographic pulmonary angiography and prognostic significance in patients with acute pulmonary embolism. Thorax. 2005;60:956–61.
62. Bach AG, Nansalmaa B, Kranz J, Taute BM, Wienke A, Schramm D, et al. CT pulmonary angiography findings that predict 30-day mortality in patients with acute pulmonary embolism. Eur J Radiol. 2015;84:332–7.
63. Lyhne MD, Kline JA, Nielsen-Kudsk JE, Andersen A. Pulmonary vasodilation in acute pulmonary embolism – a systematic review. Pulm Circ. 2020;10:2045894019899775.
64. Çildag MB, Gok M, Karaman CZ. Pulmonary artery obstruction index and right ventricular dysfunction signs in initial and follow up pulmonary computed tomography angiography in acute pulmonary embolism. J Clin Diagn Res. 2017;11:TC21–5.
65. Varol K, Gumus C, Yucel H, Sezer F, Seker E, Inci MF, et al. Correlation of right ventricular dysfunction on acute pulmonary embolism with pulmonary artery computed tomography obstruction index ratio [PACTOIR] and comparison with echocardiography. Jpn J Radiol. 2015;33:311–6.
66. Apfaltrer P, Henzler T, Meyer M, Roeger S, Haghi D, Gruettner J, et al. Correlation of CT angiographic pulmonary artery obstruction scores with right ventricular dysfunction and clinical outcome in patients with acute pulmonary embolism. Eur J Radiol. 2012;81:2867–71.
67. Akhoundi N, Sedghian S, Siami A, Yazdani Nia I, Naseri Z, Ghadiri Asli SM, et al. Does adding the pulmonary infarction and right ventricle to left ventricle diameter ratio to the Qanadli index [a combined Qanadli index] more accurately, predict short-term mortality in patients with pulmonary embolism? Indian J Radiol Imaging. 2023;33:478–83.
68. Furlan A, Patil A, Park B, Chang CCH, Roberts MS, Bae KT. Accuracy and reproducibility of blood clot burden quantification with pulmonary CT angiography. AJR Am J Roentgenol. 2011;196:516–23.
69. Shen C, Yu N, Wen L, Zhou S, Dong F, Liu M, et al. Risk stratification of acute pulmonary embolism based on the clot volume and right ventricular dysfunction on CT pulmonary angiography. Clin Respir J. 2019;13:674–82.
70. Ocak I, Fuhrman C. CT angiography findings of the left atrium and right ventricle in patients with massive pulmonary embolism. AJR Am J Roentgenol. 2008;191:1072–6.
71. Hama Y, Yakushiji T, Iwasaki Y, Kaji T, Isomura N, Kusano S. Small left atrium: an adjunctive sign of hemodynamically compromised massive pulmonary embolism. Yonsei Med J. 2005;46:733–6.
72. Aviram G, Steinvil A, Berliner S, Rosen G, Sosna J, Man A, et al. The association between the embolic load and atrial size in acute pulmonary embolism. J Thromb Haemost. 2011;9:293–9.
73. Faghihi Langroudi T, Sheikh M, Naderian M, Sanei Taheri M, Ashraf-Ganjouei A, Khaheshi I. The association between the pulmonary arterial obstruction index and atrial size in patients with acute pulmonary embolism. Radiol Res Pract. 2019;2019:6025931.
74. Aviram G, Soikher E, Bendet A, Shmueli H, Ziv-Baran T, Amitai Y, et al. Prediction of mortality in pulmonary embolism based on left atrial volume measured on CT pulmonary angiography. Chest. 2016;149:667–75.
75. Zuin M, Rigatelli G, Turchetta S, Zonzin P, Zuliani G, Roncon L. Left atrial size measured on CT pulmonary angiography: another parameter of pulmonary embolism severity? A systematic review. J Thromb Thrombolysis. 2020;50:181–9.
76. Simonneau G, Torbicki A, Dorfmüller P, Kim N. The pathophysiology of chronic thromboembolic pulmonary hypertension. Eur Respir Rev. 2017;26:160112.
77. Johnson TRC, editor. Dual energy CT in clinical practice. Heidelberg: Springer; 2011. p. 216. [Medical radiology].
78. Parakh A, Lennartz S, An C, Rajiah P, Yeh BM, Simeone FJ, et al. Dual-energy CT images: pearls and pitfalls. Radiographics. 2021;41:98–119.
79. Kalisz K, Halliburton S, Abbara S, Leipsic JA, Albrecht MH, Schoepf UJ, et al. Update on cardiovascular applications of multienergy CT. Radiographics. 2017;37:1955–74.

80. Lu GM, Zhao Y, Zhang LJ, Schoepf UJ. Dual-energy CT of the lung. AJR Am J Roentgenol. 2012;199:S40–53.
81. Yuan R, Shuman WP, Earls JP, Hague CJ, Mumtaz HA, Scott-Moncrieff A, et al. Reduced iodine load at CT pulmonary angiography with dual-energy monochromatic imaging: comparison with standard CT pulmonary angiography–a prospective randomized trial. Radiology. 2012;262:290–7.
82. Jones SE, Wittram C. The indeterminate CT pulmonary angiogram: imaging characteristics and patient clinical outcome. Radiology. 2005;237:329–37.
83. Apfaltrer P, Sudarski S, Schneider D, Nance JW, Haubenreisser H, Fink C, et al. Value of monoenergetic low-kV dual energy CT datasets for improved image quality of CT pulmonary angiography. Eur J Radiol. 2014;83:322–8.
84. Bae K, Jeon KN, Cho SB, Park SE, Moon JI, Baek HJ, et al. Improved opacification of a suboptimally enhanced pulmonary artery in chest CT: experience using a dual-layer detector spectral CT. AJR Am J Roentgenol. 2018;210:734–41.
85. Chae EJ, Seo JB, Goo HW, Kim N, Song KS, Lee SD, et al. Xenon ventilation CT with a dual-energy technique of dual-source CT: initial experience. Radiology. 2008;248:615–24.
86. Kong X, Sheng HX, Lu GM, Meinel FG, Dyer KT, Schoepf UJ, et al. Xenon-enhanced dual-energy CT lung ventilation imaging: techniques and clinical applications. AJR Am J Roentgenol. 2014;202:309–17.
87. Zhang LJ, Zhou CS, Lu GM. Dual energy computed tomography demonstrated lung ventilation/perfusion mismatch in a 19-year-old patient with pulmonary embolism. Circulation. 2012;126:2441–3.
88. Zhang LJ, Zhou CS, Schoepf UJ, Sheng HX, Wu SY, Krazinski AW, et al. Dual-energy CT lung ventilation/perfusion imaging for diagnosing pulmonary embolism. Eur Radiol. 2013;23:2666–75.
89. Otrakji A, Digumarthy SR, Lo Gullo R, Flores EJ, Shepard JAO, Kalra MK. Dual-energy CT: spectrum of thoracic abnormalities. Radiographics. 2016;36:38–52.
90. Giordano J, Khung S, Duhamel A, Hossein-Foucher C, Bellèvre D, Lamblin N, et al. Lung perfusion characteristics in pulmonary arterial hypertension [PAH] and peripheral forms of chronic thromboembolic pulmonary hypertension [pCTEPH]: dual-energy CT experience in 31 patients. Eur Radiol. 2017;27:1631–9.
91. Kröger JR, Gerhardt F, Dumitrescu D, Rosenkranz S, Schmidt M, Maintz D, et al. Diagnosis of pulmonary hypertension using spectral-detector CT. Int J Cardiol. 2019;285:80–5.
92. Pontana F, Remy-Jardin M, Duhamel A, Faivre JB, Wallaert B, Remy J. Lung perfusion with dual energy multi-detector row CT: can it help recognize ground glass opacities of vascular origin? Acad Radiol. 2010;17:587–94.
93. Clough AV, Haworth ST, Roerig DL, Hoffman EA, Dawson CA. Influence of gravity on radiographic contrast material-based measurements of regional blood flow distribution. Acad Radiol. 2003;10:128–38.
94. Wildberger JE, Schoepf UJ, Mahnken AH, Herzog P, Ditt H, Niethammer MU, et al. Approaches to CT perfusion imaging in pulmonary embolism. Semin Roentgenol. 2005;40:64–73.
95. Lu GM, Wu SY, Yeh BM, Zhang LJ. Dual-energy computed tomography in pulmonary embolism. BJR. 2010;83:707–18.
96. Ameli-Renani S, Rahman F, Nair A, Ramsay L, Bacon JL, Weller A, et al. Dual-energy CT for imaging of pulmonary hypertension: challenges and opportunities. Radiographics. 2014;34:1769–90.
97. Kim BH, Seo JB, Chae EJ, Lee HJ, Hwang HJ, Lim C. Analysis of perfusion defects by causes other than acute pulmonary thromboembolism on contrast-enhanced dual-energy CT in consecutive 537 patients. Eur J Radiol. 2012;81:e647–52.
98. Meinel FG, Graef A, Sommer WH, Thierfelder KM, Reiser MF, Johnson TRC. Influence of vascular enhancement, age and gender on pulmonary perfused blood volume quantified by dual-energy-CTPA. Eur J Radiol. 2013;82:1565–70.
99. Michel RP, Hakim TS. Increased resistance in postobstructive pulmonary vasculopathy: structure-function relationships. J Appl Physiol (1985). 1991;71:601–10.
100. Renard B, Remy-Jardin M, Santangelo T, Faivre JB, Tacelli N, Remy J, et al. Dual-energy CT angiography of chronic thromboembolic disease: can it help recognize links between the severity of pulmonary arterial obstruction and perfusion defects? Eur J Radiol. 2011;79:467–72.
101. Hong YJ, Kim JY, Choe KO, Hur J, Lee HJ, Choi BW, et al. Different perfusion pattern between acute and chronic pulmonary thromboembolism: evaluation with two-phase dual-energy perfusion CT. AJR Am J Roentgenol. 2013;200:812–7.
102. Koike H, Sueyoshi E, Sakamoto I, Uetani M. Clinical significance of late phase of lung perfusion blood volume [lung perfusion blood volume] quantified by dual-energy computed tomography in patients with pulmonary thromboembolism. J Thorac Imaging. 2017;32:43–9.
103. Bacon JL, Madden BP, Gissane C, Sayer C, Sheard S, Vlahos I. Vascular and parenchymal enhancement assessment by dual-phase dual-energy CT in the diagnostic investigation of pulmonary hypertension. Radiol Cardiothorac Imaging. 2020;2:e200009.
104. Chae EJ, Seo JB, Jang YM, Krauss B, Lee CW, Lee HJ, et al. Dual-energy CT for assessment of the severity of acute pulmonary embolism: pulmonary perfusion defect score compared with CT angiographic obstruction score and right ventricular/left ventricular diameter ratio. Am J Roentgenol. 2010;194:604–10.

105. Thieme SF, Ashoori N, Bamberg F, Sommer WH, Johnson TRC, Leuchte H, et al. Severity assessment of pulmonary embolism using dual energy CT – correlation of a pulmonary perfusion defect score with clinical and morphological parameters of blood oxygenation and right ventricular failure. Eur Radiol. 2012;22:269–78.
106. Takagi H, Ota H, Sugimura K, Otani K, Tominaga J, Aoki T, et al. Dual-energy CT to estimate clinical severity of chronic thromboembolic pulmonary hypertension: comparison with invasive right heart catheterization. Eur J Radiol. 2016;85:1574–80.
107. Apfaltrer P, Bachmann V, Meyer M, Henzler T, Barraza JM, Gruettner J, et al. Prognostic value of perfusion defect volume at dual energy CTA in patients with pulmonary embolism: correlation with CTA obstruction scores, CT parameters of right ventricular dysfunction and adverse clinical outcome. Eur J Radiol. 2012;81:3592–7.
108. Bauer RW, Frellesen C, Renker M, Schell B, Lehnert T, Ackermann H, et al. Dual energy CT pulmonary blood volume assessment in acute pulmonary embolism – correlation with D-dimer level, right heart strain and clinical outcome. Eur Radiol. 2011;21:1914–21.
109. Lee HJ, Wanderley M, da Silva Rubin VC, Alcala GC, Costa ELV, Parga JR, et al. Quantitative analysis of pulmonary perfusion with dual-energy CT angiography: comparison of two quantification methods in patients with pulmonary embolism. Int J Card Imaging. 2023;39:853–62.
110. Cao JJ, Wang Y, Schapiro W, McLaughlin J, Cheng J, Passick M, et al. Effects of respiratory cycle and body position on quantitative pulmonary perfusion by MRI. J Magn Reson Imaging. 2011;34:225–30.
111. Busse N, Erwin W, Pan T. Evaluation of a semiautomated lung mass calculation technique for internal dosimetry applications. Med Phys. 2013;40:122503.
112. Wu HW, Cheng JJ, Li JY, Yin Y, Hua J, Xu JR. Pulmonary embolism detection and characterization through quantitative iodine-based material decomposition images with spectral computed tomography imaging. Investig Radiol. 2012;47:85–91.
113. Nallasamy N, Bullen J, Karim W, Heresi GA, Renapurkar RD. Evaluation of vascular parameters in patients with pulmonary thromboembolic disease using dual-energy computed tomography. J Thorac Imaging. 2019;34:367–72.
114. Cai XR, Feng YZ, Qiu L, Xian ZH, Yang WC, Mo XK, et al. Iodine distribution map in dual-energy computed tomography pulmonary artery imaging with rapid kVp switching for the diagnostic analysis and quantitative evaluation of acute pulmonary embolism. Acad Radiol. 2015;22:743–51.
115. Abdellatif W, Ebada MA, Alkanj S, Negida A, Murray N, Khosa F, et al. Diagnostic accuracy of dual-energy CT in detection of acute pulmonary embolism: a systematic review and meta-analysis. Can Assoc Radiol J. 2021;72:285–92.
116. Okada M, Kunihiro Y, Nakashima Y, Nomura T, Kudomi S, Yonezawa T, et al. Added value of lung perfused blood volume images using dual-energy CT for assessment of acute pulmonary embolism. Eur J Radiol. 2015;84:172–7.
117. Carrier M, Klok FA. Symptomatic subsegmental pulmonary embolism: to treat or not to treat? Hematology Am Soc Hematol Educ Program. 2017;2017:237–41.
118. Weidman EK, Plodkowski AJ, Halpenny DF, Hayes SA, Perez-Johnston R, Zheng J, et al. Dual-energy CT angiography for detection of pulmonary emboli: incremental benefit of iodine maps. Radiology. 2018;289:546–53.
119. Takx RAP, Henzler T, Schoepf UJ, Germann T, Schoenberg SO, Shirinova A, et al. Predictive value of perfusion defects on dual energy CTA in the absence of thromboembolic clots. J Cardiovasc Comput Tomogr. 2017;11:183–7.
120. Pontana F, Faivre JB, Remy-Jardin M, Flohr T, Schmidt B, Tacelli N, et al. Lung perfusion with dual-energy multidetector-row CT [MDCT]: feasibility for the evaluation of acute pulmonary embolism in 117 consecutive patients. Acad Radiol. 2008;15:1494–504.
121. Geyer LL, Scherr M, Körner M, Wirth S, Deak P, Reiser MF, et al. Imaging of acute pulmonary embolism using a dual energy CT system with rapid kVp switching: initial results. Eur J Radiol. 2012;81:3711–8.
122. Meyer M, Haubenreisser H, Sudarski S, Doesch C, Ong MM, Borggrefe M, et al. Where do we stand? Functional imaging in acute and chronic pulmonary embolism with state-of-the-art CT. Eur J Radiol. 2015;84:2432–7.
123. Meinel FG, Graef A, Bamberg F, Thieme SF, Schwarz F, Sommer WH, et al. Effectiveness of automated quantification of pulmonary perfused blood volume using dual-energy CTPA for the severity assessment of acute pulmonary embolism. Investig Radiol. 2013;48:563–9.
124. Perez-Johnston R, Plodkowski AJ, Halpenny DF, Hayes SA, Capanu M, Araujo-Filho JAB, et al. Perfusion defects on dual-energy CTA in patients with suspected pulmonary embolism correlate with right heart strain and lower survival. Eur Radiol. 2021;31:2013–21.
125. Sakamoto A, Sakamoto I, Nagayama H, Koike H, Sueyoshi E, Uetani M. Quantification of lung perfusion blood volume with dual-energy CT: assessment of the severity of acute pulmonary thromboembolism. AJR Am J Roentgenol. 2014;203:287–91.
126. Miura S, Ohno Y, Kimura H, Kichikawa K. Quantitative lung perfused blood volume imaging on dual-energy CT: capability for quantitative assessment of disease severity in patients with acute pulmonary thromboembolism. Acta Radiol. 2015;56:284–93.

127. Zhou Y, Shi H, Wang Y, Kumar AR, Chi B, Han P. Assessment of correlation between CT angiographic clot load score, pulmonary perfusion defect score and global right ventricular function with dual-source CT for acute pulmonary embolism. Br J Radiol. 2012;85:972–9.
128. Zhang LJ, Yang GF, Zhao YE, Zhou CS, Lu GM. Detection of pulmonary embolism using dual-energy computed tomography and correlation with cardiovascular measurements: a preliminary study. Acta Radiol. 2009;50:892–901.
129. Foldyna B, Zangeneh FA, Wagner M, Doktorov K, Basmagi S, Matveeva A, et al. Pulmonary perfusion defect volume on dual-energy CT: prognostic marker of adverse events in patients with suspected pulmonary embolism. Int J Card Imaging. 2023;39:1333–41.
130. Im DJ, Hur J, Han K, Suh YJ, Hong YJ, Lee HJ, et al. Prognostic value of dual-energy CT-based iodine quantification versus conventional CT in acute pulmonary embolism: a propensity-match analysis. Korean J Radiol. 2020;21:1095–103.
131. Dournes G, Verdier D, Montaudon M, Bullier E, Rivière A, Dromer C, et al. Dual-energy CT perfusion and angiography in chronic thromboembolic pulmonary hypertension: diagnostic accuracy and concordance with radionuclide scintigraphy. Eur Radiol. 2014;24:42–51.
132. Le Faivre J, Duhamel A, Khung S, Faivre JB, Lamblin N, Remy J, et al. Impact of CT perfusion imaging on the assessment of peripheral chronic pulmonary thromboembolism: clinical experience in 62 patients. Eur Radiol. 2016;26:4011–20.
133. Saeedan MB, Bullen J, Heresi GA, Rizk A, Karim W, Renapurkar RD. Morphologic and functional dual-energy CT parameters in patients with chronic thromboembolic pulmonary hypertension and chronic thromboembolic disease. AJR Am J Roentgenol. 2020;215:1335–41.
134. Kroeger JR, Zöllner J, Gerhardt F, Rosenkranz S, Gertz RJ, Kerszenblat S, et al. Detection of patients with chronic thromboembolic pulmonary hypertension by volumetric iodine quantification in the lung-a case control study. Quant Imaging Med Surg. 2022;12:1121–9.
135. Meinel FG, Graef A, Thierfelder KM, Armbruster M, Schild C, Neurohr C, et al. Automated quantification of pulmonary perfused blood volume by dual-energy CTPA in chronic thromboembolic pulmonary hypertension. RöFo. 2014;186:151–6.
136. Tsutsumi Y, Iwano S, Okumura N, Adachi S, Abe S, Kondo T, et al. Assessment of severity in chronic thromboembolic pulmonary hypertension by quantitative parameters of dual-energy computed tomography. J Comput Assist Tomogr. 2020;44:578–85.
137. Eberhard M, Alkadhi H. Machine learning and deep neural networks: applications in patient and scan preparation, contrast medium, and radiation dose optimization. J Thorac Imaging. 2020;35:S17–20.
138. Abozeed M, Conic S, Bullen J, Rizk A, Saeedan MB, Karim W, et al. Dual energy CT based scoring in chronic thromboembolic pulmonary hypertension and correlation with clinical and hemodynamic parameters: a retrospective cross-sectional study. Cardiovasc Diagn Ther. 2022;12:305–13.
139. Ameli-Renani S, Ramsay L, Bacon JL, Rahman F, Nair A, Smith V, et al. Dual-energy computed tomography in the assessment of vascular and parenchymal enhancement in suspected pulmonary hypertension. J Thorac Imaging. 2014;29:98–106.
140. Bird E, Hasenstab K, Kim N, Madani M, Malhotra A, Hahn L, et al. Mapping the spatial extent of hypoperfusion in chronic thromboembolic pulmonary hypertension using multienergy CT. Radiol Cardiothorac Imaging. 2023;5:e220221.
141. Klok FA, Ageno W, Ay C, Bäck M, Barco S, Bertoletti L, et al. Optimal follow-up after acute pulmonary embolism: a position paper of the European Society of Cardiology Working Group on pulmonary circulation and right ventricular function, in collaboration with the European Society of Cardiology Working Group on atherosclerosis and vascular biology, endorsed by the European Respiratory Society. Eur Heart J. 2022;43:183–9.
142. Koike H, Sueyoshi E, Sakamoto I, Uetani M, Nakata T, Maemura K. Quantification of lung perfusion blood volume [lung PBV] by dual-energy CT in patients with chronic thromboembolic pulmonary hypertension [CTEPH] before and after balloon pulmonary angioplasty [BPA]: preliminary results. Eur J Radiol. 2016;85:1607–12.
143. Koike H, Sueyoshi E, Sakamoto I, Uetani M, Nakata T, Maemura K. Comparative clinical and predictive value of lung perfusion blood volume CT, lung perfusion SPECT and catheter pulmonary angiography images in patients with chronic thromboembolic pulmonary hypertension before and after balloon pulmonary angioplasty. Eur Radiol. 2018;28:5091–9.
144. Koike H, Sueyoshi E, Nishimura T, Iwano Y, Oka T, Uetani M, et al. Effect of balloon pulmonary angioplasty on homogenization of lung perfusion blood volume by dual-energy computed tomography in patients with chronic thromboembolic pulmonary hypertension. Lung. 2021;199:475–83.
145. Desai A, Malaisrie SC, Cuttica M, Freed BH, Rich S, Schimmel D, et al. Dual-energy computed tomography as an alternative noninvasive study for evaluation of chronic thromboembolic pulmonary hypertension postoperatively. Circ Cardiovasc Imaging. 2020;13:e010168.
146. Krissak R, Henzler T, Reichert M, Krauss B, Schoenberg SO, Fink C. Enhanced visualization of lung vessels for diagnosis of pulmonary embolism using dual energy CT angiography. Investig Radiol. 2010;45:341–6.
147. Chang S, Hur J, Im DJ, Suh YJ, Hong YJ, Lee HJ, et al. Dual-energy CT-based iodine quantification for differentiating pulmonary artery sarcoma from

pulmonary thromboembolism: a pilot study. Eur Radiol. 2016;26:3162–70.
148. Johns CS, Swift AJ, Rajaram S, Hughes PJC, Capener DJ, Kiely DG, et al. Lung perfusion: MRI vs. SPECT for screening in suspected chronic thromboembolic pulmonary hypertension. J Magn Reson Imaging. 2017;46:1693–7.
149. Rajaram S, Swift AJ, Telfer A, Hurdman J, Marshall H, Lorenz E, et al. 3D contrast-enhanced lung perfusion MRI is an effective screening tool for chronic thromboembolic pulmonary hypertension: results from the ASPIRE registry. Thorax. 2013;68:677–8.
150. Gopalan D, Blanchard D, Auger WR. Diagnostic evaluation of chronic thromboembolic pulmonary hypertension. Ann Am Thorac Soc. 2016;13 Suppl 3:S222–39.
151. Schoenfeld C, Cebotari S, Hinrichs J, Renne J, Kaireit T, Olsson KM, et al. MR imaging–derived regional pulmonary parenchymal perfusion and cardiac function for monitoring patients with chronic thromboembolic pulmonary hypertension before and after pulmonary endarterectomy. Radiology. 2016;279:925–34.
152. Schoenfeld C, Hinrichs JB, Olsson KM, Kuettner MA, Renne J, Kaireit T, et al. Cardio-pulmonary MRI for detection of treatment response after a single BPA treatment session in CTEPH patients. Eur Radiol. 2019;29:1693–702.
153. Moher Alsady T, Kaireit TF, Behrendt L, Winther HB, Olsson KM, Wacker F, et al. Comparison of dual-energy computer tomography and dynamic contrast-enhanced MRI for evaluating lung perfusion defects in chronic thromboembolic pulmonary hypertension. PLoS One. 2021;16:e0251740.
154. Thieme SF, Becker CR, Hacker M, Nikolaou K, Reiser MF, Johnson TRC. Dual energy CT for the assessment of lung perfusion—correlation to scintigraphy. Eur J Radiol. 2008;68:369–74.
155. Meysman M, Everaert H, Buls N, Nieboer K, de Mey J. Comparison of ventilation-perfusion single-photon emission computed tomography [V/Q SPECT] versus dual-energy CT perfusion and angiography [DECT] after 6 months of pulmonary embolism [PE] treatment. Eur J Radiol. 2015;84:1816–9.
156. Thieme SF, Graute V, Nikolaou K, Maxien D, Reiser MF, Hacker M, et al. Dual energy CT lung perfusion imaging—correlation with SPECT/CT. Eur J Radiol. 2012;81:360–5.
157. Masy M, Giordano J, Petyt G, Hossein-Foucher C, Duhamel A, Kyheng M, et al. Dual-energy CT [DECT] lung perfusion in pulmonary hypertension: concordance rate with V/Q scintigraphy in diagnosing chronic thromboembolic pulmonary hypertension [CTEPH]. Eur Radiol. 2018;28:5100–10.
158. Si-Mohamed S, Moreau-Triby C, Tylski P, Tatard-Leitman V, Wdowik Q, Boccalini S, et al. Head-to-head comparison of lung perfusion with dual-energy CT and SPECT-CT. Diagn Interv Imaging. 2020;101:299–310.
159. Remy-Jardin M, Ryerson CJ, Schiebler ML, Leung ANC, Wild JM, Hoeper MM, et al. Imaging of pulmonary hypertension in adults: a position paper from the Fleischner society. Radiology. 2021;298:531–49.
160. Rahaghi FN, Ross JC, Agarwal M, González G, Come CE, Diaz AA, et al. Pulmonary vascular morphology as an imaging biomarker in chronic thromboembolic pulmonary hypertension. Pulm Circ. 2016;6:70–81.
161. Matsuoka S, Kotoku A, Yamashiro T, Matsushita S, Fujikawa A, Yagihashi K, et al. Quantitative CT evaluation of small pulmonary vessels in patients with acute pulmonary embolism. Acad Radiol. 2018;25:653–8.
162. Hassan SM, Nardelli P, Minhas JK, Ash SY, Estépar RSJ, Antkowiak MC, et al. CT imaging determinants of persistent hypoxemia in acute intermediate-risk pulmonary embolism. J Thromb Thrombolysis. 2023;56:196–201.
163. Piazza G, Hohlfelder B, Jaff MR, Ouriel K, Engelhardt TC, Sterling KM, et al. A prospective, single-arm, Multicenter trial of ultrasound-facilitated, catheter-directed, low-dose fibrinolysis for acute massive and submassive pulmonary embolism: the SEATTLE II study. JACC Cardiovasc Interv. 2015;8:1382–92.
164. Rahaghi FN, San José Estépar R, Goldhaber SZ, Minhas JK, Nardelli P, Vegas Sanchez-Ferrero G, et al. Quantification and significance of pulmonary vascular volume in predicting response to ultrasound-facilitated, catheter-directed fibrinolysis in acute pulmonary embolism [SEATTLE-3D]. Circ Cardiovasc Imaging. 2019;12:e009903.

18 Quantitative Imaging in Airway Diseases

Logan Sun, Georgina Bailey, and Carole A. Ridge

Introduction

Diseases of the airway are prevalent globally and can affect any level of the tracheobronchial tree. In combination with clinical, spirometric, biochemical and histopathological tests, imaging plays a pivotal role in the detection, characterisation and management of airway diseases. Advances in imaging of airway diseases have been underutilised and have the potential to improve our understanding of disease pathophysiology, progression and treatment response. In particular, better utilisation of medical imaging enhances the diagnostic and therapeutic decision-making of early disease processes.

Quantitative imaging describes the principle of extracting data from medical imaging and measuring them to obtain numerical results. This can yield reproducible outcomes, dramatically reducing inter- and intra-observer variation, particularly in image acquisition, processing and analysis. Reasons for the growing interest in quantitative imaging are numerous. In imaging research, it allows objective measurements of imaging data sets, eliminating bias. It has already provided new insight into the understanding of well-studied diseases. In clinical practice, validated quantitative methods detect early-stage diseases and subtle temporal change on follow-up. For example, mild emphysema is seen on HRCT before it is detectable on spirometry, which underpins the current diagnostic criteria [1]. Early detection may have the greatest benefit in younger patients who could potentially avoid living with debilitating functional impairment for decades. Developing new imaging markers based on quantitative imaging provides novel ways to predict treatment response and prognosis, paving the way to personalised precision medicine. With more powerful computing power, quantitative imaging methods are also increasingly automated, improving workflow efficiency.

This chapter summarises the most prevalent chronic airway conditions—chronic obstructive pulmonary disease (COPD), asthma and bronchiectasis—and their imaging manifestations, and rarer airway diseases. The second half of the chapter delves into numerous quantitative imaging techniques, arranged by the anatomical compartment of the abnormality.

L. Sun · G. Bailey
Department of Radiology, The Royal Brompton Hospital, London, UK

C. A. Ridge (✉)
Department of Radiology, The Royal Brompton Hospital, London, UK

National Heart and Lung Institute, Imperial College London, London, UK
e-mail: c.ridge@nhs.net

R. Gill, P. Rajiah (eds.), *Quantitative Imaging in the Thorax*,
https://doi.org/10.1007/978-3-032-14103-3_18

Common Airway Diseases

Chronic Obstructive Pulmonary Disease (COPD)

COPD is characterised by chronic respiratory symptoms, predominantly due to a combination of airway and alveolar abnormalities leading to airflow obstruction. The proportion of airway versus alveolar abnormalities varies from individual to individual. The development of COPD, like many acquired conditions, represents an interplay between environmental and host factors, the most significant of which is tobacco smoking [2].

The prevalence of COPD worldwide largely reflects the heterogenous prevalence of tobacco smoking. Based on large international epidemiological studies, the global prevalence of COPD is estimated to be 10.3%. COPD was the third leading cause of death in 2019 [3]. The 2017 Global Burden of Disease study estimates nearly 3.2 million deaths caused by COPD globally, rising by 17.5% between 2007 and 2017 [4]. Further increase is expected with increasing exposures [5].

Common clinical symptoms include dyspnoea, wheeze, cough and sputum production. Increased sputum production for 3 months or more over two consecutive years is the classic definition for chronic bronchitis [6]. COPD is a diagnosis which should be considered in any patient over the age of 35, presenting with one or more of the above symptoms for a prolonged period, with a compatible exposure history [7].

To make the diagnosis of COPD, spirometry must indicate the presence of significant irreversible or at least partially irreversible airflow obstruction [2]. Disease severity is graded from 1 (mild) to 4 (severe) [5].

The pathology in COPD is a combination of two major processes—remodelling and collapse of small airways (airways under 2 mm in diameter) and the destruction of alveolar walls, with subsequent loss of the alveolar attachments to the adjacent small airways leading to the theory that emphysema is a consequence of small airway disease [8].

On a cellular level, lung specimens of COPD individuals frequently show alveolar, airway and vascular macrophage, neutrophil and lymphocyte infiltration leading to the release of proinflammatory mediators, recruiting endothelial, epithelial cells and fibroblasts [9]. The secretion of elastase and other proteolytic enzymes is thought to be contributory to the development of emphysema in combination with oxidative stress [9, 10].

Tobacco smoke directly induces excessive production of growth factors and promotes small airway fibrosis [11].

The most reliable radiographic signs are those which reflect the obstructive nature of COPD giving rise to pulmonary hyperinflation [1]. Lucent areas of lung destruction and a reduction in vascularity secondary to ventilation impairment are seen [12, 13].

Numerous radiographic signs for overinflation have been investigated against CT and pulmonary function test; specifically, diaphragmatic flattening correlates well with lung function testing in COPD patients [14] (Fig. 18.1). High-resolution computed tomography (HRCT) and pulmonary function testing are more sensitive methods of identifying COPD than radiographs, especially in mild disease [1, 13].

Emphysema is characterised on HRCT by irreversible, hypoattenuating areas, with no discernible wall [15]. Using various methods, such as edge-enhanced algorithms and minimal intensity projection images (minIP), detection can be enhanced [16, 17].

The distribution of emphysema includes three main subtypes: centrilobular, paraseptal and panlobular.

Centrilobular emphysema is characterised by clustered lucency around the centre of the secondary pulmonary lobule with an upper zone distribution [18]. Centrilobular emphysema has no visible boundary. When moderate to severe, the enlarged cystic airspaces outline the centrilobular structures, i.e. pulmonary airways and arteries [19] (Fig. 18.2).

Paraseptal emphysema is characterised by enlarged airspaces centred on the distal acinus with an upper zone predilection favouring subpleural lung [20]. These enlarged airspaces often

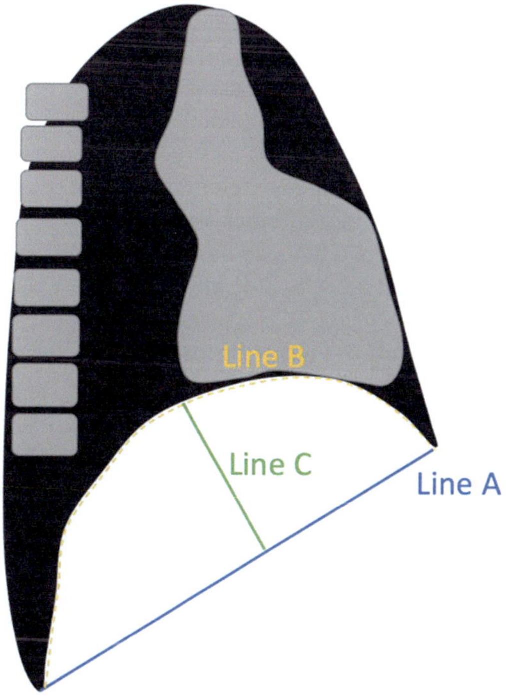

Fig. 18.1 Assessing overinflation. Line A (solid blue line) connects the anterior and posterior costophrenic recesses on a lateral chest radiograph. Line B (dotted orange line) traces the outline of the hemidiaphragm. Line C (solid green line) the perpendicular to Line A and bisected the top of the dome created by line B. The length of line C less than 2.6 cm is poorly correlated with lung function test and suggests overinflation

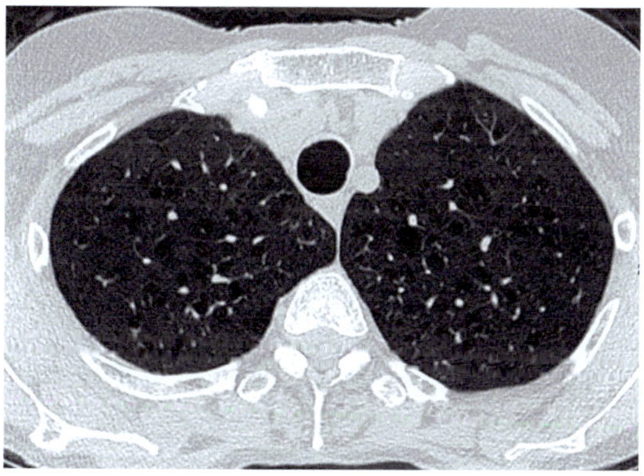

Fig. 18.2 Centrilobular emphysema. Axial CT of a 68-year-old demonstrating multiple round cystic airspaces in the upper lobes bilaterally in keeping with centrilobular emphysema. The lack of any perceptible walls gives rise to the typical moth-eaten appearance

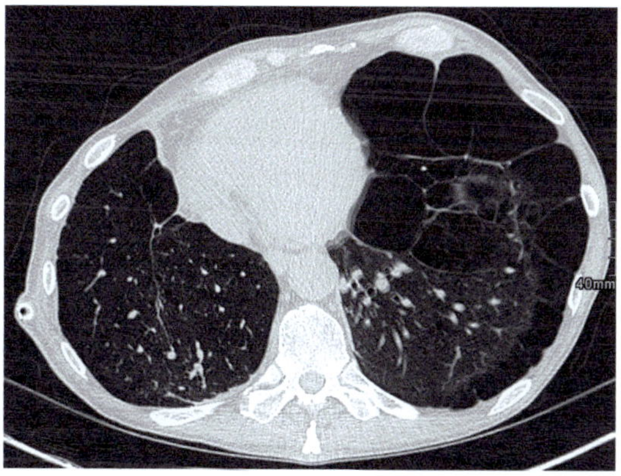

Fig. 18.3 Paraseptal emphysema. Axial CT of a 58-year-old with severe paraseptal emphysema characterised by multiple adjacent subpleural bullae in the left lower lobe separated by thin septa. The extent of disease results in hyper-expansion of the left hemithorax and mediastinal shift to the right

form a row along the pleural surface, with very thin walls, often outlining the interlobular septa (Fig. 18.3).

Panlobular emphysema is a severe extensive form of emphysema. Pathologically, the affected area stretches from the respiratory bronchioles to the alveoli. On CT, the lungs are hyperlucent with scant normal lung parenchyma (Fig. 18.4). The extent is often diffuse [18, 20]. Classically, it has been associated with alpha-1-antityrpsin deficiency, a lower zone predominant disease [21].

Large airways disease in COPD presents most commonly as tracheobronchial wall thickening. Thickened airway walls exhibit a combination of increased wall area on cross-section, as well as a reduced luminal calibre. This is in contrast to asthma, in which the bronchial wall thickening is seen without an associated reduction in the calibre of the lumen [22].

The small airways are defined as a cartilaginous airway with a diameter of 2 mm or less [23] and is the main site of airflow obstruction [8]. On conventional CT, small airways disease is seen as lobules of lower density, with reduced calibre vessels traversing through. On expiratory CT, the low-density nature of these areas is more evident [8].

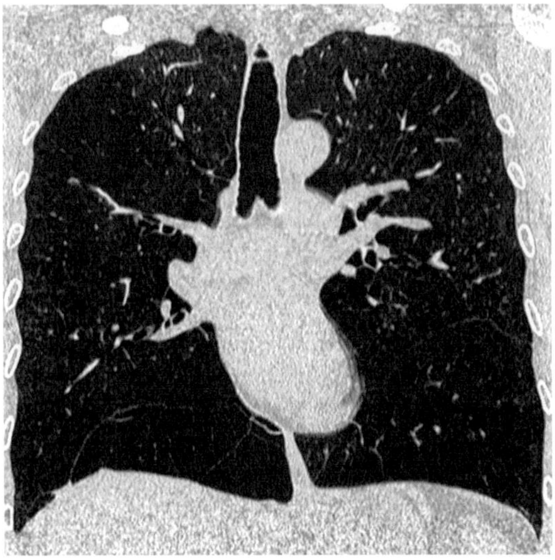

Fig. 18.4 Panlobular emphysema. Coronal CT of a 50-year-old with severe destruction of the lung parenchyma demonstrated by large swathes of hypoattenuating lung (particularly at the bases) without perceptible walls, consistent with panlobular emphysema. There is also flattening of the hemidiaphragms indicative of hyper-expansion

Asthma

Asthma is a common chronic respiratory disease, characterised by airway hyperresponsiveness, inflammation, remodelling and expiratory airflow limitation. The airflow obstruction is often reversible with treatment [24, 25]. It affects an estimated 315 million adults and children worldwide (approximately 4.5%) [25, 26].

An asthma diagnosis depends on a compatible history of clinical symptoms and evidence of expiratory airflow limitation. Sometimes, there is a recognisable exacerbating factor, such as exercise or high pollen concentration. Asthma can be subcategorised into phenotypes in order to provide individualised treatment and better predict outcomes [25, 27, 28]. Phenotypes are divided into clusters according to characteristic demographics, symptoms and/or pathophysiology [25]. Individual members within a cluster associate strongly with each other, whilst inter-cluster association is weak [29].

Acute and chronic inflammation has a central role in the pathogenesis of asthma. In allergen-induced acute exacerbations, IgE mediated mast cell degranulation causes rapid onset bronchoconstriction, smooth muscle spasm, airway oedema and subsequent airway narrowing. Over time, chronic inflammation causes structural changes to occur in airways and are felt to underly treatment resistance and disease progression [30].

Imaging has a limited role in the diagnosis and management of asthma. In children, chest radiographs rarely lead to a change in management [31]. The role of imaging in asthma is to exclude other alternative diagnoses [25, 32]. The most common CT findings are bronchial wall thickening, deceased lung attenuation. Other less common findings include bronchiectasis and bronchiolectasis and centrilobular nodules [33].

Bronchiectasis

Bronchiectasis is defined as the permanent dilatation of airways [15, 34–36]. Causes include specific gene mutations (as seen in cystic fibrosis and primary ciliary dyskinesia), immunodeficiencies, intraluminal obstruction, extrinsic airway compression, allergic airway diseases and a myriad of pulmonary infections. Idiopathic disease is also recognised [34, 36].

Affected individuals suffer from chronic cough with copious sputum production. Other common symptoms include dyspnoea, exercise intolerance, fatigue and haemoptysis. Rarely, haemoptysis is associated with hypertrophied bronchial arteries [35].

A 2013 UK study estimates 566 cases per 100,000 population, with a slight female predominance. Prevalence is increasing in the elderly [34, 37, 38].

HRCT is the most sensitive and specific tool in detecting and characterising bronchiectasis [35]. Dilated airways, sometimes within 1 cm of the pleural surface, is suggestive. Bronchiectasis is often accompanied by other signs of airway inflammation, namely, airway wall thickening and mucoid impaction [15]. The Reid classification divides the severity of bronchiectasis based on morphological descriptors—cylindrical, varicose and cystic [39] (Fig. 18.5a–e).

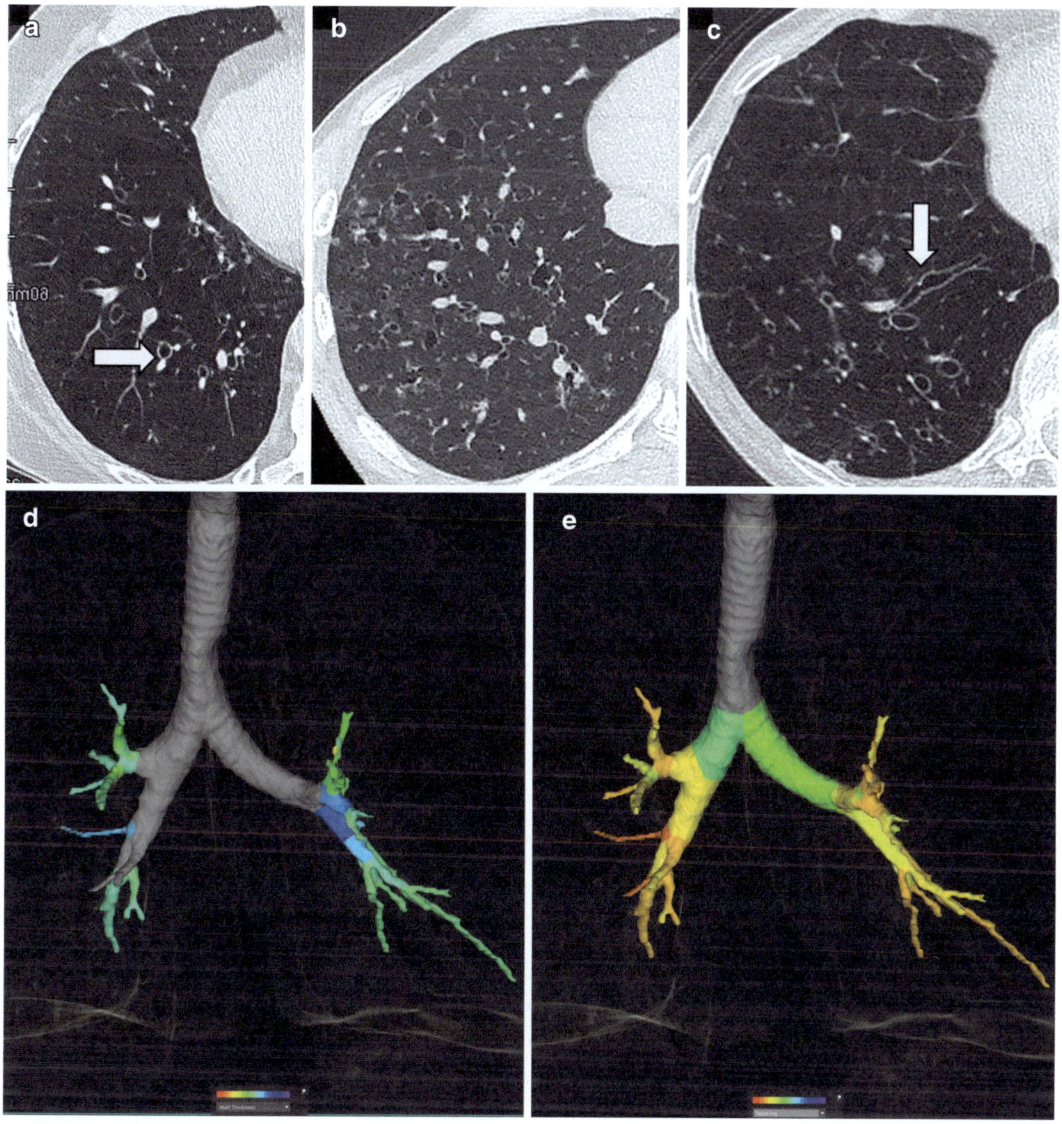

Fig. 18.5 (**a**–**e**) Bronchiectasis. Three axial CT slices demonstrating different morphological subtypes of bronchiectasis: (**a**) The airways are uniformly dilated in keeping with cylindrical bronchiectasis. The airways have a larger diameter than the accompanying pulmonary arteries on CT; the so-called signet ring sign (arrow). (**b**) Multiple thin walled, rounded lucencies give the appearance of cysts. These 'cysts' are the result of focal dilatation of the airways in a patient with cystic bronchiectasis. (**c**) An abnormal airway which is alternately dilated and stenosed (arrow) in keeping with varicose bronchiectasis. 3D volume rendered colour maps were generated using the CT as shown in **c** demonstrating airway wall thickness and non-tapering. The wall thickness colour map indicates that the bronchus intermedius and lingular bronchus are significantly thick walled, coloured in blue (**d**). The tapering colour map (**e**) confirms the presence of non-tapering airways in the left lower lobe, the lobe most affected by bronchiectasis in this patient, as shown in orange

Miscellaneous Airway Diseases

Tracheomalacia

Tracheomalacia is a condition caused by the excessive collapsibility of the trachea due to softening of the cartilaginous support. When an increase in intrathoracic pressure is transmitted to the trachea, the normally C-shaped tracheal cartilages deform—the shapes of the deformity are named crescentic, sabretooth and circumferential [40]. The transient reduction in trachea calibre occurs when intrathoracic pressure is at its greatest, such as during forced expiration or coughing (Fig. 18.6a–c). A similar entity, named excessive dynamic airway collapse (EDAC), has many clinical overlaps with tracheomalacia, but the reduction in tracheal calibre comes from excessive bowing of the posterior tracheal membrane (pars membranacea), with no collagenous abnormality [40, 41]. This distinction in the nomenclature is less clear in the paediatric population [41]. Other common symptoms include respiratory stridor, exercise intolerance, frequent respiratory infections and cyanosis [41, 42]. The frequency of excessive collapse is estimated to be 5% [40].

Causes of acquired tracheomalacia include recurrent upper respiratory tract infection, relapsing polychondritis and other inflammatory large airway diseases. External compression due to tumours and goitres have also been described. Iatrogenic causes such as tracheostomy or prolonged intubation cause focal tracheomalacia [43, 44]. However, the aetiology of excessive collapse in most adults remain unclear [40].

The most common method of assessment is flexible bronchoscopy, which allows real-time assessment of the trachea whilst performing breathing manoeuvres [41]. However, this is

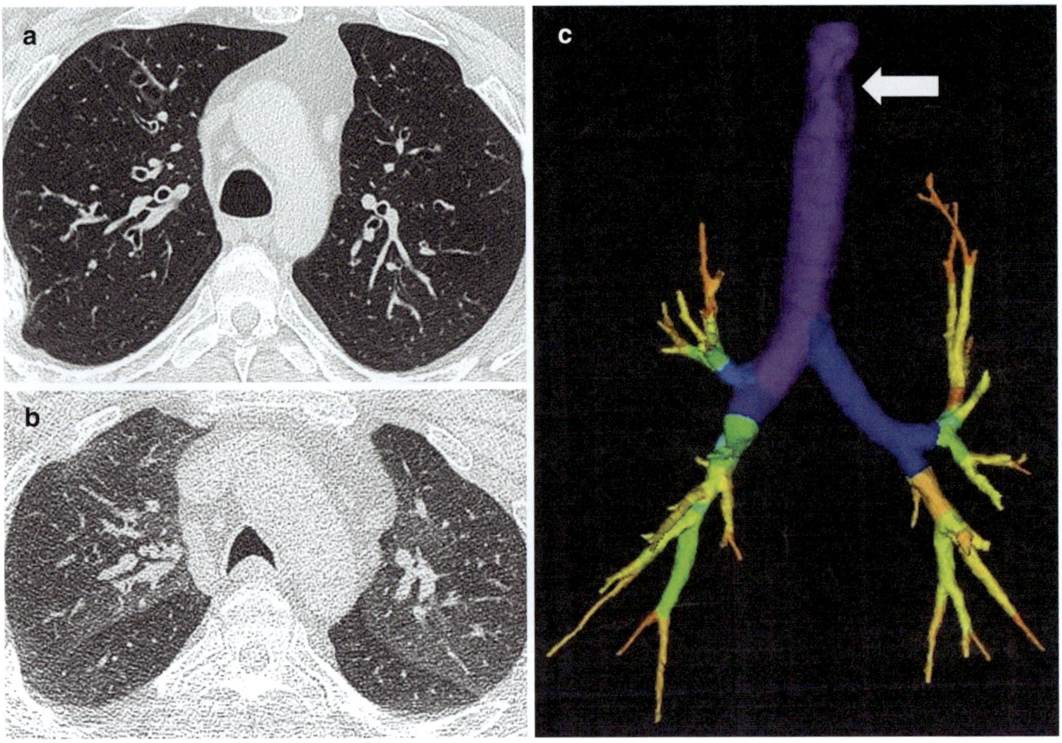

Fig. 18.6 (**a–c**) Expiratory central airway collapse. (**a**) Inspiratory axial CT of a 51-year-old with apparently normal morphology of the trachea (**b**) Axial CT of the same patient acquired during held expiration shows a significant reduction in the AP diameter of the trachea with bowing of the posterior membrane and triangular anterior cartilage. This so-called lunate morphology is typical of the cartilaginous abnormality in tracheomalacia. (**c**) A 3D reconstruction of the expiratory CT highlighting subglottic stenosis (arrow)

invasive and introduces the non-physiologic condition of a bronchoscope. CT, especially dynamic CT, is being increasingly utilised as a non-invasive tool in assessing tracheal collapse. Standard end-expiratory protocols looking for small airway disease may underestimate the severity of the collapse [40]. Dynamic CT measurements have shown to be more reproducible over time [45].

COVID-19 Pneumonia-Associated Pneumonia and ILD

COVID-19 is a clinical syndrome caused by the virus SARS-CoV-2, a novel viral agent most frequently contracted through the respiratory tract [46]. To date, it has caused seven million deaths worldwide [47]. Those with pre-existing underlying conditions, such as diabetes, cancer, hypertension and prior cardiac or pulmonary diseases have worse prognosis [48].

Patchy consolidation, often seen bilaterally with a peripheral and basal predominance, resembling those caused by other bacterial and viral pneumonias, is the most typical radiographic appearance (Fig. 18.7). HRCT is better able to distinguish specific patterns of lung injury, such as organising pneumonia and diffuse alveolar damage [49].

Long-COVID consists of a chronic form of the infection, whereby patients exhibit persistent or new symptom(s) at least 12 weeks since the initial diagnosis, without evidence of reinfection. Respiratory symptoms are the most common manifestation [50]. At 3 months, ground glass opacities (GGOs) and subpleural bands in a subset of patients have been found on one study. At 6 months, some patients develop fibrosis. Air

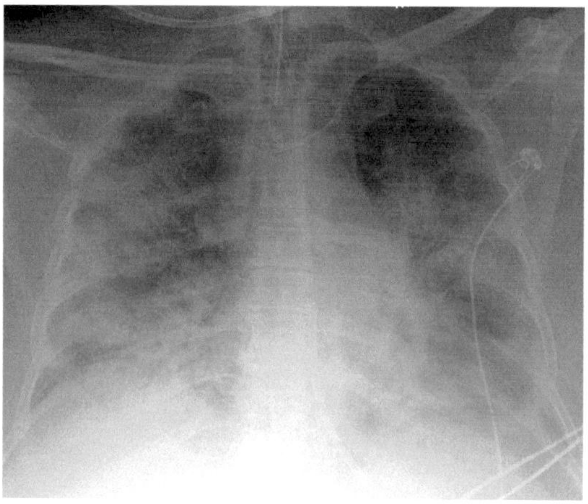

Fig. 18.7 COVID-19. Frontal chest radiograph of a 59-year-old with severe acute COVID-19 pneumonitis which demonstrates typical bilateral, lower zone predominant, peripheral consolidation. The patient is intubated and has a left sided central line and nasogastric tube in place

trapping was also noted, suggesting the development of small airway disease [50, 51].

Diffuse Idiopathic Pulmonary Neuroendocrine Cell Hyperplasia (DIPNECH)

DIPNECH is a diffuse lung disease, with scattered foci of pre-malignant neuroendocrine cells. It is a rare disease, though the estimated prevalence may be mistakenly low partly due to its under-recognised status. Even in symptomatic patients, the clinical diagnosis is often delayed, due to overlapping clinical presentation with asthma and chronic bronchitis [52, 53]. CT appearances are typically a combination of mosaic attenuation, from small airway obstruction, and multiple small solid nodules [52, 54] (Fig. 18.8)

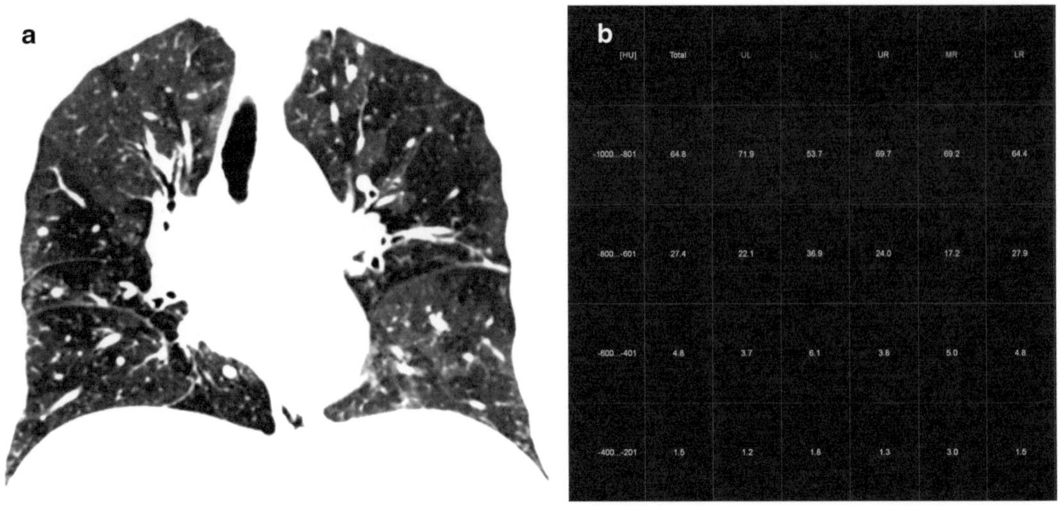

[HU]	Total	UL	LL	UR	MR	LR
-1000...-801	64.8	71.9	53.7	69.7	69.2	64.4
-800...-601	27.4	22.1	36.9	24.0	17.2	27.9
-600...-401	4.8	3.7	6.1	3.8	5.0	4.8
-400...-201	1.5	1.2	1.8	1.3	3.0	1.5

Fig. 18.8 DIPNECH. (**a**) Coronal reformatted image of a 76-year-old patient with bronchial wall thickening, mosaic attenuation and multiple lung nodules consistent with DIPNECH. (**b**) A significant portion of the pixels in the lungs are between −800 and −100 HU, in keeping with air trapping, this data can then be tabulated for quantitative purposes. The left upper lobe is worst affected (relative volume of lung less than −800 HU is 71.9%)

Current Quantitative Imaging Methods in Airway Diseases

Compared to qualitative imaging interpretation, quantitative imaging techniques have several general advantages, namely, the superior reproducibility, lack of intra- and interobserver variation, the ability to identify early or mild disease and the ability to detect subtle interval progression in follow-up imaging studies.

There are now several established and emerging techniques in quantitative imaging, which assess all imaging manifestations of airway diseases. The more basic techniques are generally more labour-intensive and rely on human effort, counting or scoring image findings. More modern techniques are often semi-automated, which is built on the foundation of accurate segmentation of the anatomy of interest. For example, segmentation of the lung parenchyma or tracheobronchial tree is required for emphysema scoring and airway wall measurements, respectively. These are performed by computer software with manual editing, when required.

Abnormalities of the Large Airways

All airway diseases exhibit degrees of bronchial wall thickening. Measuring bronchial wall thickening may seem intuitively straightforward, as abnormally thick-walled large and medium sized airways can be directly visualised on thin-section CT imaging. Earlier attempts of studying the degree of airway thickening involved manual tracing. Achieving reproducible measurements by this method proved to be difficult and time-consuming. More recently, computer algorithms, which can measure airway parameters accurately down to the fifth or sixth generation bronchi, are increasingly explored in research and clinical settings [55]. One method these algorithms are based on is the principle of full width at half maximum (FWHM).

The principle of FWHN starts by segmenting out the tracheobronchial tree from the rest of the imaged anatomy. Then, airway centrelines are delineated, which allow perpendicular cuts through an airway to obtain an orthogonal cross-sectional image. Using this cross-sectional image, an imaginary straight line is plotted from the centre of the lumen radiating outwards,

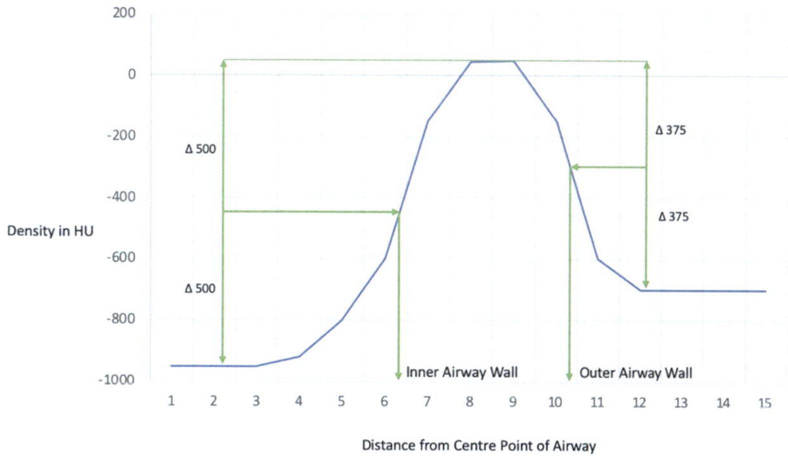

Fig. 18.9 Full width at half maximum (FWHM). By plotting the pixel density against the distance from the centre of the airway, a characteristic asymmetrical curve is drawn. From this curve and using the FWHM principle, the exact points of the inner and outer airway wall are defined

through the bronchial wall and into the adjacent lung parenchyma. The pixel density in Hounsfield units along this imaginary line is plotted against the distance from the centre point (Fig. 18.9). This line on the graph will look like a bell-shaped curve, with a sharp upstroke representing the transition from the lumen to the inner bronchial wall and then a sharp downstroke from the outer bronchial wall to the surrounding lung parenchyma. Of course, this characteristic curve depends on the absence of mucus plugging and normal aeration in the surrounding lung. The curve is not perfectly symmetrical, because lung parenchyma is not as low in density as the air inside the lumen. Using the point that is the half maximal difference in the change in density, for both the upstroke and the downstroke, the inner and outer bronchial walls are defined. All the above steps can now be automated [56]. Knowing the precise location of the inner and outer bronchial walls allows further geometric measurements to be calculated. Commonly used measurements include the inner perimeter (Pi), wall thickness (WT), airway wall area (WA), lumen area or inner airway area (Ai) and outer airway area (WA + Ai) (Fig. 18.10). To enable meaningful comparison, airway wall measurements are standardised against the size of the corresponding airway. Wall area percentage (WA%) is the airway wall area as a percentage of the outer airway area. WA% has been found to increase in COPD patients. Although both the bronchial wall area and outer airway area decrease in COPD patients, it is the latter that decreases disproportionally more [55]. Wall thickness percentage (WT%) and Pi10 (described in detail below) are two other measures used to compare bronchial wall thickness [55].

To determine Pi10, the bronchial wall area and the corresponding internal perimeter of all the segmented airways are utilised. Then, the square root of each bronchial wall area is plotted against the paired internal lumen perimeter, so that a straight line of regression could be calculated (Fig. 18.11). A Pi10 is derived from this line of regression and is defined as the square root of the bronchial wall area in a theoretical airway with a 10 mm internal perimeter [56, 57].

The potential use of Pi10 as a marker of airway wall thickening was investigated by comparing 463 COPD cases from the Norwegian GenKOLS (translates into genetic COPD) population against 431 controls (current or ex-smokers without the diagnosis of COPD). Pi10 was found to be higher in the COPD group and increased with the number of pack-years, more so in the control group. Pi10 did not significantly correlate with current number of cigarettes smoked, which may suggest that airway remodelling takes time to develop. Of note, Pi10 was higher in males and decreased slightly with age, with the authors concluding that Pi10 could be used as a marker of airway wall thickening if population characteristics were considered [57].

CT measures of airway thickening are known to be associated with airflow limitation [56, 58,

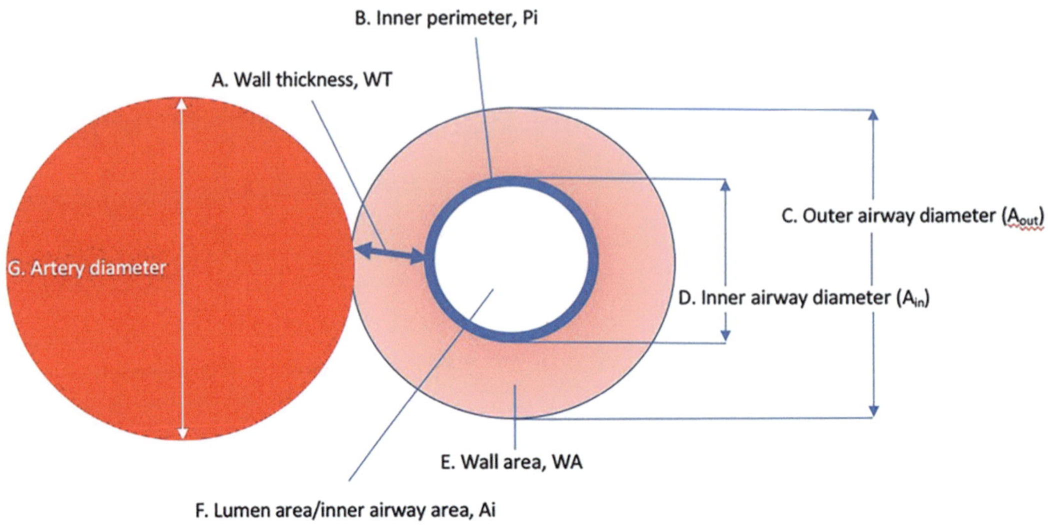

Fig. 18.10 Cross-section of an airway artery pair. The cross-section of an airway is obtained from the segmented tracheobronchial tree. The key measured parameters are labelled (**a–d**). (**a**) is the wall thickness, represented by the double-headed arrow. (**b**) is the inner perimeter, highlighted by the thick blue circular line. (**c**) is the outer airway diameter (A_{out}). (**d**) is the inner airway diameter (A_{in}). (**e**) is the wall area, WA, coloured in pink. (**f**) is the inner airway area coloured in white (Ai). (**g**) is the adjacent pulmonary artery diameter. The sum of (**e**) and (**f**) gives total airway area/outer airway area, Ao

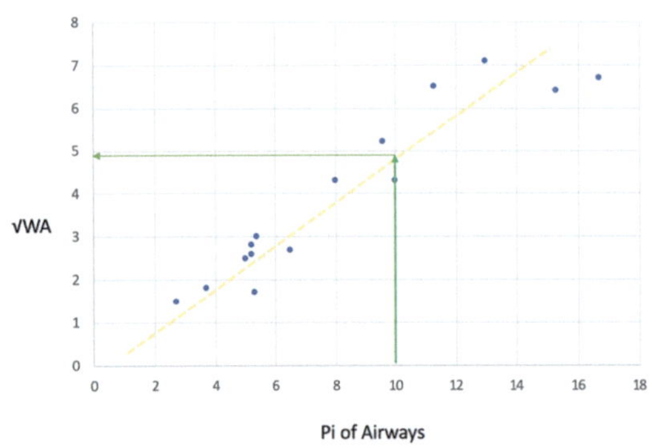

Fig. 18.11 Determining Pi10. The internal diameter of all the segmented airways are plotted against the respective square root of the bronchial wall area ($\sqrt{WA}$). A line of regression determines the value of $\sqrt{WA}$ for a theoretical airway with an inner perimeter of 10mm. This can then be used as a standardised index of bronchial wall thickness

59]. In a prospective study of 433 COPD patients from the German COPD cohort COSYCONECT (COPD and Systemic Consequences Comorbidities Network), the authors found Pi10 to negatively correlate with FEV_1 and positively with RV/TLC. Pi10 correlated with GOLD classification and was particularly high in GOLD group D. It also served as a predictor of exacerbations and mortality, independent of the degree of airflow obstruction. Thus, in COPD patients who have undergone CT imaging, Pi10 provides an opportunity to identify those who may benefit from preventative treatment escalation, independent of spirometry results. In addition, in GOLD groups C and D, Pi10 was lower in patients receiving triple therapy, which may hint toward triple therapy's postulated airway remodelling effects [56].

Other studies have validated the utility of airway morphometry on quantitative CT analysis in asthma. On study investigated how airway measurements could identify asthma phenotypes. The authors grouped 455 asthmatic individuals from the Severe Asthma Research Program (an initiative in the United States) into five clinical phenotypes—cluster 1, minimal disease; cluster 2, mild, reversible; cluster 3, obese asthma; cluster 4, severe, reversible; and cluster 5, severe, irreversible. Each participant's CT was analysed for airway morphometry, using Pi10, lumen area (Ai), wall area percentage (WA%) and wall thickness percentage (WT%). The authors found that those in clusters 4 and 5 had thicker airway walls, reduced lumen size and overall reduced airway size compared to the other clusters. The authors concluded that several airway metrics from quantitative CT can help to identify individuals with severe clinical phenotypes [60].

Another study which supports careful use of airway measurements in assessing asthma severity found significantly higher airway wall thickness (WT) and area (WA) in the severe asthmatics, both in absolute terms and as WA% and WT%. In addition to clinical phenotype, WT% and WA% also correlated positively with findings on endobronchial endothelial biopsies and treatment response with bronchodilators. However, the differences were not significant between individuals with mild to moderate asthma and healthy controls, leading the authors to downplay these measurements' potential as clinical imaging biomarkers [61].

The WA% and Pi10 methods of measuring large airway wall dimensions were later applied to a cohort of 66 confirmed cases of COVID-19 during the first half of 2020. The authors compared these bronchial wall measurements to those in non-COVID-19 individuals imaged within the year before the start of the pandemic. During the acute phase of infection, the study group had significantly higher measures of airway wall thickening down to the eighth generation subsegmental bronchi compared with the control group. The authors later also compared the initial airway measurements during the acute stage with follow-up CTs performed later in the recovery phase for the same cohort of patients. The result from 66 CT pairs revealed that the bronchial wall thickness during the recovery phase demonstrated interval improvement in most of patients. Interestingly, the degree of bronchial wall thickening was not significantly correlated with levels of CRP or length of hospitalisation, leading the authors to hypothesise that the bronchial wall thickening is a secondary phenomenon due to wider pulmonary inflammation, rather than being a primary site of infection [62]. This theory is supported by autopsy and immunological studies. It is noted that in autopsy specimens, there is increased pulmonary vascular endothelial injury compared with comparable specimens from severe influenza. In addition, widespread microangiopathy and intravascular microthrombosis are features of COVID-19, found at a ninefold increase compared to influenza cases [63]. Studies like this have led some experts to regard COVID-19 as primarily a disease of endothelial dysfunction [64, 65].

Airway Dilatation and Non-tapering

Large airway measurement leans on the traditional teaching of airway-artery pairs (AA pairs), which states that an airway should be smaller in diameter than the accompanying pulmonary artery. Indeed, this is a commonly used HRCT sign to identify bronchiectasis, so-called the signet ring sign [66, 67]. Historically, attempts to quantify bronchiectasis saw careful measurements of AA pairs performed manually, with an associated time penalty.

As with other quantification methods, accurate automated measurements of airway-arterial pairs are dependent on the correct segmentation of the relevant anatomy studied. Acquiring an accurate segmentation of the tracheobronchial tree and delineating the centrelines are crucial steps before acquiring true orthogonal cross-sectional images of AA pairs. Oblique cuts can over-estimate dimensions of tubular structures.

Using methods such as FWHM described in section "Abnormalities of the Large Airways", AA pair dimensions can be obtained. These often include airway wall thickness, lumen diameter, total/outer airway diameter, inner airway diameter and the diameter of the adjacent artery (Fig. 18.10). Key ratios between these can be used as indicators for airway dilatation and/or wall thickening, and the study of these indicators is named AA analysis. Indicators from the same airway generation should be used to ensure a fair comparison between individuals [68].

Using AA analysis, a study compared the airways of 13 children with primary ciliary dyskinesia against those of 12 healthy controls. The tracheobronchial tree of each chest CT was first reconstructed semi-automatically. Then, cross-sectional images were obtained through all the visible AA pairs. A total of 1526 AA pairs in the

PCD group and 1516 in the control group were identified and analysed. By noting down the artery wall thickness (WT), inner airway diameter (A_{in}), outer airway diameter (A_{out}) and the artery diameter (A), it was possible to derive the $A_{in}A$ ratio, $A_{out}A$ ratio, WT to Aout ratio (Awt ratio) and WT/A ratio. The authors have found that, there was clear evidence of airway dilatation, with AinA ratio and AoutA ratio significantly higher in children with PCD. However, there was no convincing evidence for significant bronchial wall thickening in PCD children, with Awt ratio significantly higher in the control group [69].

More recently, an automated airway-artery measuring method was tested against its manual counterpart in a study of 23 participants (11 CF, 12 healthy controls). The authors found that the result of the computer algorithm correlated well with manual measurements of AA pairs. This represents a significant improvement, as manual measurements are prohibitively time-consuming, taking approximately 2 days for a pre-school child and up to 1 week to measure all the visible AA pairs in an adult. The algorithm takes 20 min. This may pave the way for enhanced disease detection and longitudinal monitoring [68].

Another key feature of bronchiectasis is the lack of airway tapering. This feature was quantified in a study comprised of 12 children with CF and 12 age and sex-matched controls. To control for the differences in lung sizes, all CTs were resized to 4 L, approximately the average total lung volume in all study subjects. Using proprietary software to perform airway segmentation and centreline delineation, intra-branch tapering (amount of tapering along the branch) and inter-branch tapering (amount of tapering before and after a bifurcation) are measured. Airway diameter is measured at every 0.5 mm along the centreline. Intra-branch tapering is measured as a percentage. For example, 2% equates to a decrease in the airway diameter by 2% for every mm along the centreline. For the inter-branch measurement, the average diameter of the studied airway was compared to the average diameter of the parent airway, or the airway in the preceding generation, and the percentage decrease in the average diameter was reported. In the analysis, intra-branch and inter-branch tapering were both found to be significantly less in children with CF compared with healthy controls. This was true in airways of all sizes, which differs from the AA ratio. Concomitant analysis of AA ratios found that this was only significantly different between the study and control groups in the smallest 1/3 of airways [70]. Thus, this method may reveal the true extent of the airway involvement in CF patients, not detectable by AA analysis.

One retrospective study compared AA ratios in DIPNECH patients compared with normal healthy individuals. The authors used a software which automatically created a 3D volume rendered tracheobronchial tree from the CT dataset. The airway centrelines were also automatically delineated, which created a roadmap that the radiologist could use to 'navigate' along the tracheobronchial tree. Taking airway and artery measurements were also aided by the software. The airway diameter:artery diameter ratio (AA ratio) and airway wall thickness:artery diameter ratio (AWTA ratio) were taken at the level of the proximal segmental bronchi. In the analysis, the authors found that patients with DIPNECH had significantly greater bronchial wall thickness and AA ratio. A multivariant model, which combined AA ratio, AWTA ratio and pulmonary nodule count, was accurate in discriminating the DIPNECH and control cohorts. AA ratio also showed positive correlation with FVC, but not with FEV1 or DLCO, and had no correlation with clinical symptoms [71]. It seems AA analysis may aid the diagnosis of DIPNECH but does not provide further insight into the level of airflow obstruction or the clinical severity of the disease.

With the growing use of automation when measuring AA pairs, more data can be analysed more quickly, which could greatly benefit rarer diseases (such as PCD and DIPNECH). Given that both CF and PCD patients share bronchiectasis as one of the main disease patterns, research methodology (including image quantification methods) from the better studied condition—CF—is readily applied to those with PCD. This presents potential problems. Some authors have highlighted the need to validate research methods and disease severity scoring systems based on CF when used on other causes of bronchiectasis. This is important, given the differences in the pathophysiology and nature of airway structural changes between the different diseases [72].

Dynamic Collapse of Large Airways

The use of dynamic CT is a non-invasive method of assessing large airway collapse between inspiration and expiration. Traditionally, the diagnostic cut-off is arbitrarily set at 50% reduction in the cross-sectional area [73–75]. Using this threshold, an early small cohort study of 8 patients looked at the validity of dynamic CT in tracheomalacia. To calculate the cross-sectional area, the authors used a density threshold of −350HU to segment the lumen. They studied the temporal change in the luminal cross-sectional area at eight different levels along the trachea for each patient and compared these measurements to bronchoscopic findings. They concluded that the results correlated well with symptoms and bronchoscopy [76].

Many other studies have also used the traditional 50% threshold. Dynamic CT correctly diagnosed 28/29 patients in one study with bronchoscopy proven tracheomalacia, concluding that dynamic CT is a sensitive tool. If the cross-sectional area cannot be calculated, it is reasonable to use diameter measurements, as there is good correlation between percentage reduction in the cross-sectional area with the reduction in the inner diameter of the sagittal and coronary diameters [73].

The 50% threshold has been widely debated, as a significant proportion of asymptomatic population reach this diagnostic criterion. Moreover, not reaching this threshold may reflect patient factors, such as the expiratory effort during scanning. Healthy volunteers with no history of respiratory diseases and normal spirometry were invited to undergo dynamic CT in one study. The authors measured the degree of tracheal collapse by comparing the reduction in the cross-sectional area of the trachea at comparable points—1 cm above the carina and 1 cm above the aortic arch, arguing that the tracheal shape and size at these points were less influenced by factors other than intra-thoracic pressure, such as the adjacent thoracic aorta. Using a computerised area calculation tool, the lumen area was measured by carefully tracing around the inner tracheal wall on lung window. With these paired measurements, the authors calculated the percentage reduction using the equation $LC = 100 \times [1 - (LAee/LAei)]$, where LC is the luminal collapse, LAee the expiratory area and LAei the inspiratory area. The results showed a majority of the 51 healthy volunteers reached this threshold. Thus, the authors argued for a higher threshold of >70%, which roughly equates to 1 standard deviation above the mean [42].

Mucus Plugging

Mucus plugging is another common finding in large airway diseases. A visual scoring system was developed and evaluated for quantifying mucus plugging on HRCT. There were 122 individuals with asthma and 22 healthy controls included in the analysis. For each bronchopulmonary segment, either a score of 0 or 1 is given, depending on the absence or presence of mucus plugs, respectively. Thus, a score between 0 and 20 for each CT could be calculated. The definition of a mucus plug was defined by the authors as the total occlusion of an airway, at least 2 cm from a pleural edge, irrespective of generation or size. The authors discovered a significant between-group difference, with asthmatics receiving higher scores compared to healthy controls. Most of the plugs were found at the subsegmental level and were often observed to persist in the same locations for many years. The asthmatic group was further divided based on FEV1, and this inversely correlated with the proportion of individuals with a mucus plug score of 4 or above (considered a high burden). A high score also correlated with higher levels of sputum eosinophil and eosinophil peroxidase, which were thought to be a possible cause of mucus plug production [77]. At the time of writing, no automated method of mucus plugging has been published in the literature.

Total Airway Count

Progressive airway loss is observed in both COPD and asthma. One study investigated the relationship between the degree of total airway loss and with severity of asthma. In total, 70 pre- and post-bronchodilator CTs were analysed. Automated tracheobronchial tree segmentation and counting of the total number of airways was performed (TAC). TAC was significantly diminished in those with the most severe asthma, with severity graded according to GINA (Global Initiative for Asthma). Patients with lower TAC also demonstrated higher percentages of ventilation defect, as measured on MRI with hyperpolarised gas, and more pronounced airway remodelling. TAC was also shown to predict FEV1 to a good degree of accuracy [78].

Abnormalities of the Small Airways

Air Trapping

Small airways are defined histologically as non-cartilaginous airways, anatomically smaller than 2 mm in diameter. The small airways are a major site of airflow obstruction in many airway diseases, including COPD and asthma. The small airways are also believed to represent the initiating site of disease in COPD, before the development of emphysema. So, the correct identification and quantification of small airway disease is likely to enhance our understanding of the pathophysiology and advance the detection of early disease.

Despite the importance of the small airways, assessment using imaging has always lagged the use of spirometry, because by definition, a small airway is not discernible on HRCT when not affected by disease. This makes direct morphological assessment very challenging. In cases of exudative bronchiolitis, the invisibility of small airways is unmasked by the presence of an exudative material, forming airway plugs and soft centrilobular nodules, giving a tree-in-bud appearance. The causes include but are not limited to tuberculosis, mycoplasma and panbronchiolitis. Quantitative methods are not readily applied to this CT sign. In another form of small airway disease—obliterative bronchiolitis (OB)—the affected airways narrow or disappear, leading to hyperinflation of the distal airspaces from excessive gas retention. On HRCT, this manifests as mosaic attenuation, a patchwork of different lung densities, with hypoattenuating lobules correlating with the extent of OB (Fig. 18.12). This HRCT sign is commonly seen in airway diseases, such as asthma and COPD and becomes particularly pronounced on expiratory imaging. It is measured using several quantitative methods.

The simplest method of grading the severity of air trapping can be performed using a numeric grading. The first objective method of estimating air trapping measures the total number of voxels below a threshold on an expiratory scan, as healthy lung increases in density on expiration, and should therefore be excluded (Fig. 18.8). Another method compares the increase in mean lung density between paired inspiratory and expi-

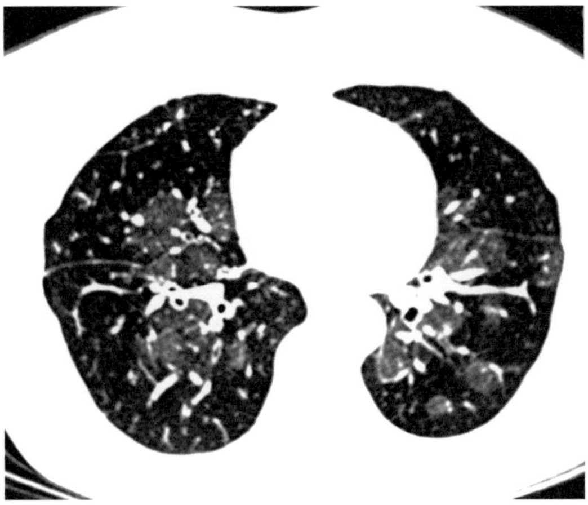

Fig. 18.12 Mosaic attenuation in obliterative bronchiolitis. Narrow window axial CT in a 68-year-old showing mosaic attenuation, whereby the lung is made up of a patchwork of hypoattenuating lung contrasting with areas of normal lung giving a mosaic pattern. The vessels within the abnormal, hypoattenuating lung are smaller in calibre

ratory scans. On the expiratory scan, mean lung density in healthy lung increases significantly more than air trapped lung [79]. However, these methods do not exclude CT voxels representing emphysema, which is a common challenge when attempting to quantify air trapping, as the two abnormalities overlap significantly in imaging appearance and often co-exist. To address this issue, a further step can be added, by excluding the voxels below −950HU and measuring the relative volume for voxels between −860 and −950HU [80]. The lower limit of −950HU provides exclusion of co-existent emphysema. The basis for this is that in normal lung, there should be a relatively large change in the proportion of voxels measured between those two values between inspiration and expiration. However, in small airway disease, as the amount of air trapping increases, more voxels between those two values would remain on the expiratory scan. In a small study cohort of 36 patients, on which this method was found, it was found that the thresholds of −860 to −950HU correlated most strongly with pulmonary function test, in both patients with severe emphysema (defined as >15% low attenuation area below −950HU) and those with mild to moderate emphysema [80]. Thus, Δvolume (−860 to −950HU) is regarded as a good imaging method of quantifying small airway disease. It seems logical that for any method to be accurate in measuring the amount of air trapping, paired inspiratory and expiratory studies should be used to exclude areas of emphysematous destruction [55].

Long COVID-19 individuals with long-lasting respiratory symptoms often exhibit persistent lung parenchymal imaging findings. One of the common abnormalities seen, air trapping, is increasingly being recognised [62, 81]. Paired inspiratory and expiratory follow-up CTs in long COVID individuals after the initial infection show a significant proportion of patients displaying air trapping [82]. Using paired CTs taken at least 30 days post-hospital discharge, a study of 48 COVID patients, who presented with persistent respiratory symptoms, was examined for the extent of air trapping. Each lung is divided into upper, mid and lower zones, thus totalling six lung zones. Each zone was visually inspected and assigned a number on a 4-point scale, with 0 representing no air trapping, 1 for 1–24%, 2 for 25–49%, 3 for 50–74% and 4 for 75% or more, to a maximum score of 24. The majority of the 48 patients had persistent parenchymal abnormality, and air trapping was the most prevalent abnormality, outnumbering ground glass opacities, reticulation, parenchymal bands, traction bronchiectasis and others. The air trapping score was associated with gender (with men worse affected), increased interval between symptom onset and hospital admission, ARDS and elevated levels of two acute phase proteins (C-reactive protein and ferritin) [82]. This suggests that air trapping is more extensive in severe COVID-19 infections.

Quantitative measures of air trapping have been applied to different asthma clusters using mean lung density (MLD) and lung volume at less than −856HU on expiratory CT performed at functional residual volume. The most clinically severe phenotype clusters showed significant differences to other clusters, having both significantly lower mean lung density and a higher proportion of the lung volume below −856 HU. The −856HU threshold was chosen as previous studies had shown good correlation with functional studies of airflow obstruction [32, 60]. Differences between the less severe clusters were not found. Furthermore, using paired inspiratory/expiratory CTs to acquire volume measurements, the authors found that the most severe clusters of asthmatics showed relatively little expiratory-to-inspiratory volume change, which led the authors to hypothesise that the impaired mechanics of breathing are important to symptoms and could be due to hyperinflation [60].

Another study investigated the between group difference in COVID-19 survivors. Two hundred five individuals were split into two groups according to their carbon monoxide diffusion capacity (DLCO). Group 1 had DLCO less than 80%, whilst the remainder made up group 2. Two methods of measuring air trapping were tested: a semiquantitative method and a quantitative method. The semi-quantitative method was based on a visual scoring system ranging from 0 to 25. The total score is the sum of five sub-scores, each out of 5, one for each lobe of the lung. The higher the percentage of air trapping visualised, the higher the score. The second method used was based on the work performed in COPD cohorts using Δvolume (−860 to −950HU) [80]. In the analysis, group 1 (reduced gas transfer) had significantly more air trapping on their 6 months follow-up CT using both quantitative methods [83].

Parametric response mapping is currently one of the most modern imaging processing techniques, whereby the expiratory acquisition is mapped onto the inspiratory acquisition, so that they overlap in geometry. Individual voxels are then compared between the paired scans, to determinate if these represent normal lung tissue, areas of air trapping or emphysema. Arbitrarily, each voxel can be assigned a different colour, depending on the category it falls into, to give a visual representation of the amount and distribution of each of these [84].

Emphysema

Emphysema is one of the most common imaging features of COPD to be assessed quantitatively. Emphysema is lower in density than normal parenchyma on CT, first described by Rosenblum et al. in 1978 [85], which is a feature that underpins how computer algorithms quantify the extent and distribution of the disease. As with other imaging features, analysing emphysema depends on accurate lung segmentation, in which the boundaries of the lungs are mapped out against adjacent structures, such as the chest wall and mediastinum. Large central bronchovascular structures are often excluded, too. It is imperative that there is no concomitant acute lung pathology, such as patches of consolidation, which would obscure any analysis.

Earlier attempts in quantifying emphysema were completed visually. For example, Bergin et al. assessed the extent of emphysema seen on pre-operative axial lung CTs in patients about to undergo lung resection. The three CT readers scored each CT based on a four-point scale, depending on the extent of the emphysema see, in 25% increments: 0–25% (1), 25–50% (2), 50–75% (3) and over 75% (4). Each of the 32 CT data was scored twice, both for the resected lung as well as their lungs overall. The results were then correlated against pathological findings in the corresponding resected specimen. The authors found significant correlation between both sets of CT scores and the pathological scoring. Furthermore, the predictive accuracy of CT scores was better than that of spirometry [86]. However, other studies have found that, whilst visual inspection positively correlates with the true extent of emphysema as measured by histological analysis, it consistently overestimates the extent of emphysema compared with quantitative methods and also resulted in greater interobserver variation [87, 88].

Computer-aided quantification of emphysema is estimated by either of two techniques. The first technique is a densitometry-based method, whereby a specific threshold is selected, and the pixels below this are labelled as emphysema. The most commonly adopted now is −950 Hounsfield unit, as it correlates well with micro- and macroscopic histopathological findings. The proportion of lung occupied by pixels below the set threshold is calculated as a percentage of the total lung volume, and a low attenuation percentage (LAA%) is derived. $LAA\%_{<950HU}$ has been shown to correlate well with FEV_1, gas transfer, 6-min walk test and BODE score [55]. The second method uses a different definition for emphysema, termed percentile densitometry. Using a frequency distribution curve for all the pixel densities, a percentile threshold is chosen. As emphysema increases, the curve plotted progressively shift towards the left, and if a fixed percentile threshold is chosen, this will also shift towards the left, to a lower density (Fig. 18.13). The most commonly used threshold is 15%, Perc15, based on work in patients with alpha-1 antitrypsin deficiency, in which this threshold correlated well with histopathology specimens. There is no consensus over which one of the methods is superior, and both are still used [55].

To gain additional insight into how the emphysema is distributed, the lungs can be further segmented using various methods. The simplest is

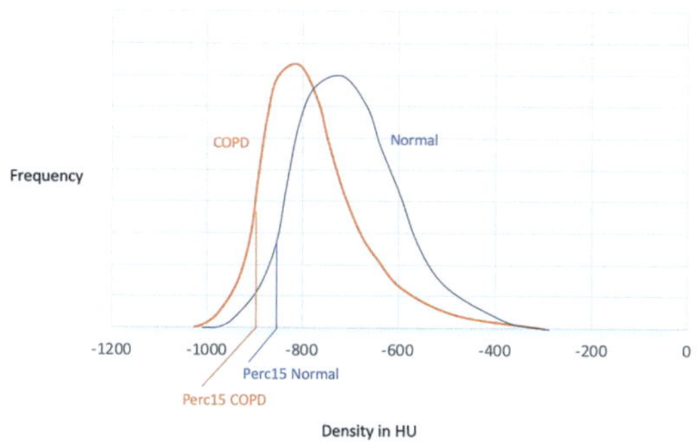

Fig. 18.13 Percentile densitometry method of estimating emphysema. The curves in the graph represent the density distribution of a normal lung (blue) and an emphysematous lung (orange). Areas of emphysema shift the orange curve to the left, so that Perc 15, the point that demarcates the limit of the lowest 15% of pixels, becomes a lower value

by dividing the lungs into equal thirds in the craniocaudal direction, between the apex and the dome of the hemidiaphragms—upper, mid and third zones. Alternatively, by identifying the course of the fissures, the lungs can be subsegmented into lobes. Lobar $LAA\%_{<950HU}$ can then be tabulated along with other useful measures such as lobar volume (Fig. 18.14b). Applying colour to the CT can assist in the visual understanding of the distribution of emphysema (Fig. 18.14a). A heterogeneity index can be given, to quantify the degree of emphysema heterogeneity. An interlobar difference of 15% in the extent of the emphysema (an index of 1.15) is a traditionally accepted threshold, which differentiates between low and high heterogeneity [89]. However, evidence is beginning to show that homogeneous disease can also have persistent symptomatic benefit after lung volume reduction surgery [90].

Whilst computer aided emphysema quantification is proven to be an indispensable tool, there are challenges to be aware of. Note that emphysema quantification on HRCT can be significantly influenced by any dose reduction techniques and reconstruction algorisms used. For example, when using a filtered back projection at reduced doses, the amount of noise in the resultant image significantly overestimates the amount of emphysema present. This is found to be the case in both emphysema quantification methods described above, LAA% and percentile densitometry [91]. This does not render emphysema quantification useless in low-dose images, but the necessary adjustments need to be in place, calibrated against full-dose imaging. Quantification in low-dose imaging is likely to become increasingly relevant, as targeted lung health check programmes are being expanded across many parts of the world, primarily screening for lung cancer.

Another area of interest is in the emerging roles of MRI. Though CT remains the cornerstone of all aspects of thoracic imaging, emerging MRI techniques provide new imaging opportunities by overcoming the inherent low proton-density nature of the lungs that has previously made MRI a challenge. One technique is by hyperpolarised gas inhalation, typically xenon (129 Xe) or helium (3 He). A mixture of the hyperpolarised gas and medical-grade nitrogen is inhaled through a mouthpiece, immediately followed by image acquisition on a breath-hold of approximately 10–20 s [92]. This allows assessment of ventilation by measuring the amount and distribution of the inhaled gas. Areas of poor ventilation show as signal voids. The extent of this abnormality can be quantified as ventilation defect percentage, which is the volume taken up by signal voids, as a percentage of the total lung capacity. The degree of heterogeneity can also be quantified. Acquiring multiple images over either a single breath or multiple breaths yields dynamic ventilation MRI, which enables detailed assessment of the rate of gas entering each lobe, the maximum intensity each lobe reaches and the heterogeneity of the distribution [92].

Many promising applications of MRI have been explored in the literature. For example, using a visual scoring system, MR with hyperpolarised gas shows good correlation with measures of asthma severity and spirometric results. Interestingly, MR ventilation defects have been shown to persist in the same location in individuals across many years and can help to predict response to bronchodilators [93].

Measuring the apparent diffusion coefficient (ADC) has been shown to detect the earli-

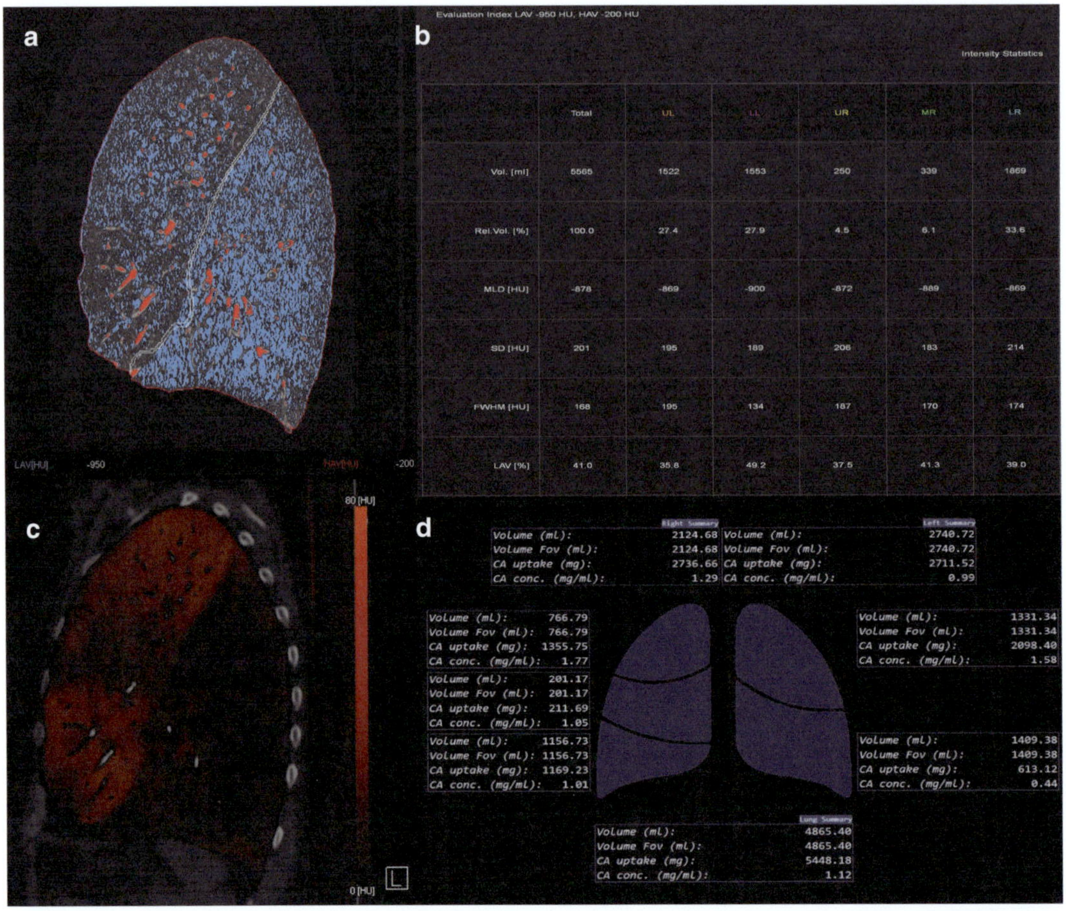

Fig. 18.14 (**a**–**d**) Imaging work-up for lung volume reduction. Quantitative imaging in lung volume reduction planning in a patient with COPD. (**a**) Sagittal density map of the left lung at a threshold of ≤950 HU showing centrilobular emphysema (blue), with basal predominance. (**b**) The associated intensity statistic table confirms that the destruction score is worst in the left lower lobe (low attenuation value (LAV%) of 49.2%). (**c**) Same day dual energy CT pulmonary angiography is used to then create a colour map of iodine distribution which confirms poor iodine perfusion of the left lower lobe. This correlates with the pictographic depiction of iodine distribution which confirms a relatively low contrast agent (CA) uptake of 613 mg of iodine compared to that of the left upper lobe—2098.4 mg iodine (**d**). These findings prompted a referral for lung volume reduction of the left lower lobe

est signs of alveolar damage in patients with a known tobacco exposure, much earlier than any functional or structural abnormality becomes apparent on spirometry or HRCT. In emphysematous lung, diffusion of inhaled gases across the alveolar-capillary membrane is impaired. This leads to excessive retention of inhaled hyperpolarised gas in these areas, and the ADC value is therefore abnormally high. Thus, ADC value serves as an imaging biomarker for subtle changes in the lung microstructure. ADC values correlate strongly with CT methods of emphysema evaluation in COPD patients without the use of ionising radiation. Work has already begun on developing a quantitative metric so that it could be validated and easily interpreted in future clinical settings [94].

Miscellaneous Quantitative Imaging Methods in Airways Disease

Fissural Integrity

In cases of severe overinflation due to COPD, lung volume reduction surgery is shown to be beneficial in the National Emphysema Treatment Trial outcomes [95]. However, patients with advanced COPD are inherently at high risk for major surgery, and many patients who would benefit from lung volume reduction are excluded based on surgical risk. Thankfully, there are now numerous endoscopic procedures that have also been shown to be therapeutically beneficial [96]. One method of achieving volume reduction is with endobronchial valves, which are well-studied. These one-way valves are implanted endoscopically, with the aim of reducing the volume of the most diseased, overinflated lobe (Fig. 18.15). The success of this procedure depends on the integrity of the fissures, as collateral interlobar ventilation is one of the main reasons for procedure failure [97]. Visual assessment of the fissures on HRCT is often fraught with inaccuracies and is being superseded by cloud-based, computer-aided assessment tools. In a retrospective study, a computer-aided assessment tool used was found to be a better predictor of procedure success than visual inspection, when success is defined by a volume reduction in the target lobe of >350 mL [98]. Examples of these fissure assessment tools are now in limited clinical use to aid patient selection prior to endobronchial valve implantation. In patients with intact fissures, measured at >95% intact, it is non-inferior to the invasive bronchoscopic method of evaluating collateral ventilation at predicting procedure success [99].

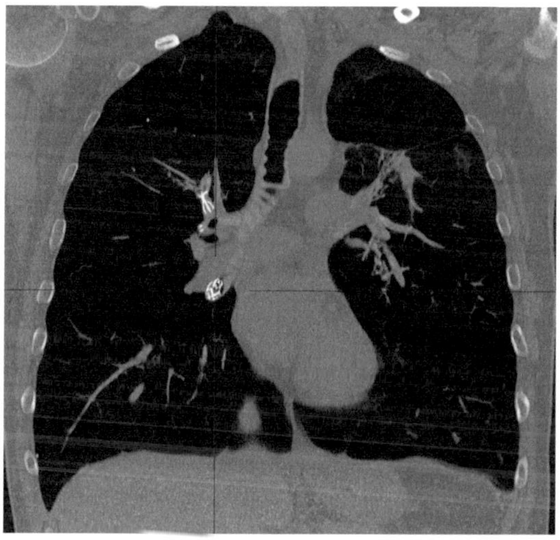

Fig. 18.15 Endobronchial valves. Reformatted maximum intensity projection (MIP) coronal CT in a 53 year-old male with panlobular emphysema. Endobronchial valves within the right middle and upper lobe bronchi. The right upper and middle lobes remain expanded, indicating failure of the valves

Dynamic MRI with hyperpolarised gas is also able to predict fissural integrity, by identifying areas of delayed ventilation. These regions are felt to represent collateral ventilation (Fig. 18.16). This represents another potential non-invasive technique to quantify the amount of collateral ventilation for the future, either as an alternative or an adjunct to HRCT fissural assessment tools described above [92].

Perfusion Abnormalities in Airway Diseases

Ventilation abnormalities associated with airway diseases are often accompanied by perfusion defects, possibly secondary to hypoxic pulmonary vasoconstriction, which is a homeostatic mechanism diverting blood to better aerated lung units for efficient gas exchange. Therefore, perfusion abnormalities could be used as a surrogate measure of ventilation and, by extension, airways disease, if some assumptions are met. For example, there should be no intrinsic pulmonary vascular disease, such as pulmonary emboli, that could influence the pattern of perfusion.

When selecting patients for lung volume reduction, clinicians often consider the lobar perfusion differential. It is used as a functional measurement; lobes with poor perfusion contribute little to gas exchange. Resection of poorly perfused lung has been shown to correlate well with a positive treatment response, measured by survival and functional improvement [100, 101].

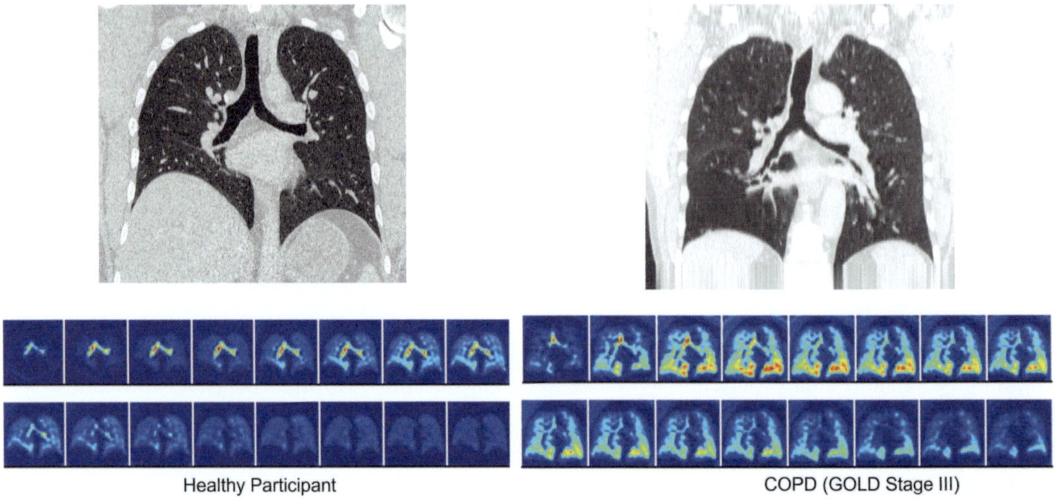

Fig. 18.16 Dynamic MRI with hyperpolarised gas. Dynamic pulmonary ventilation in a healthy participant (left) and chronic obstructive pulmonary disease (COPD) patient (right). Top figures are coronal computed tomography images of the thorax and bottom dynamic ventilation hyperpolarised Xenon-129 MRI (DXeV-MRI) images acquired during a free breathing cycle (in time steps). Delayed ventilation in the right lower (black arrow) and left lower zones (grey arrow) in the COPD patient have been demonstrated on DXeV-MRI, relative to signal change in the trachea. These might represent collateral ventilation, and useful for guiding lung volume reduction therapy in COPD. (Images curtesy of Dr Mitchell Chen, Imperial College London)

Dual energy CT (DECT) is emerging as an alternative tool, alongside SPECT perfusion scan (SPECT-PS), which is currently the established method. DECT is a paired acquisition of the same image volume at two different peak kilovoltages (kVp). Using knowledge of the attenuation properties of iodine at different kVp, a virtual non-contrast scan can be created. Then, by calculating the difference between this and the enhanced images, an iodine map of the lung can be derived. This iodine map can be illustrated using a colour scale, enhancing visual assessment [102] (Fig. 18.14c). Alternatively, by overlaying the iodine map onto the anatomical data with each lobe segmented, relative perfusion of each lobe can be estimated (Fig. 18.14d). One study found a strong linear correlation between DECT and SPECT-PS in 123 patients. The authors highlighted that patients also undergo non-contrast thoracic CT as part of the standard pre-procedural assessment, providing an opportunity for DECT to be carried out in the same appointment. Therefore, the patient selection process can be streamlined if DECT is selected in favour of SPECT-PS [103, 104].

Not only does perfusion change in physiological terms in airways disease, but vessels change anatomically, decreasing in calibre in long-standing airway disease. The association between vascular pruning with the severity of asthma was investigated in one study, using non-contrast CTs. The total pulmonary blood vessel volume (TBV), blood vessel volume of vessels less than 5 mm^2 in cross-sectional area (BV5) and blood vessel volume of vessels less than 10 mm^2 in cross-sectional area (BV10) were measured. In vascular pruning, a lower ratio of BV5/TBV and BV10/TBV would be expected. The results of the study revealed a significant difference in these ratios between asthmatics and healthy controls, with the biggest difference found in those with poorly controlled asthma. Another finding is the increased frequency of exacerbations seen in patients with higher degree of pruning, pointing towards possible prognostic value of this indicator [105]. This study provides a reminder that asthma can affect other lung compartments other than airways; lung perfusion can be significantly altered.

Mechanics of Breathing

Paired CTs taken at total lung capacity (full inspiration) and functional residual capacity (full expiration) can be analysed to give insight into the mechanism of breathing. One study found reduced volume change in the lung bases in asthmatic individuals compared to healthy controls. However, in the lung apices, the inverse was true. This is useful, as FVC in the asthmatics was shown to be 100% predicted. It seems the lack of ventilation in the bases, likely caused by air trapping is being compensated with increased ventilation at the lung apices [106].

Anisotropic deformation index (ADI) measures the strength of the directionality during lung deformation. An ADI value of 0 means perfect isometric deformation, where the change in volume in all three axis is equal. It is independent to the magnitude of the volume change. Indeed, the net volume change may be zero. For example, if a unit of lung increases in one axis, but decreases in equal measure in another, the net volume change may be zero, but the ADI would be greater than 0 [107]. In severe asthma, ADI values change significantly, particularly on expiration, which could in future provide another quantitative measure to identify disease phenotype and assess severity [60, 108].

Summary and Future Perspectives

There are now more quantitative imaging methods to investigate airway diseases than ever before, offering new possibilities in the management of conditions, such as COPD and asthma, which did not traditionally depend on imaging. Thus, quantitative imaging is providing a new perspective on the role of imaging in the diagnosis and management of airway diseases. The examples provided in this chapter are the most well studied but by no means represent an exhaustive list. These methods have facilitated the design and development of new imaging bio markers, with many showing promise for future clinical use. However, additional longitudinal studies are required to validate their utility to phenotype diseases, predict treatment response and disease outcomes.

As discussed in this chapter, some quantitative methods can be labour intensive and time-consuming. However, newer methods are increasingly automated, and the rate of change is accelerating. It will be interesting to discover how artificial intelligence will change the way quantitative imaging is utilised. Knowledge about pitfalls is important, but with each successive generation, artificial intelligence and quantitative imaging are likely to open new possibilities.

References

1. Sanders C. The radiographic diagnosis of emphysema. Radiol Clin North Am. 1991;29:1019–30.
2. Vogelmeier CF, Criner GJ, Martinez FJ, Anzueto A, Barnes PJ, Bourbeau J, et al. Global strategy for the diagnosis, management, and prevention of chronic obstructive lung disease 2017 report. GOLD executive summary. Am J Respir Crit Care Med. 2017;195:557–82.
3. World Health Organization. Global Health Estimates 2020: deaths by cause, age, sex, by country and by region, 2000–2019. [Internet]. 2020 [cited 2023 Sept 21]. Available from: https://www.who.int/data/gho/data/themes/mortality-and-global-health-estimates/ghe-leading-causes-of-death
4. GBD 2017 Causes of Death Collaborators. Global, regional, and national age-sex-specific mortality for 282 causes of death in 195 countries and territories, 1980–2017: a systematic analysis for the Global Burden of Disease Study 2017. Lancet. 2018;392:1736–88.
5. Agustí A, Celli BR, Criner GJ, Halpin D, Anzueto A, Barnes P, et al. Global initiative for chronic obstructive lung disease 2023 report: GOLD executive summary. Eur Respir J. 2023;61:2300239.
6. Definition and classification of chronic bronchitis for clinical and epidemiological purposes. A report to the Medical Research Council by their committee on the aetiology of chronic bronchitis. Lancet. 1965;1:775–9.
7. National Institute for Health and Care Excellence. Diagnosis of chronic obstructive pulmonary disease. 2023.
8. McDonough JE, Yuan R, Suzuki M, Seyednejad N, Elliott WM, Sanchez PG, et al. Small-airway obstruction and emphysema in chronic obstructive pulmonary disease. N Engl J Med. 2011;365:1567–75.
9. Barnes PJ. Inflammatory mechanisms in patients with chronic obstructive pulmonary disease. J Allergy Clin Immunol. 2016;138:16–27.

10. Stockley RA. Neutrophils and protease/antiprotease imbalance. Am J Respir Crit Care Med. 1999;160:S49–52.
11. Churg A, Tai H, Coulthard T, Wang R, Wright JL. Cigarette smoke drives small airway remodeling by induction of growth factors in the airway wall. Am J Respir Crit Care Med. 2006;174:1327–34.
12. Pratt PC. Role of conventional chest radiography in diagnosis and exclusion of emphysema. Am J Med. 1987;82:998–1006.
13. Webb WR. Radiology of obstructive pulmonary disease. AJR Am J Roentgenol. 1997;169:637–47.
14. Reich SB, Weinshelbaum A, Yee J. Correlation of radiographic measurements and pulmonary function tests in chronic obstructive pulmonary disease. AJR Am J Roentgenol. 1985;144:695–9.
15. Hansell DM, Bankier AA, MacMahon H, McLoud TC, Müller NL, Remy J. Fleischner society: glossary of terms for thoracic imaging. Radiology. 2008;246:697–722.
16. Remy-Jardin M, Remy J, Gosselin B, Copin MC, Wurtz A, Duhamel A. Sliding thin slab, minimum intensity projection technique in the diagnosis of emphysema: histopathologic-CT correlation. Radiology. 1996;200:665–71.
17. Aziz ZA, Wells AU, Desai SR, Ellis SM, Walker AE, MacDonald S, et al. Functional impairment in emphysema: contribution of airway abnormalities and distribution of parenchymal disease. AJR Am J Roentgenol. 2005;185:1509–15.
18. Anderson AE, Foraker AG. Centrilobular emphysema and panlobular emphysema: two different diseases. Thorax. 1973;28:547–50.
19. Litmanovich D, Boiselle PM, Bankier AA. CT of pulmonary emphysema–current status, challenges, and future directions. Eur Radiol. 2009;19:537–51.
20. Takahashi M, Fukuoka J, Nitta N, Takazakura R, Nagatani Y, Murakami Y, et al. Imaging of pulmonary emphysema: a pictorial review. Int J Chron Obstruct Pulmon Dis. 2008;3:193–204.
21. Guest PJ, Hansell DM. High resolution computed tomography (HRCT) in emphysema associated with alpha-1-antitrypsin deficiency. Clin Radiol. 1992;45:260–6.
22. Nakano Y, Müller NL, King GG, Niimi A, Kalloger SE, Mishima M, et al. Quantitative assessment of airway remodeling using high-resolution CT. Chest. 2002;122:271S–5S.
23. Allen TC. Small airways disease. Surg Pathol Clin. 2010;3:171–86.
24. Papi A, Brightling C, Pedersen SE, Reddel HK. Asthma. Lancet. 2018;391:783–800.
25. Venkatesan P. 2023 GINA report for asthma. Lancet Respir Med. 2023;11:589.
26. To T, Stanojevic S, Moores G, Gershon AS, Bateman ED, Cruz AA, et al. Global asthma prevalence in adults: findings from the cross-sectional world health survey. BMC Public Health. 2012;19:204.
27. Bourdin A, Chanez P. Clustering in asthma: why, how and for how long? Eur Respir J. 2013;41:1247–8.
28. Holgate ST, Polosa R. The mechanisms, diagnosis, and management of severe asthma in adults. Lancet. 2006;368:780–93.
29. Haldar P, Pavord ID, Shaw DE, Berry MA, Thomas M, Brightling CE, et al. Cluster analysis and clinical asthma phenotypes. Am J Respir Crit Care Med. 2008;178:218–24.
30. National Asthma Education and Prevention Program, Third Expert Panel on the Diagnosis and Management of Asthma. Expert panel report 3: guidelines for the diagnosis and management of asthma. Bethesda: National Heart, Lung, and Blood Institute (US); 2007.
31. Hederos CA, Janson S, Andersson H, Hedlin G. Chest x-ray investigation in newly discovered asthma. Pediatr Allergy Immunol. 2004;15:163–5.
32. Verschakelen JA. Quantitative CT of the lung to study asthma. Radiology. 2022;304:460–1.
33. Grenier P, Mourey-Gerosa I, Benali K, Brauner MW, Leung AN, Lenoir S, et al. Abnormalities of the airways and lung parenchyma in asthmatics: CT observations in 50 patients and inter- and intraobserver variability. Eur Radiol. 1996;6:199–206.
34. Chalmers JD, Polverino E, Crichton ML, Ringshausen FC, De Soyza A, Vendrell M, et al. Bronchiectasis in Europe: data on disease characteristics from the European Bronchiectasis registry (EMBARC). Lancet Respir Med. 2023;11:637–49.
35. Milliron B, Henry TS, Veeraraghavan S, Little BP. Bronchiectasis: mechanisms and imaging clues of associated common and uncommon diseases. Radiographics. 2015;35:1011–30.
36. Bush A, Floto RA. Pathophysiology, causes and genetics of paediatric and adult bronchiectasis. Respirology. 2019;24:1053–62.
37. Quint JK, Millett ERC, Joshi M, Navaratnam V, Thomas SL, Hurst JR, et al. Changes in the incidence, prevalence and mortality of bronchiectasis in the UK from 2004 to 2013: a population-based cohort study. Eur Respir J. 2016;47:186–93.
38. Mayor S. Bronchiectasis is increasing in the UK, study shows. BMJ. 2015;351:h5916.
39. Reid LM. Reduction in bronchial subdivision in bronchiectasis. Thorax. 1950;5:233–47.
40. Aslam A, De Luis CJ, Morrison RJ, Lagisetty KH, Litmanovich D, Sella EC, et al. Tracheobronchomalacia and excessive dynamic airway collapse: current concepts and future directions. Radiographics. 2022;42:1012–27.
41. Wallis C, Alexopoulou E, Antón-Pacheco JL, Bhatt JM, Bush A, Chang AB, et al. ERS statement on tracheomalacia and bronchomalacia in children. Eur Respir J. 2019;54:1900382.
42. Boiselle PM, O'Donnell CR, Bankier AA, Ernst A, Millet ME, Potemkin A, et al. Tracheal collapsibility in healthy volunteers during forced expiration: assessment with multidetector CT. Radiology. 2009;252:255–62.

43. Fraser RS, Müller NL, Colman N, Paré PD. Diagnosis of diseases of the chest. 4th ed. Philadelphia: WB Saunders; 2001. p. 2042–6.
44. Buitrago DH, Wilson JL, Parikh M, Majid A, Gangadharan SP. Current concepts in severe adult tracheobronchomalacia: evaluation and treatment. J Thorac Dis. 2017;9:E57–66.
45. Boiselle PM, O'Donnell CR, Loring SH, Bankier AA. Reproducibility of forced expiratory tracheal collapse: assessment with MDCT in healthy volunteers. Acad Radiol. 2010;17:1186–9.
46. Ochani R, Asad A, Yasmin F, Shaikh S, Khalid H, Batra S, et al. COVID-19 pandemic: from origins to outcomes. A comprehensive review of viral pathogenesis, clinical manifestations, diagnostic evaluation, and management. Infez Med. 2021;29:20–36.
47. World Health Organisation. WHO coronarvirus (COVID-19) dashboard.
48. Long B, Carius BM, Chavez S, Liang SY, Brady WJ, Koyfman A, et al. Clinical update on COVID-19 for the emergency clinician: presentation and evaluation. Am J Emerg Med. 2022;54:46–57.
49. Toussie D, Voutsinas N, Chung M, Bernheim A. Imaging of COVID-19. Semin Roentgenol. 2022;57:40–52.
50. Daines L, Zheng B, Pfeffer P, Hurst JR, Sheikh A. A clinical review of long-COVID with a focus on the respiratory system. Curr Opin Pulm Med. 2022;28:174–9.
51. Solomon JJ, Heyman B, Ko JP, Condos R, Lynch DA. CT of post-acute lung complications of COVID-19. Radiology. 2021;301:E383–95.
52. Mengoli MC, Rossi G, Cavazza A, Franco R, Marino FZ, Migaldi M, et al. Diffuse idiopathic pulmonary neuroendocrine cell hyperplasia (DIPNECH) syndrome and carcinoid tumors with/without NECH. Am J Surg Pathol. 2018;42:646–55.
53. Little BP, Junn JC, Zheng KS, Sanchez FW, Henry TS, Veeraraghavan S, et al. Diffuse idiopathic pulmonary neuroendocrine cell hyperplasia: imaging and clinical features of a frequently delayed diagnosis. Am J Roentgenol. 2020;215:1312–20.
54. Chassagnon G, Favelle O, Marchand-Adam S, De Muret A, Revel MP. DIPNECH: when to suggest this diagnosis on CT. Clin Radiol. 2015;70:317–25.
55. Ostridge K, Wilkinson TMA. Present and future utility of computed tomography scanning in the assessment and management of COPD. Eur Respir J. 2016;48:216–28.
56. Kahnert K, Jörres RA, Kauczor HU, Alter P, Trudzinski FC, Herth F, et al. Standardized airway wall thickness Pi10 from routine CT scans of COPD patients as imaging biomarker for disease severity, lung function decline, and mortality. Ther Adv Respir Dis. 2023;17:17534666221148664.
57. Grydeland TB, Dirksen A, Coxson HO, Pillai SG, Sharma S, Eide GE, et al. Quantitative computed tomography: emphysema and airway wall thickness by sex, age and smoking. Eur Respir J. 2009;34:858–65.
58. Nakano Y, Muro S, Sakai H, Hirai T, Chin K, Tsukino M, et al. Computed tomographic measurements of airway dimensions and emphysema in smokers. Correlation with lung function. Am J Respir Crit Care Med. 2000;162:1102–8.
59. Arakawa H, Fujimoto K, Fukushima Y, Kaji Y. Thin-section CT imaging that correlates with pulmonary function tests in obstructive airway disease. Eur J Radiol. 2011;80:e157–63.
60. Trivedi AP, Hall C, Goss CW, Lew D, Krings JG, McGregor MC, et al. Quantitative CT characteristics of cluster phenotypes in the severe asthma research program cohorts. Radiology. 2022;304:450–9.
61. Aysola RS, Hoffman EA, Gierada D, Wenzel S, Cook-Granroth J, Tarsi J, et al. Airway remodeling measured by multidetector CT is increased in severe asthma and correlates with pathology. Chest. 2008;134:1183–91.
62. Xu J, Liang Z, Jian W, Li J, Tang G, Mo X, et al. Changes of quantitative CT-based airway wall dimensions in patients with COVID-19 during early recovery. J Thorac Dis. 2021;13:1517–30.
63. Ackermann M, Verleden SE, Kuehnel M, Haverich A, Welte T, Laenger F, et al. Pulmonary vascular endothelialitis, thrombosis, and angiogenesis in Covid-19. N Engl J Med. 2020;383:120–8.
64. Bonaventura A, Vecchié A, Dagna L, Martinod K, Dixon DL, Van Tassell BW, et al. Endothelial dysfunction and immunothrombosis as key pathogenic mechanisms in COVID-19. Nat Rev Immunol. 2021;21:319–29.
65. Nägele MP, Haubner B, Tanner FC, Ruschitzka F, Flammer AJ. Endothelial dysfunction in COVID-19: current findings and therapeutic implications. Atherosclerosis. 2020;314:58–62.
66. Hansell DM. Bronchiectasis. Radiol Clin North Am. 1998;36:107–28.
67. Ouellette H. The signet ring sign. Radiology. 1999;212:67–8.
68. Lv Q, Gallardo-Estrella L, Andrinopoulou ER, Chen Y, Charbonnier JP, Sandvik RM, et al. Automatic analysis of bronchus-artery dimensions to diagnose and monitor airways disease in cystic fibrosis. Thorax. 2023;79:13–22.
69. Ferraro V, Andrinopoulou ER, Sijbring AMM, Haarman EG, Tiddens HAWM, Pijnenburg MWH. Airway–artery quantitative assessment on chest computed tomography in paediatric primary ciliary dyskinesia. ERJ Open Res [Internet]. 2020;6:00210–2019. Available from: http://openres.ersjournals.com/content/6/3/00210-2019.abstract.
70. Kuo W, Perez-Rovira A, Tiddens H, de Bruijne M. Airway tapering: an objective image biomarker for bronchiectasis. Eur Radiol. 2020;30:2703–11.
71. O'Brien C, Duignan JA, Gleeson M, O'Carroll O, Franciosi AN, O'Toole D, et al. Quantitative airway assessment of diffuse idiopathic pulmonary neuroendocrine cell hyperplasia (DIPNECH) on CT as a novel biomarker. Diagnostics. 2022;12:3096.

72. Robinson P, Morgan L. Bronchiectasis in PCD looks different to CF on CT scan. Multidiscip Respir Med. 2018;13:24.
73. Stern EJ, Graham CM, Webb WR, Gamsu G. Normal trachea during forced expiration: dynamic CT measurements. Radiology. 1993;187:27–31.
74. Bezuidenhout AF, Boiselle PM, Heidinger BH, Alape D, Buitrago DH, Majid A, et al. Longitudinal follow-up of patients with tracheobronchomalacia after undergoing tracheobronchoplasty: computed tomography findings and clinical correlation. J Thorac Imaging. 2019;34:278–83.
75. Mitropoulos A, Song WJ, Almaghlouth F, Kemp S, Polkey M, Hull JH. Detection and diagnosis of large airway collapse: a systematic review. ERJ Open Res. 2021;7:00055-2021.
76. Hein E, Rogalla P, Hentschel C, Taupitz M, Hamm B. Dynamic and quantitative assessment of tracheomalacia by electron beam tomography: correlation with clinical symptoms and bronchoscopy. J Comput Assist Tomogr. 2000;24:247–52.
77. Dunican EM, Elicker BM, Gierada DS, Nagle SK, Schiebler ML, Newell JD, et al. Mucus plugs in patients with asthma linked to eosinophilia and airflow obstruction. J Clin Invest. 2018;128:997–1009.
78. Eddy RL, Svenningsen S, Kirby M, Knipping D, McCormack DG, Licskai C, et al. Is computed tomography airway count related to asthma severity and airway structure and function? Am J Respir Crit Care Med. 2020;201:923–33.
79. Kubo K, Eda S, Yamamoto H, Fujimoto K, Matsuzawa Y, Maruyama Y, et al. Expiratory and inspiratory chest computed tomography and pulmonary function tests in cigarette smokers. Eur Respir J. 1999;13:252–6.
80. Matsuoka S, Kurihara Y, Yagihashi K, Hoshino M, Watanabe N, Nakajima Y. Quantitative assessment of air trapping in chronic obstructive pulmonary disease using inspiratory and expiratory volumetric MDCT. AJR Am J Roentgenol. 2008;190:762–9.
81. Huang R, Zhu J, Zhou J, Shang Y, Lin X, Gong S, et al. Inspiratory and expiratory chest high-resolution CT: small-airway disease evaluation in patients with COVID-19. Curr Med Imaging. 2021;17:1299–307.
82. Franquet T, Giménez A, Ketai L, Mazzini S, Rial A, Pomar V, et al. Air trapping in COVID-19 patients following hospital discharge: retrospective evaluation with paired inspiratory/expiratory thin-section CT. Eur Radiol. 2022;32:4427–36.
83. Jia X, Han X, Cao Y, Fan Y, Yuan M, Li Y, et al. Quantitative inspiratory–expiratory chest CT findings in COVID-19 survivors at the 6-month follow-up. Sci Rep. 2022;12:7402.
84. Galbán CJ, Han MK, Boes JL, Chughtai KA, Meyer CR, Johnson TD, et al. Computed tomography-based biomarker provides unique signature for diagnosis of COPD phenotypes and disease progression. Nat Med. 2012;18:1711–5.
85. Rosenblum LJ, Mauceri RA, Wellenstein DE, Bassano DA, Cohen WN, Heitzman ER. Computed tomography of the lung. Radiology. 1978;129:521–4.
86. Bergin C, Müller N, Nichols DM, Lillington G, Hogg JC, Mullen B, et al. The diagnosis of emphysema. A computed tomographic-pathologic correlation. Am Rev Respir Dis. 1986;133:541–6.
87. Desai SR, Hansell DM, Walker A, MacDonald SLS, Chabat F, Wells AU. Quantification of emphysema: a composite physiologic index derived from CT estimation of disease extent. Eur Radiol. 2007;17:911–8.
88. Bankier AA, De Maertelaer V, Keyzer C, Gevenois PA. Pulmonary emphysema: subjective visual grading versus objective quantification with macroscopic morphometry and thin-section CT densitometry. Radiology. 1999;211:851–8.
89. Valipour A, Shah PL, Gesierich W, Eberhardt R, Snell G, Strange C, et al. Patterns of emphysema heterogeneity. Respiration. 2015;90:402–11.
90. Weder W, Tutic M, Lardinois D, Jungraithmayr W, Hillinger S, Russi EW, et al. Persistent benefit from lung volume reduction surgery in patients with homogeneous emphysema. Ann Thorac Surg. 2009;87:229–37.
91. den Harder AM, de Boer E, Lagerweij SJ, Boomsma MF, Schilham AMR, Willemink MJ, et al. Emphysema quantification using chest CT: influence of radiation dose reduction and reconstruction technique. Eur Radiol Exp. 2018;2:30.
92. Foo CT, Langton D, Thompson BR, Thien F. Functional lung imaging using novel and emerging MRI techniques. Front Med (Lausanne). 2023;10:1060940.
93. Eddy RL, Svenningsen S, Licskai C, McCormack DG, Parraga G. Hyperpolarized helium 3 MRI in mild-to-moderate asthma: prediction of postbronchodilator reversibility. Radiology. 2019;293:212–20.
94. Tafti S, Garrison WJ, Mugler JP, Shim YM, Altes TA, Mata JF, et al. Emphysema index based on hyperpolarized 3He or 129Xe diffusion MRI: performance and comparison with quantitative CT and pulmonary function tests. Radiology. 2020;297:201–10.
95. Fishman A, Martinez F, Naunheim K, Piantadosi S, Wise R, Ries A, et al. A randomized trial comparing lung-volume-reduction surgery with medical therapy for severe emphysema. N Engl J Med. 2003;348:2059–73.
96. Shah PL, Herth FJ, van Geffen WH, Deslee G, Slebos DJ. Lung volume reduction for emphysema. Lancet Respir Med. 2017;5:147–56.
97. Garner JL, Desai SR. Lung fissural integrity: it's written in the genes. Am J Respir Crit Care Med. 2021;204:750–2.
98. Fiorelli A, Poggi C, Anile M, Cascone R, Carlucci A, Cassiano F, et al. Visual analysis versus quantitative CT analysis of interlobar fissure integrity in selecting emphysematous patients for endobronchial valve treatment. Interact Cardiovasc Thorac Surg. 2019;28:751–9.

99. Fiorelli A, Santini M, Shah P. When can computed tomography-fissure analysis replace Chartis collateral ventilation assessment in the prediction of patients with emphysema who might benefit from endobronchial valve therapy? Interact Cardiovasc Thorac Surg. 2018;26:313–8.
100. Chandra D, Lipson DA, Hoffman EA, Hansen-Flaschen J, Sciurba FC, Decamp MM, et al. Perfusion scintigraphy and patient selection for lung volume reduction surgery. Am J Respir Crit Care Med. 2010;182:937–46.
101. Huebner RH, Theilig D, Herzog D, Poellinger A, Doellinger F, Schreiter N, et al. Lung perfusion and emphysema distribution affect the outcome of endobronchial valve therapy. Int J Chron Obstruct Pulmon Dis. 2016;1245:1245–59.
102. Vlahos I, Jacobsen MC, Godoy MC, Stefanidis K, Layman RR. Dual-energy CT in pulmonary vascular disease. Br J Radiol. 2022;95:20210699.
103. Si-Mohamed S, Moreau-Triby C, Tylski P, Tatard-Leitman V, Wdowik Q, Boccalini S, et al. Head-to-head comparison of lung perfusion with dual-energy CT and SPECT-CT. Diagn Interv Imaging. 2020;101:299–310.
104. Jeyin N, Desai SR, Padley SPG, Wechalekar K, Gregg S, Sousa T, et al. Dual-energy computed tomographic pulmonary angiography accurately estimates lobar perfusion before lung volume reduction for severe emphysema. J Thorac Imaging. 2023;38:104–12.
105. Ash SY, Rahaghi FN, Come CE, Ross JC, Colon AG, Cardet-Guisasola JC, et al. Pruning of the pulmonary vasculature in asthma. The Severe Asthma Research Program (SARP) cohort. Am J Respir Crit Care Med. 2018;198:39–50.
106. Choi S, Hoffman EA, Wenzel SE, Tawhai MH, Yin Y, Castro M, et al. Registration-based assessment of regional lung function via volumetric CT images of normal subjects vs. severe asthmatics. J Appl Physiol. 2013;115:730–42.
107. Amelon R, Cao K, Ding K, Christensen GE, Reinhardt JM, Raghavan ML. Three-dimensional characterization of regional lung deformation. J Biomech. 2011;44:2489–95.
108. Jahani N, Choi S, Choi J, Haghighi B, Hoffman EA, Comellas AP, et al. A four-dimensional computed tomography comparison of healthy and asthmatic human lungs. J Biomech. 2017;56:102–10.

19 Quantitative Imaging of Interstitial Lung Disease

Raquelle El Alam, Aparna Singh, and Mark M. Hammer

Introduction

While diffuse lung diseases, particularly interstitial lung disease (ILD) and pulmonary fibrosis, have traditionally been assessed qualitatively by radiologists, recently developed quantitative methods for assessment of ILD have drawn great interest [11]. These show promise in several important tasks, from diagnosis (e.g., idiopathic pulmonary fibrosis versus connective tissue disease-associated interstitial lung disease) to prognosis and monitoring of disease response to therapy. Quantitative methods may also serve as radiologist assistants, particularly for parts of the United States or around the world where subspecialty-trained thoracic radiologists are not easily available. However, the field is still in its early stages, and while many promising techniques have been developed, the optimal technique for each particular disease has yet to be established. In this chapter, we will review the various quantitative algorithms that have been applied to diffuse lung diseases and some of the early results that have been demonstrated.

R. El Alam · A. Singh · M. M. Hammer (✉)
Brigham and Women's Hospital, Department of Radiology, Boston, MA, USA
e-mail: mhammer@bwh.harvard.edu

Overview of Different Techniques

Several quantitative techniques have been developed for the characterization and assessment of lung diseases by CT. They can be grouped into three broad categories: lung density analysis, local texture analysis, and deep learning approaches. In this section we will briefly introduce each category before delving in greater detail in the following sections.

Lung Density Analysis

Lung density analysis, the simplest quantification technique, simply relies on the global distribution of X-ray attenuation values in the lungs. Thin-section CT images of the chest are passed to the algorithm, which initially segments (isolates) the lung parenchyma and then obtains a histogram of attenuation values (in Hounsfield units). This histogram may be analyzed in several ways.

Threshold-based measures involve counting pixels that are either above or below a specific attenuation value and combining these counts to determine the absolute or relative volume of certain features. This technique is useful when evaluating diseases characterized by reduced lung density, such as emphysema [46]. It is also useful for assessing diseases that result in increased lung density, such as interstitial lung disease (ILD), for example, in systemic sclerosis (SSc)

R. Gill, P. Rajiah (eds.), *Quantitative Imaging in the Thorax*,
https://doi.org/10.1007/978-3-032-14103-3_19

patients [8]. Note that the simplistic lung density analysis cannot distinguish between different patterns of disease or even different causes for increased or decreased lung density (e.g., air trapping versus emphysema, or inflammation versus fibrosis).

Texture Analysis

Lung texture analysis is a fully automated method that processes images, conducts analyses, and provides output without the need for clinician involvement. Texture analysis begins by dividing the lung into small regions. It then maps a "texture pattern" for each region by using various statistical properties of the gray values in that region, such as run-length matrices, fractal measures, and gray-level co-occurrence matrices. The texture analysis software then provides a quantitative report with color-coded images and data to aid in diagnosing and monitoring interstitial lung disease, enhancing diagnostic accuracy and reader agreement. Image filtration techniques can be utilized to remove noise, enhance edges, and highlight specific features [25]. Integration of multiple textural features allows for the development of a detection and prediction model, enabling objective and reproducible evaluations of lung parenchymal changes in diffuse lung diseases. For instance, texture analysis can be used to classify interstitial lung disease (i.e., UIP versus other pattern), potentially serving as a diagnostic aid [14].

Local texture analysis techniques provide valuable insights for diagnosing and monitoring lung diseases. They capture fine-grained spatial patterns, detecting subtle changes in texture that may not be visible. These techniques are particularly useful in challenging cases like idiopathic pulmonary fibrosis (IPF) prognosis, where radiological and physiological factors vary [28]. One of the best known texture analysis tools for interstitial lung disease is CALIPER. Developed at Mayo Clinic Rochester, CALIPER analyzes spatial patterns and textures within lung images using computational algorithms, providing quantitative metrics that aid in the detection and classification of lung diseases. The histogram signature mapping techniques used in CALIPER are trained based on expert radiologist consensus assessments of pathologically confirmed training sets obtained from the Lung Tissue Research Consortium. CALIPER shows promise in diagnosing and staging interstitial lung diseases and in COPD by differentiating between normal and abnormal lung tissue.

Deep Learning

Machine learning is a field of artificial intelligence where an algorithm can analyze a dataset and extract important features through complex computational techniques [12]. The so-called deep learning is a category of machine learning algorithms that are based on convolutional neural networks. These algorithms are loosely based on how neurons are connected in the brain: there are multiple layers of individual elements. Each element has an activation threshold, below which no "signal" is transmitted to the next layer. The successive layers can detect increasingly complex patterns in the underlying data. All machine learning algorithms, including convolutional neural networks, need to be trained, i.e., provided a large set of data to establish the connections within the network. There are two types of training: supervised and unsupervised. In supervised learning, the algorithm is provided with labeled data and learns to predict labels for new input. On the other hand, unsupervised learning involves working with unlabeled data, where the algorithm must find its own patterns and groupings [11]. Depending upon how they are trained, deep learning algorithms may be used to diagnose the pattern of interstitial lung disease or predict patient prognosis.

Lung Density Analysis

As discussed above, lung density analysis focuses on evaluating the distribution and extent of abnormal lung parenchymal density. Lung densitometry offers several advantages over visual assessment [29]. Firstly, visual assessment is subjective and shows only moderate reproducibility among observers. Additionally, densitometry allows for a complete evaluation of the entire lung parenchyma, whereas visual assessment may be limited by radiologist focus on a subset of CT slices. Lung densitometry also requires less time compared to a formal visual scoring system. Densitometry measurements can provide a quantitative assessment that can be correlated with pathology, pulmonary function tests, dyspnea and quality of life measurements, and other parameters in various lung diseases. Finally, density measurements can provide a quantitative measure that can be tracked over time to show progression of disease or response to therapy. These advantages make lung densitometry a valuable tool for quantitative assessment and monitoring of lung changes.

Lung density analysis employs various thresholds to delineate areas of abnormal density within the lung parenchyma. These thresholds are crucial for distinguishing between healthy and diseased lung tissue, enabling quantitative assessment. Typically, thresholds are expressed in Hounsfield units (HU), which quantify radiodensity. The range of normally attenuated lung is usually defined as −950 HU to −701 HU [33]. Mean lung attenuation (MLA) is a straightforward measurement used for quantifying pulmonary fibrosis and estimating the extent of emphysema [29]. However, MLA is not sensitive for abnormalities, given that lung diseases are often heterogeneous, and other histogram-based indexes are typically employed for emphysema and fibrosis assessment. Emphysema is primarily evaluated using relative areas (RAs) and percentiles (PI), while fibrosis is often assessed using skewness and kurtosis. RA represents the percentage of lung with density values below or above a specific threshold; for example, RA <−950 refers to the fraction of lung tissue below −950 HU, with higher values indicating increased emphysema extent [26]. RA <−950 may also be referred to as low-attenuation area (LAA). Percentile indexes (often abbreviated PercX, where X is a number) indicate the Hounsfield unit (HU) value below which a given percentage of voxels is distributed [27]. In emphysema, various percentile indexes have shown significant correlations with microscopic and macroscopic measurements of emphysema, with Perc1 and Perc15 being commonly used. The 15th percentile point (Perc15) is a threshold in Hounsfield units (HU) below which the 15% of voxels with the lowest density are distributed [29].

While some studies looking at pulmonary fibrosis have used threshold-based high-attenuation area (HAA), most densitometric studies quantifying pulmonary fibrosis have utilized the measures of skewness and kurtosis in the density histogram. Skewness indicates the asymmetry of the histogram, while kurtosis measures the peakedness compared to a normal distribution.

Low-Attenuation Diseases

Several diseases may produce low-attenuation regions in the lung, including emphysema (most common), air trapping, and cystic lung disease. Emphysema is identified through thin section CT scans by alveolar destruction, which results in decreased vascularity and non-circumscribed "empty spaces" in the lung. Decreased lung density, measured using threshold-based methods, indicates the extent of emphysema. Perc15 serves as a valuable indicator for identifying the severity of emphysema as well as measuring the effectiveness of emphysema reduction [38]. Lower Perc15 values, indicating more extensive emphysema, are associated with decreased lung function [31]. Perc15 can also be used to measure emphysema in α-1 antitrypsin deficiency [35].

A greater amount of LAA is associated with reduced pulmonary function, accelerated decline, and increased risk of airway obstruction [31]. These indexes can also be assessed at a lobar or subsegmental level, which can be used for pre-surgical planning prior to lung resection. Greater LAA correlates with increased risk of postoperative pulmonary complications [20]. Interestingly, quantitative CT using lobar volumes and LAA can also be used to predict postoperative pulmonary function [34].

Quantitative assessment of emphysema is also critical to lung volume reduction procedures. Lung volume reduction is a palliative treatment for patients with severe COPD, designed to improve lung function and reduce oxygen dependence. While initially performed surgically, lung volume reduction is increasingly being performed bronchoscopically (abbreviated BLVR) by placing one-way endobronchial valves [23]. Quantitative CT analysis is used to identify which patients are eligible for BLVR and which lobe(s) to target. The emphysema score, calculated as the percentage of voxels with values below a certain threshold (e.g., −910 HU or −950 HU), helps assess the severity of emphysema in each lobe. Lobes with an emphysema score greater than 50% are often targeted for treatment [23]. The heterogeneity score, which represents the difference in emphysema scores between lobes, is often used to identify which patients are eligible: those that benefit most would have worse involvement of one lobe than the other on each side.

Air trapping can also produce low-attenuation areas in the lung and is generally not distinguishable from emphysema by simple density analysis. Differentiating between air trapping and emphysema can be challenging, but texture-based analysis can help distinguish causes of low-attenuation areas [45]. On the other hand, quantitative measure of air trapping can be performed directly if paired inspiratory and expiratory CT images are available. Quantitative CT metrics, including lung volumes and air trapping volumes (volume of lung regions with attenuation values <856 HU (excluding central airways)) have been found to detect air trapping on expiratory imaging, which correlated with pulmonary function testing metrics for bronchiolitis obliterans syndrome (BOS) diagnosis in lung transplant recipients [5]. Quantitative air trapping metrics were also stronger predictors for PFTs than semiquantitative scores such as mosaic attenuation [32].

Lymphangioleiomyomatosis (LAM), one of the most common cystic lung diseases, is an uncommon pulmonary condition marked by the presence of thin-walled cysts within the lung tissue caused by the abnormal growth of cells resembling smooth muscle [11]. In LAM patients, the RA <−950 HU correlated with pulmonary function test (PFT) results. Quantitative algorithms, such as automated segmentation and watershed techniques, have been used to assess cyst volume, distribution, and boundaries [4]. Quantitative CT analysis has helped in understanding LAM treatment and disease mechanisms. For instance, the watershed algorithm analysis of CT data from the Multicenter International Lymphangioleiomyomatosis Efficacy and Safety of Sirolimus Trial (MILES) trial indicated that sirolimus, a medication used in LAM, may stabilize pulmonary function decline by improving expiratory cyst emptying and reducing air trapping [4]. Additionally, quantitative analysis has shown that differences in small pulmonary vessel density can help distinguish LAM from other lung diseases with cystic destruction like COPD [2].

Fibrotic Lung Diseases

Lung density analysis may also be used to quantify pulmonary fibrosis, which leads to areas of increased lung density (Fig. 19.1). Idiopathic pulmonary fibrosis (IPF) is a disease with an unpredictable but poor prognosis [11]. Thin-section CT scans play a crucial role in assessing the severity of the disease and predicting its progression. Quantifying fibrotic changes in IPF is more complicated than density analysis in emphysema, where disease progression is reflected in simply decreased lung density. Various approaches have been developed, including histogram-based analysis focusing on kurtosis, which measures the sharpness of the attenuation distribution peak. Densitometric parameters, including mean lung density, standard deviation of lung density, kurtosis, and skewness, have been shown to predict survival in IPF patients and correlate with PFTs [42]. Kurtosis has been identified as the strongest predictor of mortality in fibrotic interstitial pneumonia [41].

HAA represents a measurable characteristic associated with subclinical interstitial lung disease [14]. HAA (in one study defined as −600 to

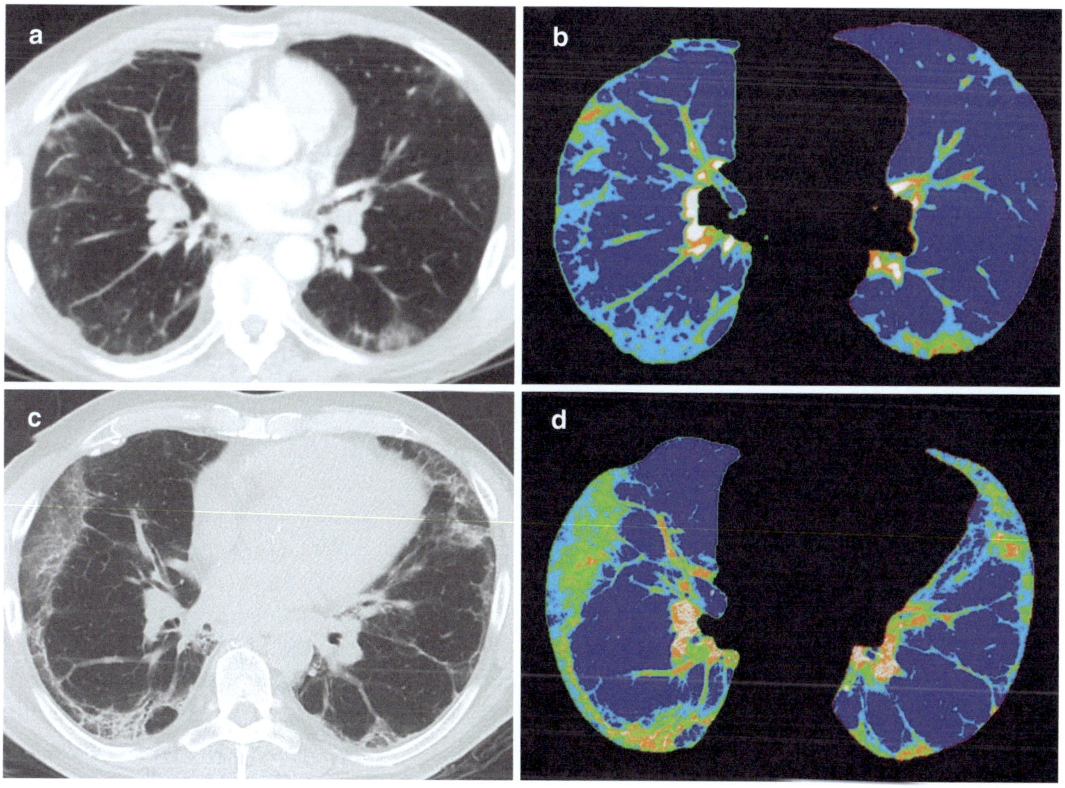

Fig. 19.1 Lung density analysis of a patient with interstitial lung disease from myositis. (**a**) CT and (**b**) corresponding density map performed at the initial timepoint and (**c**) CT and (**d**) corresponding density map performed at 2-year follow-up show progression of fibrosis with increasing high-attenuation areas

−250 Hounsfield units) has been associated with increased levels of lung remodeling biomarkers, a higher risk of interstitial lung abnormalities (ILA) and all-cause mortality, and decreased lung function [49]. The presence of high-attenuation areas is associated with an increased risk of hospitalization and mortality due to interstitial lung disease in the general population [50]. Quantitative assessment of HAA has also been used to quantify ILD associated with systemic sclerosis and monitor its progression [8, 51]. Greater HAA correlates with lower forced vital capacity (FVC) and diffusion capacity of carbon monoxide (DLCO), as well as reduced total lung volume.

However, lung density analysis is likely not sufficiently complex to differentiate between UIP pattern fibrosis/IPF and other forms of ILD. In a study with NSIP and UIP patients without honeycombing on CT, in which lung parenchyma was divided into four density ranges, NSIP patients showed higher fractions of ground-glass and reticular density compared to UIP patients [15]. NSIP also had less skewed density histograms with wider peaks than UIP. These results were, however, not reproducible in differentiating between UIP pattern fibrosis/IPF patients and patients with hypersensitivity pneumonitis or unclassifiable interstitial pneumonia [39, 40].

These simple density-based measures lack the ability to assess morphology or spatial relationships at a local level, making it challenging to distinguish between different diseases that exhibit similar attenuation values but possess distinct morphological or pathological characteristics. Consequently, such measures have limited usefulness in distinguishing discerning reticular fibrosis from ground-glass opacities and consolidations in interstitial lung disease (ILD) [11].

Texture Analysis

Imaging follow-up of patients with ILD is performed by chest CT and helps determine whether patients need treatment and whether the treatment is working. However, it is still performed qualitatively in clinical practice and hence somewhat subjective [46]. Quantitative assessment may objectively assess subtle changes in disease extent or character that can assist in efficacy of antifibrotic therapy or detecting early drug-induced pneumonitis [46].

Texture analysis refers to an automated assessment of global and regional CT pixel values to generate quantitative metrics [46]. Texture analysis methods may use different approaches, but many use statistical analysis of a local region of pixels in the image; using one or multiple statistical parameters, the algorithm then attempts to classify that region into one of several categories (e.g., in the context of interstitial lung disease, emphysema, ground glass, or honeycombing). In a given area of interest, the gray level frequency distribution will be evaluated from the pixel intensity histogram by first-order statistics, including the mean intensity, the percentage of pixels in a range (threshold), the irregularity (entropy), the standard deviation, the asymmetry (skewness), and the peakedness (kurtosis) [25]. Thus, automated assessment is performed for the type of abnormality (emphysema, honeycombing, or ground glass) and its severity (fine or coarse reticulations) using texture analysis, resulting in overall assessment of disease extent [46]. In this section, we will discuss the following texture analysis algorithms: the adaptive multiple feature method (AMFM), the Gaussian histogram normalized correlation (GHNC), data-driven textural analysis (DTA), and computer-aided lung informatics for pathology evaluation and rating (CALIPER).

AMFM uses statistical texture analysis combined with a Bayesian classifier to recognize and quantify the volume of a variety of radiological patterns [46]. It can identify normal lung as well as ground-glass opacity, and it can distinguish emphysema from fibrosis [22, 46] but performed poorly in identifying honeycombing [22, 46]. However, a more advanced form of AMFM with three-dimensional assessment was able to identify honeycombing, with sensitivity of 100% for consolidation and emphysema and 95% for honeycombing, while their specificity was 100% and 97%, respectively [46, 48].

GHNC is another texture analysis algorithm that uses local histograms of CT attenuation to classify regions of the lungs into normal, ground glass, consolidation, emphysema, and fibrosis [17, 18, 46]. This algorithm performed well, with no significant differences in the sensitivity, specificity, and accuracy between GHNC analysis, visual CT score, and radiologist interpretation [18]. In addition, the volumes of normal and fibrotic lung measured by GHNC correlated with diffusing capacity of carbon monoxide (DLCO), showing its ability to correlate with real patient outcomes [17].

The above texture analysis methods rely on prespecified statistical features. This approach can be limited because the features are based on assumptions regarding which imaging characteristics are helpful; they also rely on model parameters that must be tuned by trial and error. On the other hand, DTA is based on an unsupervised feature learning paradigm. Unsupervised learning extracts features directly from the data, potentially avoiding biases and therefore possibly performing better than models developed with prespecified features [16]. DTA was developed using clustering to find common regional imaging features. This technique produces a sort of "dictionary" of normal and abnormal regions that can be applied to analyze a new image. Dictionary entries tend to be simple elements like directed edges or blobs. In a study of 280 patients with IPF, the fibrosis score derived from DTA correlated with pulmonary function tests (PFTs) at baseline, and worsening fibrosis score correlated with declining PFTs [16].

CALIPER is another texture analysis algorithm that uses both morphological analysis and

3D histogram analysis to characterize CT images of the lungs. In comparison to the previously described techniques, CALIPER was built by providing training voxels to radiologists to determine the appropriate morphological label [7, 21]. A retrospective study of 55 patients with IPF showed an association between CALIPER-measured percent ILD and survival at multivariate analysis [28]. One interesting finding from use of CALIPER is that the area of the lung occupied by vessels is prognostically important. Indeed, increased pulmonary vessel volume (an output of CALIPER) is associated with decline in PFTs, independent of pulmonary hypertension [6] [19]. Pulmonary vessel volume was more prognostic than age, gender, and physiology in predicting mortality in patients with ILD [19]. Since the volumetric assessment of the morphology and size of the pulmonary vessels is substantially difficult for a radiologist, machine learning techniques can detect important features imperceptible by humans [46].

In summary, CT texture analysis shows promise in quantifying the extent of ILD, measuring its progression, and predicting patient outcomes. Although these techniques are not yet externally validated for clinical use, they may eventually become complementary to radiologist visual assessment for ILD diagnosis and follow-up.

Deep Learning

In contrast to CT texture analysis, which generally focuses on small regions of the lungs that are then summed to provide an overall assessment, deep learning techniques are more holistic. Deep learning is a type of machine learning using convolutional neural networks consisting of hierarchical layers of interconnected nonlinear processing units; each successive layer receives the output from previous layers. Conceptually, one may imagine that each successive layer provides increasing levels of data abstraction (i.e., higher level features) This is inspired by how neurons are connected in the human brain. When an excitation threshold is achieved, an activating signal is released through the axon toward the synapses with surrounding neurons, and a complex signal can be encoded [9].

There are a number of commonly used (and publicly available) architectures for deep learning algorithms. These networks have multiple uses in the radiology field, including in image classification, object detection, and semantic and instance segmentation [12]. The simplest deep learning task is classification, with the goal simply to predict a category for an image. Detection architectures incorporate the backbone of a trained classification network, not only classifying the objects in an image but also predicting the coordinates that localize the detected objects. Architectures for segmentation tasks must label each pixel in the image [12].

However, in order for a deep learning algorithm to work for a particular task, it must be trained, usually on a large number of examples. The training algorithm simultaneously optimizes the layers responsible for feature extraction, selection, classification, or regression [1]. Deep learning is able to discover intricate patterns in complex data such as images and map them into simple classifications such as a disease entity or patient outcomes like mortality. This approach has several benefits: new disease phenotypes linked to prognosis may be identified, and subtle/complex imaging features that are not obvious visually may be discovered [6]. However, it is prone to several biases including selection/sampling biases caused by bias in training data fed to the model. There are several factors that may predispose to bias and other training errors, including the choice of a single/unrepresentative source of data, improper identification of the dataset, and inadequate exploratory data analysis [36].

For ILD, deep learning algorithms may be used for several tasks: (1) diagnosis of ILD (i.e., UIP versus non-UIP pattern), (2) disease prognosis, and (3) ILD severity. There are several examples of deep learning algorithms applied for ILD diagnosis. The Systematic Objective Fibrotic Imaging Analysis Algorithm (SOFIA) is a deep convolutional neural network trained to provide diagnostic probabilities for usual interstitial pneumonia based on current practice guidelines criteria in the Australian IPF Registry [6]. SOFIA was also able to provide disease prognosis in patients with progressive fibrotic lung disease which was better than guideline-based histologic pattern or expert radiologist evaluation. In fact, in multivariable analysis after adjustment for sex, age, guideline-based radiological diagnosis, and disease severity, only SOFIA UIP probability categories predicted survival [44].

In another deep learning study performed by Walsh et al., a dataset of 1157 high-resolution CT scans with diffuse lung disease was gathered [43]. Scans were classified according to Fleischner Society diagnostic criteria for idiopathic pulmonary fibrosis. On a test set of 75 patients with fibrotic lung disease, the algorithm performed better than 66% of the thoracic radiologists. The algorithm and the thoracic radiologists had similar discrimination between usual interstitial pneumonia and non-usual interstitial pneumonia diagnoses.

Content-based image retrieval (CBIR) is a type of deep learning algorithm that acts as an image search engine that attempts to retrieve images from its database that have similar appearances to the current case [24]. This algorithm does not come up with a list of differential diagnoses; instead, it presents a series of selected cases with similar imaging patterns with a corresponding diagnosis for the reader's reference [47]. In a study by Choe et al., CBIR was successful in improving the diagnostic accuracy of interstitial lung disease from 46.1% to 60.9% in a sample of 288 patients, as well as improving agreement between readers with different levels of experience [13]. Without artificial intelligence support, the performance of a general radiologist for the top differential diagnosis of interstitial lung disease was merely 60%. But with support from artificial intelligence, the performance was about 80% [47].

While the algorithms described above are primarily for diagnosis, several algorithms can also quantify extent of disease. One study developed a deep learning algorithm that evaluated patients with interstitial lung disease related to systemic sclerosis [10]. There were significant correlations between extent of disease obtained from the algorithm and pulmonary function tests results including total lung capacity, forced vital capacity, and diffusion lung capacity for carbon monoxide.

In a study by Aoki et al., evaluation of ILD using a new deep learning-based method was compared to evaluation using patients' clinical outcome and traditional computer-aided diagnosis (CAD) [3]. The authors demonstrated significant correlations between deep learning-based quantification and PFTs as well as patient prognosis.

Another study used not only CT images but also clinical information to develop a convolutional neural network model to diagnose the type of ILD [30]. This model had a sensitivity of 82.4% and specificity of 68.1%, outperforming in sensitivity a senior pulmonologist (55.9%) and a senior thoracic radiologist (41.2%) in diagnosing true UIP cases. In this same study, the authors extended their model using a Transformer to predict 3-year survival analysis based on patient disease progression. The model integrates information from each patient visit and predicts the efficacy of current and future treatment.

Finally, a recent systematic review of 19 studies was published on the use of artificial intelligence (AI) for analysis of ILD, with most studies focusing on ILD classification [37]. Of the 19 studies, 2 demonstrated accuracy almost identical to expert chest radiologists, and accuracies of AI were between 78% and 91% in the other studies. However, there was a high risk of bias in 15 out of the 19 studies. Thus, existing research in the accuracy of deep learning algorithms for ILD is limited by few, low-moderate quality retrospective studies, and to our knowledge, there are no well-designed, prospective studies proving the utility of AI in classifying and quantifying ILD.

In conclusion, evaluation of high-resolution CT with deep learning algorithms may provide a more reproducible way to classify and quantify fibrotic lung disease. In the near future, algorithms may be able to achieve accuracy greater than human experts. The algorithms may also be able to provide prognostication that goes beyond what human observers are able to do. While there is still a lack of standardization of algorithms and, as of yet, few to no prospective confirmatory trials, deep learning algorithms have the potential to revolutionize evaluation of ILD. The biggest potential lies in centers where thoracic imaging expertise is scarce.

Conclusion

While three categories of quantitative techniques have been developed to assess interstitial lung diseases by CT, the greatest amount of data is available for texture analysis, specifically the CALIPER algorithm. Newly developed deep learning methods hold promise to surpass the performance of texture analysis, but only limited data is available so far on their performance. The next few years will likely see an explosion of more deep learning algorithms, as well as more rigorous studies evaluating those algorithms that have been developed. It is likely that quantitative assessments of some sort will become commonplace as adjuncts to radiologist visual assessment for diagnosis and monitoring of patients with interstitial lung disease in the future.

References

1. Alzubaidi L, Zhang J, Humaidi AJ, et al. Review of deep learning: concepts, CNN architectures, challenges, applications, future directions. J Big Data. 2021;8:53. https://doi.org/10.1186/s40537-021-00444-8.
2. Ando K, Tobino K, Kurihara M, et al. Quantitative CT analysis of small pulmonary vessels in lymphangioleiomyomatosis. Eur J Radiol. 2012;81:3925–30. https://doi.org/10.1016/j.ejrad.2012.05.033.
3. Aoki R, Iwasawa T, Saka T, et al. Effects of automatic deep-learning-based lung analysis on quantification of interstitial lung disease: correlation with pulmonary function test results and prognosis. Diagnostics. 2022;12:3038. https://doi.org/10.3390/diagnostics12123038.
4. Argula RG, Kokosi M, Lo P, et al. A novel quantitative computed tomographic analysis suggests how sirolimus stabilizes progressive air trapping in lymphangioleiomyomatosis. Ann Am Thorac Soc. 2016;13:342–9. https://doi.org/10.1513/AnnalsATS.201509-631OC.
5. Barbosa EM, Simpson S, Lee JC, et al. Multivariate modeling using quantitative CT metrics may improve accuracy of diagnosis of bronchiolitis obliterans syndrome after lung transplantation. Comput Biol Med. 2017;89:275–81. https://doi.org/10.1016/j.compbiomed.2017.08.016.
6. Barnes H, Humphries SM, George PM, et al. Machine learning in radiology: the new frontier in interstitial lung diseases. Lancet Digit Health. 2023;5:e41–50. https://doi.org/10.1016/S2589-7500(22)00230-8.
7. Bartholmai BJ, Raghunath S, Karwoski RA, et al. Quantitative computed tomography imaging of interstitial lung diseases. J Thorac Imaging. 2013;28:298–307. https://doi.org/10.1097/RTI.0b013e3182a21969.
8. Carvalho ARS, Guimarães AR, Sztajnbok FR, et al. Automatic quantification of interstitial lung disease from chest computed tomography in systemic sclerosis. Front Med. 2020;7:577739.
9. Chartrand G, Cheng PM, Vorontsov E, et al. Deep learning: a primer for radiologists. Radiographics. 2017;37:2113–31. https://doi.org/10.1148/rg.2017170077.
10. Chassagnon G, Vakalopoulou M, Régent A, et al. Deep learning–based approach for automated assessment of interstitial lung disease in systemic sclerosis on CT images. Radiol Artif Intell. 2020;2:e190006. https://doi.org/10.1148/ryai.2020190006.
11. Chen A, Karwoski RA, Gierada DS, et al. Quantitative CT analysis of diffuse lung disease. Radiographics. 2020;40:28–43. https://doi.org/10.1148/rg.2020190099.
12. Cheng PM, Montagnon E, Yamashita R, et al. Deep learning: an update for radiologists. Radiographics. 2021;41:1427–45. https://doi.org/10.1148/rg.2021200210.
13. Choe J, Hwang HJ, Seo JB, et al. Content-based image retrieval by using deep learning for interstitial lung disease diagnosis with chest CT. Radiology. 2022;302:187–97. https://doi.org/10.1148/radiol.2021204164.
14. Depeursinge A, Chin AS, Leung AN, et al. Automated classification of usual interstitial pneumonia using regional volumetric texture analysis in high-resolution CT. Investig Radiol. 2015;50:261–7. https://doi.org/10.1097/RLI.0000000000000127.
15. Do K-H, Lee JS, Colby TV, et al. Nonspecific interstitial pneumonia versus usual interstitial pneumonia: differences in the density histogram of high-resolution CT. J Comput Assist Tomogr. 2005;29:544–8. https://doi.org/10.1097/01.rct.0000164255.43859.96.
16. Humphries SM, Yagihashi K, Huckleberry J, et al. Idiopathic pulmonary fibrosis: data-driven textural analysis of extent of fibrosis at baseline and 15-month follow-up. Radiology. 2017;285:270–8. https://doi.org/10.1148/radiol.2017161177.
17. Iwasawa T, Asakura A, Sakai F, et al. Assessment of prognosis of patients with idiopathic pulmonary fibrosis by computer-aided analysis of CT images. J Thorac Imaging. 2009;24:216–22. https://doi.org/10.1097/RTI.0b013e3181a6527d.
18. Iwasawa T, Ogura T, Sakai F, et al. CT analysis of the effect of pirfenidone in patients with idiopathic pul-

monary fibrosis. Eur J Radiol. 2014;83:32–8. https://doi.org/10.1016/j.ejrad.2012.02.014.
19. Jacob J, Bartholmai BJ, Rajagopalan S, et al. Evaluation of computer-based computer tomography stratification against outcome models in connective tissue disease-related interstitial lung disease: a patient outcome study. BMC Med. 2016;14:190. https://doi.org/10.1186/s12916-016-0739-7.
20. Kaplan T, Atac GK, Gunal N, et al. Quantitative computerized tomography assessment of lung density as a predictor of postoperative pulmonary morbidity in patients with lung cancer. J Thorac Dis. 2015;7:1391–7. https://doi.org/10.3978/j.issn.2072-1439.2015.07.26.
21. Karwoski RA, Bartholmai B, Zavaletta VA, et al. Processing of CT images for analysis of diffuse lung disease in the lung tissue research consortium. Medical Imaging 2008: Physiology, Function, and Structure from Medical Images In: Hu XP, Clough AV, editors. San Diego; Society of Photo-Optical Instrumentation Engineers (SPIE), 2008. p. 691614.
22. Kim EJ, Elicker BM, Maldonado F, et al. Usual interstitial pneumonia in rheumatoid arthritis-associated interstitial lung disease. Eur Respir J. 2010;35:1322–8. https://doi.org/10.1183/09031936.00092309.
23. Klooster K, ten Hacken NHT, Hartman JE, et al. Endobronchial valves for emphysema without interlobar collateral ventilation. N Engl J Med. 2015;373:2325–35. https://doi.org/10.1056/NEJMoa1507807.
24. Latif A, Rasheed A, Sajid U, et al. Content-based image retrieval and feature extraction: a comprehensive review. Math Probl Eng. 2019;2019:1–21. https://doi.org/10.1155/2019/9658350.
25. Lubner MG, Smith AD, Sandrasegaran K, et al. CT texture analysis: definitions, applications, biologic correlates, and challenges. Radiographics. 2017;37:1483–503. https://doi.org/10.1148/rg.2017170056.
26. Madani A, Zanen J, de Maertelaer V, Gevenois PA. Pulmonary emphysema: objective quantification at multi-detector row CT—comparison with macroscopic and microscopic morphometry. Radiology. 2006;238:1036–43. https://doi.org/10.1148/radiol.2382042196.
27. Madani A, De Maertelaer V, Zanen J, Gevenois PA. Pulmonary emphysema: radiation dose and section thickness at multidetector CT quantification—comparison with macroscopic and microscopic morphometry. Radiology. 2007;243:250–7. https://doi.org/10.1148/radiol.2431060194.
28. Maldonado F, Moua T, Rajagopalan S, et al. Automated quantification of radiological patterns predicts survival in idiopathic pulmonary fibrosis. Eur Respir J. 2014;43:204–12. https://doi.org/10.1183/09031936.00071812.
29. Mascalchi M, Camiciottoli G, Diciotti S. Lung densitometry: why, how and when. J Thorac Dis. 2017;9:3319–45. https://doi.org/10.21037/jtd.2017.08.17.
30. Mei X, Liu Z, Singh A, et al. Interstitial lung disease diagnosis and prognosis using an AI system integrating longitudinal data. Nat Commun. 2023;14:2272. https://doi.org/10.1038/s41467-023-37720-5.
31. Mohamed Hoesein FAA, De Hoop B, Zanen P, et al. CT-quantified emphysema in male heavy smokers: association with lung function decline. Thorax. 2011;66:782–7. https://doi.org/10.1136/thx.2010.145995.
32. Mortani Barbosa EJ, Shou H, Simpsom S, et al. Quantitative computed tomography metrics from the transplanted lung can predict forced expiratory volume in the first second after lung transplantation. J Thorac Imaging. 2018;33:112–23. https://doi.org/10.1097/RTI.0000000000000307.
33. Ohkubo H, Kanemitsu Y, Uemura T, et al. Normal lung quantification in usual interstitial pneumonia pattern: the impact of threshold-based volumetric CT analysis for the staging of idiopathic pulmonary fibrosis. PLoS One. 2016;11:e0152505. https://doi.org/10.1371/journal.pone.0152505.
34. Ohno Y, Koyama H, Nogami M, et al. State-of-the-art radiological techniques improve the assessment of postoperative lung function in patients with non-small cell lung cancer. Eur J Radiol. 2011;77:97–104. https://doi.org/10.1016/j.ejrad.2009.07.024.
35. Parr DG, Stoel BC, Stolk J, Stockley RA. Validation of computed tomographic lung densitometry for monitoring emphysema in α1-antitrypsin deficiency. Thorax. 2006;61:485–90. https://doi.org/10.1136/thx.2005.054890.
36. Rouzrokh P, Khosravi B, Faghani S, et al. Mitigating bias in radiology machine learning: 1. Data handling. Radiol Artif Intell. 2022;4:e210290. https://doi.org/10.1148/ryai.210290.
37. Soffer S, Morgenthau S. A, Shimon O, et al. Artificial intelligence for interstitial lung disease analysis on chest computed tomography: a systematic review. 2021. https://doi.org/10.1016/j.acra.2021.05.014.
38. Stolk J, Versteegh MIM, Montenij LJ, et al. Densitometry for assessment of effect of lung volume reduction surgery for emphysema. Eur Respir J. 2007;29:1138–43. https://doi.org/10.1183/09031936.00056206.
39. Sverzellati N, Zompatori M, De Luca G, et al. Evaluation of quantitative CT indexes in idiopathic interstitial pneumonitis using a low-dose technique. Eur J Radiol. 2005;56:370–5. https://doi.org/10.1016/j.ejrad.2005.05.012.
40. Sverzellati N, Calabrò E, Chetta A, et al. Visual score and quantitative CT indices in pulmonary fibrosis: relationship with physiologic impairment. Radiol Med (Torino). 2007;112:1160–72. https://doi.org/10.1007/s11547-007-0213-x.
41. Tanizawa K, Handa T, Nagai S, et al. Clinical impact of high-attenuation and cystic areas on computed tomography in fibrotic idiopathic interstitial pneumonias. BMC Pulm Med. 2015;15:74. https://doi.org/10.1186/s12890-015-0069-0.

42. Torrisi SE, Palmucci S, Stefano A, et al. Assessment of survival in patients with idiopathic pulmonary fibrosis using quantitative HRCT indexes. Multidiscip Respir Med. 2018;13:43. https://doi.org/10.1186/s40248-018-0155-2.
43. Walsh SLF, Calandriello L, Silva M, Sverzellati N. Deep learning for classifying fibrotic lung disease on high-resolution computed tomography: a case-cohort study. Lancet Respir Med. 2018;6:837–45. https://doi.org/10.1016/S2213-2600(18)30286-8.
44. Walsh SLF, Mackintosh JA, Calandriello L, et al. Deep learning–based outcome prediction in progressive fibrotic lung disease using high-resolution computed tomography. Am J Respir Crit Care Med. 2022;206:883–91. https://doi.org/10.1164/rccm.202112-2684OC.
45. Wang Z, Gu S, Leader JK, et al. Optimal threshold in CT quantification of emphysema. Eur Radiol. 2013;23:975–84. https://doi.org/10.1007/s00330-012-2683-z.
46. Weatherley ND, Eaden JA, Stewart NJ, et al. Experimental and quantitative imaging techniques in interstitial lung disease. Thorax. 2019;74:611–9. https://doi.org/10.1136/thoraxjnl-2018-211779.
47. Wielpütz MO. Artificial intelligence for interstitial lung disease: proudly supporting radiologists since 2021. Radiology. 2022;302:198–9. https://doi.org/10.1148/radiol.2021210731.
48. Xu Y, van Beek EJR, Hwanjo Y, et al. Computer-aided classification of interstitial lung diseases via MDCT: 3D adaptive multiple feature method (3D AMFM). Acad Radiol. 2006;13:969–78. https://doi.org/10.1016/j.acra.2006.04.017.
49. Bina Choi Steven M, Kawut Ganesh, Raghu Eric, Hoffman Russell, Tracy Purnema, Madahar Elana J, Bernstein R. Graham, Barr David J, Lederer Anna, Podolanczuk (2020). Regional distribution of high-attenuation areas on chest computed tomography in the Multi-Ethnic Study of Atherosclerosis ERJ Open Research 6(1) 00115-2019-10.1183/23120541.00115-2019
50. Kenneth K, Lau Dee, Nandurkar (2020) High attenuation areas in pulmonary computed tomography: Their meaning and use in interstitial lung disease Respirology 25(8):787–789 https://doi.org/10.1111/resp.v25.8 10.1111/resp.13820
51. Faisal Jamal Kumar, Shashi Nuno, Vaz Tracy, Doyle Paul, Dellaripa Mark, Hammer (2024) Quantitative Chest Computed Tomography for Progression of Interstitial Lung Disease in Antisynthetase Patients Journal of Thoracic Imaging 39(5):281–284. https://doi.org/10.1097/RTI.0000000000000770

20 Quantitative Assessment of Lung Nodule: Deep Learning and Radiomics

Eui Jin Hwang and Jin Mo Goo

Introduction

Evaluation of lung nodules is a vital component of chest imaging since lung nodules are frequently encountered and may represent lung cancer. Traditionally, lung nodule evaluation on chest radiography or chest computed tomography (CT) has been based on visual evaluation by human readers such as radiologists. Visual evaluation of lung nodules on chest radiography and CT has substantially contributed to the diagnosis of lung cancer, outcome prediction of patients with lung cancer, monitoring the response to the treatment for lung cancer, and decision-making for the management of patients with lung nodules or lung cancer. However, visual evaluation of human readers is susceptible to errors and inter-reader variability. Furthermore, the incidence of lung nodules is increasing [1, 2], and the corresponding growth of the demand for the imaging evaluation of lung nodules may significantly burden radiologists and clinicians. In this regard, computerized evaluation of lung nodules has been investigated for decades to reduce the burden, error, and variability of visual interpretation. Recently, deep learning-based artificial intelligence (AI) has been making a breakthrough in the computerized imaging evaluation of lung nodules. Deep learning algorithms have demonstrated expert-level or beyond performance in detecting and characterizing lung nodules and have begun to be used in actual clinical practice [3–5].

Meanwhile, the extraction of relevant information for patients' diagnosis and prognosis from images that are difficult to obtain with visual assessment is another important research task in the era of precision medicine [6]. This is particularly true in the imaging evaluation of lung nodules and lung cancer, since it would be an essential component of personalized management and treatment of patients. Radiomics, a method that extracts a large number of imaging features by high-throughput image analysis to predict the diagnosis or outcome of patients, has achieved considerable achievements since the 2010s [6, 7]. More recently, deep learning approaches also exhibited astonishing potential in predicting diagnosis or outcome from medical images [8, 9].

In this chapter, we will introduce the potential roles of deep learning and radiomics in imaging evaluation of lung nodule and lung cancer. We will also discuss the current status of clinical utilization of deep learning and radiomics for lung nodule evaluation and practical considerations and challenges for the clinical implementation (Fig. 20.1).

E. J. Hwang · J. M. Goo (✉)
Department of Radiology, Seoul National University Hospital, Seoul National University College of Medicine, Seoul, South Korea
e-mail: jmgoo@snu.ac.kr

R. Gill, P. Rajiah (eds.), *Quantitative Imaging in the Thorax*,
https://doi.org/10.1007/978-3-032-14103-3_20

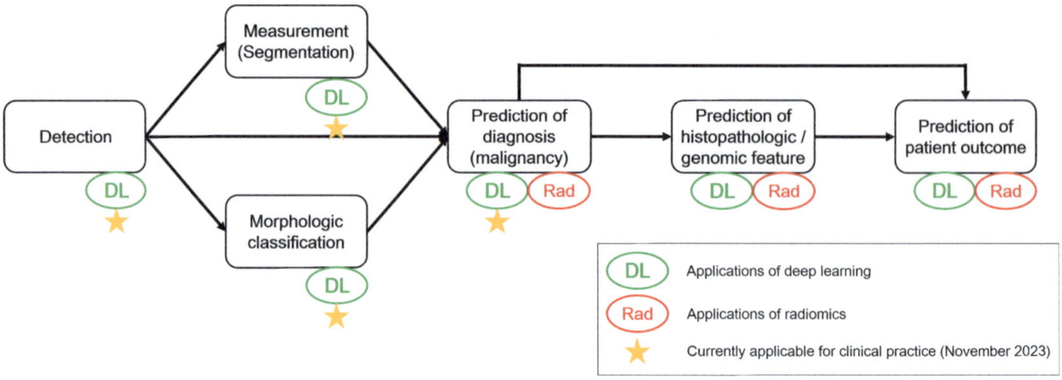

Fig. 20.1 Schematic flow for image evaluation of lung nodules and applications of deep learning and radiomics

Applications of Deep Learning and Radiomics

Lung Nodule Detection in Chest Radiography

Chest radiography is the most commonly conducted radiologic examination. It is used to evaluate various diseases of the lungs and heart. Among them, detecting lung nodule is one of the most important and difficult tasks in the interpretation of chest radiographs; retrospectively visible lung cancer nodules are sometimes overlooked by radiologists [10, 11]. Therefore, computer-aided detection (CAD) of lung nodules on chest radiographs has been investigated since the 1960s [12].

Since the early phase of the rise of deep learning, many researchers have developed and evaluated deep learning algorithms for the automated detection of lung nodules on chest radiographs [13–15]. Deep learning algorithms exhibited radiologist-level performance and enhanced radiologists' sensitivity in multiple early studies evaluating their performance and efficacy [13–15]. Retrospective diagnostic cohort studies also reported that deep learning algorithms could identify lung cancers in chest radiographs of asymptomatic health checkup participants [16] and high-risk lung cancer screening participants [17] with radiologist-level sensitivity and specificity. Studies also reported that deep learning-based CAD tool can detect lung cancer nodules that were initially overlooked by radiologists' interpretation [18, 19]. A study by Hwang et al. [20] reported that the use of a deep learning-based CAD tool for lung nodules led to improved detection yield of new metastatic nodules in chest radiographs of oncologic patients. In a parallel randomized controlled trial by Nam et al. [21], the interpretation of chest radiographs using a deep learning-based CAD tool increased the detection of clinically relevant lung nodules. Accumulating evidence suggests that deep learning-based CAD tools for lung nodules on chest radiographs can improve the sensitivity of lung nodule detection and prevent overlooking lung nodules. Further research would be required to confirm whether the deep learning-based CAD tool can help early diagnosis of lung cancers.

Lung Nodule Detection in Chest CT

Chest CT is the standard modality for imaging evaluation of lung nodules, and detection of lung nodule is the initial step for the full evaluation and characterization of lung nodules. Although the sensitivity of chest CT for lung nodule detection is much higher than that of chest radiography, scrutinizing chest CTs to identify small lung nodules is a time-consuming task for radiologists. In addition to the increasing number of CT examinations and incidence of lung nodules, the implementation of lung cancer screening using low-dose chest CT in high-risk populations may increase the burden of lung nodule detection for radiologists. In this regard, a CAD tool for the detection of lung nodules on chest CT has the potential to improve the quality and efficiency of chest CT interpretation.

Automated detection of lung nodules using a deep learning technique has been an active target of research and development. In 2016, there was a competition called LUNA 16 challenge [22], comparing deep learning algorithms for the automated detection of 1186 nodules in 888 chest CTs. The first-place deep learning algorithm exhibited 97% sensitivity at one false-positive per examination. A retrospective observer study reported that the interpretation of screening low-dose chest CTs using a CAD tool led to decreased interpretation time and improved inter-reader agreement. Another study compared deep learning-based CAD and double reading by radiologists for the detection of lung nodules in screening CTs [23]. As a result, the CAD-assisted reading exhibited higher sensitivity for lung nodule detection than double reading (86.2% vs. 79.2%); however, it also resulted in more false-positive results (1.53 vs. 0.13 per examination). It has not yet been sufficiently investigated whether the interpretation of chest CTs using a deep learning-based CAD tool can improve the radiologists' performance of lung nodule detection or the diagnostic accuracy for lung cancer. Compared to chest radiography, establishing solid evidence for the improved sensitivity of lung nodule or lung cancer detection using a deep learning-based CAD tool would be practically difficult since the margin for the sensitivity improvement would be relatively narrow.

Segmentation and Size Measurement of Lung Nodules

Measuring the size of lung nodule is the cornerstone for the evaluation of the malignancy risk of nodules since larger nodule has a higher risk for lung cancer compared to smaller nodules. Therefore, the size of the lung nodule is a key component in all of the available guidelines for the management of lung nodules. Conventional manual measurement of lung nodule is prone to intra- and inter-reader variability and may lead to unnecessary variability in the risk estimation and management of lung nodules.

Reliable measurement of a lung nodule is also important for the determination of its growth. Considering the variability of manual measurement, current guidelines suggest that an increased average nodule diameter greater than 1.5 or 2 mm is a threshold for the determination of nodule growth [24, 25]. Volumetric measurement of lung nodules would be a more sensitive method for the detection of growth compared to the diametric measurement [26]. For example, even if the volume of a nodule doubles, the diametric growth of the nodule would be only 26%. In this background, volumetric measurement of lung nodules has been implemented in multiple lung cancer screening trials [27–29] and nodule management guidelines [30, 31]. Segmentation of a lung nodule is an initial step for volumetric measurement, while manual segmentation in daily practice is practically impossible.

Lung nodule segmentation based on a deep learning technique exhibited better accuracy than conventional semiautomated methods [32]. Another study reported that automated lung nodule segmentation was successful for most nodules detected on screening CTs, while manual modification of segmentation was required for 28% of nodules [33]. Automated measurement of lung nodules may help reduce not only the variability in lung nodule measurement but also the burden of CT interpretation by radiologists.

Subsolid lung nodules that contain an area of ground-glass opacity in CT may represent a spectrum of pulmonary adenocarcinoma, including premalignant lesions (atypical adenomatous hyperplasia), preinvasive malignancy (adenocarcinoma in situ), or invasive adenocarcinoma. Measurement and determination of growth are essential components for the evaluation and management of subsolid nodules, which are prone to intra- or inter-reader variability due to relatively low contrast with the normal lung [34]. In the study by Kim et al. [35], semiautomated measurement of subsolid nodules led to improved and reproducible diagnosis of invasive adenocarcinoma. In another study by Ahn et al. [36], automated measurement of solid component of subsolid nodules on CT using a deep learning algorithm exhibited excellent agreement with manual measurement (intraclass correlation coefficient, 0.82–0.89) and good agreement with the size of invasive component in pathologic examination (intraclass correlation coefficient, 0.67).

Classification of Lung Nodules

Classification of lung nodules according to their consistency and features would be another important component for the nodule evaluation. It is well known that the risk of lung cancer would be different across the consistency of lung nodules. Nodules showing ground-glass opacity components on CT have a higher probability of malignancy. In this regard, consistency of lung nodules is the key component for lung nodule management guidelines, along with nodule size. In addition, nodules with specific calcifications and polygonal or lentiform shape nodule adjacent to the pleura (e.g., perifissural and juxtapleural nodules) may indicate benign nature. A study by Ciompi et al. [37] reported that a deep-learning algorithm can classify screening-detected lung nodules into solid, part-solid, non-solid, calcified, perifissural, and spiculated nodules. The agreement of nodule classification between the algorithm and radiologists was similar to that between radiologists. Automated types of lung nodules based on their radiologic characteristics can help decision-making for lung nodule management based on existing guidelines.

Prediction of Lung Cancer Diagnosis

Differentiating patients with and without lung cancer is the ultimate goal of imaging evaluation of lung nodules. Several early deep-learning studies focused on the classification of examinations with and without lung cancer. In 2017, a competition called Data Science Bowl 2017 was held to evaluate deep learning algorithms for the classification of screening low-dose chest CTs with and without lung cancers [38]. The task for algorithms in the competition was predicting lung cancer diagnosis within 1 year in 500 low-dose CTs screening. The top 10 deep learning algorithms exhibited an area under the receiver operating characteristic curves (AUC) between 0.849 and 0.883 [38]. Two of the top three algorithms (AUCs, 0.900 and 0.902) exhibited similar classification accuracy with radiologists (AUC, 0.917). Researchers at Google reported a deep learning algorithm that can evaluate a single low-dose chest CT exam or two CT exams, including prior exams, to predict lung cancer diagnosis within 1 or 2 years. The algorithm exhibited higher accuracy compared to CT interpretation by radiologists using the lung CT screening reporting and data system [39]. Huang et al. [40] developed a deep learning model to predict 3-year lung cancer risk using two low-dose CT exams. The deep learning model demonstrated 1-, 2-, and 3-year time-dependent AUCs of 0.968, 0.946, and 0.899, respectively. Despite their excellent performances, those deep learning models did not appropriately provide localization or explanation for the predicted risk of lung cancer, limiting their clinical applicability.

There has also been an effort to predict lung cancer risk from chest radiographs. Lu et al. [41] reported a deep learning-based prediction model that can predict 12-year lung cancer risk from chest radiographs. The model exhibited higher predictive accuracy compared to the existing eligibility criteria for lung cancer screening. The result suggests that a deep learning model can help optimize candidate selection for lung cancer screening. When the deep learning model developed in the USA was applied to chest radiographs of asymptomatic current or former smokers in South Korea, the model could successfully stratify lung cancer risks and exhibited potential to reduce the number of lung cancer screening participants while maintaining inclusion of lung cancer patients [42].

Differentiation of Benign from Malignant Lung Nodules

Prediction of malignancy risk for individual lung nodules would be a more practical approach compared to the examination-level classification.

Although there are multiple established clinical (e.g., age, sex, cigarette smoking, family history of lung cancer) and radiological factors (e.g., nodule size, consistency, location, presence of emphysema), it is difficult for radiologists to assess the risk of malignancy objectively and reproducibly for individual lung nodules detected on CTs. Risk prediction models were developed using data from incidentally detected pulmonary nodules [43] or lung cancer screening participants [44]. With multiple input clinical and radiological variables, these prediction models can provide objective probability of malignancy risk for a nodule. The Brock University model (also known as McWilliams model or PanCan model) [44] was incorporated in the British Thoracic Society nodule management guideline [30] and used in the International Lung Screening Trial for the management of screening participants [45]. However, those prediction models cannot fully utilize the information in CT images, since only a limited number of specific radiological variables can be integrated into the prediction models. Researchers have tried to classify benign versus malignant lung nodules on CT images, using deep learning or radiomics.

Several studies have reported that deep learning-based models can accurately differentiate benign and malignant lung nodules on CTs. In a study by Massion et al. [46], a deep learning model can predict the malignancy risk of lung nodules with higher performance than existing prediction models (Brock University model and Mayo Clinic model). In another study by Kim et al. [47], the performances of radiologists and pulmonologists for the prediction of malignant nodule were improved after the assessment of the prediction by deep learning model. The inter-reader agreement was also improved with the use of models. Radiomic models also exhibited potential to classify benign and malignant lung nodules [48–51]. For example, Beig et al. [49] reported that radiomic models using both intranodular and perinodular features exhibited excellent performance for the differentiation of adenocarcinoma from granulomas (AUC, 0.80), showing higher performance than radiologists' interpretation (AUC, 0.60–0.61) and a radiomic model using only intranodular features (AUC, 0.75).

Prediction of Histopathologic and Genomic Features

Histopathologic morphology and microscopic invasion of adjacent structures by lung cancer are not only important prognostic factors but also essential information for therapeutic decision making. Since histopathologic evaluation of tissue specimen obtained by minimally invasive sampling before surgery has limitations in full characterization of lung cancer, imaging features can be an important surrogate for the histopathologic features. However, conventional visual assessment has limited accuracy and inter-reader agreement for the prediction of histopathologic features [52–55]. Many radiomic and deep learning studies investigated the prediction of various histopathologic features, such as invasiveness of adenocarcinomas appearing as subsolid nodules [56–58], visceral pleural invasion of lung cancer [59–61], and lymph node metastasis of lung cancer [62–64].

Multiple established genetic alterations play a crucial role in the development and progression of lung cancer (e.g., epidermal growth factor receptor [*EGFR*] mutation, Kirsten rat sarcoma viral oncogene homolog [*KRAS*] mutation, anaplastic lymphoma kinase [*ALK*] rearrangement) [65]. Identification of these "oncogenic driver mutations" is a key component for therapeutic decision-making, since targeted therapy for specific driver mutations can improve patients' prognosis. Since obtaining adequate cancer tissue for the molecular diagnosis of lung cancer is not always possible, the prediction of the genetic status of cancer from images, called radio-genomics, has been investigated by many researchers. There are numerous studies regarding radiomic models for the prediction of specific genetic alterations in lung cancer from CT images. Deep learning technique has also been applied to the prediction of genetic alterations, including EGFR mutation [66–68], ALK rearrangement [66, 69], and KRAS [70]. For example, a study by Wang et al. [67] reported that a deep learning-based model can predict *EGFR* mutation status of lung cancer using CT images (AUC, 0.81), with better predictive performance than a radiomic model (AUC, 0.64).

Immune checkpoint inhibitors (ICIs) have opened a new horizon in the treatment of lung cancer. Based on results of randomized controlled trials reporting survival benefits of using ICIs not only as first- [71, 72] or second-line treatment for advanced lung cancers [73, 74] but also as perioperative treatment for resectable lung cancers [75, 76], it is now widely used in the treatment of patients with lung cancers. The degree of programmed death ligand-1 (PD-L1) expression of lung cancer is a key component for the decision to treat patient with ICIs, since higher degree of expression of PD-L1 in cancer cells is associated with higher response rate to ICIs. Several proof-of-concept studies have suggested that radiomic and deep learning models can predict PD-L1 expression from CT images in patients with lung cancers [67, 77–79]. Tumor mutation burden (TMB) is another important biomarker for the prediction of response to ICIs. A study by He et al. [80] reported that deep learning-based model can predict TMB with higher accuracy (AUC, 0.81) than radiomic model (0.74) and can stratify patients' overall survival.

Prediction of Patient Outcome

Several imaging features of lung cancer, including size, consistency, location, and margin characteristics, are established as important predictors of patient outcome. Those features are incorporated in the staging system and management guidelines and utilized to guide clinical decision-making. Deep learning or radiomics may help extract valuable quantitative prognostic biomarkers from CT images of lung cancer, which cannot be obtained by conventional visual evaluation. Reproducible assessment of conventional radiologic features, such as nodule size [36, 81] and prediction of relevant histopathologic or molecular features [61, 82], as well as direct prediction of prognosis from images, may have prognostic implications.

Many studies reported that deep learning and radiomic models can predict the prognosis of lung cancer after surgery [83–86], radiotherapy [87, 88], and systemic treatment [89–91]. A study by Nam et al. [92] reported that the results of a deep learning model to predict survival of lung adenocarcinoma patients from CT images were associated with histopathologic risk factors such as microscopic invasion and aggressive histopathologic subtype. The result suggests that deep learning can extract surrogate information for the histopathologic risk factors from CT images. A landmark study in the field of radiomics by Aerts et al. [93] reported that the radiomic model can stratify the prognosis of lung cancer patients, and the radiomic features had association with genomic profile of lung cancers.

Prediction of response to specific treatment, including cytotoxic chemotherapy [94], targeted agents [95–97], and ICI [80, 82], would be another promising application of deep learning and radiomics, since molecular biomarkers obtained by minimally invasive tissue sampling cannot represent the entire cancer biology in a patient because of intra-tumoral and inter-tumoral heterogeneities.

Linkage Between Deep Learning and Radiomics

Although deep learning and radiomics need different process of development for the prediction of clinically relevant feature or outcomes, they may have a synergetic effect in several aspects. First, deep learning algorithm can provide reproducible segmentation of lung nodules for the radiomic analysis. Segmentation of lung nodules is an initial key step for radiomics, since many radiomic features can be extracted from the segmented nodules. A study by Parmar et al. [98] reported that radiomic features derived using semiautomated lung nodule segmentation exhibited better reproducibility.

Second, deep learning can help reduce the heterogeneity of image characteristics before radiomic analysis. Heterogeneities in scanning and reconstruction parameters, such as scanner, reconstruction kernel, and slice thickness, are important hurdles for the generalizability of radiomics [99–101]. In addition to classification of images and detection of specific findings in images, deep learning technology can be used to generate new images with different styles and preserved image content. A study by Choe et al. [102] reported that a deep learning algorithm can generate CT images simulating images from different reconstruction kernels. The variability of radiomic features was significantly reduced by using the kernel conversion technique. Another study by Park et al. [103] used a deep learning model to generate CT images with 1-mm thickness from 3- or 5-mm thickness CT images. Utilization of generated images significantly reduced the variability of radiomic features.

Third, radiomic features and deep learning techniques can be combined for the prediction of relevant outcomes. Several studies reported that the inclusion of radiomic features in the deep learning model can enhance the predictive performance of the model [104–106].

Utilization in Clinical Practice and Challenges

Based on their excellent performance in early studies, deep learning-based algorithms for lung nodule detection in chest radiographs (Fig. 20.2) and lung nodule detection and characterization in CTs (Fig. 20.3) have begun to be used in actual clinical practice [4, 107]. All currently used deep learning-based software medical devices are approved as an assistant tool for physicians' interpretation and decision making, rather than a stand-alone interpretation tool. Efficacy of deep learning software for lung nodule detection in chest radiographs (i.e., improved lung nodule detection accuracy by radiologists using deep learning software) in an actual practice situation has been demonstrated in before-and-after study [20] and randomized clinical trial [21]. However, efficacy evaluation of deep learning tools for lung nodule detection and classification in CTs was not demonstrated in the situation of usual clinical practice. Furthermore, clinical impact of using deep learning beyond the image interpretation has not been reported yet. Further research may be needed to investigate the clinical impact and value of deep learning-based tools for lung nodule detection and classification.

Recently, a deep learning-based clinical decision support system that can predict risk of lung cancer for indeterminate pulmonary nodules received US Food and Drug Administration clearance. However, applications of deep learning beyond the detection and classification of lung nodules, especially those for prediction of histopathologic diagnosis or future outcomes, have been rarely utilized in daily practice. The most important hurdle for the clinical utilization of these deep learning-based prediction tools might be the limited explainability. Limited logical explanation for the background of its output is a well-known limitation of deep learning-based models [108]. The most widely used method to solve this issue is saliency map [109]. The saliency map can display which area of image has affected the output of deep learning algorithm. In the case of algorithm for lung nodule detection, a saliency map can highlight the location of the nodule and persuade the readers. However, in cases of algorithms for less-intuitive tasks, such as predicting future outcomes, it is difficult to provide the user with a logical explanation for deep learning model's output with the saliency map alone. Continuous technological investigation to solve this explainability issue would be required to promote clinical utilization of deep learning for tasks other than lung nodule detection/classification.

Other important obstacles to the clinical implementation of deep learning-based AI include (a) difficulty in seamless integration with legacy practice systems, such as picture archiving and communication system and electronic health record system; (b) limited reimbursement for using deep learning-based AI in practice; (c) concerns regarding the legal liability associated with the use of deep learning-based AI; and (d) practical limited access to deep learning tools in resource-limited areas. To overcome these hurdles, not only technical and clinical research for the development and evaluation of deep learn-

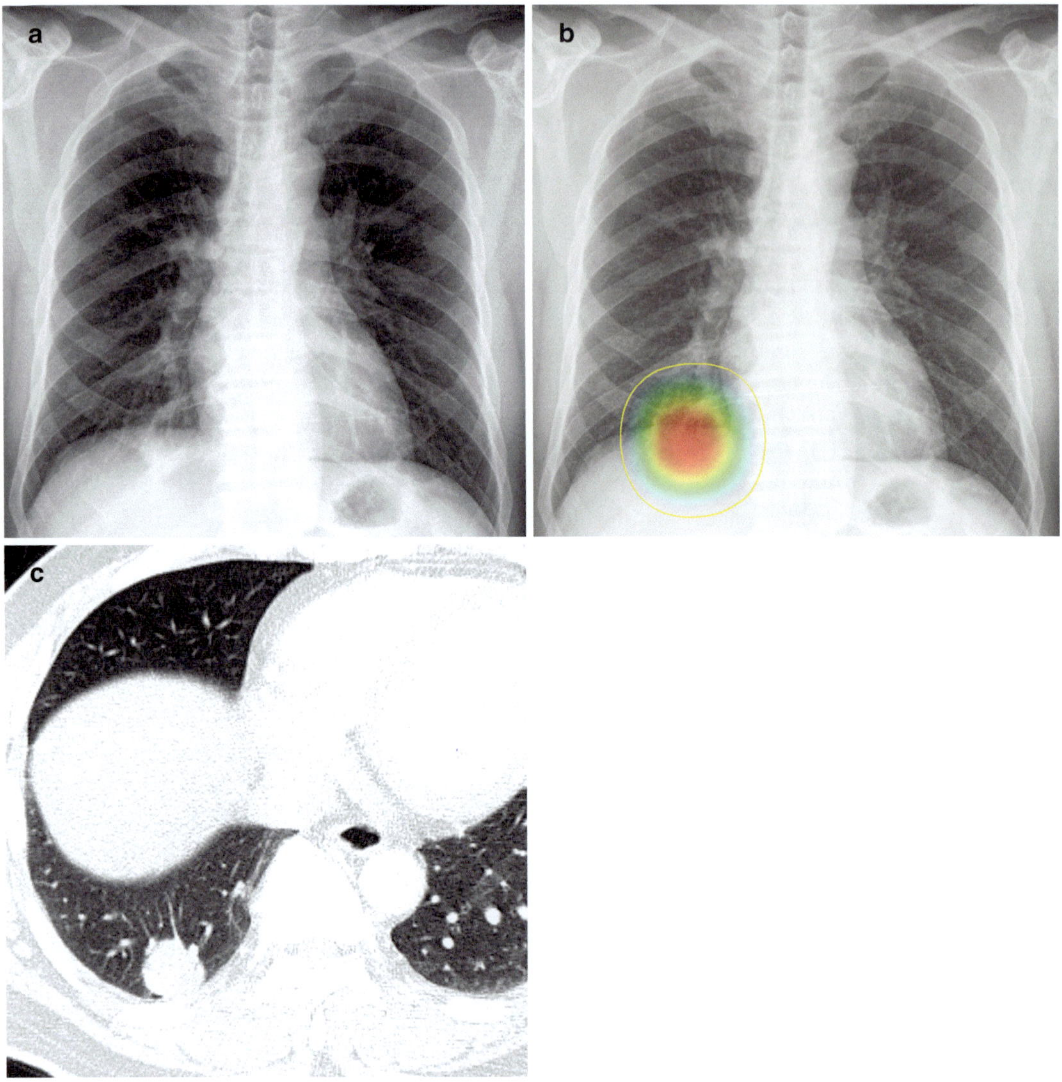

Fig. 20.2 Automated detection of lung nodules in chest radiographs using a commercially available deep learning software. (**a**) Chest radiography shows nodular opacity at the right basal lung near the diaphragm. (**b**) A commercialized deep learning software successfully detected and annotated the lesion with a heat map overlaid on the chest radiographic image. (**c**) Corresponding chest CT image shows a pulmonary nodule in the right lower lobe of the lung, which was diagnosed as lung cancer

ing algorithms but also multidisciplinary cooperation of various stakeholders and policy support would be required.

When it comes to the radiomics, the situation is worse than deep learning. As mentioned earlier, various studies have shown the potential of radiomics for the evaluation of lung nodules. However, radiomics has not yet been used in actual clinical practice [110]. It might be attributable to several following limitations of radiomics. First of all, radiomic features are largely influenced by various technical factors, such as image acquisition and reconstruction parameters, and segmentation of lung nodule [99–101]. Therefore, reproducible performance of a radiomic model in a new clinical setting is hard to achieve. Standardization of image acquisition and reconstruction parameters would be an ideal solution,

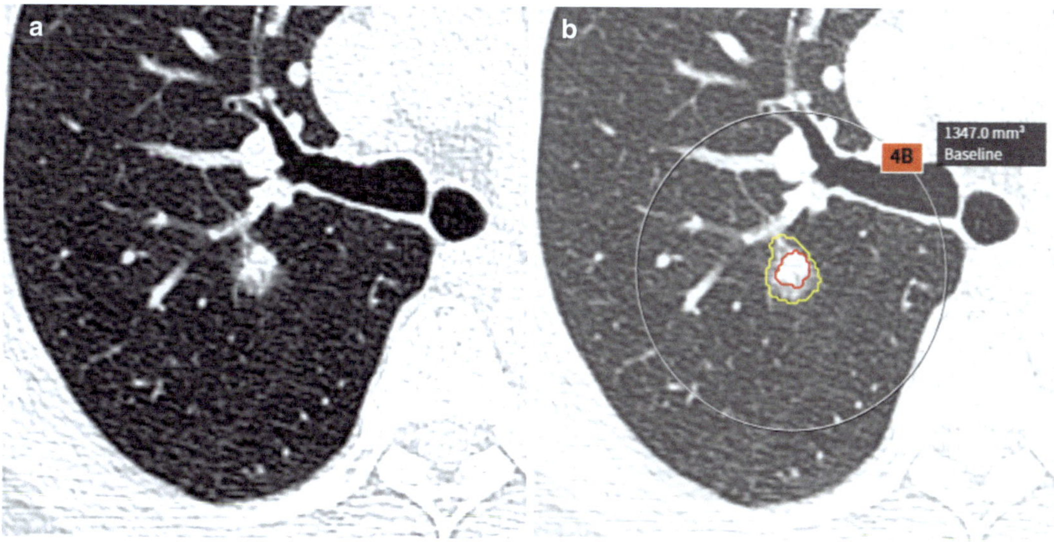

Fig. 20.3 Automated measurement and classification of lung nodules in chest CT using a commercially available deep learning software. (**a**) Chest CT image shows a part-solid nodule in the right upper lobe of the lung, which was diagnosed as lung cancer after surgical resection. (**b**) A commercialized deep learning software automatically segmented the entire nodule and internal solid component, to measure and classify the nodule according to the existing criteria (lung CT screening reporting and data system [Lung-RADS], category 4B)

but it would be practically very difficult. As mentioned above, utilization of deep learning-based technologies for image preprocessing for the neutralization of heterogeneous image textures and automated and reproducible segmentation can be a potential solution. Second, similar to deep learning, logical interpretation for the relationship between radiomic features and clinical outcomes is often challenging. This limited explainability would be an important hurdle for physicians to understand and trust the model's prediction. Third, despite many studies suggesting the potential of radiomics, studies that demonstrated reproducible performance in multiple datasets and clinical usefulness and value of radiomic model have been extremely rare. Further studies would be required to generate firm evidence for the reproducible performance and clinical effectiveness of radiomic models.

Finally, both deep learning and radiomics are data-driven methodologies, and large-scale imaging data with corresponding clinical information is an essential component for the development of deep learning or radiomic models. Since it is difficult for individual researchers to collect large-scale data directly, data sharing and making open-source data repository are important tasks to facilitate the development of deep learning and radiomic models. Open-source datasets may also promote transparent evaluation of developed models.

Conclusion

In this chapter, we described various applications of deep learning and radiomics in the imaging evaluation of lung nodule and lung cancer. Many studies have shown the potential of deep learning and radiomics as a valuable tool for lung nodule evaluation. However, except for deep learning-based tools for lung nodule detection on chest radiographs or CTs, the application of deep learning or radiomics to actual clinical practice is extremely limited. Multidisciplinary efforts need to be continued to facilitate the clinical implementation of deep learning and radiomics and guide them to improve practice quality and patient health: (a) development of deep learning and radiomic models with high accuracy and reproducibility, (b) evaluation of deep learning and radiomic models in terms of not only technical performance but also clinical impact and generalizability in various real-world situations, (c) seamless integration with legacy clinical workflow and discovering ideal method of utilization in practice, and (d) establishment of standardized large-scale, high-quality imaging data for the continuous development and evaluation of deep learning and radiomic models.

References

1. Gould MK, Tang T, Liu IL, Lee J, Zheng C, Danforth KN, et al. Recent trends in the identification of incidental pulmonary nodules. Am J Respir Crit Care Med. 2015;192:1208–14.
2. Hendrix W, Rutten M, Hendrix N, van Ginneken B, Schaefer-Prokop C, Scholten ET, et al. Trends in the incidence of pulmonary nodules in chest computed tomography: 10-year results from two Dutch hospitals. Eur Radiol. 2023;33:8279–88.
3. European Society of R. Current practical experience with artificial intelligence in clinical radiology: a survey of the European Society of Radiology. Insights Imaging. 2022;13:107.
4. Hwang EJ, Goo JM, Yoon SH, Beck KS, Seo JB, Choi BW, et al. Use of artificial intelligence-based software as medical devices for chest radiography: a position paper from the Korean Society of Thoracic Radiology. Korean J Radiol. 2021;22:1743–8.
5. Allen B, Agarwal S, Coombs L, Wald C, Dreyer K. 2020 ACR Data Science Institute Artificial Intelligence Survey. J Am Coll Radiol. 2021;18:1153–9.
6. Lambin P, Leijenaar RTH, Deist TM, Peerlings J, de Jong EEC, van Timmeren J, et al. Radiomics: the bridge between medical imaging and personalized medicine. Nat Rev Clin Oncol. 2017;14:749–62.
7. Lee G, Park H, Bak SH, Lee HY. Radiomics in lung cancer from basic to advanced: current status and future directions. Korean J Radiol. 2020;21:159–71.
8. Kim H, Park CM. Tumor-associated prognostic factors extractable from chest CT scans in patients with lung cancer. Transl Lung Cancer Res. 2023;12:1133–9.
9. Lee JH, Hwang EJ, Kim H, Park CM. A narrative review of deep learning applications in lung cancer research: from screening to prognostication. Transl Lung Cancer Res. 2022;11:1217–29.
10. Austin JH, Romney BM, Goldsmith LS. Missed bronchogenic carcinoma: radiographic findings in 27 patients with a potentially resectable lesion evident in retrospect. Radiology. 1992;182:115–22.
11. Gavelli G, Giampalma E. Sensitivity and specificity of chest X-ray screening for lung cancer: review article. Cancer. 2000;89:2453–6.
12. Lodwick GS, Keats TE, Dorst JP. The coding of roentgen images for computer analysis as applied to lung cancer. Radiology. 1963;81:185–200.
13. Nam JG, Park S, Hwang EJ, Lee JH, Jin KN, Lim KY, et al. Development and validation of deep learning-based automatic detection algorithm for malignant pulmonary nodules on chest radiographs. Radiology. 2019;290:218–28.
14. Sim Y, Chung MJ, Kotter E, Yune S, Kim M, Do S, et al. Deep convolutional neural network-based software improves radiologist detection of malignant lung nodules on chest radiographs. Radiology. 2020;294:199–209.
15. Cha MJ, Chung MJ, Lee JH, Lee KS. Performance of deep learning model in detecting operable lung cancer with chest radiographs. J Thorac Imaging. 2019;34:86–91.
16. Lee JH, Sun HY, Park S, Kim H, Hwang EJ, Goo JM, et al. Performance of a deep learning algorithm compared with radiologic interpretation for lung cancer detection on chest radiographs in a health screening population. Radiology. 2020;297:687–96.
17. Yoo H, Kim KH, Singh R, Digumarthy SR, Kalra MK. Validation of a deep learning algorithm for the detection of malignant pulmonary nodules in chest radiographs. JAMA Netw Open. 2020;3:e2017135.
18. Nam JG, Hwang EJ, Kim DS, Yoo SJ, Choi H, Goo JM, et al. Undetected lung cancer at posteroanterior chest radiography: potential role of a deep learning-based detection algorithm. Radiol Cardiothorac Imaging. 2020;2:e190222.
19. Jang S, Song H, Shin YJ, Kim J, Kim J, Lee KW, et al. Deep learning-based automatic detection algorithm for reducing overlooked lung cancers on chest radiographs. Radiology. 2020;296:652–61.
20. Hwang EJ, Lee JS, Lee JH, Lim WH, Kim JH, Choi KS, et al. Deep learning for detection of pulmonary metastasis on chest radiographs. Radiology. 2021;301:455–63.
21. Nam JG, Hwang EJ, Kim J, Park N, Lee EH, Kim HJ, et al. AI improves nodule detection on chest radiographs in a health screening population: a randomized controlled trial. Radiology. 2023;307:e221894.
22. Setio AAA, Traverso A, de Bel T, Berens MSN, Bogaard CVD, Cerello P, et al. Validation, comparison, and combination of algorithms for automatic detection of pulmonary nodules in computed tomography images: the LUNA16 challenge. Med Image Anal. 2017;42:1–13.
23. Li L, Liu Z, Huang H, Lin M, Luo D. Evaluating the performance of a deep learning-based computer-aided diagnosis (DL-CAD) system for detecting and characterizing lung nodules: comparison with the performance of double reading by radiologists. Thorac Cancer. 2019;10:183–92.
24. Chelala L, Hossain R, Kazerooni EA, Christensen JD, Dyer DS, White CS. Lung-RADS version 1.1: challenges and a look ahead, from the AJR special series on radiology reporting and data systems. AJR Am J Roentgenol. 2021;216:1411–22.

25. Bankier AA, MacMahon H, Goo JM, Rubin GD, Schaefer-Prokop CM, Naidich DP. Recommendations for measuring pulmonary nodules at CT: a statement from the Fleischner Society. Radiology. 2017;285:584–600.
26. Nair A, Dyer DS, Heuvelmans MA, Mashar M, Silva M, Hammer MM. Contextualizing the role of volumetric analysis in pulmonary nodule assessment: AJR expert panel narrative review. AJR Am J Roentgenol. 2023;220:314–29.
27. de Koning HJ, van der Aalst CM, de Jong PA, Scholten ET, Nackaerts K, Heuvelmans MA, et al. Reduced lung-cancer mortality with volume CT screening in a randomized trial. N Engl J Med. 2020;382:503–13.
28. Field JK, Duffy SW, Baldwin DR, Brain KE, Devaraj A, Eisen T, et al. The UK Lung Cancer Screening Trial: a pilot randomised controlled trial of low-dose computed tomography screening for the early detection of lung cancer. Health Technol Assess. 2016;20:1–146.
29. Pastorino U, Silva M, Sestini S, Sabia F, Boeri M, Cantarutti A, et al. Prolonged lung cancer screening reduced 10-year mortality in the MILD trial: new confirmation of lung cancer screening efficacy. Ann Oncol. 2019;30:1162–9.
30. Callister ME, Baldwin DR, Akram AR, Barnard S, Cane P, Draffan J, et al. British Thoracic Society guidelines for the investigation and management of pulmonary nodules. Thorax. 2015;70 Suppl 2:ii1–ii54.
31. Oudkerk M, Devaraj A, Vliegenthart R, Henzler T, Prosch H, Heussel CP, et al. European position statement on lung cancer screening. Lancet Oncol. 2017;18:e754–e66.
32. Bianconi F, Fravolini ML, Pizzoli S, Palumbo I, Minestrini M, Rondini M, et al. Comparative evaluation of conventional and deep learning methods for semi-automated segmentation of pulmonary nodules on CT. Quant Imaging Med Surg. 2021;11:3286–305.
33. Jacobs C, Schreuder A, van Riel SJ, Scholten ET, Wittenberg R, Wille MMW, et al. Assisted versus manual interpretation of low-dose CT scans for lung cancer screening: impact on lung-RADS agreement. Radiol Imaging Cancer. 2021;3:e200160.
34. Austin JH, Garg K, Aberle D, Yankelevitz D, Kuriyama K, Lee HJ, et al. Radiologic implications of the 2011 classification of adenocarcinoma of the lung. Radiology. 2013;266:62–71.
35. Kim H, Park CM, Hwang EJ, Ahn SY, Goo JM. Pulmonary subsolid nodules: value of semi-automatic measurement in diagnostic accuracy, diagnostic reproducibility and nodule classification agreement. Eur Radiol. 2018;28:2124–33.
36. Ahn Y, Lee SM, Noh HN, Kim W, Choe J, Do KH, et al. Use of a commercially available deep learning algorithm to measure the solid portions of lung cancer manifesting as subsolid lesions at CT: comparisons with radiologists and invasive component size at pathologic examination. Radiology. 2021;299:202–10.
37. Ciompi F, Chung K, van Riel SJ, Setio AAA, Gerke PK, Jacobs C, et al. Towards automatic pulmonary nodule management in lung cancer screening with deep learning. Sci Rep. 2017;7:46479.
38. Jacobs C, Setio AAA, Scholten ET, Gerke PK, Bhattacharya H, et al. Deep learning for lung cancer detection on screening CT scans: results of a large-scale public competition and an observer study with 11 radiologists. Radiol Artif Intell. 2021;3:e210027.
39. Ardila D, Kiraly AP, Bharadwaj S, Choi B, Reicher JJ, Peng L, et al. End-to-end lung cancer screening with three-dimensional deep learning on low-dose chest computed tomography. Nat Med. 2019;25:954–61.
40. Huang P, Lin CT, Li Y, Tammemagi MC, Brock MV, Atkar-Khattra S, et al. Prediction of lung cancer risk at follow-up screening with low-dose CT: a training and validation study of a deep learning method. Lancet Digit Health. 2019;1:e353–e62.
41. Lu MT, Raghu VK, Mayrhofer T, Aerts H, Hoffmann U. Deep learning using chest radiographs to identify high-risk smokers for lung cancer screening computed tomography: development and validation of a prediction model. Ann Intern Med. 2020;173:704–13.
42. Lee JH, Lee D, Lu MT, Raghu VK, Park CM, Goo JM, et al. Deep learning to optimize candidate selection for lung cancer CT screening: advancing the 2021 USPSTF recommendations. Radiology. 2022;305:209–18.
43. Swensen SJ, Silverstein MD, Ilstrup DM, Schleck CD, Edell ES. The probability of malignancy in solitary pulmonary nodules. Application to small radiologically indeterminate nodules. Arch Intern Med. 1997;157:849–55.
44. McWilliams A, Tammemagi MC, Mayo JR, Roberts H, Liu G, Soghrati K, et al. Probability of cancer in pulmonary nodules detected on first screening CT. N Engl J Med. 2013;369:910–9.
45. Tammemagi MC, Schmidt H, Martel S, McWilliams A, Goffin JR, Johnston MR, et al. Participant selection for lung cancer screening by risk modelling (the Pan-Canadian Early Detection of Lung Cancer [PanCan] study): a single-arm, prospective study. Lancet Oncol. 2017;18:1523–31.
46. Massion PP, Antic S, Ather S, Arteta C, Brabec J, Chen H, et al. Assessing the accuracy of a deep learning method to risk stratify indeterminate pulmonary nodules. Am J Respir Crit Care Med. 2020;202:241–9.
47. Kim RY, Oke JL, Pickup LC, Munden RF, Dotson TL, Bellinger CR, et al. Artificial intelligence tool for assessment of indeterminate pulmonary nodules detected with CT. Radiology. 2022;304:683–91.
48. Alilou M, Beig N, Orooji M, Rajiah P, Velcheti V, Rakshit S, et al. An integrated segmentation and shape-based classification scheme for distinguishing

adenocarcinomas from granulomas on lung CT. Med Phys. 2017;44:3556–69.
49. Beig N, Khorrami M, Alilou M, Prasanna P, Braman N, Orooji M, et al. Perinodular and intranodular radiomic features on lung CT images distinguish adenocarcinomas from granulomas. Radiology. 2019;290:783–92.
50. He L, Huang Y, Ma Z, Liang C, Liang C, Liu Z. Effects of contrast-enhancement, reconstruction slice thickness and convolution kernel on the diagnostic performance of radiomics signature in solitary pulmonary nodule. Sci Rep. 2016;6:34921.
51. Lu CY, Tsao PN, Ke YY, Lin YH, Lin YH, Hung CC, et al. Concurrent hearing, genetic, and cytomegalovirus screening in newborns. Taiwan J Pediatr. 2018;199:144–50 e1.
52. Kim H, Goo JM, Kim YT, Park CM. CT-defined visceral pleural invasion in T1 lung adenocarcinoma: lack of relationship to disease-free survival. Radiology. 2019;292:741–9.
53. Lim WH, Lee KH, Lee JH, Park H, Nam JG, Hwang EJ, et al. Diagnostic performance and prognostic value of CT-defined visceral pleural invasion in early-stage lung adenocarcinomas. Eur Radiol. 2023;34:1934–45.
54. Lin JT, Yang XN, Zhong WZ, Liao RQ, Dong S, Nie Q, et al. Association of maximum standardized uptake value with occult mediastinal lymph node metastases in cN0 non-small cell lung cancer. Eur J Cardiothorac Surg. 2016;50:914–9.
55. Wang L, Jiang W, Zhan C, Shi Y, Zhang Y, Lin Z, et al. Lymph node metastasis in clinical stage IA peripheral lung cancer. Lung Cancer. 2015;90:41–6.
56. Kim H, Lee D, Cho WS, Lee JC, Goo JM, Kim HC, et al. CT-based deep learning model to differentiate invasive pulmonary adenocarcinomas appearing as subsolid nodules among surgical candidates: comparison of the diagnostic performance with a size-based logistic model and radiologists. Eur Radiol. 2020;30:3295–305.
57. Chae HD, Park CM, Park SJ, Lee SM, Kim KG, Goo JM. Computerized texture analysis of persistent part-solid ground-glass nodules: differentiation of preinvasive lesions from invasive pulmonary adenocarcinomas. Radiology. 2014;273:285–93.
58. Park S, Park G, Lee SM, Kim W, Park H, Jung K, et al. Deep learning-based differentiation of invasive adenocarcinomas from preinvasive or minimally invasive lesions among pulmonary subsolid nodules. Eur Radiol. 2021;31:6239–47.
59. Zuo Z, Li Y, Peng K, Li X, Tan Q, Mo Y, et al. CT texture analysis-based nomogram for the preoperative prediction of visceral pleural invasion in cT1N0M0 lung adenocarcinoma: an external validation cohort study. Clin Radiol. 2022;77:e215–e21.
60. Wei SH, Zhang JM, Shi B, Gao F, Zhang ZX, Qian LT. The value of CT radiomics features to predict visceral pleural invasion in ≤3 cm peripheral type early non-small cell lung cancer. J Xray Sci Technol. 2022;30:1115–26.
61. Choi H, Kim H, Hong W, Park J, Hwang EJ, Park CM, et al. Prediction of visceral pleural invasion in lung cancer on CT: deep learning model achieves a radiologist-level performance with adaptive sensitivity and specificity to clinical needs. Eur Radiol. 2021;31:2866–76.
62. Zhong Y, She Y, Deng J, Chen S, Wang T, Yang M, et al. Deep learning for prediction of N2 metastasis and survival for clinical stage I non-small cell lung cancer. Radiology. 2022;302:200–11.
63. Ma X, Xia L, Chen J, Wan W, Zhou W. Development and validation of a deep learning signature for predicting lymph node metastasis in lung adenocarcinoma: comparison with radiomics signature and clinical-semantic model. Eur Radiol. 2023;33:1949–62.
64. Zhong Y, Yuan M, Zhang T, Zhang YD, Li H, Yu TF. Radiomics approach to prediction of occult mediastinal lymph node metastasis of lung adenocarcinoma. AJR Am J Roentgenol. 2018;211:109–13.
65. Tan AC, Tan DSW. Targeted therapies for lung cancer patients with oncogenic driver molecular alterations. J Clin Oncol. 2022;40:611–25.
66. Tan X, Li Y, Wang S, Xia H, Meng R, Xu J, et al. Predicting EGFR mutation, ALK rearrangement, and uncommon EGFR mutation in NSCLC patients by driverless artificial intelligence: a cohort study. Respir Res. 2022;23:132.
67. Wang C, Xu X, Shao J, Zhou K, Zhao K, He Y, et al. Deep learning to predict EGFR mutation and PD-L1 expression status in non-small-cell lung cancer on computed tomography images. J Oncol. 2021;2021:5499385.
68. Wang S, Shi J, Ye Z, Dong D, Yu D, Zhou M, et al. Predicting EGFR mutation status in lung adenocarcinoma on computed tomography image using deep learning. Eur Respir J. 2019;53:1800986.
69. Song Z, Liu T, Shi L, Yu Z, Shen Q, Xu M, et al. The deep learning model combining CT image and clinicopathological information for predicting ALK fusion status and response to ALK-TKI therapy in non-small cell lung cancer patients. Eur J Nucl Med Mol Imaging. 2021;48:361–71.
70. Dong Y, Hou L, Yang W, Han J, Wang J, Qiang Y, et al. Multi-channel multi-task deep learning for predicting EGFR and KRAS mutations of non-small cell lung cancer on CT images. Quant Imaging Med Surg. 2021;11:2354–75.
71. Reck M, Rodriguez-Abreu D, Robinson AG, Hui R, Csoszi T, Fulop A, et al. Pembrolizumab versus chemotherapy for PD-L1-positive non-small-cell lung cancer. N Engl J Med. 2016;375:1823–33.
72. Socinski MA, Jotte RM, Cappuzzo F, Orlandi F, Stroyakovskiy D, Nogami N, et al. Atezolizumab for first-line treatment of metastatic nonsquamous NSCLC. N Engl J Med. 2018;378:2288–301.
73. Herbst RS, Baas P, Kim DW, Felip E, Perez-Gracia JL, Han JY, et al. Pembrolizumab versus docetaxel for previously treated, PD-L1-positive, advanced non-small-cell lung cancer (KEYNOTE-010): a randomised controlled trial. Lancet. 2016;387:1540–50.

74. Rittmeyer A, Barlesi F, Waterkamp D, Park K, Ciardiello F, von Pawel J, et al. Atezolizumab versus docetaxel in patients with previously treated non-small-cell lung cancer (OAK): a phase 3, open-label, multicentre randomised controlled trial. Lancet. 2017;389:255–65.
75. Wakelee H, Liberman M, Kato T, Tsuboi M, Lee SH, Gao S, et al. Perioperative pembrolizumab for early-stage non-small-cell lung cancer. N Engl J Med. 2023;389:491–503.
76. Provencio M, Nadal E, Gonzalez-Larriba JL, Martinez-Marti A, Bernabe R, Bosch-Barrera J, et al. Perioperative nivolumab and chemotherapy in stage III non-small-cell lung cancer. N Engl J Med. 2023;389:504–13.
77. Shao J, Ma J, Zhang S, Li J, Dai H, Liang S, et al. Radiogenomic system for non-invasive identification of multiple actionable mutations and PD-L1 expression in non-small cell lung cancer based on CT images. Cancers (Basel). 2022;14:4823.
78. Tian P, He B, Mu W, Liu K, Liu L, Zeng H, et al. Assessing PD-L1 expression in non-small cell lung cancer and predicting responses to immune checkpoint inhibitors using deep learning on computed tomography images. Theranostics. 2021;11:2098–107.
79. Wang C, Ma J, Shao J, Zhang S, Li J, Yan J, et al. Non invasive measurement using deep learning algorithm based on multi-source features fusion to predict PD-L1 expression and survival in NSCLC. Front Immunol. 2022;13:828560.
80. He B, Dong D, She Y, Zhou C, Fang M, Zhu Y, et al. Predicting response to immunotherapy in advanced non-small-cell lung cancer using tumor mutational burden radiomic biomarker. J Immunother Cancer. 2020;8:e000550.
81. Kawaguchi Y, Shimada Y, Murakami K, Omori T, Kudo Y, Makino Y, et al. Prognostic impact of artificial intelligence-based volumetric quantification of the solid part of the tumor in clinical stage 0-I adenocarcinoma. Lung Cancer. 2022;170:85–90.
82. Sun R, Limkin EJ, Vakalopoulou M, Dercle L, Champiat S, Han SR, et al. A radiomics approach to assess tumour-infiltrating CD8 cells and response to anti-PD-1 or anti-PD-L1 immunotherapy: an imaging biomarker, retrospective multicohort study. Lancet Oncol. 2018;19:1180–91.
83. Huang Y, Liu Z, He L, Chen X, Pan D, Ma Z, et al. Radiomics signature: a potential biomarker for the prediction of disease-free survival in early-stage (I or II) non-small cell lung cancer. Radiology. 2016;281:947–57.
84. Kim H, Goo JM, Lee KH, Kim YT, Park CM. Preoperative CT-based deep learning model for predicting disease-free survival in patients with lung adenocarcinomas. Radiology. 2020;296:216–24.
85. Kinoshita F, Takenaka T, Yamashita T, Matsumoto K, Oku Y, Ono Y, et al. Development of artificial intelligence prognostic model for surgically resected non-small cell lung cancer. Sci Rep. 2023;13:15683.
86. Wang T, She Y, Yang Y, Liu X, Chen S, Zhong Y, et al. Radiomics for survival risk stratification of clinical and pathologic stage IA pure-solid non-small cell lung cancer. Radiology. 2022;302:425–34.
87. Jacobs CD, Mehta K, Gao J, Wang X, Salama JK, Kelsey CR, et al. Nomogram predicting overall survival benefit of stereotactic ablative radiotherapy for early-stage non-small cell lung cancer. Clin Lung Cancer. 2022;23:177–84.
88. Kim H, Lee JH, Kim HJ, Park CM, Wu HG, Goo JM. Extended application of a CT-based artificial intelligence prognostication model in patients with primary lung cancer undergoing stereotactic ablative radiotherapy. Radiother Oncol. 2021;165:166–73.
89. Deng K, Wang L, Liu Y, Li X, Hou Q, Cao M, et al. A deep learning-based system for survival benefit prediction of tyrosine kinase inhibitors and immune checkpoint inhibitors in stage IV non-small cell lung cancer patients: a multicenter, prognostic study. EClinicalMedicine. 2022;51:101541.
90. Saad MB, Hong L, Aminu M, Vokes NI, Chen P, Salehjahromi M, et al. Predicting benefit from immune checkpoint inhibitors in patients with non-small-cell lung cancer by CT-based ensemble deep learning: a retrospective study. Lancet Digit Health. 2023;5:e404–e20.
91. Wang TW, Hsu MS, Lin YH, Chiu HY, Chao HS, Liao CY, et al. Application of radiomics in prognosing lung cancer treated with epidermal growth factor receptor tyrosine kinase inhibitors: a systematic review and meta-analysis. Cancers (Basel). 2023;15:3542.
92. Nam JG, Park S, Park CM, Jeon YK, Chung DH, Goo JM, et al. Histopathologic basis for a chest CT deep learning survival prediction model in patients with lung adenocarcinoma. Radiology. 2022;305:441–51.
93. Aerts HJ, Velazquez ER, Leijenaar RT, Parmar C, Grossmann P, Carvalho S, et al. Decoding tumour phenotype by noninvasive imaging using a quantitative radiomics approach. Nat Commun. 2014;5:4006.
94. Wei H, Yang F, Liu Z, Sun S, Xu F, Liu P, et al. Application of computed tomography-based radiomics signature analysis in the prediction of the response of small cell lung cancer patients to first-line chemotherapy. Exp Ther Med. 2019;17:3621–9.
95. Qureshi R, Basit SA, Shamsi JA, Fan X, Nawaz M, Yan H, et al. Machine learning based personalized drug response prediction for lung cancer patients. Sci Rep. 2022;12:18935.
96. Song J, Shi J, Dong D, Fang M, Zhong W, Wang K, et al. A new approach to predict progression-free survival in stage IV EGFR-mutant NSCLC patients with EGFR-TKI therapy. Clin Cancer Res. 2018;24:3583–92.
97. Song J, Wang L, Ng NN, Zhao M, Shi J, Wu N, et al. Development and validation of a machine learning model to explore tyrosine kinase inhibitor response in patients with stage IV EGFR variant-positive non-small cell lung cancer. JAMA Netw Open. 2020;3:e2030442.

98. Parmar C, Rios Velazquez E, Leijenaar R, Jermoumi M, Carvalho S, Mak RH, et al. Robust radiomics feature quantification using semiautomatic volumetric segmentation. PLoS One. 2014;9:e102107.
99. Berenguer R, Pastor-Juan MDR, Canales-Vazquez J, Castro-Garcia M, Villas MV, Mansilla Legorburo F, et al. Radiomics of CT features may be nonreproducible and redundant: influence of CT acquisition parameters. Radiology. 2018;288:407–15.
100. Kim H, Park CM, Lee M, Park SJ, Song YS, Lee JH, et al. Impact of reconstruction algorithms on CT radiomic features of pulmonary tumors: analysis of intra- and inter-reader variability and inter-reconstruction algorithm variability. PLoS One. 2016;11:e0164924.
101. Meyer M, Ronald J, Vernuccio F, Nelson RC, Ramirez-Giraldo JC, Solomon J, et al. Reproducibility of CT radiomic features within the same patient: influence of radiation dose and CT reconstruction settings. Radiology. 2019;293:583–91.
102. Choe J, Lee SM, Do KH, Lee G, Lee JG, Lee SM, et al. Deep learning-based image conversion of CT reconstruction kernels improves radiomics reproducibility for pulmonary nodules or masses. Radiology. 2019;292:365–73.
103. Park S, Lee SM, Do KH, Lee JG, Bae W, Park H, et al. Deep learning algorithm for reducing CT slice thickness: effect on reproducibility of radiomic features in lung cancer. Korean J Radiol. 2019;20:1431–40.
104. Paul R, Hawkins SH, Schabath MB, Gillies RJ, Hall LO, Goldgof DB. Predicting malignant nodules by fusing deep features with classical radiomics features. J Med Imaging (Bellingham). 2018;5:011021.
105. Zhang B, Qi S, Pan X, Li C, Yao Y, Qian W, et al. Deep CNN model using CT radiomics feature mapping recognizes EGFR gene mutation status of lung adenocarcinoma. Front Oncol. 2020;10:598721.
106. Paul R, Kariev S, Cherezov D, Schabath MB, Gillies RJ, Hall LO, et al. Deep radiomics: deep learning on radiomics texture images. In: Mazurowski MA, Drukker K, editors. Medical imaging 2021: computer-aided diagnosis. SPIE; 2021.
107. Schreuder A, Scholten ET, van Ginneken B, Jacobs C. Artificial intelligence for detection and characterization of pulmonary nodules in lung cancer CT screening: ready for practice? Transl Lung Cancer Res. 2021;10:2378–88.
108. Razzak MI, Naz S, Zaib A. Deep learning for medical image processing: overview, challenges and the future. In: Classification in BioApps. Cham: Springer; 2018. p. 323–50.
109. Selvaraju RR, Cogswell M, Das A, Vedantam R, Parikh D, Batra D. Grad-CAM: visual explanations from deep networks via gradient-based localization. In: Proceedings of the IEEE international conference on computer vision. Venice: IEEE; 2017.
110. Shaikh FA, Kolowitz BJ, Awan O, Aerts HJ, von Reden A, Halabi S, et al. Technical challenges in the clinical application of radiomics. JCO Clin Cancer Inform. 2017;1:1–8.

21 Perfusion, Diffusion, and Metabolism of Pulmonary Nodules, Masses, and Lung Cancer

Yoshiyuki Ozawa, Takahiro Ueda, Masahiko Nomura, Takeshi Yoshikawa, Daisuke Takenaka, and Yoshiharu Ohno

Introduction

Quantitative imaging modalities constitute promising methods for improving lung cancer identification and follow-up, as they use more accurate parameters than subjective analyses for assessment and prediction of treatment response, thus optimizing care for individual patients [1]. Lung nodule measurement using computed tomography (CT) is an important quantitative marker for predicting likelihood of malignancy as well as progression of disease [2]. Moreover, fluorine-18-fluorodeoxyglucose positron emission tomography/computed tomography (FDG-PET/CT) provides information on a tumor's morphology, extension, and glucose metabolism, outperforming CT or PET alone for nodule evaluation and lung cancer staging [3–5].

Since the introduction of magnetic resonance imaging (MRI) for the assessment of thoracic and lung diseases, various limitations of this procedure, mostly related to the relatively low proton density of lung parenchyma, the presence of cardiac and respiratory motion artifacts, and long acquisition time, have hampered the clinical application of this technique. During the last few decades, however, the introduction of technical advancements in MR systems or sequences as well as clinical application of gadolinium (Gd) contrast media in routine clinical practice has frequently resulted in solutions for some of the limitations of MRI, although the Radiology Diagnostic Oncology Group (RDOG) of the Radiological Society of North America (RSNA) reported in 1991 that, in comparison with CT, MRI is of limited clinical relevance for tumor classification and assessment of mediastinal node metastases [6]. Moreover, it has been suggested that recent advances in MRI techniques, such as dynamic first-pass contrast-enhanced (CE)-perfusion MRI, diffusion-weighted imaging (DWI), or chemical exchange saturation transfer (CEST) imaging, may be suitable for nodule assessment, tumor staging, and therapeutic effect prediction or evaluation in routine clinical practice or for academic studies. Furthermore, based on findings obtained with perfusion matrixes, dynamic first-pass CE-perfusion imaging with

Y. Ozawa · T. Ueda · T. Yoshikawa · D. Takenaka
Department of Diagnostic Radiology, Fujita Health University School of Medicine,
Toyoake, Aichi, Japan
e-mail: yoshiyuki.ozawa@fujita-hu.ac.jp; t-ueda@fujita-hu.ac.jp; takeshi.yoshikawa@fujita-hu.ac.jp; daisuke.takenaka.fr@fujita-hu.ac.jp

M. Nomura · Y. Ohno (✉)
Department of Diagnostic Radiology, Fujita Health University School of Medicine,
Toyoake, Aichi, Japan

Joint Research Laboratory of Advanced Medical Imaging and Artificial Intelligence, Fujita Health University School of Medicine, Toyoake, Aichi, Japan
e-mail: nomura@fujita-hu.ac.jp; yohno@fujita-hu.ac.jp

R. Gill, P. Rajiah (eds.), *Quantitative Imaging in the Thorax*,
https://doi.org/10.1007/978-3-032-14103-3_21

MRI or area-detector CT (ADCT) is reportedly a promising imaging technique for differentiating malignant from benign nodules or distinguishing nodules requiring further intervention or treatment from nodules with no need for further evaluation [7–20]. However, some dynamic CE-perfusion MDCT studies, whose scanning technique could not assess the actual first-pass component of time-CT number changes based on contrast enhancement course curves, used quantitative analysis for nodule enhancement evaluation by non-appropriately assessed perfusion indexes [21–28]. Moreover, some software for quantitative perfusion evaluation has also been used more often for automating quantitative analyses and reducing intra- and inter-reader variability. In contrast to dynamic first-pass CE-perfusion imaging, DWI is also reportedly useful for nodule evaluation or TNM staging of not only lung cancer but also other thoracic tumors [4, 5, 29–41]. Furthermore, CEST imaging has been introduced as a technique for providing additional physiological and functional information for conventional MRI and has become prominent in the field of molecular imaging since the mid-2010s [42–52]. CEST imaging is performed by applying multiple magnetization transfer pulses to the resonance frequency of slow- to intermediate-rate exchanging protons (NH-, OH-, or metal-bound water molecule) of endogenous or exogenous agents [44–46]. Moreover, amide proton transfer (APT) imaging is a subset of CEST imaging that applies specifically to chemical exchange between protons of bulk water and amide groups (-NH) of endogenous mobile proteins and peptides. It has been reported that such exchangeable protons are more abundant in tumors than in healthy tissues [47–52], and it has been demonstrated in in vitro and in vivo studies that there is a significant difference in the APT between malignant and benign or healthy tissues [42, 43, 47–52]. In addition, in vitro or in vivo studies found APT-weighted (APTw) imaging to be potentially effective for distinguishing lung cancer from other thoracic tumors or organizing pneumonia, characterizing subtypes of non-small cell lung cancer (NSCLC), or predicting therapeutic effect [49, 50, 52].

This chapter deals with the basics of perfusion imaging, DWI, and CEST imaging as well as clinical applications of quantitative assessment using these three MR methods for patients with pulmonary nodules, masses, or lung cancer.

Basics of Quantitative MR Imaging

Basics of Dynamic First-Pass CE-Perfusion Imaging

During the late 1990s and in 2000, the use of quantitatively analyzed dynamic first-pass contrast-enhanced-perfusion CT by means of electron-beam CT was reported for not only animals but also for normal individuals and/or patients with pulmonary thromboembolism [53]. However, after the introduction of multidetector row CT (MDCT) for clinical use, electron-beam CT used for dynamic first-pass contrast-enhanced-perfusion CT changed to MDCT, and a few investigators have reported on the latter's potential for quantitative assessment of tumors or nodule perfusion assessment for diagnosis of pulmonary nodules or lung cancer, or for therapeutic effect assessment for lung cancer patients undergoing conservative therapy [21–28]. However, the number of detector rows of MDCT used in these studies ranged from only 4 to 64. Therefore, the limited scan range attainable with dynamic scanning at the same table position or the mixture of a variety of perfusion data obtained at different time points and positions within the scan range due to the helical scanning method were major drawbacks of this technique [21–28]. These studies had suggested that use of the MDCT technique could not assess the actual first-pass entry of contrast media within nodules or lung cancer. Since 2007, however, ADCT with a 320-detector row has been used in routine clinical practice for not only morphological examinations but also functional assessments, especially the use of mathematical models for real first-pass evaluation of perfusion of a pulmonary nodule or mass as well as of lung cancer [12–20].

Unlike dynamic first-pass CE-perfusion CT, MRI features three general types of CE-MRI for academic and clinical purposes: conventional CE-MRI, dynamic CE-MRI, and dynamic first-pass CE-perfusion MRI, which have been in use since the 1990s [7–20, 54–63]. Although unenhanced MRI has both more advantages and disadvantages than dynamic first-pass CE-perfusion MRI, quantitatively and qualitatively assessed dynamic first-pass CE-perfusion MRI has been more frequently and widely used for assessments due to its simpler clinical settings. With dynamic first-pass CE-perfusion MRI, multiple images can be acquired during the first passage using an intravascular contrast agent for identification within the lung of nodules, masses, or lung cancer. The images are generally obtained by using a three-dimensional (3D) or two-dimensional (2D) dynamic gradient-echo sequence with ultrashort echo time (TE). Multiple images are acquired rapidly during a bolus intravenous administration of gadolinium contrast media, which also function as T1-shortening contrast agents. Images can be acquired either at multiple levels to evaluate the whole lung on 3D sequences or at a single anatomic level on 2D sequences. In addition, images can be evaluated repeatedly during the passage of contrast material. Temporal resolution of dynamic first-pass CE-perfusion MRI is recommended for dynamic series using temporal resolution equal to or less than 1.2 s. This temporal resolution assists clinicians to clearly differentiate pulmonary arterial, parenchymal, pulmonary venous, and systemic arterial phases.

Although dynamic first-pass contrast-enhanced-perfusion MRI or ADCT data can be obtained in routine clinical practice, it is difficult to qualitatively evaluate nodules, masses, or tumor perfusion. Therefore, dynamic first-pass contrast-enhanced-perfusion data has been evaluated by means of semiquantitative perfusion matrixes such as maximum relative enhancement or the ratio and slope of enhancement or quantitative perfusion matrixes by using various mathematical models such as the deconvolution, single- and dual-input maximum slope, and single-input Patlak plot models [12–20]. The details of these mathematical models are not included in this chapter, but several experts have suggested that the Patlak plot method is not well suited for dynamic first-pass CE-perfusion data assessment for diagnosing pulmonary nodules or masses nor for therapeutic effect assessment for patients with lung cancer following conservative therapy [12, 18]. Clinicians should therefore gain a clear understanding of these mathematical models for the analysis of perfusion matrixes for various academic or clinical purposes.

Basics of Diffusion-Weighted Imaging (DWI)

Conventional DWI

During the last few decades, DWI has been used for assessment of not only intracranial but also extracranial diseases including thoracic oncology. DWI measurements can be quickly performed and do not need contrast media administration. These imaging sequences can thus be added to existing imaging protocols without a significant increase in examination time. Furthermore, DWI yields both qualitative and quantitative information that can be helpful for tumor assessment.

DWI explores the random motion of water molecules in the body. Water molecules held in a container outside the body are in constant random Brownian motion. This uninhibited motion of water molecules represents free diffusion; in contrast, the movement of water molecules in biologic tissues is restricted because their motion is modified and limited by interactions with cell membranes and macromolecules [64–72].

In biologic tissue, the DWI signal is derived from the motion of water molecules in the extracellular space, the intracellular space, and the intravascular space [64–72]. Within a given unit of time, water molecules in the intravascular space will have to cover a greater diffusion distance because of blood flow than those in the extracellular and intracellular spaces. The contribution of intravascular water diffusion to the measured DWI signal can thus clearly vary among tissues. In fact, a significant proportion of tumors showing increased vascularity may be accounted for by the contribution of intravascular water diffusion to the MR signal [73–76].

The degree to which water diffusion in biologic tissue is restricted is inversely correlated to the tissue cellularity and the integrity of cell membranes [64–72]. For example, the motion of water molecules is more restricted in tissues with a high cellular density associated with numerous intact cell membranes (i.e., tumor tissue). Moreover, the lipophilic cell membranes act as barriers to the motion of water molecules in both the extracellular and intracellular spaces. By contrast, in areas of low cellularity or where the cellular membrane has been breached, the motion of water molecules is less restricted. A less cellular environment thus provides a larger extracellular space for diffusion of water molecules, and these molecules may also freely transgress defective cell membranes to move from the extracellular into the intracellular compartment.

The apparent diffusion coefficient (ADC) is currently frequently used for the detection and quantification of water diffusion by using T2-weighted spin-echo-type echo-planar imaging (EPI), turbo spin-echo (TSE), or fast advanced spin-echo (FASE) sequences with the aid of a symmetric pair of diffusion-sensitizing (bipolar) gradients around the 180° refocusing pulse [38, 64–77]. Static molecules acquire phase information from the first diffusion gradient, but this information will be rephased by the second diffusion gradient without a significant change in the measured signal intensity. By comparison, moving water molecules acquire different phase information from the first gradient, but because of their motion, their signal will not be completely rephased by the second gradient, thus leading to signal loss. Hence, the motion of water molecules is detected as attenuation of the measured signal intensity at DWI, while the degree of water motion has been found to be proportional to the degree of signal attenuation [70].

The sensitivity of the DWI sequence to water motion can be altered by changing the gradient amplitude, the duration of the applied gradient, and the time interval between the paired gradients. On clinical MR scanners, the diffusion sensitivity is easily altered by changing the parameter known as the b value, which is proportional to these three factors. When the b value is changed, it is usually the gradient amplitude, rather than the duration or time intervals between gradients, that is also altered [70].

Water molecules with a large degree of motion or a great diffusion distance, which is mainly observed within the intravascular space, will show signal attenuation with small b values equal to or less than100 s/mm^2. In contrast, large b values equal to or higher than 600 s/mm^2 are usually required to perceive slow-moving water molecules or small diffusion distances because these show more gradual signal attenuation with an increase in b values. The root mean square displacement of water molecules that occurs during a diffusion measurement is estimated to be approximately 8 μm, while the mean size of cells in the human body measures about 10 μm. Hence, the information provided by DWI reflects changes that are occurring at a cellular spatial scale. For this reason, DWI is considered to be a valuable tool for evaluating changes in the tumor microenvironment, both before and after treatment [70].

Generally speaking, the differential signal attenuation at different b values can be used to calculate the ADC from DWIs with at least two diffusion weightings, or b values. In its simplest form, the slope of the line that describes the relationship between the logarithm of the signal intensity and the b value is the ADC. When the calculation is performed within the entire DWI voxels, the ADC value for every image voxel can be derived and displayed as a parametric ADC map. Thus, voxels that show a steeper slope of signal attenuation with an increase in b values will have higher ADC values indicating higher water diffusivity than voxels that show a gradual slope of signal attenuation. Cellular or tumor tissues often return lower ADC values than native or benign tissues, which facilitates their detection and characterization. Although an ADC map may be generated under optimal measurement conditions by using just two b values, DWI using more than two b values for image acquisition generally yields more accurate ADC values or ADC maps for use in routine clinical practice [70].

Intravoxel Incoherent Motion on DWI

The wide use of DWI for various academic or clinical aims has led many investigators to suggest that the calculated ADC value is sensitive to capillary perfusion, which represents the bulk motion of intravascular water protons within imaging voxels [64–68, 71, 72]. In 1986, Le Bihan et al. [64] proposed the principles of intravoxel incoherent motion (IVIM) and suggested that using a more sophisticated approach to describe the relationship between signal attenuation in tissues with an increase in the b value would make it possible to estimate the quantitative parameters that separately reflect tissue diffusivity and tissue microcapillary perfusion. Many investigators have therefore become interested during the past few decades in applying the suggested analytic techniques beyond simple ADC calculations to tease out the effects of microcapillary perfusion from DWI data for not only intracranial but also extracranial diseases [71, 72]. This interest is also driven by the realization that the assumption of a simple exponential relationship between signal attenuation and b value for ADC calculation is simplistic, as is the perceived value of obtaining perfusion-related data from a relatively simple measurement. However, to do this in a meaningful way demands insight into the approach and a clear understanding of the strengths and limitations of the method.

When DWI is performed using well-perfused body tissues with b values ranging from 0 to 1000 s/mm^2, which are usually applied for body imaging, the measured signal attenuation at low b values of 100 s/mm^2 or less results not only from water diffusion in tissues but also from microcirculation within the normal capillary network. Both these processes result in phase dispersion on DWI, leading to signal attenuation. Le Bihan et al. [64] characterized the behavior of protons that display signal attenuation at DWI as showing IVIM.

Microcirculatory perfusion within capillaries has no specific orientation and can be considered pseudo diffusion, which depends on the velocity of the flowing blood and the vascular architecture. The effect of pseudo diffusion on the signal attenuation for each imaging voxel is also b value dependent. However, the rate of signal attenuation resulting from pseudo diffusion is typically greater than tissue diffusion because of the larger distances of proton displacement during the application of the motion-probing gradients. Therefore, in normal perfused tissue at higher b values, pseudo diffusion accounts for only a small proportion of the measured signal from each imaging voxel, while this relative contribution to the DWI signal becomes significant only at lower b values [64–68, 71, 72].

Plotting of the signal attenuation of a well-perfused tissue with increasing b values from a healthy individual on DWI with b values equal to or less than 100 s/mm^2 shows that protons associated with flowing blood feature relatively large diffusion distances, and that the signal is suppressed by small diffusion weightings. The slope of signal attenuation for b values near zero is therefore steeper, which can be attributed to microcapillary perfusion. On the other hand, larger b values are less sensitive to the impact of microcapillary perfusion because the signal attenuation of the perfusing protons is essentially complete. At larger b values of more than 100 s/mm^2, the slope of signal attenuation becomes less steep, which is more reflective of tissue diffusivity. In this case, a line drawn to best fit all the data points has the shape of a hockey stick, which is indeed shown by the IVIM model. The IVIM approach uses a biexponential function to describe the DWI data and is based on the assumption that the measured signal attenuation on DWI comprises a mixture of tissue perfusion and tissue diffusivity effects. Using IVIM-based analysis, it is therefore possible to derive other quantitative indexes that describe tissue water diffusivity, tissue perfusion (pseudo-diffusion coefficient: D*), as well as for these indexes to be displayed as parametric maps [64–68, 71, 72].

For most commercial MRI systems, the ADC value is currently calculated automatically and by default all available b-value images are used with a mono-exponential function. Thus, depending on the range and number of b values used for imaging, the calculation of ADC using this approach is, to various extents, influenced by microcapillary perfusion. The preceding discussion should therefore make it clear that the ADC values of perfused tissues calculated from only images with low b values equal to or less than 100 s/mm^2 (ADC_{low}) would be perfusion sensitive, whereas the ADC values calculated from images with higher b values of more than 100 s/mm^2 (ADC_{high}) and excluding lower b values would be relatively perfusion insensitive. It can also be argued that ADC_{high} values are likely to be very similar to the diffusion coefficient (D) derived by IVIM-based analysis for any particular tissue, although ADC_{low} is perfusion sensitive and very similar to the pseudo perfusion (D*) and also affected by diffusion effects in tissues. In addition, perfusion fraction (f) is generally also determined from data obtained with IVIM-based analysis [64–68, 71, 72].

Computed DWI

Computed DWI is a mathematical computation technique which builds on previously described principles [41, 78–81] and calculates a high b-value (or any b-value) image from actually acquired DWIs (i.e., actual DWIs) with at least two different b values [41, 78–81]. One of the disadvantages of actual DWI with high b values is generally considered to yield a lower image quality such as poor SNR and image distortion, but this disadvantage may be avoided when computed DWI is used for oncologic patients. Imaging with two or more b values allows for the calculation of ADC of tissues on a voxel-by-voxel basis by using the following equation [41, 79–81]:

$$S(b) = S(0)e^{-b \cdot \mathrm{ADC}} \quad (21.1)$$

where $S(0)$ is the signal intensity at a b value (b) of 0 sec/mm^2. Once the ADC is known, it can be used to extrapolate the expected signal intensity for each image voxel to any computed b value, b_c, as follows:

$$S(b_c) = S^*(0)e^{-b \cdot \mathrm{ADC}*} \quad (21.2)$$

where S*(0) and ADC* are the per-voxel estimates of S(0) and ADC, respectively, thus generating a computed DW MR image. DWI images, typically obtained at b values between 0 and 1000 sec/mm^2, are used to calculate tissue ADC maps in accordance with Eq. (21.1), from which mathematically computed images at higher b values are generated. It has been suggested that, in comparison with actual DWI, computed DWI has superior potential for malignant lesion detection, differentiation of malignant from benign lesions, or N-stage classification for a variety of oncologic patients in routine clinical practice [41, 79–81].

Basics of CEST Imaging

Contrast agents are widely used in MR imaging for signal enhancement. They allow for better differentiation between normal or healthy tissue and diseased tissue, as well as better visualization of different structures. Most of the agents in clinical use today are Gd contrast media that shorten the relaxation time of the free water protons. Since these agents are not selective, they are delivered uniformly throughout the extracellular space after intravenous injection [82].

In addition to the use of relaxation-based contrast agents, MR imaging offers a variety of contrast techniques based on the intrinsic properties of tissue, such as coupling to neighboring nuclei, chemical exchange saturation transfer, or flow [46]. Magnetization transfer (MT) contrast uses an off-resonance RF pulse to saturate a broad water signal that lies beneath a sharper bulk water signal in many tissues [83]. This method employs a technique utilizing saturation transfer (ST) mainly via dipolar exchange and has been widely used to produce modified tissue contrast for MR imaging in clinical settings. In the early 1990s, chemical exchange saturation transfer (CEST) was introduced as a new type of method, which has drawn considerable attention as a novel mechanism yielding modified tissue contrast for MR imaging based upon exchangeable protons (-NH, -OH, -SH, etc.) on endogenous or exogenous molecules. Since this method is also a technique utilizing ST but via chemical exchange, it uses an RF pulse at a specific frequency so that the target molecule is selectively saturated, and the saturation is transferred to the bulk water [84]. This method provides more detailed physiological and functional information such as pH and metabolite levels than conventional MR imaging and has gained prominence in the field of molecular imaging [44, 85–90]. This method is a current topic of interest for research using in vivo and in vitro studies into various disorders in addition to oncologic diseases [43, 47–52, 91–95].

CEST Mechanism

Exchangeable solute protons (s) that resonate at a frequency different from the bulk water protons (w) are selectively saturated using an RF pulse. This saturation is subsequently transferred to bulk water where proton exchange between water and solutes takes place (exchange rate) and the water signal becomes slightly attenuated. In view of the low concentration of solute protons (μM to mM range), a single saturation transfer would be insufficient to show any discernable effect on water protons with their concentration of about 110 M. However, because the water pool is much larger than the saturated solute proton pool, each exchanged saturated solute proton is replaced by a non-saturated water proton. If the solute protons have a relatively fast exchange rate (residence time in the millisecond range) and the saturation time is sufficiently long (in the second range), prolonged irradiation leads to substantial enhancement of the saturation effect, which eventually becomes visible on the water signal, thus allowing for indirect imaging of the presence of low-concentration solutes. These frequency-dependent saturation effects are visualized by plotting the water saturation (S_{sat}) normalized by the signal without saturation (S_0) as a function of saturation frequency. This yields what has been named a Z-spectrum or CEST spectrum [47–52, 96]. Such a spectrum is assumed to be symmetrical and is characterized by the magnetization transfer ratio (MTR) at each frequency adjacent to the water frequency, with 0 ppm assigned to the water frequency. The effect of CEST is addressed by employing the symmetry of the water saturation through an MT ratio asymmetry analysis with respect to the water frequency [97]. Such an analysis inherently assumes independent contributions of solute and water protons, which is satisfactory as a first approximation, but need not always be the case. Using the definition in the literature of MTR (= 1 − S_{sat}/S_0), this process is characterized by subtracting MTRs at the negative ($-\Delta\omega$) and positive ($\Delta\omega$) side of frequencies [97]:

$$\begin{aligned}\mathrm{MTR}_{\mathrm{asym}}(\Delta\omega) &= \mathrm{MTR}(\Delta\omega) - \mathrm{MTR}(-\Delta\omega) \\ &= S_{\mathrm{sat}}(-\Delta\omega)/S_0 - S_{\mathrm{sat}}(\Delta\omega)/S_0\end{aligned} \tag{21.3}$$

in which $\Delta\omega$ is the difference between radiation and water frequency. It should be noted that this asymmetry analysis is based on an inherent assumption of symmetry of non-CEST contributions adjacent to the water signal, which often is incorrect, especially in vivo but also in vitro. Therefore, the magnitude of the CEST effect is often determined from the difference in $\mathrm{MTR}_{\mathrm{asym}}$ between the target tissue (e.g., lesion) and the reference tissue (e.g., normal tissue) in many studies [47]. Further, as in the case of MT imaging, it has to be realized that results obtained with this type of quantification are often difficult to reproduce in other research laboratories because, unless saturation efficiency is 100%, the effect depends on the strength of the applied RF field (B1), generally referred to as "power" in MR jargon. This difficulty can be somewhat ameliorated by taking left/right ratios of the signal attenuation but doing this complicates quantification in terms of exchange rates and concentrations.

CEST Classification

CEST constitutes a powerful sensitivity enhancement mechanism in which low-concentration solutes can be visualized through the water signal as described in the preceding section on CEST mechanism. This enhancement, which depends on the agent proton concentration and the rate of exchange, makes the specific design of agents, constructs, and MRI pulse sequences possible for optimization of the contrast based on the two parameters pertinent for enhancement. CEST is therefore inherently suitable as a molecular and cellular imaging approach and can employ both paramagnetic species (exogenous agents) and diamagnetic species (endogenous agents), which has resulted in the names paraCEST and diaCEST, respectively [42, 84–87, 89, 98–100].

This useful classification relates mostly to the magnitude of the difference between chemical shift and that of water, which can be greatly enlarged when using paramagnetic shift agents, thereby allowing for much higher exchange rates to be used while maintaining the slow-intermediate MR exchange regime. For diaCEST compounds the range is generally 0–7 ppm from water (hydroxy [-OH], amine [-NH_2], amide [-NH], and imino [=NH] groups), but this can be extended to 18–19 ppm or even much higher (>50 ppm) through hydrogen bonding or exchange of water molecules. As for nomenclature, early classifications were made on the basis of molecular size, endogenous occurrence, and type of molecular construct, and these characteristics are reflected in the names [101, 102]. In addition, many approaches have been named specifically for the target molecule or mechanism involved by adding CEST to the name, e.g., glycoCEST for glycogen, gagCEST for glycosaminoglycans, and lipoCEST for liposomes [44, 94, 103]. As many of the proposed methods target the same exchange groups, it probably would have been more appropriate to base the names on the type of exchange group, i.e., glycoCEST (i.e., -OH group), gagCEST (i.e., -OH and/or -NH groups), gluCEST (-NH_2 group), and APT (-$CONH_2$ group). However, the types overlap since there are both macromolecular and liposome applications for paraCEST and diaCEST agents and many of the same approaches can be applied to either group. An additional issue is that saturation transfer is only one of many possible magnetic label-transfer approaches, so that the inclusion of "CEST" in the names of the agents is technically incorrect. Although a classification based on the exchange mechanism, namely, atomic (protonic) exchange, molecular exchange, and compartmental exchange, has been proposed, only atomic (protonic) exchange has been tested for other organs than the brain, such as the thorax [48–50, 52, 104–111].

Amide Proton Transfer-Weighted (APTw) Imaging

APTw imaging is one subset of CEST imaging that applies specifically to the chemical exchange between protons of free tissue water (bulk-water) and amide (-NH) groups. It is assumed that amide protons of endogenous mobile proteins and peptides in the cytoplasm are the major source of the APT signal in tissues [87]. This assumption was supported by the finding of a nuclear magnetic resonance (NMR) study that the amide protons of mobile protein/peptide sidechains (Gln, Asn) and backbone amides resonate at 6.8 ppm and 8.2–8.4 ppm (2.1 ppm and 3.5–3.7 ppm downfield of water resonance), respectively [112]. The effect of APT strongly correlates with pH because proton exchange in -NH groups slows dramatically with a decrease in pH [46]. The relationship between pH and the CEST effect (MTR_{asym}) can be expressed in the following equation, which was derived using phosphorus spectroscopy to determine intracellular pH values:

$$pH = 9.4 + \log\left[\frac{MTR_{asym}}{5.73}\right] \tag{21.4}$$

Many studies have used APTw imaging to study ischemia in animal as well as human stroke studies [87, 92, 113]. It has also been reported that such exchangeable protons are more abundant in tumor tissues than in healthy tissues [42, 87]. When applied to rats implanted with 9 L gliosarcoma tumors in the brain, APTw imaging could distinguish between pathology-confirmed regions of tumor and tissue edema, whereas standard T1W, T2W, and FLAIR imaging or DWI could not. Other previous studies have demonstrated that the APT signal increased by 3–4% in tumors compared to peritumoral brain tissue in an experimental rat glial tumor at 4.7 T and human brain tumors at 3 T [112, 114]. Another study of patients with diffuse glioma showed that the APT signal increased with the WHO grade (II to IV) and thus resulted in a clear distinction between low-grade (II) and high-grade (III and IV) tumors [48]. Moreover, Zhou et al. demonstrated in orthotopic murine models that APTw imaging could clearly differentiate viable glioma tissue (hyperintense) from radiation necrosis (hypointense to isointense), as well as that the APT signal of the tumor decreased substantially after radiation [115]. Furthermore, Sagiyama et al. used mouse models of human glioma and found that APTw imaging can detect early tumor response to therapy, which precedes morphological changes [90]. Although the method is sensitive to motion and B0 inhomogeneity, a few studies have applied APTw imaging to the thorax. Togao et al. conducted an animal study and reported that APTw imaging can be used to quantify lung tumors in the moving lung. They reported that the measured APT effect was higher in tumors showing more active proliferation than others and suggested that APTw imaging has the potential to serve as a characterization test to differentiate type or grade of lung cancer noninvasively, which may eventually reduce the need for invasive needle biopsy or resection for lung cancer [47].

Clinical Application of Quantitative MR Imaging for Pulmonary Nodules, Masses, or Lung Cancer

Quantitative Management for Pulmonary Nodules or Masses

Unenhanced MRI

Pulmonary nodule or mass characterizations are still major challenges for clinicians. Currently, chest radiography or CT is utilized worldwide for lung cancer or nodule detection in routine clinical practice or lung cancer screening. After detection, however, characterization of the potential of the nodules or masses for malignancy is crucial. Assessments of a variety of MR sequences for pulmonary nodule characterization [5, 11, 14, 16, 34–36, 39, 116–118] have determined that only two different ways for nodule characterization are effective, one unenhanced and the other using CE-MRI methods. Some nodules or masses such as hamartomas, bronchial atresia, or aspergillomas show typical signal intensities on T1- and T2-weighted spin-echo (SE) or turbo SE imaging and are easily differentiated from other nodules [5, 11, 14, 16, 34–36, 39, 116–118]. In the early 1990s and thereafter, however, most nodules have been found to show low signal intensity on T1-weighted images and intermediate or relatively high signal intensity on T2-weighted images. Moreover, it has been determined that two other proposed MR sequences, CE-T1-weighted SE and turbo SE imaging, have limited utility for differentiating malignant from benign nodules such as tuberculomas or hamartomas [5, 11, 14, 16, 34–36, 39, 116–118]. Conventional MRI was therefore considered to have limited clinical utility until new unenhanced or dynamic CE-MRI was introduced in the 2000s.

During the last few decades, three types of unenhanced MRI for pulmonary nodule or mass assessments have been introduced and recommended: DWI, T1-weighted short inversioin time (TI) or Tau inversion recovery (STIR) turbo SE imaging, and APTw imaging, which is a type of CEST imaging. DWI has become the most widely used method for a variety of oncologic patients, and many investigators have referred in their publications to its capability for distinguishing malignant from benign nodules or masses [5, 11, 14, 16, 34–36, 39, 116–118]. A meta-analysis revealed that DWI yielded pooled sensitivity and specificity of 83% and 80%, respectively, for differentiating malignant from benign lesions [119], while another meta-analysis compared the differentiation capabilities of DWI and FDG-PET/CT [120]. The latter study determined that the pooled sensitivity and specificity of DWI were 0.85 (95% confidence interval [CI] 0.77–0.90) and 0.91 (95% CI 0.82–0.96), while those of FDG-PET/CT were 0.82 (95% CI 0.70–0.90) and 0.81 (95% CI 0.72–0.87), respectively. Moreover, the area under the ROC curve (AUC) of DWI was 0.94 (95% CI 0.91–0.96), which was not significantly different although slightly larger than that of 0.87 (95% CI 0.84–0.90) for PET/CT ($Z = 1.58$, $p > 0.05$). The potential of DWI for differentiating malignant from benign pulmonary lesions may thus be similar to that of FDG-PET/CT and render it suitable for use in routine clinical practice.

T1-weighted STIR turbo SE imaging was also introduced as a promising approach, whether or not in direct comparison with DWI, and with superior potential for differentiating malignant from benign nodules or subtyping lung cancer [5, 11, 14, 16, 34–36, 39, 116–118, 121–123]. The nodule detection capability of STIR turbo SE imaging had been frequently compared with that of other MR sequences as well as of multidetector row computed tomography (MDCT), but Koyama et al. were the first to directly compare the nodule detection rates and quantitative differentiation capabilities of STIR turbo SE imaging, other MR sequences, and MDCT [121]. Their study found the overall detection rate of each of the MR sequences (82.5%) was significantly lower than that of MDCT (97.0%, $p < 0.05$), although the detection rate for malignant nodules showed no significant difference ($p > 0.05$). Moreover, the diagnostic capability of STIR turbo SE imaging was found to be significantly higher than that of other MR sequences ($p < 0.05$). Although STIR uses semiquantitative analysis methods, it has been suggested that it is very sensitive to changes in T1 and T2 and makes it possible for some T1-dependent decay to be substituted for T2-dependent decay in equivalent SE or turbo SE sequences [121–123]. Because many pathological lesions show an increase in both T1 and T2, the addition of these two types of contrasts to the STIR sequence yields a higher net tissue contrast [121–123]. Therefore, STIR turbo SE imaging should be considered to function as an unenhanced and quantitative MRI in this setting.

A comparison of the capabilities of DWI and STIR turbo SE imaging for detection and subtype classification of non-small cell lung cancer (NSCLC) showed that the detection rate of DWI was significantly lower than that of STIR turbo SE imaging ($p < 0.05$). Although the ADC values showed no significant difference regarding subtype classification, the contrast ratios (CRs) on STIR turbo SE imaging of bronchioalveolar carcinomas (BACs) were significantly lower than those of other types ($p < 0.05$). When threshold values for differentiating BACs from others were adopted, the sensitivity and accuracy of DWI proved to be significantly lower than those of STIR turbo SE imaging ($P < 0.05$) [122]. Moreover, Koyama et al. found to be more effective than STIR turbo SE imaging for differentiation of small cell lung cancer (SCLC) from NSCLC [123]. This study found significant differences between mean ADC values ($p < 0.001$) and mean CRs ($p = 0.003$). With the adoption of feasible threshold values, the specificity (85.7%) and accuracy (85.7%) of DWI turned out to be higher than those of STIR turbo SE imaging (specificity, 63.3%, $p = 0.001$, and accuracy, 66.1%, $p = 0.001$). Moreover, the accuracy of the combination of the two indexes (94.6%; $p = 0.04$) could be significantly improved as compared with DWI alone. Therefore, this study suggested that DWI should be considered more suitable for the differentiation of SCLC from NSCLC than STIR turbo SE imaging, while their combination can significantly improve accuracy in this setting [123].

The third type of unenhanced MRI, first reported in 2016, is APTw imaging for evaluation of pulmonary nodules or masses using a novel contrast enhancement method based on the CEST effect [49, 50]. The first clinical study using APTw imaging for differentiating malignant from benign thoracic lesions was published in 2016 [49]. In this study, measurements on APTw imaging with a magnetization transfer ratio asymmetry (MTR_{asym}) at 3.5 ppm of malignant tumors were significantly larger than those for benign lesions ($p = 0.008$). Moreover, measurements of other thoracic malignancies on APTw imaging obtained with MTR_{asym} at 3.5 ppm were significantly larger than those of lung cancer ($p = 0.005$), while MTR_{asym} at 3.5 ppm of adenocarcinoma was significantly higher than that of squamous cell carcinoma ($p = 0.02$). Furthermore, the threshold values for differentiation between malignant and benign thoracic lesions, sensitivity, specificity, and accuracy, were 100%, 75.0%, and 90.5% (19 of 21 lesions), respectively. Finally, for the threshold values for differentiation of lung cancer from other thoracic malignancies, the corresponding values were 100%, 75.0%, and 92.3%, while those for the threshold values for differentiation of adenocarcinoma and squamous cell carcinoma were all 100%. The aforementioned results has led to the suggestion that APTw imaging may constitute the next promising technique for management of thoracic lesions by using quantitatively assessed unenhanced MRI in routine clinical practice [49].

A comparison of APTw imaging, DWI, FDG-PET/CT, and combined methods for differentiation of malignant from benign pulmonary nodules has resulted in another paper with productive results published in 2018 [50]. This study determined that the specificity of MTR_{asym} at 3.5 ppm and SUV_{max} was significantly higher than that of ADC ($p < 0.05$), although the sensitivity of ADC was significantly higher than that of MTR_{asym} at 3.5 ppm ($p = 0.002$) and SUV_{max} ($p = 0.004$). Moreover, sensitivity of MTR_{asym} at 3.5 ppm combined with SUV_{max} was significantly higher than that of MTR_{asym} at 3.5 ppm ($p = 0.001$) and of SUV_{max} ($p = 0.002$) alone. In addition, specificity and accuracy of the combination of MTR_{asym} at 3.5 ppm and SUV_{max} were significantly higher than those of ADC (specificity, $p = 0.002$; accuracy, $p = 0.008$). APTw imaging thus appears to be as effective as DWI and FDG-PET/CT for differentiation of malignant from benign nodules and should be combined with other metabolic information provided by FDG-PET/CT, although further investigations are warranted to determine the real significance of APTw imaging in routine clinical practice [50] (Fig. 21.1). Therefore, unenhanced MRI should be considered effective, primarily for evaluating pulmonary nodules or masses, and further investigations using MRI are being planned for the use of appropriate contrast media administration.

Dynamic CE-MRI

A comparison with unenhanced MRI resulted in dynamic CE-MRI with conventional SE, turbo SE, or gradient-echo (GRE) sequences being deemed effective until the early 1990s [54–63]. However, these techniques were comparatively time-consuming and had less temporal or spatial resolution than 3D dynamic first-pass CE-MR imaging with ultrafast echo time (TE), which has been in use together with the dynamic first-pass CE-perfusion MRI technique since 2002 [7–11, 15, 16, 20]. The findings of a meta-analysis indicated the diagnostic performance of semiquantitatively evaluated dynamic CT and MRI was not significantly different from that of FDG-PET, although studies included for meta analysis for PET were too much and previous manuscripts in comparison with dynamic CT or MRI [63]. Semiquantitative and quantitative dynamic CE-MRI with ultrashort TE have therefore been undergoing tests during the last few decades and reportedly feature greater specificity and accuracy than dynamic CT or FDG-PET/CT [10, 15, 19] (Fig. 21.2). However, a study that directly compared the capability for differentiating malignant from benign nodules of dynamic first-pass CE-perfusion ADCT using the quantitative method with that of MRI using the semiquantitative method as well as that of FDG-PET/CT found that all indexes showed significant differences between malignant and benign nodules with low biologic activity ($p = 0.0001$). The AUC for total perfusion on dynamic first-pass CE-perfusion ADCT was significantly larger than that for other indexes ($0.0006 \leq p \leq 0.04$). The specificity and accuracy of total perfusion obtained with dynamic first-pass CE-perfusion ADCT were significantly higher than those attained with the maximum relative enhancement ratio from dynamic first-pass CE-perfusion MRI with ultrashort TE (specificity, $p < 0.0001$; accuracy, $p < 0.0001$), slope of enhancement ratio (specificity, $p < 0.0001$; accuracy, $p < 0.0001$), or with SUV_{max} (specificity, $p < 0.0001$; accuracy, $p < 0.0001$). These findings therefore determined that quantitatively analyzed dynamic first-pass CE-perfusion ADCT was more specific and accurate than semiquantitatively analyzed dynamic first-pass CE-perfusion MRI or FDG-PET/CT for the diagnosis of solitary pulmonary nodules in routine clinical practice [15]. On the other hand, when the same mathematical model was used for quantitative evaluation of dynamic first-pass CE-perfusion ADCT and for MRI with ultrashort TE, another study [19] demonstrated that AUCs of total perfusion on dynamic first-pass CE-perfusion ADCT (AUC = 0.89) and of MRI with ultrashort TE (AUC = 0.88) were significantly larger than those of systemic arterial perfusion ADCT and of MRI with ultrashort TE ($p < 0.05$). Moreover, the accuracy of total perfusion for dynamic first-pass CE-perfusion ADCT (87.3%) and of dynamic first-pass CE-perfusion MRI with ultrashort TE (87.3%) was significantly higher than that of systemic arterial perfusion for the two methods (77.5%, $p = 0.02$) and of SUV_{max} (78.9%, $p = 0.03$). Furthermore,

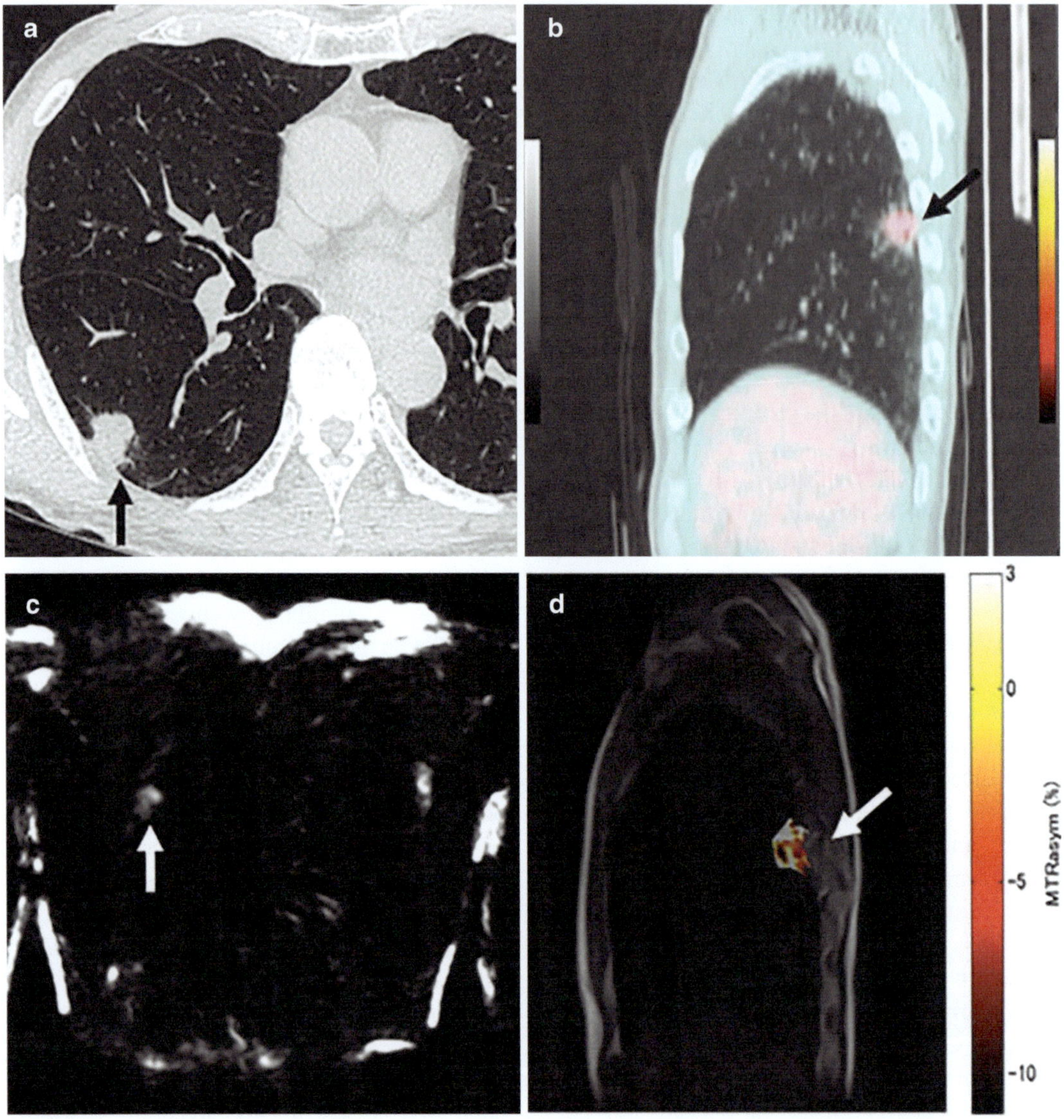

Fig. 21.1 A 69-year-old female with invasive adenocarcinoma. (Permission obtained from reference [50]). (**a**) Thin-section CT shows a nodule (arrow) with pleural indentation, notch, and spicula in the right lower lobe. (**b**) FDG-PET/CT (L, PET/CT without ROI; R, PET/CT with ROI) shows a nodule with high FDG uptake (arrow). SUV_{max} of this nodule measured 2.6. This case was assessed as false-negative on PET/CT. However, when combined with MTR_{asym} at 3.5 ppm, this case was reevaluated as true-positive. (**c**) DWI obtained with a FASE sequence with b value of 1000s/ mm^2 (L, DWI without ROI; R, DWI with ROI) shows the nodule with a high signal intensity (arrow). ADC of this nodule was 1.18×10^{-3} mm^2/sec. This case was evaluated as true-positive on DWI. (**d**) APTw imaging (L, APTw image without ROI; R, APTw image with ROI) shows the nodule with a high MTR_{asym} of 3.5 ppm (arrow), which was 1.99%. This case was assessed as true-positive on APTw imaging. In addition, these findings could improve the diagnostic performance of PET/CT for this case

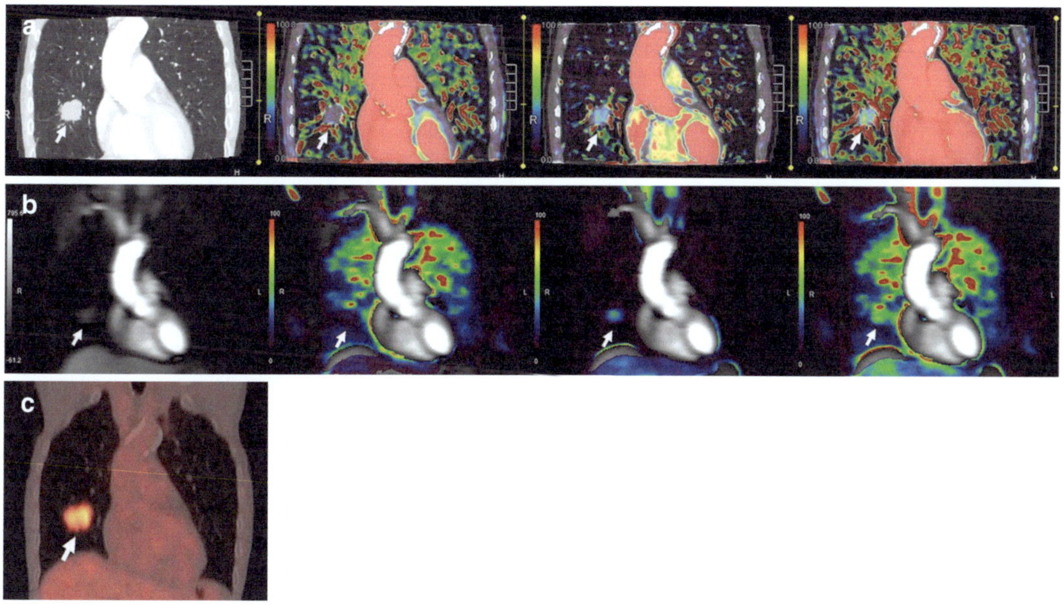

Fig. 21.2 An 80-year-old female patient with adenocarcinoma showing a lepidic pattern. (Permission obtained from reference [19]). (**a**) (L to R: thin-section multiplanar reformatted (MPR) image from thin-section CT data and from pulmonary arterial perfusion, systemic arterial perfusion, and total perfusion maps, respectively). Thin-section MPR image shows a nodule (arrow) with a diameter of 21 mm in the right middle lobe. Dynamic first-pass CE-perfusion ADCT assessed with the dual-input maximum slope method yielded perfusion maps which also show a nodule (arrow). Pulmonary arterial perfusion, systemic arterial perfusion, and total perfusion were 13.0 ml/100 ml/min, 25.9 ml/100 ml/min, and 39.0 ml/100 ml/min, respectively. Application of the three feasible threshold values led to an assessment of this nodule as malignant or as requiring further intervention and treatment. This case was determined to be true-positive for all perfusion indices. (**b**) (L to R: source image, pulmonary arterial perfusion, systemic arterial perfusion, and total perfusion maps). Dynamic first-pass CE-perfusion MRI with ultrashort TE assessed with the same dual-input maximum slope method produced perfusion maps, which also show a nodule (arrow). Pulmonary arterial perfusion, systemic arterial perfusion, and total perfusion were 11.0 ml/100 ml/min, 31.4 ml/100 ml/min, and 42.5 ml/100 ml/min, respectively. Application of the three feasible threshold values led to an assessment of this nodule as malignant or as requiring further intervention and treatment. This case was found to be true-positive for all perfusion indices. (c) FDG-PET/CT shows a nodule (arrow) with high uptake of FDG and SUV_{max} evaluated as 4.0. Application of the feasible threshold value led to assessment of this nodule as malignant or as requiring further intervention and treatment. This case was true-positive based on high SUV_{max}

determination of the diagnostic capability of each radiological index for differentiating nodules requiring aggressive intervention and treatment from nodules needing only follow-up examination showed that the accuracy of total perfusion for dynamic first-pass CE-perfusion ADCT (90.1%) and of MRI with ultrashort TE (88.7%) was significantly higher than that of systemic arterial perfusion for the two methods (80.3%, $p < 0.05$) and of SUV_{max} (78.9%, $p < 0.05$). These findings suggest that, when the same quantitative analysis method dynamic is used for both techniques, first-pass CE-perfusion ADCT and MRI with ultrashort TE should be considered as having similar potential capabilities or being superior to FDG-PET/CT in these settings [19]. Moreover, quantitatively assessed dynamic first-pass CE-perfusion matrixes from ADCT or MRI with ultrashort TE are currently considered as equal or superior to FDG-PET/CT in its potential for differentiating malignant from benign nodules or distinguishing nodules requiring aggressive intervention and treatment from nodules needing only follow-up examination [7–19]. Therefore, dynamic first-pass CE perfusion ADCT or MRI with ultrashort TE can be expected to be more frequently used for management of pulmonary nodules or masses in routine clinical practice.

Quantitative Assessment of N-Stage in Lung Cancer

Since the RDOG report was published in 1991, determining the superiority of T-category evaluation for conventional T1-weighted SE imaging to that of CT was inadequate [6], CT and FDG-PET or PET/CT have come into use for lung cancer staging (tumor, node, metastasis, or TNM system), while MRI has been rarely employed in routine clinical practice. Although MRI had originally been recommended as superior to CT for T-category assessments [5, 11, 34–37, 39, 116–118, 124–128], quantitatively or semiquantitatively assessed STIR turbo SE imaging or FASE imaging and DWI are now seen as game changers for N-stage evaluation with a better diagnostic performance than FDG-PET or PET/CT, not only for NSCLC but also for SCLC and other thoracic tumors such as thymic epithelial tumors or malignant mesotheliomas [30–39, 129–137]. Moreover, it has been determined that STIR turbo SE imaging or FASE imaging is more sensitive and accurate than DWI or FDG-PET/CT, and these techniques have been recommended for detection of metastatic lymph nodes as a preoperative examination procedure for NSCLC patients [30–39, 129–137]. In addition, when MRI and PET/CT data can be used, inclusive criteria (positive for nodal metastasis on either MRI or PET/CT) improve the sensitivity for detecting lymph node metastasis compared with that of PET/CT alone and may thus reduce the number of unnecessary open thoracotomies, mediastinoscopies, or other interventions [133]. Finally, several meta-analyses have ascertained that the diagnostic performance of MRI is superior to that of PET/CT on a per-node and per-patient basis [138–141]. Table 21.1 shows a summary of diagnostic performances for N-category evaluations on STIR turbo SE imaging or DWI. In addition, research results reported thus far suggest that MRI can function as a substitute or in a complementary role for lung cancer staging, especially N-category evaluation, with FDG-PET/CT in routine clinical practice.

Evaluation or Prediction of Therapeutic Effect of Conservative Therapy for Lung Cancer

Currently, the evaluation of treatment response in oncology depends on the response evaluation criteria in solid tumors (RECIST), which in turn is based on changes in size [142]. CE-T1-weighted imaging, dynamic CE-MRI including dynamic first-pass CE-perfusion MRI with ultrashort TE, and DWI are alternative procedures which have been found to be effective for predicting and evaluating treatment response in patients with lung cancer [9, 34–36, 39, 142–152]. Therapeutic effect prediction and evaluation were first performed in 2000 using CE-T1-weighted imaging to assess the importance of tumor necrosis for prognosis [143]. In a study of 90 patients with NSCLC, changes in tumor necrosis or cavity size concurrently with a reduction in tumor size showed better correlation with prognosis than did a reduction in size only [143]. Dynamic CE-perfusion MRI for evaluation of tumor angiogenesis is another potentially effective technique for patients with NSCLC. In a study by Fujimoto and colleagues [144], a statistically significant difference was established between the slope values of vascular endothelial growth factor (VEGF)-positive and VEGF-negative tumors ($p < 0.01$), while overall survival of patients with VEGF-positive tumors was found to be significantly shorter than that of patients with VEGF-negative tumors ($p < 0.01$). A study to evaluate the role of dynamic CE-MRI in a hybrid 3 T PET/MRI system for assessment of response in patients with NSCLC receiving radiation therapy found that the percentage reduction in K_{trans} at a mean of 6 weeks after stereotactic body radiation therapy (SBRT) correlated with the percentage reduction in tumor size 3 months after SBRT [152]. Dynamic first-pass CE-perfusion MRI with ultrashort TE may also play a possible role in the detection of tumor recurrence [9]. In a

Table 21.1 Summary of diagnostic performance by N-category evaluation for quantitatively and semiquantitatively assessed MRI

Author	Field strength (Tesla)	Imaging method	Analysis	MRI			FDG-PET/CT			CT		
				SE (%)	SP (%)	AC (%)	SE (%)	SP (%)	AC (%)	SE (%)	SP (%)	AC (%)
Takenaka [129]	1.5	STIR	Per node	100	96	96	N/A			52	91	83
		T1WI		52	91	83						
		STIR	Per patient	100	75	88				46	75	60
		T1WI		46	75	60						
Ohno [130]		STIR	Per patient	88 or 93	86 or 87	86 or 89	N/A			53	83	72
Ohno [131]		STIR	Per node	86.3 or 89	97.2 or 99	96.3 or 98.2	80.8 or 82.3	95.8 or 96.2	65.9 or 94.6	N/A		
			Per patient	83.7 or 90.1	90.3 or 93.1	87.8 or 92.2	74.4 or 76.7	87.5	82.6 or 83.5			
Morikawa [132]		STIR	Per node	93.9 or 96.3	67.3 or 70.9	84.7	86.6 or 90.2	65.5 or 94.5	80.3 or 89.8	N/A		
			Per patient	N/A	N/A	N/A	86.9 or 90.2	65.6 or 96.9	81.7 or 90.3			
Nakayama [30]		STIR	Per patient	61.5	98.1	91	N/A					
		DWI	Per patient	69.2	100	94						
Usuda [31]		DWI	Per node	75	99	95	48	97	90	N/A		
			Per patient	N/A		71	N/A		65			
Ohno [32]		STIR	Per node	80, 81.5 or 83.7	84.4, 85.9 or 86.7	82.2, 83.7 or 85.1	71.9 or 75.6	88.8 or 88.9	80.4 or 82.2	N/A		
		DWI		72.6 or 74.8	87.4	80 or 81.1						
		STIR	Per patient	77.4 or 82.8	88.5 or 89.2	84.4 or 86.8	69.9 or 74.2	91.7 or 92.4	83.6 or 85.6			
		DWI		71 or 74.2	89.8 or 90.4	82.8 or 84.4						
Kim [33]		Combined DWI, T2WI, or PET/CT	Per node	44 or 69	93 or 99	89	46	96	87	N/A		
			Per patient	N/A		71	N/A		63			

(continued)

Table 21.1 (continued)

Author	Field strength (Tesla)	Imaging method	Analysis	MRI SE (%)	MRI SP (%)	MRI AC (%)	FDG-PET/CT SE (%)	FDG-PET/CT SP (%)	FDG-PET/CT AC (%)	CT SE (%)	CT SP (%)	CT AC (%)
Ohno [38]	3	STIR	Per node	82.1	98.7	90.4	57.7	97.4	77.6	N/A		
		FASE-DWI		82.1	98.7	90.4						
		EPI-DWI		60.3	98.7	79.5						
		STIR	Operative vs. inoperative	100	88	89.5	50	89.2	84.2			
		FASE-DWI		100	88	89.5						
		EPI-DWI		75	89.2	87.4						
Ohno [41]		STIR	Per node	86.8	60.5 or 66.7	73.7 or 76.8	78.9 or 85.1	57 or 71.1	71 or 75	N/A		
		Actual DWI		82.5 or 83.3	60.5 or 66.7	71.5 or 75						
		ADC map from aDWI		81 or 82.5	60.5 or 71.9	71.5 or 76.8						
		cDWI		86.8 or 87.7	60.5 or 71.9	74.1 or 79.4						
		STIR	N-category	N/A		86.9 or 90.6	N/A		82.9 or 85.3			
		aDWI				84.5 or 86.9						
		ADC map from aDWI				84.5 or 86.9						
		cDWI				86.5 or 90.2						

SE sensitivity, *SP* specificity, *AC* accuracy, *STIR* short inversion time (TI) or Tau inversion recovery, *T1WI* T1-weighted imaging, *DWI* diffusion-weighted imaging, *FASE-DWI* DWI obtained with FASE sequence, *EPI-DWI* DWI obtained with EPI sequence, *aDWI* actual DWI, *ADC* apparent diffusion coefficient (ADC), *cDWI* computed DWI, *N/A* not applicable

study of 114 patients with NSCLC treated with chemoradiotherapy, semiquantitatively assessed indexes for dynamic first-pass CE-perfusion MRI with ultrashort TE showed significant differences between the local control and the local failure group ($p < 0.05$). Application of the feasible threshold value resulted in values of 90.9% for sensitivity and 91.3% for specificity for differentiation between the two groups. Moreover, when the same threshold value was used for estimating progression after therapy, the mean survival period of patients whose slope of enhancement was equal to or less than 0.08/s was significantly longer than that of patients with a slope of enhancement greater than 0.08/s ($p < 0.01$) [9]. Furthermore, Seki et al. directly compared therapeutic effect prediction capability of quantitatively assessed dynamic first-pass CE-perfusion ADCT and MRI with ultrashort TE, which were analyzed using the same mathematical model, and of FDG-PET/CT for NSCLC patients treated with conservative therapy [20]. This study found that the AUCs for total perfusion on ADCT and on MRI with ultrashort TE were significantly larger than that for pulmonary arterial perfusion ($P < 0.05$). Moreover, mean PFS and OS of the responder and nonresponder groups were significantly different for total and systemic arterial perfusions using each of the dynamic first-pass CE-perfusion methods ($p < 0.05$), although FDG-PET/CT showed a significant difference only in mean OS between the two groups ($p < 0.05$). Therefore, quantitatively assessed dynamic first-pass CE-perfusion ADCT and MR imaging are equally or more effective for early prediction of treatment response in NSCLC patients treated with chemoradiotherapy [20] (Fig. 21.3).

In addition to dynamic CE-MRI with ultra-short TE, DWI with quantitative evaluation with ADC may also be useful for the evaluation or prediction of therapeutic response or prognosis for lung cancer patients treated with conservative therapy [146, 147]. Yabuuchi et al. directly compared the capability of dynamic CE-MRI and DWI for early response evaluation after chemotherapy of NSCLC and determined that there was significant correlation only between early changes on ADC and final tumor size reduction rate ($r^2 = 0.41$, $p = 0.00025$) [146]. Moreover, the median progression-free survival (PFS) period for the group showing a satisfactory increase in ADC was 12.1 months, and that for the group with no major change or a decrease of ADC was 6.67 months ($p = 0.021$), while median overall survival (OS) for the two groups was 22.4 and 12.3 months, respectively ($p = 0.048$) [146]. They therefore concluded that ADC seems to be a promising tool for monitoring early response to or predicting prognosis after chemotherapy for NSCLC [146]. These results have been recently confirmed in another study by Weiss and colleagues [150], who found that, after serial DWI performed during chemoradiotherapy, the increase seen on ADC for patients with OS of

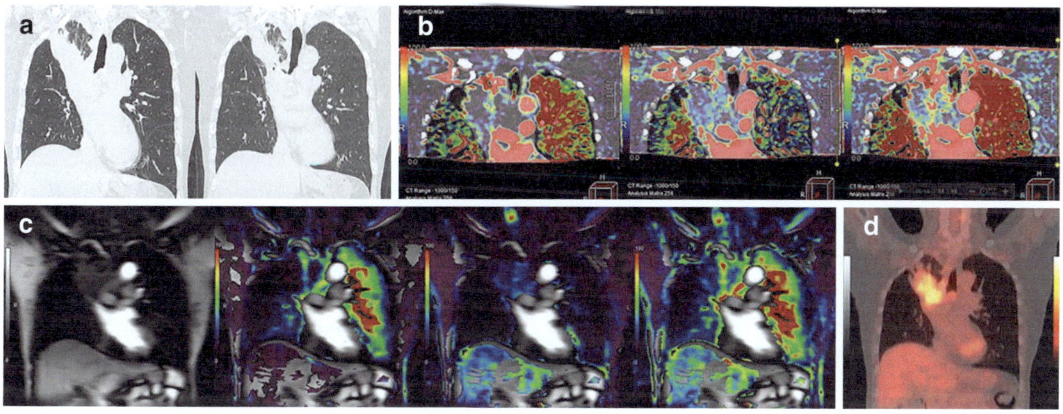

Fig. 21.3 An 81-year-old male patient with squamous cell carcinoma treated with chemoradiotherapy and assessed as NC. Progression-free and overall survival of 15 and 24 months, respectively. (Permission obtained from reference [20]). (**a**) Thin-section MPR images from thin-section CT data obtained (L) pre- and (R) post-treatment at lung window settings show lung cancer in the right upper lobe. This case was assessed as NC based on response evaluation criteria in solid tumors (RECIST ver.1.1). (**b**) Perfusion maps derived from dynamic first-pass CE-perfusion area-detector CT assessed with the dual-input maximum slope method (L to R: pulmonary arterial perfusion, systemic arterial perfusion, and total perfusion maps) for the same targeted lesion. Pulmonary arterial perfusion, systemic arterial perfusion, and total perfusion were 13.6, 18.9, and 32.5 ml/100 ml/min, respectively. This case was assessed as a RECIST-based nonresponder for systemic arterial and total perfusions, and as true-positive. (**c**) Source image and perfusion maps derived from dynamic first-pass CE-perfusion MR imaging assessed with the dual-input maximum slope method (L to R: source image, pulmonary arterial perfusion, systemic arterial perfusion, and total perfusion maps) for the same targeted lesion. Pulmonary arterial perfusion, systemic arterial perfusion, and total perfusion were 9.2, 28.9, and 38.1 ml/100 ml/min, respectively. This case was also assessed as a RECIST-based nonresponder for systemic arterial and total perfusions, and as true-positive. However, this case was evaluated as responder and as false-positive on the basis of pulmonary arterial perfusion findings. (**d**) FDG PET/CT shows high uptake of FDG, and SUV_{max} was evaluated as 4.7. This case was evaluated as a RECIST responder and assessed as false-negative. PR, partial response; MPR, multiplanar reformatted; RECIST, response evaluation criteria in solid tumor; CE, contrast enhanced; SUV, standardized uptake value; PET, positron emission tomography

less than 12 months was lower than that for patients with longer survival ($p < 0.05$).

In another study of therapeutic evaluation, an assessment of therapeutic effect prediction based on findings from DWI and FDG-PET/CT reported that the performance of ADC for distinguishing partial response (PR) from stable disease or progressive disease (SD or PD) in NSCLC patient groups was better than that based on the maximum standardized uptake value (SUV_{max}) obtained with FDG-PET/CT [147]. Moreover, the AUC for ADC (AUC = 0.84) was significantly larger than that for SUV_{max} (AUC = 0.64, $p < 0.05$). The application of feasible threshold values resulted in specificity (44.4%) and accuracy (76.6%) of DWI becoming significantly higher than those of FDG-PET/CT (specificity, 11.1%, $p < 0.05$, and accuracy, 67.2%, $p < 0.05$). This suggests that DWI may have superior potential to that of FDG-PET/CT for prediction of tumor response in NSCLC patients to conservative therapy before chemoradiotherapy [147].

In addition to quantitatively assessed dynamic first-pass CE-perfusion MRI with ultrashort TE and DWI, the capability of APTw imaging for prediction of therapeutic effect was also directly compared with that of DWI and FDG-PET/CT to identify significant predictors for PFS and OS of stage III NSCLC patients treated with chemoradiotherapy [51] (Fig. 21.4). In this study [51], MTR_{asym} at 3.5 ppm (hazard ratio [HR] = 0.70) and SUV_{max} (HR = 1.41) were identified as significant predictors for PFS, while tumor staging (HR = 0.57) was also found to be a significant predictor for OS. This led to the conclusion that the performance of APTw imaging was potentially as good as that of DWI or FDG-PET/CT for predicting the therapeutic effect of chemoradiotherapy for stage III NSCLC patients [51].

Although the potential of each quantitative method for therapeutic effect evaluation or prediction as well as recurrence prediction has been established during the last few decades, further investigations with larger prospective cohorts or stronger evidence are warranted for future applications of the method for lung cancer patients treated with conservative therapies.

Conclusion

During the last few decades, advancements of MR systems, sequences and reconstruction methods, utilization of contrast media, and application of various software for quantitative or semiquantitative analyses have improved the efficacy of lung MRI for various pulmonary diseases. The Fleischner Society as well as the Japanese Society of Magnetic Resonance in Medicine recently published new reposition papers for encouraging the use of lung MRI in routine clinical practice. Moreover, lung cancer is considered one of the most suitable clinical indications for lung MRI, and many investigators are attempting to provide clinical evidence for the efficacy of various MR techniques with and without the use of quantitative methods. In addition, recent advances in MRI as well as dealing with a limited number of clinical problems for physicians have resulted in more opportunities than for CT or FDG-PET/CT for clinical applications of lung MRI as a substitute or in complementary roles for management of lung cancer patients. Although CT has so far remained the principal imaging tool for routine radiological examination of lung cancer patients, quantitatively assessed MRI may emerge in certain situations as the clinical standard or show major potential for changing patient care. Therefore, MRIs with and without quantitative analyses should be considered important tools capable of providing unique physiological, pathophysiological, and morphological information about relaxation time or water molecule diffusion-based imaging as well as metabolic information concerning patients with lung cancer.

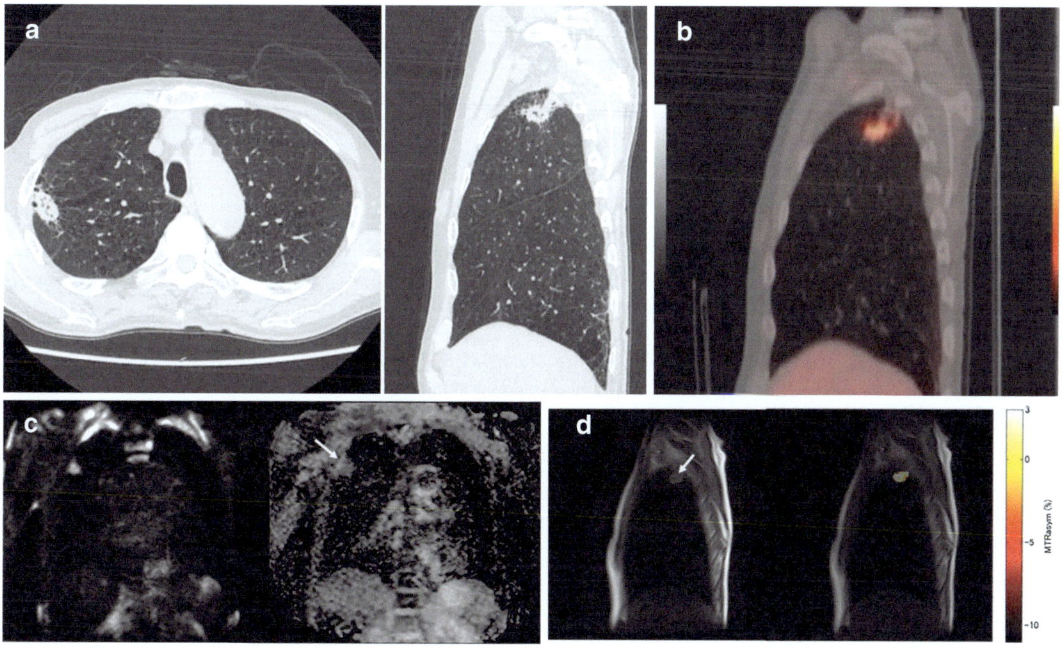

Fig. 21.4 A 62-year-old male with invasive adenocarcinoma and classified as responder. (Permission obtained from reference [52]). (**a**) Thin-section CT shows a nodule with a notch and spicula in the right upper lobe. This nodule was pathologically diagnosed as an invasive adenocarcinoma. (**b**) FDG-PET/CT shows a nodule with high FDG uptake in the right upper lobe. (**c**) (L, diffusion-weighted image obtained by FASE sequence at a b value of 1000 s/mm^2; R, ADC map): The nodule showed high signal intensity and relatively low ADC. (**d**) (L, original image for CEST imaging; R, MTR_{asym} at 3.5 ppm map): Original image for APTw imaging of the nodule (arrow) in the right upper lobe. APTw/CEST image for MTR_{asym} on the 3.5 ppm map shows the nodule with a high MTR_{asym} of 3.5 ppm

References

1. Yankeelov TE, Mankoff DA, Schwartz LH, et al. Quantitative imaging in cancer clinical trials. Clin Cancer Res. 2016;22(2):284–90.
2. UyBico SJ, Wu CC, Suh RD, Le NH, Brown K, Krishnam MS. Lung cancer staging essentials: the new TNM staging system and potential imaging pitfalls. Radiographics. 2010;30(5):1163–81.
3. Halpern BS, Schiepers C, Weber WA, et al. Presurgical staging of non-small cell lung cancer: positron emission tomography, integrated positron emission tomography/CT, and software image fusion. Chest. 2005;128(4):2289–97.
4. Ohno Y, Koyama H, Lee HY, Yoshikawa T, Sugimura K. Magnetic resonance imaging (MRI) and positron emission tomography (PET)/MRI for lung cancer staging. J Thorac Imaging. 2016;31(4):215–27.
5. Ohno Y, Ozawa Y, Koyama H, et al. State of the art MR imaging for lung cancer TNM stage evaluation. Cancers (Basel). 2023;15(3):950.
6. Webb WR, Gatsonis C, Zerhouni EA, et al. CT and MR imaging in staging non-small cell bronchogenic carcinoma: report of the Radiologic Diagnostic Oncology Group. Radiology. 1991;178(3):705–13.
7. Ohno Y, Hatabu H, Takenaka D, Adachi S, Kono M, Sugimura K. Solitary pulmonary nodules: potential role of dynamic MR imaging in management initial experience. Radiology. 2002;224(2):503–11.
8. Ohno Y, Hatabu H, Takenaka D, et al. Dynamic MR imaging: value of differentiating subtypes of peripheral small adenocarcinoma of the lung. Eur J Radiol. 2004;52(2):144–50.
9. Ohno Y, Nogami M, Higashino T, et al. Prognostic value of dynamic MR imaging for non small-cell lung cancer patients after chemoradiotherapy. J Magn Reson Imaging. 2005;21(6):775–83.
10. Ohno Y, Koyama H, Takenaka D, et al. Dynamic MRI, dynamic multidetector-row computed tomography (MDCT), and coregistered 2-[fluorine-18]-fluoro 2 deoxy-D-glucose-positron emission tomography (FDG-PET)/CT: comparative study of capability for management of pulmonary nodules. J Magn Reson Imaging. 2008;27(6):1284–95.

11. Sieren JC, Ohno Y, Koyama H, Sugimura K, McLennan G. Recent technological and application developments in computed tomography and magnetic resonance imaging for improved pulmonary nodule detection and lung cancer staging. J Magn Reson Imaging. 2010;32(6):1353–69.
12. Ohno Y, Koyama H, Matsumoto K, et al. Differentiation of malignant and benign pulmonary nodules with quantitative first-pass 320-detector row perfusion CT versus FDG PET/CT. Radiology. 2011;258(2):599–609.
13. Ohno Y, Nishio M, Koyama H, et al. Comparison of quantitatively analyzed dynamic area-detector CT using various mathematic methods with FDG PET/CT in management of solitary pulmonary nodules. AJR Am J Roentgenol. 2013;200(6):W593–602.
14. Ohno Y, Nishio M, Koyama H, et al. Dynamic contrast-enhanced CT and MRI for pulmonary nodule assessment. AJR Am J Roentgenol. 2014;202(3):515–29.
15. Ohno Y, Nishio M, Koyama H, et al. Solitary pulmonary nodules: comparison of dynamic first-pass contrast-enhanced perfusion area-detector CT, dynamic first-pass contrast-enhanced MR imaging, and FDG PET/CT. Radiology. 2015;274(2):563–75.
16. Ohno Y, Koyama H, Lee HY, Miura S, Yoshikawa T, Sugimura K. Contrast-enhanced CT- and MRI-based perfusion assessment for pulmonary diseases: basics and clinical applications. Diagn Interv Radiol. 2016;22(5):407–21.
17. Ohno Y, Koyama H, Fujisawa Y, et al. Dynamic contrast-enhanced perfusion area detector CT for non-small cell lung cancer patients: influence of mathematical models on early prediction capabilities for treatment response and recurrence after chemoradiotherapy. Eur J Radiol. 2016;85(1):176–86.
18. Ohno Y, Fujisawa Y, Koyama H, et al. Dynamic contrast-enhanced perfusion area-detector CT assessed with various mathematical models: its capability for therapeutic outcome prediction for non-small cell lung cancer patients with chemoradiotherapy as compared with that of FDG-PET/CT. Eur J Radiol. 2017;86:83–91.
19. Ohno Y, Fujisawa Y, Yui M, et al. Solitary pulmonary nodule: comparison of quantitative capability for differentiation and management among dynamic CE-perfusion MRI at 3 T system, dynamic CE-perfusion ADCT and FDG-PET/CT. Eur J Radiol. 2019;115:22–30.
20. Seki S, Fujisawa Y, Yui M, et al. Dynamic contrast-enhanced area-detector CT vs dynamic contrast-enhanced perfusion MRI vs FDG-PET/CT: comparison of utility for quantitative therapeutic outcome prediction for NSCLC patients undergoing chemoradiotherapy. Magn Reson Med Sci. 2020;19(1):29–39.
21. Miles KA, Griffiths MR, Fuentes MA. Standardized perfusion value: universal CT contrast enhancement scale that correlates with FDG PET in lung nodules. Radiology. 2001;220(2):548–53.
22. Sitartchouk I, Roberts HC, Pereira AM, Bayanati H, Waddell T, Roberts TP. Computed tomography perfusion using first pass methods for lung nodule characterization. Investig Radiol. 2008;43(6):349–58.
23. Li Y, Yang ZG, Chen TW, Chen HJ, Sun JY, Lu YR. Peripheral lung carcinoma: correlation of angiogenesis and first-pass perfusion parameters of 64-detector row CT. Lung Cancer. 2008;61(1):44–53.
24. Wang J, Wu N, Cham MD, Song Y. Tumor response in patients with advanced non-small cell lung cancer: perfusion CT evaluation of chemotherapy and radiation therapy. AJR Am J Roentgenol. 2009;193(4):1090–6.
25. Lee YH, Kwon W, Kim MS, et al. Lung perfusion CT: the differentiation of cavitary mass. Eur J Radiol. 2010;73(1):59–65.
26. Li Y, Yang ZG, Chen TW, Yu JQ, Sun JY, Chen HJ. First-pass perfusion imaging of solitary pulmonary nodules with 64-detector row CT: comparison of perfusion parameters of malignant and benign lesions. Br J Radiol. 2010;83(993):785–90.
27. Fraioli F, Anzidei M, Zaccagna F, et al. Whole-tumor perfusion CT in patients with advanced lung adenocarcinoma treated with conventional and antiangiogenetic chemotherapy: initial experience. Radiology. 2011;259(2):574–82.
28. Tacelli N, Santangelo T, Scherpereel A, et al. Perfusion CT allows prediction of therapy response in non-small cell lung cancer treated with conventional and anti-angiogenic chemotherapy. Eur Radiol. 2013;23(8):2127–36.
29. Ohno Y, Koyama H, Onishi Y, et al. Non-small cell lung cancer: whole-body MR examination for M-stage assessment--utility for whole-body diffusion-weighted imaging compared with integrated FDG PET/CT. Radiology. 2008;248(2):643–54.
30. Nakayama J, Miyasaka K, Omatsu T, et al. Metastases in mediastinal and hilar lymph nodes in patients with non-small cell lung cancer: quantitative assessment with diffusion-weighted magnetic resonance imaging and apparent diffusion coefficient. J Comput Assist Tomogr. 2010;34(1):1–8.
31. Usuda K, Zhao XT, Sagawa M, et al. Diffusion-weighted imaging is superior to positron emission tomography in the detection and nodal assessment of lung cancers. Ann Thorac Surg. 2011;91(6):1689–95.
32. Ohno Y, Koyama H, Yoshikawa T, et al. N stage disease in patients with non-small cell lung cancer: efficacy of quantitative and qualitative assessment with STIR turbo spin-echo imaging, diffusion-weighted MR imaging, and fluorodeoxyglucose PET/CT. Radiology. 2011;261(2):605–15.
33. Kim YN, Yi CA, Lee KS, et al. A proposal for combined MRI and PET/CT interpretation criteria for preoperative nodal staging in non-small-cell lung cancer. Eur Radiol. 2012;22(7):1537–46.
34. Koyama H, Ohno Y, Seki S, et al. Magnetic resonance imaging for lung cancer. J Thorac Imaging. 2013;28(3):138–50.

35. Ohno Y. New applications of magnetic resonance imaging for thoracic oncology. Semin Respir Crit Care Med. 2014;35(1):27–40.
36. Ohno Y, Koyama H, Yoshikawa T, Matsumoto S, Sugimura K. Lung cancer assessment using MR imaging: an update. Magn Reson Imaging Clin N Am. 2015;23(2):231–44.
37. Kim HS, Lee KS, Ohno Y, van Beek EJ, Biederer J. PET/CT versus MRI for diagnosis, staging, and follow-up of lung cancer. J Magn Reson Imaging. 2015;42(2):247–60.
38. Ohno Y, Koyama H, Yoshikawa T, et al. Diffusion-weighted MR imaging using FASE sequence for 3T MR system: preliminary comparison of capability for N-stage assessment by means of diffusion-weighted MR imaging using EPI sequence, STIR FASE imaging and FDG PET/CT for non-small cell lung cancer patients. Eur J Radiol. 2015;84(11):2321–31.
39. Ciliberto M, Kishida Y, Seki S, Yoshikawa T, Ohno Y. Update of MR imaging for evaluation of lung cancer. Radiol Clin North Am. 2018;56(3):437–69.
40. Machado Medeiros T, Altmayer S, et al. 18F-FDG PET/CT and whole-body MRI diagnostic performance in M staging for non-small cell lung cancer: a systematic review and meta-analysis. Eur Radiol. 2020;30(7):3641–9.
41. Ohno Y, Yui M, Takenaka D, et al. Computed DWI MRI results in superior capability for N-stage assessment of non-small cell lung cancer than that of actual DWI, STIR imaging, and FDG-PET/CT. J Magn Reson Imaging. 2023;57(1):259–72.
42. Zhou J, Lal B, Wilson DA, Laterra J, van Zijl PC. Amide proton transfer (APT) contrast for imaging of brain tumors. Magn Reson Med. 2003;50(6):1120–6.
43. Jones CK, Schlosser MJ, van Zijl PC, Pomper MG, Golay X, Zhou J. Amide proton transfer imaging of human brain tumors at 3T. Magn Reson Med. 2006;56(3):585–92.
44. van Zijl PC, Jones CK, Ren J, Malloy CR, Sherry AD. MRI detection of glycogen in vivo by using chemical exchange saturation transfer imaging (glycoCEST). Proc Natl Acad Sci USA. 2007;104(11):4359–64.
45. van Zijl PC, Yadav NN. Chemical exchange saturation transfer (CEST): what is in a name and what isn't? Magn Reson Med. 2011;65(4):927–48.
46. Vinogradov E, Sherry AD, Lenkinski RE. CEST: from basic principles to applications, challenges and opportunities. J Magn Reson. 2013;229:155–72.
47. Togao O, Kessinger CW, Huang G, et al. Characterization of lung cancer by amide proton transfer (APT) imaging: an in-vivo study in an orthotopic mouse model. PLoS One. 2013;8(10):e77019.
48. Togao O, Yoshiura T, Keupp J, et al. Amide proton transfer imaging of adult diffuse gliomas: correlation with histopathological grades. Neuro-Oncology. 2014;16(3):441–8.
49. Ohno Y, Yui M, Koyama H, et al. Chemical exchange saturation transfer MR imaging: preliminary results for differentiation of malignant and benign thoracic lesions. Radiology. 2016;279(2):578–89.
50. Ohno Y, Kishida Y, Seki S, et al. Amide proton transfer-weighted imaging to differentiate malignant from benign pulmonary lesions: comparison with diffusion-weighted imaging and FDG-PET/CT. J Magn Reson Imaging. 2018;47(4):1013–21.
51. Desmond KL, Mehrabian H, Chavez S, et al. Chemical exchange saturation transfer for predicting response to stereotactic radiosurgery in human brain metastasis. Magn Reson Med. 2017;78(3):1110–20.
52. Ohno Y, Yui M, Yamamoto K, et al. Chemical exchange saturation transfer MRI: capability for predicting therapeutic effect of chemoradiotherapy on non-small cell lung cancer patients. J Magn Reson Imaging. 2023;58(1):174–86.
53. Schoepf UJ, Bruening R, Konschitzky H, et al. Pulmonary embolism: comprehensive diagnosis by using electron-beam CT for detection of emboli and assessment of pulmonary blood flow. Radiology. 2000;217(3):693–700.
54. Kono M, Adachi S, Kusumoto M, Sakai E. Clinical utility of Gd-DTPA-enhanced magnetic resonance imaging in lung cancer. J Thorac Imaging. 1993;8(1):18–26.
55. Kusumoto M, Kono M, Adachi S, et al. Gadopentetate-dimeglumine-enhanced magnetic resonance imaging for lung nodules. Differentiation of lung cancer and tuberculoma. Investig Radiol. 1994;29(Suppl 2):S255–6.
56. Gückel C, Schnabel K, Deimling M, Steinbrich W. Solitary pulmonary nodules: MR evaluation of enhancement patterns with contrast-enhanced dynamic snapshot gradient-echo imaging. Radiology. 1996;200(3):681–6.
57. Schaefer JF, Vollmar J, Schick F, et al. Solitary pulmonary nodules: dynamic contrast-enhanced MR imaging--perfusion differences in malignant and benign lesions. Radiology. 2004;232(2):544–53.
58. Kim JH, Kim HJ, Lee KH, Kim KH, Lee HL. Solitary pulmonary nodules: a comparative study evaluated with contrast-enhanced dynamic MR imaging and CT. J Comput Assist Tomogr. 2004;28(6):766–75.
59. Tozaki M, Ichiba N, Fukuda K. Dynamic magnetic resonance imaging of solitary pulmonary nodules: utility of kinetic patterns in differential diagnosis. J Comput Assist Tomogr. 2005;29(1):13–9.
60. Schaefer JF, Schneider V, Vollmar J, et al. Solitary pulmonary nodules: association between signal characteristics in dynamic contrast enhanced MRI and tumor angiogenesis. Lung Cancer. 2006;53(1):39–49.
61. Kono R, Fujimoto K, Terasaki H, et al. Dynamic MRI of solitary pulmonary nodules: comparison of enhancement patterns of malignant and benign small peripheral lung lesions. AJR Am J Roentgenol. 2007;188(1):26–36
62. Donmez FY, Yekeler E, Saeidi V, Tunaci A, Tunacı M, Acunas G. Dynamic contrast enhancement patterns of solitary pulmonary nodules on 3D

gradient-recalled echo MRI. AJR Am J Roentgenol. 2007;189(6):1380–6.
63. Cronin P, Dwamena BA, Kelly AM, Carlos RC. Solitary pulmonary nodules: meta-analytic comparison of cross-sectional imaging modalities for diagnosis of malignancy. Radiology. 2008;246(3):772–82.
64. Le Bihan D, Breton E, Lallemand D, Grenier P, Cabanis E, Laval-Jeantet M. MR imaging of intravoxel incoherent motions: application to diffusion and perfusion in neurologic disorders. Radiology. 1986;161(2):401–7.
65. Le Bihan D, Breton E, Lallemand D, Aubin ML, Vignaud J, Laval-Jeantet M. Separation of diffusion and perfusion in intravoxel incoherent motion MR imaging. Radiology. 1988;168(2):497–505.
66. Le Bihan D, Turner R, Moonen CT, Pekar J. Imaging of diffusion and microcirculation with gradient sensitization: design, strategy, and significance. J Magn Reson Imaging. 1991;1(1):7–28.
67. Le Bihan D, Turner R, Douek P, Patronas N. Diffusion MR imaging: clinical applications. AJR Am J Roentgenol. 1992;159(3):591–9.
68. Le Bihan D. Molecular diffusion, tissue microdynamics and microstructure. NMR Biomed. 1995;8(7-8):375–86.
69. Thoeny HC, De Keyzer F, Vandecaveye V, et al. Effect of vascular targeting agent in rat tumor model: dynamic contrast-enhanced versus diffusion-weighted MR imaging. Radiology. 2005;237(2):492–9.
70. Koh DM, Collins DJ. Diffusion-weighted MRI in the body: applications and challenges in oncology. AJR Am J Roentgenol. 2007;188(6):1622–35.
71. Le Bihan D. Intravoxel incoherent motion perfusion MR imaging: a wake-up call. Radiology. 2008;249(3):748–52.
72. Koh DM, Collins DJ, Orton MR. Intravoxel incoherent motion in body diffusion-weighted MRI: reality and challenges. AJR Am J Roentgenol. 2011;196(6):1351–61.
73. Lang P, Wendland MF, Saeed M, et al. Osteogenic sarcoma: noninvasive in vivo assessment of tumor necrosis with diffusion-weighted MR imaging. Radiology. 1998;206(1):227–35.
74. Sugahara T, Korogi Y, Kochi M, et al. Usefulness of diffusion-weighted MRI with echo-planar technique in the evaluation of cellularity in gliomas. J Magn Reson Imaging. 1999;9(1):53–60.
75. Gauvain KM, McKinstry RC, Mukherjee P, et al. Evaluating pediatric brain tumor cellularity with diffusion-tensor imaging. AJR Am J Roentgenol. 2001;177(2):449–54.
76. Guo Y, Cai YQ, Cai ZL, et al. Differentiation of clinically benign and malignant breast lesions using diffusion-weighted imaging. J Magn Reson Imaging. 2002;16(2):172–8.
77. Mikayama R, Yabuuchi H, Sonoda S, et al. Comparison of intravoxel incoherent motion diffusion-weighted imaging between turbo spin-echo and echo-planar imaging of the head and neck. Eur Radiol. 2018;28(1):316–24.
78. Riederer SJ, Suddarth SA, Bobman SA, Lee JN, Wang HZ, MacFall JR. Automated MR image synthesis: feasibility studies. Radiology. 1984;153(1):203–6.
79. Blackledge MD, Leach MO, Collins DJ, Koh DM. Computed diffusion-weighted MR imaging may improve tumor detection. Radiology. 2011;261(2):573–81.
80. Ueno Y, Takahashi S, Kitajima K, et al. Computed diffusion-weighted imaging using 3-T magnetic resonance imaging for prostate cancer diagnosis. Eur Radiol. 2013;23(12):3509–16.
81. Ueno YR, Tamada T, Takahashi S, et al. Computed diffusion-weighted imaging in prostate cancer: basics, advantages, cautions, and future prospects. Korean J Radiol. 2018;19(5):832–7.
82. Caravan P, Ellison JJ, McMurry TJ, Lauffer RB. Gadolinium(III) chelates as MRI contrast agents: structure, dynamics, and applications. Chem Rev. 1999;99(9):2293–352.
83. Henkelman RM, Stanisz GJ, Graham SJ. Magnetization transfer in MRI: a review. NMR Biomed. 2001;14(2):57–64.
84. Ward KM, Aletras AH, Balaban RS. A new class of contrast agents for MRI based on proton chemical exchange dependent saturation transfer (CEST). J Magn Reson. 2000;143(1):79–87.
85. Aime S, Barge A, Delli Castelli D, et al. Paramagnetic lanthanide (III) complexes as pH-sensitive chemical exchange saturation transfer (CEST) contrast agents for MRI applications. Magn Reson Med. 2002;47(4):639–48.
86. Aime S, Delli Castelli D, Terreno E. Novel pH-reporter MRI contrast agents. Angew Chem Int Ed Engl. 2002;41(22):4334–6.
87. Zhou J, Payen JF, Wilson DA, Traystman RJ, van Zijl PC. Using the amide proton signals of intracellular proteins and peptides to detect pH effects in MRI. Nat Med. 2003;9(8):1085–90.
88. Aime S, Delli Castelli D, Fedeli F, Terreno E. A paramagnetic MRI-CEST agent responsive to lactate concentration. J Am Chem Soc. 2002;124(32):9364–5.
89. Zhang S, Trokowski R, Sherry AD. A paramagnetic CEST agent for imaging glucose by MRI. J Am Chem Soc. 2003;125(50):15288–9.
90. Sagiyama K, Mashimo T, Togao O, et al. In vivo chemical exchange saturation transfer imaging allows early detection of a therapeutic response in glioblastoma. Proc Natl Acad Sci USA. 2014;111(12):4542–7.
91. McMahon MT, Gilad AA, Zhou J, Sun PZ, Bulte JW, van Zijl PC. Quantifying exchange rates in chemical exchange saturation transfer agents using the saturation time and saturation power dependencies of the magnetization transfer effect on the magnetic resonance imaging signal (QUEST and QUESP): Ph calibration for poly-L-lysine and a starburst dendrimer. Magn Reson Med. 2006;55(4):836–47.

92. Sun PZ, Zhou J, Sun W, Huang J, van Zijl PC. Detection of the ischemic penumbra using pH-weighted MRI. J Cereb Blood Flow Metab. 2007;27(6):1129–36.
93. McMahon MT, Gilad AA, DeLiso MA, Berman SM, Bulte JW, van Zijl PC. New "multicolor" polypeptide diamagnetic chemical exchange saturation transfer (DIACEST) contrast agents for MRI. Magn Reson Med. 2008;60(4):803–12.
94. Ling W, Regatte RR, Navon G, Jerschow A. Assessment of glycosaminoglycan concentration in vivo by chemical exchange-dependent saturation transfer (gagCEST). Proc Natl Acad Sci USA. 2008;105(7):2266–70.
95. Sheth VR, Li Y, Chen LQ, Howison CM, Flask CA, Pagel MD. Measuring in vivo tumor pHe with CEST-FISP MRI. Magn Reson Med. 2012;67(3):760–8.
96. Bryant RG. The dynamics of water-protein interactions. Annu Rev Biophys Biomol Struct. 1996;25:29–53.
97. Guivel-Scharen V, Sinnwell T, Wolff SD, Balaban RS. Detection of proton chemical exchange between metabolites and water in biological tissues. J Magn Reson. 1998;133(1):36–45.
98. Zhang S, Merritt M, Woessner DE, Lenkinski RE, Sherry AD. PARACEST agents: modulating MRI contrast via water proton exchange. Acc Chem Res. 2003;36(10):783–90.
99. Ward KM, Balaban RS. Determination of pH using water protons and chemical exchange dependent saturation transfer (CEST). Magn Reson Med. 2000;44(5):799–802.
100. Snoussi K, Bulte JW, Guéron M, van Zijl PC. Sensitive CEST agents based on nucleic acid imino proton exchange: detection of poly(rU) and of a dendrimer-poly(rU) model for nucleic acid delivery and pharmacology. Magn Reson Med. 2003;49(6):998–1005.
101. Terreno E, Castelli DD, Aime S. Encoding the frequency dependence in MRI contrast media: the emerging class of CEST agents. Contrast Media Mol Imaging. 2010;5(2):78–98.
102. Terreno E, Castelli DD, Viale A, Aime S. Challenges for molecular magnetic resonance imaging. Chem Rev. 2010;110(5):3019–42.
103. Aime S, Delli Castelli D, Terreno E. Highly sensitive MRI chemical exchange saturation transfer agents using liposomes. Angew Chem Int Ed Engl. 2005;44(34):5513–5.
104. Donahue MJ, Donahue PC, Rane S, et al. Assessment of lymphatic impairment and interstitial protein accumulation in patients with breast cancer treatment-related lymphedema using CEST MRI. Magn Reson Med. 2016;75(1):345–55.
105. Yuan J, Chen S, King AD, et al. Amide proton transfer-weighted imaging of the head and neck at 3T: a feasibility study on healthy human subjects and patients with head and neck cancer. NMR Biomed. 2014;27(10):1239–47.
106. Nishie A, Takayama Y, Asayama Y, et al. Amide proton transfer imaging can predict tumor grade in rectal cancer. Magn Reson Imaging. 2018;51:96–103.
107. Ishimatsu K, Nishie A, Takayama Y, et al. Amide proton transfer imaging for differentiating benign ovarian cystic lesions: potential of first time right. Eur J Radiol. 2019;120:108656.
108. Goldenberg JM, Cárdenas-Rodríguez J, Pagel MD. Machine learning improves classification of preclinical models of pancreatic cancer with chemical exchange saturation transfer MRI. Magn Reson Med. 2019;81(1):594–601.
109. Wamelink IJHG, Kuijer JPA, Padrela BE, et al. Reproducibility of 3 T APT-CEST in healthy volunteers and patients with brain glioma. J Magn Reson Imaging. 2023;57(1):206–15.
110. Wada T, Togao O, Tokunaga C, et al. Grading of gliomas using 3D CEST imaging with compressed sensing and sensitivity encoding. Eur J Radiol. 2023;158:110654.
111. Murayama K, Ohno Y, Yui M, et al. Three-dimensional gradient-Echo-based amide proton transfer-weighted imaging of brain tumors: comparison with two-dimensional spin-Echo-based amide proton transfer-weighted imaging. J Comput Assist Tomogr. 2023;47(3):494–9.
112. van Zijl PC, Zhou J, Mori N, Payen JF, Wilson D, Mori S. Mechanism of magnetization transfer during on-resonance water saturation. A new approach to detect mobile proteins, peptides, and lipids. Magn Reson Med. 2003;49(3):440–9.
113. Sun PZ, Zhou J, Huang J, van Zijl P. Simplified quantitative description of amide proton transfer (APT) imaging during acute ischemia. Magn Reson Med. 2007;57(2):405–10.
114. Gillies RJ, Bhujwalla ZM, Evelhoch J, et al. Applications of magnetic resonance in model systems: tumor biology and physiology. Neoplasia. 2000;2(1–2):139–51.
115. Zhou J, Tryggestad E, Wen Z, et al. Differentiation between glioma and radiation necrosis using molecular magnetic resonance imaging of endogenous proteins and peptides. Nat Med. 2011;17(1):130–4.
116. Hatabu H, Ohno Y, Gefter WB, Fleischner Society, et al. Expanding applications of pulmonary MRI in the clinical evaluation of lung disorders: Fleischner society position paper. Radiology. 2020;297(2):286–301.
117. Schiebler ML, Parraga G, Gefter WB, et al. Synopsis from expanding applications of pulmonary MRI in the clinical evaluation of lung disorders: Fleischner society position paper. Chest. 2021;159(2):492–5.
118. Tanaka Y, Ohno Y, Hanamatsu S, et al. State-of-the-art MR imaging for thoracic diseases. Magn Reson Med Sci. 2022;21(1):212–34
119. Li B, Li Q, Chen C, Guan Y, Liu S. A systematic review and meta-analysis of the accuracy of diffusion-weighted MRI in the detection of malig-

nant pulmonary nodules and masses. Acad Radiol. 2014;21(1):21–9.
120. Liu J, Xia X, Zou Q, et al. Diagnostic performance of diffusion-weighted imaging versus 18F-FDG PET/CT in differentiating pulmonary lesions: an updated meta-analysis of comparative studies. BMC Med Imaging. 2023;23(1):37.
121. Koyama H, Ohno Y, Kono A, et al. Quantitative and qualitative assessment of non-contrast-enhanced pulmonary MR imaging for management of pulmonary nodules in 161 subjects. Eur Radiol. 2008;18(10):2120–31.
122. Koyama H, Ohno Y, Aoyama N, et al. Comparison of STIR turbo SE imaging and diffusion-weighted imaging of the lung: capability for detection and subtype classification of pulmonary adenocarcinomas. Eur Radiol. 2010;20(4):790–800.
123. Koyama H, Ohno Y, Nishio M, et al. Diffusion-weighted imaging vs STIR turbo SE imaging: capability for quantitative differentiation of small-cell lung cancer from non-small-cell lung cancer. Br J Radiol. 2014;87(1038):20130307.
124. Sakai S, Murayama S, Murakami J, Hashiguchi N, Masuda K. Bronchogenic carcinoma invasion of the chest wall: evaluation with dynamic cine MRI during breathing. J Comput Assist Tomogr. 1997;21(4):595–600.
125. Takahashi K, Furuse M, Hanaoka H, et al. Pulmonary vein and left atrial invasion by lung cancer: assessment by breath-hold gadolinium-enhanced three-dimensional MR angiography. J Comput Assist Tomogr. 2000;24(4):557–61.
126. Ohno Y, Adachi S, Motoyama A, et al. Multiphase ECG-triggered 3D contrast-enhanced MR angiography: utility for evaluation of hilar and mediastinal invasion of bronchogenic carcinoma. J Magn Reson Imaging. 2001;13(2):215–24.
127. Ohno Y, Nishio M, Koyama H, et al. Journal Club: comparison of assessment of preoperative pulmonary vasculature in patients with non-small cell lung cancer by non-contrast- and 4D contrast-enhanced 3-T MR angiography and contrast-enhanced 64-MDCT. AJR Am J Roentgenol. 2014;202(3):493–506.
128. Tang W, Wu N, OuYang H, Huang Y, Liu L, Li M. The presurgical T staging of non-small cell lung cancer: efficacy comparison of 64-MDCT and 3.0 T MRI. Cancer Imaging. 2015;15(1):14.
129. Takenaka D, Ohno Y, Hatabu H, et al. Differentiation of metastatic versus non-metastatic mediastinal lymph nodes in patients with non-small cell lung cancer using respiratory-triggered short inversion time inversion recovery (STIR) turbo spin-echo MR imaging. Eur J Radiol. 2002;44(3):216–24.
130. Ohno Y, Hatabu H, Takenaka D, et al. Metastases in mediastinal and hilar lymph nodes in patients with non-small cell lung cancer: quantitative and qualitative assessment with STIR turbo spin-echo MR imaging. Radiology. 2004;231(3):872–9.
131. Ohno Y, Koyama H, Nogami M, et al. STIR turbo SE MR imaging vs. coregistered FDG-PET/CT: quantitative and qualitative assessment of N-stage in non-small-cell lung cancer patients. J Magn Reson Imaging. 2007;26(4):1071–80.
132. Morikawa M, Demura Y, Ishizaki T, et al. The effectiveness of 18F-FDG PET/CT combined with STIR MRI for diagnosing nodal involvement in the thorax. J Nucl Med. 2009;50(1):81–7.
133. Ohno Y, Koyama H, Yoshikawa T, et al. Three-way comparison of whole-body MR, Coregistered whole-body FDG PET/MR, and integrated whole-body FDG PET/CT imaging: TNM and stage assessment capability for non-small cell lung cancer patients. Radiology. 2015;275(3):849–61.
134. Ohno Y, Yui M, Aoyagi K, et al. Whole-body MRI: comparison of its capability for TNM staging of malignant pleural mesothelioma with that of Coregistered PET/MRI, integrated FDG PET/CT, and conventional imaging. AJR Am J Roentgenol. 2019;212(2):311–9.
135. Ohno Y, Takeshi Y, Takenaka D, Koyama H, Aoyagi K, Yui M. Comparison of diagnostic accuracy for TNM stage among whole-body MRI and Coregistered PET/MRI using 1.5-T and 3-T MRI systems and integrated PET/CT for non-small cell lung cancer. AJR Am J Roentgenol. 2020;215(5):1191–8.
136. Ohno Y, Kishida Y, Seki S, et al. Comparison of Interobserver agreement and diagnostic accuracy for IASLC/ITMIG Thymic epithelial tumor staging among co-registered FDG-PET/MRI, whole-body MRI, integrated FDG-PET/CT, and conventional imaging examination with and without contrast media administrations. Acad Radiol. 2022;29(Suppl 3):S122–31.
137. Ohno Y, Yoshikawa T, Takenaka D, et al. Small cell lung cancer staging: prospective comparison of conventional staging tests, FDG PET/CT, whole-body MRI, and Coregistered FDG PET/MRI. AJR Am J Roentgenol. 2022;218(5):899–908.
138. Shen G, Hu S, Deng H, Kuang A. Performance of DWI in the nodal characterization and assessment of lung cancer: a meta-analysis. AJR Am J Roentgenol. 2016;206(2):283–90.
139. Peerlings J, Troost EG, Nelemans PJ, et al. The diagnostic value of MR imaging in determining the lymph node status of patients with non-small cell lung cancer: a meta-analysis. Radiology. 2016;281(1):86–98.
140. Shen G, Lan Y, Zhang K, Ren P, Jia Z. Comparison of 18F-FDG PET/CT and DWI for detection of mediastinal nodal metastasis in non-small cell lung cancer: a meta-analysis. PLoS One. 2017;12(3):e0173104.
141. Brea TP, Raviña AR, Villamor JMC, Gómez AG, de Alegría AM, Valdés L. Use of magnetic resonance imaging for N-staging in patients with non-small cell lung cancer. A systematic review. Arch Bronconeumol (Engl Ed). 2019;55(1):9–16.
142. Eisenhauer EA, Therasse P, Bogaerts J, et al. New response evaluation criteria in solid tumours: revised

RECIST guideline (version 1.1). Eur J Cancer. 2009;45(2):228–47.
143. Ohno Y, Adachi S, Kono M, Kusumoto M, Motoyama A, Sugimura K. Predicting the prognosis of non-small cell lung cancer patient treated with conservative therapy using contrast-enhanced MR imaging. Eur Radiol. 2000;10(11):1770–81.
144. Fujimoto K, Abe T, Müller NL, et al. Small peripheral pulmonary carcinomas evaluated with dynamic MR imaging: correlation with tumor vascularity and prognosis. Radiology. 2003;227(3):786–93.
145. de Langen AJ, van den Boogaart V, Lubberink M, et al. Monitoring response to antiangiogenic therapy in non-small cell lung cancer using imaging markers derived from PET and dynamic contrast-enhanced MRI. J Nucl Med. 2011;52(1):48–55.
146. Yabuuchi H, Hatakenaka M, Takayama K, et al. Non-small cell lung cancer: detection of early response to chemotherapy by using contrast-enhanced dynamic and diffusion-weighted MR imaging. Radiology. 2011;261(2):598–604.
147. Ohno Y, Koyama H, Yoshikawa T, et al. Diffusion-weighted MRI versus 18F-FDG PET/CT: performance as predictors of tumor treatment response and patient survival in patients with non-small cell lung cancer receiving chemoradiotherapy. AJR Am J Roentgenol. 2012;198(1):75–82.
148. Nishino M, Hatabu H, Johnson BE, McLoud TC. State of the art: response assessment in lung cancer in the era of genomic medicine. Radiology. 2014;271(1):6–27.
149. Kumar S, Liney G, Rai R, Holloway L, Moses D, Vinod SK. Magnetic resonance imaging in lung: a review of its potential for radiotherapy. Br J Radiol. 2016;89(1060):20150431.
150. Weiss E, Ford JC, Olsen KM, et al. Apparent diffusion coefficient (ADC) change on repeated diffusion-weighted magnetic resonance imaging during radiochemotherapy for non-small cell lung cancer: a pilot study. Lung Cancer. 2016;96:113–9.
151. Weller A, O'Brien MER, Ahmed M, et al. Mechanism and non-mechanism based imaging biomarkers for assessing biological response to treatment in non-small cell lung cancer. Eur J Cancer. 2016;59:65–78.
152. Huang YS, Chen JL, Hsu FM, et al. Response assessment of stereotactic body radiation therapy using dynamic contrast-enhanced integrated MR-PET in non-small cell lung cancer patients. J Magn Reson Imaging. 2018;47(1):191–9.

Quantitative Imaging in Response Assessment of Lung Neoplasms

22

Shane M. Crilly, Desmond Killick, and David J. Murphy

Introduction

Lung cancer is the second most common cancer worldwide and the leading cause of cancer-related death worldwide. In 2020, it accounted for 11.4% of all cancer diagnoses and 18.0% of all cancer-related deaths globally [1, 2]. The epidemiology of lung cancer is multifactorial, with several risk factors contributing to its development including smoking, exposure to secondhand smoke, radon, air pollution, occupational exposures (such as asbestos, arsenic, and diesel exhaust), and genetic predisposition. Smoking is the most significant risk factor for lung cancer, accounting for 85% of cases in the United States [3, 4]. Lung cancer is classified into two major types based on histology: non-small cell lung cancer (NSCLC) and small-cell lung cancer (SCLC). NSCLC accounts for approximately 85% of all lung cancer cases and includes three main subtypes: adenocarcinoma, squamous cell carcinoma, and large cell carcinoma. Adenocarcinoma is the most common subtype and accounts for approximately 40% of NSCLC cases, while squamous cell carcinoma accounts for approximately 25%.

Surgery remains the primary curative treatment for early-stage localized NSCLC, but the majority of patients are diagnosed at a more advanced stage, precluding surgical resection—in 2021 only 21% of lung cancer cases in the United States underwent surgical treatment [5]. Therefore, for the majority of patients with NSCLC, and for almost all patients with small cell carcinoma, non-surgical treatments are the mainstay of therapies.

In NSCLC, traditional cytotoxic chemotherapy regimens have revolved around platinum-based therapies, with at best modest survival benefits [6]. Advances in therapeutics and molecular tumor profiling have enabled a transition from empiric chemotherapy to a more personalized approach based on individual tumor biology. The era of personalized medicine in lung cancer started with the discovery of epidermal growth factor receptor mutation (EGFR) mutations in NSCLC and the development of tyrosine kinase inhibitors (TKIs) to successfully target these mutations [7]. Other targetable driver mutations have since been discovered, and tumor genomic characterization is now recommended at diagnosis by the World Health Organization (WHO) and National Comprehensive Cancer Network (NCCN)

S. M. Crilly · D. Killick
Department of Radiology, St. Vincent's University Hospital, Dublin, Ireland

D. J. Murphy (✉)
Department of Radiology, St. Vincent's University Hospital, Dublin, Ireland

School of Medicine University College Dublin, Dublin, Ireland

R. Gill, P. Rajiah (eds.), *Quantitative Imaging in the Thorax*,
https://doi.org/10.1007/978-3-032-14103-3_22

before the treatment of advanced adenocarcinoma [8, 9]. Targetable agents are more likely to be found in adenocarcinomas than other NSCLC subtypes, particularly among never smokers—when no actionable mutation is identified, chemotherapy and/or immunotherapy can be administered [10]. Resistance is a frequent problem in patients treated with targeted therapy, often requiring switching to second- and third-generation targeted therapies [11].

SCLC is an extremely aggressive form of lung cancer originating from neuroendocrine precursor cells. It grows extremely rapidly and metastasizes early, with greater than 70% of patients having metastatic disease at the time of diagnosis [12]. Although SCLC is now staged according to the Union for International Cancer Control tumor-nodes-metastasis (TNM) staging system eighth edition, the traditional classification into limited disease (LD-SCLC) and extensive disease (ED-SCLC) is still useful when discussing therapeutic approach [13]. LD-SCLC was described as disease confined to a single hemithorax that can be safely covered by a single radiation field [14]. The standard treatment for LD-SCLC with curative intent consists of platinum-doublet chemotherapy with concurrent radiotherapy [15, 16]. For patients with metastatic, ED-SCLC platinum-based chemotherapy is the first-line treatment, with a growing role for immunotherapy.

Chemotherapy

Before the advent of targeted therapy and immunotherapy regimens in advanced NSCLC, chemotherapy was the only treatment option, with combination, platinum-based treatment helping improve patient symptoms with modest survival benefit. Now, chemotherapy regimens are recommended for patients not eligible for targeted or immunotherapies, with platinum-based doublet combinations preferred, for example, combinations of cisplatin or carboplatin with either pemetrexed (non-squamous) or gemcitabine/docetaxel (squamous) as first-line agents, with various other recommended regimens (see Table 22.1) [16].

Chemotherapy remains an essential component of treatment of patients with SCLC. For patients with advanced extensive-stage SCLC, a combination of chemotherapy and immunotherapy is preferable. Platinum agents plus etoposide are frequently combined with programmed death ligand (PD-L1) target immune checkpoint inhibitors (ICIs), with carboplatin, etoposide, and atezolizumab, among recommended first-line systemic therapy options [18].

Table 22.1 Commonly used approved drugs for the treatment of lung cancer and their main complications

Drug class	Example	Major complication
Chemotherapy	Cisplatin Carboplatin Gemcitabine Docetaxel	Non-specific interstitial pneumonitis (NSIP) Hypersensitivity pneumonitis (HP) Organizing pneumonia (OP) Arterial thromboembolism
Targeted therapy		
Tyrosine kinase inhibitors (epidermal growth factor receptor (EGFR) mutations)	Erlotinib Gefitinib Afatinib Dacomitinib Osimertinib	Organizing pneumonia (OP) NSIP HP Diffuse alveolar damage (DAD) Simple pulmonary eosinophilia
Tyrosine kinase inhibitors (anaplastic lymphoma kinase (ALK) rearrangements)	Crizotinib Alectinib Loratinib	OP DAD

(continued)

Table 22.1 (continued)

Drug class	Example	Major complication
Tyrosine kinase inhibitors (BRAF V600E proto-oncogene)	Dabrafenib Trametinib	OP DAD Sarcoid-like reaction
Tyrosine kinase inhibitors (Kiersten rat sarcoma (KRAS) mutation)	Sotorasib	Pneumonitis (pattern not yet described
Angiogenesis inhibitors (VEGF/VEGF receptor monoclonal antibodies)	Bevacizumab Ramucirumab	Pulmonary hemorrhage Arterial thromboembolism
Immunotherapy		
Immune checkpoint inhibitors (CTLA-4 monoclonal antibodies)	Ipilimuma	Pleural effusion Myocarditis
Immune checkpoint inhibitors (anti-PD1 agents)	Nivolumab pembrolizumab	
Immune checkpoint inhibitors (anti-PDL1 agents)	Durvalumab Atezolizumab	OP HP DAD NSIP Sarcoid-like reaction

Adapted from Murphy et al. [17]

Targeted Therapy

Targeted therapies are engineered to attack a specific tumor protein or structure, such as blood vessel, and offer a more refined treatment method than chemotherapy (see Table 22.1). The choice of agent depends on individual tumor biology and the presence of specific oncogenic drivers. Activating EGFR mutations are frequent actionable targets for patients with non-squamous NSCLC, in particular non-mucinous adenocarcinomas. TKIs such as erlotinib and gefitinib were among the first targeted lung cancer therapies developed to successfully target tumors with these mutations [19]. Multiple discrete EGFR mutations have subsequently been identified, some of which are responsive to TKIs, while others confer resistance. For example, the T790M EFGR mutation confers resistance to first-generation TKIs but can be successfully targeted with second-generation TKIs such as afatinib and dacomitinib. Osimertinib is a third-generation TKI which can be effective for patients with a T790M mutation that have progressed on first- and second-generation TKIs [20]. Approximately 5% of NSCLC have ALK gene rearrangements, in particular adenocarcinomas. These NSCLCs are usually sensitive to treatment with TKIs, such as the first-generation crizotinib and second-generation TKIs such as alectinib and lorlatinib [16]. ROS1 rearrangement is structurally similar to ALK and is highly sensitive to certain TKIs. The BRAF pV600E mutation is another mutation present in approximately 1–2% of adenocarcinomas with available targetable therapy, dabrafenib and trametinib.

KRAS is a G protein involved in transduction of growth signals from receptor tyrosine kinases. Mutations in KRAS genes are present in approximately 25–30% of adenocarcinomas in a North American population [21]. KRAS mutations are associated with cigarette smoking, unlike many of the other targetable adenocarcinoma mutations. Until recently there were no specific agents, but sotorasib has now been approved as an oral TKI that targets tumors with a KRAS p.G12C mutation [22]. There are other driver mutations that are less common and can be treated, such as METex14 skipping mutations, NTRK 1/2/3 gene fusions and RET rearrangements.

Angiogenesis inhibitors are targeted anti-cancer treatments that inhibit vascular endothelial growth factors (VEGF) or VEGF receptors. For example, bevacizumab is a monoclonal antibody to VEGF that can be added to chemotherapy regimens for advanced non-squamous NSCLC in the absence of targetable driver mutation [16]. Ramucirumab is a monoclonal antibody agent that targets VEGF receptors and can be used in combination with chemotherapy for metastatic non-squamous NSCLC with disease progression after platinum-based chemotherapy.

Immunotherapy

ICIs have dramatically improved the treatment of several cancers, chiefly melanoma, renal cell carcinoma, and NSCLC (see Table 22.1). Programmed cell death protein-1 (PD-1) and cytotoxic T-lymphocyte-associated protein 4 (CTLA-4) are produced by certain types of cancer cells to prevent host immune cytotoxic T-lymphocytes [23]. ICIs are monoclonal antibodies that specifically target the CTLA-4 and PD-1 molecules involved in the tumor-related signaling, reactivating the host adaptive anti-cancer immune response. One of the earliest clinical trials investigating immunotherapy in lung cancer was a phase I study of the anti-CTLA-4 monoclonal antibody ipilimumab, demonstrating promising efficacy in advanced NSCLC, with a disease control rate of 24% and a median overall survival (OS) of 12.2 months [24]. Since then, multiple clinical trials have demonstrated the efficacy of various ICIs in the treatment of advanced NSCLC, such as the anti-PD1 agents nivolumab and pembrolizumab and the anti-PDL1 treatments durvalumab and atezolizumab [25].

Imaging Follow-Up

CT is the main imaging modality used in imaging follow-up lung cancer, either to assess for recurrence in the case of definitive initial treatment or to restage in advanced disease. For patients with NSCLC treated with curative intent, chest CT (with or without IV contrast) is recommended by the National Cancer Control Network (NCCN) as the modality of choice for disease surveillance [16]. 18F-fluorodeoxyglucose (FDG) PET/CT is recommended in cases of equivocal disease recurrence/progression on CT and brain MRI when there is a high suspicion of intracranial disease. For patients with Stage I–II NSCLC treated with surgery +/− adjuvant chemotherapy, the recommended CT interval is every 6 months for 2–3 years, then switching to a low-dose annual non-contrast CT thereafter. For Stage I–II disease where the primary treatment modality is radiotherapy or for Stage III–IV oligometastatic disease where all sites are treated with curative intent, the recommended CT interval is shorter at 3–6 months for 3 years, then moving out to a 6-monthly interval for the subsequent 2 years followed by low-dose annual non-contrast CT. FDG PET/CT and brain MRI are not routinely recommended in asymptomatic patients. PET is recommended in cases of equivocal disease recurrence/progression on CT and brain MRI when there is a high suspicion of intracranial disease.

For patients with advanced NSCLC receiving systemic therapy, the NCCN recommends response assessment with CT after the initial two cycles, followed by every two to four cycles of therapy, but these schedules are often individualized. In general, it is not recommended to continue chemotherapy beyond four to six cycles. Most patients with advanced NSCLC undergo four cycles of initial chemotherapy (e.g., carboplatin/pemetrexed/pembrolizumab for non-squamous NSCLC) followed by maintenance therapy. If treatment is well tolerated, an addition of two extra cycles (a total of six) is considered. Patients with disease progression after initial systemic treatment receive subsequent therapy, the regimen of which depends on the tumor histology, specific genetic variant, initial systemic therapy regimen, and the presence of symptoms. Response assessment is often performed every 6–12 weeks in patients receiving subsequent or maintenance therapy due to the high risk of progression [16].

For patients with limited-stage SCLC undergoing adjuvant therapy, NCCN guidelines recommended that response assessment is performed with CT chest, abdomen, and pelvis (CAP) with contrast and brain MRI with gadolinium, only after the completion of adjuvant therapy [18]. For patients receiving systemic therapy alone, or systemic therapy followed by radiation, repeat CT CAP is recommended after the initial two cycles and at the end of therapy. In cases of extensive-stage SCLC, response assessment by CT is recommended after two to three cycles of systemic therapy and at completion of therapy. Brain MRI is preferred to CT in patients with brain metastasis.

Imaging Response Assessment

The fundamental purpose of imaging for treatment response assessment is to assess whether a given treatment is having the desired effect or not and to inform the treating physician whether the treatment strategy needs to be altered. It also offers the chance to assess for any treatment-related complications that may occur. The WHO criteria [26] and later the Response Evaluation Criteria in Solid Tumors (RECIST) were developed for objective response assessment for solid tumors from cytotoxic chemotherapy, based mainly on anatomic imaging with CT [27]. These criteria, in particular the updated RECIST 1.1, have formed the basis of objective response assessment in chemotherapy clinical trials over the past number of decades [28]. As the use of novel targeted agents and immune checkpoint inhibitors has increased new and modified objective response criteria, biologic agents and immunotherapy have been proposed to reflect the different mechanisms of action of these agents compared to platinum based cytotoxic chemotherapy (see Table 22.2) [29, 30].

Anatomic imaging with CT with diameter measurements still forms the backbone of response assessment in lung cancer, but there is an increasing focus on more advanced techniques with volumetric analysis, automatic segmentation, radiomics, and artificial intelligence all potentially playing a future role (Fig. 22.1). The increased use of FDG PET/CT and advanced MRI as imaging modalities in response assessment also informs a different perspective to standard anatomic imaging.

Table 22.2 Summary and comparison of the main response assessment criteria after lung cancer therapy

Criteria	Main imaging modality & measurement	Complete response (CR)	Partial response (PR)	Stable disease (SD)	Unconfirmed progressive disease (UPD)	Progressive disease (PD)
WHO	CT Change in sum of products of the LD and greatest perpendicular diameters No maximal number of lesions specified	Disappearance of all known disease, confirmed at ≥4 weeks	≥50% decrease from baseline, confirmed at ≥4 weeks	Neither PR nor PD criteria met	Not described	≥25% increase of one or more lesions or appearance of new lesions
RECIST 1.1	CT Maximum of five target lesions Based on sum of unidimensional diameters	Complete resolution of non-nodal lesions Reduction in size of all pathologic nodes to <1 cm in short axis	≥30% reduction in disease burden	Neither CR, PR, or PD	Not described	≥20% increase in disease burden compared to nadir Minimum increase of 5 mm New target or non-target lesions

(continued)

Table 22.2 (continued)

Criteria	Main imaging modality & measurement	Complete response (CR)	Partial response (PR)	Stable disease (SD)	Unconfirmed progressive disease (UPD)	Progressive disease (PD)
iRECIST	Same as RECIST 1.1	Same as RECIST 1.1	Same as RECIST 1.1	Neither CR, PR, PD, or UPD	Same as PD by RECIST 1.1	>5 mm increase in size of sum of target lesions/any increase in size of non-target lesions/ appearance of new lesions on a follow-up CT 4–8 weeks following UPD
EORTC PET	FDG PET/CT Based on SUVmax	Complete resolution of all FDG uptake in all lesions	≥30% reduction in sum of SUVmax	Neither CMR, PMR, or PMD	Not described	≥20% increase in the sum of SUV_{max} Appearance of new FDG-avid lesions typical for tumor
PERCIST	FDG PET/CT Based on sum of SULpeak Five or fewer target lesions	Complete resolution of all FDG uptake in all lesions	≥30% reduction in SULpeak and ≥0.8 absolute decrease in SULpeak	Neither CMR, PMR, or PMD	Not described	≥30% increase in SULpeak or >0.8 increase in SULpeak Appearance of new FDG-avid lesions typical for tumor
imPERCIST	FDG PET/CT Based on sum of SULpeak Five or fewer target lesions	Resolution of all metabolically active lesions	Reduction in sum of SULpeak by ≥30% and absolute reduction in SULpeak by ≥0.8	Neither CMR, PMR, or PMD	Not described	≥30% increase in sum of SULpeak after at least 3 months
iPERCIST	FDG PET/CT Based on sum of SULpeak Five or fewer target lesions	Complete disappearance of any uptake in target lesions	Reduction in SULpeak in target lesions ≥30%	Neither CMR, PMR, or PMD	New lesions or increase in > 30% in sum of SULpeak or of the SULpeak of the most intense lesion classified as immune unconfirmed disease progression (iuPMD)	Persistent changes on PET 4–8 weeks following iuPMD

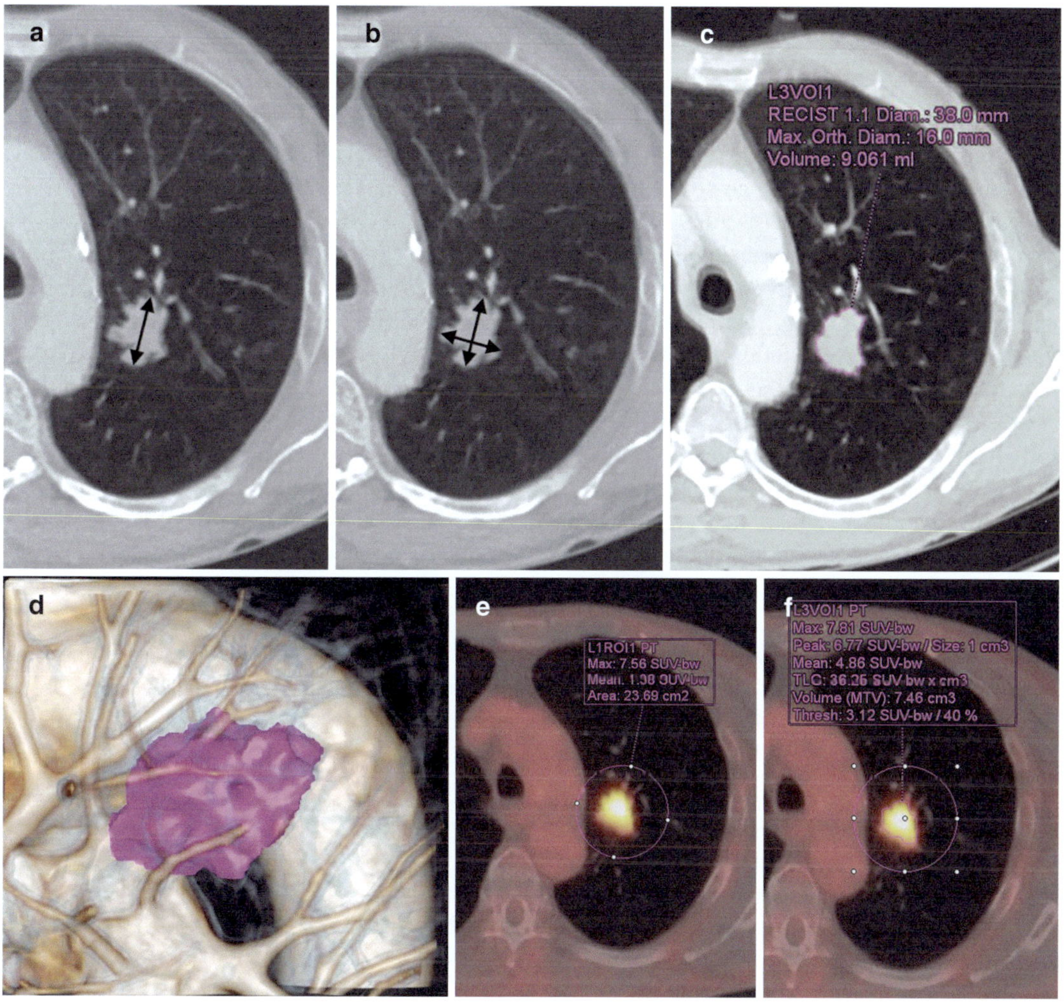

Fig. 22.1 Measurement techniques. (**a**, **b**) Axial CT images showing unidimensional (**a**) and bidimensional measurements of a 36-mm adenocarcinoma in the left upper lobe. (**c**) CT volumetric measurement of the same tumor. (**d**) 3D volume rendered image showing the tumor in purple. (**e**) Fused axial FDG PET/CT image demonstrates increased metabolic uptake with measurement of SUV_{max}. (**f**) FDG PET/CT volumetric measurements of MTV and TLG

FDG PET/CT provides an excellent assessment of disease extent and metabolic signature. The measurement of the standardized uptake value (SUV) of FDG, a semiquantitative measure of the amount of radiotracer uptake in a given region of interest (ROI), is commonly performed in clinical staging. Lung tumor SUVmax has been found to correlate with the pathological stage of the disease [31]. Changes in the SUVmax or SUVmean of FDG in lung tumors over time can also be used to monitor treatment response and predict patient outcomes. Several studies have demonstrated that a decrease in SUVmax of more than 30% after the first cycle of chemotherapy or radiation therapy is associated with a better prognosis and longer progression-free survival [32–34]. Indeed, in a study published in 2021 by Ke et al., it was found using RECIST criteria to evaluate treatment response in 120 patients with advanced lung cancer patients on combined immune checkpoint inhibitors and chemotherapy that tumor SUVmax and serum lactate dehydrogenase best predicted median survival time [35]. In addition, quantitative PET/CT imaging has been shown to be useful in distinguishing between post-treatment inflammation and residual tumor, which is helpful in guiding further treatment decisions [36, 37].

Treatment response criteria mainly assess changes in tumor size using CT imaging [38]. However, these changes can potentially lag behind molecular and biological changes [39]. The use of dynamic contrast-enhanced (DCE)-MRI is being explored as a method for investigating the tumor microenvironment using perfusion and capillary permeability [40]. Parameters that reflect tumor blood flow and blood volume can be used as biomarkers in the assessment of tumor vascularity, which is relevant in the assessment of chemotherapy response [41]. The analysis of DCE-MRI data ranges from observation of signal intensity variation after contrast delivery to more complex methods involving theoretical pharmacokinetic analysis [42]. The majority of more recent studies have focused on the relationship between tumor response to therapy and quantitative parameters that have been retrieved from the pharmacokinetic analysis of DCE-MRI. In the field of neurooncology, semiquantitative parameters such as positive enhancement integral, signal enhancement ratio, maximum slope of increase, and time to peak have been demonstrated to correlate with the antiangiogenic treatment of recurrent glioma [43], and more recently they have been shown to strongly correlate with quantitative parameters generated from DCE-MRI. Moreover, semiquantitative parameters have at times been shown to be superior to quantitative parameters in assessing tumor response [44].

While current response criteria are widely validated, there are important limitations to assessing tumor response based solely on size [45]. For example, accurate and consistent measurements can be difficult to obtain in the likes of ground-glass opacities and semi-solid nodules [46]. Other markers of tumor response such as functional, density, and metabolic changes are not evaluated by criteria such as RECIST 1.1. Metabolic responses may precede changes in tumor size, particularly in the setting of immunotherapy. Imaging techniques such as DCE-MRI and diffusion-weighted imaging (DWI)-MRI can provide more functional and metabolic information in both the predication and assessment of treatment response [47]. DWI measures the movement of water molecules (Brownian motion) using magnetic field gradients. Lesions that have a higher cell density, such as tumors, appear bright on DWI due to decreased diffusion. When tumors respond positively to treatment, a reduction in their cellularity is expected which is measurable as an increase in apparent diffusion coefficient (ADC) on DWI-MRI. Regier et al. demonstrated that ADC could potentially be used as a marker of response of NSCLC to treatment with a potential to assess for early response before there is a change in tumor size [48]. In addition, Fleckenstein et al. report that DWI can potentially distinguish tumor recurrence, atelectasis, and radiation-induced lung toxicity, something conventional CT and FDG PET/CT cannot reliably do [49]. In turn, this could reduce the number of patients subjected to unnecessary invasive diagnostic procedures for benign changes. DWI through ADC values can possibly distinguish between benign and malignant lymph nodes, with the former having higher ADC values [49].

Imaging Response Assessment Criteria (Tables 22.2 and 22.3)

The accurate radiologic assessment of tumor response is pivotal for both effective treatment and also for the development of new therapies. There has been great development and expansion of image-based tumor response criteria over recent decades with the purpose of achieving objective assessment of treatment response in oncologic clinical trials. Response criteria were principally designed for use in clinical trials and are not generally formally used by radiologists in clinical practice, but they still provide a good overall framework for response assessment. Quantitative response assessment is often absent from the clinical radiology report, which can lead to problems for the referring physician ascertaining response status, which can hinder treatment decision-making, and has the potential to adversely impact patient care [50]. There are

Table 22.3 Proposed targeted response assessment criteria after lung cancer therapy

Criteria	Main imaging modality and measurement	Complete response (CR)	Partial response (PR)	Stable disease (SD)	Progressive disease (PD)
Choi	CT Lesion diameter and density (HU)	Disappearance of all lesions No new lesions	Decrease in size of ≥10% or decrease in HU of ≥15% on CT No new lesions No obvious progression of non-targeted lesions	Neither CR, PR, or PD	(a) Increase of tumor size of ≥10% and does not meet the criteria of PR according to tumor density (HU) on CT (b) New lesions
"New CT Criteria" (Lee criteria)	CT Only solid component of target lesion measured When lesion cavitation is present, the cavity size is subtracted from lesion diameter	Disappearance of all lesions No new lesions	(a) If solid portion of tumor ≤5 mm^2: Decrease in size of ≥30% in diameter No new lesions No progression of target lesions (b) If solid portion of tumor >5 mm^2: Decrease in size of ≥10% in diameter or a reduction in tumor HU of ≥15% No new lesions No progression of target lesions	Neither CR, PR, or PD	(a) Increase in tumor size ≥10%20% in diameter and by at least 5 mm Does not meet PR criteria by HU changes No cavitation (b) New lesion(s)

many potential explanations for this, including lack of disease-specific and therapy-specific knowledge. Having a working knowledge of response assessment criteria is helpful in performing accurate response assessment.

WHO Criteria

In 1979, the WHO published the first response criteria using bidimensional measurements of tumors [26]. The WHO outlined the requirement for essential data recording, criteria for response assessment, and reporting guidelines. These criteria for solid tumors were developed in an effort to standardize the characterization of chemotherapeutic efficacy and also to facilitate comparisons between studies and historical data [51]. The WHO criteria was developed during an era of cytotoxic chemotherapeutic agents and are still in use [52].

The initial WHO methods involved classifying lesions into two groups as measurable and non-measurable depending upon the ability to accurately and reproducibly measure a lesion on imaging. The size of the lesion was derived as a two-dimensional diameter caliper measurement with multiplication of the longest diameter by its perpendicular diameter. In certain circumstances and conditions, such as hepatomegaly or mediastinal adenopathy, unidimensional measurements were allowed [53]. The aforementioned dimensions were then summed over all lesions and the changes categorized for the summed products. The categorizations included complete response (CR) = tumor has disappeared for at least 4 weeks; partial response (PR) = 50% or greater reduction in the sum of tumor size products from the baseline confirmed at 4 weeks; progressive disease (PD) = at least a 25% increase in tumor size in one or more lesions with no complete response, partial response, or stable disease (SD) documented before the increase in size or development of new tumor sites; and no change = neither complete response nor partial response nor progressive disease [54]. Complete response, partial response, no change, and progressive disease were defined separately for measurable and non-measurable disease, as well as for bone metastasis.

The WHO criteria were validated in prospective randomized trials and enjoyed the status of most widely used criteria for a significant period of time [55]. Despite the best efforts however, the WHO criteria failed to fully standardize response assessment. The details of measurement rules were inadequately described, as were the handling of exceptions. In turn, this led to the eventual development of several modifications to the criteria across various trials leading to the loss of comparability. The WHO criteria were unclear as to how many tumor lesions should be measured, how small a lesion could be measured, and how disease progression should be defined. That said, the WHO criteria are the criteria used to define clinical response rates in many trials over the past several decades which act as important reference studies. Although not as commonly used at present, familiarity with the WHO response criteria is helpful, as many of the subsequent response criteria were derived from the principles pioneered by the WHO criteria.

RECIST

The RECIST are based on the sum of unidimensional longest diameter of target lesions to determine the overall tumor response [56]. RECIST 1.0 was initially developed in 2000 and is based on the sum of the longest diameter of the target lesion. The updated RECIST 1.1 criteria were published in 2009 and include additional guidelines for the assessment of non-target lesions.

RECIST criteria require the identification of at least one target lesion, which is the largest measurable lesion in a patient. The longest diameter of target lesions is measured (except lymph nodes where short axis diameter is used), and the sum of target lesion diameters is then used to calculate a percentage difference. Resulting percentage changes compared to baseline (or from nadir in the context of progression after initial shrinkage) along with any supporting evidence from non-target lesions allow the use of categorically defined response categories as follows: PD with a ≥20% increase in the sum of target lesions compared with nadir/one or more new lesions/definite progression of non-target lesions (Fig. 22.2); PR where there is ≥30% decrease in the sum of target lesions compared with baseline (Figs. 22.3 and 22.4); CR defined as the disappearance of all target and non-target lesions (Fig. 22.5); and SD where there is neither PR nor PD [57]. RECIST 1.1 also includes an assessment of non-target lesions, which are not included in the overall response calculation. Non-target lesions are assessed based on their presence or absence and are reported separately from the target lesion.

There are however limitations of RECIST when it comes to solid tumors in general and also more specifically regarding lung cancer. RECIST focuses mainly on lesion diameter, but this can be challenging in lung cancers with irregular or infiltrative margins and in subsolid lesions with a large ground-glass component. Other morphological criteria such as cavitation, change in density, and enhancement are not incorporated [58]. Measurement variability is a well-documented problem that has been shown to potentially lead to incorrect classification of progressive lung cancer by RECIST1.0 of up to 30% [59]. Significant variations in measured lung tumor diameters of up to 22.8% was reported in a study by Zhao et al. of same-day repeat CTs in patients with NSCLC [60]. This variability is reproducible within the partial response range in RECIST 1.1 but is above the greater than 20% cutoff for progressive disease, which could potentially result in response misclassification. Unidimensional size measurement assumes equal radial tumor growth, but this can often be more heterogeneous due to internal variation in tumor biology-tumor volumetry, discussed in further detail later on in this chapter, has been shown to be accurate and reproducible, and will likely be incorporated into future RECIST iterations [61].

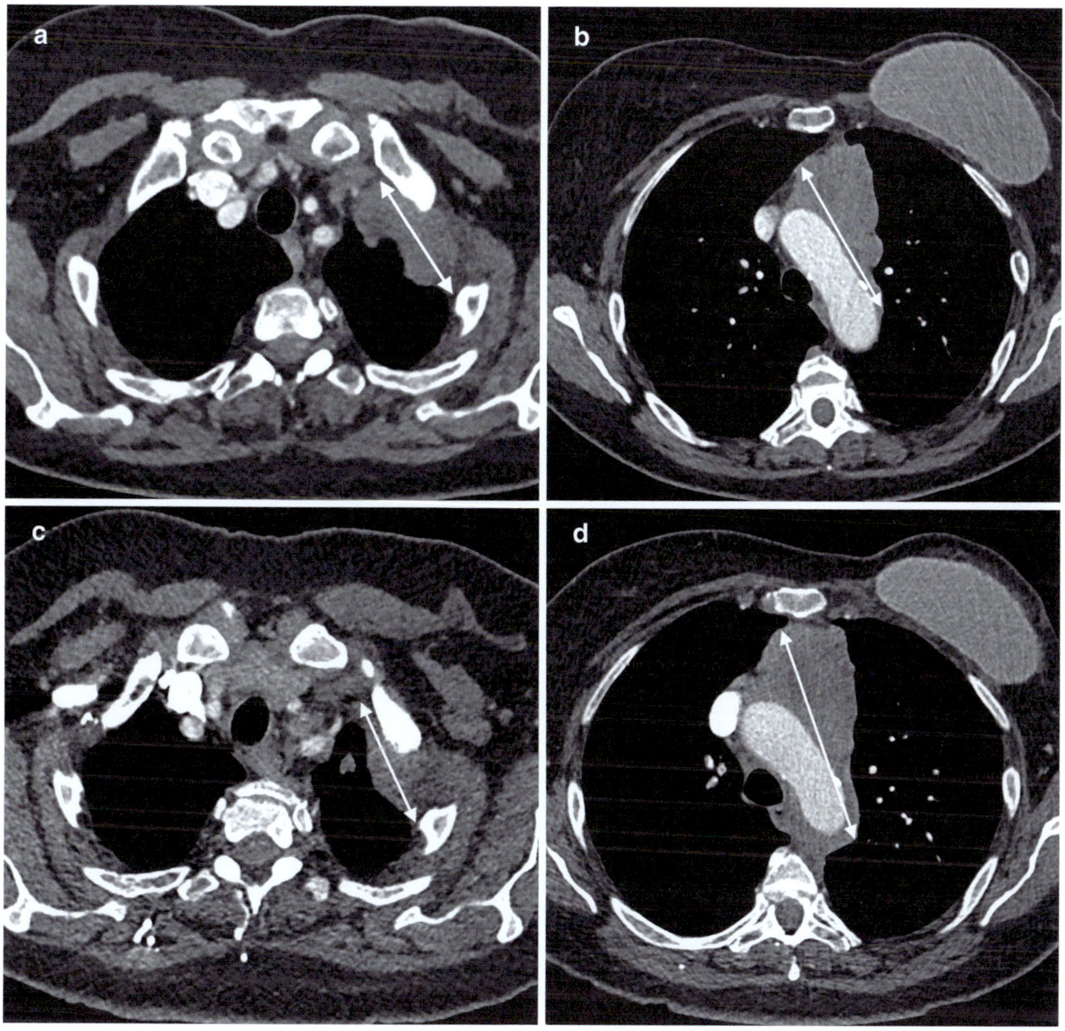

Fig. 22.2 Disease progression in a patient with metastatic adenocarcinoma on chemotherapy. (**a**) Initial CT demonstrates a 5.5-cm left apical primary (double arrows) and (**b**) a 7.7-cm anterior mediastinal nodal mass (double arrows). (**c**) Restaging CT after completion of chemotherapy with stable left apical primary (double arrows) but (**d**) enlarging mediastinal disease, now measuring 11.5 cm and extending posterior to the aortic arch (double arrows)

Response Assessment with 18F-FDG PET/CT

Quantitative FDG PET/CT imaging is a valuable modality in the management of lung cancer, providing valuable information for diagnosis, staging, and treatment response evaluation, providing both functional and anatomical information. Technical factors that can affect lesion SUV values need to be considered especially when performing serial FDG PET/CTs, as they may lead to spurious measurements. These include performing PETs on the same camera with the same reconstruction algorithm where possible and using similar radiotracer dose injected radioactivity and uptake times [62]. In general, there should be a gap of at least 10 days between chemotherapy administration and FDG PET to avoid tumor stunning which can artificially reduce metabolic activity.

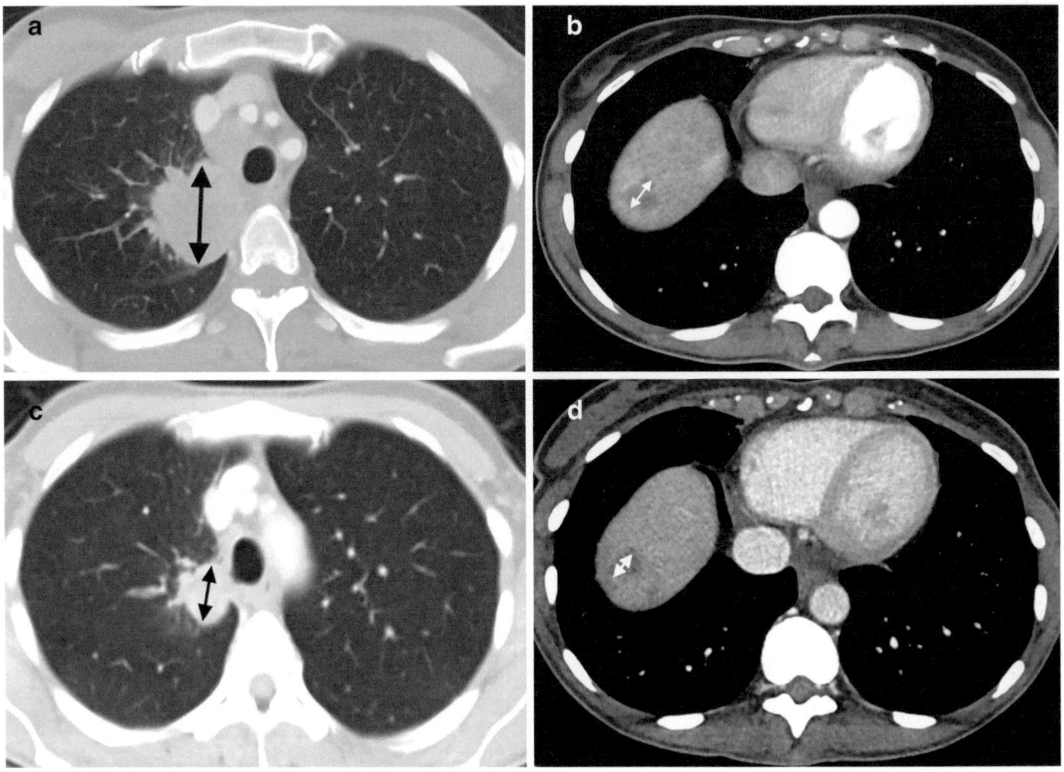

Fig. 22.3 A patient with metastatic adenocarcinoma (T2bN2M1c) with a partial response on platinum-based chemotherapy. (**a**) Axial CT thorax with a 44-mm right upper lobe tumor (double arrows). Note also the enlarged station 4R lymph node. There was multiple liver metastasis at presentation (**b**), the largest at the hepatic dome measuring 21 mm (double arrows). (**c**) Restaging CT post chemotherapy shows reduction of the right upper lobe mass (now 23 mm, double arrows) and of the liver metastasis (**d**), with the hepatic dome lesion now 13 mm (double arrows). Appearances are consistent with a partial disease response

European Organization for Research and Treatment of Cancer Criteria

The European Organization for Research and Treatment of Cancer (EORTC) criteria were the original metabolic response assessment criteria proposed for solid tumors [63]. They have been widely considered useful in assessing both tumor response and predicting patient outcome, focusing on the measurement of lesion-specific ROIs that are then followed up on each subsequent scan [64]. EORTC defines four response categories: complete metabolic response (CMR), partial metabolic response (PMR), stable metabolic disease (SMD), and progressive metabolic disease (PMD) (Fig. 22.6). It is useful in assessing both tumor response and predicting patient outcome. However, since their publication, studies have largely investigated the use of FDG PET for treatment monitoring, with an emphasis on whole-body imaging mostly using hybrid PET/CT imaging and not standalone PET. As a result, this prompted the development of the PET Response Criteria in Solid Tumors (PERCIST) criteria which provides more detailed guidance on treatment monitoring with hybrid PET/CT.

PERCIST Criteria

The PERCIST criteria uses target lesion peak SUL (SUV normalized to lean body mass) to measure tumor metabolic activity [54].

PERCIST defines CMR as a complete resolution of abnormal FDG uptake within target lesions; PMR, a reduction of at least 30% in tar-

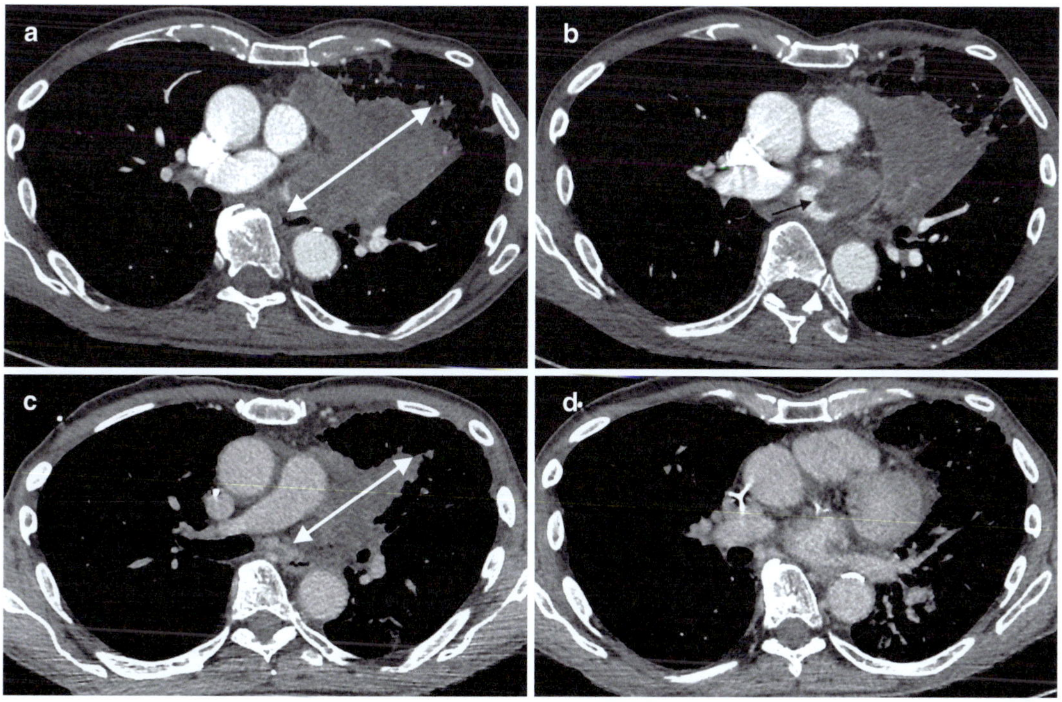

Fig. 22.4 A patient with a locally invasive T4 squamous cell carcinoma with a partial response on chemotherapy and radiotherapy. (**a**) Staging CT thorax with a 10.3 cm left upper lobe mass (double arrows) with mediastinal invasion and (**b**) tumor thrombus invading in the left atrium via the left superior pulmonary vein (arrow). (**c**) Restaging CT shows a reduction in LUL tumor (7.6 cm, double arrows) with (**d**) resolution of the left atrial tumor thrombus consistent with a partial treatment response

get lesion peak SUL in the absence of new sites of disease; PMD, an increase of at least 30% in peak lesion SUL (compared to baseline FDG PET in a pattern typical for tumor) and/or the presence of new sites of metabolically active disease; SMD, as neither CMR, PMR, nor PMD. For definitive characterization of PMD, it is important that the pattern of increased FDG uptake is typical for tumor, as treatment effect and/or superimposed infection may also manifest as areas if increased FDG uptake.

PERCIST uses a change in SULpeak of 30% as a cutoff for tumor response and progression. This threshold has been supported by a number of studies since its development [65]. In addition, to avoid labeling minor absolute changes in FDG uptake as a response, PERCIST requires a minimum absolute difference in SUL of 0.8, as well as a minimum tumor SUL in order to consider a lesion measurable for response [65]. Under the EORTC criteria, target lesions are selected on imaging before therapy and then reidentified on follow-up imaging with their subsequent change in size or FDG uptake recorded. However, in the PERCIST criteria, baseline and follow-up imaging are reviewed, and the lesion with the highest FDG uptake on each scan is identified. The change in SULpeak is then calculated to assess for response.

Several studies have evaluated the role of the PERCIST criteria in the evaluation of response to targeted therapies in lung cancer patients. A 2016 pooled analysis comparing.

RECIST 1.1 and PERCIST criteria in 268 patients with solid organ tumors, of which 60 had lung cancer, found that the concordance of tumor responses between RECIST and PERCIST was moderate, and the authors concluded that PERCIST might be more suitable for assessing tumor response than the RECIST [66]. Additionally it has been demonstrated that the PERCIST criteria has higher accuracy and prog-

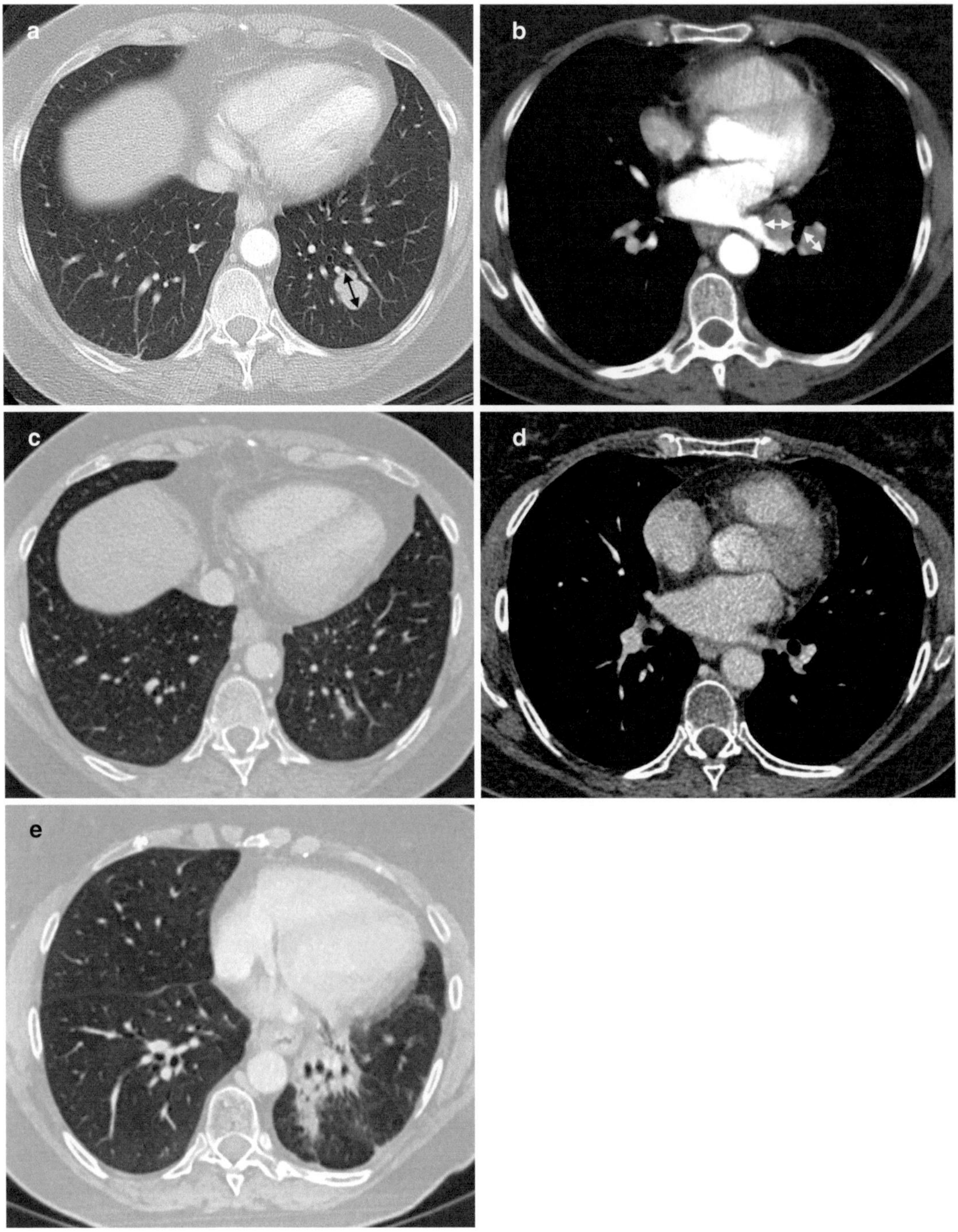

Fig. 22.5 A patient with limited-stage small-cell lung cancer treated with combination chemotherapy and radiotherapy with complete treatment response. (**a**) CT thorax with a 2 cm left lower lobe primary tumor (double arrows) with (**b**) two enlarged ipsilateral left hilar lymph nodes measuring up to 1.5 cm in short axis (double arrows). (**c**) Restaging CT post-treatment with no residual measurable lesion in the left lower lobe with minor linear peribronchial consolidation at the site of the previous tumor and (**d**) resolution of left hilar lymphadenopathy consistent with complete treatment response. (**e**) Surveillance CT 9 years post treatment with sustained complete response, with established post-radiation fibrosis at the site of treated tumor

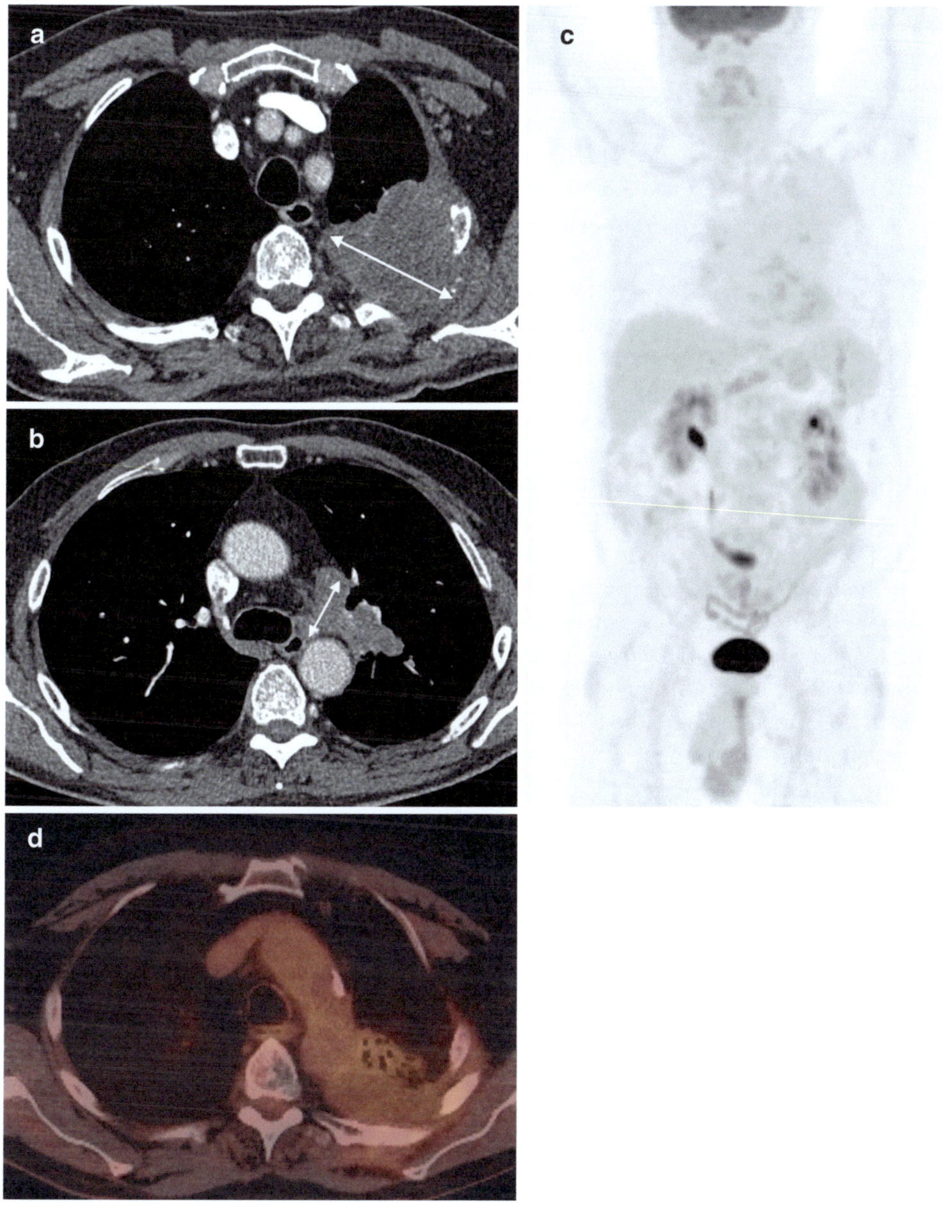

Fig. 22.6 A patient with a locally invasive squamous cell carcinoma with complete metabolic response on FDG PET/CT post chemotherapy and radiotherapy. (**a**) Staging CT thorax demonstrates an 8 cm left upper lobe mass with local chest wall invasion and (**b**) bulky ipsilateral mediastinal nodal (N2) disease. This was intensely metabolically active on FDG PET/CT (not shown). End-of-treatment FDG PET/CT maximal intensity projection (**c**) and fused axial image (**d**) shows no residual FDG-avid disease consistent with a complete metabolic response

nostic value than RECIST in predicting progression-free survival and OS [67].

The use of PERCIST criteria has also been investigated in the evaluation of response to targeted therapies in lung cancer. PERCIST criteria were used to evaluate response to crizotinib, an ALK inhibitor, in 15 patients with advanced non-small cell lung cancer, and were able to detect progression earlier than CT in 10/22 (45%) events of progression, with the other disease progression events detected simultaneously [68]. Tiwary et al. used

PERCIST to perform metabolic response assessment of the ALK inhibitor crizotinib in 22 patients with metastatic ALK-positive lung adenocarcinoma; 8 of the 22 patients demonstrated partial metabolic response, 12 out of 22, stable metabolic disease; and 2 of the 22 patients, disease progression (new brain metastases in both) [69–71].

PERCIST criteria have been assessed for response assessment of ICIs in solid organ tumors, including lung cancer. Beer et al. compared RECIST, Immunotherapy Response Evaluation Criteria in Solid Tumors (iRECIST), and PERCIST in the evaluation of response to ICI PD-1/PD-L1 therapy in patients with NSCLC [72]. The study demonstrated that RECIST 1.1 and PERCIST 1.0 showed only moderate agreement but that both can predict treatment response to ICI therapy. PERCIST has the potential to identify treatment response early after treatment initiation but cannot reliably differentiate pseudoprogression from disease progression. In order to overcome this shortcoming of the criteria, the immunotherapy-modified PET response criteria in solid tumors (imPERCIST) were introduced.

Hopkins Criteria

The Hopkins qualitative PET response assessment criteria are different to both the EORTC-PET and PERCIST in that they are based on a visual assessment of FDG uptake relative to background mediastinal blood pool and liver activity rather than semiquantitative SUV measurements. Proposed initially as a response assessment PET score for head and neck cancers, it has since been validated for use in NSCLC [73]. A score of 1–5 is assigned based on a visual assessment of lesion uptake relative to mediastinal blood pool and hepatic activity as follows: 1 = FDG uptake less than the mediastinal blood pool; 2 = uptake greater than the mediastinal blood pool but less than the liver; 3 = diffuse FDG uptake greater than the liver; 4 = focal FDG uptake greater than the liver; and 5 = focal FDG uptake two to three times greater than the liver. A score of 1 or 2 is considered negative for residual disease, with a score of 4/5 positive for persistent metabolically active disease. A score of 3 is often considered indeterminate and requires more frequent imaging follow-up.

Response Assessment for Targeted Therapies (Table 22.3)

Response criteria limitations have become apparent in the era of precision lung cancer therapy. For example, patients with advanced NSCLC with EGFR mutation treated with TKIs often show an initial reduction in tumor size followed by prolonged stability or slow regrowth over months or sometimes even years (Figs. 22.7 and 22.8). Often oncologists will continue treatment in these patients despite the presence of disease progression by RECIST 1.1, as the slow growth trajectory is suggestive that at least some of the tumor cells remain sensitive to the targeted therapy. This has been shown to be an effective approach in clinical practice and can delay the need for salvage therapy, especially in patients with late-onset progression in the absence of extra-thoracic metastatic disease [74]. Sustained stable disease is a common pattern seen with targeted therapies, reflecting effective anti-tumor activity, in contradistinction to cytotoxic chemotherapy where stable disease is often a marker of ineffective treatment. Discontinuing TKI therapy in EGFR-mutated NSCLCs is associated with a risk of accelerated disease progression (flare phenomenon) in up to 23% of patients [75]. Antiangiogenic therapy (e.g., bevacizumab) often causes cavitation of the lung tumour, without a change in overall lesion diameter. It has been proposed that excluding the zone of cavitation when performing response assessment in these circumstances can alter response classification compared to the standard unidimensional lesion diameter in RECIST [76]. In order to account for the different mechanism of action and response kinetics of targeted therapies in lung cancer, changes to the quantitative evaluation of disease response have been evaluated.

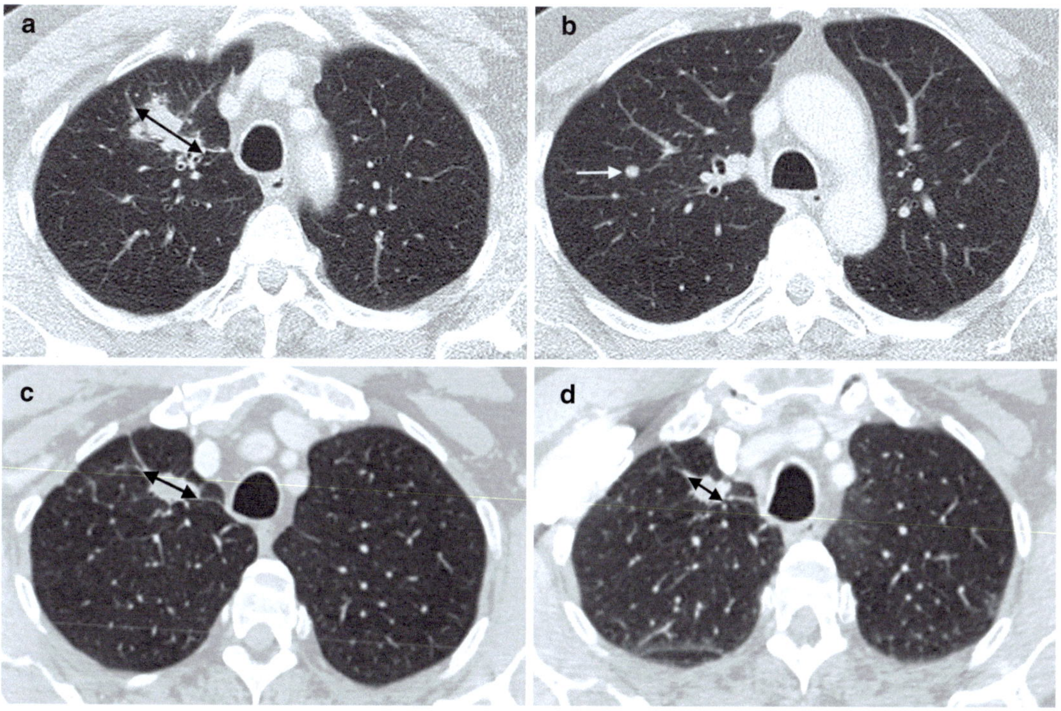

Fig. 22.7 A patient with EGFR-mutated adenocarcinoma, initially treated with chemotherapy followed by a TKI with a prolonged partial disease response. (**a**) Initial CT with a 5.1 cm irregular right upper lobe primary tumor (double arrows) with surrounding tumor nodules and a (**b**) 8 mm separate right upper lobe nodule (arrow). (**c**) Restaging CT post chemotherapy with a reduction in the right upper lobe mass (now 31 mm, double arrows) and resolution of the surrounding nodules. The patient was switched to maintenance TKI therapy, and a restaging CT 7 years (**d**) later shows a further reduction in the right upper lobe nodule to 25 mm (double arrows) consistent with a prolonged partial response

Choi Criteria

Reduction in lesion density on CT, as measured by Hounsfield units (HU), is a potential marker of disease response that has been most evaluated based on studies on gastrointestinal stromal tumors treated with TKIs—the Choi criteria define response in these tumors as a 10% reduction in size or 15% reduction in lesion density [77]. Several studies have evaluated the efficacy of the Choi criteria in assessing response to targeted therapy in lung cancer. In one study, the Choi criteria was compared to RECIST in patients with NSCLC treated with the TKI gefitinib, finding that the Choi criteria were more accurate than RECIST in predicting both progression-free and OS [70, 71]. The Choi criteria have also been shown to be superior to RECIST in predicting overall and progression-free survival in patients with advanced NSCLC response treated with the VEGF inhibitor bevacizumab [69, 78].

New CT Response Criteria

Lee et al have attempted to combine the various specific differences of targeted therapies compared to cytotoxic chemotherapy into a specific response criteria for NSCLC treated with TKIs [79]. The “new CT response criteria” (also known as the Lee criteria) incorporates lesion attenuation (measured with HU), presence of cavitation, and measurement of the solid component of subsolid lesions and showed better performance than RECIST1.1 in prediction of patient survival. RECIST measurements of a lung target lesion include both the solid and

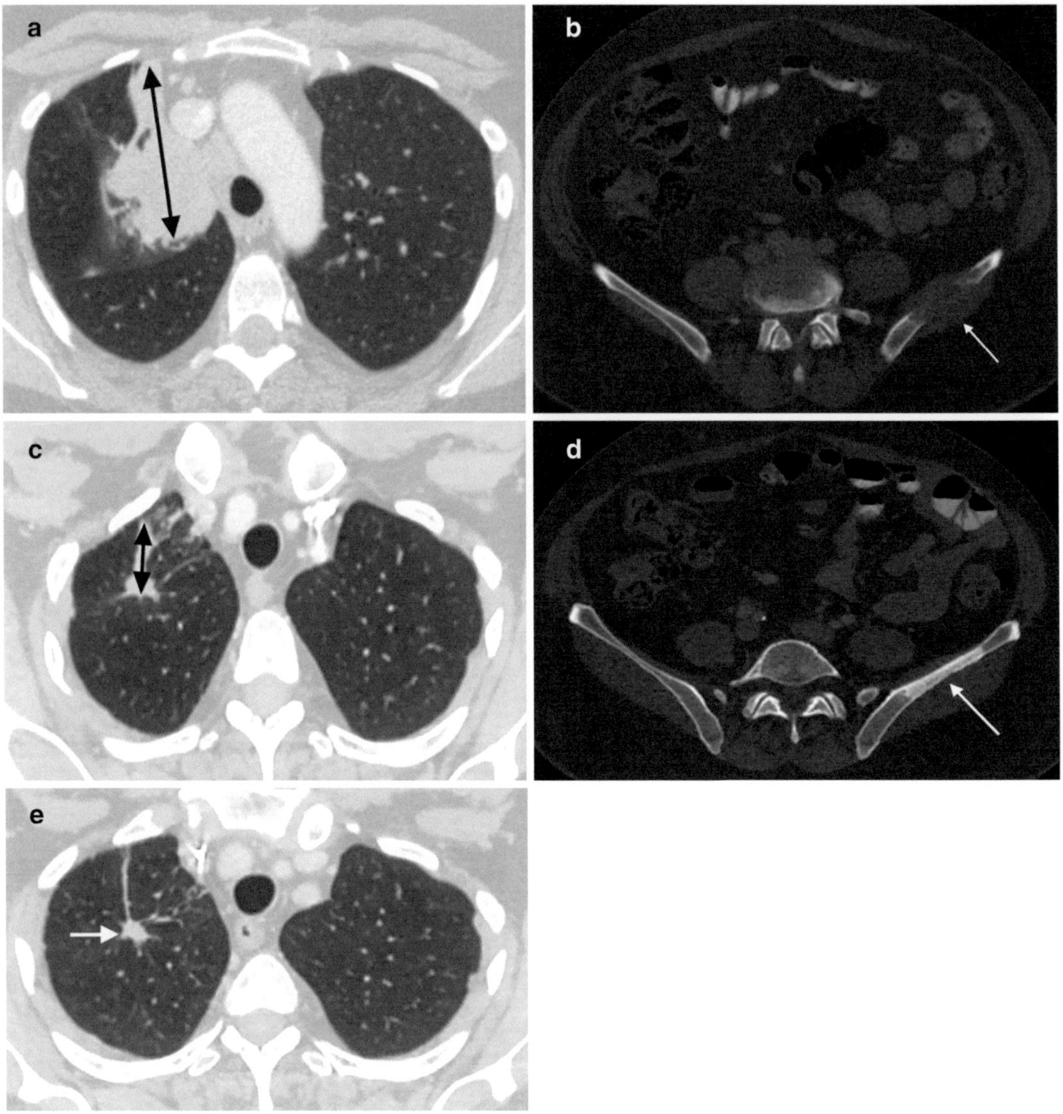

Fig. 22.8 A patient with EGFR-mutant metastatic adenocarcinoma, prolonged partial disease response on TKI-targeted therapy. (**a**) CT thorax with a 6.2 cm right upper lobe mass (double arrows), station 4R lymphadenopathy, and (**b**) a lytic metastasis the left iliac bone (arrow). (**c**) Restaging CT after treatment with platinum-based chemotherapy with a reduction in the right upper lobe tumor (15 mm, double arrows) and (**d**) sclerosis in the left iliac bone metastasis consistent with partial treatment response. The patient was switched to maintenance TKI-targeted therapy, with a subsequent restaging CT 7 years later (**e**) showing further slight reduction in the right upper lobe tumor (arrow) consistent with persistent partial response

ground-glass components. Lee et al. propose to only record the size of the solid component as the size of the target lesion (measured on mediastinal windows). When internal cavitation is present, such as in tumors treated with antiangiogenic therapies, the cavity size is subtracted from tumor diameter [77]. Partial response is defined for tumors greater than 5 mm^2 as either a decrease in size of greater than or equal to 10% or a reduction in tumor HU of greater than or equal to 15%. Decrease in tumor burden in patents with EFGR mutant adenocarcinomas on TKI therapy as measured by the Lee criteria is associated with longer progression-free survival and OS than standard response assessment by RECIST [80, 81]. The Lee criteria have also been shown to be more accurate than RECIST in predicting progression-free survival and OS in patients with EGFR-mutant lung adenocarcinoma receiving TKIs [82, 83].

Immunotherapy Response Assessment (Table 22.2)

Immunotherapy has revolutionized the treatment of several types of cancer, including lung cancer. RECIST and other response criteria were designed and validated principally for cytotoxic chemotherapy; however, immune checkpoint inhibitors have different mechanisms of action, and it may take longer for patients to respond, or they may have atypical responses. ICIs can cause lesion enlargement due to tumor infiltration by inflammatory cells, indistinguishable from disease progression on CT. This response pattern is called pseudoprogression and can be seen in 0.6–5% of patients with NSCLC on immunotherapies [84]. New criteria, specifically designed to assess the response to immunotherapy, have therefore been developed.

iRECIST

Immunotherapy Response Evaluation Criteria in Solid Tumors (iRECIST) was first introduced in 2017 by the iRECIST Working Group, a multidisciplinary group composed of oncologists, radiologists, and statisticians, who aimed to standardize the assessment of response to immunotherapy [85]. The major difference between iRECIST and RECIST 1.1 is in the assessment of progressive disease. iRECIST has two new response categories, unconfirmed progression of disease (UPD) and confirmed progressive disease (PD). If a target lesion increases in size by greater than 30% or if new lesions appear, then this should be categorized as UPD and follow-up imaging performed in 4–8 weeks. If the follow-up scan (usually CT) shows further target lesion growth (increase in sum of target lesions greater than 5 mm), growth of any new lesions that had appeared, any increase in the size of non-target lesions, or additional new lesions, then disease progression is confirmed. If any lesions demonstrate partial or complete response on this short interval CT, then pseudoprogression can be retrospectively diagnosed. Hyperprogression of disease is a rare pattern described in patients treated with immunotherapy where there is a dramatic increase in tumor burden over a very short period, although this is not as of yet a universally accepted pattern [86]. iRECIST also includes the assessment of immune-related lesions (IRLs), defined as new lesions or enlargement of previously stable lesions with typical radiological features of immune-related adverse events (irAEs). IRLs are identified and evaluated separately from target and non-target lesions, and their response is measured independently [87]. The iRECIST criteria have been shown to improve the accuracy and consistency of response assessment in several studies. Hodi et al. compared the response assessment of advanced melanoma patients treated with immunotherapy using both RECIST and iRECIST criteria, finding that iRECIST improved the prediction of both overall and progression-free survival [88–90].

Immunotherapy PET Response

Immune checkpoint inhibitors stimulate host antitumor response, and a positive response can present on FDG PET/CT as an increase in the volume of metabolic activity in the existing tumors, as well as in the development of new inflammatory lesions which may incorrectly be viewed as progressive disease based on PERCIST [91]. The immunotherapy-modified PERCIST (imPERCIST) criteria has been proposed to improve discriminating between pseudoprogression and actual disease progression on FDG PET/CT. Contrary to PERCIST, imPERCIST differs in that the appearance of new lesions is not sufficient to diagnose progressive metabolic disease; new lesions are included in the sum of SULpeak only if their uptake is greater than pre-existing target lesions, or if there were fewer than five lesions on the baseline PET. The imPERCIST criteria adapt the PERCIST criteria along the lines of iRECIST in terms of the classification of unconfirmed progression of disease and the need to re-evaluate with further FDG PET/CT in 4–8 weeks; for patients with metastatic lung cancer on immunotherapy, up to one-third with unconfirmed disease progression on the first interim PET are shown to have an atypical response pattern on a subsequent short interval PET, underlying the importance of not incorrectly confirming disease progression on the first interim PET in patients on ICIs who are clinically well [92].

The clinical benefit of immunotherapy-modified classifications is still under investigation. To date, some studies have shown an improved accuracy in response assessment using the newer modified criteria, although other clinical trials evaluating ICIs have questioned the benefit of iRECIST and imPERCIST due to the uncertain incidence of immunotherapy-related pseudoprogression [93–95]. In addition, it remains unclear whether the immune response to PD-1 inhibitors follows the same pattern in all solid tumors.

In 2021, Ayati et al. compared the correlation between survival outcome and response assessment by PERCIST, imPERCIST, RECIST 1.1, and iRECIST in NSCLC patients on ICI treatment [95]. This study demonstrated comparable results using five lesions with the highest metabolic activity for both PERCIST and imPERCIST and suggest that an interval change in the metabolic activity of the most metabolically active lesion can accurately reflect the overall metabolic response to PD-1 inhibitors. When classifying patients as controlled disease or progressive disease, imPERCIST accurately recategorized 20% of pseudoprogression patients into the controlled-disease category, having been initially categorized as progressive disease [95].

Treatment Complications (Table 22.1)

As well as performing accurate response assessment, early recognition of recognized treatment-related complications is an important role of imaging follow-up in lung cancer. Understanding the common treatment-related adverse events, along with a high index of suspicion, is important, enabling prompt recognition and institution of appropriate therapy.

Chemotherapy

Drug-related pneumonitis (DRP) is a well-described complication of cytotoxic chemotherapy. The clinical presentation is often non-specific, with symptoms including dyspnea, cough, and low-grade fever. Suspicion for a DRP should be raised when there is a close temporal association between receiving a chemotherapy drug known to cause pneumonitis and symptom onset. CT features are often non-specific, including bilateral patchy ground-glass opacities, consolidation, nodules,reticulation, and occasionally signs of overt fibrosis including traction bronchiectasis and honeycombing [96]. DRP is graded clinically by the Common Terminology Criteria for Adverse Events into five categories, with grade 1 DRP classified as asymptomatic with radiology features only up to death (grade 5) [96]. Each individual drug can be associated with a number of different imaging patterns of DRP, with a hypersensitivity pneumonia (HP), organizing pneumonia (OP), and non-specific interstitial pneumonia (NSIP) patterns the most common. Patients are at risk for developing chemotherapy-related pneumonitis 5–10 days after cycle 1 or 2. The main differential diagnosis is usually pneumonia (typical or atypical) and pulmonary edema. Distinguishing between these entities and DRP based solely on CT appearances is difficult and requires a significant input from the multidisciplinary team considering clinical, radiological, and laboratory findings to make a firm diagnosis. Pulmonary embolism is a life-threatening complication of chemotherapy for lung cancer which is associated with specific chemotherapy agents used in lung cancer, in particular cisplatin [97].

Targeted Therapies

Targeted therapies are associated with a number of specific complications. TKI toxicity most frequently affects the skin and the GI tract, with

DRP a rarer occurrence. TKI pneumonitis imaging findings include ground-glass opacities, consolidation, and reticulation, with the CT patterns of lung injury including OP, NSIP, HP, diffuse alveolar damage, and simple pulmonary eosinophilia [98]. The risk of pneumonitis is higher in patients with a history of smoking, pre-existing lung disease, and those receiving concurrent radiation therapy. Transient asymptomatic opacities are a mild form of DRP described in EGFR-TKIs, especially osimertinib, where new focal pulmonary opacities appear on CT in an asymptomatic patient [99]. These are, by definition, transient and will usually resolve within 12 weeks without any additional treatment. Pulmonary hemorrhage is a described complication in antiangiogenic therapies, such as the anti-VEGF agents, and typically present on CT with mixed areas of consolidation, ground glass, and interlobular septal thickening, with or without frank hemoptysis. Targeted therapies are also associated with multisystem complications. Anti-VEGF therapies have been associated with an increased risk of cardiovascular events, including hypertension, congestive heart failure, and arterial thrombotic events [100–102]. Sorafenib and regorafenib have been associated with an increased risk of hepatotoxicity [103, 104].

Immune-Related Adverse Events

Immunotherapy has revolutionized the treatment of lung cancer, but it is associated with a unique spectrum of side effects, known as irAEs, that can affect multiple organ systems. The imaging findings of irAEs can be variable and nonspecific, making it challenging to differentiate them from disease progression or other causes. The incidence of irAEs is 30–66%, and manifestations can range from abnormal laboratory tests or imaging studies without symptoms to life-threating conditions [105]. Most irAEs will resolve after stopping immunotherapy, with steroids required for the more severe cases. DRP is one of the most common irAEs in patients receiving immunotherapy for lung cancer, typically presenting as bilateral ground-glass opacities and consolidation often with a peripheral or subpleural distribution, usually displaying either a hypersensitivity or organizing pneumonia pattern of lung injury on CT (Figs. 22.9, 22.10, and 22.11) [106–108]. The incidence of pneumonitis varies depending on the type of immunotherapy and the presence of pre-existing pulmonary disease, with higher rates reported for anti-PD-1/PD-L1 agents [109].

Another important irAE affecting the thorax is sarcoid-like reactions, which are characterized by the formation of non-caseating granulomas in various organs, including the lungs. These granulomas may be detected incidentally in imaging or may present with symptoms such as cough and dyspnea. On CT, sarcoid-like reactions typically manifest as nodules or masses with a perilymphatic distribution, as well as mediastinal and hilar lymphadenopathy [110]. Other less common pulmonary irAEs include diffuse alveolar hemorrhage and acute respiratory distress syndrome, manifesting as confluent areas of consolidation and ground glass often with an anteroposterior gradient [111, 112].

ICI-related myopericarditis is a potentially fatal adverse event caused by T cell-mediated attack on cardiac myocytes and/or the pericardium (Fig. 22.12) [113]. Myocarditis can present with a wide range of symptoms, including chest pain, dyspnea, palpitations, and fatigue. Early detection is crucial as severe cases can progress rapidly to heart failure and cardiogenic shock. Diagnosis is often challenging, as symptoms may overlap with other cardiac conditions or side effects of cancer treatments. The diagnosis of myocarditis that is dependent on a comprehensive evaluation is necessary, including electrocardiogram, cardiac troponin levels, echocardiography, and cardiac MRI [114]. Early recognition and prompt management of myocarditis are essential to prevent severe complications. Treatment often involves discontinuation of immunotherapy and initiation of high-dose corticosteroids to suppress the immune response. In severe cases, additional immunosuppressive agents like infliximab (anti-TNF-α antibody) may be considered [115]. Thyroiditis is a relatively common thoracic irAE that can manifest

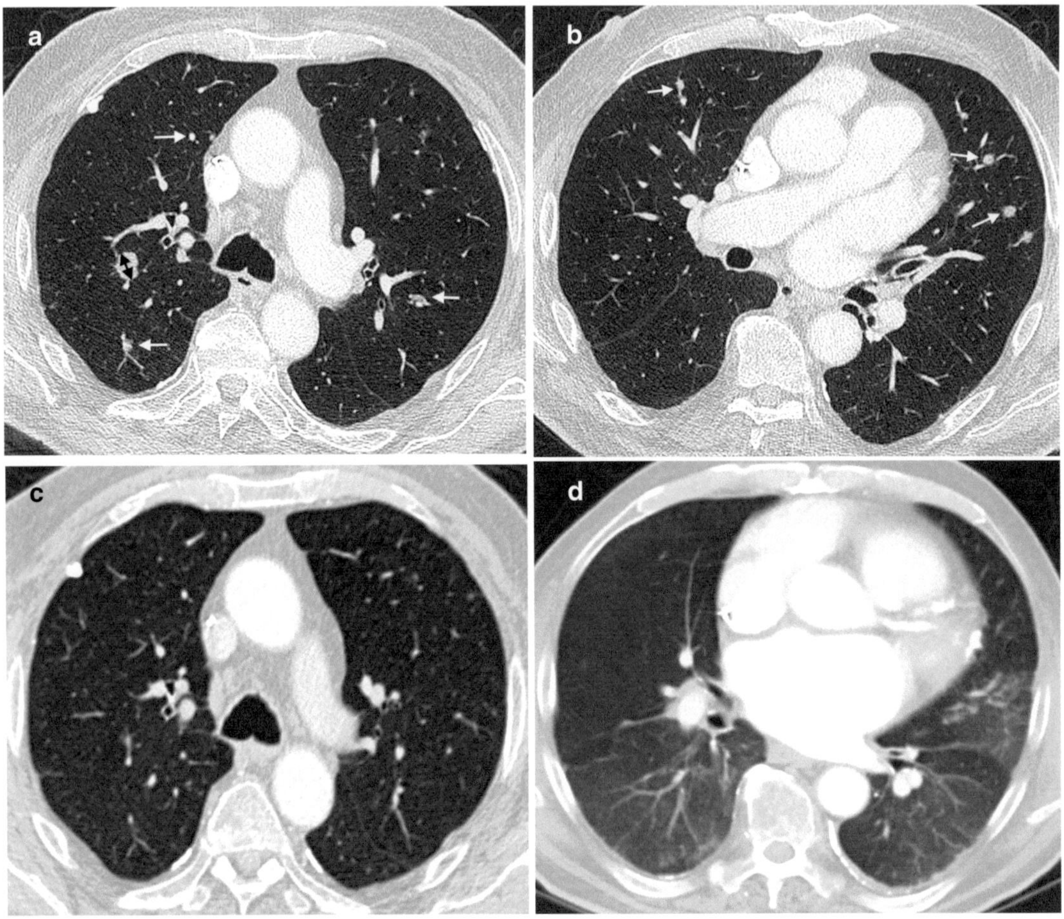

Fig. 22.9 A patient with metastatic squamous cell carcinoma with a complete response on immune checkpoint inhibitors (CI) and subsequently developed a drug-related pneumonitis. (**a**, **b**) Initial CT demonstrates multiple bilateral pulmonary metastasis (arrows) with a dominant 14 mm right upper lobe nodule (double arrows). (**c**) Restaging CT on immunotherapy shows a complete treatment response with no residual measurable nodules. (**d**) Subsequent CT on ICI with acute shortness of breath demonstrates new confluent bilateral ground-glass opacities compatible with drug-related pneumonitis

clinically with either hyper- or hypothyroidism (Fig. 22.13).

Extra-thoracic irAEs can manifest as dermatologic, gastrointestinal, endocrine, neurological, renal, or musculoskeletal disorders, among others. Examples include skin rashes, colitis, hypophysitis, neuropathies, glomerulonephritis, colitis, and arthritis (Figs. 22.14 and 22.15). These manifestations can significantly impact patients' quality of life and treatment outcomes. Diagnosing extra-thoracic irAEs requires a high index of suspicion, as symptoms may be nonspecific. The management of extra-thoracic irAEs depends on the affected organ system and the severity of the adverse event. Treatment typically involves immune suppression using corticosteroids or other immunosuppressive agents. In severe or refractory cases, infliximab, mycophenolate mofetil, or rituximab may be considered [116].

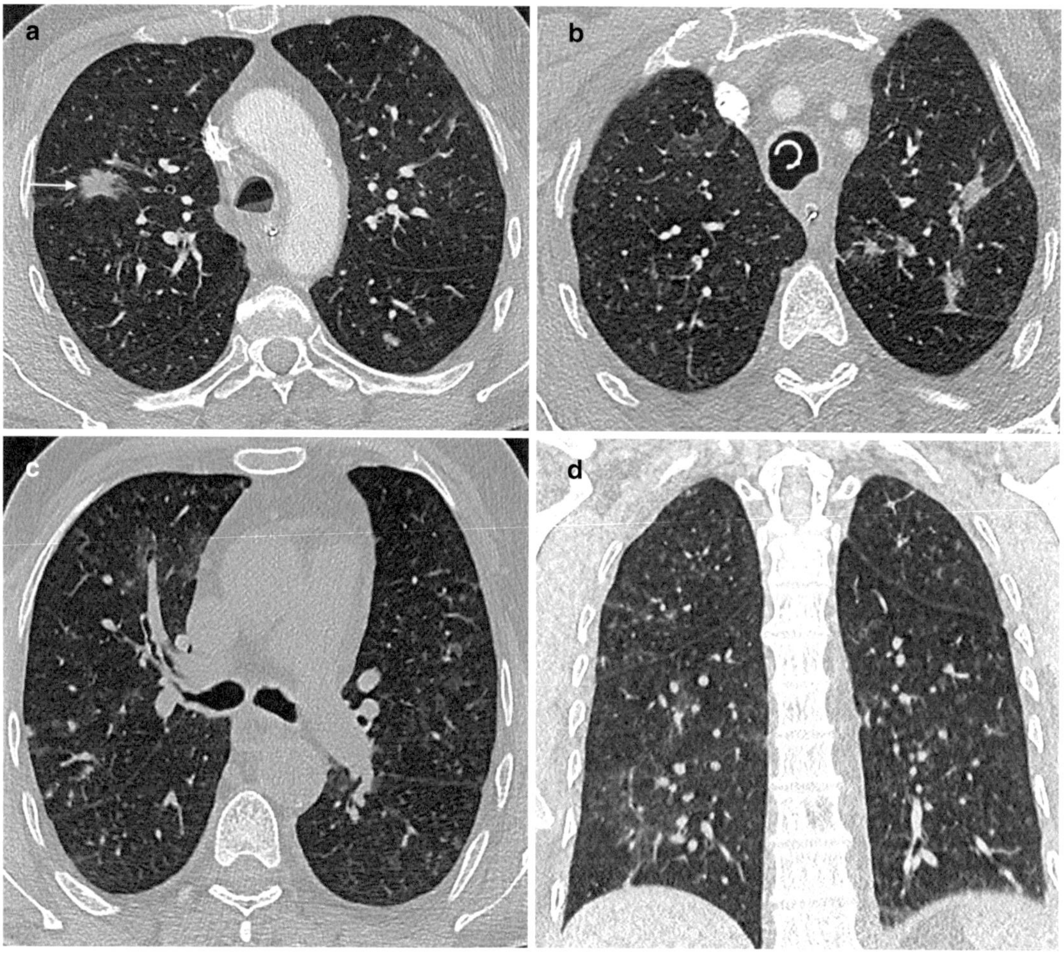

Fig. 22.10 A patient with metastatic adenocarcinoma treated with immunotherapy complicated by drug-related pneumonitis. (**a**) Initial CT shows a spiculated 17 mm primary tumor in the right upper lobe with bone metastasis (not shown). The patient was treated with nivolumab and developed severe respiratory distress requiring intubation, with CT thorax at that time (**b**–**d**) with patchy bilateral ground-glass opacities and left upper lobe perilobular consolidation. There were no clinical signs of infection. The patient was treated for drug-related pneumonitis with corticosteroids and immunotherapy cessation but unfortunately passed away

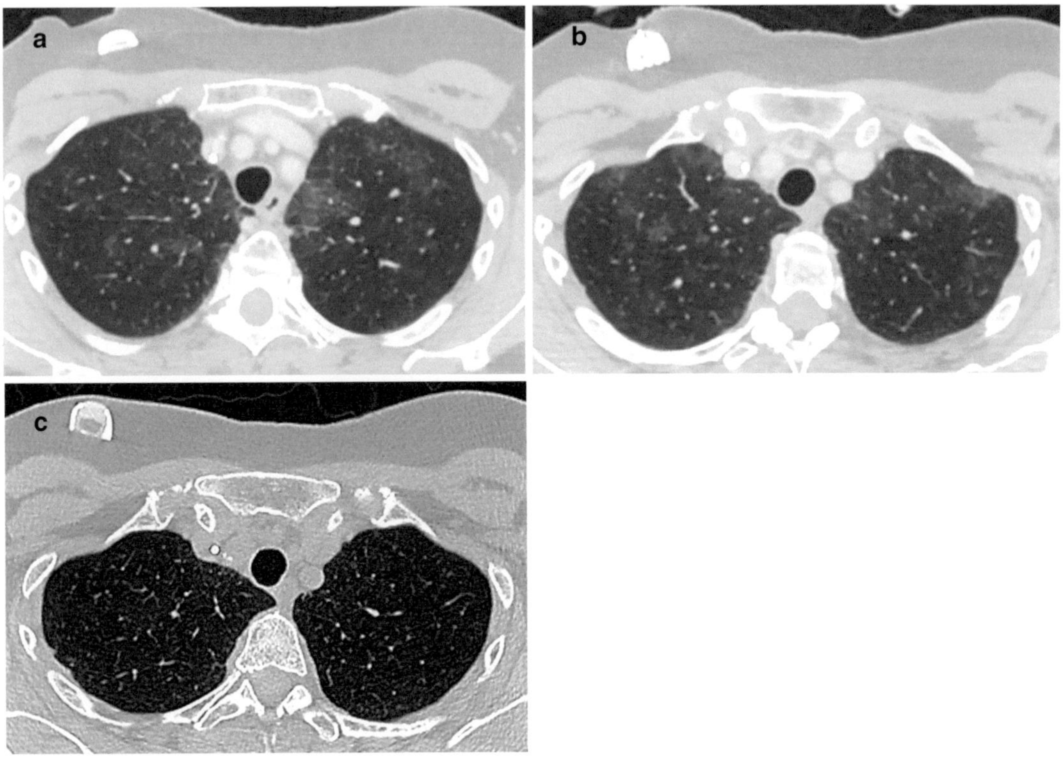

Fig. 22.11 A patient with metastatic non-small cell lung cancer, not otherwise specified (NSCLC, NOS) treated with an ICI with a mild dug-related pneumonitis. (**a**, **b**) CT performed when the patient developed acute, mild shortness of breath with new patchy bilateral upper lobe ground-glass opacities. The ICI treatment was paused with resolution of symptoms and a subsequent CT 6 weeks later (**c**) showing resolution of the ground glass

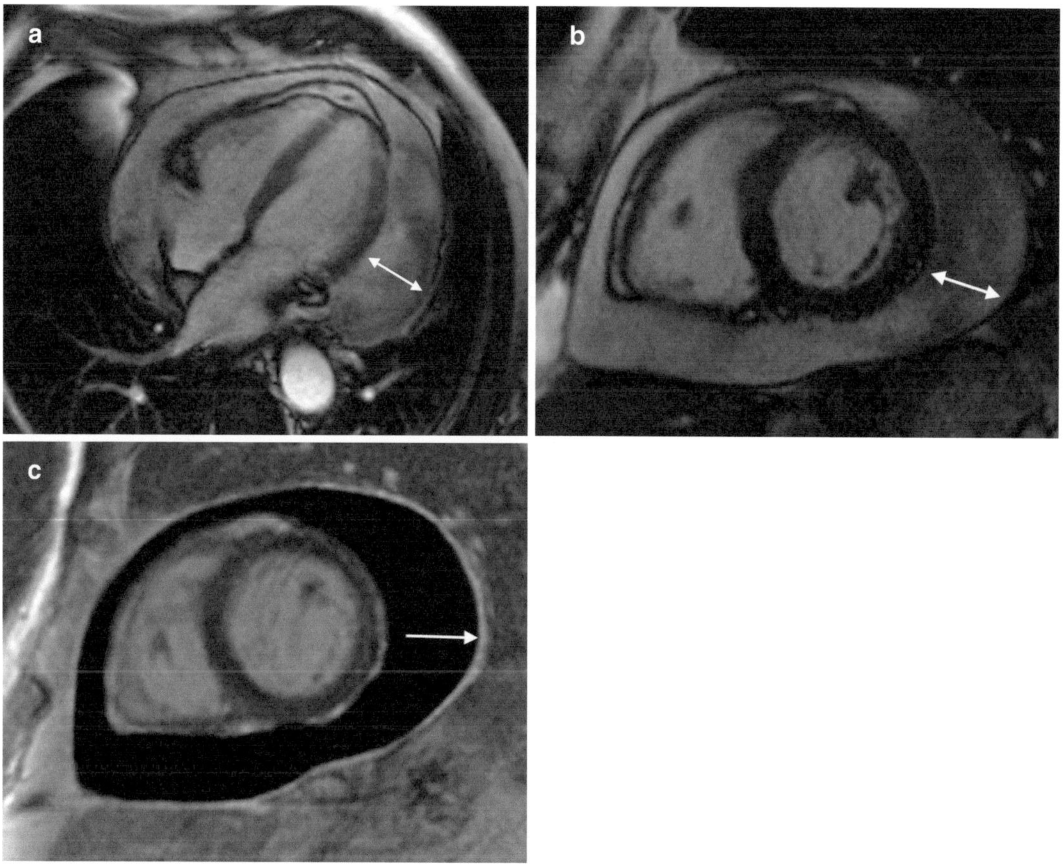

Fig. 22.12 A patient with metastatic non-small cell carcinoma treated with immunotherapy complicated by pericarditis. (**a**) Cardiac MRI SSFP four-chamber and short-axis (**b**) images show a large pleural effusion (double arrows), with (**c**) pericardial late gadolinium enhancement on PSIR (arrow)

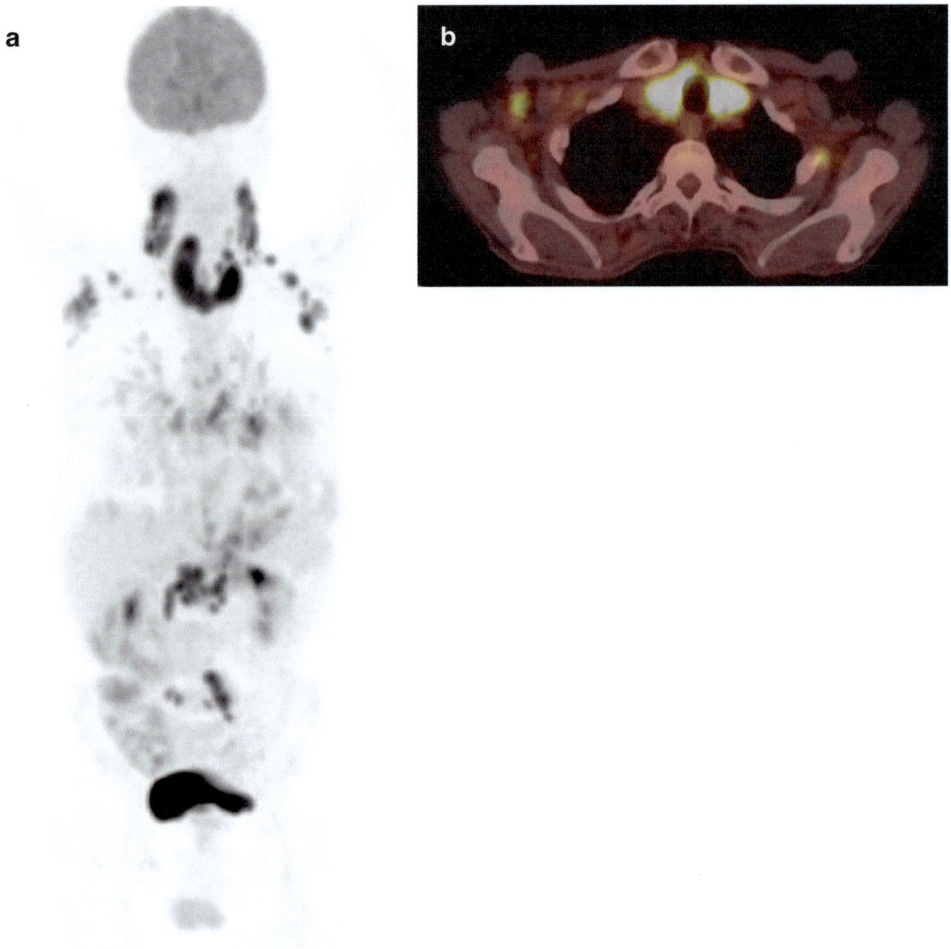

Fig. 22.13 A patient with metastatic NSCLC on immunotherapy with treatment thyroiditis on PET. Restaging FDG PET/CT PET maximal intensity projection (**a**) and fused axial (**b**) images show diffuse intense thyroid uptake compatible with immunotherapy-related thyroiditis

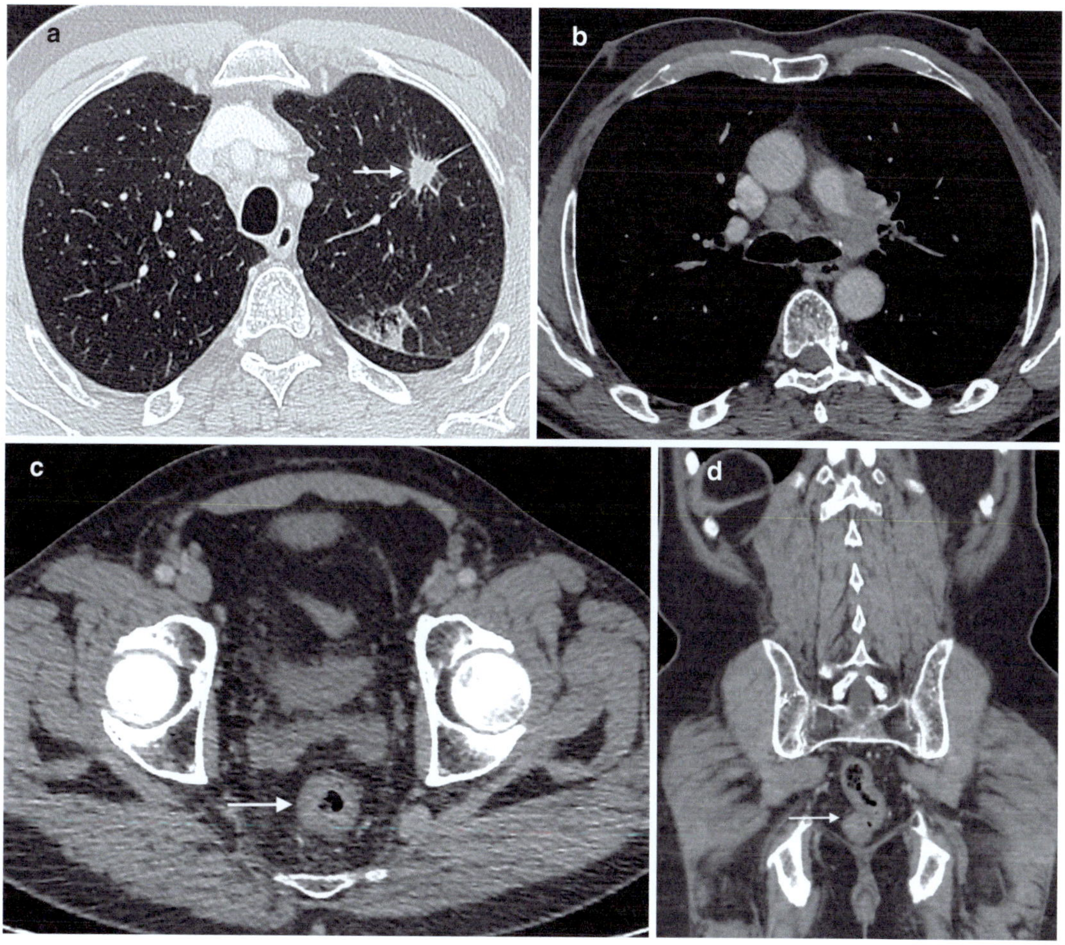

Fig. 22.14 A patient with metastatic squamous cell carcinoma on immunotherapy presented complicated by proctitis. (**a**) Initial CT thorax shows the 1.6 cm left upper lobe primary tumor (arrow) with (**b**) bilateral mediastinal lymphadenopathy. The patient was treated with immunotherapy and presented with diarrhea and acute abdominal pain. CT abdomen axial (**c**) and coronal (**d**) images show rectal thickening (arrow) with mild mesorectal fat stranding, consistent with immunotherapy-related proctitis

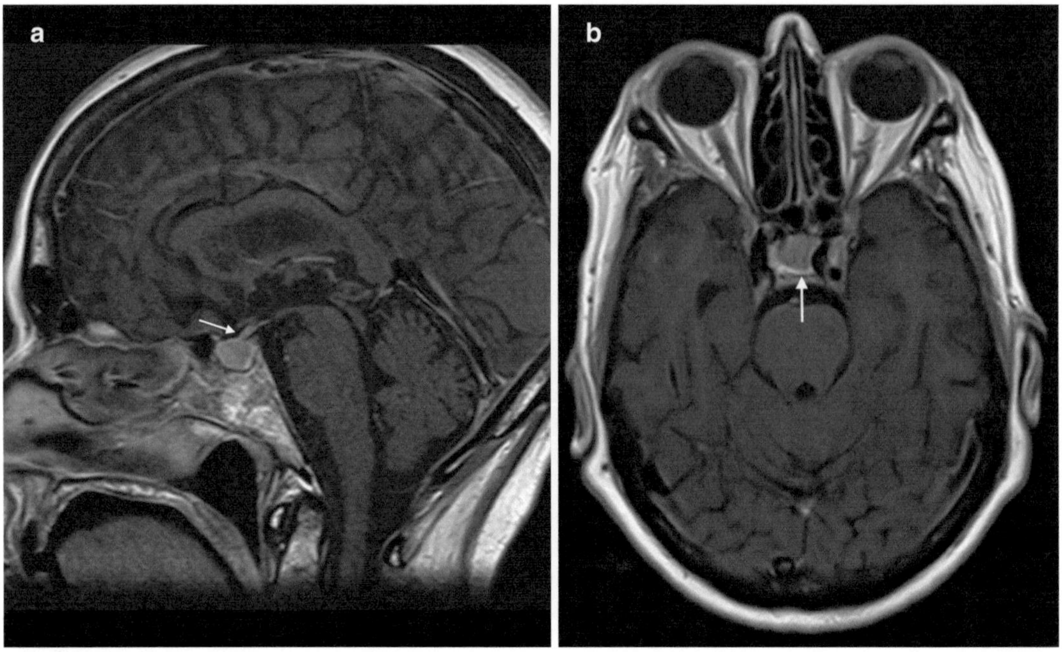

Fig. 22.15 A patient with metastatic adenocarcinoma on immunotherapy presented with headaches and newly reduced cortisol. Brain MRI T1w sagittal (**a**) and axial (**b**) post-contrast images show enlargement and enhancement of pituitary and stalk (arrow) compatible with immunotherapy-related hypophysitis

Advanced Response Assessment Techniques

Volumetric Evaluation

Volumetric tumor assessment is potentially more sensitive and accurate than conventional diameter measurements, such as unidimensional measurements used in RECIST, as it takes into account changes in three-dimensional lesion volume, which may be a more sensitive assessment of lesion growth (Fig. 22.1) [117, 118]. Hayes et al. found volumetric response assessment of lung adenocarcinoma on first follow-up CT better predicted OS than RECIST [117]. Kamran et al. evaluated the predictive value of volumetric assessment in patients with limited-stage SCLC, comparing quantitative CT-based volumetric tumor assessment with TNM Classification in 105 patients [119]. Interestingly, these results demonstrated that T-stage and N-stage were not associated with clinical outcome; however, that tumor volume at diagnosis was found to be a significant predictor of locoregional recurrence, distant metastasis, future progression, and OS. This suggests that tumor volume may be a better predictor of outcome than TNM stage in LS-SCLC, as is the case in other thoracic malignancies such as malignant pleural mesothelioma [119]. Unidimensional size measurement assumes equal radial tumor growth, but this can often be more heterogeneous due to internal variation in tumor biology-tumor volumetry that has been shown to be accurate and reproducible and will likely be incorporated into future iterations of RECIST, as access to robust and validated software for semiautomated and fully automated lesion volumetric segmentation becomes more widespread [120, 121]. Variations in CT acquisition and analysis can lead to inconsistencies in measurements and affect the accuracy of volumetric assessment, and this will need to be minimized before volumetric response assessment becomes routine.

Liu et al. demonstrated that a clinical and PET/CT volumetric prognostic index, generated using a Cox regression model from a cohort which included pretreatment variables (whole-body metabolic tumor volume [MTVwb], clinical TNM stage, tumor histology, performance status, age, race, gender, smoking history, and treatment) for NSCLC patients, has moderately strong prognostic power and is more prognostic than its individual prognostic variables and other indices [122]. A meta-analysis on volumetric parameters from 18F-FDG PET (metabolic tumor volume [MTV] and total lesion glycolysis [TLG]) in patients with lung cancer demonstrated that they are significant prognostic factors (Fig. 22.1) [123]. Patients with a high tumor MTV and/or TLG have been shown to be at higher risk of adverse events and death; in a meta-analysis published by Wen et al., stage I/II NSCLC cases with increased TLG and MTV had a higher risk of side effects, and the authors found that TLG related to increased mortality risk [124].

Automated Segmentation

Automated segmentation involves the use of software algorithms to segment and measure the volume of a tumor on CT, MRI, or PET/CT images, with minimal or no user input.

Automated segmentation techniques have the potential to improve the accuracy and reproducibility of tumor response assessment in lung cancer patients. These techniques offer several advantages over manual measurements of tumor size, including potentially improved prognostic value and the ability to monitor changes in tumor burden over time. As previously described, tumor volume is prognostic and can be used to assess disease response. Primakov et al. report a prospective in silico clinical trial of 1328 thoracic CTs demonstrating that the performance of an automatic segmentation model for NSCLC is acceptable and that radiologists and radiation oncologists preferred automatic segmentations in 56% of the cases, rather than the manual contours [125]. The authors then calculated the RECIST diameter and tumor volume for both the expert and the automatic segmentation and found that for both metrics the automatically generated segmentations had greater prognostic power. Automatically generated segmentations had the power to stratify patients into low and high survival groups with a higher significance than those methods based on expert manual contours. The use of the automated segmentation technique demonstrated a trend toward better performance and less variability for larger and less complex tumors with superior reproducibility and significant time-saving benefits compared to manual segmentation [125].

Several studies have investigated the potential of automated segmentation techniques for assessing other solid cancer responses to therapy. For example, a study of 74 pediatric patients with Ewing's sarcoma that volumetric assessment of tumor response was a more significant predictor of OS in patients than RECIST or WHO measurements [126]. Similarly, a study by Lee et al. demonstrated that MTV, a measure of tumor burden on FDG PET imaging, was significantly associated with worse OS and progression-free survival [127].

In addition to predicting patient outcomes, automated segmentation techniques may also improve the accuracy and reproducibility of tumor response assessment. Zhang et al. assessed the use of a modified version of ResNet (a residual neural network deep learning model) for automated segmentation of gross target volume in CTs of patients with NSCLC with a view to radiotherapy volume planning [128]. ResNet was able to perform automatic segmentation quickly and accurately, although many of the datasets required additional manual alteration prior to the final clinical implementation. Manual measurements of tumor size were less reliable and subject to interobserver variability [128]. Jiang et al. evaluated automated segmentation techniques under the umbrella of multiple resolution residually connected network formulations to detect and segment lung tumors in patients from three datasets consisting of 377 tumors from an open-source cancer archive, 304 advanced stage NSCLC treated with anti-PD-1 checkpoint immunotherapy, and 529 lung nodules from a large consortium [129]. The authors utilized a multi-scale convolutional neural network (CNN) approach for volumetrically segmenting lung tumors which enabled accurate, automated identification of and serial measurement of tumor volumes in the lung, with the potential to quicken and enhance clinical decision-making and better predict response to treatment [129].

Despite these promising results, there are several challenges associated with the use of automated segmentation techniques. One is the need for standardized imaging protocols to ensure consistent and accurate segmentation across different imaging modalities and institutions [130]. Another challenge is the need for validation of automated segmentation techniques against gold standard measurements of tumor size and response.

Radiomics

Advances in CT allows for a complex lesion assessment, enabling a computerized feature-based analysis of imaging features that are not visually apparent including lesion texture, density, and shape. These features can be quantified using image analysis software, and statistical models can be developed to correlate imaging features with clinical outcomes, such as tumor stage, prognosis, and response to therapy. This process of radiomics begins with acquisition of high-quality, three-dimensional volumetric imaging usually, but not limited to, CT. The lesion is then segmented, whether manually or increasingly using automated software, and quantitative features are extracted using high-throughput computing. Texture analysis, density analysis, and shape analysis are among the most widely studied radiomics techniques and have shown promise in predicting tumor stage, invasiveness, prognosis, and response to therapy.

Texture analysis quantifies the heterogeneity of a lung lesion by analyzing the gray-level intensity patterns within the tumor. It can be performed using various proprietary software packages, and different texture features can be extracted, including first-order statistics, second-order statistics, and higher-order statistics [131]. Texture analysis has been shown to be useful for differentiating benign from malignant lung nodules, predicting tumor recurrence, and assessing treatment response. For example, Palumbo et al. found that adding shape and texture features increased the performance of both CT-based and PET-based prediction models, with an overall improvement in accuracy of 3.4–11.2% and 2.2–10.2%, respectively [132]. They found that shape and texture features from 18F-FDG PET/CT can lead to a better discrimination between benign and malignant lung nodules by increasing the accuracy of the prediction models by an appreciable margin [132].

Another CT-based quantitative imaging technique is density analysis, which quantifies the voxel intensity values within a lung lesion. This can be done using histogram analysis, where the distribution of voxel intensity values is plotted as a histogram, and various parameters, including mean, standard deviation, skewness, and kurtosis, can be calculated. Density analysis has been shown to be useful for predicting tumor invasiveness and prognosis. Ganeshan et al. demonstrated that the quantification of attenuation heterogeneity using CT texture analysis methods can provide valuable information in the domains of disease severity and prognosis and in treatment and planning response [133]. Shape analysis quantifies the geometric features of the lung lesion, including volume, surface area, and sphericity. Tumor contour analysis has been shown to be useful for predicting tumor aggressiveness and prognosis. Bianconi et al. assessed 203 patients with NSCLC, finding that a combination of tumor volume and gray-level run-length matrix (a surrogate marker of contour smoothness and average pixel signal intensity along the periphery of the lesion) provided the best prognostic prediction value over other three-dimensional and texture features [134]. Further research is needed to validate these techniques and to establish their clinical utility in routine lung cancer imaging.

Artificial Intelligence

Artificial intelligence (AI) algorithms have the potential to significantly impact and improve cancer imaging. They are mainly derived from analysis of pre-existing data with the purpose of predicting or classifying objects [135]. AI algorithms are capable of handling large volumes of computational and repetitive labor work, making it a suitable tool for assisting radiologists in oncology imaging. The main components of an AI model include the dataset used for training, an algorithm that is used to generate the prediction model, the pretreatment method and the pre-trained model used to enhance the speed of building models and inherit previous experience [135]. A subset of AI, machine learning (ML), involves gathering algorithms to solve problems but without being explicitly programmed. This includes support vector machines, decision trees, and Bayesian networks. A further subclass of ML is deep learning, which achieves both feature selection and model fitting simultaneously. The heterogeneity of lung cancer makes it potentially amenable to AI application, with several studies already reporting on the application of AI in lung nodule detection, disease risk stratification, drug development, diagnostic application in histopathology, and prognosis prediction [135].

For the most part, AI models can be divided into categories: supervised learning, unsupervised learning, semi-supervised learning, and reinforcement learning. Supervised learning requires preparation of the labeled dataset with the inputs and desired outputs in order to train the algorithm. Supervised learning has the capability of solving prediction problems such as regression and classification. The majority of AI models that are aimed at predicting cancer risk and survival, as well as nodule detection and characteristics, are based on supervised learning [135]. Unsupervised learning does not require labeled data, with the algorithm dividing samples by itself according to inputs, and is capable of finding association between samples. Unsupervised learning provides a less accurate algorithm but avoids the labor-intensive process of labeling datasets for model training. Reinforcement learning involves a reward function that is used to adjust the algorithm, with the algorithm evolving as it interacts with the dataset—this model has the potential to develop a self-evolving AI application, for example, for lung nodule detection.

With an ever-increasing workload coupled with the repetitive nature of imaging, there is room for AI to participate greatly in lung cancer imaging. Human error is inevitable, with anything up to 25% of lung nodules going undetected on CXR [136]. Deep learning models have further displayed the power of AI in CXR analysis. A deep learning application, known as "CheXNet," was trained and developed on "Chest-Xray14" which is one of the largest CXR databases in the world. "CheXNet" was shown to exceed radiologist performance in detecting lung nodules and masses [137]. When used in low-dose chest CT, the primary objective of AI is nodule detection, classification, and malignancy prediction. As with AI applications in CXR, AI has been shown to increase the sensitivity of nodule detection while also decreasing interpretation time, with one study demonstrating computer-aided detection (CAD) systems to detect up to 70% of lung cancers not picked up by a radiologist [138]. Initial CAD tools developed for the detection of nodules on thoracic CT were based on ML models and were found to have up to 96.7% sensitivity but encountered a high number of false positives and poor performance in detecting subsolid nodules [138]. More recently however, CAD tools have been based on deep learning methods and continue to display a high sensitivity rate but also continue to be limited by false-positive reporting despite these rates decreasing when compared to earlier ML based tools [139].

Deep learning tools have been shown to automatically detect and measure nodules while also suggesting a Lung-RADS classification in low-dose lung cancer screening CTs [140]. These tools have been demonstrated to have fewer negative misclassifications than radiologists but did result in more positive misclassifications. With regard to malignancy risk prediction, AI applications can analyze a nodule's global characteristics and not just its size. This can be achieved using radiomics or a deep learning method and has been proven to be very successful. For example, using a radiomics approach on a subset of NLST participants with lung nodules, one model was shown to be capable of predicting which nodules would become malignant at 1 and 2 years with an accuracy of 80% [141].

The development of rigorous and clinically relevant AI techniques to help lung cancer response assessment has the potential to advance cancer care. Quantitative assessment through manual measurement is time-consuming, tedious, and prone to a degree of interobserver variability. Xu et al. employed a deep neural network using transfer learning of CNN with recurrent neural networks on 179 patients with stage III NSCLC treated with chemoradiotherapy, analyzing pre- and post-treatment CT scans [142]. They found that the model using predefined cancer-specific outcomes (progression, distant metastases, and local-regional recurrence) had the ability to stratify patients into low- and high-risk mortality groups (hazard ratio = 6.16, $p < 0.001$) and could predict response in a subset of the patients. The authors also found that the model performance in determining cancer-specific outcomes like 2-year survival was enhanced on each additional study which was introduced to CNN. Several studies have developed AI models to predict lung cancer response to treatment. Trebeschi et al. developed an AI model to predict treatment outcomes to immunotherapy in NSCLC [143]. Their lesion-level performance in NSCLC yielded an AUC of 0.83, whereas the best patient-level prediction models had an AUC of 0.76. CD8 cell infiltration within NSCLC tumors has been associated with response to immunotherapy—a model employed by Sun et al. used an eight radiomic features to discriminate inflamed tumors from immune desert tumors, with an AUC of 0.76 [144]. Tunali et al. developed a radiomic clinical model to predict rapid disease progression in NSCLC patients treated with immunotherapy, including hyperprogression under immunotherapy, with an AUC of 0.81–0.85 [144]. In a follow-up study, the same authors using a radiomics model utilizing using gene expression data from a radiogenomics dataset stratified patients undergoing immunotherapy into risk groups; low, moderate, high, and very high [145]. They demonstrated that the very high-risk group was associated with very poor OS. Mu et al. extracted the radiomic features from PET/CTs of 194 patients with stage IIIB–IV NSCLC to train a multiparametric radiomics signature (mpRS) model to predict clinical benefit in a training, retrospective and prospective patient cohorts using a binary cutoff of progression-free survival at 6 months [146]. The authors found that the mpRS could predict durable clinical benefit with AUCs of 0.81–0.86 and could predict progression-free and OS. These studies suggest that AI has an important role to play in the near future in the assessment of response to treatment in lung cancer and has efficacy in predicting both patients who are likely to respond to and garner benefit from targeted therapy but also has an evolving role in predicting overall disease survival.

Conclusion

In conclusion, lung cancer remains a significant global health challenge, ranking as the second most common cancer worldwide and the leading cause of cancer-related mortality. Its prevalence underscores the need for innovative treatment strategies, particularly as surgical intervention is limited to early-stage disease. While traditional cytotoxic chemotherapy has been the mainstay, the advent of personalized medicine has ushered in a new era of targeted and immunotherapies therapies based on molecular tumor profiling. Accurate disease response assessment with multi-modality imaging and early recognition of treatment-related adverse events play a crucial role in the clinical care of patients with lung cancer. Ongoing rapid advances in computing and imaging technology underpinning the artificial intelligence revolution will likely significantly alter and improve how we perform lung cancer response assessment in the future.

References

1. Siegel RL, Miller KD, Jemal A. Cancer statistics, 2020. CA Cancer J Clin. 2020;70:7–30.
2. Bray F, Ferlay J, Soerjomataram I, Siegel RL, Torre LA, Jemal A. Global cancer statistics 2018: GLOBOCAN estimates of incidence and mortal-

ity worldwide for 36 cancers in 185 countries. CA Cancer J Clin. 2018;68:394–424.
3. American Cancer Society. Cancer facts & figures. 2019. Available from: https://www.cancer.org/content/dam/cancer-org/research/cancer-facts-and-statistics/annual-cancer-facts-and-figures/2019/cancer-facts-and-figures-2019.pdf. Last accessed 31 Aug 2023.
4. WHO. Lung cancer factsheet. 2023. Available from: https://www.who.int/news-room/fact-sheets/detail/lung-cancer. Last accessed 31 Aug 2023.
5. American Lung Association. State of lung cancer. 2022. Available from: https://www.lung.org/research/state-of-lung-cancer/key-findings. Last accessed 31 Aug 2023.
6. Breathnach OS, Freidlin B, Conley B, Green MR, Johnson DH, Gandara DR, et al. Twenty-two years of phase III trials for patients with advanced non-small-cell lung cancer: sobering results. J Clin Oncol. 2001;19:1734–42.
7. Lynch TJ, Bell DW, Sordella R, Gurubhagavatula S, Okimoto RA, Brannigan BW, et al. Activating mutations in the epidermal growth factor receptor underlying responsiveness of non-small-cell lung cancer to gefitinib. N Engl J Med. 2004;350:2129–39.
8. Travis WD, Brambilla E, Nicholson AG, Yatabe Y, Austin JHM, Beasley MB, et al. The 2015 World Health Organization classification of lung tumors: impact of genetic, clinical and radiologic advances since the 2004 classification. J Thorac Oncol. 2015;10:1243–60.
9. Ettinger DS, Wood DE, Aisner DL, Akerley W, Bauman J, Chirieac LR, et al. Non-small cell lung cancer, version 5.2017, NCCN clinical practice guidelines in oncology. J Natl Compr Cancer Netw. 2017;15:504–35.
10. Pao W, Miller V, Zakowski M, Doherty J, Politi K, Sarkaria I, et al. EGF receptor gene mutations are common in lung cancers from "never smokers" and are associated with sensitivity of tumors to gefitinib and erlotinib. Proc Natl Acad Sci USA. 2004;101:13306–11.
11. Gonzalez de Castro D, Clarke PA, Al-Lazikani B, Workman P. Personalized cancer medicine: molecular diagnostics, predictive biomarkers, and drug resistance. Clin Pharmacol Ther. 2013;93:252–9.
12. Slotman B, Faivre-Finn C, Kramer G, Rankin E, Snee M, Hatton M, et al. Prophylactic cranial irradiation in extensive small-cell lung cancer. N Engl J Med. 2007;357:664–72.
13. Nicholson AG, Chansky K, Crowley J, Beyruti R, Kubota K, Turrisi A, et al. The International Association for the Study of Lung Cancer lung cancer staging project: proposals for the revision of the clinical and pathologic staging of small cell lung cancer in the forthcoming eighth edition of the TNM classification for lung cancer. J Thorac Oncol. 2016;11:300–11.
14. Spiro SG, Silvestri GA. One hundred years of lung cancer. Am J Respir Crit Care Med. 2005;172:523–9.
15. Hiddinga BI, Raskin J, Janssens A, Pauwels P, Van Meerbeeck JP. Recent developments in the treatment of small cell lung cancer. Eur Respir Rev. 2021;30:210079.
16. Ettinger DS, Wood DE, Aisner DL, Akerley W, Bauman JR, Bharat A, et al. Non-small cell lung cancer, version 3.2022, NCCN clinical practice guidelines in oncology. J Natl Compr Cancer Netw. 2022;20:497–530.
17. Murphy DJ, Mayoral M, Larici AR, Ginsberg MS, Cicchetti G, Fintelmann FJ, et al. Imaging follow-up of nonsurgical therapies for lung cancer: AJR expert panel narrative review. AJR Am J Roentgenol. 2023;9:1–16.
18. National Cancer Control Network. NCCN clinical practice guidelines in oncology. Small cell lung cancer version 3. 2023. Available from: www.nccn.org. Last accessed 31 Aug 2023.
19. Rosell R, Carcereny E, Gervais R, Vergnenegre A, Massuti B, Felip E, et al. Erlotinib versus standard chemotherapy as first-line treatment for European patients with advanced EGFR mutation-positive non-small-cell lung cancer (EURTAC): a multicentre, open-label, randomised phase 3 trial. Lancet Oncol. 2012;13:239–46.
20. Remon J, Steuer CE, Ramalingam SS, Felip E. Osimertinib and other third-generation EGFR TKI in EGFR-mutant NSCLC patients. Ann Oncol. 2018;29:i20-i7.
21. Sequist LV, Heist RS, Shaw AT, Fidias P, Rosovsky R, Temel JS, et al. Implementing multiplexed genotyping of non-small-cell lung cancers into routine clinical practice. Ann Oncol. 2011;22:2616–24.
22. Skoulidis F, Li BT, Dy GK, Price TJ, Falchook GS, Wolf J, et al. Sotorasib for lung cancers with KRAS p.G12C mutation. N Engl J Med. 2021;384:2371–81.
23. Halpenny D, O'Dwyer E, Camacho Vasquez J, Shaverdian N, Girshman J, Ginsberg MS. Imaging of novel oncologic treatments in lung cancer part 2: local ablative therapies. J Thorac Imaging. 2020;35:37–48.
24. Tanvetyanon T, Creelan BC, Antonia SJ. The safety and efficacy of nivolumab in advanced (metastatic) non-small cell lung cancer. Expert Rev Anticancer Ther. 2016;16:903–10.
25. Costa LB, Queiroz MA, Barbosa FG, Nunes RF, Zaniboni EC, Ruiz MM, et al. Reassessing patterns of response to immunotherapy with PET: from morphology to metabolism. Radiographics. 2021;41:120–43.
26. Palmer M. WHO handbook for reporting results of cancer treatment. Br J Cancer. 1982;45:484–5.
27. Therasse P, Arbuck SG, Eisenhauer EA, Wanders J, Kaplan RS, Rubinstein L, et al. New guidelines to evaluate the response to treatment in solid tumors. European Organization for Research and Treatment of Cancer, National Cancer Institute of the United States, National Cancer Institute of Canada. J Natl Cancer Inst. 2000;92:205–16.

28. Eisenhauer EA, Therasse P, Bogaerts J, Schwartz LH, Sargent D, Ford R, et al. New response evaluation criteria in solid tumours: revised RECIST guideline (version 1.1). Eur J Cancer. 2009;45:228–47.
29. Nishino M, Jagannathan JP, Krajewski KM, O'Regan K, Hatabu H, Shapiro G, et al. Personalized tumor response assessment in the era of molecular medicine: cancer-specific and therapy-specific response criteria to complement pitfalls of RECIST. AJR Am J Roentgenol. 2012;198:737–45.
30. Somarouthu B, Lee SI, Urban T, Sadow CA, Harris GJ, Kambadakone A. Immune-related tumour response assessment criteria: a comprehensive review. Br J Radiol. 2018;91:20170457.
31. Li H, Gao L, Ma H, Arefan D, He J, Wang J, et al. Radiomics-based features for prediction of histological subtypes in central lung cancer. Front Oncol. 2021;11:658887.
32. Gillies RJ, Kinahan PE, Hricak H. Radiomics: images are more than pictures, they are data. Radiology. 2016;278:563–77.
33. Lubner MG, Smith AD, Sandrasegaran K, Sahani DV, Pickhardt PJ. CT texture analysis: definitions, applications, biologic correlates, and challenges. Radiographics. 2017;37:1483–503.
34. Volpi S, Ali JM, Tasker A, Peryt A, Aresu G, Coonar AS. The role of positron emission tomography in the diagnosis, staging and response assessment of non-small cell lung cancer. Ann Transl Med. 2018;6:95.
35. Ke L, Wang L, Yu J, Meng X. Prognostic significance of SUVmax combined with lactate dehydrogenase in advanced lung cancer patients treated with immune checkpoint inhibitor plus chemotherapy: a retrospective study. Front Oncol. 2021;11:652312.
36. Lardinois D, Weder W, Hany TF, Kamel EM, Korom S, Seifert B, et al. Staging of non-small-cell lung cancer with integrated positron-emission tomography and computed tomography. N Engl J Med. 2003;348:2500–7.
37. Zhao K, Wang C, Shi F, Huang Y, Ma L, Li M, et al. Combined prognostic value of the SUVmax derived from FDG-PET and the lymphocyte-monocyte ratio in patients with stage IIIB-IV non-small cell lung cancer receiving chemotherapy. BMC Cancer. 2021;21:66.
38. Tirkes T, Hollar MA, Tann M, Kohli MD, Akisik F, Sandrasegaran K. Response criteria in oncologic imaging: review of traditional and new criteria. Radiographics. 2013;33:1323–41.
39. Gao Y, Wang K, Tang XX, Niu JL, Wang J. A pilot study of prognostic value of metastatic lymph node count and size in patients with different stages of gastric carcinoma. Cancer Manag Res. 2022;14:2055–64.
40. Lawson CE, Marti JM, Radivojevic T, Jonnalagadda SVR, Gentz R, Hillson NJ, et al. Machine learning for metabolic engineering: a review. Metab Eng. 2021;63:34–60.
41. Nensa F, Stattaus J, Morgan B, Horsfield MA, Soria JC, Besse B, et al. Dynamic contrast-enhanced MRI parameters as biomarkers for the effect of vatalanib in patients with non-small-cell lung cancer. Future Oncol. 2014;10:823–33.
42. Zhu J, Yun J, Wang K, Liu L, Zheng J, Mei L, et al. Assessment of early response to lung cancer chemotherapy by semiquantitative analysis of dynamic contrast-enhanced MRI. Dis Markers. 2022;2022:2669281.
43. Lavini C, Verhoeff JJ, Majoie CB, Stalpers LJ, Richel DJ, Maas M. Model-based, semiquantitative and time intensity curve shape analysis of dynamic contrast-enhanced MRI: a comparison in patients undergoing antiangiogenic treatment for recurrent glioma. J Magn Reson Imaging. 2011;34:1303–12.
44. Li X, Arlinghaus LR, Ayers GD, Chakravarthy AB, Abramson RG, Abramson VG, et al. DCE-MRI analysis methods for predicting the response of breast cancer to neoadjuvant chemotherapy: pilot study findings. Magn Reson Med. 2014;71:1592–602.
45. Owens C, Hindocha S, Lee R, Millard T, Sharma B. The lung cancers: staging and response, CT, (18) F-FDG PET/CT, MRI, DWI: review and new perspectives. Br J Radiol. 2023;96:20220339.
46. Coche E. Evaluation of lung tumor response to therapy: current and emerging techniques. Diagn Interv Imaging. 2016;97:1053–65.
47. Jagoda P, Fleckenstein J, Sonnhoff M, Schneider G, Ruebe C, Buecker A, et al. Diffusion-weighted MRI improves response assessment after definitive radiotherapy in patients with NSCLC. Cancer Imaging. 2021;21:21.
48. Regier M, Derlin T, Schwarz D, Laqmani A, Henes FO, Groth M, et al. Diffusion weighted MRI and 18F-FDG PET/CT in non-small cell lung cancer (NSCLC): does the apparent diffusion coefficient (ADC) correlate with tracer uptake (SUV)? Eur J Radiol. 2012;81:2913–8.
49. Fleckenstein J, Jelden M, Kremp S, Jagoda P, Stroeder J, Khreish F, et al. The impact of diffusion-weighted MRI on the definition of gross tumor volume in radiotherapy of non-small-cell lung cancer. PLoS One. 2016;11:e0162816.
50. Gill RR. Tumor metrics standardization and integration with electronic health records: a step forward on a long road. Acad Radiol. 2021;28:1408–9.
51. Travis WD, Brambilla E, Burke AP, Marx A, Nicholson AG. Introduction to the 2015 World Health Organization classification of Tumors of the lung, pleura, thymus, and heart. J Thorac Oncol. 2015;10:1240–2.
52. Miller AB, Hoogstraten B, Staquet M, Winkler A. Reporting results of cancer treatment. Cancer. 1981;47:207–14.
53. Wolchok JD, Hoos A, O'Day S, Weber JS, Hamid O, Lebbe C, et al. Guidelines for the evaluation of immune therapy activity in solid tumors: immune-related response criteria. Clin Cancer Res. 2009;15:7412–20.
54. Wahl RL, Jacene H, Kasamon Y, Lodge MA. From RECIST to PERCIST: evolving considerations for

PET response criteria in solid tumors. J Nucl Med. 2009;50 Suppl 1:122S–50S.
55. Subbiah V, Chuang HH, Gambhire D, Kairemo K. Defining clinical response criteria and early response criteria for precision oncology: current state-of-the-art and future perspectives. Diagnostics (Basel). 2017;7:10.
56. Nishino M, Jackman DM, Hatabu H, Yeap BY, Cioffredi LA, Yap JT, et al. New Response Evaluation Criteria in Solid Tumors (RECIST) guidelines for advanced non-small cell lung cancer: comparison with original RECIST and impact on assessment of tumor response to targeted therapy. AJR Am J Roentgenol. 2010;195:W221–8.
57. Nishino M, Hatabu H, Johnson BE, McLoud TC. State of the art: response assessment in lung cancer in the era of genomic medicine. Radiology. 2014;271:6–27.
58. Hwang JK, Lee SH, Song YB, Ahn J, Carriere K, Jang MJ, et al. Response by Hwang et al to letter regarding article, "Glycemic control status after percutaneous coronary intervention and long-term clinical outcomes in patients with type 2 diabetes mellitus". Circ Cardiovasc Interv. 2017;10:e004157.
59. Erasmus JJ, Gladish GW, Broemeling L, Sabloff BS, Truong MT, Herbst RS, et al. Interobserver and intraobserver variability in measurement of non-small-cell carcinoma lung lesions: implications for assessment of tumor response. J Clin Oncol. 2003;21:2574–82.
60. Zhao B, James LP, Moskowitz CS, Guo P, Ginsberg MS, Lefkowitz RA, et al. Evaluating variability in tumor measurements from same-day repeat CT scans of patients with non-small cell lung cancer. Radiology. 2009;252:263–72.
61. Nishino M. Tumor response assessment for precision cancer therapy: response evaluation criteria in solid Tumors and beyond. Am Soc Clin Oncol Educ Book. 2018;38:1019–29.
62. Murphy DJ, Royle L, Chalampalakis Z, Alves L, Martins N, Bassett P, et al. The effect of a novel Bayesian penalised likelihood PET reconstruction algorithm on the assessment of malignancy risk in solitary pulmonary nodules according to the British Thoracic Society guidelines. Eur J Radiol. 2019;117.149–55.
63. Kim JH. Comparison of the EORTC criteria and PERCIST in solid tumors: a pooled analysis and review. Oncotarget. 2016;7:58105–10.
64. Young H, Baum R, Cremerius U, Herholz K, Hoekstra O, Lammertsma AA, et al. Measurement of clinical and subclinical tumour response using [18F]-fluorodeoxyglucose and positron emission tomography: review and 1999 EORTC recommendations. European Organization for Research and Treatment of Cancer (EORTC) PET study group. Eur J Cancer. 1999;35:1773–82.
65. de Langen AJ, Vincent A, Velasquez LM, van Tinteren H, Boellaard R, Shankar LK, et al. Repeatability of 18F-FDG uptake measurements in tumors: a metaanalysis. J Nucl Med. 2012;53:701–8.
66. Min SJ, Jang HJ, Kim JH. Comparison of the RECIST and PERCIST criteria in solid tumors: a pooled analysis and review. Oncotarget. 2016;7:27848–54.
67. Pinker K, Riedl C, Weber WA. Evaluating tumor response with FDG PET: updates on PERCIST, comparison with EORTC criteria and clues to future developments. Eur J Nucl Med Mol Imaging. 2017;44:55–66.
68. Kerner GS, Koole MJ, Bongaerts AH, Pruim J, Groen HJ, Consortium CAF. Total body metabolic tumor response in ALK positive non-small cell lung cancer patients treated with ALK inhibition. PLoS One. 2016;11:e0149955.
69. Ou SH, Bartlett CH, Mino-Kenudson M, Cui J, Iafrate AJ. Crizotinib for the treatment of ALK-rearranged non-small cell lung cancer: a success story to usher in the second decade of molecular targeted therapy in oncology. Oncologist. 2012;17:1351–75.
70. van Gool MH, Aukema TS, Hartemink KJ, Valdes Olmos RA, van Tinteren H, Klomp HM. FDG-PET/CT response evaluation during EGFR-TKI treatment in patients with NSCLC. World J Radiol. 2014;6:392–8.
71. Tiwary A, Goyal H, Goel D. Metabolic response assessment of ALK inhibitor crizotinib by F18 FDG PET-CT in ALK positive metastatic adenocarcinoma lung. J Cancer Res Therapeut. 2017;13: pS410.
72. Beer L, Hochmair M, Haug AR, Schwabel B, Kifjak D, Wadsak W, et al. Comparison of RECIST, iRECIST, and PERCIST for the evaluation of response to PD-1/PD-L1 blockade therapy in patients with non-small cell lung cancer. Clin Nucl Med. 2019;44:535–43.
73. Sheikhbahaei S, Mena E, Marcus C, Wray R, Taghipour M, Subramaniam RM. 18F-FDG PET/CT: therapy response assessment interpretation (Hopkins criteria) and survival outcomes in lung cancer patients. J Nucl Med. 2016;57:855–60.
74. Park K, Yu CJ, Kim SW, Lin MC, Sriuranpong V, Tsai CM, et al. First-line erlotinib therapy until and beyond response evaluation criteria in solid tumors progression in Asian patients with epidermal growth factor receptor mutation-positive non-small-cell lung cancer: the ASPIRATION study. JAMA Oncol. 2016;2:305–12.
75. Chaft JE, Oxnard GR, Sima CS, Kris MG, Miller VA, Riely GJ. Disease flare after tyrosine kinase inhibitor discontinuation in patients with EGFR-mutant lung cancer and acquired resistance to erlotinib or gefitinib: implications for clinical trial design. Clin Cancer Res. 2011;17:6298–303.
76. Crabb SJ, Patsios D, Sauerbrei E, Ellis PM, Arnold A, Goss G, et al. Tumor cavitation: impact on objective response evaluation in trials of angiogenesis inhibitors in non-small-cell lung cancer. J Clin Oncol. 2009;27:404–10.
77. Choi H, Charnsangavej C, Faria SC, Macapinlac HA, Burgess MA, Patel SR, et al. Correlation of

computed tomography and positron emission tomography in patients with metastatic gastrointestinal stromal tumor treated at a single institution with imatinib mesylate: proposal of new computed tomography response criteria. J Clin Oncol. 2007;25:1753–9.
78. Huang Z, Xiong Q, Cui Z, Tao H, Zhang S, Wang L, et al. Efficacy and safety of crizotinib plus bevacizumab in ALK/ROS-1/c-MET positive non-small cell lung cancer: an open-label, single-arm, prospective observational study. Am J Transl Res. 2021;13:1526–34.
79. Lee HY, Lee KS, Ahn MJ, Hwang HS, Lee JW, Park K, et al. New CT response criteria in non-small cell lung cancer: proposal and application in EGFR tyrosine kinase inhibitor therapy. Lung Cancer. 2011;73:63–9.
80. Lee HY, Lee KS, Hwang HS, Lee JW, Ahn MJ, Park K, et al. Molecularly targeted therapy using bevacizumab for non-small cell lung cancer: a pilot study for the new CT response criteria. Korean J Radiol. 2010;11:618–26.
81. Lucidarme O, Wagner M, Gillard P, Kim S, Bachet JB, Rousseau B, et al. RECIST and CHOI criteria in the evaluation of tumor response in patients with metastatic colorectal cancer treated with regorafenib, a prospective multicenter study. Cancer Imaging. 2019;19:85.
82. Lee HY, Jeong JY, Lee KS, Kim HJ, Han J, Kim BT, et al. Solitary pulmonary nodular lung adenocarcinoma: correlation of histopathologic scoring and patient survival with imaging biomarkers. Radiology. 2012;264:884–93.
83. Lee HY, Jeong JY, Lee KS, Yi CA, Kim BT, Kang H, et al. Histopathology of lung adenocarcinoma based on new IASLC/ATS/ERS classification: prognostic stratification with functional and metabolic imaging biomarkers. J Magn Reson Imaging. 2013;38:905–13.
84. Tazdait M, Mezquita L, Lahmar J, Ferrara R, Bidault F, Ammari S, et al. Patterns of responses in metastatic NSCLC during PD-1 or PDL-1 inhibitor therapy: comparison of RECIST 1.1, irRECIST and iRECIST criteria. Eur J Cancer. 2018;88:38–47.
85. Ferte C, Marabelle A. iRECIST: a clarification of tumour response assessment in the immunotherapy era. Eur J Cancer. 2017;77:165–7.
86. Borcoman E, Kanjanapan Y, Champiat S, Kato S, Servois V, Kurzrock R, et al. Novel patterns of response under immunotherapy. Ann Oncol. 2019;30:385–96.
87. Travis WD, Brambilla E, Noguchi M, Nicholson AG, Geisinger KR, Yatabe Y, et al. International Association for the Study of Lung Cancer/American Thoracic Society/European Respiratory Society international multidisciplinary classification of lung adenocarcinoma. J Thorac Oncol. 2011;6:244–85.
88. Schmid-Bindert G, Engel-Riedel W, Reck M, Schuette W, Stohlmacher J, Fischer JR, et al. A randomized phase 2 study of pemetrexed in combination with cisplatin or carboplatin as adjuvant chemotherapy in patients with completely resected stage IB or II non-small-cell lung cancer. Lung Cancer. 2015;90:397–404.
89. Hodi FS, Hwu WJ, Kefford R, Weber JS, Daud A, Hamid O, et al. Evaluation of immune-related response criteria and RECIST v1.1 in patients with advanced melanoma treated with pembrolizumab. J Clin Oncol. 2016;34:1510–7.
90. Rheinheimer S, Christopoulos P, Erdmann S, Saupe J, Golpon H, Vogel-Claussen J, et al. Dynamic contrast enhanced MRI of pulmonary adenocarcinomas for early risk stratification: higher contrast uptake associated with response and better prognosis. BMC Med Imaging. 2022;22:215.
91. Suresh K, Voong KR, Shankar B, Forde PM, Ettinger DS, Marrone KA, et al. Pneumonitis in non-small cell lung cancer patients receiving immune checkpoint immunotherapy: incidence and risk factors. J Thorac Oncol. 2018;13:1930–9.
92. Lopci E, Hicks RJ, Dimitrakopoulou-Strauss A, Dercle L, Iravani A, Seban RD, et al. Joint EANM/SNMMI/ANZSNM practice guidelines/procedure standards on recommended use of [(18)F]FDG PET/CT imaging during immunomodulatory treatments in patients with solid tumors version 1.0. Eur J Nucl Med Mol Imaging. 2022;49:2323–41.
93. Chiou VL, Burotto M. Pseudoprogression and immune-related response in solid Tumors. J Clin Oncol. 2015;33:3541–3.
94. Ishiwata T, Ebata T, Iwasawa S, Matsushima J, Ota S, Nakatani Y, et al. Nivolumab-induced acute fibrinous and organizing pneumonia (AFOP). Intern Med. 2017;56:2311–5.
95. Ayati N, Lee ST, Zakavi SR, Cheng M, Lau WFE, Parakh S, et al. Response evaluation and survival prediction after PD-1 immunotherapy in patients with non-small cell lung cancer: comparison of assessment methods. J Nucl Med. 2021;62:926–33.
96. Tvsvgk T, Handa A, Kumar K, Mutreja D, Subramanian S. Chemotherapy-associated pulmonary toxicity-case series from a single center. South Asian J Cancer. 2021;10:255–60.
97. Ryu JH. Chemotherapy-induced pulmonary toxicity in lung cancer patients. J Thorac Oncol. 2010;5:1313–4.
98. Torrisi JM, Schwartz LH, Gollub MJ, Ginsberg MS, Bosl GJ, Hricak H. CT findings of chemotherapy-induced toxicity: what radiologists need to know about the clinical and radiologic manifestations of chemotherapy toxicity. Radiology. 2011;258:41–56.
99. Ohmori T, Yamaoka T, Ando K, Kusumoto S, Kishino Y, Manabe R, et al. Molecular and clinical features of EGFR-TKI-associated lung injury. Int J Mol Sci. 2021;22:792.
100. Eremina V, Jefferson JA, Kowalewska J, Hochster H, Haas M, Weisstuch J, et al. VEGF inhibition and renal thrombotic microangiopathy. N Engl J Med. 2008;358:1129–36.
101. Vaklavas C, Lenihan D, Kurzrock R, Tsimberidou AM. Anti-vascular endothelial growth factor ther-

apies and cardiovascular toxicity: what are the important clinical markers to target? Oncologist. 2010;15:130–41.
102. Lee H, Lee HY, Sun JM, Lee SH, Kim Y, Park SE, et al. Transient asymptomatic pulmonary opacities during Osimertinib treatment and its clinical implication. J Thorac Oncol. 2018;13:1106–12.
103. Advani A, Kelly DJ, Advani SL, Cox AJ, Thai K, Zhang Y, et al. Role of VEGF in maintaining renal structure and function under normotensive and hypertensive conditions. Proc Natl Acad Sci USA. 2007;104:14448–53.
104. Zhao B, Zhao H. Incidence and risk of regorafenib-induced hepatotoxicity. Oncotarget. 2017;8:84102–11.
105. AlAsmari AF, Ali N, AlAsmari F, AlAnazi WA, Alqahtani F, Alharbi M, et al. Elucidation of the molecular mechanisms underlying sorafenib-induced hepatotoxicity. Oxidative Med Cell Longev. 2020;2020:7453406.
106. Lim GI, Lee KH, Jeong SW, Uh ST, Jin SY, Lee DH, et al. Clinical features of interstitial lung diseases. Korean J Intern Med. 1996;11:113–21.
107. Antoniou KM, Margaritopoulos GA, Tomassetti S, Bonella F, Costabel U, Poletti V. Interstitial lung disease. Eur Respir Rev. 2014;23:40–54.
108. Owen DH, Wei L, Bertino EM, Edd T, Villalona-Calero MA, He K, et al. Incidence, risk factors, and effect on survival of immune-related adverse events in patients with non-small-cell lung cancer. Clin Lung Cancer. 2018;19:e893–900.
109. Nishino M, Ramaiya NH, Awad MM, Sholl LM, Maattala JA, Taibi M, et al. PD-1 inhibitor-related pneumonitis in advanced cancer patients: radiographic patterns and clinical course. Clin Cancer Res. 2016;22:6051–60.
110. Tiu BC, Zubiri L, Iheke J, Pahalyants V, Theodosakis N, Ugwu-Dike P, et al. Real-world incidence and impact of pneumonitis in patients with lung cancer treated with immune checkpoint inhibitors: a multi-institutional cohort study. J Immunother Cancer. 2022;10:e004670.
111. Garanzini EM, Scaramuzza D, Spadarella G, Di Guardo L, Marchiano A. Sarcoidosis-like disease mimicking metastases during adjuvant ipilimumab therapy in advanced melanoma patient: CT scan and MRI help in managing difficult clinical decision. BJR Case Rep. 2020;6:20190065.
112. Kanaoka K, Ikebe S, Ihara S, Tsuji H, Yasuoka H, Minami S. Durvalumab-induced diffuse alveolar hemorrhage: an autopsy case report. Case Rep Oncol. 2020;13:696–701.
113. Moslehi J, Salem JE. Immune checkpoint inhibitor myocarditis treatment strategies and future directions. JACC Cardio Oncol. 2022;4:704–7.
114. Miyauchi Y, Naito H, Tsunemori H, Tani R, Hasui Y, Miyake Y, et al. Myocarditis as an immune-related adverse event following treatment with ipilimumab and nivolumab combination therapy for metastatic renal cell carcinoma: a case report. J Med Case Rep. 2021;15:508.
115. Arcari L, Tini G, Camastra G, Ciolina F, De Santis D, Russo D, et al. Cardiac magnetic resonance imaging in immune check-point inhibitor myocarditis: a systematic review. J Imaging. 2022;8:99.
116. Haanen J, Carbonnel F, Robert C, Kerr KM, Peters S, Larkin J, et al. Management of toxicities from immunotherapy: ESMO clinical practice guidelines for diagnosis, treatment and follow-up. Ann Oncol. 2017;28:iv119–iv42.
117. Hayes SA, Pietanza MC, O'Driscoll D, Zheng J, Moskowitz CS, Kris MG, et al. Comparison of CT volumetric measurement with RECIST response in patients with lung cancer. Eur J Radiol. 2016;85:524–33.
118. Devaraj A, van Ginneken B, Nair A, Baldwin D. Use of volumetry for lung nodule management: theory and practice. Radiology. 2017;284:630–44.
119. Kamran SC, Coroller T, Milani N, Agrawal V, Baldini EH, Chen AB, et al. The impact of quantitative CT-based tumor volumetric features on the outcomes of patients with limited stage small cell lung cancer. Radiat Oncol. 2020;15:14.
120. Zhao B, Oxnard GR, Moskowitz CS, Kris MG, Pao W, Guo P, et al. A pilot study of volume measurement as a method of tumor response evaluation to aid biomarker development. Clin Cancer Res. 2010;16:4647–53.
121. Murphy DJ, Gill RR. Volumetric assessment in malignant pleural mesothelioma. Ann Transl Med. 2017;5:241.
122. Liu L, Zhang J, Ferguson MK, Appelbaum D, Zhang JX, Pu Y. Developing a clinical and PET/CT volumetric prognostic index for risk assessment and management of NSCLC patients after initial therapy. Front Biosci (Landmark Ed). 2022;27:16.
123. Im HJ, Pak K, Cheon GJ, Kang KW, Kim SJ, Kim IJ, et al. Prognostic value of volumetric parameters of (18)F-FDG PET in non-small-cell lung cancer: a meta-analysis. Eur J Nucl Med Mol Imaging. 2015;42:241–51.
124. Wen W, Piao Y, Xu D, Li X. Prognostic value of MTV and TLG of (18)F-FDG PET in patients with stage I and II non-small-cell lung cancer: a meta-analysis. Contrast Media Mol Imaging. 2021;2021:7528971.
125. Primakov SP, Ibrahim A, van Timmeren JE, Wu G, Keek SA, Beuque M, et al. Automated detection and segmentation of non-small cell lung cancer computed tomography images. Nat Commun. 2022;13:3423.
126. Aghighi M, Boe J, Rosenberg J, Von Eyben R, Gawande RS, Petit P, et al. Three dimensional radiologic assessment of chemotherapy response in Ewing sarcoma can be used to predict clinical outcome. Radiology. 2016;280:905–15.
127. Lee P, Bazan JG, Lavori PW, Weerasuriya DK, Quon A, Le QT, et al. Metabolic tumor volume is an independent prognostic factor in patients treated defini-

tively for non-small-cell lung cancer. Clin Lung Cancer. 2012;13:52–8.
128. Zhang F, Wang Q, Li H. Automatic segmentation of the gross target volume in non-small cell lung cancer using a modified version of ResNet. Technol Cancer Res Treat. 2020;19:1533033820947484.
129. Jiang J, Hu YC, Liu CJ, Halpenny D, Hellmann MD, Deasy JO, et al. Multiple resolution residually connected feature streams for automatic lung tumor segmentation from CT images. IEEE Trans Med Imaging. 2019;38:134–44.
130. Li XT, Huang RY. Standardization of imaging methods for machine learning in neuro-oncology. Neurooncol Adv. 2020;2:iv49–55.
131. Litvin AA, Burkin DA, Kropinov AA, Paramzin FN. Radiomics and digital image texture analysis in oncology (review). Sovrem Tekhnologii Med. 2021;13:97–104.
132. Palumbo B, Bianconi F, Palumbo I, Fravolini ML, Minestrini M, Nuvoli S, et al. Value of shape and texture features from (18)F-FDG PET/CT to discriminate between benign and malignant solitary pulmonary nodules: an experimental evaluation. Diagnostics (Basel). 2020;10:696.
133. Ganeshan B, Miles KA. Quantifying tumour heterogeneity with CT. Cancer Imaging. 2013;13:140–9.
134. Bianconi F, Fravolini ML, Bello-Cerezo R, Minestrini M, Scialpi M, Palumbo B. Evaluation of shape and textural features from CT as prognostic biomarkers in non-small cell lung cancer. Anticancer Res. 2018;38:2155–60.
135. Chiu HY, Chao HS, Chen YM. Application of artificial intelligence in lung cancer. Cancers (Basel). 2022;14:1370.
136. Onishi Y, Teramoto A, Tsujimoto M, Tsukamoto T, Saito K, Toyama H, et al. Automated pulmonary nodule classification in computed tomography images using a deep convolutional neural Network trained by generative adversarial networks. Biomed Res Int. 2019;2019:6051939.
137. Rajpurkar P, Irvin J, Ball RL, Zhu K, Yang B, Mehta H, et al. Deep learning for chest radiograph diagnosis: a retrospective comparison of the CheXNeXt algorithm to practicing radiologists. PLoS Med. 2018;15:e1002686.
138. Liang M, Tang W, Xu DM, Jirapatnakul AC, Reeves AP, Henschke CI, et al. Low-dose CT screening for lung cancer: computer-aided detection of missed lung cancers. Radiology. 2016;281:279–88.
139. Zhao Y, de Bock GH, Vliegenthart R, van Klaveren RJ, Wang Y, Bogoni L, et al. Performance of computer-aided detection of pulmonary nodules in low-dose CT: comparison with double reading by nodule volume. Eur Radiol. 2012;22:2076–84.
140. Lancaster HL, Zheng S, Aleshina OO, Yu D, Yu Chernina V, Heuvelmans MA, et al. Outstanding negative prediction performance of solid pulmonary nodule volume AI for ultra-LDCT baseline lung cancer screening risk stratification. Lung Cancer. 2022;165:133–40.
141. Hawkins S, Wang H, Liu Y, Garcia A, Stringfield O, Krewer H, et al. Predicting malignant nodules from screening CT scans. J Thorac Oncol. 2016;11:2120–8.
142. Xu Y, Hosny A, Zeleznik R, Parmar C, Coroller T, Franco I, et al. Deep learning predicts lung cancer treatment response from serial medical imaging. Clin Cancer Res. 2019;25:3266–75.
143. Sun R, Limkin EJ, Vakalopoulou M, Dercle L, Champiat S, Han SR, et al. A radiomics approach to assess tumour-infiltrating CD8 cells and response to anti-PD-1 or anti-PD-L1 immunotherapy: an imaging biomarker, retrospective multicohort study. Lancet Oncol. 2018;19:1180–91.
144. Tunali I, Gray JE, Qi J, Abdalah M, Jeong DK, Guvenis A, et al. Novel clinical and radiomic predictors of rapid disease progression phenotypes among lung cancer patients treated with immunotherapy: an early report. Lung Cancer. 2019;129:75–9.
145. Mu W, Tunali I, Gray JE, Qi J, Schabath MB, Gillies RJ. Radiomics of (18)F-FDG PET/CT images predicts clinical benefit of advanced NSCLC patients to checkpoint blockade immunotherapy. Eur J Nucl Med Mol Imaging. 2020;47:1168–82.
146. Trebeschi S, Drago SG, Birkbak NJ, Kurilova I, Calin AM, Delli Pizzi A, et al. Predicting response to cancer immunotherapy using noninvasive radiomic biomarkers. Ann Oncol. 2019;30:998–1004.

23 Quantitative Imaging in Pleura

Thomas Frauenfelder and Yalynska Tetyana

Introduction

Pleural disease is affecting ~300 people per 100,000 population annually and is associated with essential morbidity and mortality [1]. Radiological investigation of pleural pathologies is key in establishing a diagnosis, primary management, and follow-up. Initial modality for the determination of pleural disease is chest X-ray (CXR). Further, when pleural abnormalities are detected, thoracic ultrasound, computed tomography (CT), magnetic resonance imaging (MRI), and positron emission tomography (PET) can each play an important role in radiological management, but appropriate modality selection is critical [2]. With the recent development of radiological technologies, there have appeared a variety of new imaging tools such as QI which has become available for use in the management of pleural disease.

The QI by the Quantitative Imaging Biomarkers Alliance (QIBA) is defined as "the extraction of quantifiable features from medical images for the assessment of normal or the severity, degree of change, or status of a disease, injury, or chronic condition relative to normal" [3]. Pleural thickness, percentage circumferential pleural involvement, and the number of foci of rounded atelectasis at anatomically defined levels are all metrics of imaging in pleural disease [2, 4].

There are potential caveats in the quantitative assessment of the pleural diseases; it could be difficult to delineate indistinct pleural boundaries and reliably distinguish PE from thickening fibrosis [5].

Current Imaging Methods and Their Quantitative Parameter Related to Pleural Disease

CXR

Accurate description of the size of pleural effusion (PE) is important for patient management including urgency of intervention [6, 7]. Quantitative assessment of PE volume is crucial when it comes to identification of thoracentesis in critically ill patients [7, 8].

Precise positioning and amount of fluid play an important role in clinical diagnosis of PE. Since fluid will be dispersed posteriorly on supine CXR, this position is less useful for the evaluation of the PE.

However, there is no consensus on whether the posterior-anterior (PA), lateral, anterior-posterior (AP), or supine CXR is superior in its diagnostic accuracy of PE. The sensitivity of identifying a parapneumonic PE (PPE) for lat-

T. Frauenfelder (✉) · Y. Tetyana
University Hospital Zurich, Institute of Diagnostic and Interventional Radiology, Zurich, Switzerland
e-mail: thomas.frauenfelder@usz.ch

R. Gill, P. Rajiah (eds.), *Quantitative Imaging in the Thorax*,
https://doi.org/10.1007/978-3-032-14103-3_23

eral, PA, and AP CXRs was 86%, 82%, and 78%, respectively. All three CXR views combined missed 13% of effusions of a size significant enough to warrant diagnostic thoracentesis [9]. Large effusions are detected with a sensitivity of 92% and a specificity of 89%, on AP CXRs, whereas small and medium effusions are often misdiagnosed of completely unrecognised [10]. Compared to frontal CXRs, lateral CXRs have a higher sensitivity for detecting small PEs (mean of 26 ml) [11]. The sensitivity of CXR in detection of PE decreases in the supine position [9]. Digital supine CXRs, performed at the bedside of intensive care unit (ICU) patients and interpreted by experienced radiologists, have not been able to provide reliable quantitative evaluation of pleural effusions [12]. Nonetheless, ICU patients are diagnosed with PE based on imaging obtained from a supine AP CXR, conducted at the bedside [8].

There is currently no standardized measurement system for assessment of PE size. The terms "small, moderate, and large" are often used. However, because there is no consensus of size limits for these terms, there is significant variability in size description [7, 13]. CXR in an erect PA position can be used to evaluate the size of pleural effusions by the recognized method of counting intercostal spaces (ICS) from costophrenic angle (CPA): small, localized to 1 ICS (effusion <500 ml); medium, 2–3 ICS (500–1000 mL); and large, 4 ICS (>1000 ml) [13]. The severity of the pleural effusion is determined based on the size and the height range of the shadow on the CXR [8]. A prediction rule, which was established based on the gold standard of CT volumetric measurements, has been developed to help estimate PE volume from PA or lateral radiographs. This prediction rule is based on the absence or presence of meniscus on CXR [6, 11]. At a volume of 50 ml, PE becomes visible as a meniscus on a lateral CXR. On a PA CXR, a PE is visible as a meniscus at 200 ml, and at 500 ml, the meniscus obscures the hemidiaphragm (HD) [6, 11].

CXR can reveal PE in patients in the orthostatic position if the volume of effusion is equal to or greater than 200 ml [11]. Further studies have demonstrated large standard deviations for PE volume estimation in the lateral and posterior CPAs on CXR. This led to an updated model for PE volume estimation, where the HD in either the lateral or posterior CPA on CXR was correlated with nearly 100 ml, while a meniscus occurring at the HD in either CPA and completely obstructed the HD was correlated with about 250 ml and a mean of approximately 650 ml, respectively [11].

Despite the improvement in CXR quality over the last years, it's important to note that the absence of visible meniscus on either the frontal or lateral CXR cannot exclude the presence of PE. There is speculation that some subpulmonic effusions don't produce the characteristic lateral shift on the HD of the frontal CXR; this can go unrecognized. Moreover, scarring or muscle slips of the HD level can lead to artifacts, which influence the visibility of menisci within the CPAs. Thus, when used in a clinical setting, the visual prediction rule should be used with caution [11].

There are models of deep learning (DL) which can classify the PE grades on CXR, thus allowing clinicians to compare CXR images using quantitative and objective measurements [8]. A universal DL model, which automatically extracts data from radiology reports, has recently been developed. Clinically, this tool helps accurately quantify PE severity [8]. DL is a form of artificial intelligence (AI) which can self-learn a task without explicit programing [8]. This allows for the severity of PE to be accurately detected, leading to fast and reliable diagnosis and reduced work pressure for radiologists [8].

It is worth mentioning that pleural abnormalities according to the International Labour Organization Classification 2000 include the following:

- Localized pleural thickening (represents localized pleural thickening, generally of the parietal pleura, and a minimum width of about 3 mm is required for an in-profile plaque to be recorded as present)
- CPA obliteration (may occur without diffuse pleural thickening, if the pleural thickening extends up the lateral chest wall from the

obliterated CPA, the thickening should be classified as diffuse pleural thickening)
- Diffuse pleural thickening (represents thickening of the visceral pleura; a minimum width of about 3 mm is required for in-profile diffuse pleural thickening to be recorded as present) [14]

Pleural disease is suggestive of malignancy if there is mediastinal pleural involvement, nodular and/or circumferential pleural thickening (more than 1 cm), or nodularity and/or infiltration of the chest wall or diaphragm [15].

Ultrasound

Thoracic ultrasound (TUS) is a routine tool in the clinical visualization of PE for diagnosis, management, and follow-up [16, 17].

Ultrasound (US) can accurately detect PE with 93% accuracy, while bedside chest X-rays are only 47% accurate [18]. During the initial TUS examination, usually a curvilinear probe (2.5–5 MHz) with a dynamic range of 60 dBs and depth of 8 cm is used [16]. In the sitting position, the free fluid will accumulate in the dependent space of the pleural cavity; therefore an ultrasound evaluation in this position is preferable because it allows to achieve a more precise quantification of PE. US is an accurate diagnostic method in recognition of PE (which is characterized as echogenic or anechoic) and is also potentially reliable for the identification of fibrin and loculations which may or may not be present [16, 19].

The PE according to the US characteristics of the PE can appear as anechoic (black), complex non-septated (black with white strands), complex septated (black with white septa), or homogeneously echogenic (white). Semiquantitative assessment of PE volume can be done using US and transesophageal echocardiography (TEE). Small volumes of pleural fluid can be detected bilaterally using TEE [4, 20, 21].

TUS assessment of PE by measuring its posterior depth has been reported to be correlated with drained pleural effusion volume (PEV) [20]. Several equations for estimating PEV have been presented in literature. Most commonly, patients are evaluated in the sitting position, as this position allows to easily examine the effusion at the posterior axillary line. To assess the reliability of US measurements of PE, equations with simple measurements were compared for accuracy. The most accurate formula for predicting PE was (lateral height of effusion + distance between lung and diaphragm) × 70, whereas $H \times 100$ was the simplest yet accurate equation [22].

Bedsides, US is an effective method of quantitatively assessing unloculated PE in ICU patients [17]. There is a significant correlation between the US measurement of the maximal interpleural distance, measured at the level of both the base and apex of the thorax, and the actual volume of PE obtained by thoracentesis. When maximal end-expiratory interpleural distance was measured to be >45 mm (right) or >50 mm (left), a PE of >800 mL was predicted with a sensitivity of 94% and 100% and specificity of 76% and 67%, respectively [12].

US helps select a proper spot for a successful thoracentesis [12], consequently reducing the risk of pneumothorax and/or hemothorax [17, 23].

Hypoechogenicity index (HI) was proposed as a quantitative, objective image marker to evaluate the echogenicity of pleural effusions of various causes [16]. The HI reflects the summary of pixels that a pleural effusion can generate; it is a simple and quick marker of pleural effusion density. The HI can be calculated as the mean echo level of all pixels of the rib divided by the mean echo levels of all pixels of pleural effusion. The expressive pathophysiological stages of a PPE may be reflected by the HI index. During a US exam, the PPE is usually anechoic or hypoechoic because it has a low content of cell counts and fibrin. This results in higher HI values. HI demonstrates a significant correlation with the biochemical biomarkers that reflect the intensity of pleural inflammation during the course of PPE such as pH, glucose, and lactate dehydrogenase [16].

The discreet vertical reverberation artifacts originating from the pleural line extend to the depth of the image without diminishing in intensity and move synchronously with lung sliding known as B-lines or ultrasound lung comets [24]. Due to the replacement of air by exudate, transudate, collagen, and blood, the density of the underlying lung is increased, and the acoustic mismatch between the pleura and the underlying structures is lowered. Comet tail artifacts occur due to the back-and-forth reflection of the ultrasound beam between the transducer and the object [25].

It should be noted that occasionally, up to two B-lines can be seen at the base of normal lungs. The presence of B-lines becomes significant when three or more are seen in a single image between two ribs. The number of B-lines increases in the air content of the lung decreases, suggesting an increase in lung density. B-lines appear confluent when spaced closer than 3 mm, due to subpleural fluid-filled alveoli [26].

With the help technological advances such as elastography and contrast-enhanced TUS, recent research has focused on the differentiation between benign and malignant pleural disease and assistance with biopsy site selection in cases of suspected thoracic malignancy [27].

MRI

An MRI can help develop a differential diagnosis for a known soft tissue lesion, due to its excellent contrast resolution, multiple sequences, and potential for dynamic contrast enhancement. Nonetheless, it is rarely superior to a CT for this purpose [28]. At present, diffusion-weighted magnetic resonance imaging (DWI) is widely used in both research and clinical applications. DWI is based on the diffusivity of water molecules in different tissues and as a functional MRI technique allows for qualitative and quantitative characterization of tissues. The quantitative data is obtained through the measurement of the apparent diffusion coefficient (ADC) [29].

The usefulness of ADC measurements in the evaluation of pleura has been explored [30]. A study of DWI's ability to differentiate between transudates and exudative PE showed a significant difference between the mean ADC of transudates and exudates ($3.42 \pm 0.76 \times 10^{-3}$ mm^2/s versus $3.18 \pm 1.82 \times 10^{-3}$ mm^2/s); using an optimum cutoff of 3.38×10^{-3} mm^2/s gave a sensitivity and specificity of 90.6% and 85.0%, respectively [31]. Similar data of average ADC for exudative and transudative effusion was obtained in an earlier study with the cutoff value of 3.6×10^{-3} mm^2/s (specificity and sensitivity, 63% and 71%, respectively) [32]. Lately, the optimum cutoff point of 3.51×10^{-3} mm^2/s yielded a sensitivity of 90.4% and specificity of 78% [33].

It is important to note that the mean ADCs of exudative effusions are significantly lower than those of the transudative effusions [31–33].

However, the mean ADC of malignant effusion was not significantly different from benign PE [29, 34]. Inflammatory-infectious and inflammatory-malignant effusions are difficult to differentiate using DWI-MRI. More accurate differentiation between these two conditions can be achieved from ADC values obtained by DWI using the pulse-triggering technique [35].

An ADC value as a quantitative parameter of DWI can be used to differentiate malignant pleural diseases from benign lesions [29, 34] as well as to predict a malignant transformation of solitary fibrous tumors (SFT) of the pleura and in the characterization of PE. ADC values of pleural malignancies are usually significantly lower than for benign lesion [29, 36].

A study of DWI's ability to differentiate between benign and malignant pleural thickening in asbestos-related pleural diseases revealed a significant difference between the mean ADC of benign and malignant pleural thickening with an optimum cutoff of 1.28×10^{-3} mm^2/s (sensitivity, specificity, negative and positive predictive values (NPV and PPV), and the diagnostic accuracy of 92.6%, 85%, 84%, 87%, and 86%, respectively) [36].

The assessment of the diagnostic value of DWI-MRI in detection and characterization of pleural diseases and its capability in differentiating benign from malignant pleural lesions showed that using a mean ADC value of 1.68×10^{-3} mm^2/s as a cutoff can differentiate malignant from benign pleural diseases with a sensitivity of 89.3%, specificity of

100%, positive predictive value of 100%, negative predictive value of 81.2%, and an accuracy of 92.68% [29]. In another study a mean ADC value of 1.52×10^{-3} mm^2/s was suggested as an optimal cutoff with 100% specificity and PPV, 71.4% sensitivity, and 87.1% accuracy [37]. The mean ADC values for malignant pleural disease were significantly lower than ADC values for benign lesions ($1.10 \pm 0.53 \times 10^{-3}$ mm^2/s and $2.19 \pm 0.42 \times 10^{-3}$ mm^2/s, respectively) [29]. Despite the high specificity and accuracy, of ADC in the differentiation between malignant and benign pleural lesions, the sensitivity is relatively low [29].

To measure ADC of pleural disease, different methods of region-of-interest (ROI) positioning can be used [13]. There are several factors, which affect the measurements and can lead to unreliable values. One of these factors is the manual method of ROI positioning for measuring the ADC [38, 39]. Using different ROI methods in the same tumor showed significant differences in ADC values, suggesting that this method of measurement significantly affects the ADC [40].

Intravenous contrast administration is mandatory for the assessment of pleural disease. Pleural enhancement and pleural nodularity can be demonstrated using pre- and postcontrast fast gradient echo (GRE) sequences. It is best to evaluate tumor deposits in the pleura in the portal venous phase [28]. MRI with contrast media can differentiate between transudative and exudative pleural effusions [28]. In exudative effusions, on delayed-phase images, the third spacing of the contrast agent can occur, resulting in diffuse non-mass-like enhancement, while transudative pleural effusions have no contrast enhancement [28].

A peak mean signal intensity (SI) which occurs shortly after the injection of contrast media (≤4.5 min or 280 s) is defined as early contrast enhancement (ECE). If at least one ROI shows ECE, the images are classified as malignant. It is suggested that ECE appeared to be an accurate and reproducible, perfusion-based biomarker of pleural malignancy. The sensitivity, specificity, and positive and negative predictive values of ECE in pleural malignancy were 91%, 86%, 91%, and 85%, respectively. Since ECE assessment can be performed in patients with minimal pleural thickening, this suggests that ECE can potentially assist with early-stage mesothelioma detection [41].

Dynamic contrast-enhanced (DCE)-MRI involves repeated imaging of the same anatomical area following injection of gadolinium contrast media (Fig. 23.1). The calculation of the pharmacokinetic parameters that reflect tumor perfusion, vascularity, and vascular permeability is based on the uptake and subsequent washout of contrast in the tissue [4].

Compared to FLASH and TWIST sequencing, radial DCE-MRI sequencing demonstrated optimal motion robustness in thoracic imaging with a minimum decrease in signal-to-noise ratio [42].

CT

Today, computed tomography is a routine diagnostic method of pleural disease.

Since the tissue phase of imaging is of interest when examining the pleura, thoracic CT is routinely performed in an arterial phase of enhancement [4].

Recently, a 3D semiautomatic method and a novel fully automated AI method have been developed for quantitative assessment of the pleural plaque volume and its reproducibility in patients with pleural plaques [43, 44]. It was demonstrated that noninvasive 3D semiautomated quantification of pleural plaques is both possible and reproducible with very good to almost perfect agreement at interobserver and intraobserver evaluations. It is important to highlight that it is not possible to differentiate between pleural plaques and other peripheral structures such as extrapleural fat, veins, muscle, or some osteophytes when their shape was directed inward from the pleural surface, due to the propagation of voxel attenuation [43]. Therefore, the volumetric analysis of using 3D-CT semiautomatic quantification and a novel automated AI method has demonstrated good feasibility and reproducibility in patients with occupational exposure to asbestos and can help correlate with

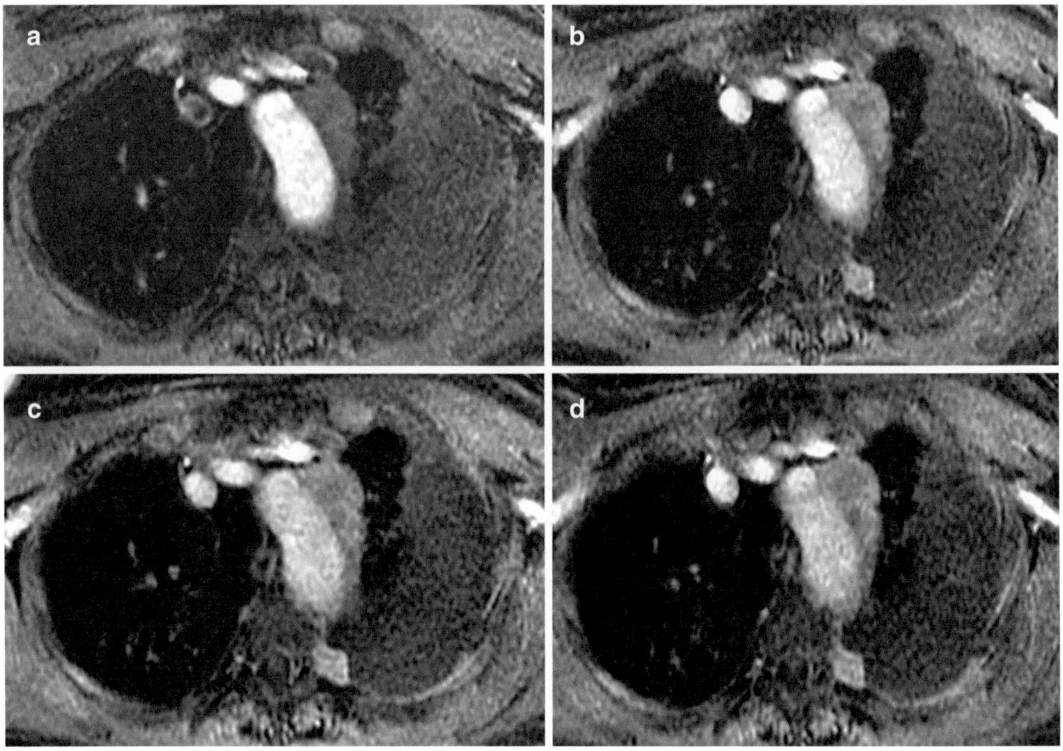

Fig. 23.1 Example of DCE-MRI. A 72-year-old man with malignant pleural mesothelioma on the left. T1W 3D GRE (LAVA) with 2-point Dixon fat/water separation (FLEX) after 20/60 s (**a**), 120 s (**b**), 4 min (**c**), and 5 min (**d**) after contrast media injection

other asbestos-related disease outcomes and prognosis [43, 44].

Recently, CT measurements of tumor thickness (cTT) and tumor volume (cTV) were used to identify CT-based tumor burden. These values were then compared to actual tumor size, to assess the prognostic value of CT-based measurements in relation to the actual all tumor burden. The sum of the two thickest spots on the axial section plane (perpendicular to the chest wall or mediastinum) at three representative different levels (optimally at the lower, middle, and upper levels if feasible) was defined as tumor thickness (given in mm) [45, 46]. Over the past few years, many algorithms have been developed to calculate the TV as well as other quantitative characteristics, including the extraction of statistical or radiomics features [47]. Radiomics is a quantitative approach to medical imaging with the goal of extracting, quantifying, and analyzing specific features such as shape, intensity, and texture of tumor images. Radiomics provide objective and reproducible quantitative information which can assist in the interpretation of these complex findings including pleural thickening of effusion in patients with malignant pleural mesothelioma (MPM) or benign pleural disease [47], and it can be a tool to aid clinical decision support systems for the treatment of MPM in the future [48]. The quantitative analysis of textural and shape features on CT and MRI can help differentiate benign pleural disease from malignant. In addition, it was established that a radiomics model can improve diagnostic confidence in the evaluation of pleural diseases characterized by MRI [49].

The novel DL models use an artificial neural network to extract higher-level features from images through multiple interconnected layers [44, 47, 50].

Spectral CT was evaluated for the ability to differentiate between benign and malignant

PE. CT values at different photon energy levels and material density values from different material bases were the quantitative measurements of interest. No difference was noted in the CT values in the polychromatic 140 kVp images. However, in monochromatic images at 40 keV, there was a significant difference between benign and malignant PE. No difference was observed in the water density, fat density, blood density, and the spectral curve slope measurements in the material decomposition images [51].

Nonetheless, CT values for benign and malignant PE were statistically different at both 40 keV and 100 keV monochromatic spectral images. Using 38.4 HU and 6.32 HU as the threshold value for CT value measurement at 40 keV and 100 keV and an effective atomic number of 7.885, a sensitivity of 92.5%, 100%, and 80% and a specificity of 53.5%, 66.7%, and 71.4% with an area under curve of 0.795, 0.843, and 0.740 for differentiating benign from malignant PE were attained. Despite that no difference was noted in the slopes of the spectral curve of benign and malignant PE, the overall spectral curve of the benign PE was lower than the malignant. A difference was also observed in the effective atomic number value between the benign and malignant PE [51].

Thus, the combination of the effective atomic number and the CT value measurement at both high and low energy levels obtained in a single scan can aid in the differential diagnosis of benign from malignant PE. When combined with disease history and patient's age, special CT imaging can significantly assist in the understanding of the nature of PE [51]. Photon-counting CT as an advanced and promising technique for tissue characterization is expected to be markedly better in the evaluation of pleural diseases [52].

As known, the Response Evaluation Criteria in Solid Tumors (RECIST) is limited in use for MPM because of the unique morphology and growth pattern of this tumor. The modified RECIST (mRECIST) for MPM has been developed to minimize the limitations of RECIST and specifically has changed the approach to tumor measurement (or measure the tumor thickness perpendicular to the chest wall (or mediastinum) and limited the number (to 6) of measured sites of pleura [53]. In patients with MPM, mRECIST 1.1 recommends to measure up to three sites of disease greater than 7 mm in thickness across three CT sections on the baseline and follow-up scans [54].

PET/CT

A combination of two methods (PET and CT) in one (PET/CT) allows for the visualization of metabolically active tissue by increased update of a radiolabeled glucose isotope (^{18}fluorodeoxyglucose (FDG)). The quantitative value of FDG PET/CT is the maximal standardized uptake value (SUV_{max}) Patients with malignant PE showed significantly higher SUV_{max} than those with benign PE (1.84 ± 0.37 and 1.39 ± 0.62, respectively); therefore, this parameter can also be used for the differentiation of malignant and benign PE [55]. In addition, a target tissue-to-normal tissue ratio threshold TNR (SUV_{max} PE divided by SUV_{mean} Th12) >0.95 on PET images may be the most accurate parameter for identifying malignant PE [55]. The SUV normalized for body weight can be the best parameter for identifying malignant PE [55].

Recently, a scoring system based on PET/CT (the PET/CT score) has been established as a means of differentiating between malignant PE and benign effusions. The proposed scoring system includes 29 PET/CT parameters, based on increased ^{18}F-FDG uptake by the pleura, pleural thickening, and PE. This PET/CT score can discriminate malignant PE from benign with a sensitivity of 83.3% and specificity of 92.2% [56].

Thicker sections of MPMs are generally better detected than thinner sections by FDG PET/CT. Using the receiver operating characteristics curve, an optimal cutoff value of (SUV_{max}) for diagnosing malignancy in FDG PET/CT was established to be of 4.45 [57].

Malignant Pleural Mesothelioma

MPM is a primary aggressive malignancy of the pleura with poor prognosis and responsive to therapy. Noninvasive imaging is inappreciable in providing quantitative assessment of tumor response in patients with unresectable disease [58]. Currently, diagnosis and staging of MPM require multimodality visualization [52, 59]. Multimodality visualization includes CT, MRI, and hybrid imaging—PET/CT or PET/MRI—and allows obtaining a comprehensive assessment of MPM (Figs. 23.2 and 23.3). The modality of choice for staging and evaluation of therapy

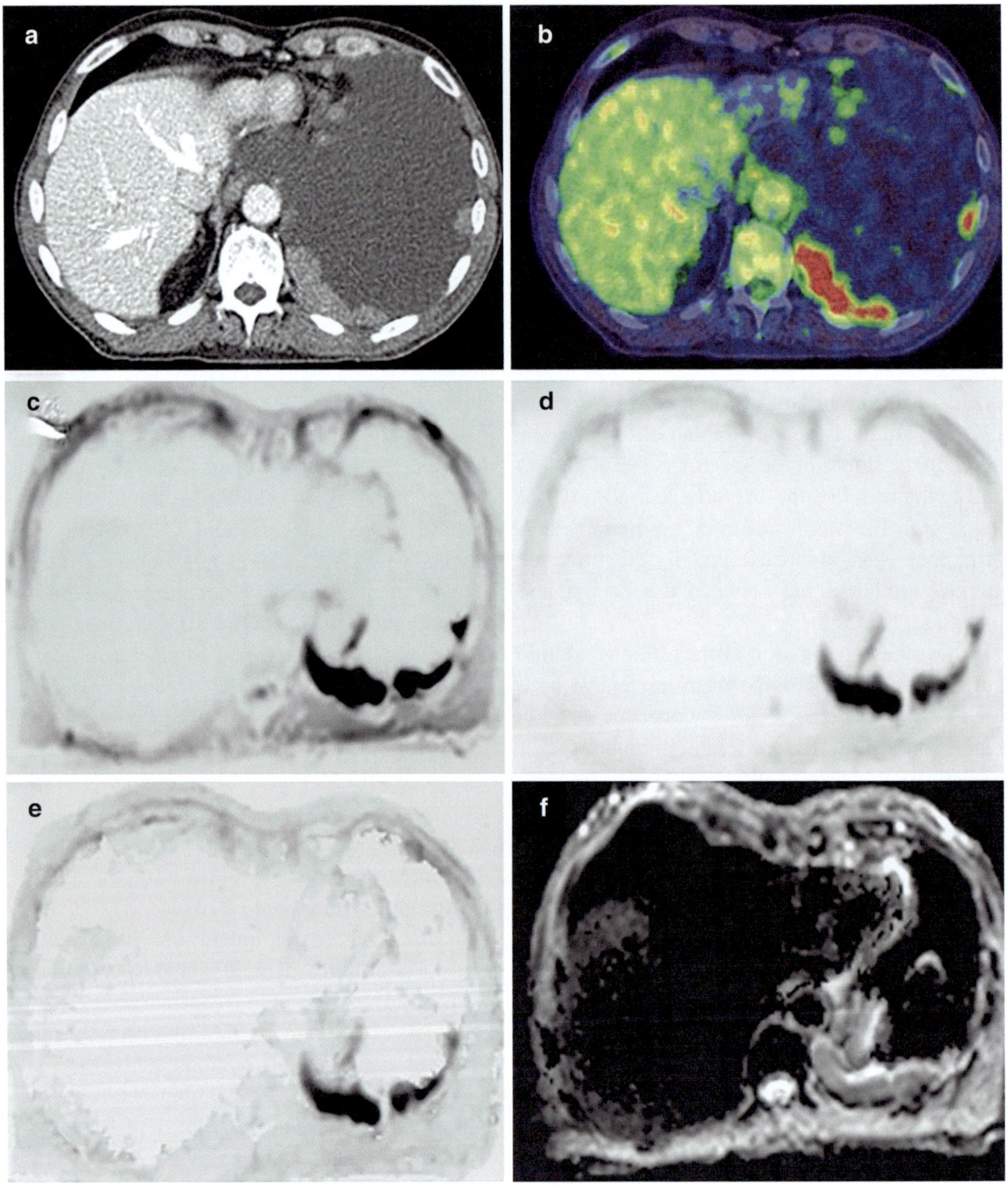

Fig. 23.2 A 70-year-old man with the epithelioid type of MPM on the left. Multimodality visualization of the tumor: CT in axial plane (**a**), PET/CT (**b**), DWI STIR with different *b* values, namely, $b = 100$ (**c**), $b = 1500$ (**d**), $b = 2000$ (**e**), and ADC map (**f**). T2 blade WI (**g**) and T1 vibe_ Dixon WI post contrast (**h**) in the coronal plane. WI weighted image

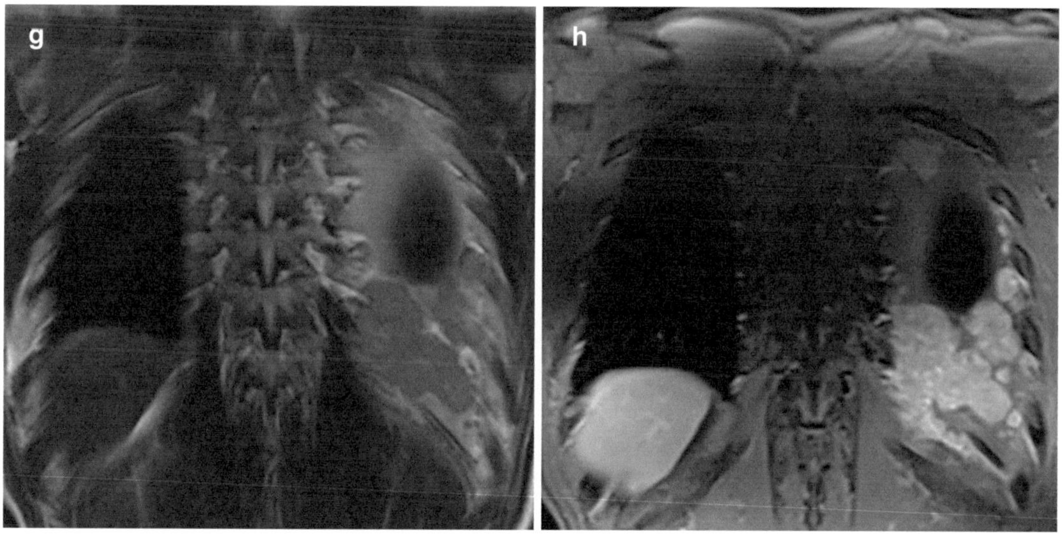

Fig. 23.2 (continued)

response is CT, whereas MRI is commonly used to screen the adjacent tissues, such as the diaphragm, mediastinum, and chest wall for tumor invasion.

New predicting features of patient survival can be identified by using DL models, and it can potentially help discover new biomarkers [60]. It is highly desirable to identify biomarkers that could help guide the most effective individualized therapy approach [61]. The clinical staging of MPM can be improved by a quantitative assessment which has demonstrated low interobserver variability and can yield a criterion of tumor size [62].

US in MM diagnosis with PE can be used to guide biopsy to the thickened pleura [63]. A recent single-center preliminary study evaluated the diagnostic accuracy of a TUS in the identification of malignant pleural involvement, with the goal of helping guide pleural biopsies to differentiate between primary and secondary pleural malignancies [64]

The localization of pleural thickening, local infiltration, mass extent, mass nature, and ultrasound features were all easily defined by TUS. The sensitivity, PPV, NPV, and accuracy in US presentation of MPM was 97%, 95%, 93%, and 94%, respectively. Hence, US is an important component of the diagnostic procedure when detecting a safe entry site for biopsies of MPMs [64].

In the detection, staging, and follow-up of MPM, a thoracic contrast-enhanced multidetector computed tomography (CE-MDCT) is the imaging modality of choice [52, 65, 66]. Quantitative analysis can be carried out by measuring HU in MPM lesions and in the surrounding tissue in both phases. The differences of contrast between phases can be determined by subtracting HU in the surrounding tissue from HU in the lesion [65].

Recently, the visibility of MPM in CE-MDCT was analyzed and compared in the arterial and late phase intraindividually by subjective and objective analysis. Subjective assessment of MPM was better visualized by both the experienced and the unexperienced radiologist in the late phase. The same finding was confirmed by objective measurements of tumor density as well as contrast to the surrounding tissue [65].

Both in late-phase MPM and in contrast to the surrounding tissue, late-phase MPM demonstrated significantly higher absolute HU values [65]. Late-phase scanning in contrast enhanced thoracic CE-MDCT can improve diagnostic accuracy in the detection of MPM. In cases where MPM is suspected, it is worth considering modifying routine arterial-phase imaging to a late-phase scan [65].

Dual-energy CT scanning allows to quantify iodine concentration in the tissue and, accord-

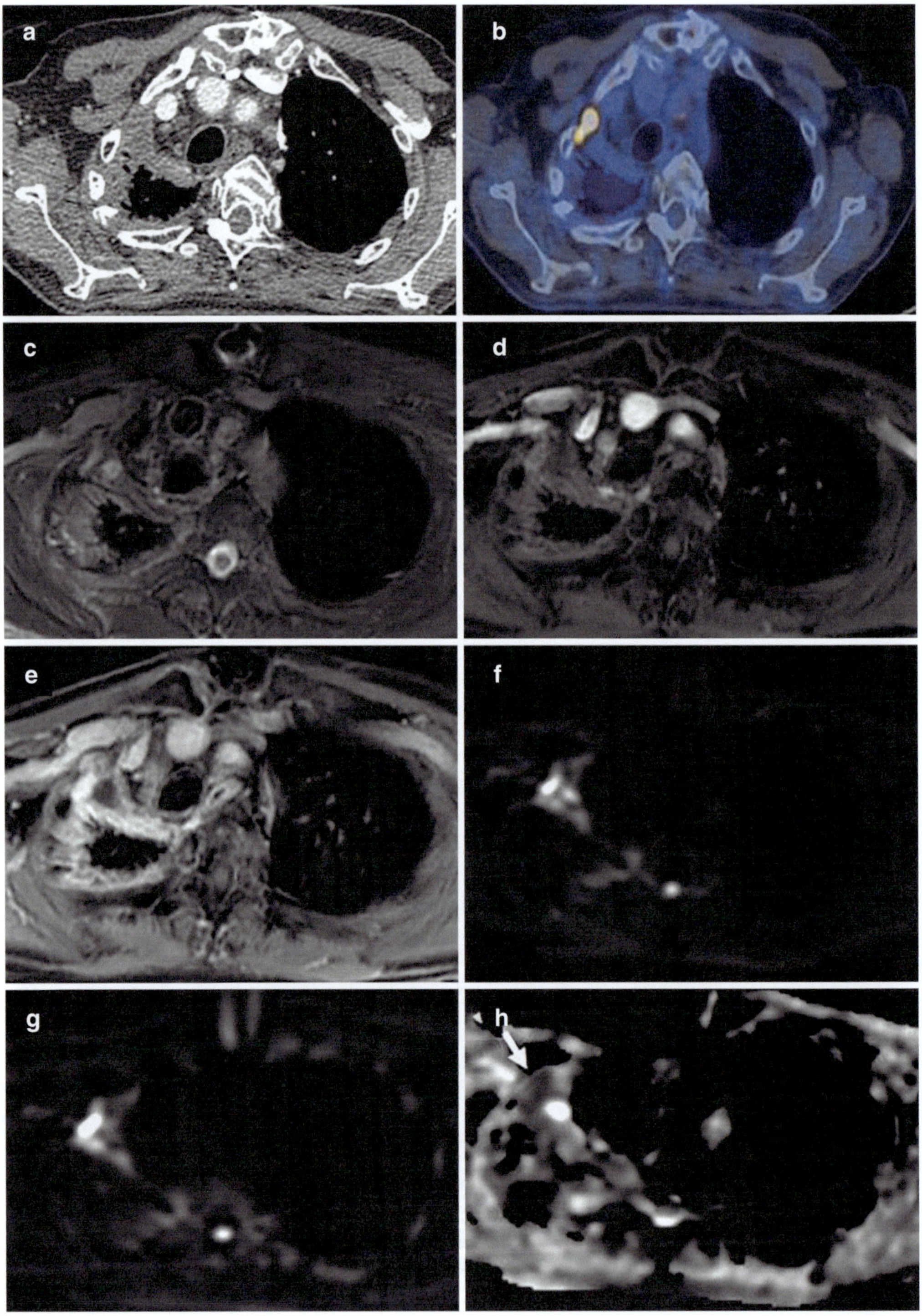

Fig. 23.3 An 86-year-old man with the sarcomatoid type of MPM on the right. Multimodality visualization of the tumor in the axial plane: arterial phase of CT (**a**), PET/CT (**b**), T2 FS (**c**), 3D LAVA with contrast media, namely, 20/60 sec (**d**) and 8 min (**e**) after contrast media injection. DWI with two different *b* values: $b = 500$ (**f**), $b = 1500$ (**g**), and ADC map (**h**). Highly active tumor on PET/CT demonstrates a hyperintensity signal on DWI and low apparent diffusion coefficient on the ADC map (white arrow)

ingly, characterize the tissue as well as evaluate the perfusion [52]. Recently, DCE-CT has shown the potential value of a 2–4-min delay added as a second phase of enhancement to routine chest CT to achieve optimal MPM enhancement [67]. However, further study of the delayed phase is required for accurate MPM staging and assessment of response to therapy [67].

The quantitative perfusion parameters at DCE-CT have demonstrated a positive correlation with tumor micro-vessel density (MVD). There is a knowledge gap in perfusion CT, with reference to differentiation between benign pleural disease and PM. ECE can help fill this gap in cases where MPM is suspected. The combination of SI measurements and assessment of ECE behavior across the entire pleura using a volumetric approach could guide further research in this field [68].

To date, volumetry is very important for assessing tumor volume and is a reliable, reproducible, and sensitive method for measuring tumor volume and response to treatment after induction chemotherapy (Fig. 23.4).

The combination of two quantitative parameters: tumor volume assessed from CT scans and maximal fissural thickness has been proposed as alternative clinical staging model. Quantitative staging of the MPM can improve prognostic performance and provide a cost-effective and clinically relevant surrogate for clinical TNM staging [69].

The largest volumetry study fulfilled in MPM with the first description of a fully automated and externally validated AI segmentation tool was presented [70]. MRI as well as CT can be used for automatic segmentation techniques (Fig. 23.5).

Tumor volume measurement allows for a quantitative assessment of MPM tumor burden and has prognostic significance [71]. The combination of TV and number of pleural sites (NPS) on CT as a prognostic classifier for MPM has been shown to be superior to TV, NPS, and TNM alone [72].

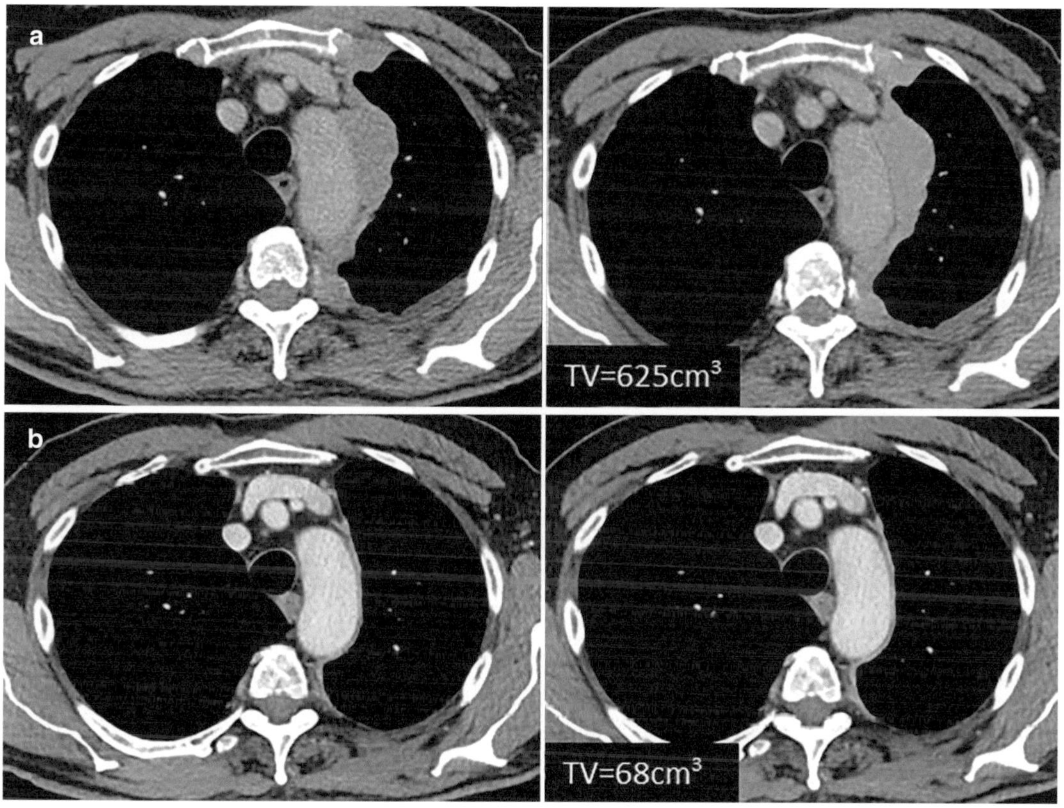

Fig. 23.4 CT images of a 72-year-old man with the epithelioid type of MPM on the left. Volumetric measurement before (**a**) and after (**b**) three cycles of chemotherapy. TV tumor volume

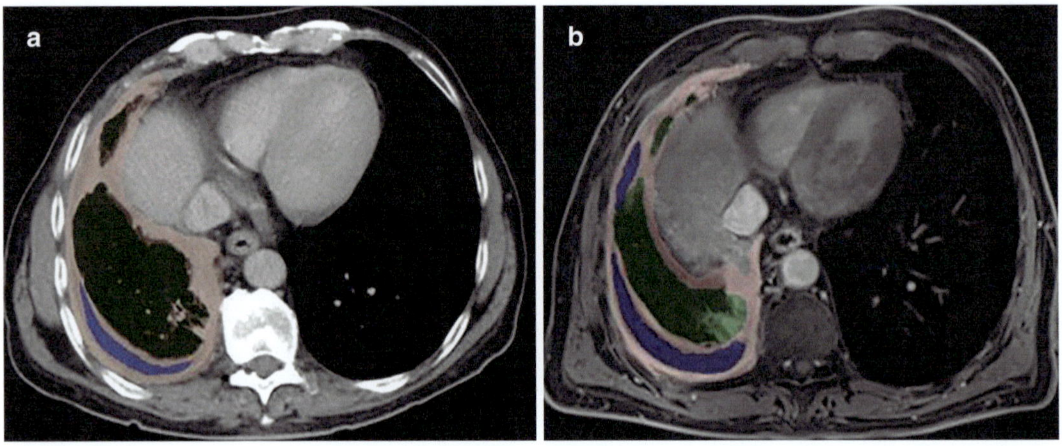

Fig. 23.5 AI segmentation. CT (**a**) and MRI (**b**) images of a 77-year-old man with the epithelioid type of MPM on the right. AI artificial intelligence

Time limitations and interobserver variability make the task of segmenting MPM from surrounding structures difficult to conduct without computer assistance. Semiautomatic or automatic computer-based methods can decrease the time burden and improve the reproducibility of the process [47, 73]. Automatic segmentation of the MPM and measurement of the detection of the volume require special software.

Modified RECIST criteria became the standard for MPM because it takes into account the rind-like growth of the tumor. Response to chemotherapy of the MPM can be evaluated by mRECIST criteria and tumor volumetry [46, 74]. The robustness of volumetric measurement of MPM before as well as after chemotherapy to mRECIST has been evaluated using different approaches [73, 75]. In an evaluation of tumor response after therapy, volumetric approaches and mRECIST have provided the most accurate scores in comparison to CT [47] and conventional RECIST [74].

A volumetric approach intends to use dedicated software featuring semiautomatic [73] or automatic segmentation with linear interpolation, which allows for manual adjustments. The thickness of the tumor can be measured perpendicular to the chest wall and mediastinum at two positions on three different levels [46] with a minimal craniocaudal distance of 1 cm according to the mRECIST criteria.

The software, which was previously developed for liver segmentation and volumetry, can also easily be used for other types of volumetries using the linear interpolation segmentation algorithm [75]. Furthermore, it demonstrated a high intraclass correlation and interobserver agreement for the absolute tumor volumes measured by specialized software. Therefore, the volumetry is useful for the assessment of chemotherapy response by using volumetric measurement in CT scans, because it is highly reliable, reproducible, and reader independent compared with the mRECIST criteria [75].

It is very important to note that mRECIST has a greater variability compared to volumetry. Based on the difference of the sum, tumor progression is either defined as partial response, stable disease, or progressive disease. However, this measurement method can be interpreted very broadly, leading to a wide range of results (Fig. 23.6).

The MPM demonstrates an inhomogeneous hypointense to isointense signal on T1W MRI and hyperintense signal on T2W sequences and enhancement after contrast administration [76].

Both DWI and ADC maps can be used for the assessment of MPM [29, 74]. The mean ADCs of MPM in different studies were similar ($0.84 \pm 0.22 \times 10^{-3}$ mm²/s [29], $0.84 \pm 0.05 \times 10^{-3}$ mm²/s [36]).

In one study the average ADC of the epithelioid subtype of MM was significantly higher than

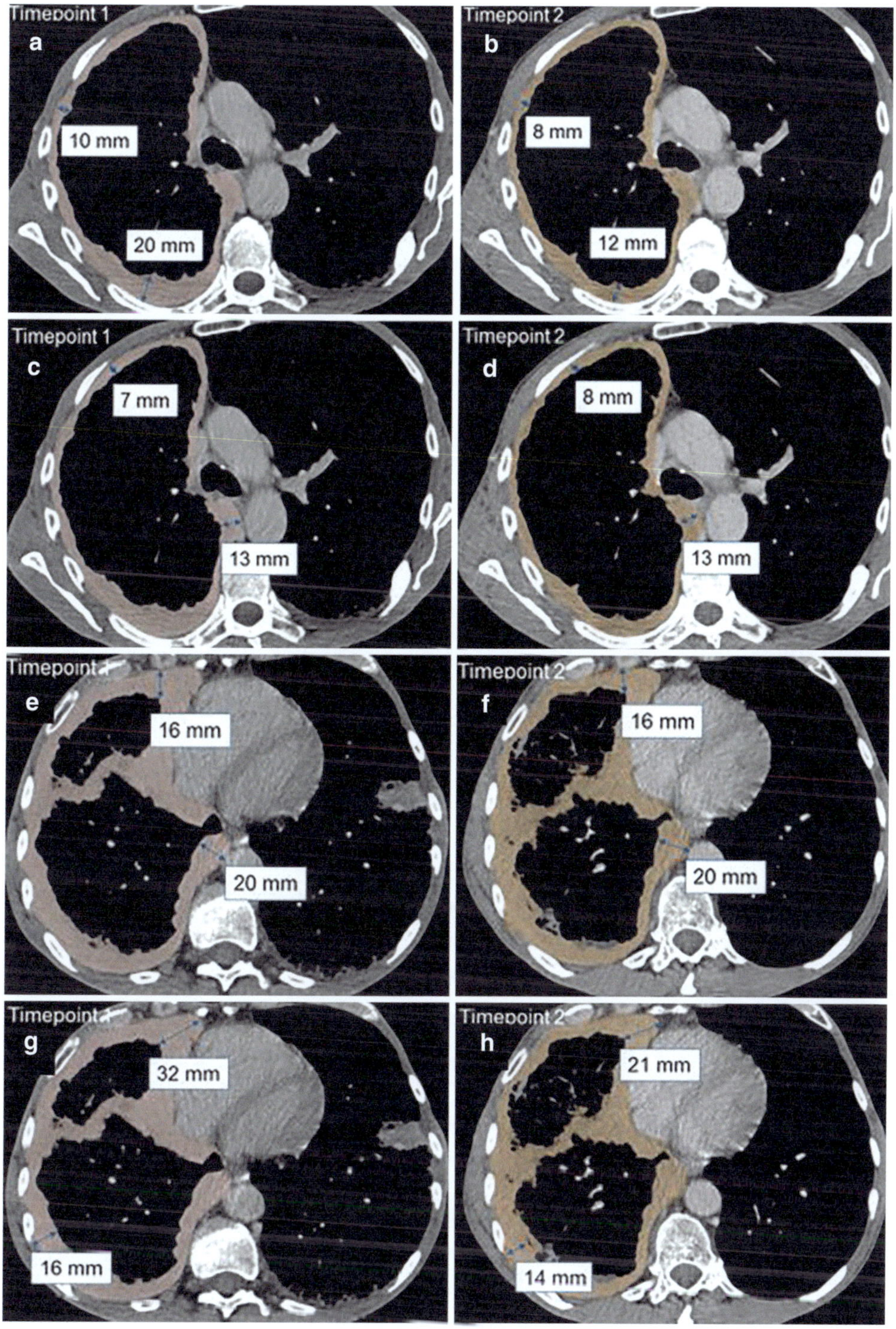

Fig. 23.6 CT images of a 59-year-old man with the epithelioid type of MPM on the right. Example using mRECIST for tumor response assessment after induction chemotherapy. Three types of tumor response in one case, namely, partial response (difference, −33%) (**a**, **b**); only a slightly different position of the measures leads to a stable disease (difference, +5%) (**c**, **d**); looks as a stable disease (difference, 0%) (**e**, **f**); when slightly changing the direction, still being perpendicular to the pleural surface can be defined as a progressive disease (difference, +28%) (**g**, **h**)

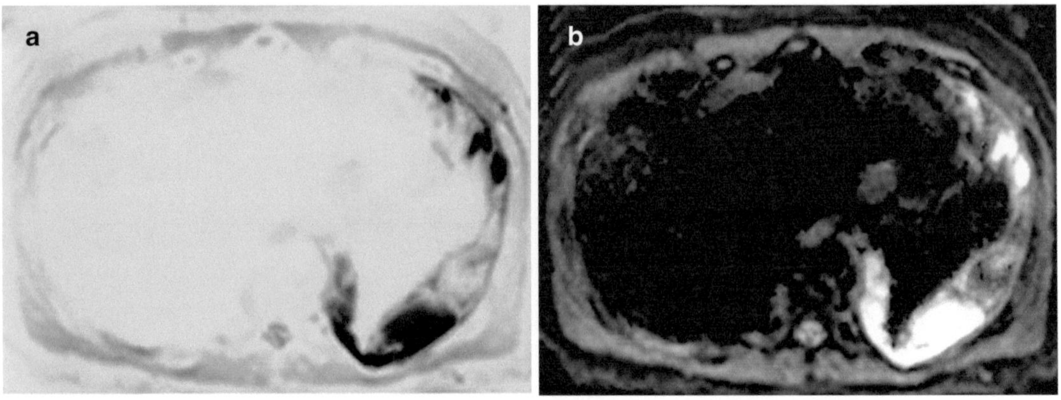

Fig. 23.7 A 59-year-old man with the epithelioid type of MPM on the left. DWI STIR with *b* value 100 (**a**) and ADC map (**b**). The tumor has a heterogeneous signal on both DWI and ADC maps

the ADC of the sarcomatoid subtype ($1.31 \pm 0.15 \times 10^{-3}$ mm²/s versus $0.99 \pm 0.07 \times 10^{-3}$ mm²/s, respectively) [77]. In another study, the ADC value for epithelioid MPMs was not significantly higher than the ADC for biphasic MPMs ($1.23 \pm 0.26 \times 10^{-3}$ mm²/s and $1.17 \pm 0.21 \times 10^{-3}$ mm²/s, respectively) [36]. The presence of necrosis or inflammation in the tumor can explain a misclassification of lesions in an ADC range between 1.52 and 2.00×10^{-3} mm²/s [37]. Therefore, DWI and ADC not always clearly demonstrate diffusion restriction in MPM (Fig. 23.7), especially in the presence of PE. The combination of DWI with DCE (Fig. 23.8) as well as PET with MRI or CT (Fig. 23.9) allows for a comprehensive assessment of the tumor. Addition of DCE can improve the sensitivity and accuracy to 92.8% and 93.5%, respectively; however the specificity is decreased to 94.1% [37].

It is important to underline that something new and useful has been described in the diagnosis and guide-for-biopsy MRI sign in DWI called "pleural pointillism" or "pointillism signal" which was defined as multiple (two or more) hyperintense areas visible by using a *b* value of 1000 in the pleura not identifiable with lower *b* values [78]. These multiple hyperintense foci have a high predictive value for malignancy, and it was noticed that they are more relevant than circumferential pleural thickening [30, 78].

DWI and DCE-MRI can be used to assess histological subtypes of MPM as well as the response to therapy [71].

Additional information, concerning chest wall invasion and mediastinal and nervous structures, especially before surgical treatment of MPM, can be obtained using contrast-enhanced MRI [52, 59]. The optimal mesothelioma contrast enhancement on MRI is not typical for the routine clinical imaging because it occurs at a longer time delay [79]. It has recently been found that the optimal enhancement of MPM on contrast-enhanced MRI occurs between 150 and 300 s after contrast injection [79]. However, further studies of the delayed phase on DCE-MRI are required [74, 79].

DCE-MRI provides quantitative, noninvasive, and longitudinal data on tumor vascularization characteristics. Thus, it can improve individual therapeutic prognostication [61].

Due to increased neo-angiogenesis and vascular permeability during DCE-MRI, MPM demonstrates a rapid uptake and washout of the contrast agent [47]. Biological effects in patients undergoing chemotherapy may be assessed using DCE-MRI and the pharmacokinetic parameters of MPM enhancement post-contrast administration [80]. A two-component pharmacokinetic model was established for the DCE-MRI analysis. The pharmacokinetic parameters amplitude (Amp), redistribution rate constant (kep), and

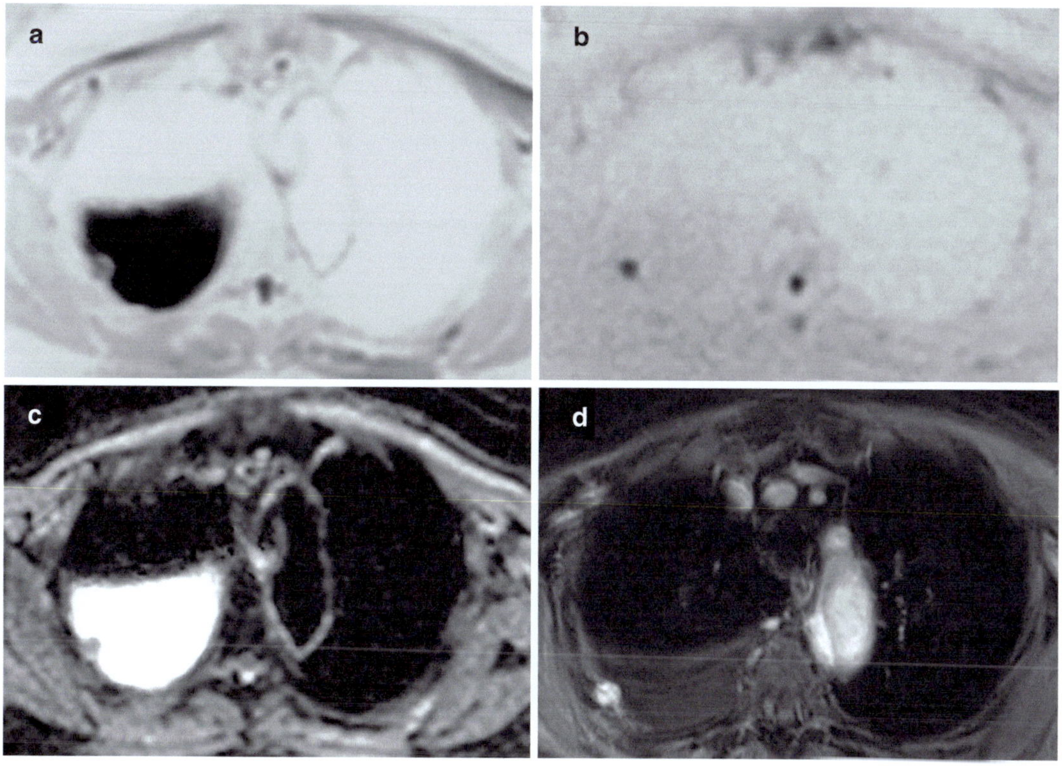

Fig. 23.8 A 78-year-old man with the epithelioid type of MPM on the right. DWI STIR with two different *b* values: b = 100 (**a**), b = 1500 (**b**), and ADC map (**c**). T1 vibe_ Dixon WI image: 2 min after contrast media injection (**d**) demonstrates homogeneous tumor contrast enhancement. WI weighed image

elimination rate constant (kel) were used to characterize tumor regions. Amp and kel can distinguish between normal and tumor tissues ($p \leq 0.001$). A positive correlation was found between lower kep values and response to therapy, where the median kep value within the tumor for clinical responders and nonresponders was 2.6 min and 3.6 min, respectively, which coincide with longer survival (780 days versus 460 days). DCE-MRI and its parameters in MPM patients can help in the identification of microscopic features and tumor heterogeneity for therapy monitoring [80].

A quantitative analysis of tumor enhancement by DCE-MRI parameters can be also evaluated using two different kinetic models: the extended Tofts model (ET) and the adiabatic approximation of tissue homogeneity (AATH) model [61, 81]. The mRECIST criteria was used to correlate chemotherapy treatment response with DCE parameters. High pretreatment efflux rate constant between extravascular, extracellular space, and plasma (kep) values suggested better treatment response [81]. In patients with MPM who were treated with cisplatin-based chemotherapy, DCE-MRI parameters were evaluated as predictors for the progression-free survival (PFS) and overall survival (OS). The most favorable parameter was the K^{trans} value, where higher pretreatment ET-calculated (ET-extended Tofts) K^{trans} values were associated with longer OS, with an estimated sensitivity of 89% and specificity of 78%. DCE-MRI can therefore assist in predicting patient response to chemotherapy. K^{trans} values reflect blood flow or vessel wall permeability, depending on predominant effect, suggesting that increased vascular perfusion or permeability may provide superior access to chemotherapy [61].

Recently, the flowing five single- or dual-input tracer kinetic models, namely, Tofts-Kety (TK),

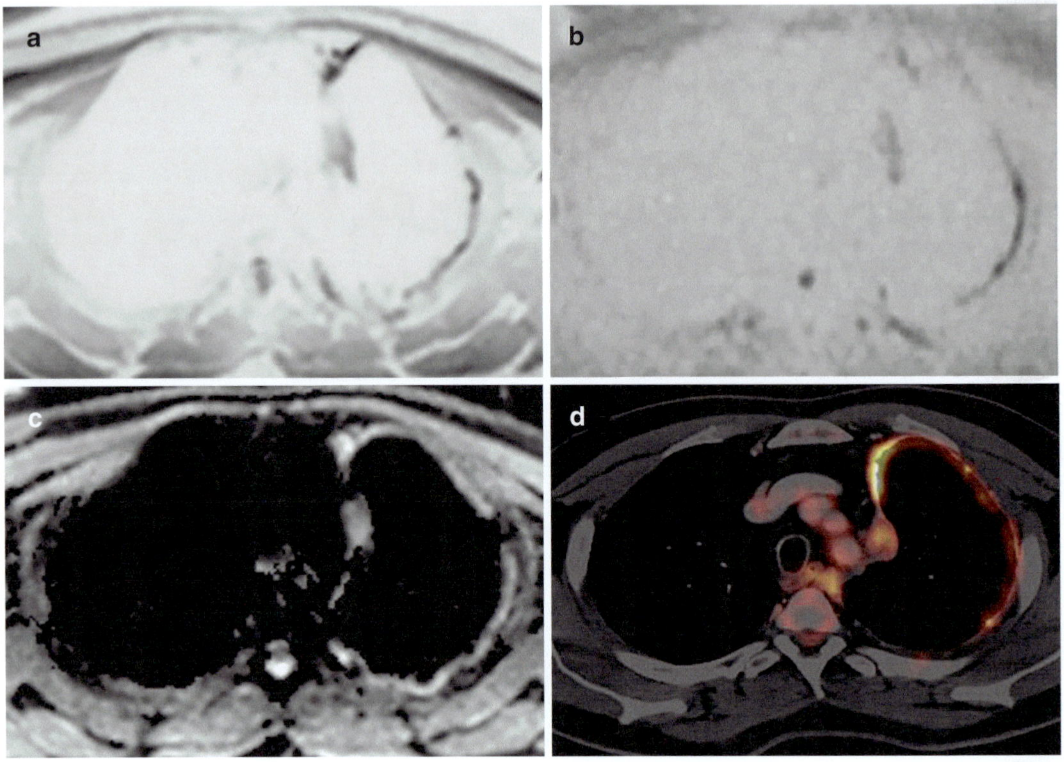

Fig. 23.9 A 59-year-old man with the epithelioid type of MPM on the left. DWI STIR with two different *b* values: *b* = 100 (**a**), *b* = 1500 (**b**), and ADC map (**c**). Highly active tumor on PET/CT (**d**)

extended TK (ETK), two-compartment exchange (2CX), AATH, and distributed parameter (DP) models, were used to analyze the DCE-MRI data. A coronal four-dimensional (4D) T1-weighted high-resolution imaging method with volume excitation (4D THRIVE) sequence during free breathing was used to obtain DCE-MRI data. The five different dual-input AQ10 tracer kinetic models, implemented with a continuous-time formalism, are able to fit the DCE-MRI data in MPM to varying degrees, fit the DCE-MRI data in MPM. With the exception of the TK model, the four other models demonstrated higher pulmonary arterial contribution to MPM compared to systemic arterial contribution. This suggests that MPM may derive a significant portion of its blood supply from the pulmonary circulation. However, there is a lack of consensus regarding the source of blood supply to the visceral pleura. Of the five single and dual kinetic models, the dual-input 2CX model showed to be the best fit in the voxel-based analysis for MPM. The 2CX model described tracer kinetic behavior most optimally, allowing for assessment of microvascular properties in MPM. The contribution of pulmonary versus systemic arterial flow to the total pulmonary perfusion in the tumors varied among the different kinetic models. Overall, arterial flow was higher than systemic arterial flow in MPM. However, the systemic arterial contribution to tumor perfusion is not negligible and could significantly impact the prognostic and predictive value of DCE-MRI metrics for thoracic malignancies [82].

A new method of MRI that aimed to identify an increase in MVD was proposed as a means of identifying patients with PM of any pleural thickening. ECE was the novel semi-objective, perfusion-based biomarker used, which was targeted to areas with increased MVD [68]. ECE has an optimal diagnostic value at a peak in signal intensity, occurring at or before 4.5 min

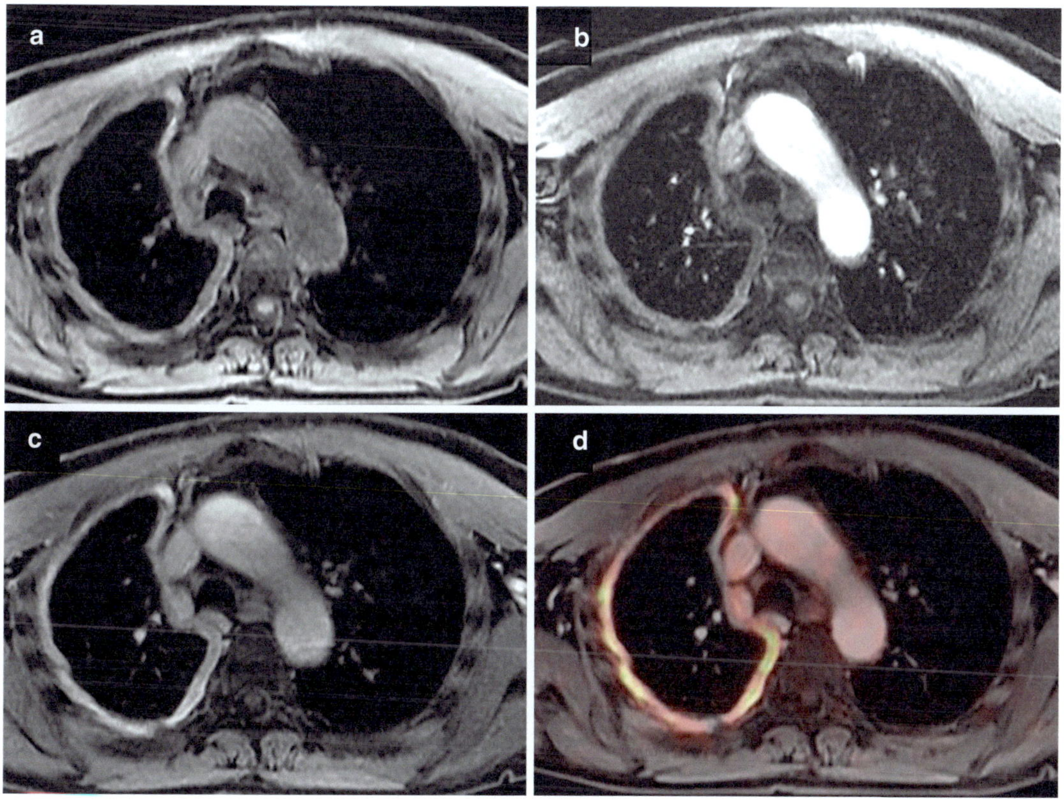

Fig. 23.10 MRI images (**a–c**) and PET/MRI (**d**) of a 66-year-old man with the epithelioid type of MPM on the right. T1W 3D GRE (LAVA) with 2-point Dixon fat/water separation (FLEX) without contrast (**a**); 60 s (**b**) and 4 min—early contrast enhancement (**c**) after contrast media injection. Malignancy of tumor is confirmed by PET/MRI (**d**)

(270 s) post-gadolinium contrast. The timing here is later than the currently recommended time of 60 s post-iodinated contrast. When ECE was compared to subjective MRI and CT morphology results, ECE performance was comparable or superior to subjective MRI and CT and yielded a sensitivity of 83% (95% CI 61–94%), specificity of 83% (95% CI 68–91%), positive predictive value of 68% (95% CI 47–84%), and negative predictive value of 92% (78–97%) [68].

In this manner, ECE can be measured in areas with minimal pleural thickening and demonstrates higher diagnostic sensitivity and negative predictive value than subjective CT morphology without perfusion analysis (56% and 67%, respectively) and MRI morphology (68% and 78%, respectively). ECE also demonstrated a superior interobserver agreement of κ 0.784, whereas this value for CT was κ 0.65 and MRI morphology κ 0.593; the median pleural thickness in this study was 5 mm. Quantitative perfusion parameters at DCE-CT have been shown to correlate with tumor MVD [68].

ECE is a promising biomarker for pleural malignancy diagnosis, with early studies demonstrating sensitive, specific, and reproducible results (Fig. 23.10). ECE is likely a biomarker which reflects increased MVD in patients with MPM, making it applicable to patients with minimal pleural thickening. ECE can also help identify effusion dominant, low-volume PM, including early-stage MPM [68].

The evaluation of lymph node involvement as well as detection of metastatic lesions in patients with MPM can be more complete with the help of PET/CT [52, 59]. PET/MRI is a promising

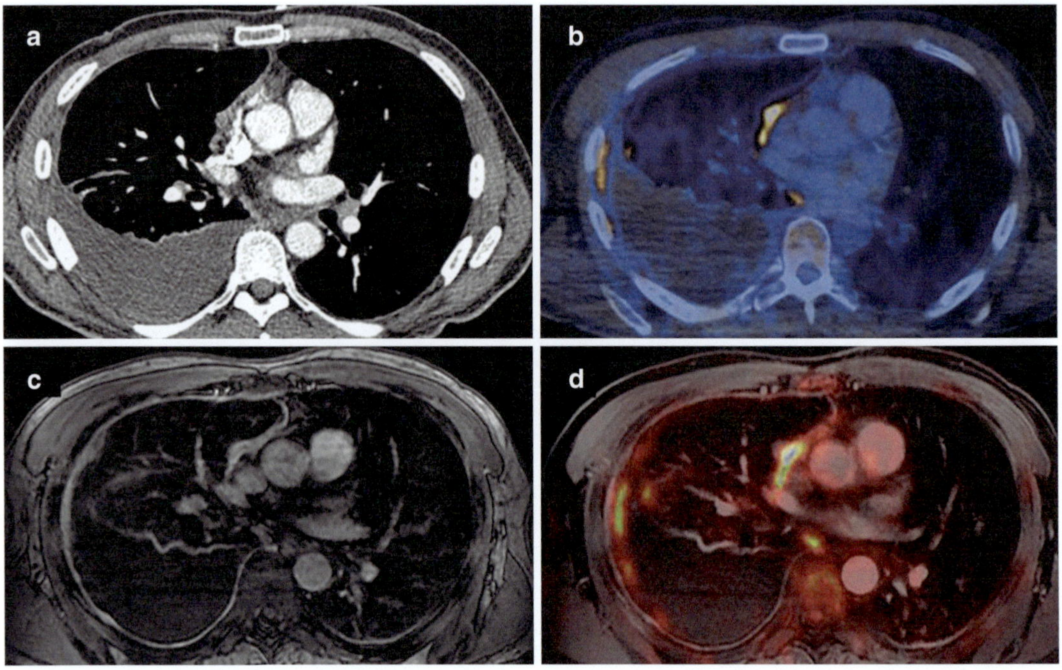

Fig. 23.11 A 75-year-old man with MPM and pleural effusion on the right. Hybrid visualization of the MPM: CT (**a**), PET/CT (**b**), MRI (**c**), and PET/MRI (**d**) images

modality; it's comparable with PET/CT for MPM assessment (Fig. 23.11).

Recently, the investigation of the diagnostic utility of a deep learning method based on 3D deep convolutional neural network (DCNN) for differentiation of MPM from benign pleural disease using FDG PET/CT imaging has found a significantly greater mean SUV_{max} value when compared to benign pleural disease [50]. TLG (total lesion glycolysis) as pretreatment volume-based quantitative parameter of ^{18}F-FDG PET/CT has been shown to be the better potential surrogate markers for MPM prognosis [83]. Lately, the investigation of the diagnostic utility of a deep learning method based on 3D DCNN in combination with the results of FDG PET/CT imaging includes a novel potential tool that has established flexibility for differentiation of MPM. The mean SUV_{max} value for MPM was significantly greater compared to benign pleural disease. A protocol which incorporated an SUV_{max} value for discrimination between MPM and benign pleural lesion has demonstrated an optimal SUV_{max} cutoff of 2.23 with a sensitivity, specificity, and accuracy of 85.6%, 75.0%, and 81.3%, respectively [50]. Although the volume can be a prognostic factor for the OS, it has shown a lower c-index compared with the FDG PET radiomics-based PFS model. Nevertheless, a successful FDG PET radiomics model for the prediction of PFS in MPM patients on pretreatment images was created. However, it was established that radiomics models based on CT, SUV_{max}, and SUV_{mean} with a good prognostic ability could not be generated [48].

New, constantly developing methods of post-processing analysis, particularly volumetry or texture analysis, will further help improve patient-specific treatment strategies [52].

Pleural Effusion/Empyema

Pleural thickening, pleural enhancement, micro-bubbles, extrapleural fat stranding, and loculation are important findings in the visualization of empyema [84]. It is important to emphasize that when pleural empyema is suspected, better dif-

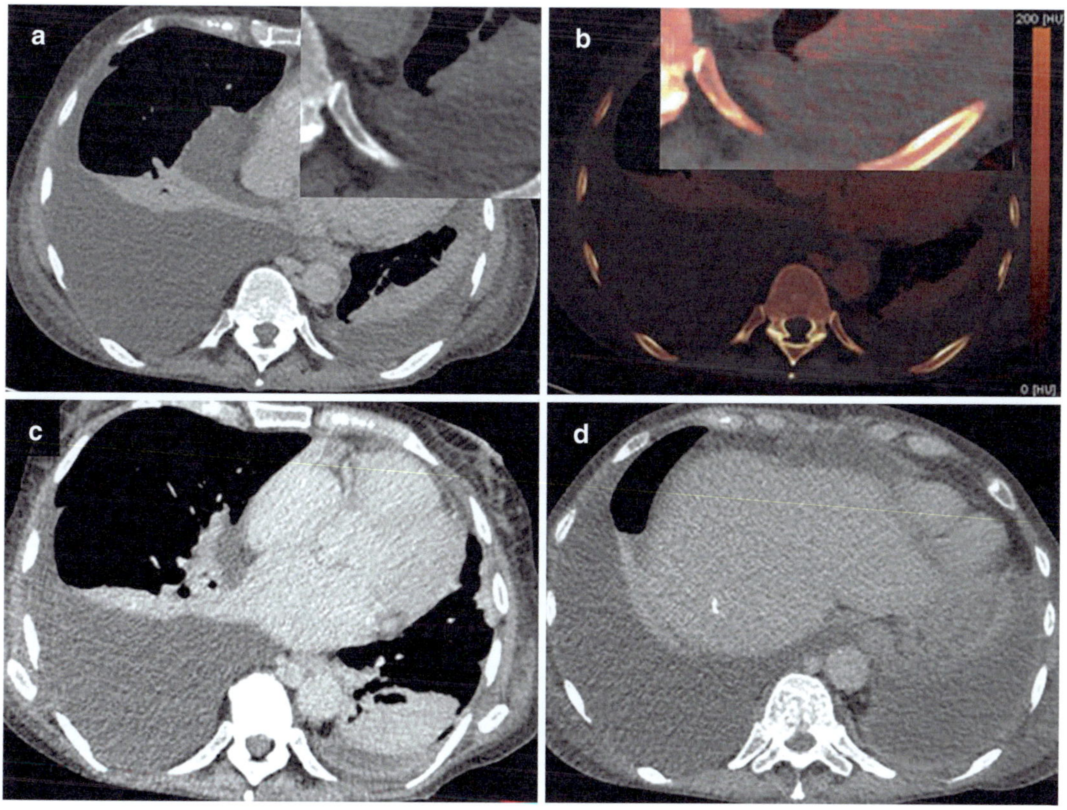

Fig. 23.12 PCD-CT images in the axial plane of a 53-year-old woman with pleural effusion on the right and empyema on the left. All energy spectra images (**a**, **c**, **d**) and iodine map (**b**). Pleural empyema on the left with pleural thickening, marginal contrast enhancement, and gentle septations. Partial atelectasis of the lower lobes adjacent to the pleural effusion and empyema. W/L, 150/600 Hounsfield units

ferentiation between non-infectious pleural effusion and pleural empyema can be achieved by optimizing CT protocols (Fig. 23.12).

The diagnosis of empyema requires administration of a contrast media. All typical signs of empyema can be more clearly visualized on the arterial phase of CT (Fig. 23.13).

The enhancement of the pleura by MRI was revealed to be comparable to contrast-enhanced CT [85]. The ADC of the PE in cases of empyema often decreases due to the presence of pus. In empyema, the ADC of pleural fluid was significantly lower than the ADC of the MPMs, the pleural disseminations, and the pleural effusions. The ADC value of empyema was thus significantly lower without significant decrease in diffusion of the pleura. The ADC value of pleura and pleural cavity should be closely considered when diagnosing empyema [34]. Pleura in patients with empyema has revealed significantly higher mean attenuation values when compared with non-infectious pleural effusion (85.1 ± 20.6 and 15.5 ± 3.4, respectively) [86]. A recent meta-analysis of the diagnostic capabilities of CT scans in diagnosing empyema revealed a combined specificity of 90% and sensitivity of 62%. Advanced imaging and implementation of CT-optimized protocols of contrast media administration can improve the sensitivity and make CT more reliable and useful for pleural empyema management decision-making [87].

In recent years, empyema diagnosis by CT has demonstrated a sensitivity of 72.84% and a specificity of 90.94% with moderate to almost perfect interrater agreement for pleural empyema-associated findings, with the highest accuracy for

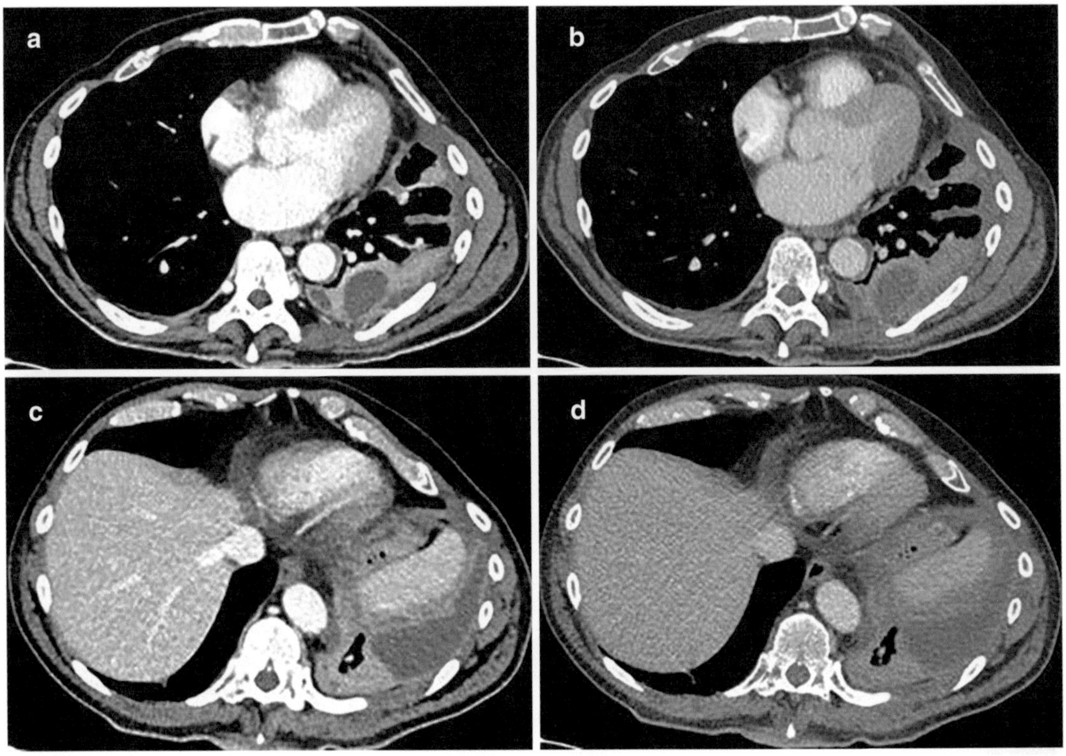

Fig. 23.13 CT images of a 66-year-old man with pleural empyema on the left. Arterial phase (**a**, **c**) and venous phase (**b**, **d**). The arterial phase demonstrates better pleural thickening, marginal contrast enhancement, and loculations

pleural enhancement (87%) and thickening (81,9%). AI has demonstrated a sensitivity of 74.41% and specificity of 77.78%. Actively developing AI-based algorithms for diagnostic imaging can become increasingly relevant in the diagnosis, classification, and evaluation of disease outcome [84].

Recently, the impact of different virtual monoenergetic image (VMI) energies and iodine maps of PCD-CT on the diagnostic accuracy and confidence to differentiate pleural empyema from non-infectious pleural effusion has been presented. Diagnostic accuracy and confidence at lower VMI energies were significantly higher with the highest accuracy at 40 keV (Fig. 23.14). In addition, the use of iodine maps has improved the diagnostic accuracy at higher VMI energies (60–70 keV) and still remained high enough at low VMI energies (Fig. 23.15). Thus, higher diagnostic accuracy and diagnostic confidence in the diagnosis of pleural empyema can be achieved at low VMI energies, and iodine maps have been shown to be effective in diagnosing empyema only at high VMI energies [86].

Fibroma

SFT is a rare and, in most cases, benign primary neoplasm of the pleura [88]. CT and MRI can be valuable tools in the diagnosis of SFTs. Sometimes, SFT can demonstrate variable radiological features that mimic a variety of other intrathoracic lesions. Although there are some radiological findings that suggest the presence of SFT malignancy, currently radiological methods are not able to accurately distinguish between benign and malignant subtypes of pleural SFTs [89].

A recent study has revealed a little enhancement in the early phase and progressive enhancement in the delayed phase on DCE-MRI for fibrous SFTs, while cellular SFTs demonstrated rapid initial enhancement [90]. Thus, variable

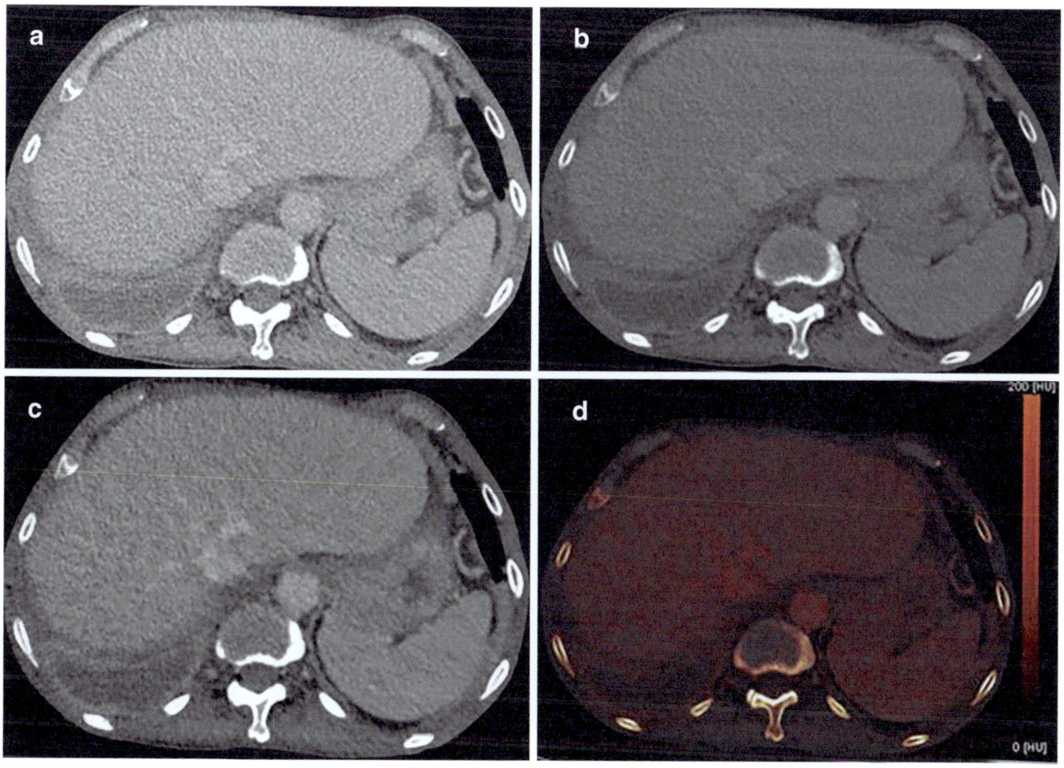

Fig. 23.14 PCD-CT images in the axial plane of a 68-year-old man with pleural empyema on the right. The multi-energy reconstruction, including all energy spectra (**a**), VMI energies: 40 keV (**b**), 70 keV (**c**), and iodine map (**d**). Imaging features of pleural empyema including pleural enhancement and pleural thickening. W/L, 150/600 Hounsfield units

contrast enhancement patterns on MRI are caused by morphological heterogeneity of the tumor [91]. Nevertheless, the mean ADC value for cellular and fibrous solid tumors has not shown a significant difference [90].

Currently, the utility of FDG PET and FDG PET/CT in the differentiation of benign and malignant SFTs is still controversial. An earlier study showed a significant difference between the mean SUV_{max} of the malignant and benign SFTs (3.6 and 2.0, respectively) [92]; meanwhile, the median SUV_{max} value 4.35 for primary pulmonary synovial sarcoma has been reported [93]. Therefore, malignant SFTs have demonstrated the tendency to be strongly hypermetabolic and homogeneous at PET, while the benign SFTs had low-grade activity [94]. The mean HU of malignant SFTs has been shown to be lower than for benign. Low ^{18}F-FDG uptake has been revealed for both benign and malignant SFTs; however, higher ^{18}F-FDG uptake with significant difference exhibited malignant SFT [95]. In the detection of the malignant SFT, the following threshold values were established ≤39.81 HU for density and ≥3.47 for SUV_{max} [95]. However, it has been noted that when using SUV_{max} individually in the identification of malignant SFSs, the utility of ^{18}F-FDG PET/CT is limited due to their low values, whereas the combined interpretation of both CT images and ^{18}F-FDG PET/CT findings can be useful in the detection of malignancy [95]. In a recent single-institution study, it has been shown that there is a significant difference in metabolic parameters of a malignant SFT compared with benign SFT; in addition to higher SUV_{max} values, malignant SFTs also often demonstrated higher SUV_{mean} values, higher TLG values, and higher maximum standardized uptake lean body mass

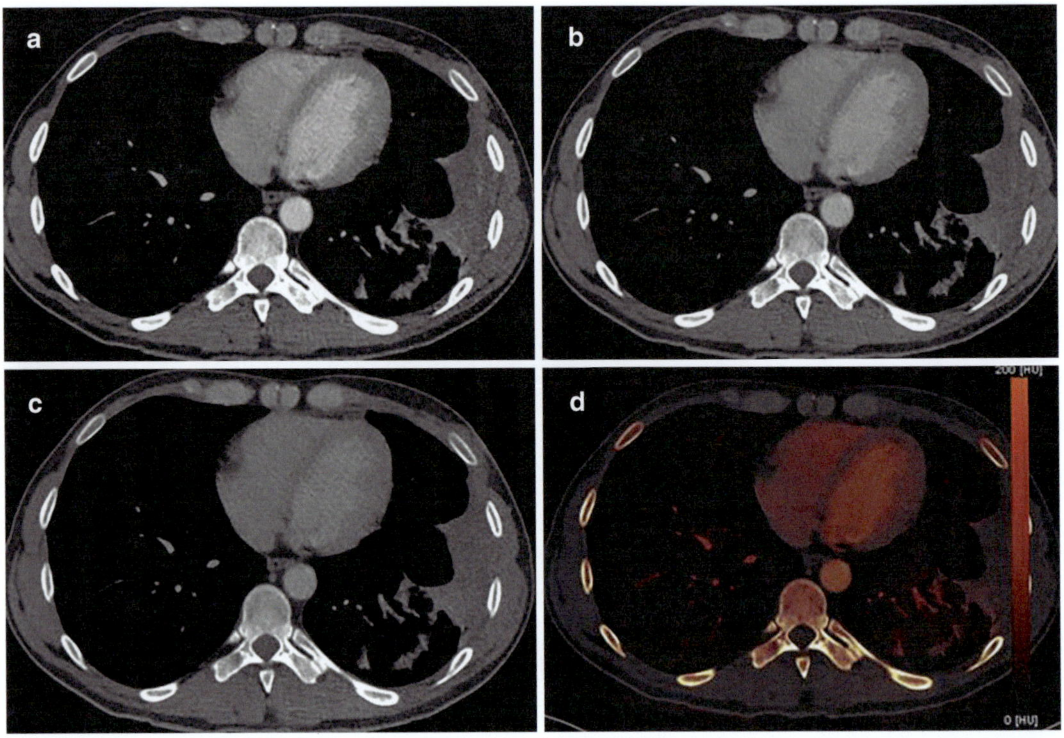

Fig. 23.15 PCD-CT images in the axial plane of a 48-year-old man with pleural empyema on the left. The multi-energy reconstruction, including VMI energies: 40 keV (a), 70 keV (**b**), 80 keV (**c**), and iodine map (**d**). Pleural enhancement and pleural thickening are easily seen at 40 keV (**a**) and become less visible with increasing VMI energies. W/L, 150/600 Hounsfield units

(SUL_{max}) values. Accordingly, in the detection of malignant SFT, the SUV_{max} can achieve an accuracy of 87.5%, and the SUL_{max} and SUV_{mean} exceed the accuracy of 90%. However, at the same time, metabolic tumor volume and TLG volumetric parameters were less useful in the differentiation malignant versus benign SFTs [96].

MRI Protocols

Pleural thoracic MRI protocols are widely available across vendor platforms and can easily be created with standard sequences. In addition, the necessary sequences can be extracted from other protocols and applied to the thorax. It is most preferable to use sequences of 20 s (or less) with breath-hold. In cases where a patient cannot hold their breath or a longer sequence is used, respiratory triggering can be implemented.

The pleural MRI protocol includes the following sequences: multiplane T2W with and without fat suppression (T2W-IR and SSFSE, respectively), which can help recognize the subpleural fat or determine its an invasion or obliteration), and axial T1W with and without fat suppression (precontract fast GRE and simple fast spin echo, respectively). It is recommended that dynamic postcontrast fast GRE sequences are performed in arterial, portal venous, 3-min, and 5-min delayed phases (parameters on the pre- and postcontrast fast GRE images must be identical in order to allow for subtraction) (Fig. 23.16).

Coronal and sagittal fast GRE sequences can be performed during the interval between the portal venous and 5-min delayed images. DWI with *b* values of 0, 100, and 800–1000 sec/mm^2 with ADC map should be added. The coronal and sagittal real-time balanced SSFP imaging can be

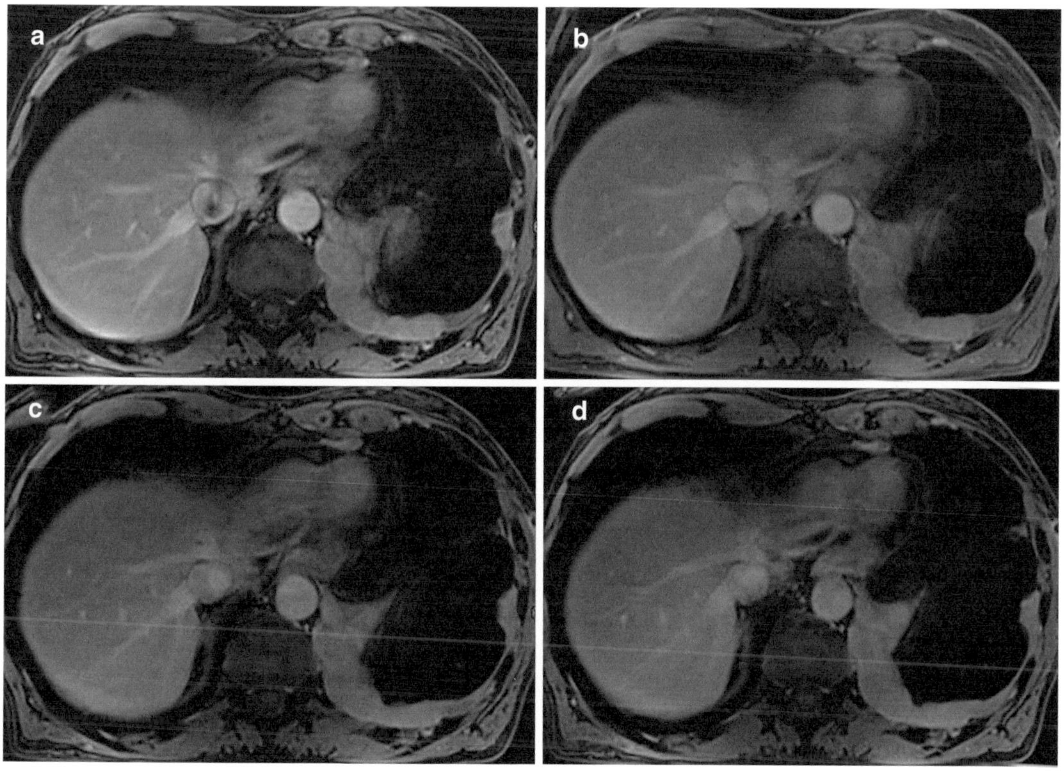

Fig. 23.16 MRI images in the axial plane of a 70-year-old man with the epithelioid type of MPM on the left. T1 vibe_Dixon WI after contrast media injection: 2 min (**a**), 3 min (**b**), 4 min (**c**), and 6 min (**d**). Optimal contrast is achieved after 4 min. WI weighted images

added as a routine component of pleural MRI protocol using a field of view that encompasses the diaphragm [28].

References

1. Bodtger U, Hallifax RJ. Epidemiology: why is pleural disease becoming more common? In: Maskell NA, Laursen CB, Lee YCG, et al., editors. Pleural disease (ERS monograph). Sheffield. European Respiratory Society; 2020. p. 1–12.
2. Hallifax RJ, Talwar A, Wrightson JM, Edey A, Gleeson FV. State-of-the-art: radiological investigation of pleural disease. Respir Med. 2017;124:88–99. https://doi.org/10.1016/j.rmed.2017.02.013.
3. Radiological Society of North America (RSNA). Quantitative Imaging Biomarkers Alliance (QIBA). 2017. Quantitative Imaging Biomarkers Alliance RSNA. Accessed 13 July 2023.
4. Helm EJ, Matin TN, Gleeson FV. Imaging of the Pleura. J Magn Reson Imaging. 2010;32:1275–86. https://doi.org/10.1002/jmri.22372.
5. Hsia CCW, Bates JHT, Driehuys B, Fain SB, Goldin JG, Hoffman EA, et al. Quantitative imaging metrics for the assessment of pulmonary pathophysiology: an official American Thoracic Society and Fleischner Society Joint Workshop Report. Ann Am Thorac Soc. 2023;20(2):161–95. https://doi.org/10.1513/AnnalsATS.202211-915ST.
6. Blackmore CC, Black WC, Dallas RV, Crow HC. Pleural fluid volume estimation: a chest radiograph prediction rule. Acad Radiol. 1996;3:103–9.
7. Moy MP, Levsky JM, Berko NS, Godelman A, Jain VR, Haramati LB. A new, simple method for estimating pleural effusion size on CT scans. Chest. 2013;143(4):1054–9. https://doi.org/10.1378/chest.12-1292.
8. Huang T, Yang R, Shen L, Feng A, Li L, He N, et al. Deep transfer learning to quantify pleural effusion severity in chest X-rays. BMC Med Imaging. 2022;22:100. https://doi.org/10.1186/s12880-022-00827.
9. Brixey AG, Luo Y, Skouras V, Awdankiewicz A, Light RW. The efficacy of chest radiographs in detecting parapneumonic effusions. Respirology. 2011;16(6):1000–4. https://doi.org/10.1111/j.1440-1843.2011.02006.x.

10. Kitazono MT, Lau CT, Parada AN, et al. Differentiation of pleural effusions from parenchymal opacities: accuracy of bedside chest radiography. AJR. 2010;194:407–12. https://doi.org/10.2214/AJR.09.2950.
11. Mammarappallil JG, Sarah A, Anderson SA, Danelson KA, Stitzel JA, Chiles C. Estimation of pleural fluid volumes on chest radiography using computed tomography volumetric analysis. An update of the visual prediction rule. J Thorac Imaging. 2015;30:336–9.
12. Vignon P, Chastagner C, Berkane V, Chardac E, François B, Normand S, et al. Quantitative assessment of pleural effusion in critically ill patients by means of ultrasonography. Crit Care Med. 2005;33:1757–63. https://doi.org/10.1097/01.CCM.0000171532.02639.08.
13. Brockelsby C, Ahmed M, Gautam M. Pleural effusion size estimation: US, CXR OR CT? Thorax. 2016;71(Suppl 3):A1–A288.
14. ILO Guidelines for the use of the ILO International Classification of Radiographs of Pneumoconioses. Revised Geneva. 2011. International Labour Office, 2002 (Occupational Safety and Health Series, No. 22 (rev. 2011).
15. Volpi F, D'Amore CA, Colligiani L, Milazzo A, Cavaliere S, De Liperi A, et al. The use of chest magnetic resonance imaging in malignant pleural mesothelioma diagnosis. Diagnostics. 2022;12(3):750. https://doi.org/10.3390/diagnostics12030750.
16. Varsamas C, Kalkanis A, Gourgoulianis KI, Malli F. The use of a novel quantitative marker of echogenicity of pleural fluid in parapneumonic pleural effusions. Can Respir J. 2020:1283590. https://doi.org/10.1155/2020/1283590.
17. Soni NJ, Franco R, Velez MI, Schnobrich D, Dancel R, Restrepo MI, et al. Ultrasound in the diagnosis and management of pleural effusions. J Hosp Med. 2015;10(12):811–6. https://doi.org/10.1002/jhm.2434.
18. Lichtenstein D, Goldstein I, Mourgeon E, Cluzel P, Grenier P, Rouby JJ. Comparative diagnostic performances of auscultation, chest radiography, and lung ultrasonography in acute respiratory distress syndrome. Anesthesiology. 2004;100(1):9–15. https://doi.org/10.1097/00000542-200401000-00006.
19. Mercer RM, Psallidas I, Rahman NM. Ultrasound in the management of pleural disease. Expert Rev Respir Med. 2017;11(4):323–31. https://doi.org/10.1080/17476348.2017.1300531.
20. Remerand F, Dellamonica J, Mao Z, Ferrari F, Bouhemad B, Jianxin Y, et al. Multiplane ultrasound approach to quantify pleural effusion at the bedside. Intensive Care Med. 2010;36:656–664. https://doi.org/10.1007/s00134-010-1769-9.
21. Capper SJ, Ross JJ, Sandström E, Braidley PC, Morgan-Hughes NJ. Transoesophageal echocardiography for the detection and quantification of pleural fluid in cardiac surgical patients. Br J Anaesth. 2007;98:442–6. https://doi.org/10.1093/bja/aem010.
22. Hassan M, Rizk R, Essam H, Abouelnour A. Validation of equations for pleural effusion volume estimation by ultrasonography. J Ultrasound. 2017;20:267–71. https://doi.org/10.1007/s40477-017-0266-1.
23. Corcoran JP, Tazi-Mezalek R, Maldonado F, Yarmus LB, Annema JT, Koegelenberg CFN, et al. State of the art thoracic ultrasound: intervention and therapeutics. Thorax. 2017;72(9):840–9. https://doi.org/10.1136/thoraxjnl-2016-209340.
24. Lichtenstein DA, Mezière GA, Lagoueyte JF, Biderman P, Goldstein I, Gepner A. A-lines and B-lines: lung ultrasound as a bedside tool for predicting pulmonary artery occlusion pressure in the critically ill. Chest. 2009;136:1014–20. https://doi.org/10.1378/chest.09-0001.
25. Vieira JR, Castro MR, Guimarães TP, Pinheiro AJ, Figueiredo AC, Martins BJ, et al. Evaluation of pulmonary B lines by different intensive care physicians using bedside ultrasonography: a reliability study. Rev Bras Ter Intensiva. 2019;31(3):354–60. https://doi.org/10.5935/0103-507X.20190058.
26. Bhoil R, Ahluwalia A, Chopra R, Surya M, Bhoil S. Signs and lines in lung ultrasound. J Ultrason. 2021;21(86):e225–33. https://doi.org/10.15557/JoU.2021.0036.
27. Hassan M, Mercer RM, Rahman NM. Thoracic ultrasound in the modern management of pleural disease. Eur Respir Rev. 2020;29(156):190136. https://doi.org/10.1183/16000617.0136-2019.
28. Raptis CA, McWilliams SR, Ratkowski KL, Broncano J, Green DB, Bhalla S. Mediastinal and pleural MR imaging: practical approach for daily practice. Radiographics. 2018;38(1):37–55. https://doi.org/10.1148/rg.2018170091.
29. Sabri YY, Mahmoud IH, El-Gendy LT, Abd El-Mageed MR, Tadros SF. Added value of diffusion-weighted MRI in assessment of pleural lesions. Egypt J Radiol Nucl Med. 2021;52:184. https://doi.org/10.1186/s43055-021-00557-3.
30. Coolen J, Verschakelen J, De Wever W. MRI of pleural diseases. Curr Opin Pulm Med. 2015;21:399–406. https://doi.org/10.1097/MCP.0000000000000177.
31. Baysal T, Bulat T, Gokirmak M, Kalkan S, Dusak A, Dogan M. Diffusion-weighted MR imaging of pleural fluid: differentiation of transudative vs exudative pleural effusions. Eur Radiol. 2004;14:890–6. https://doi.org/10.1007/s00330-003-1995-4.
32. İnan N, Arslan A, Akansel G, Arslan Z, Eleman L, Demirci A. Diffusion weighted MRI in the characterization of pleural effusions. Diagn Interv Radiol. 2009;15(1):13–8.
33. Keskin Z, Yesildag M, Alkan E, Kayhan A, Tolu I, Keskin S. Differentiation between transudative and exudative pleural effusions by diffusion weighted magnetic resonance imaging. Iran J Radiol. 2019;16(2):e78775. https://doi.org/10.5812/iranjradiol.78775.
34. Usuda K, Iwai S, Funasaki A, Sekimura A, Motono N, Matoba M, et al. Diffusion-weighted imaging can differentiate between malignant and Benign pleural

diseases. Cancers (Basel). 2019;11(6):811. https://doi.org/10.3390/cancers11060811.
35. Karatag O, Alar T, Kosar S, Ocakoglu G, Yildiz Y, Gedik E, et al. Can diffusion weighted MRI differentiate between inflammatory-infectious and malignant pleural effusions? JBR-BTR. 2015;98(2):63–7. https://doi.org/10.5334/jbr-btr.767.
36. Koç M, Poyraz AK. The role of diffusion-weighted MR imaging in detecting malignant and benign pleural thickening in asbestos-related pleural diseases. Erciyes Med J. 2017;39(2):44–7. https://doi.org/10.5152/etd.2017.16045.
37. Coolen J, De Keyzer F, Nafteux P, De Wever W, Dooms C, Vansteenkiste J, et al. Malignant pleural disease: diagnosis by using diffusion-weighted and dynamic contrast-enhanced MR imaging—initial experience. Radiology. 2012;263:884–92. https://doi.org/10.1148/radiol.12110872.
38. Priola AM, Gned D, Veltri A, Priola SM. Chemical shift and diffusion-weighted magnetic resonance imaging of the anterior mediastinum in oncology: current clinical applications in qualitative and quantitative assessment. Crit Rev Oncol Hematol. 2016;98:335–57. https://doi.org/10.1016/j.critrevonc.2015.11.012.
39. Schmidt H, Gatidis S, Schwenzer NF, Martirosian P. Impact of measurement parameters on apparent diffusion coefficient quantification in diffusion-weighted-magnetic resonance imaging. Investig Radiol. 2015;50:46–56. https://doi.org/10.1097/RLI.0000000000000095.
40. Priola AM, Priola SM, Parlatano D, Gned D, Giraudo MT, Giardino R, et al. Apparent diffusion coefficient measurements in diffusion-weighted magnetic resonance imaging of the anterior mediastinum: interobserver reproducibility of five different methods of region-of-interest positioning. Eur Radiol. 2017;27:1386–94. https://doi.org/10.1007/s00330-016-4527-8.
41. Armato SG, Blyth KG, Keating JJ, Katz S, Tsim S, Coolen J, et al. Imaging in pleural mesothelioma: a review of the 13th international conference of the International Mesothelioma Interest Group. Lung Cancer. 2016;101:48–58. https://doi.org/10.1016/j.lungcan.2016.09.003.
42. Ng TSC, Seethamraju RT, Bueno R, Gill RR. Clinical implementation of a free-breathing, motion-robust dynamic contrast-enhanced MRI protocol to evaluate pleural tumors. Am J Roentgenol. 2020;215:94–104. https://doi.org/10.2214/AJR.19.21612.
43. Dournes G, Dubois A, Benlala I, Lacourt A, Paris C, Gislard A, et al. 3-dimensional quantification of composite pleural plaque volume in patients exposed to Asbestos using high-resolution computed tomography. A validation study. J Thorac Imaging. 2019;34:320–5. https://doi.org/10.1097/RTI.0000000000000377.
44. Benlala I, De Senneville BD, Dournes G, Menant M, Gramond C, Thaon I, et al. Deep learning for the automatic quantification of pleural plaques in Asbestos-exposed subjects. Int J Environ Res Public Health. 2022;19(3):1417. https://doi.org/10.3390/ijerph19031417.
45. Lauk O, Patella M, Neuer T, Battilana B, Frauenfelder T, Nguyen-Kim TDL, et al. Implementing CT tumor volume and CT pleural thickness into future staging systems for malignant pleural mesothelioma. Cancer Imaging. 2021;21:48. https://doi.org/10.1186/s40644-021-00415-5.
46. Armato SG, Nowak AK, Francis RJ, Katz SI, Kholmatov M, Blyth KG, et al. Imaging in pleural mesothelioma: a review of the 15th international conference of the International Mesothelioma Interest Group. Lung Cancer. 2022;164:76–83. https://doi.org/10.1016/j.lungcan.2021.12.008.
47. Romei C, Fanni SC, Volpi F, Milazzo A, D'Amore CA, Colligiani L, et al. New updates of the imaging role in diagnosis, staging, and response treatment of malignant pleural mesothelioma. Cancer. 2021;13:4377. https://doi.org/10.3390/cancers13174377.
48. Pavic M, Bogowicz M, Kraft J, Vuong D, Mayinger M, Kroeze SGC, et al. FDG PET versus CT radiomics to predict outcome in malignant pleural mesothelioma patients. EJNMMI Res. 2020;10(1):81. https://doi.org/10.1186/s13550-020-00669-3.
49. Pena E, Ojiaku M, Inacio JR, Gupta A, Macdonald DB, Shabana W, et al. Can CT and MR shape and textural features differentiate Benign versus malignant pleural lesions? Acad Radiol. 2017;24(10):1277–87. https://doi.org/10.1016/j.acra.2017.03.006.
50. Kitajima K, Matsuo H, Kono A, Kuribayashi K, Kijima T, Hashimoto M, et al. Deep learning with deep convolutional neural network using FDG-PET/CT for malignant pleural mesothelioma diagnosis. Oncotarget. 2021;12(12):1187–96. https://doi.org/10.18632/oncotarget.27979.
51. Zhang X, Duan H, Yu Y, Ma C, Ren Z, Lei Y, et al. Differential diagnosis between benign and malignant pleural effusion with dual-energy spectral CT. PLoS One. 2018;13(4):e0193714. https://doi.org/10.1371/journal.pone.0193714.
52. Martini K, Frauenfelder T. Old Borders and New Horizons in multimodality imaging of malignant pleural mesothelioma. Thorac Cardiovasc Surg. 2022;70(8):677–83. https://doi.org/10.1055/s-0041-1728714.
53. Byrne MJ, Nowak AK. Modified RECIST criteria for assessment of response in malignant pleural mesothelioma. Ann Oncol. 2004;15(2):257–60.
54. Armato SG, Nowak AK. Revised modified response evaluation criteria in solid tumors for assessment of response in malignant pleural mesothelioma (version 1.1). J Thorac Oncol. 2018;13(7):1012–21. https://doi.org/10.1016/j.jtho.2018.04.034.
55. Nakajima R, Abe K, Sakai S. Diagnostic ability of FDG-PET/CT in the detection of malignant pleural effusion. Medicine. 2015;94(29):1–6.
56. Yang M-F, Tong Z-H, Wang Z, Zhang Y-Y, Xu L-L, Wang X-J, et al. Development and validation of the PET-CT score for diagnosis of malignant pleural effu-

sion. Eur J Nucl Med Mol Imaging. 2019;46:1457–67. https://doi.org/10.1007/s00259-019-04287-7.
57. Usuda K, Sagawa M, Motono N, Ueno M, Tanaka M, Machida Y, et al. Advantages of diffusion-weighted imaging over positron emission tomography-computed tomography in assessment of hilar and mediastinal lymph node in lung cancer. Ann Surg Oncol. 2013;20:1676–83. https://doi.org/10.1245/s10434-012-2799-z.
58. Bonde A, Singh R, Prasad SR, Kamireddy D, Aggarwal A, Ramani N, et al. Mesotheliomas and Benign Mesothelial tumors: update on pathologic and imaging findings. Radiographics. 2022;43(3):e220128. https://doi.org/10.1148/rg.220128.
59. Strange CD, Shroff GS, Ahuja J, Vlahos I, Benveniste MFK, Truong MT. Imaging of malignant pleural mesothelioma: pearls and pitfalls. Semin Ultrasound CT MR. 2021;42(6):542–51.39. https://doi.org/10.1053/j.sult.2021.04.011.
60. Courtiol P, Maussion C, Moarii M, Pronier E, Pilcer S, Sefta M, et al. Deep learning-based classification of mesothelioma improves prediction of patient outcome. Nat Med. 2019;25(10):1519–25. https://doi.org/10.1038/s41591-019-0583-3.
61. Vivoda Tomšič M, Korošec P, Kovač V, Bisdas S, Šurlan PK. Dynamic contrast-enhanced MRI in malignant pleural mesothelioma: prediction of outcome based on DCE-MRI measurements in patients undergoing cytotoxic chemotherapy. BMC Cancer. 2022;22(1):191. https://doi.org/10.1186/s12885-022-09277-x.
62. Gill RR, Murphy DJ, Seethamraju RT, Mazzola E, Bueno R, Richards WG. Interobserver variability of quantitative and qualitative assessment using MRI in malignant pleural mesothelioma. Radiol Cardiothorac Imaging. 2020;2(2):e190066. https://doi.org/10.1148/ryct.2020190066.
63. De Paoli L, Quaia E, Poillucci G, Gennari A, Cova MA. Imaging characteristics of pleural tumours. Insights Imaging. 2015;6:729–40. https://doi.org/10.1007/s13244-015-0441-x.
64. Messina G, Bove M, Natale G, Di Filippo V, Opromolla G, Rainone A, et al. Diagnosis of malignant pleural disease: ultrasound as "a detective probe". Thorac Cancer. 2023;14(3):223–30. https://doi.org/10.1111/1759-7714.14735.
65. Luerken L, Thurn FL, Zeman F, Stroszczynski C, Hamer OW. Conspicuity of malignant pleural mesothelioma in contrast enhanced MDCT—arterial phase or late phase? BMC Cancer. 2021;21:1144. https://doi.org/10.1186/s12885-021-08842-0.
66. Gill RR, Gerbaudo VH, Jacobson FL, Trotman-Dickenson B, Matsuoka S, Hunsaker A, et al. MR imaging of Benign and malignant pleural disease. Magn Reson Imaging Clin N Am. 2008;16(2):319–39. https://doi.org/10.1016/j.mric.2008.03.004.
67. Patel A, Roshkovan L, McNulty S, Alley E, Torigian DA, Nachiappan AC, et al. Delayed-phase enhancement for evaluation of malignant pleural mesothelioma on computed tomography: a prospective Cohort Study. Clin Lung Cancer. 2021;22(3):210–217.e1. https://doi.org/10.1016/j.cllc.2020.06.002.
68. Tsim S, Humphreys CA, Cowell GW, Stobo DB, Noble C, Woodward R, et al. Early Contrast Enhancement: a novel magnetic resonance imaging biomarker of pleural malignancy. Lung Cancer. 2018;118:48–56. https://doi.org/10.1016/j.lungcan.2018.01.014.
69. Gill RR, Yeap BY, Bueno R, Richards WG. Quantitative clinical staging for patients with malignant pleural mesothelioma. J Natl Cancer Inst. 2017;110:258–64. https://doi.org/10.1093/jnci/djx175.
70. Kidd AC, Anderson O, Cowell GW, Weir AJ, Voisey JP, Evison M, et al. Fully automated volumetric measurement of malignant pleural mesothelioma by deep learning AI: validation and comparison with modified RECIST response criteria. Thorax. 2022;77:1251–9. https://doi.org/10.1136/thoraxjnl-2021-217808.
71. Murphy DJ, Gill RR. Volumetric assessment in malignant pleural mesothelioma. Ann Transl Med. 2017;5(11):241. https://doi.org/10.21037/atm.2017.05.23.
72. Proto C, Signorelli D, Mallone S, Prelaj A, Lo Russo G, Imbimbo M, et al. The prognostic role of TNM staging compared with tumor volume and number of pleural sites in malignant pleural mesothelioma. Clin Lung Cancer. 2019;20(6):e652–60. https://doi.org/10.1016/j.cllc.2019.06.019.
73. Chen M, Helm E, Joshi N, Gleeson F, Brady M. Computer-aided volumetric assessment of malignant pleural mesothelioma on CT using a random walk-based method. Int J Comput Assist Radiol Surg. 2017;12(4):529–38. https://doi.org/10.1007/s11548-016-1511-3.
74. Cheng L, Tunariu N, Collins DJ, Blackledge MD, Riddell AM, Leach MO, et al. Response evaluation in mesothelioma: beyond RECIST. Lung Cancer. 2015;90(3):433–41. https://doi.org/10.1016/j.lungcan.2015.08.012.
75. Frauenfelder T, Tutic M, Weder W, Gotti RP, Stahel RA, Seifert B, et al. Volumetry: an alternative to assess therapy response for malignant pleural mesothelioma? Eur Respir J. 2011;38:162–8. https://doi.org/10.1183/09031936.00146110.
76. Carter BW, Betancourt SL, Shroff GS, Lichtenberger JP 3rd. MR imaging of pleural neoplasms. Top Magn Reson Imaging. 2018;27(2):73–82. https://doi.org/10.1097/RMR.0000000000000162.
77. Gill RR, Umeoka S, Mamata H, Tilleman TR, Stanwell P, Woodhams R, et al. Diffusion-weighted MRI of malignant pleural mesothelioma: preliminary assessment of apparent diffusion coefficient in histologic subtypes. AJR Am J Roentgenol. 2010;195(2):w125–30. https://doi.org/10.2214/AJR.09.3519.
78. Coolen J, De Keyzer F, Nafteux P, De Wever W, Dooms C, Vansteenkiste J, et al. Malignant pleural mesothelioma: visual assessment by using pleural pointillism at diffusion-weighted MR imaging. Radiology. 2015;274(2):576–84. https://doi.org/10.1148/radiol.14132111.

79. Patel AM, Berger I, Wileyto EP, Khalid U, Torigian DA, Nachiappan AC, et al. The value of delayed phase enhanced imaging in malignant pleural mesothelioma. J Thorac Dis. 2017;9(8):2344–9. https://doi.org/10.21037/jtd.2017.07.86.
80. Giesel FL, Bischoff H, von Tengg-Kobligk H, Weber M-A, Zechmann CM, Kauczor H-U, et al. DynamicContrast-enhanced MRI of malignant pleural mesothelioma. Chest. 2006;129:1570–6. https://doi.org/10.1378/chest.129.6.1570.
81. Vivoda Tomšič M, Bisdas S, Kovač V, Serša I, Šurlan PK. Dynamic contrast-enhanced MRI of malignant pleural mesothelioma: a comparative study of pharmacokinetic models and correlation with mRECIST criteria. Cancer Imaging. 2019;19(1):10. https://doi.org/10.1186/s40644-019-0189-5.
82. Lee SH, Rimner A, Deasy JO, Hunt MA, Tyagi N. Dual-input tracer kinetic modeling of dynamic contrast-enhanced MRI in thoracic malignancies. J Appl Clin Med Phys. 2019;20(11):169–88. https://doi.org/10.1002/acm2.12740.
83. Kitajima K, Doi H, Kuribayashi K, Hashimoto M, Tsuchitani T, Tanooka M, et al. Prognostic value of pretreatment volume-based quantitative ^{18}F-FDG PET/CT parameters in patients with malignant pleural mesothelioma. Eur J Radiol. 2017;86:176–83. https://doi.org/10.1016/j.ejrad.2016.11.019.
84. Sexauer R, Stieltjes B, Bremerich J, D'Antonoli TA, Schmidt N. Considerations on baseline generation for imaging AI studies illustrated on the CT-based prediction of Empyema and outcome assessment. J Imaging. 2022;8(3):50. https://doi.org/10.3390/jimaging8030050.
85. Sodhi KS, Bhatia A, Nichat V, Mathew JL, Saxena AK, Samujh R, et al. Chest MRI as an emerging modality in the evaluation of empyema in children with specific indications: Pilot study. Pediatr Pulmonol. 2021;56(8):2668–75. https://doi.org/10.1002/ppul.25457.
86. Jungblut L, Abel F, Nakhostin D, Mergen V, Sartoretti T, Euler A, et al. Impact of photon counting detector CT derived virtual monoenergetic images and iodine maps on the diagnosis of pleural empyema. Diagn Interv Imaging. 2023;104(2):84–90. https://doi.org/10.1016/j.diii.2022.09.006.
87. Zettinig D, D'Antonoli TA, Wilder-Smith A, Bremerich J, Roth JA, Sexauer R. Diagnostic accuracy of imaging findings in pleural Empyema: systematic review and meta-analysis. J Imaging. 2021;8(1):3. https://doi.org/10.3390/jimaging8010003.
88. Abu AW. Solitary fibrous tumours of the pleura. Eur J Cardiothorac Surg. 2012;41(3):587–97. https://doi.org/10.1093/ejcts/ezr009.
89. Chick JF, Chauhan NR, Madan R. Solitary fibrous tumors of the thorax: nomenclature, epidemiology, radiologic and pathologic findings, differential diagnoses, and management. AJR Am J Roentgenol. 2013;200(3):W238–48. https://doi.org/10.2214/AJR.11.8430.
90. Nagata S, Nishimura H, Amrami KK, Akiba J, Tonan T, Fujimoto K, et al. The value of MRI and clinical features in differentiating between cellular and fibrous solitary fibrous Tumors. AJR Am J Roentgenol. 2017;208(1):10–7. https://doi.org/10.2214/AJR.16.16423.
91. Tateishi U, Nishihara H, Morikawa T, Miyasaka K. Solitary fibrous tumor of the pleura: MR appearance and enhancement pattern. J Comput Assist Tomogr. 2002;26(2):174–9. https://doi.org/10.1097/00004728-200203000-00002.
92. Yeom YK, Kim MY, Lee HJ, Kim SS. Solitary fibrous tumors of the pleura of the thorax: CT and FDG PET characteristics in a Tertiary Referral Center. Medicine (Baltimore). 2015;94(38):e1548. https://doi.org/10.1097/MD.0000000000001548.
93. Kim GH, Kim MY, Koo HJ, Song JS, Choi CM. Primary pulmonary synovial sarcoma in a tertiary referral center: clinical characteristics, CT, and ^{18}F-FDG PET findings, with pathologic correlations. Medicine (Baltimore). 2015;94(34):e1392. https://doi.org/10.1097/MD.0000000000001392.
94. Ginat DT, Bokhari A, Bhatt S, Dogra V. Imaging features of solitary fibrous tumors. AJR Am J Roentgenol. 2011;196(3):487–95. https://doi.org/10.2214/AJR.10.4948.
95. Tazeler Z, Tan G, Aslan A, Tan S. The utility of 18F-FDG PET/CT in solitary fibrous tumors of the pleura. Rev Esp Med Nucl Imagen Mol. 2016;35(3):165–70. https://doi.org/10.1016/j.remn.2015.10.003.
96. Zhao L, Wang H, Shi J. ^{18}F-FDG PET/CT characteristics of solitary fibrous tumour of the pleura: single institution experience. Ann Nucl Med. 2022;36(5):429–38. https://doi.org/10.1007/s12149-022-01723-x.

24 Quantitative Imaging of Mediastinal Masses

Constance de Margerie-Mellon, Caroline Caramella, Estelle Blanc-Autran, and Laetitia Vercellino

Introduction

Mediastinum is a complex anatomical area composed of various organs, vessels, nerves, and lymphatic system of the surrounding soft tissue. The mediastinum is usually divided into three compartments, anterior or prevascular, middle or visceral, and posterior or paravertebral, according to the International Thymic Malignancy Interest Group (ITMIG) classification, admitted as the most recent standard [1]. Mediastinal lesions are rare, with an estimated prevalence lower than 1% [2]. They can arise from all these compartments and organs; however most of them are located in the prevascular compartment, and thymomas, lymphomas, and benign mediastinal cysts represent the main causes [2]. There are multiple other causes of tumoral, lymphatic, congenital, or vascular origins.

Imaging plays a central role in the management of mediastinal masses, and various techniques are used [3]. Mediastinal lesions may be discovered on the frontal and/or lateral chest X-rays; however, X-ray performances for localization and characterization of mediastinal masses are very low. More advanced techniques are usually necessary, and imaging reports can rely on both qualitative and quantitative features. Chest-computed tomography is often the first-line imaging technique for mediastinal mass characterization, due to its widespread availability [4]. It allows us to determine the exact location of the mass that provides a preliminary orientation for its nature and to measure it with precision. It also offers information on the mass composition with attenuation measurements (fatty, cystic, or tissular attenuations). In recent years, CT-derived radiomics features have been also tested for tumor characterization [5]. Mediastinal MRI is usually a second-line imaging technique, when additional information is needed for adequate characterization. MRI is especially useful to identify intracellular fat in thymic hyperplasia, cystic nature of remodeled cyst, or tissular areas in mostly cystic masses [6].

C. de Margerie-Mellon (✉)
Hôpital Saint-Louis APHP, Radiology Department, Paris, France

INSERM UMR_S970, PARCC, Université Paris Cité, Paris, France
e-mail: constance.de-margerie@aphp.fr

C. Caramella
Hôpital Marie Lannelongue, Radiology Department, Le Plessis-Robinson, France
e-mail: ca.caramella@ghpsj.fr

E. Blanc-Autran
Hôpital Marie Lannelongue, Nuclear Medicine department, Le Plessis-Robinson, France

L. Vercellino
Hôpital Saint-Louis APHP, Nuclear Medicine department, Paris, France

INSERM UMR_S942, Université Paris Cité, Paris, France
e-mail: laetitia.vercellino@aphp.fr

R. Gill, P. Rajiah (eds.), *Quantitative Imaging in the Thorax*,
https://doi.org/10.1007/978-3-032-14103-3_24

MRI also offers quantitative data through diffusion-weighted (DW) sequences and can be used for staging of mediastinal neoplasms. Finally, ^{18}FDG PET/CT (abbreviated in PET/CT) is used in prognosis, staging, and/or follow-up objectives, rather than for characterization, using different PET-derived metrics, especially in lymphomas [7].

The aim of this chapter is to review the role of quantitative imaging with CT, MRI, and PET/CT for the management of mediastinal lesions, including thymic abnormalities, mediastinal lymphomas, mediastinal cysts, and other less common mediastinal masses.

Thymic Lesions

Normal Thymus

The thymus is a lymphatic organ that grows during infancy and childhood and then slowly decreases in size after puberty with a typic replacement of the soft tissue by fat. However, thymic remnants can be observed in the adult population, especially with the increase in the number of chest CT performed for any cause worldwide. A semi-quantitative scoring system has been described by Ackman et al., depending on the composition of the thymus [8] (Fig. 24.1):

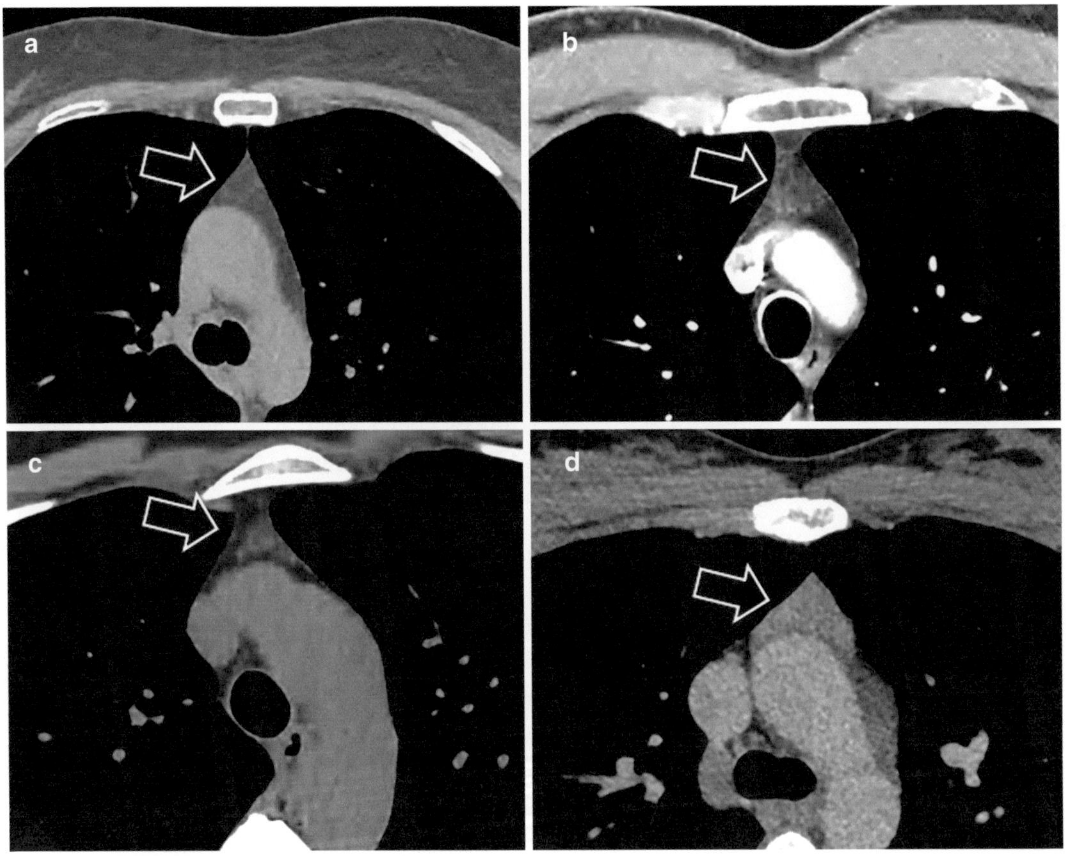

Fig. 24.1 Semi-quantitative scoring system for thymus composition. Fat content in the thymic gland (arrows) on axial CT sections using Ackman et al.'s 4-point scale scoring system. (**a**) Score 0: complete fatty replacement. (**b**) Score 1: predominantly fatty thymus. (**c**) Score 2: approximately one-half fatty and one-half soft tissue-attenuated thymus. (**d**) Score 3: predominantly soft tissue-attenuated thymus

- Score 0: complete fatty replacement
- Score 1: predominantly fatty thymus
- Score 2: approximately one-half fatty and one-half soft tissue-attenuated thymus
- Score 3: predominantly soft tissue-attenuated thymus

In an observational study of 2580 healthy participants (mean age 58.9 year olds), Araki et al. showed in 2016 that 8% of the population still exhibit a score 3 or 4 component in the thymic area, especially in never smokers and in women with lower body mass index [9]. In those cases, the size and shape of the thymus are an important information: the thickness of the thymus never exceeds 10 mm in women and 14 mm in men. In most cases, thymus had a pyramidal shape with straight or convex margins.

On PET/CT, the size and FDG uptake of the normal thymus vary with age and correlate with fatty infiltration. In case of complete fatty involution, no uptake is seen within the thymus area [10].

Thymic Hyperplasia

Histologically, two types of thymic hyperplasia are described: true thymic hyperplasia and lymphoid follicular hyperplasia. In true thymic hyperplasia, also called thymic rebound, the normal architecture of the thymus is preserved, and there is an increase in the number of both thymic epithelial cells and lymphoid germinal centers throughout the gland. This can be observed in several contexts such as steroid treatment (including inhaled steroids), chemotherapy, transplantation, or surgery. The thymus enlargement can be observed several weeks to months after the supposed causal event. In lymphoid follicular hyperplasia, there is an isolated enlargement of the lymphoid germinal centers. This can be seen in contexts such as chronic inflammatory or autoim mune disorders and is especially common in myasthenia gravis [11]. These two entities cannot be differentiated on imaging.

While CT can correctly highlight the presence of large fatty trabeculae in thymic hyperplasia, which rules out the presence of a tumor, there are still challenging cases, especially in younger patients, and the fear of missing either a thymoma or a lymphoma can remain. CT-derived radiomics features associated with clinical parameters have been used in one study to differentiate mass-like thymic hyperplasia and low-risk thymoma with promising results [12].

However, most studies have focused on MRI, as it is able to better characterize the composition of the thymus gland, especially the presence of fat, thanks to the chemical-shift sequence. Chemical-shift imaging is based on the difference in the relative precessional frequencies of water and fat protons. When comparing the in-phase and opposed-phase sequences, there is a signal intensity drop on opposed-phase images in case of tissues composed of a fat-water mixture. On the other hand, there is no signal change in case of the tissue composed solely by either water or fat [13]. The visual assessment of the loss of signal is sufficient in most cases and indicates thymic hyperplasia. However, a quantitative assessment can be used in doubtful situations. The signal intensity index (SII) is the most recommended technique. A region of interest (ROI) is drawn in the same area of the thymic tissue on both in-phase and opposed-phased sequences, and the SII is calculated from the following equation (Figs. 24.2 and 24.3):

$$\mathrm{SII} = \left[\frac{\mathrm{tSIin} - \mathrm{tSIop}}{\mathrm{tSIin}}\right] \times 100\%$$

where in = in phase, opp = opposed phase, SI = signal intensity, and t = thymus.

A cut off value of 9% is generally used for distinguishing hyperplasia from thymoma [14]. Another more complex technique has been proposed: the chemical-shift ratio (CSR), which explores the relative change in the ratio of signal intensity of the thymic tissue to that of the muscles with the following formula [15]:

$$\mathrm{CSR} = \frac{\mathrm{tSIop}/\mathrm{mSIop}}{\mathrm{tSIin}/\mathrm{mSIin}}$$

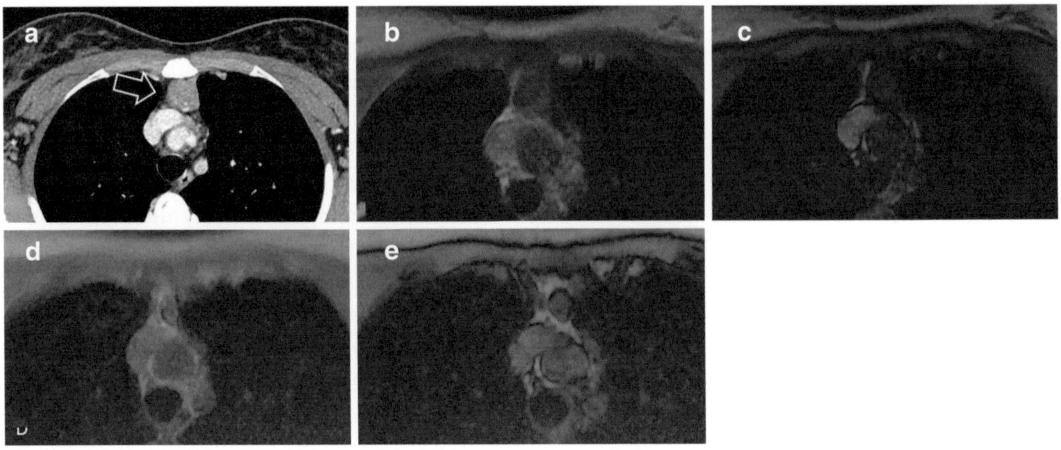

Fig. 24.2 Thymic hyperplasia as a differential diagnosis of thymoma. A 33-year-old woman with a history of hyperthyroidism. (**a**) CT, axial enhanced image: round prevascular mediastinal mass (arrow). (**b**, **c**) MR, axial T1 in-phase (**b**) and out-phase (**c**) images: subtle loss of signal within the mediastinal mass on the out-phase image (mean signal intensity measure: 255) compared to the in-phase image (mean signal intensity measure: 324). The signal intensity index was 21%, in favor of thymic hyperplasia. (**d**, **e**) MR, axial T1 in-phase (**d**) and out-phase (**e**) images 1 year later: spontaneous shrinkage of the mediastinal mass, with persistent loss of signal between (**d**) and (**e**)

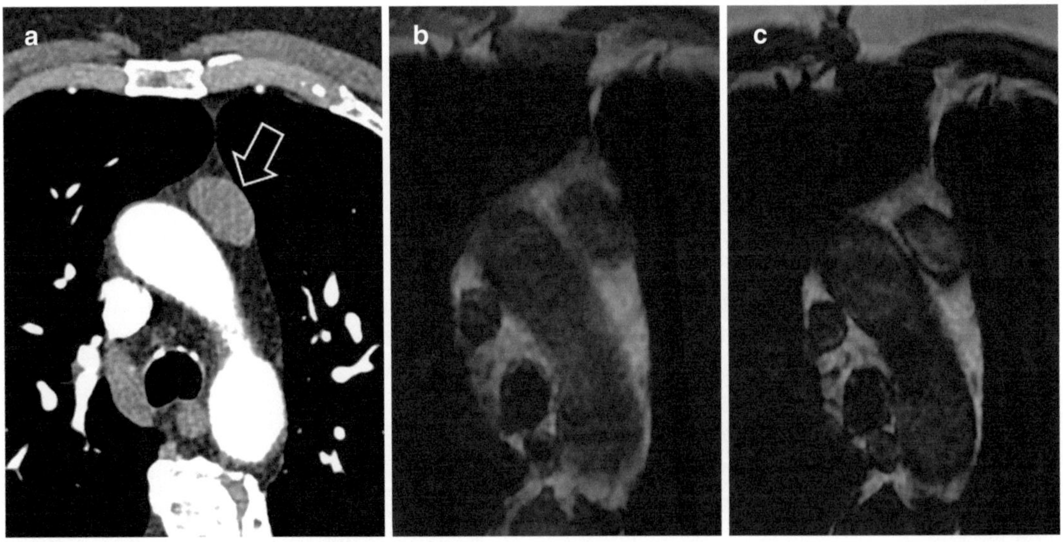

Fig. 24.3 Thymoma as a differential diagnosis of thymic hyperplasia. A 56-year-old man with a history of myasthenia gravis. (**a**) CT, axial enhanced image: round prevascular mediastinal mass (arrow). (**b**, **c**) MR, axial T1 in-phase (**b**) and out-phase (**c**) images: no loss of signal within the mediastinal mass on the out-phase image (mean signal intensity measure: 354) compared to the in-phase image (mean signal intensity measure: 377). The signal intensity index was 6%, not in favor of thymic hyperplasia. Surgery revealed thymoma type B2

where in = in phase, m = muscle, opp = opposed phase, SI = signal intensity, and t = thymus.

Used with a cut-off of 0.849, this formula does not seem to add more information than SII and may be less specific in young patients with a limited amount of intramuscular fat [16].

DW imaging is another technique that could help distinguish normal thymus from malignant lesion. Priola et al. compared in 2018 a group of

40 subjects with normal thymus and 33 patients with anterior mediastinal lymphomas of the similar ages (9–29 years old) [17]. SII on chemical-shift imaging was not able to differentiate healthy and lymphoma subjects; however, the apparent diffusion coefficient (ADC) was significantly different between both groups (mean ADC of normal thymus $2.48 \pm 0.38 \times 10^{-3}$ mm^2/s versus $1.24 \pm 0.23 \times 10^{-3}$ mm^2/s in the lymphoma group). The same study also showed that ADC of normal thymus is age dependent and increases with age.

Thymic hyperplasia can manifest with an uptake on PET/CT, which is classically diffuse, contrary to thymomas which tend to have more heterogeneous hypermetabolism (Fig. 24.4). In young patients with lymphoma, the differentiation between recurrent lymphoma and thymic hyperplasia is often challenging. Gawande et al. showed that, in a cohort of 218 pediatric oncology patients, a maximum standard uptake value (SUV_{max}) of more than 3.4 was highly predictive of lymphoma [18].

Thymomas and Thymic Carcinomas

Thymomas and thymic carcinoma are tumors arising from the epithelial cells of the thymus. They are rare tumors with a reported incidence of 1.7 per million per year in Europe [19]. They more likely occur in adult patients around 50–60 years of age. Thymic tumors are subdivided into thymomas types A, AB, B1, B2, and B3 and thymic carcinoma according to the WHO histological classification based on the morphology of the epithelial cells and the ratio of lymphocytes to epithelial cells [20]. Thymoma types A, AB, and B1 are generally considered as low-risk tumors, whereas B2 and B3 thymomas are considered as high-risk ones. The Masaoka-Koga classification is used to define the stadification of the tumor and relies on the examination of both imaging and the surgical specimen [21]. More recently, a tumor, node, and metastasis classification type of thymic neoplasms was proposed by the International Association for the Study of Lung Cancer and the ITMIG [22]. This classification is based on the retrospective analysis of a large multicenter cohort of patients and better correlates with prognosis.

Clinically, one-third of patients harboring these tumors is asymptomatic, one-third presents with symptoms related to local compression, and one-third with symptoms related to autoimmune disorders (myasthenia gravis, Good syndrome, aplasia, etc.) [19].

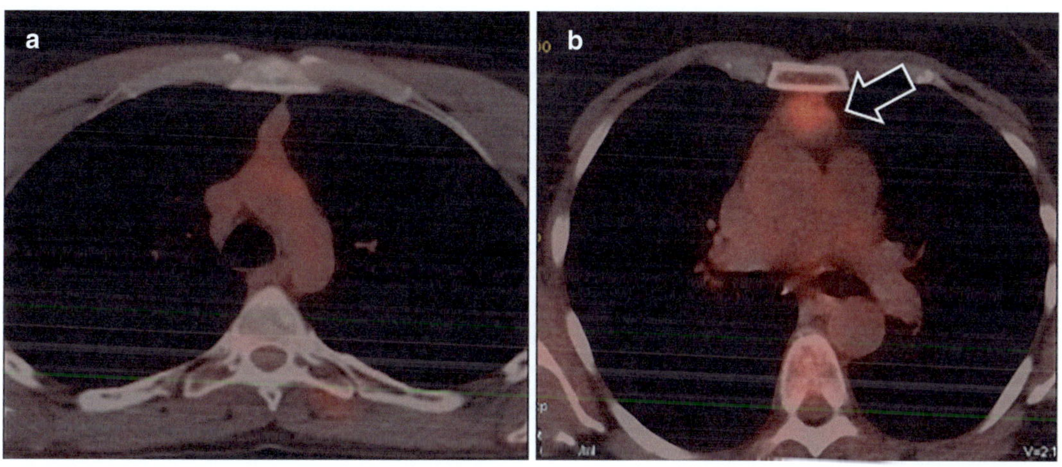

Fig. 24.4 ^{18}FDG PET/CT uptake in thymic hyperplasia. A 35-year-old man with a recent history of chemotherapy for mediastinal seminoma, end-of-treatment ^{18}FDG PET/CT (axial PET/CT-fused images (**a**) and (**b**)). Round prevascular mediastinal mass (arrow) with a homogeneous moderate uptake (SUV_{max} of 5.2). The patient underwent surgery. Histological diagnosis: thymic hyperplasia

On CT, thymomas usually appear as a round or oval mass in the prevascular compartment of the mediastinum, typically with well-defined margins and homogeneous enhancement, especially in low-grade tumors. However, it can also be heterogeneous, with cystic, necrotic, hemorrhagic areas or focal calcifications, more likely in high-risk lesions [23]. Thymomas rarely spread to the lymph node or lungs but are likely to develop pleural metastasis or pericardial invasion. Thymic carcinomas are more aggressive tumors that tend to have more irregular contours and heterogeneous enhancement and may be associated with great vessel invasion, enlarged lymph nodes, and distant lesions such as liver, lung, or bone metastases.

MRI is not always performed for thymomas and thymic carcinomas but can help in the assessment of local invasiveness. Thymomas usually appear with a low-to-intermediate signal intensity on T1-weighted imaging and a high signal intensity on T2-weighted imaging, to the muscle. A well-defined capsule and a homogeneous enhancement are more likely in low-risk thymomas than in high-risk thymomas and thymic carcinomas.

Several CT or MRI-based studies have investigated the possibility of differentiation between histological subtypes of thymic epithelial tumors with quantitative parameters (Figs. 24.5 and 24.6). Using the WHO histologic classification of thymomas in a series of 99 patients, Marom et al. showed that thymomas ≥7 cm were more likely to be of B3 WHO type [24]. Several studies used DWI to attempt a distinction between subtypes, showing lower ADC values in high-risk thymo-

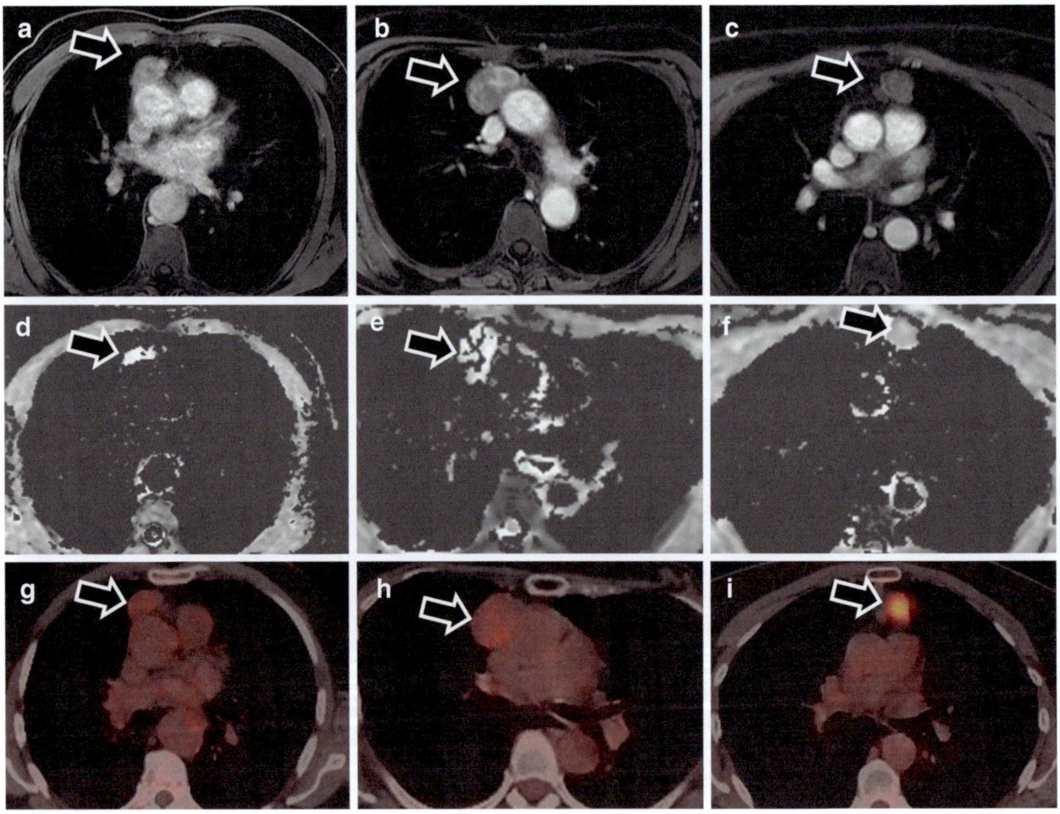

Fig. 24.5 Thymomas with decreasing apparent diffusion coefficients (ADC) and increasing SUV_{max} according to histological subtypes. (**a–c**) MRI T1-enhanced axial images. (**d–f**) MRI ADC maps. (**g–i**) ^{18}FDG PET/CT (axially fused images). (**a**, **d**, **g**) Thymoma type A (arrow). ADC was 2.8×10^{-3} mm^2/s and SUV_{max} was 2.8. (**b**, **e**, **h**) Thymoma type AB (arrow). ADC was 2.3×10^{-3} mm^2/s and SUV_{max} was 3.3. (**c**, **f**, **i**) Thymoma type B3 (arrow). ADC was 1.9×10^{-3} mm^2/s and SUV_{max} was 6.2

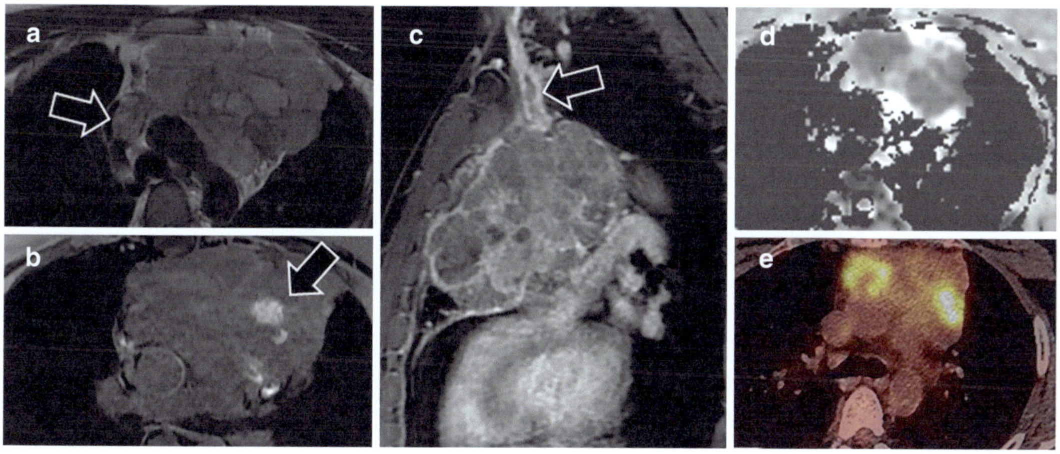

Fig. 24.6 Thymic carcinoma. (**a**) MR, axial T2 image: large hyperintense heterogeneous mass of the prevascular mediastinum, with invasion of the superior vena cava (arrow). (**b**) MR, unenhanced axial T1 image: the mass is predominantly hypointense, with spots of hyperintense corresponding to hemorrhagic changes (arrow). (**c**) MR, enhanced sagittal T1 image. Heterogeneous contrast enhancement, excellent visibility of the superior vena cava invasion (arrow). (**d**) MR, apparent diffusion coefficient map. Heterogeneous mass, with ADC values ranging from 0.8 to 2×10^{-3} mm^2/s. (**e**) Axial ^{18}FDG PET/CT-fused image. $SUV_{max} = 6.9$

mas and thymic carcinomas than in low-risk carcinomas [25–27]. Using a multiparametric model based on both DWI and dynamic contrast-enhanced MRI, Shen et al. reached an AUC of 0.925 to distinguish thymomas versus high-risk thymomas and thymic carcinomas [27]. Kong et al. used the 10th percentile of ADC, a parameter derived from the histogram analysis of ADC maps as a cut-off value to discriminate between the same two groups and obtained an AUC of 0.957 [26]. Other researchers used more advanced quantitative techniques such as texture analysis or radiomics of MRI-derived parameters and obtained AUCs over 0.87 to distinguish low-risk from high-risk tumors [28, 29].

On PET/CT, thymomas usually show an uptake which increases with the WHO classification (lower uptake in low-grade thymomas, higher uptake in thymic carcinomas), but there are large overlaps observed in the different subtypes [30, 31] (Figs. 24.5 and 24.6). Contrary to the diffuse uptake that can be observed in thymic hyperplasia, thymomas often have a heterogeneous presentation on PET imaging with areas of more intense hypermetabolism. Overall intensity does predict the prognosis, and PET/CT is also useful in the detection of distant metastasis, especially in thymic carcinomas [32].

Lymphomas

Overview

Mediastinal lymphomas account for 50–60% of mediastinal malignancies and encompass several common and uncommon histological types, such as primary B-cell lymphoma (PMBL), Hodgkin lymphoma (HL), diffuse large B-cell lymphoma (DLBCL), and mediastinal "gray-zone" lymphoma (GZL) [33, 34]. The mediastinal involvement can either be primary or secondary to a systemic disease.

MRI

Few studies have investigated the role of DWI in the context of mediastinal lymphomas. Gumustas et al. studied the differentiation between lymphoma and sarcoidosis in cases of enlarged mediastinal lymph nodes and demonstrated that an optimal ADC threshold of 1.266×10^3 mm^2/s enabled a 100% sensitivity and an 81% specificity for the differentiation between the two diseases [35]. Liao et al. studied DWI in lymphomatous nodes after chemotherapy and showed that mean ADC was lower in the nodes of patients with partial response compared to patients with complete response [36].

PET/CT

PET/CT quantitative analysis include basic quantification with SUV, volumetric indices such as total metabolic tumor volume (total MTV (TMTV), sum of all metabolically active lesions) and total lesion glycolysis (TLG, product of total MTV by the mean SUV in this volume), and more refined analyses such as radiomics (especially textural analysis). PET/CT can have a role at diagnosis, for prognosis determination, for staging, and for therapeutic response evaluation.

Diagnosis

FDG PET/CT can be useful for diagnostic purposes, for the differentiation between lymphoma and other mediastinal diseases (such as thymoma), and between lymphoma histological subtypes.

Differentiation from Thymic Epithelial Lesions

The aim of differentiating thymic epithelial lesions from primary mediastinal lymphomas is mostly to avoid unnecessary mediastinal surgeries. PET/CT metabolic parameters and radiomics feature analysis, alongside clinical and biological data, can contribute to this differential diagnosis.

Zhu et al. showed that in 136 patients SUV_{max}, SUV_{mean}, MTV, and TLG, were higher in lymphomas than in thymic epithelial tumors. Combining SUV_{max} (with a cut-off value of 12.3) and patient age (with a cut-off of 40 years old, younger age for patient with lymphoma) yielded an AUC of 0.908 [37].

Wang et al. found that in a cohort of 173 patients the best metabolic parameter was tumor-to-normal liver standard uptake value ratio, with a cut-off of 6.2. When this parameter was combined with clinical data (age and clinical symptoms), an excellent AUC of 0.964 was reached [38].

Li et al. derived from a study on 89 patients a PET/CT-based radiomics nomogram to help differentiate thymic epithelial tumors and mediastinal lymphomas, in order to avoid unnecessary surgery [39]. Beside the predictive value of LDH, patient age, $SUV_{average}$, a "rad score" based on several radiomics features could contribute to classify the patients. They thus proposed nomograms with and without rad score, with good diagnostic accuracy, the best clinical efficacy being achieved by the combined model (combination of clinical, metabolic, and radiomics data).

Differentiation Between Lymphoma Types

Abenavoli et al. performed a volumetric and textural analysis (with first- and second-order features) of bulky mediastinal masses of different histological types of lymphoma: HL, PMBL, and GZL (a rare, unclassifiable lymphoma with characteristics of both other histological types) in 117 patients [40]. SUV and TLG significantly differed across these three groups of lymphomas (with lower values for HL and higher for PMBL), and MTV was significantly higher in PMBL and GZL compared with HL. Besides, there was a significant difference between several textural features.

Prognosis

Once the accurate diagnosis of lymphoma is established, quantification can be of use for prognosis and staging values. Total MTV can be used to stratify patients for the risk of treatment failure and relapse and to tailor the therapeutic strategy.

Total MTV has been validated as a predictive and prognostic factor across many different types of lymphomas (Fig. 24.7) [41, 42]. Ceriani et al. evaluated the prognostic value of metabolic heterogeneity (MH) in 103 patients with PMBL [43]. MH was determined using the area under curve of cumulative SUV-volume histogram method. Dichotomizing MH between low and high, it was significantly associated with progression-free survival (PFS). Among different parameters including MH, MTV, TLG, international prognostic index, tumor bulk (mediastinal mass >10 cm), and age as a continuous variable, TLG and MH had statistical significance for prediction of PFS. Combining these two features identified patients at high risk for progression, leading to the possibility of risk-stratified treatments.

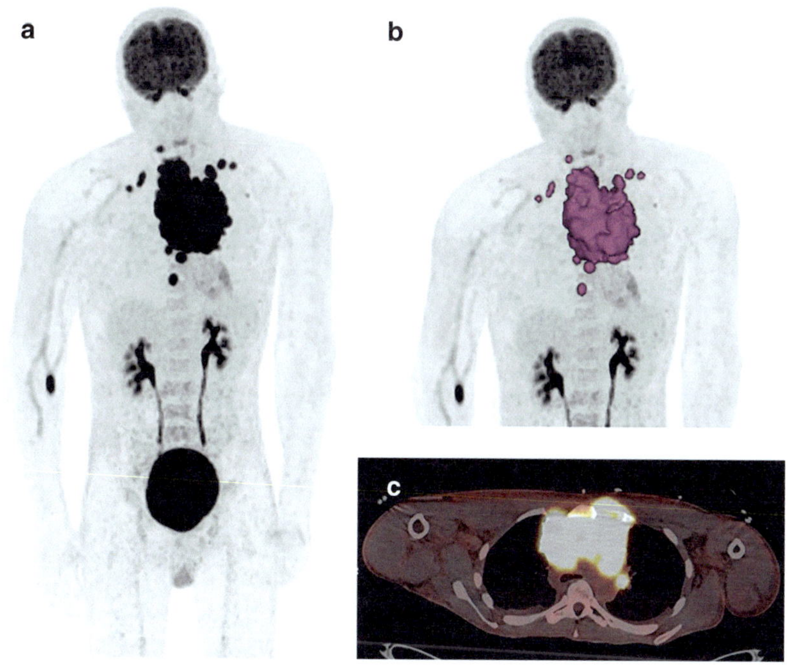

Fig. 24.7 TMTV. Primary B-cell lymphoma in a 24-year-old man. (**a**) ^{18}FDG PET maximal intensity projection. (**b**) Determination of TMTV using a fixed threshold of SUV4. (**c**) Axial PET/CT-fused image showing intensely hypermetabolic large mediastinal lesion. SUV_{max} = 31.2, TMTV (>SUV4) = 630 ml, total lesion glycolysis = 6758 g

Table 24.1 The 5-point scale or Deauville score, derived from Barrington et al. [46]

Deauville score	Visual analysis	Semi-quantitative
1	No uptake	No significant uptake
2	Uptake ≤ mediastinum uptake	Uptake < SUV_{max} of the mediastinum blood pool
3	Uptake > mediastinum uptake but ≤ liver uptake	Uptake < SUV_{max} in a large region of the normal liver
4	Uptake moderately higher than liver uptake	Uptake > SUV_{max} in a large region of the normal liver
5	Uptake markedly higher than liver uptake and/or new lesions	Uptake 2x to 3x > SUV_{max} in the liver

There are several delineation techniques, among the most common are a percentage of SUV_{max} (usually 41% of the SUV_{max} of the most intense lesion), a fixed SUVmax threshold (e.g., lesions with SUV_{max} > 4), or a region-growing automatic software. For mediastinal involvement some specific study addressed this issue. They found that the different methods yielded significant different results, but all could stratify patients according to treatment failure. However the best prediction accuracy was provided by a fixed threshold >25% SUV_{max} [44].

Therapeutic Response

In FDG-avid lymphomas, PET/CT is the gold standard for the assessment of therapeutic response. In the above-mentioned histological subtypes, it is recommended for interim and end-of-treatment evaluation [45]. The 5-point scale score (5 PS), also known as Deauville score (DS), is recommended for a standardized interpretation of PET/CT after treatment for any type of FDG-avid lymphoma, whatever the location (Table 24.1) [46]. Though this scale was initially meant to be obtained through a visual analysis, it clearly relies on semi-quantitative data, with reference to mediastinal and hepatic background [47, 48] (Fig. 24.8). In particular, Hasenclever et al. proposed a quantitative DS for HL, corresponding to the quotient of SUV_{peak} of residual tumors by the average uptake of the liver (Table 24.2).

The interpretation does not differ for mediastinal lymphomas, but this group of lymphomas

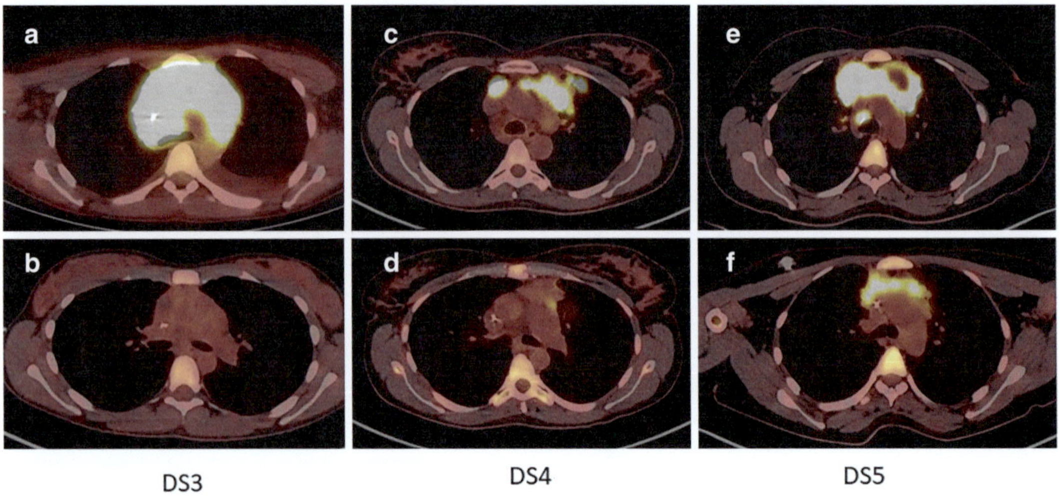

Fig. 24.8 Metabolic response with Deauville score. Examples of metabolic response on interim PET for primary B-cell lymphomas. Axial [18]FDG PET/CT-fused images. (**a**) Pre-treatment and (**b**) interim PET/CT: $SUV_{max} = 2.7$ vs 24 (hepatic $SUV_{max} = 2.8$), DS3. (**c**) Pre-treatment and (**d**) PET/CT: $SUV_{max} = 4.9$ vs 24.1 (hepatic $SUV_{max} = 2.8$), DS4, $\Delta SUV_{max} = -80\%$. (**e**) Pre-treatment and (**f**) interim PET/CT: $SUV_{max} = 12.4$ vs 24.5 (hepatic $SUV_{max} = 3.2$), DS5, $\Delta SUV_{max} = -49\%$

often present with residual masses of various sizes: metabolic response evaluation is therefore essential. DS is used for all histological subtypes, but Delta SUV_{max} (difference between initial and current SUV_{max}) has now been validated in DLBCL.

While DS1–DS3 patterns are usually considered to be consistent with complete metabolic response, the value of DS4 and DS5 patterns depends on the timepoint of PET evaluation and the comparison with baseline imaging [45]. A PET classified as DS4 or DS5 with decreased SUV_{max} compared with baseline is consistent with partial metabolic response: at interim PET it suggests responding disease, while at end of the treatment, it is associated with residual disease.

The value of the variation or SUV_{max} between baseline and interim PET/CT has been mostly studied in DLBCL [49, 50]. In several reports it seems that a Delta SUV_{max} of more than 66% after two cycles of chemotherapy and 70% after four cycles is associated with better response and outcome. The report from the GAINED study that evaluated a PET-driven strategy in 581 patients provided strong evidence that when baseline SUV_{max} was over 10, Delta SUV_{max} was a better predictor of patient outcome than DS. A radiomics study from this trial concluded that there was no added value of PET features and radiomics in this PET-driven strategy based on Delta SUV_{max} [51].

Finally, several reports proposed a combination of baseline characteristics (TMTV, TLG) and interim PET response to stratify patients for the risk of relapse. In a report by Ceriani et al. in patients with PMBL, patients with a TLG superior to the cut-off and a DS4–D5 on interim PET had a poor outcome compared with all the other groups of patients [52].

Table 24.2 Definition of qPET, from Georgi et al. [47, 48] qPET definition has been established for Hodgkin lymphoma

qDS	qPET value of the lesion with the highest residual uptake
1	0 (no uptake)
2	<0.95
3	≥0.95 but <1.30
4	≥1.30 but <2.00
4	≥2.00

Other Mediastinal Lesions

Benign Cysts

Benign cysts represent approximately 20% of mediastinal lesions and can arise from the three mediastinal compartments, with a predominance in the prevascular area [2]. The most common causes of benign cysts are pericardial cysts (in the anterior cardiophrenic angles), thymic cysts (in the prevascular compartment), bronchogenic cysts (close to the tracheobronchial tree), and duplication cysts (adjacent to the esophageal wall).

On CT, benign cysts are characterized by imperceptible or thin walls and homogeneous attenuation without contrast enhancement [53]. This homogeneous attenuation is usually that of water (between 0 and 20 HU); in that case the purely cystic nature of the lesion can be confirmed (Fig. 24.9). However, some mediastinal cysts are spontaneously hyperattenuating (because of hemorrhagic or proteinaceous contents), with attenuation measurements up to 100 HU, and/or even pseudo-enhancement due to beam-hardening artifacts from neighboring major vessels and can be misinterpreted as tissular lesions on enhanced CT images [54, 55] (Fig. 24.10). In the case of round or oval well-circumscribed mediastinal lesions with homogeneous attenuation, MR should be considered to distinguish between a cystic and a solid lesion. More specifically, the ITMIG suggested the use of MRI for work-up of suspected anterior medi-

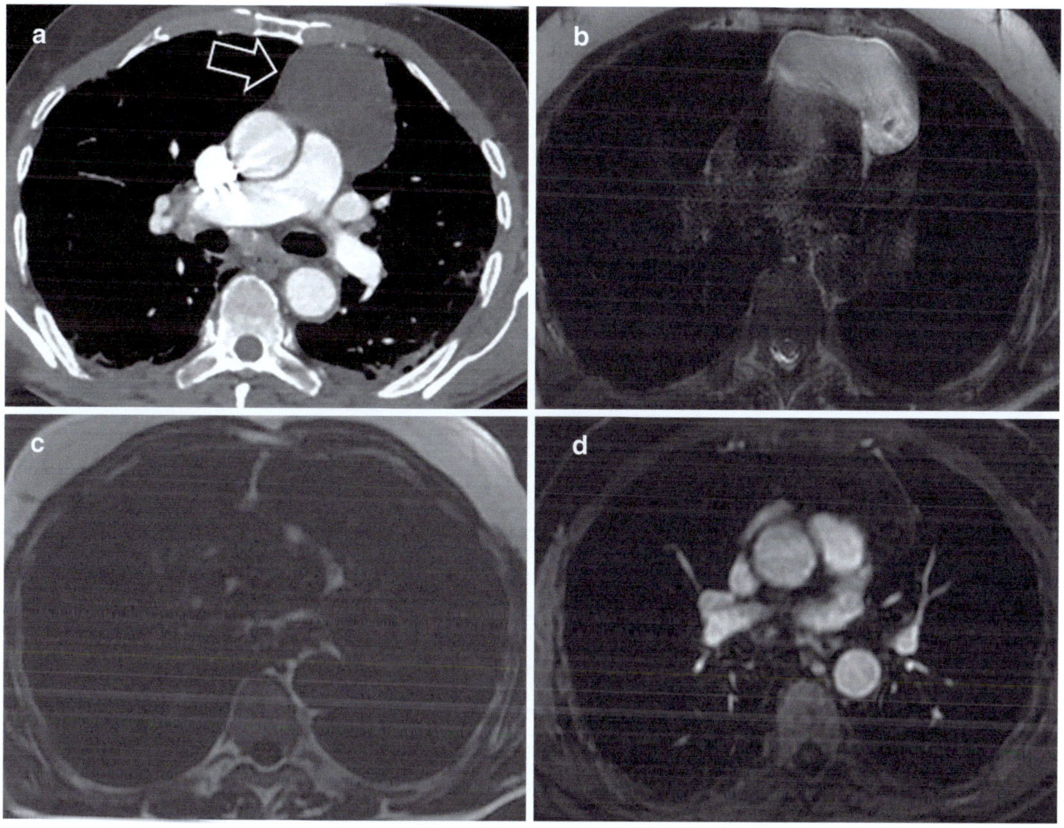

Fig. 24.9 Thymic cyst. A 54-year-old man. (**a**) CT-enhanced axial section. Round, homogeneous mass of the prevascular mediastinum (arrow). Measured attenuation: 7 HU. (**b**) MR, axial T2 image: diffuse hyperintense signal of the mass. (**c**) MR, axial unenhanced T1 image: diffuse hypointense signal of the mass. (**d**) MR, axial enhanced T1 image: no contrast enhancement of the mass

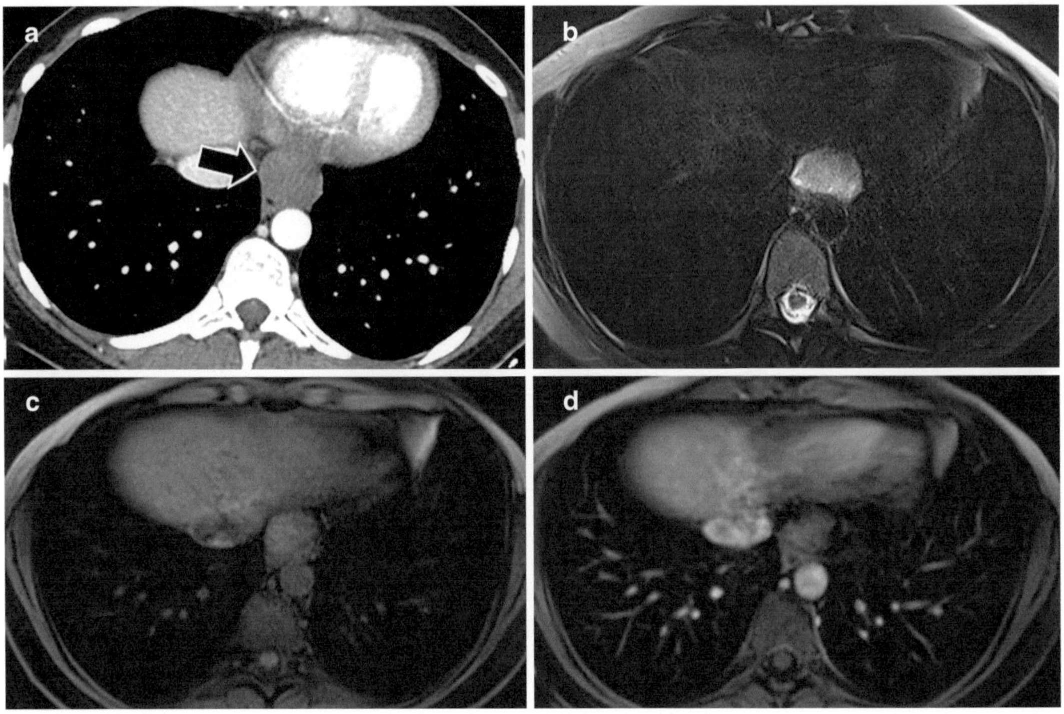

Fig. 24.10 Bronchogenic cyst. A 23-year-old woman. CT-enhanced axial section. (**a**) Round, homogeneous mass of the visceral mediastinum (arrow). Measured attenuation: 57 HU. (**b**) MR, T2 axial image. Diffuse hyperintense signal of the mass. (**c**) MR, unenhanced T1 axial image. Diffuse hyperintense signal. (**d**) MR, enhanced T1 axial image: no contrast enhancement within the mass, confirmed by subtraction images (not shown)

astinal cystic lesion because of the possible confusion between thymic cyst and cystic thymoma [56] (Fig. 24.11).

On MRI, benign cystic masses harbor various signals, depending on their content. Cysts with purely serous content show low signal intensity on T1-weighted images and high signal intensity similar to cerebrospinal fluid on T2-weighted images (Fig. 24.9). When the cyst content is proteinaceous or hemorrhagic, T1 signal is iso- or hyperintense to the muscle, and T2 signal is usually hyperintense [57]. After contrast injection, enhancement is always absent except for a possible thin rim uptake (Fig. 24.10). In some cases, authentic solid tumors can show features similar to benign cysts on morphological sequences. DW imaging offers additional information in these questionable lesions, by showing signal suppression on high-b-value images or high apparent diffusion coefficient ($>2.5 \times 10^{-3}$ mm^2/s) in benign cystic lesions, as opposed to solid lesions [58]. The combined analysis of both contrast-enhanced and DW images is recommended, especially for prevascular mediastinal masses [59] (Fig. 24.11).

Germ Cell Tumors

Germ cell tumors (GCTs) are a group of neoplasms usually arising in the testes or in the ovaries. Rarely, germ cell tumors arise outside the gonads, from primitive germ cells that have failed to migrate to the gonads [60]. The main extragonadal sites include the retroperitoneum, the anterior mediastinum, and the pineal gland. Germ cell tumors account for approximately 4% of mediastinal masses and are mainly distributed in the prevascular compartment; they mainly affect

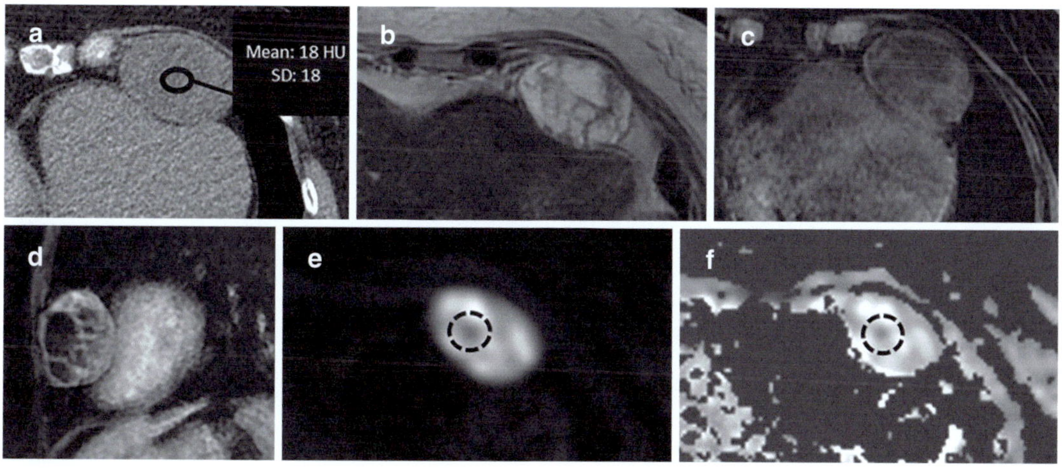

Fig. 24.11 Cystic thymoma (type A). A 68-year-old woman. (**a**) CT, axial unenhanced section: a well-defined mass with homogeneous low attenuation (mean: 18 HU) in the prevascular mediastinum. (**b**) MR, axial T2 image: presence of multiple thin inner walls within the hyper intense signal, predominantly cystic mass. (**c**) MR, axial unenhanced T1 image: predominant hypointense signal of the mass. (**d**) MR, sagittal enhanced T1 image: heterogeneous enhancement of the mass. (**d**, **e**) MR, diffusion b800 (**e**) and apparent diffusion coefficient map (**f**) images: the mass shows predominant hyperintense signal, and ADC is mainly not restricted (1.97×10^{-3} mm^2/cm), but some areas show a restriction down to 1.3×10^{-3} mm^2/cm (circle)

children and young adults [2]. Histologically, these tumors are divided into teratomas, seminomas, and nonseminomatous germ cell tumors (NSGCTs). Teratomas are further divided into mature and immature. Mature teratomas represent the most common type of mediastinal GCT. They are composed of well-differentiated tissues derived from more than one of the three embryonic germ cell layers (ectoderm, mesoderm, and endoderm).

Mature teratomas harbor various associations of soft tissue, fat, cystic, and calcium components [61]. On CT or MRI, a well-defined, round, or lobulated prevascular mass containing soft tissue, fluid, and fat attenuations (confirmed by attenuation measurements) or signal favors the diagnosis [62] (Fig. 24.12). The fat-fluid level is uncommon but highly evocative. Calcifications may also be present, and rarely, bone or tooth can be identified within the mass. Immature teratomas, seminomas, and NSGCTs are malignant GSTs that have less distinctive imaging features. They present as large prevascular lobulated masses, with soft tissue attenuation or signal and possible areas of necrosis or hemorrhage, more commonly in NSGSTs [63, 64]. Invasion of adjacent structures, lymph nodes, or distant metastases may be present.

PET/CT can be used in mediastinal GCTs in various contexts: to explore ambiguous findings identified during tumoral extension assessment on CT, to identify sites of recurrence in case of elevated circulating markers, or to predict the presence of viable tumoral tissue post-chemotherapy. More recently, some researchers showed that, based on SUV_{max}, PET/CT could discriminate between malignant and benign mediastinal GCTs (median SUV_{max} 10.3 versus 2.5) and between seminomas and NSGCTs (median SUV_{max} 6.3 versus 12.5) [65].

Other Mediastinal Lesions

The main diagnoses of other mediastinal masses include small cell carcinomas, neurogenic tumors, benign thyroid lesions, and lymphatic

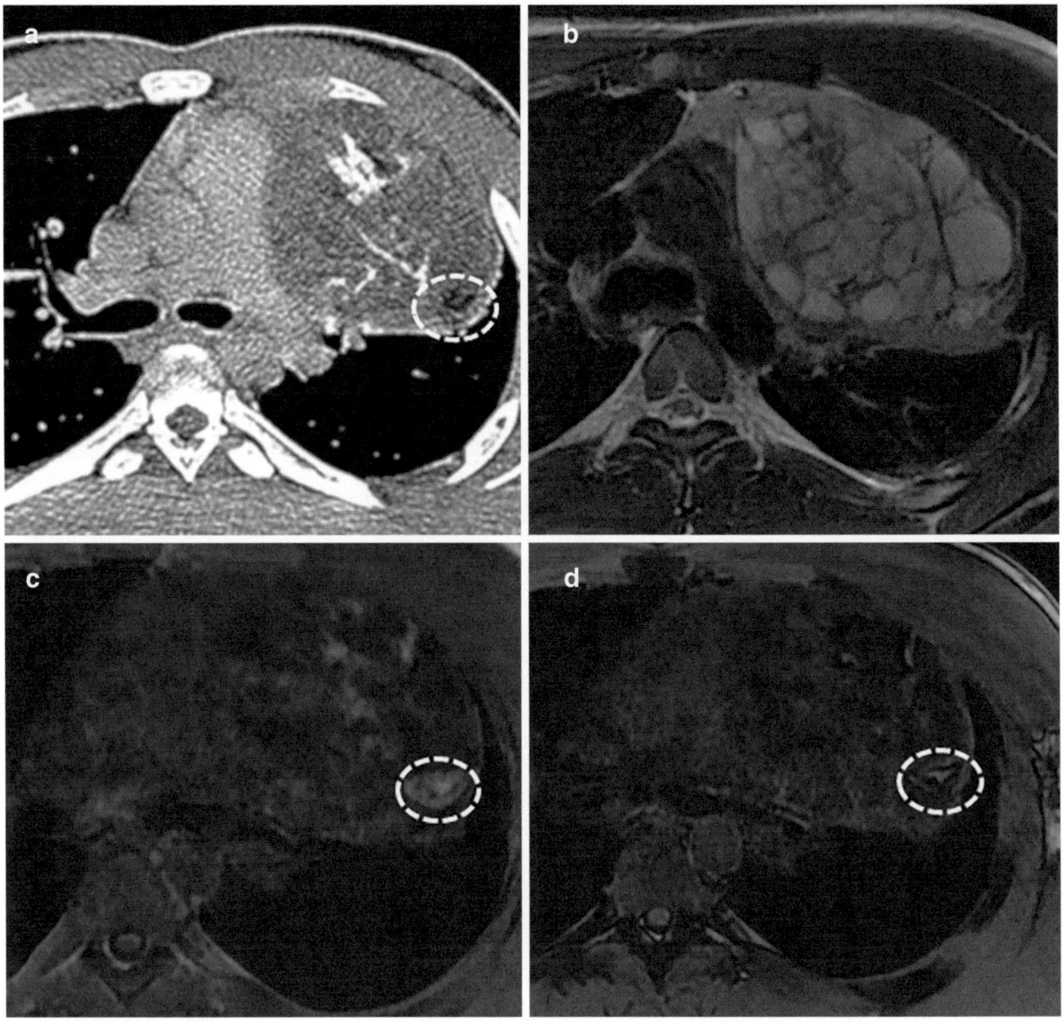

Fig. 24.12 Mature teratoma. A 17-year-old man. (**a**) CT, axial enhanced section: prevascular mediastinal mass harboring soft tissue attenuation, calcified and fatty (circle: measured attenuation of −51 HU) components. (**b**) MR, T2 axial image: hypointense signal areas with multiple inner walls within the mass. (**c**, **d**) MR, T1 in-phase (**c**) and out-phase (**d**) axial images. Loss of signal inside the fatty component identified on CT (circles)

metastasis. Each of these entities present with evocative morphological imaging features, and some of them occur in specific clinical contexts. Small cell carcinomas usually present as a large hilar or perihilar mass associated with mediastinal lymphadenopathies in patients with smoking history. Neurogenic tumors are round or elongated tumors that are mostly seen in the posterior mediastinum, in paraspinal locations. Benign thyroid lesions are usually seen in continuity of the normal thyroid gland and harbor density or signal similar to that of the gland. Lymphatic metastases often occur in the context of a previously known cancer. However, there is a very limited amount of quantitative data for these lesions.

Synthesis and Conclusion

As seen in this chapter, quantitative analysis of thoracic CT, mediastinal MRI, and PET/CT has been used in specific contexts, based on identical morphological imaging findings and/or on common histology.

The role of quantitative imaging has also been studied in broader contexts. Some MRI-based studies have investigated the role of DWI for the overall differentiation between benign and malignant mediastinal tumors [66–68]. The authors identified optimal ADC thresholds varying between 1.11 and 1.56 × 10^{-3} mm^2/s, with sensitivity and specificity ranging from 91% to 96% and from 87% to 100%, respectively. In a more specific context of mediastinal lymphadenopathies, Ramamoorthy found an optimal ADC threshold of 1.10 × 10^{-3} mm^2/s to distinguish benign and malignant causes [69]. These different thresholds can be explained by the inclusion of various tumor types in the studies and by the use of distinct technical DWI parameters and ROI positioning methods. It illustrates however the difficulty of identifying one universal threshold to perform an accurate distinction between benign and malignant lesions. Of note, Priola et al. reported that, when measuring ADC, positioning a ROI that encompasses the lesion volume is more reproducible than one small round ROI in the lesion [70].

Combining different imaging techniques is an interesting method to improve the discrimination performances. Yabuuchi et al. included dynamic contrast-enhanced MRI, diffusion-weighted MRI, and PET/CT, for the characterization of prevascular solid mediastinal masses. They showed that combining the techniques allowed to reach an accuracy of 91% to distinguish between lymphoma, germ cell tumor, and thymic epithelial tumors [71].

Overall, there are a significant number of studies dedicated to quantitative imaging of mediastinal masses, for the characterization, the follow-up, and the prognosis of mediastinal lesions. Some methods are now used in clinical routine. For instance, mediastinal MRI with the in-phase and out-phase sequences is now a widely accepted method for the identification of thymic hyperplasia, and PET/CT is recognized as essential for the prognostic assessment in mediastinal lymphoma. Other quantitative techniques, such as the use of radiomic features, or DWI or PET/CT data with predetermined thresholds to distinguish between histological subtypes, although promising, suffer from the possible overlaps between quantitative values across different tumor groups. They are also limited by the lack of external validity that limits their use in routine practice. Further research work dedicated to quantitative imaging standardization may help improve the reproducibility of such findings.

References

1. Carter BW, Tomiyama N, Bhora FY, de Christenson MLR, Nakajima J, Boiselle PM, et al. A modern definition of mediastinal compartments. J Thorac Oncol. 2014;9(9):S97–S101. https://doi.org/10.1097/jto.0000000000000292. PubMed PMID: WOS:000341688800006.
2. Roden AC, Fang W, Shen Y, Carter BW, White DB, Jenkins SM, et al. Distribution of mediastinal lesions across multi-institutional, International, Radiology Databases. J Thorac Oncol. 2020;15(4):568–79. https://doi.org/10.1016/j.jtho.2019.12.108. Epub 2019/12/25. PubMed PMID: 31870881
3. Carter BW, Benveniste MF, Madan R, Godoy MC, de Groot PM, Truong MT, et al. ITMIG classification of mediastinal compartments and multidisciplinary approach to mediastinal masses(1). Radiographics. 2017;37(2):413. https://doi.org/10.1148/rg.2017160095. PubMed PMID: WOS:000398133500004.
4. Archer JM, Ahuja J, Strange CD, Shroff GS, Gladish GW, Sabloff BS, Truong MT. Multimodality imaging of mediastinal masses and mimics. Media. 2023;7:27. https://doi.org/10.21037/med-22-53. Epub 2023/09/13. PubMed PMID: 37701642; PubMed Central PMCID: PMC10493620.
5. Zhou Z, Qu Y, Zhou Y, Wang B, Hu W, Cao Y. Development and validation of a CT-based radiomics nomogram in patients with anterior mediastinal mass: individualized options for preoperative patients. Front Oncol. 2022;12:869253. https://doi.org/10.3389/fonc.2022.869253. Epub 2022/07/26. PubMed PMID: 35875092; PubMed Central PMCID: PMC9304864.
6. Ackman JB. MR imaging of mediastinal masses. Magn Reson Imaging Clin N Am. 2015;23(2):141–64. https://doi.org/10.1016/j.mric.2015.01.002. Epub 2015/05/09. PubMed PMID: 25952512.
7. Barrington SF, Johnson PWM. (18)F-FDG PET/CT in lymphoma: has imaging-directed personalized medicine become a reality? J Nucl Med. 2017;58(10):1539–44. https://doi.org/10.2967/jnumed.116.181347. Epub 2017/08/12. PubMed

PMID: 28798034; PubMed Central PMCID: PMC5632732.
8. Ackman JB, Kovacina B, Carter BW, Wu CC, Sharma A, Shepard JA, Halpern EF. Sex difference in normal thymic appearance in adults 20-30 years of age. Radiology. 2013;268(1):245–53. https://doi.org/10.1148/radiol.13121104. Epub 2013/02/27. PubMed PMID: 23440318.
9. Araki T, Nishino M, Gao W, Dupuis J, Hunninghake GM, Murakami T, et al. Normal thymus in adults: appearance on CT and associations with age, sex, BMI and smoking. Eur Radiol. 2016;26(1):15–24. https://doi.org/10.1007/s00330-015-3796-y. Epub 2015/05/01. PubMed PMID: 25925358; PubMed Central PMCID: PMC4847950.
10. Sharma P, Singhal A, Kumar A, Bal C, Malhotra A, Kumar R. Evaluation of thymic tumors with 18F-FDG PET-CT: a pictorial review. Acta Radiologica (Stockholm, Sweden: 1987). 2013;54:14–21. https://doi.org/10.1258/ar.2012.120536.
11. Goldstein AJ, Oliva I, Honarpisheh H, Rubinowitz A. A tour of the thymus: a review of thymic lesions with radiologic and pathologic correlation. Can Assoc Radiol J. 2015;66(1):5–15. https://doi.org/10.1016/j.carj.2013.09.003. Epub 2014/04/17. PubMed PMID: 24736228.
12. Dong W, Xiong S, Wang X, Hu S, Liu Y, Liu H, et al. Development and validation of a contrast-enhanced CT-based radiomics nomogram for differentiating mass-like thymic hyperplasia and low-risk thymoma. J Cancer Res Clin Oncol. 2023;149(16):14901–10. https://doi.org/10.1007/s00432-023-05263-3. Epub 2023/08/22. PubMed PMID: 37604939.
13. Shetty AS, Sipe AL, Zulfiqar M, Tsai R, Raptis DA, Raptis CA, Bhalla S. In-phase and opposed-phase imaging: applications of chemical shift and magnetic susceptibility in the chest and abdomen. Radiographics. 2019;39(1):115–35. https://doi.org/10.1148/rg.2019180043. Epub 2018/12/15. PubMed PMID: 30547731.
14. Priola AM, Priola SM, Gned D, Giraudo MT, Fornari A, Veltri A. Comparison of CT and chemical-shift MRI for differentiating thymoma from non-thymomatous conditions in myasthenia gravis: value of qualitative and quantitative assessment. Clin Radiol. 2016;71(3):e157–69. https://doi.org/10.1016/j.crad.2015.12.009. Epub 2016/01/18. PubMed PMID: 26774127.
15. Takahashi K, Inaoka T, Murakami N, Hirota H, Iwata K, Nagasawa K, et al. Characterization of the normal and hyperplastic thymus on chemical-shift MR imaging. AJR Am J Roentgenol. 2003;180(5):1265–9. https://doi.org/10.2214/ajr.180.5.1801265. Epub 2003/04/22. PubMed PMID: 12704035.
16. Priola AM, Priola SM, Ciccone G, Evangelista A, Cataldi A, Gned D, et al. Differentiation of rebound and lymphoid thymic hyperplasia from anterior mediastinal tumors with dual-echo chemical-shift MR imaging in adulthood: reliability of the chemical-shift ratio and signal intensity index. Radiology. 2015;274(1):238–49. https://doi.org/10.1148/radiol.14132665. Epub 2014/08/12. PubMed PMID: 25105246.
17. Priola AM, Priola SM, Gned D, Giraudo MT, Veltri A. Nonsuppressing normal thymus on chemical-shift MR imaging and anterior mediastinal lymphoma: differentiation with diffusion-weighted MR imaging by using the apparent diffusion coefficient. Eur Radiol. 2018;28(4):1427–37. https://doi.org/10.1007/s00330-017-5142-z. Epub 2017/11/17. PubMed PMID: 29143106.
18. Gawande RS, Khurana A, Messing S, Zhang D, Castaneda RT, Goldsby RE, et al. Differentiation of normal thymus from anterior mediastinal lymphoma and lymphoma recurrence at pediatric PET/CT. Radiology. 2012;262(2):613–22. https://doi.org/10.1148/radiol.11110715. Epub 2011/12/14. PubMed PMID: 22157202.
19. Scorsetti M, Leo F, Trama A, D'Angelillo R, Serpico D, Macerelli M, et al. Thymoma and thymic carcinomas. Crit Rev Oncol Hematol. 2016;99:332–50. https://doi.org/10.1016/j.critrevonc.2016.01.012. Epub 2016/01/29. PubMed PMID: 26818050.
20. Marx A, Strobel P, Badve SS, Chalabreysse L, Chan JK, Chen G, et al. ITMIG consensus statement on the use of the WHO histological classification of thymoma and thymic carcinoma: refined definitions, histological criteria, and reporting. J Thorac Oncol. 2014;9(5):596–611. https://doi.org/10.1097/JTO.0000000000000154. Epub 2014/04/12. PubMed PMID: 24722150.
21. Koga K, Matsuno Y, Noguchi M, Mukai K, Asamura H, Goya T, Shimosato Y. A review of 79 thymomas: modification of staging system and reappraisal of conventional division into invasive and non-invasive thymoma. Pathol Int. 1994;44(5):359–67. https://doi.org/10.1111/j.1440-1827.1994.tb02936.x. Epub 1994/05/01. PubMed PMID: 8044305.
22. Detterbeck FC, Stratton K, Giroux D, Asamura H, Crowley J, Falkson C, et al. The IASLC/ITMIG Thymic Epithelial Tumors Staging Project: proposal for an evidence-based stage classification system for the forthcoming (8th) edition of the TNM classification of malignant tumors. J Thorac Oncol. 2014;9(9 Suppl 2):S65–72. https://doi.org/10.1097/JTO.0000000000000290. Epub 2014/11/15. PubMed PMID: 25396314.
23. Benveniste MF, Rosado-de-Christenson ML, Sabloff BS, Moran CA, Swisher SG, Marom EM. Role of imaging in the diagnosis, staging, and treatment of thymoma. Radiographics. 2011;31(7):1847–61; discussion 61-3. https://doi.org/10.1148/rg.317115505. Epub 2011/11/16. PubMed PMID: 22084174.
24. Marom EM, Milito MA, Moran CA, Liu PM, Correa AM, Kim ES, et al. Computed tomography findings predicting invasiveness of Thymoma. J Thorac Oncol. 2011;6:1274–81. https://doi.org/10.1097/JTO.0b013e31821c4203.
25. Razek A, Khairy M, Nada N. Diffusion-weighted MR imaging in Thymic epithelial tumors: correlation with

World Health Organization classification and clinical staging. Radiology. 2014;273(1):268–75. https://doi.org/10.1148/radiol.14131643. PubMed PMID: WOS:000344232100029.
26. Kong LY, Zhang W, Zhou Y, Xu H, Shi HB, Feng Q, et al. Histogram analysis of apparent diffusion coefficient maps for assessing thymic epithelial tumours: correlation with world health organization classification and clinical staging. Br J Radiol. 2018;91(1084) https://doi.org/10.1259/bjr.20170580. PubMed PMID: WOS:000432582900015.
27. Shen J, Zhang W, Zhu JJ, Xue L, Yuan M, Xu H, et al. Multiparametric magnetic resonance imaging for assessing Thymic epithelial tumors: correlation with pathological subtypes and clinical stages. J Magn Reson Imaging. 2022;56(5):1487–96. https://doi.org/10.1002/jmri.28198. PubMed PMID: WOS:000783688800001.
28. Xiao G, Hu YC, Ren JL, Qin P, Han JC, Qu XY, et al. MR imaging of thymomas: a combined radiomics nomogram to predict histologic subtypes. Eur Radiol. 2021;31(1):447–57. https://doi.org/10.1007/s00330-020-07074-3. Epub 2020/07/24. PubMed PMID: 32700020.
29. Li B, Xin YK, Xiao G, Li GF, Duan SJ, Han Y, et al. Predicting pathological subtypes and stages of thymic epithelial tumors using DWI: value of combining ADC and texture parameters. Eur Radiol. 2019;29(10):5330–40. https://doi.org/10.1007/s00330-019-06080-4. Epub 2019/03/17. PubMed PMID: 30877464.
30. Sung YM, Lee KS, Kim BT, Choi JY, Shim YM, Yi CA. 18F-FDG PET/CT of thymic epithelial tumors: usefulness for distinguishing and staging tumor subgroups. J Nucl Med. 2006;47(10):1628–34. Epub 2006/10/04. PubMed PMID: 17015898.
31. Kumar A, Regmi SK, Dutta R, Kumar R, Gupta SD, Das P, et al. Characterization of thymic masses using (18)F-FDG PET-CT. Ann Nucl Med. 2009;23(6):569–77. https://doi.org/10.1007/s12149-009-0283-z. Epub 2009/07/09. PubMed PMID: 19585212.
32. Lococo F, Chiappetta M, Triumbari EKA, Evangelista J, Congedo MT, Pizzuto DA, et al. Current roles of PET/CT in Thymic epithelial tumours: which evidences and which prospects? A pictorial review. Cancer. 2021;13(23) https://doi.org/10.3390/cancers13236091. Epub 2021/12/11. PubMed PMID. 34885200; PubMed Central PMCID: PMC8656753.
33. Pina-Oviedo S. Mediastinal lymphoproliferative disorders. Adv Anat Pathol. 2021;28(5):307–34. https://doi.org/10.1097/pap.0000000000000305. PubMed PMID: WOS:000685228100004.
34. Johnson PWM. Masses in the mediastinum: primary mediastinal lymphoma and intermediate types. Hematol Oncol. 2015;33:29–32. https://doi.org/10.1002/hon.2212. PubMed PMID: WOS:000356094300003.
35. Gümüştaş S, Inan N, Akansel G, Başyiğit I, Ciftçi E. Differentiation of lymphoma versus sarcoidosis in the setting of mediastinal-hilar lymphadenopathy: assessment with diffusion-weighted MR imaging. Sarcoidosis Vasc Diffuse Lung Dis. 2013;30(1):52–9. PubMed PMID: 24003535
36. Liao CC, Qin YY, Tang Q, Tan XH, Ke Q, Rong Y, et al. Multi-b value diffusion-weighted magnetic resonance imaging and intravoxel incoherent motion modeling: differentiation of aggressive lymphoma lesions on initial treatment and activity assessment after chemotherapy. Medicine (Baltimore). 2019;98(6):e14459. https://doi.org/10.1097/MD.0000000000014459. PubMed PMID: 30732212; PubMed Central PMCID: PMC6380798.
37. Zhu L, Li X, Wang J, Fu Q, Liu J, Ma W, et al. Value of metabolic parameters in distinguishing primary mediastinal lymphomas from thymic epithelial tumors. Cancer Biol Med. 2020;17(2):468–77. https://doi.org/10.20892/j.issn.2095-3941.2019.0428. PubMed PMID: WOS:000541560900016.
38. Wang G, Du L, Lu X, Liu J, Zhang M, Pan Y, et al. Multiparameter diagnostic model based on ¹⁸F-FDG PET and clinical characteristics can differentiate thymic epithelial tumors from thymic lymphomas. BMC Cancer. 2022;22(1) https://doi.org/10.1186/s12885-022-09988-1. PubMed PMID: WOS:000841266900001.
39. Li J, Cui N, Jiang Z, Li W, Liu W, Wang S, Wang K. Differentiating thymic epithelial tumors from mediastinal lymphomas: preoperative nomograms based on PET/CT radiomic features to minimize unnecessary anterior mediastinal surgery. J Cancer Res Clin Oncol. 2023;149(15):14101–12. https://doi.org/10.1007/s00432-023-05054-w. PubMed PMID: WOS:001044722900004.
40. Abenavoli EM, Barbetti M, Linguanti F, Mungai F, Nassi L, Puccini B, et al. Characterization of mediastinal bulky lymphomas with FDG-PET-based radiomics and machine learning techniques. Cancer. 2023;15(7) https://doi.org/10.3390/cancers15071931. PubMed PMID: WOS:000969544200001.
41. Cottereau A-S, Lanic H, Mareschal S, Meignan M, Vera P, Tilly H, et al. Molecular profile and FDG-PET/CT total metabolic tumor volume improve risk classification at diagnosis for patients with diffuse large B-cell lymphoma. Clin Cancer Res. 2016;22(15):3801–9. https://doi.org/10.1158/1078-0432.ccr-15-2825. PubMed PMID: WOS:000382265600013.
42. Cottereau A-S, Versari A, Loft A, Casasnovas O, Bellei M, Ricci R, et al. Prognostic value of baseline metabolic tumor volume in early-stage Hodgkin lymphoma in the standard arm of the H10 trial. Blood. 2018;131(13):1456–63. https://doi.org/10.1182/blood-2017-07-795476. PubMed PMID. WOS.000430687900011
43. Ceriani L, Milan L, Martelli M, Ferreri AJM, Cascione L, Zinzani PL, et al. Metabolic heterogeneity on baseline 18FDG-PET/CT scan is a predictor of outcome in primary mediastinal B-cell

lymphoma. Blood. 2018;132(2):179–86. https://doi.org/10.1182/blood-2018-01-826958. PubMed PMID: WOS:000439130200012.
44. Ceriani L, Milan L, Johnson PWM, Martelli M, Presilla S, Giovanella L, Zucca E. Baseline PET features to predict prognosis in primary mediastinal B cell lymphoma: a comparative analysis of different methods for measuring baseline metabolic tumour volume. Eur J Nucl Med Mol Imaging. 2019;46(6):1334–44. https://doi.org/10.1007/s00259-019-04286-8. PubMed PMID: WOS:000466188800018.
45. Cheson BD, Fisher RI, Barrington SF, Cavalli F, Schwartz LH, Zucca E, Lister TA. Recommendations for initial evaluation, staging, and response assessment of Hodgkin and non-Hodgkin lymphoma: the Lugano classification. J Clin Oncol. 2014;32(27):3059. https://doi.org/10.1200/jco.2013.54.8800. PubMed PMID: WOS:000342062200020.
46. Barrington SF, Mikhaeel NG, Kostakoglu L, Meignan M, Hutchings M, Mueeller SP, et al. Role of imaging in the staging and response assessment of lymphoma: consensus of the international conference on Malignant Lymphomas Imaging Working Group. J Clin Oncol. 2014;32(27):3048. https://doi.org/10.1200/jco.2013.53.5229. PubMed PMID: WOS:000342062200019.
47. Georgi TW, Kurch L, Hasenclever D, Warbey VS, Pike L, Radford J, et al. Quantitative assessment of interim PET in Hodgkin lymphoma: an evaluation of the qPET method in adult patients in the RAPID trial. PLoS One. 2020;15(4) https://doi.org/10.1371/journal.pone.0231027. PubMed PMID: WOS:000535945000082.
48. Hasenclever D, Kurch L, Mauz-Koerholz C, Elsner A, Georgi T, Wallace H, et al. qPET - a quantitative extension of the Deauville scale to assess response in interim FDG-PET scans in lymphoma. Eur J Nucl Med Mol Imaging. 2014;41(7):1301–8. https://doi.org/10.1007/s00259-014-2715-9. PubMed PMID: WOS:000337286200005.
49. Lin C, Itti E, Haioun C, Petegnief Y, Luciani A, Dupuis J, et al. Early ¹⁸F-FDG PET for prediction of prognosis in patients with diffuse large B-cell lymphoma:: SUV-based assessment versus visual analysis. J Nucl Med. 2007;48(10):1626–32. https://doi.org/10.2967/jnumed.107.042093. PubMed PMID: WOS:000252894800032.
50. Itti E, Blanc-Durand P, Berriolo-Riedinger A, Kanoun S, Kraeber-Bodéré F, Meignan M, et al. Validation of the ΔSUV. J Nucl Med. 2023;64(11):1706–11. https://doi.org/10.2967/jnumed.123.265871. Epub 20230921. PubMed PMID: 37734837.
51. Carlier T, Frécon G, Mateus D, Rizkallah M, Kraeber-Bodéré F, Kanoun S, et al. Prognostic value of. J Nucl Med. 2023; https://doi.org/10.2967/jnumed.123.265872. Epub 20231109. PubMed PMID: 37945379.
52. Ceriani L, Martelli M, Conconi A, Zinzani PL, Ferreri AJM, Botto B, et al. Prognostic models for primary mediastinal (thymic) B-cell lymphoma derived from 18-FDG PET/CT quantitative parameters in the International Extranodal Lymphoma Study Group (IELSG) 26 study. Br J Haematol. 2017;178(4):588–91. https://doi.org/10.1111/bjh.14728. PubMed PMID: WOS:000406911500012.
53. Jeung MY, Gasser B, Gangi A, Bogorin A, Charneau D, Wihlm JM, et al. Imaging of cystic masses of the mediastinum. Radiographics. 2002;22:Spec No:S79-93. https://doi.org/10.1148/radiographics.22.suppl_1.g02oc09s79. Epub 2002/10/12. PubMed PMID: 12376602.
54. Ackman JB, Verzosa S, Kovach AE, Louissaint A Jr, Lanuti M, Wright CD, et al. High rate of unnecessary thymectomy and its cause. Can computed tomography distinguish thymoma, lymphoma, thymic hyperplasia, and thymic cysts? Eur J Radiol. 2015;84(3):524–33. https://doi.org/10.1016/j.ejrad.2014.11.042. Epub 2015/01/13. PubMed PMID: 25575742.
55. Lee SH, Yoon SH, Nam JG, Kim HJ, Ahn SY, Kim HK, et al. Distinguishing between Thymic epithelial tumors and benign cysts via computed tomography. Korean J Radiol. 2019;20(4):671–82. https://doi.org/10.3348/kjr.2018.0400. Epub 2019/03/20. PubMed PMID: 30887749; PubMed Central PMCID: PMC6424822.
56. Carter BW, Okumura M, Detterbeck FC, Marom EM. Approaching the patient with an anterior mediastinal mass: a guide for radiologists. J Thorac Oncol. 2014;9(9):S110–S8. https://doi.org/10.1097/jto.0000000000000295. PubMed PMID: WOS:000341688800008.
57. Madan R, Ratanaprasatporn L, Ratanaprasatporn L, Carter BW, Ackman JB. Cystic mediastinal masses and the role of MRI. Clin Imaging. 2018;50:68–77. https://doi.org/10.1016/j.clinimag.2017.12.011. Epub 2018/01/13. PubMed PMID: 29324329.
58. Shin KE, Yi CA, Kim TS, Lee HY, Choi YS, Kim HK, Kim J. Diffusion-weighted MRI for distinguishing non-neoplastic cysts from solid masses in the mediastinum: problem-solving in mediastinal masses of indeterminate internal characteristics on CT. Eur Radiol. 2014;24(3):677–84. https://doi.org/10.1007/s00330-013-3054-0. Epub 2013/11/02. PubMed PMID: 24177751.
59. Kim JH, Choe J, Kim HK, Lee HY. MRI-based stepwise approach to anterior mediastinal cystic lesions for diagnosis and further management. Korean J Radiol. 2023;24(1):62–78. https://doi.org/10.3348/kjr.2022.0606. Epub 2023/01/07. PubMed PMID: 36606621; PubMed Central PMCID: PMC9830146.
60. Rosti G, Secondino S, Necchi A, Fornarini G, Pedrazzoli P. Primary mediastinal germ cell tumors. Semin Oncol. 2019;46(2):107–11. https://doi.org/10.1053/j.seminoncol.2019.04.001. Epub 2019/05/12. PubMed PMID: 31076171.
61. Moeller KH, Rosado-de-Christenson ML, Templeton PA. Mediastinal mature teratoma: imaging features. AJR Am J Roentgenol. 1997;169(4):985–90. https://

doi.org/10.2214/ajr.169.4.9308448. Epub 1997/10/06. PubMed PMID: 9308448.
62. Drevelegas A, Palladas P, Scordalaki A. Mediastinal germ cell tumors: a radiologic-pathologic review. Eur Radiol. 2001;11(10):1925–32. https://doi.org/10.1007/s003300000725. Epub 2001/11/10. PubMed PMID: 11702124.
63. Tian L, Liu LZ, Cui CY, Zhang WD, Kuang YL. CT findings of primary non-teratomatous germ cell tumors of the mediastinum—a report of 15 cases. Eur J Radiol. 2012;81(5):1057–61. https://doi.org/10.1016/j.ejrad.2011.02.005. Epub 2011/03/01. PubMed PMID: 21353416.
64. De Giorgi U, Pupi A, Fiorentini G, Rosti G, Marangolo M. FDG-PET in the management of germ cell tumor. Ann Oncol. 2005;16 Suppl 4:iv90–4. https://doi.org/10.1093/annonc/mdi915. Epub 2005/06/01. PubMed PMID: 15923438.
65. Lee K, Kim YI, Oh JS, Seo SY, Yun JK, Lee GD, et al. [(18)F]fluorodeoxyglucose positron emission tomography/computed tomography characteristics of primary mediastinal germ cell tumors. Sci Rep. 2023;13(1):17619. https://doi.org/10.1038/s41598-023-44913-x. Epub 2023/10/18. PubMed PMID: 37848723; PubMed Central PMCID: PMC10582033.
66. Thuy TTM, Trang NTH, Vy TT, Duc VT, Nam NH, Chien PC, et al. Role of diffusion-weighted MRI in differentiation between benign and malignant anterior mediastinal masses. Front Oncol. 2022;12:985735. https://doi.org/10.3389/fonc.2022.985735. Epub 2022/11/01. PubMed PMID: 36313699; PubMed Central PMCID: PMC9606681.
67. Gumustas S, Inan N, Sarisoy HT, Anik Y, Arslan A, Ciftci E, et al. Malignant versus benign mediastinal lesions: quantitative assessment with diffusion weighted MR imaging. Eur Radiol. 2011;21(11):2255–60. https://doi.org/10.1007/s00330-011-2180-9. Epub 2011/06/24. PubMed PMID: 21698463.
68. Razek AA, Elmorsy A, Elshafey M, Elhadedy T, Hamza O. Assessment of mediastinal tumors with diffusion-weighted single-shot echo-planar MRI. J Magn Reson Imaging. 2009;30(3):535–40. https://doi.org/10.1002/jmri.21871. PubMed PMID: 19630080.
69. Ramamoorthy E, Garg M, Singh P, Aggarwal AN, Gupta N. Role of diffusion-weighted magnetic resonance imaging for characterization of mediastinal lymphadenopathy. Diagnostics (Basel). 2023;13(4) https://doi.org/10.3390/diagnostics13040706. Epub 20230213. PubMed PMID: 36832194; PubMed Central PMCID: PMC9955495.
70. Priola AM, Priola SM, Parlatano D, Gned D, Giraudo MT, Giardino R, et al. Apparent diffusion coefficient measurements in diffusion-weighted magnetic resonance imaging of the anterior mediastinum: inter-observer reproducibility of five different methods of region-of-interest positioning. Eur Radiol. 2017;27(4):1386–94. https://doi.org/10.1007/s00330-016-4527-8. Epub 2016/08/16. PubMed PMID: 27516357.
71. Yabuuchi H, Matsuo Y, Abe K, Baba S, Sunami S, Kamitani T, et al. Anterior mediastinal solid tumours in adults: characterisation using dynamic contrast-enhanced MRI, diffusion-weighted MRI, and FDG-PET/CT. Clin Radiol. 2015;70(11):1289–98. https://doi.org/10.1016/j.crad.2015.07.004. Epub 2015/08/15. PubMed PMID: 26272529.

25 Quantitative Thoracic Imaging with Nuclear Medicine

Merissa N. Zeman, Benjamin Auer, Sedra Mohammadi, Fangchao Jiang, Neha Kwatra, and Thomas S. C. Ng

Nuclear medicine has played a pivotal role in the evaluation of the thorax for decades. Recent advances in nuclear medicine and molecular imaging now provide a comprehensive toolbox to characterize oncologic and nononcologic thoracic conditions. The availability of novel imaging systems, coupled with novel targeted molecular imaging agents, enables quantitative evaluation of disease and monitoring of therapeutic response. Moreover, the emergence of the theranostics paradigm presents a unique opportunity for targeted image-guided systemic radiotherapy. Herein, we provide an overview of nuclear medical applications for extracardiac thoracic imaging and therapy. Nuclear cardiology is an extensive and specialized discipline in its

M. N. Zeman
Division of Nuclear Medicine and Molecular Imaging, Department of Radiology, Massachusetts General Hospital, Harvard Medical School, Boston, MA, USA

Joint Program in Nuclear Medicine, Department of Radiology, Brigham and Women's Hospital, Harvard Medical School, Boston, MA, USA
e-mail: mzeman@bwh.harvard.edu

B. Auer
Joint Program in Nuclear Medicine, Department of Radiology, Brigham and Women's Hospital, Harvard Medical School, Boston, MA, USA
e-mail: bauer@bwh.harvard.edu

S. Mohammadi
Division of Nuclear Medicine and Molecular Imaging, Department of Radiology, Massachusetts General Hospital, Harvard Medical School, Boston, MA, USA
e-mail: smohammadi4@mgh.harvard.edu

F. Jiang
Center for Systems Biology, Massachusetts General Hospital, Harvard Medical School, Boston, MA, USA
e-mail: fjiang4@mgh.harvard.edu

N. Kwatra
Joint Program in Nuclear Medicine, Department of Radiology, Brigham and Women's Hospital, Harvard Medical School, Boston, MA, USA

Division of Nuclear Medicine and Molecular Imaging, Department of Radiology, Boston Children's Hospital, Harvard Medical School, Boston, MA, USA
e-mail: Neha.Kwatra@childrens.harvard.edu

T. S. C. Ng (✉)
Division of Nuclear Medicine and Molecular Imaging, Department of Radiology, Massachusetts General Hospital, Harvard Medical School, Boston, MA, USA

Joint Program in Nuclear Medicine, Department of Radiology, Brigham and Women's Hospital, Harvard Medical School, Boston, MA, USA

Center for Systems Biology, Massachusetts General Hospital, Harvard Medical School, Boston, MA, USA
e-mail: scng@mgb.org

R. Gill, P. Rajiah (eds.), *Quantitative Imaging in the Thorax*,
https://doi.org/10.1007/978-3-032-14103-3_25

own right—the reader is referred to the accompanying chapter on this topic and several excellent texts examining this field [109, 165].

In this chapter, we first review the imaging modalities and physical principles pertinent to quantitative nuclear medicine of the thorax. We then describe the current nononcologic and oncologic applications of nuclear medicine for thoracic imaging. Finally, novel nuclear medicine techniques with the potential to revolutionize noninvasive assessment of the chest will be discussed.

Physics of Quantitative Thoracic Imaging

Introduction to Nuclear Medicine Physics

Nuclear medicine imaging aims to estimate the in vivo distribution of a radiotracer by detecting gamma rays emerging from the patient using external detectors. Radiotracers can act as markers for a great variety of substances that are of physiological importance in health and disease. The radiotracers (i.e., imaging agents) consist of two parts: the radioactive element that emits the actual radiation and the pharmaceutical compound that probes the biological behavior in vivo. The radioisotopes used in nuclear medicine imaging directly or indirectly emit gamma rays that can be detected outside the patient. Gamma and X-rays share similar basic properties but differ in origin. X-rays originate from the atomic cloud of the atom, whereas gamma rays are generated from nucleus decay. Photons are particles of choice for imaging, as these can emerge from the patient without being absorbed.

The radionuclides used in nuclear medicine have an unstable nucleus and release excess energy by emitting one or more particles to become more stable, thus reaching a lower energy state. Radioactivity describes the rate at which radionuclides decay and emit radiation. It measures the number of radioactive decays occurring per unit time. The international unit of radioactivity is the becquerel and reflects 1 disintegration (i.e., one or more particle emissions) per second. In North America, the curie unit system is still used mainly for historical and practical reasons.

Radioactivity in curie can be easily converted to becquerel via the following:

$$1\,\text{millicurie}\left(\text{mCi} = 10^{-3}\,\text{Ci}\right)\text{equals}\,37\,\text{megabecquerel}\left(\text{MBq} = 10^{6}\,\text{Bq}\right).$$

Radioactivity administered for diagnostic imaging falls within tens of millicuries (mCi) or hundreds of megabecquerel (MBq). Radioactive decay can be characterized by the physical half-life, which represents the period of time over which half of the radionuclides in the sample have disintegrated. It is unique for each radionuclide isotope. Thus, if the original activity of the sample and the half-life are known, the number of radionuclides remaining in the sample at any time can be determined.

The radionuclides used for imaging should provide useful clinical information while exposing the patient to a minimal radiation dose. Ideally, the radionuclides should be pure direct or indirect gamma-ray emitters without alpha or electron emissions to minimize patient radiation exposure.

There exist multiple modes of radioactive decay. Nuclear medicine uses radionuclides that decay via positron emission for positron emission tomography (PET) and direct gamma-ray emission for planar imaging and single-photon computed tomography (SPECT). For a given radionuclide, decay schemes and emission characteristics can be found on the International Atomic Energy Agency (IAEA) website (https://www-nds.

iaea.org/relnsd/vcharthtml/VChartHTML.html). For example, ^{177}Lu decays with a 6.6-day half-life by emitting electrons via β^- (beta minus) decay in addition to low-energy gamma rays of 113 keV (6%-abundant[1]) and 208 keV (10%-abundant). During β^- decay, a neutron is transformed into a proton and an electron plus an antineutrino that does not interact with matter. Electrons are charged particles that can travel only a very short distance in tissues depending on their energies before being absorbed and are therefore unsuited for imaging but remain of great interest for targeted radionuclide therapy (TRT). ^{177}Lu is a radionuclide of choice for TRT as it can be used for both therapy and diagnostic imaging (i.e., theranostic), where the electrons are used for treating neuroendocrine or prostate cancers, for example, while the gamma rays can be used for imaging to monitor the course of the treatment [62, 96]. The clinical application of ^{177}Lu-labeled radiotracers in the context of thoracic imaging is discussed later in this chapter. ^{99m}Tc is the most used radionuclide in clinical planar and SPECT gamma-ray imaging, such as lung perfusion and ventilation, and thoracic infection and inflammation studies. ^{99m}Tc decays with a 6-h half-life by isomeric transition of a nucleus in an excited state, resulting in the emission of 89%-abundant gamma rays of 140.5 keV. The term "m" added to the mass number indicates a metastable state where the excited state of the nucleus exists for a measurable time. This form of radioactive decay is ideal because only gamma rays are emitted, thus allowing minimal radiation dose to the patient.

Positron emitter radionuclides used in PET imaging have a neutron-deficient nucleus. The excess proton is converted via β^+ decay into a neutron plus a positron, which is the antiparticle of an electron (i.e., same basic properties but opposite charge) and a neutrino. The positron can travel only a short distance into tissue depending on its energy before it combines with an electron. The electron–positron pair annihilates, and their mass is converted into two 511-keV gamma rays emitted about 180 degrees apart. PET imaging relies on detecting these annihilation gamma rays in coincidence using short timing windows, which is discussed below. Radionuclides used in PET imaging can replace natural atoms entering the human body composition, such as carbon, nitrogen, and oxygen, to track various biological functions. ^{18}F is by far the most used radionuclide in PET imaging, for example, in oncologic studies where it acts as a marker of glucose metabolism when incorporated into the fluorodeoxyglucose (FDG). Other positron emitter radionuclides are commonly used in PET, including ^{15}O, ^{11}C, ^{13}N, and ^{68}Ga. The half-lives of radionuclides used in planar and SPECT imaging are longer (hours-days) than the ones used in PET imaging (minutes-hours). For example, ^{18}F, ^{11}C, ^{15}O, ^{13}N, and ^{68}Ga have a half-life of 110, 20, 2, 10, and 68 min, respectively. These radionuclides have a positron decay abundance of nearly 100%, except for ^{68}Ga (88%), making them particularly attractive for imaging.

The radionuclides used in diagnostic and therapeutic nuclear medicine are all artificially produced, using nuclear reactors, cyclotrons, or generators. Nuclear reactors are used to produce radionuclides with an excess of neutrons, which will decay via electron capture or β^- decay, whereas a cyclotron will generate positron emitter radionuclides used for PET imaging. ^{99m}Tc is produced on-site in a generator from long-lived radionuclide (^{99}Mo, 66 hrs half-life) decay. Following production, radionuclides are attached to vector molecules to form radiotracers, which are then administered to patients via injection, oral administration, or inhalation, depending on the specific procedure. The radiotracer circulates within the body and accumulates in the target structures or organs of interest. Gamma rays emitted by the radiotracer are detected externally using specialized instruments to track various physiological functions. Planar, SPECT, and PET imaging are discussed below. For further reading, we recommend the following recent books for a basic (see [68]) and a more comprehensive [261–263] overview of nuclear medicine physics.

[1] Branching ratio or abundance refers to the fractional yield of a particular radiation emitted during decay.

Planar and Tomographic Gamma Imaging

Physics

Two-dimensional planar imaging and three-dimensional SPECT are based on detecting gamma rays with certain energy emitted from the patient via radionuclide decays (Fig. 25.1). The gamma rays are emitted isotopically (i.e., equally in all directions) and can come from any location in the patient. Unlike X-ray computed tomography (CT), the gamma-ray emission locations are unknown. The fundamental concept of planar and SPECT imaging relies on estimating these locations. To establish a spatial correlation between source and detection locations, a collimator, consisting of a highly dense material, is used. It acts similarly to an optical lens, with the principal aim of stopping undesired photons. The detector behind the collimator consists generally of a scintillator, photomultiplier tubes, and processing electronics. The detection is most commonly done in two parts. The scintillator will emit light pulses in response to the energy deposited by the gamma rays accepted by the collimator. The photomultiplier tubes (PMTs) will convert the light into an amplified electrical signal, which will be processed, and the position of interactions within the scintillator determined.

The accumulation of these measurements forms a projection or planar view, which represents the superimposition of radioactivity through the patient defined by the detection geometry for the gamma camera being placed at a given angle around the patient. SPECT relies on acquiring multiple planar views by rotating the gamma cameras around the patient to estimate the three-dimensional biodistribution of the radiotracer. For thoracic imaging, the projections are acquired over 360 degrees in small angular increments (5.6 degrees typically). These sets of planar views will be used in a reconstruction algorithm to estimate the three-dimensional (3D) radiotracer distribution.

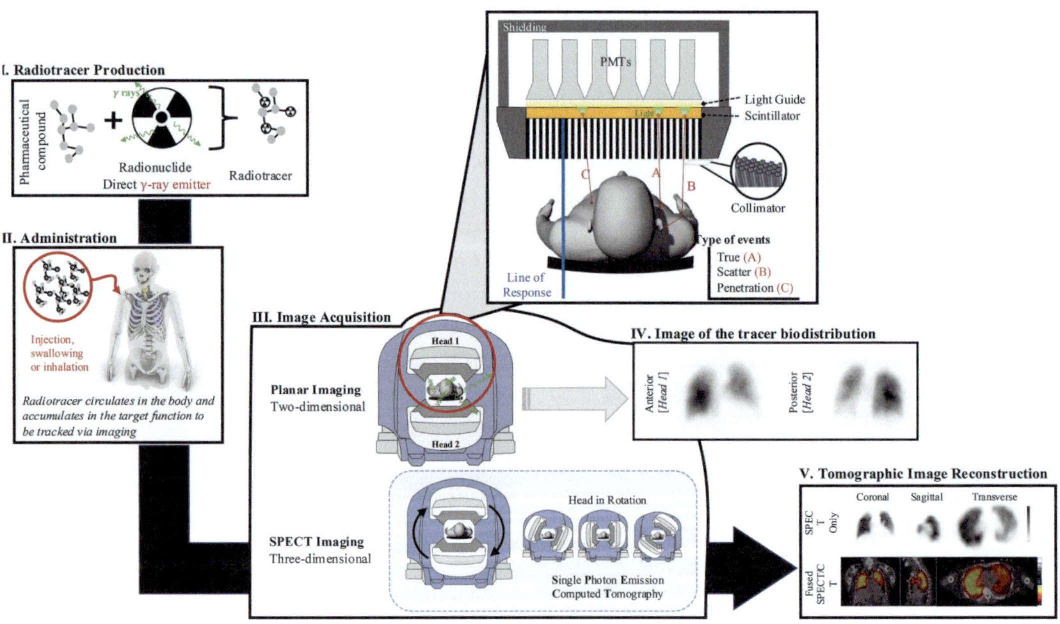

Fig. 25.1 Overview of planar and single-photon emission computed tomography (SPECT) imaging. This consists of (I) radiotracer production and (II) administration, followed by (III) image acquisition when the radiotracer has accumulated in the structure of interest(s). On the top right, the types of events and the different units of a conventional SPECT head are illustrated. (I) Planar imaging does not require data reconstruction. By contrast, (V) reconstructed SPECT provides an image reflecting the 3D distribution of the radiotracer

The collimator rejects many gamma rays with inadequate characteristics; thus, the number of counts available to estimate the radiotracer biodistribution remains limited. Furthermore, radionuclides will decay, which will even further decrease the signal available (i.e., gamma rays) for imaging over time with a rate characterized by its specific half-life. Therefore, the detection rate remains low, and planar and SPECT imaging can require a long acquisition time to achieve adequate image quality. In addition, as radioactive decay is a random process, the number of gamma rays contributing to any image region fluctuates, introducing statistical noise into the image. Image statistical noise and overall quality can be improved by collecting more gamma rays. This can be achieved by increasing the duration of the image acquisition or the administrated activity, or both. However, in practice, acquisition duration cannot be too long to limit patient discomfort, resource utilization, and financial considerations. The administrated activity is limited as well to minimize patient radiation exposure. There is thus always in every planar and SPECT imaging study a trade-off between acquisition time, administrated activity, patient comfort, and image quality, which needs to be suited for adequate diagnosis. The sensitivity, which refers to the system's capability to detect the gamma rays efficiently, should be as high as possible to reduce the statistical noise in the image for a given acquisition time.

A single set of planar views at a unique angular position can be completed relatively quickly, typically within minutes. A whole-body planar scan with multiple bed positions takes longer, often exceeding 30 min, depending on the collimator and radiotracer used. A single-bed position SPECT study requires the acquisition of multiple views and image processing and reconstruction, resulting in a total time of 10–30 min to complete the procedure. For further reading, we refer to the following review article (see [175]) describing the origins of gamma-ray imaging and the following books (see [261–263]).

Instrumentation

SPECT systems, capable of planar and tomographic imaging, generally consist of two cameras mounted on a rotating gantry. Each camera relies on the collimator, the detector, and the processing electronics. The collimator forms the image and acts as a lens. The detector detects gamma rays and consists most commonly of a continuous inorganic scintillation crystal, PMTs, preamplifiers, and amplifiers. The detector is shielded from background radiation (i.e., cosmic and patient radiation). Proximity sensors and touch-sensitive panels are present to avoid collision between the patient or the scanner bed and the camera heads.

The scintillation crystal, most commonly made of a 9.5-mm block of sodium iodide (NaI), transforms the energy deposited by the gamma rays into light pulses. NaI is sensitive to the humidity in the air (i.e., hygroscopic) and is therefore encompassed into an aluminum container, which improves the light collection as well by the PMTs. It is relatively dense and provides good stopping power and energy resolution (8–10% at 140 keV), and it is feasible to grow large crystal arrays at a reasonable cost. The NaI crystal is doped with a small amount of thallium (Tl) to create activation sites that improve light production. The number of light photons generated (38 light photons per keV) is directly proportional to the energy deposited by the gamma ray in the crystal. These light photons are then converted by an array, usually hexagonal, of ~60 PMTs, to an amplified electrical signal. The electrical signal generated from each PMT is proportional to the amount of light it detects (i.e., gamma-ray energy). The PMTs closest to the interaction location in the crystal will receive the greatest amount of light. The electrical signals from the PMTs are processed by the position/energy electronics, which estimate the location of the gamma-ray interaction, and the energy deposited within the crystal. The energy of each detected photon is processed by a pulse-height analyzer, which rejects events with energies outside of a selected energy range (i.e., photopeak). This is done to reduce contamination from Compton scatter, downscatter from higher energy gamma emissions emitted by some radionuclides (e.g., ^{123}I), or crosstalk in multi-radionuclide studies (e.g., ^{99m}Tc/^{111}In in infection studies).

The latest generation of SPECT systems incorporates an alternative detector technology based on cadmium zinc telluride (CZT) semiconductors. CZT detector offers direct conversion of the energy deposited by the gamma rays into an electrical current. This direct transfer of energy and location information results in improved performance, including energy resolution (5–6% vs. 8–10% with NaI-based technology), intrinsic spatial resolution (2.5 mm vs. 3.5–4 mm), and count rate performance (>1000 kcps vs. 135 kcps) [177]. CZT detectors are small and compact and have changed the way SPECT systems have been built, facilitating the emergence of more efficient camera design for gamma-ray imaging.

The collimator forms the image by restricting the gamma rays emitted from the patient. It establishes a spatial correlation between the source location within the patient and the detection position in the detector. The collimator most commonly used for thoracic imaging, the parallel-hole collimator, consists of a thick sheet of a highly attenuating material, usually lead-antimony, pierced by an array of a few thousand hexagonal holes. It is fabricated by stacking together sheets of lead foil to form a honeycomb structure [426]. Each hexagonal hole of the collimator, parallel to each other, acts as a collimated channel, restricting the path of the detected photons to originate from any location in the patient along a line [i.e., line of response (LOR)] perpendicular to the collimator surface defined at the center of the hole (Fig. 25.1). A parallel-hole collimator allows only the gamma rays moving perpendicular to the collimator surface to strike the detector. The other gamma rays with angled directions are stopped and therefore do not participate in the imaging process. The sensitivity of a parallel-hole collimator is thus relatively low as most of the gamma rays emerging from the patient are absorbed by the collimator. The parallel-hole collimator provides a direct planar image of the radiotracer's activity distribution onto the crystal without any image distortion (i.e., magnification or inversion). In practice, certain photons may penetrate the septa (i.e., the thickness of lead between the channels) without any energy loss, resulting in their detection within the photopeak. This effect, named penetration, degrades the image quality and can result in activity reconstructed outside the patient's body as these photons carry erroneous spatial information. As penetration and scatter in the collimator are more likely to occur for higher-energy radionuclides, such as ^{111}In or ^{177}Lu, several parallel-hole collimators exist to image at different gamma-ray energy. For example, low-energy high-resolution (LEHR) collimators are used for ^{99m}Tc imaging. For ^{111}In or ^{177}Lu imaging, a medium-energy general purpose (MEGP) collimator with wider holes and thicker septa is used to improve stopping power. Spatial resolution is the ability of the system to differentiate spatially between two sources positioned close to each other, thus reflecting the capability of the system to discern fine image details. It is governed primarily by the collimator and detector characteristics, the photon energy, and the distance from the source to the collimator. A unique feature of a parallel-hole collimator is that the sensitivity remains constant with the collimator–patient distance. However, the spatial resolution worsens with increasing the collimator–patient distance, and it is thus essential to move the camera heads as close as possible to the patient.

In practice, an infrared proximity sensor can contour the detector more closely around the patient during SPECT acquisition. SPECT imaging can separate radioactivity distributions that superimpose on top of each other on planar imaging. For thoracic imaging, typically, a total of 64 views of 128 by 128 pixels over 360 degrees are acquired with noncircular orbit enabling close patient contouring. Nowadays, SPECT imaging is generally combined with CT, which provides anatomic information that can be used mainly to improve the spatial resolution in some structures and linear attenuation coefficients for attenuation and scatter correction

[353]. SPECT makes use of iterative reconstruction to estimate the 3D distribution of the radiotracers from the sets of planar views acquired around the patient. All the underlying physics of imaging can be incorporated and corrected for during reconstruction [58].

Example of Commercial Clinical Systems

The major vendors provide conventional dual-head SPECT systems with similar features and multiple collimator sets for various clinical studies. It is worth mentioning that one vendor (Mediso Medical System) offers a triple SPECT/PET/ CT modality system (AnyScan®) combined into one unit. The NM 830® system from General Electric Healthcare consists of two gamma cameras with a 54 × 40-cm² NaI(Tl) crystal available in two thicknesses (9.5 mm and 15.9 mm) and associated with an array of 59 circular PMTs of 76 × 38 mm² (Fig. 25.2). The 15.9-mm crystal thickness provides improved stopping power for higher energy radionuclides at the expense of poorer intrinsic spatial resolution. This system has a maximum count rate of 460 kilo counts per second (kcps) with the high-count rate mode. Different parallel-hole collimator sets are available, including low-energy high-resolution and

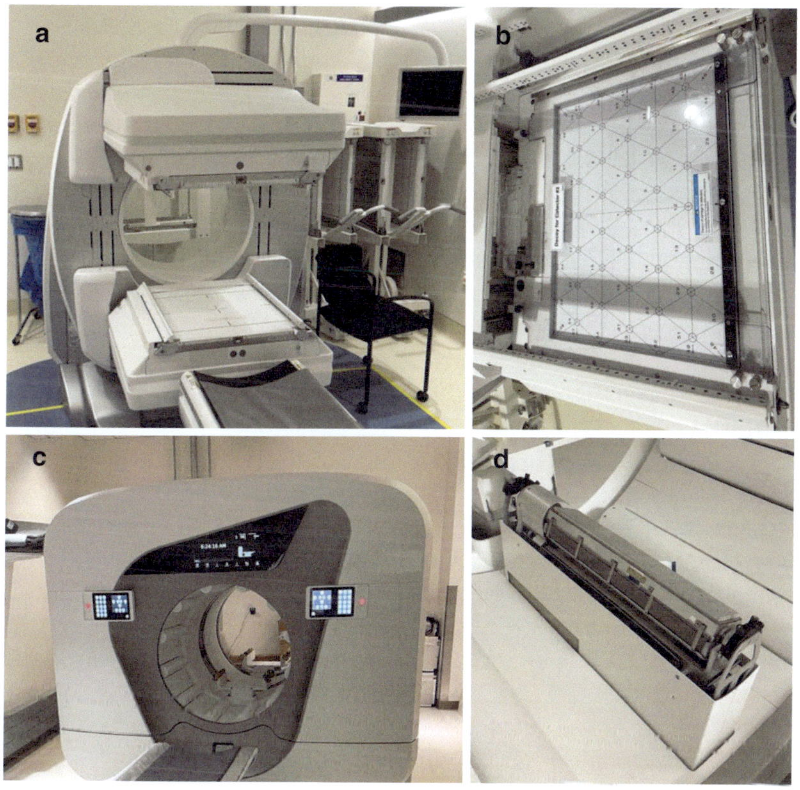

Fig. 25.2 Examples of clinical SPECT systems (**a**, **b**) NM830® SPECT-only system from General Electric Healthcare equipped with LEHRS collimators and based upon NaI(Tl) + PMT technology. On the far right, we can observe the HEGP (left) and MEGP (right) collimator carts. Collimators are exchanged manually by docking the carts and sliding the collimator sets into the heads. (**b**) Front face of the plastic cover encloses the light guide, NaI(Tl) scintillator and PMTs. The collimator is removed. The circular PMT layout can be seen on the picture, where each circled number reflects one PMT position, for a total of 59 per head. (**c**, **d**) VERITON-CT® SPECT/CT 200 series from Spectrum Dynamics with a ring of 12 CZT-detector modules arranged around 360 degrees. Each head can move in and out, and swivel around their own axis. The CT can be seen in the back of the gantry. (**d**) View of a CZT detector head, with the pressure-sensitive cover and capacitance board removed. The tungsten parallel-hole collimator can be seen. There are 2048 sensitive pixels of 2.46 × 2.46 × 6 mm³

sensitivity (LEHRS) and medium-energy general purpose (MEGP). The LEHRS collimator has a 1.43-mm channel diameter, 0.13-mm septa size, 32-mm thickness, and weight 43 kg. This results in sensitivity and spatial resolution of 92 cps/MBq and 7.4 mm for ^{99m}Tc with a 20% photopeak window at 100 mm from the collimator front face, respectively. The percentage of penetration represents 2.3% of the total counts. The MEGP collimator, designed to image ^{177}Lu, ^{67}Ga or ^{111}In, has a larger channel diameter (3 mm), septa size (1.05 mm), and thickness (58 mm) than the LEHRS collimator. This results in improved stopping power and increased weight (103 kg). For ^{67}Ga[2] with 20% energy windows centered at 93 keV, 185 keV, and 300 keV, the sensitivity, spatial resolution, and penetration fraction at 100 mm from the collimator front face are 65 cps/MBq, 9.4 mm, and 2%, respectively. This SPECT system can be combined with a CT in several configurations, eight 0.625-mm thick slices (NM 860®) and sixteen 0.625-mm thick slices (NM 870 DR®) CT scanners. The NM 870® SPECT/CT system is available with CZT detectors as well, resulting in improved imaging performance, such as energy resolution (5.6% compared to 9.5% for ^{99m}Tc), count rate capability, and tomographic spatial resolution [179]. Different parallel-hole collimator sets for ^{99m}Tc and ^{177}Lu were specifically designed to provide a one-to-one match between the CZT pixels and the collimator channels.

CZT detector technology has more recently facilitated the implementation of more efficient camera designs with high-performance imaging geometries. An example of such innovative system designs are 360-degree CZT SPECT/CT systems with a ring of cameras around 360 degrees. There are currently two systems available: the VERITON-CT® from Spectrum Dynamics and the STARGUIDE® from General Electric Healthcare. The VERITON-CT® consists of a circular ring of 12 CZT detector columns associated to a high-end CT (Fig. 25.2). Each detector column can rotate on its own axes (swivel) to focus on a given organ or structure and can move in and out to be positioned quite close to the patient for high-performance imaging. These capabilities offer flexible organ-specific acquisition providing "adaptive" SPECT imaging. The detector column uses tungsten collimators offering higher stopping power than lead alloy conventionally used. In total, there are 2048 pixels of 2.46 by 2.46 mm^2 per detector column, 6 mm thick for the 200 series and 7.3 mm for the latest release 400 series, capable of imaging up to 400 keV. Each collimator opening is registered to a single CZT pixel with square hole size of 2.46 mm and a septa thickness of 0.2 mm, and a long hole length of 24.5 mm. Such a system can offer 3D dynamic SPECT imaging with a 3–10 sec framing rate thanks to no gantry rotation, and improved sensitivity, and count rate capabilities. The VERITON-CT® was reported to provide slightly improved spatial resolution compared to conventional systems. For a point source in air, the sensitivity of the VERITON-CT® system with and without focus mode was reported to be 8 times and 1.6 times higher than conventional systems (1159 cps/MBq and 236 cps/MBq versus 144 cps/MBq) [107].

360 CZT SPECT systems are of great interest for theranostics as they can alleviate the limitation of conventional scanners for rapid whole-body SPECT imaging to assess the extent of the disease and monitor treatment via personalized dosimetry. For example, there has been a rapid growth of TRT, such as ^{177}Lu-DOTATATE for neuroendocrine tumors and ^{177}Lu-PSMA for prostate cancer. SPECT has major advantages over PET for image-based dosimetry due to its capability to image directly ^{177}Lu. There is thus a growing need for high-speed whole-body SPECT/CT imaging, for which conventional SPECT is hampered by long acquisition because of poor sensitivity. 360 CZT SPECT/CT can overcome these challenges with improved imaging performance. It has been reported recently that a ^{177}Lu whole-body SPECT/CT image can be acquired in about 10 min with such a system with decent image quality [77, 90, 195, 386, 435]. By comparison, using a conventional system, a

[2] ^{67}Ga has three gamma ray emission peaks at 93 keV (39% abundant), 185 keV (21.4% abundant), and 300 keV (16% abundant).

whole planar image for 30–40 min in combination with two 10-min one bed-position SPECT are required for whole-body imaging, resulting in 40–60 min imaging time [386].

Positron Emission Tomography

Physics

As described above, PET imaging uses unstable radionuclides emitting positrons with the same rest mass (511 keV) as electrons but with opposite charge. Following emission, positrons travel a short distance, depending on their initial kinetic energy, through tissue before annihilating with an electron from the surrounding matter to generate two 511-keV gamma rays traveling in (nearly) opposite directions (i.e., 180 ± 0.5 degrees apart). Detecting these annihilation photons is the fundamental basis of PET imaging (Fig. 25.3). This photon pair can be detected in coincidence by two opposite detectors using narrow detection timing windows of a few nanoseconds (i.e., 4–12 ns) [261]. This assumes that both photons reach the detectors simultaneously. Thus, detecting one photon by the first detector triggers the coincidence circuit. If a second photon is detected in any other detectors within the short timing window, the system identifies a coincidence event. The principle of collinearity then assumes that the position of the annihilation (i.e., where the gamma rays were emitted) relates somewhere along the line connecting the two detectors (i.e., line of response or LOR) (Fig. 25.3).

A typical PET system consists of a stationary, fully enclosed ring of such detectors surrounding the patient over 360 degrees, to maximize coincidence detection. In contrast to SPECT imaging, which can operate at different radionuclide energy, in PET, the gamma rays have a constant energy of 511 keV. The fundamental difference is that there is no use of a physical collimator absorbing a large fraction of the incident gamma rays in PET, where the collimation of the gamma rays to accept valid events is done electronically. This results in much higher sensitivity, typically by two orders of magnitude, compared to a con-

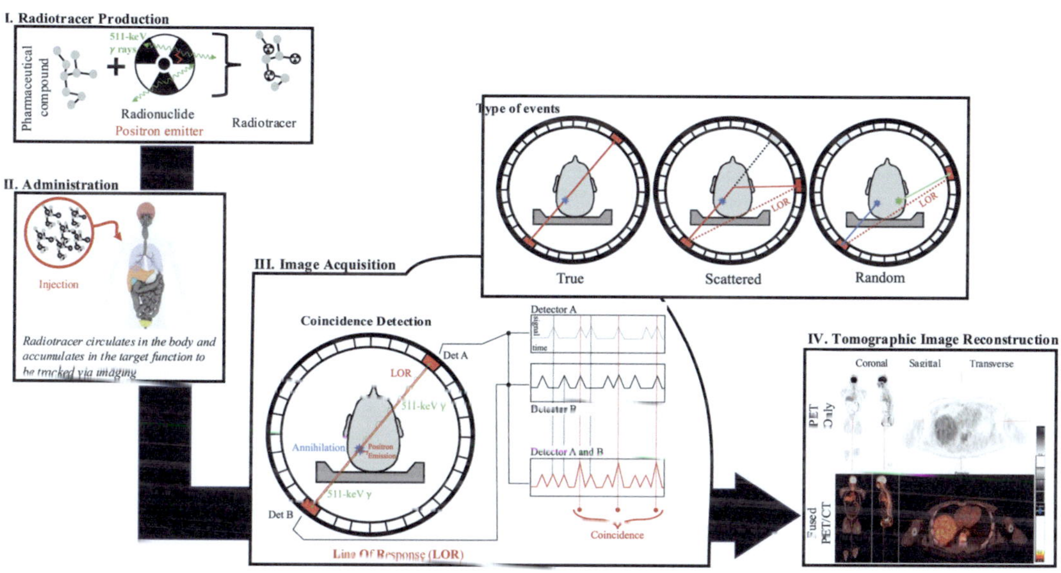

Fig. 25.3 Overview of the steps of positron emission tomography (PET) consisting of (I) radiotracer production and (II) administration followed by (III) image acquisition when the radiotracer has accumulated in the structure of interest. The last step is (IV) reconstruction of the 3D images reflecting the 3D distribution of the annihilation locations. The locations where the positrons are emitted cannot be retrieved, resulting in a fundamental limit for PET imaging dictated by the positron range

ventional dual-head SPECT system equipped with LEHR collimator.

The projections are formed by the acquisition of a multitude of these lines of response, and most commonly, an iterative reconstruction algorithm will be used to estimate the distribution of the annihilation photons. However, the actual locations where the positrons were emitted cannot be retrieved. The positron range in tissue results in a loss of spatial information, thus resulting in a blurring of the final reconstructed image. The spatial resolution in PET is thus fundamentally limited by the positron range. For ^{18}F, the average and maximal positron range in water is 0.44 mm and 2.32 mm, respectively [122]. For higher energy positron emitters, such as ^{82}Rb, the average and maximal positron range in water is 5.03 mm and 16.8 mm, respectively [122]. It is important to note that planar and SPECT imaging does not suffer from such limitation and can, therefore, in theory, achieve superior spatial resolution, which primarily depends on the collimator.

Multiple types of events can occur in PET imaging. Single events represent the total of all events detected by the PET system. A true coincidence event occurs when the system detects two annihilation photons resulting from a unique location within the coincidence time window. Random or accidental coincidences refer to erroneous and unrelated events that the system records when single photons from different annihilation locations are detected and accepted as coincidences. At a high-count rate, the number of random coincidences can exceed the true coincidence rate, and it is possible for three or more detectors to be involved. Random coincidences can also result from the emission of additional gamma rays, not generated by positron decay, with energy falling into the photopeak window. One or both annihilation photons may scatter in the patient via Compton interaction and retain sufficient energy to fall within the photopeak, thus being identified by the system as a true coincidence. This results in inaccurate positioning as the annihilation location is no longer along the LOR connecting the two-detector pair because of the change in the scattered photon direction.

Recent PET systems equipped with fast detectors can estimate the time difference between detecting the two annihilation photons, referred to as time of flight (TOF). TOF information can be used to determine the annihilation location, which, in theory, could be estimated directly without the need for image reconstruction. However, the limited timing resolution of the current detector technology (200–300 ps) results in coarse TOF-derived spatial resolution of about 5 mm [401]. However, the TOF information can be included in iterative reconstruction to improve the image quality, particularly the noise. A recent overview of the history and future technical innovation in PET imaging can be found here [194].

Instrumentation

The performance of a PET system relies on fast and accurate detection of the 511-keV annihilation photons. The detector used in PET consists of an inorganic scintillator, a light conversion unit, and processing electronics. The higher energy of the photons (i.e., 511 keV) implies that the detection technologies developed for SPECT imaging (i.e., mainly 140 keV) are inadequate. The inorganic scintillator should provide high stopping power at 511 keV and fast scintillation response for TOF. The light yield is less important since the 511-keV annihilations photons will generate more light than the lower energy photons used in conventional SPECT system with NaI(Tl)-based detectors. Bismuth germanate (BGO) was used in the early generation of PET system as it provides high stopping power with 94% of the 511-keV photons interacting within a 30-mm thick array compared to only 36% for a similar thickness of NaI(Tl) [261]. However, its performance is limited by low light production (15–20% of NaI(Tl)), resulting in poorer energy resolution (25% at 511 keV) and intrinsic spatial resolution [261]. In addition, BGO is not capable of TOF imaging due to its long scintillation time (300 ns). Nowadays, cerium-doped lutetium oxyorthosilicate (LSO) and cerium-doped lutetium yttrium oxyorthosilicate (LYSO) are used in modern TOF-PET systems. LYSO and LSO provide similar stopping power as BGO while generating much more light (75% of NaI(Tl)) in a shorter time (40–50 ns) [261]. This results in improved energy resolution (10–15% at 511 keV) to reduce scatter coincidences, timing resolution to facilitate rejection of random coincidences, and intrinsic spatial resolution. The scintillator is divided into small pixels, while SPECT system typically uses a continuous scintillator. Pixelated scintillator improves intrinsic spatial and timing resolutions.

In modern PET systems, the light emitted by the scintillator is converted into an electrical signal via silicon photomultipliers (SiPM), which are small solid-state semiconductors operating in discrete counting mode. SiPM provides multiple advantages over PMT, including better light detection, high compacity facilitating integration into large arrays, low power consumption, and fast timing response particularly suited for TOF. SiPM are also not sensitive to magnetic fields up to 1.5T, facilitating their inclusion in PET/magnetic resonance imaging (MRI) systems. A one-to-one match between scintillator pixels and SiPM elements would lead to prohibitive cost and increase the technical complexity of a PET system. To alleviate these limitations, detector blocks are used, where grooves are cut normal to the front face in the scintillator to create typically an array of 8 by 8 elements coupled optically via glue or light guide to a small array of SiPM pixels placed behind the crystal. The detector block design improves spatial resolution while decreasing the sensitivity due to the less active scintillator surface. Modern PET systems use multiple of these detector blocks arranged in rings and placed along the axial direction (i.e., patient height), resulting typically in more than 20,000 detector elements.

Similarly, to SPECT/CT systems, PET systems are usually combined with a CT scanner [45, 94]. The integration of a CT scanner provides the same advantages as SPECT imaging, enabling attenuation correction of the PET data by modeling attenuation derived from CT attenuation map in reconstruction and providing anatomical information. Even if the likelihood for photons of being attenuated increases with the gamma-ray energy, attenuation has a greater effect in PET, as the two annihilation photons need to be detected to form a coincidence instead of a single photon in SPECT. The CT scanner can also enable scout acquisition to guide the PET acquisition by facilitating the definition of the region of interest from the patient's anatomy.

The past decade has seen the emergence of combined PET/MR as a new hybrid modality. Magnetic resonance imaging (MRI) provides superior differentiation in soft tissues and can provide functional information compared to CT, without additional ionizing radiation exposure. SiPMs are usually preferred in modern PET/MR systems as they demonstrate reliable and good performance under strong static and varying magnetic fields while enabling TOF imaging. The first TOF PET/MR system, SIGNA®, was released by General Electric Healthcare in 2013 (see next section). A comprehensive overview of PET/MR was recently published [280]. MR-based attenuation correction is more challenging than PET/CT as MRI does not directly provide the linear attenuation coefficients (see below). Recent publications discuss the promising clinical applications of PET/MR, for example, in the context of respiratory diseases or breast cancer imaging where improved soft tissue contrast is critical to evaluate response to chemotherapy [115, 226, 424].

Another promising modality recently developed is total-body PET/CT. Multiple total-body TOF PET/CT systems have been introduced for clinical use by United Imaging Healthcare, the uEXPLORER®, and more recently, by Siemens Healthineers, the Biograph Vision Quadra®. These systems enable static and dynamic imaging of the total body without bed translation, resulting in a considerable increase in sensitivity of up to 40 [402, 430]. However, they remain very expensive (~3 times increase in cost) due to the utilization of more detectors to cover an extended axial length (>100 cm). Most recently, the feasibility of multiplexed PET combining iodine labeled agents with other PET radiotracers was demonstrated, enabling two separate physiological processes to be probed concurrently by PET [343]. A comprehensive overview of the new technologies in PET imaging can be found in the following paper (see [7]).

Example of Commercial Clinical Systems

The major vendors offer whole-body TOF PET/CT scanners; this section will describe selected TOF PET/CT, total-body PET/CT, and TOF PET/MR systems. The Discovery MI PET/CT® from General Electric Healthcare is built around lutetium-based scintillator plus SiPM detector blocks, named LightBurst®, in multiple axial field-of-view (FOV) configurations (4 rings [20 cm], 5 rings [25 cm], and 6 rings [30 cm]) (Fig. 25.4). The transaxial FOV is 70 cm. There is a total of 136 detector blocks per ring. A detector block combines a 4 by 9 array of lutetium-based scintillators with three 3 by 2 arrays of SiPM detectors. This results in 19,584 and 29,376 crystal pixels and 9792 and 14,688 SiPM channels for the 4 and 6 axial ring configurations, respectively. The crystal pixel size is 3.95 × 5.3 × 25 mm^3. This detection technology provides timing resolution of 380 ps [402, 430, 466]. The system incorporates an improved iterative reconstruction (Q.Clear™) that controls via a penalized factor, the relative strength of the noise propagated into the reconstructed image [417].

Another example of a commercially available system is the latest generation of TOF PET/CT from Siemens Healthineers, the Biograph Vision®. The system consists of 38 LSO scintillator plus SiPM detector blocks per axial ring and 8 axial detector rings. The transaxial FOV is 82 cm. Each detector block contains a 4 by 2 arrangement of 5 × 5 LSO crystal array coupled to a 4 × 4 SiPM array of 16 × 16 mm^2. This configuration results in 60,800 crystal pixels of 3.2 × 3.2 × 20 mm^3 and 38,912 SiPM elements. The axial FOV is 26.3 cm. The small pixel size enables superior spatial resolution, while the full crystal coverage by SiPM channels improves light collection and timing resolution (210 ps) [402, 430, 466]. Recently, Siemens Healthineers released the Biograph Vision Quadra® total-body PET/CT system, based on the same detector tech-

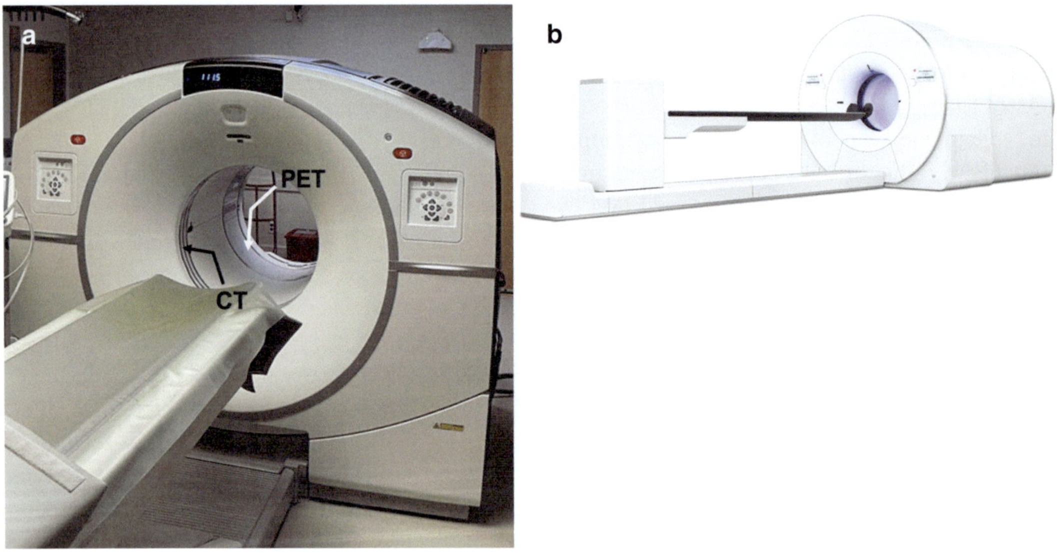

Fig. 25.4 (**a**) Image of the Discovery MI PET/CT® from General Electric Healthcare, with the CT located in the front and the four-axial ring PET in the back of the gantry. The transaxial and axial field of view is 20 cm and 70 cm, respectively. (**b**) Detailed view of the detection technology of the Discovery MI PET/CT® from General Electric Healthcare. There are a total of 136 detector blocks per ring and 3 (on the figure) blocks along the axial direction. A detector block combines a 4 by 9 array of lutetium-based scintillators with three 3 by 2 arrays of SiPM detectors. This results in a total number of 19,584 crystal pixels and 9792 SiPM channels for the four-axial ring configurations illustrated in (**a**). (Courtesy of General Electric Healthcare.)

nology [344]. It combines axially 4 of the 26.3-mm Vision® detector blocks, to increase the axial FOV to 106 cm, resulting in a total of 243,200 crystal elements associated to 155,648 SiPM channels. United Imaging Healthcare released the first commercial total-body PET/CT system, the uEXPLORER®, with a larger axial FOV of 194 cm combined to a 68.6-cm transaxial FOV (Fig. 25.4). The detector block is built around an array of 7 × 6 pixelated LYSO crystal, 2.76 × 2.76 × 18.1 mm^3, combined with 6 × 6 SiPM channels. The system utilizes 13,440 detector blocks, resulting in a total of 564,480 crystal pixels associated to 53,760 SiPM channels [390]. An overview of the clinical perspectives of total-body PET systems was recently published (see [2]).

The first commercially available TOF-PET/MRI system, SIGNA®, incorporating a 3T-MRI system (Discovery 750w®) was released by General Electric Healthcare [153, 251]. The detector block consists of an array of 4 by 9 LYSO scintillators, 4 × 5.3 × 25 mm^3 in size, coupled to a 1 × 3 arrays of SiPMs. The transaxial FOV is 62.4 cm. The 25-cm axial FOV PET system comprises a total of 20,160 crystal pixels. Each detector unit, consisting of four detector blocks, is enclosed in electromagnetically shielding to minimize interference of the MRI signal on the PET detector operation. Dedicated MR sequences and deep-learning-based [368] strategies are being developed for better MR-derived attenuation correction [251].

Considerations for Quantitative Imaging

Sources of Image Degradation

In planar, SPECT, and PET imaging, many factors impact the accuracy and precision with which the images reflect the true radiotracer concentrations in structures of interest. In this section, we will provide an overview of the main sources of image degradation in thoracic imaging, which include attenuation and scatter effects in the patient, patient respiratory motion, and limitations of the imaging instrument, such as spatial resolution, sensitivity, and dead time. In the context of quantitative imaging, it remains important to estimate their influence and implement effective corrections accurately. A comprehensive overview of the sources of image degradation and their correction can be found in Boellaard 2009; [27, 28, 110, 264]. The IAEA has released atlases describing the different artifacts occurring with gamma and PET imaging, as well as their quality control [479, 480].

Requirements for Quantitative Imaging

Detector Calibration and Quality Control

Adequate operation and calibration of SPECT and PET systems are crucial factors that heavily influence quantitative accuracy and overall image quality. Frequent testing and calibration procedures are essential to ensure that the imaging instruments maintain acceptable performance and that any issues or artifacts are detected before affecting patient studies. These include energy, linearity, uniformity, and center-of-rotation calibration, as well as multihead alignment in SPECT, and detector normalization in PET. A detailed overview of routine quality control and calibration procedures can be found in [372, 465].

Dead-Time Correction

Detectors used in SPECT and PET imaging are affected by the dead time, which refers to the minimum time interval for the system to distinguish between two separate events. During this period, the system may not be able to process further events or may merge all further events as one (i.e., pulse pile-up), thus resulting in apparent count losses and inaccurate quantitation, especially in dynamic studies. It is worth mentioning that in SPECT, CZT-based detectors provide higher count rate capability (much shorter dead time) than conventional NaI-based technology. Correction for such count rate-dependent effects is based on estimating the dead time at the anticipated count rate and applying mathematically a correction factor to retrieve the true count rate.

Random Correction for PET

The limited timing resolution and the use of a coincidence window of PET system result in the acquisition of random coincidences, where two annihilation photons originating from two different locations are detected and accepted by the coincidence algorithm. Random coincidences are estimated via a delayed coincidence window and typically subtracted from the acquired data prior to reconstruction. However, a better approach is to include (thus correct for) the random coincidence estimate in an iterative reconstruction to improve the noise texture in the reconstructed image.

Attenuation Correction

Attenuation refers to the loss of photons through the patient, depending on photon energy and source depth, due to photon interaction (predominantly Compton scatter in tissue). It can result in underestimation of true radiotracer concentration and image artifacts [94]. In planar imaging, attenuation is typically compensated by combining the geometric mean of the anterior/posterior views with a transmission measurement done with a ^{57}Co sheet source. For SPECT and PET, the most commonly used approach relies on modeling (and correcting for) the attenuation effect in an iterative reconstruction based on the inclusion of a map of attenuation coefficients derived from a CT. A detailed overview of the strategies to correct for attenuation can be found in [28, 48]. Recently, artificial intelligence (AI)-based approaches have been proposed to derive the attenuation map directly from the SPECT/PET data, resulting in lower radiation exposure [44, 76, 247]. In PET/MR, the linear attenuation coefficient of the tissues cannot be directly obtained as is the case with CT, as MRI does not measure tissue nor electron density. Several methods exist to derive the attenuation map from MR images, which include use of special MR sequences to distinguish between tissue types and then segment the anatomical structures, registered CT/MRI atlas-based approach, or more recently AI-based methods. A comprehensive overview of the different strategies can be found in [180, 233].

Scatter Correction

Compton scatter changes the photon direction and energy, which can remain high enough to be accepted within the photopeak window due to the limited energy resolution of SPECT and PET systems. It causes misplacement of the photon emitted positions, thus resulting in an increased blurry background that reduces image contrast and skews the quantitative accuracy. Most commonly, scatter is compensated by estimating the scatter from the acquisition data and removing the scatter estimate before reconstruction. The scatter contribution can be estimated from the data acquisition by placing two or more narrow energy windows adjacent to the photopeak [178, 382]. A more accurate alternative relies on direct modeling by Monte Carlo simulations [33] or by analytic calculation [431] of the scattering effect in the patient into an iterative reconstruction. Recently, AI-based scatter correction methods have been proposed [17, 288]. A recent comprehensive overview of the multiple scatter correction approaches can be found in [176].

Partial Volume Correction

Due to the imaging system limitation, spatial resolution remains relatively poor, typically of 8–12 mm for SPECT and of 4–6 mm for PET for thoracic application. This induces the partial volume effect (PVE), which led to a reduction in apparent radiotracer concentration for small structures and can also result in an apparent increase in concentration for structures surrounded by higher-uptake regions. A recent review of the multiple methods to compensate for PVE can be found in [125]. One commonly used method is utilizing correction coefficients for different sphere sizes derived from phantom study studies. The magnitude of PVE can be reduced by directly modeling in iterative reconstruction the acquisition parameters degrading the spatial resolution, particularly the collimator response in

SPECT, and by including anatomic information derived from CT or MRI to constrain the reconstruction.

Motion Correction

Motion can be of multiple types, including cardiac, respiratory, gastrointestinal, and physical or bulk movement (i.e., head or body movement). Motion can result in loss of spatial resolution due to the spatial dispersion of the radiotracer concentration, the mismatch between SPECT/PET and CT images leading to errors in attenuation and scatter correction, image artifacts, and quantitative inaccuracies (Fig. 25.5). It is critical to minimize motion during image acquisition. However, respiratory or cardiac motion is unavoidable. There are multiple methods available to correct for such motion that rely on first estimating the motion from the data itself or using a motion-tracking device and then incorporating the motion parameters into reconstruction. A recent overview of the different motion correction strategies can be found in [230].

Quantitative Imaging in Practice

Quantitative imaging, achieved by correcting for the multiple effects described above, can be used to assess activity concentration in organs or tissues of interest or alternatively to evaluate certain

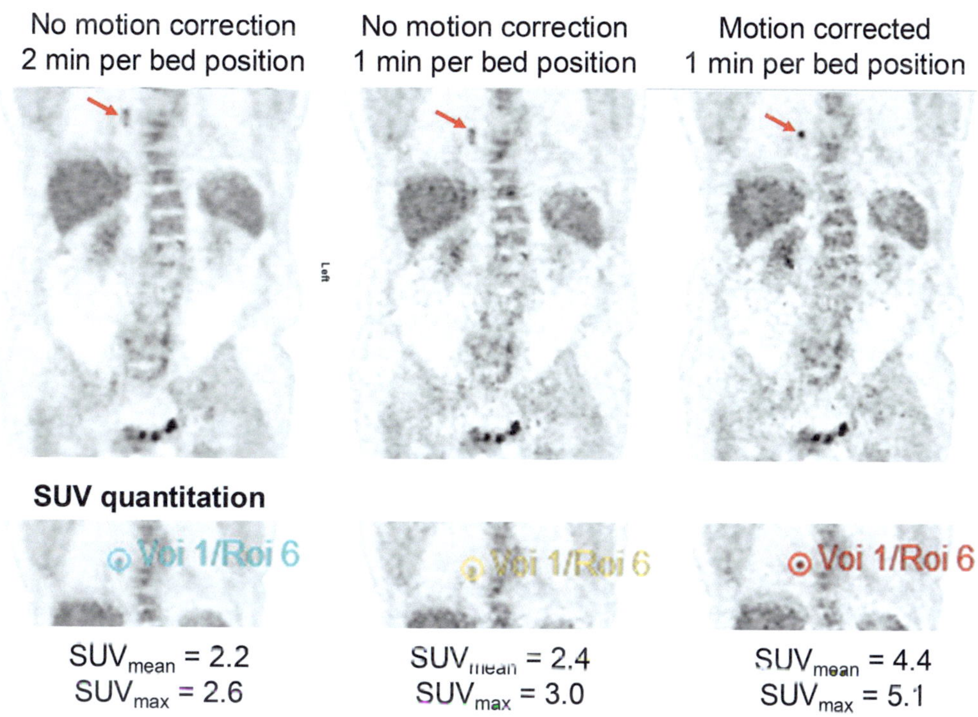

Fig. 25.5 The benefit of motion correction in FDG-PET, where activity recovery of a pulmonary lesion (red arrow) was strongly improved by the use of motion correction. The data-driven motion correction technique (Q.Static from GE Healthcare) estimates the motion from the data itself and rejects the counts at the beginning of the breathing cycle. Only the data state acquired during the quiescent period of the respiratory cycle in a similar motion are kept and used for reconstruction (50% of the data available). (Left) Original reconstruction and SUV-quantitation without motion correction applied (2 min per bed position). (Middle) Half-scan time reconstruction without motion correction to match the noise level of the Q.Static motion-corrected images seen on the right. The SUV mean and max values are also considerably higher when motion correction is applied. The nonmotion correction reconstruction suffers from the spread of activity due to respiratory motion. We can also note the improvement visually in the kidney regions

physiological parameters, such as the metabolic rate of glucose in different regions.

In contemporary clinical practice, planar gamma-ray imaging is used mainly for multiple studies where qualitative or simplistic semi-quantitative evaluation is sufficient. In contrast to absolute quantitation, semi-quantitation does not require any particular form of calibration to transform image counts into activity levels as it is based on relative measurements obtained from the same image (e.g., tissue-to-background or tissue-to-blood ratio). Overall, for quantitative studies, SPECT imaging is preferred as it provides more accurate quantitation due to its three-dimensional nature and the ability to correct for multiple effects degrading the image quality in reconstruction. Quantification of activity from planar imaging suffers mainly from the superimposition of radiotracer activity from regions located at different depths in the patient and the inability to accurately compensate for the source of image degradation, and thus remains limited. However, owing to its simplicity and speed for whole-body acquisition, planar imaging is still in use, for example, for ^{177}Lu-DOTATATE and ^{177}Lu-PSMA radionuclide therapies, when the whole-body radiotracer distribution needs to be examined [62, 400]. In this context, quantitative imaging at multiple time points can be performed to monitor the treatment by evaluating the absorbed dose in different tissues of interest. Most commonly, hybrid approaches combine whole-body planar images to localize the lesions with SPECT-based activity quantification for tissue-absorbed dose estimation. Planar images at different imaging time points can also be used to scale the activity values obtained from the SPECT image(s) [218, 359]. In this context, quantitative planar imaging consists of correcting for source depth, attenuation, and scatter and applying a calibration factor to convert image total counts in a structure of interest into activity value. Compensation for attenuation and source depth relies most commonly on estimating the geometric mean of conjugate views (i.e., anterior/posterior) in combination with a transmission measurement obtained with a ^{57}Co flood source (i.e., acquisition repeated with and without the patient to obtain the attenuation coefficients). Scatter can be corrected by subtracting the scatter estimate obtained from the dual or triple-energy window-based method. The calibration factor is specific to the acquisition parameters (e.g., collimator, system settings, and radionuclides) and relates image counts to a known amount of activity measured with a reference instrument, most commonly a dose calibrator. In practice, the calibration factor is derived from acquiring a source of known activity (i.e., standard) with the same imaging parameters as the clinical study [264].

SPECT and PET imaging can achieve far superior quantitative accuracy than planar imaging once adequate corrections for the effects degrading the image quality are applied. PET imaging provides better quantitative precision than SPECT due to its improved sensitivity and spatial resolution. However, it has been demonstrated that SPECT can approach the accuracy of PET imaging to measure in vivo quantification of radionuclide concentration within 5–10% of the true value [27, 28, 110].

Quantitative SPECT imaging has promising applications for internal dosimetry in the context of theranostics, where imaging can be used to monitor the course of the treatment. Absorbed dose estimation requires an absolute estimation of the radiotracer biodistribution, as opposed to semi-quantitation. The system thus needs to be calibrated to convert image count per unit volume into radiotracer concentration. The most used calibration procedure, named cross-calibration, is analogous to that used for PET/CT. The calibration factor can be derived from acquiring a cylindrical uniform phantom with the same acquisition and reconstruction parameters used for the patient study [264]. The standardized uptake value (SUV) has been widely used in PET and, more recently, in SPECT to quantify the radiotracer uptake in tissues in disease staging and treatment response evaluation, for example, in oncology or cardiac imaging. Following adequate cross-calibration, the SUV based on the patient weight can be evaluated for a given tissue as the radiotracer/activity concentration divided by the total administrated activity per unit weight.

Activity values are decay-corrected to the same time. Evaluation of the kinetic of the radiotracer in vivo implies converting absolute activity concentrations to biochemical measures. This requires additional information on the physiology of the tracer in vivo, such as arterial blood concentration of the radiotracer over time, that can serve as an input function to a compartmental model that characterizes the tracer kinetic (i.e., delivery, uptake, and washout). Tracer kinetic analysis has mainly been used with PET, capable of rapid dynamic acquisition needed to track in vivo the radiotracer concentration over time. However, there is a growing interest in such studies with 360 CZT SPECT/CT systems capable of 3D dynamic imaging.

Current Clinical Applications of Nuclear Medicine for Evaluation of the Thorax

Quantitative thoracic nuclear medicine imaging has nononcologic and oncologic indications, which will be explored below.

Nononcologic Conditions

Quantitative Functional Lung Scintigraphy

While global measures of pulmonary function like FEV_1 and DLCO are indispensable in the diagnosis and monitoring of various lung diseases, they are limited in their ability to localize regional areas of relatively poor or highly functioning lungs and assess the overall heterogeneity of lung function. By contrast, functional lung imaging creates a spatially oriented 3D map of altered lung mechanics. While other imaging modalities like CT and MRI have some capability to perform functional lung imaging, nuclear medicine is considered the well-validated gold standard.

Nuclear medicine functional lung imaging consists of both ventilation and perfusion scans, though, depending on the indication, institutional imaging protocol, and individual preference, patients may either undergo a combined ventilation and perfusion (V/Q) scan or a perfusion- or ventilation-only scan. The ventilation portion of the exam is obtained following patient inhalation of either an inert gas, like ^{133}xenon, or radiolabeled aerosol, like ^{99m}Tc-DTPA aerosol or ^{99m}Tc-Technegas. The latter is standard in most of Europe [265] and in 2023 was FDA-approved for use in the United States. The perfusion portion of the exam is acquired following intravenous injection of ^{99m}Tc-labeled macroaggregated albumin (MAA) particles, which subsequently become lodged in a minority of pre-capillary alveolar arterioles [104].

Quantitative analysis of functional lung imaging complements traditional visual assessment, playing an important role in the diagnosis and monitoring of various lung diseases and treatment responses. It consists of drawing regions of interest around each lung on the ventilation and perfusion scans, further dividing the lung into three equal vertical volumes, which are referred to as upper, middle, and lower lung zones (Fig. 25.6). Note that these zones do not necessarily represent lobar anatomy. The percentage of the total counts that are contained within each lung zone on both the ventilation and perfusion scans are calculated and displayed as measures of regional ventilation and perfusion.

The current clinical applications of quantitative perfusion and/or ventilation scans are wide-ranging, with both oncologic and nononcologic indications. This section will explore the latter, specifically as it relates to acute and chronic vascular and lung disease in both the adult and pediatric populations. The emerging use of other nuclear medicine imaging modalities for these applications, most notably FDG-PET, is also reviewed.

Acute Pulmonary Conditions

Pulmonary Embolism

Despite advances in diagnostic imaging, pulmonary embolism (PE) remains difficult to detect in clinical practice. Both overdiagnosis and missed diagnosis can be detrimental. The mortality rate of untreated PE can be as high as 30% [418]. In patients with high clinical probability and in

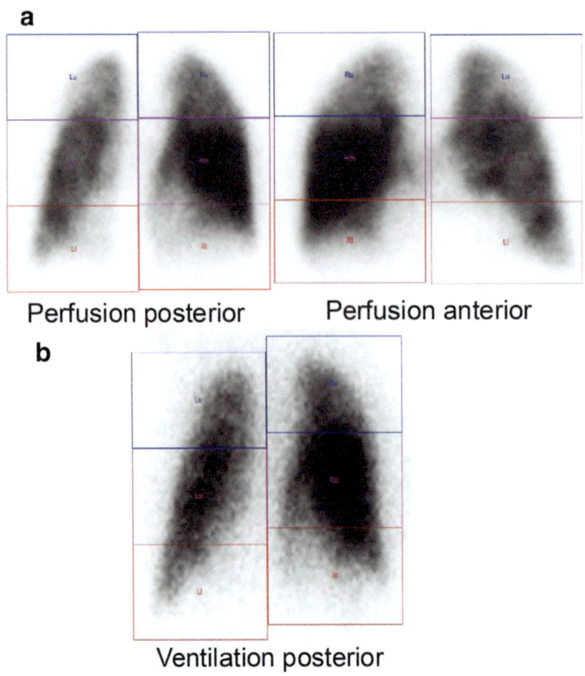

Perfusion geometric mean kct			
Left lung		Right lung	
%	kct		kct
9.0	63.62	11.2	78.99
21.0	148.64	37.0	261.56
8.8	62.14	12.9	91.18
38.9	274.41	61.1	431.73

Ventilation geometric mean kct			
Left lung		Right lung	
%	kct		kct
12.2	34.88	14.1	40.34
18.6	55.94	36.3	100.96
6.9	19.63	12.0	34.30
38.6	110.45	61.4	175.89

Fig. 25.6 Quantitative V/Q scintigraphy in a patient with COPD who presents for preoperative evaluation for lung resection following the discovery of multifocal lung nodules concerning for malignancy. (**a**) Posterior and anterior images of the lungs from ^{99m}Tc-MAA perfusion scintigraphy show the lungs being divided into three equally sized regions of interest: upper (purple outline), middle (pink outline), and lower (red outline) lung fields. The geometric mean of counts from anterior and posterior projections for each zone per lung is then used to calculate relative perfusion, which is displayed as a percentage of relative perfusion (top right). (**b**) Posterior image of the lungs from ^{133}Xe ventilation scintigraphy. The lungs are similarly divided into three equally sized regions of interest for quantification. The counts from the posterior image are used to quantify relative regional ventilation, again provided as a percentage

those with positive D-dimer but low or intermittent clinical probability, lung imaging is immensely useful [31]. Quantification of PE can help manage these patients, and V/Q scintigraphy is a reliable method for achieving this goal [118]. One of the main limitations of V/Q planar imaging is the lack of anatomical correlation, often presenting interpretation challenges. This has led to a decreasing demand for V/Q scintigraphy in favor of computed tomography pulmonary angiography (CTPA).

Nevertheless, CTPA has some disadvantages, including allergy to iodine contrast media, renal insufficiency, and risk of excessive diagnosis and overtreatment of clinically irrelevant PE [13, 449]. Furthermore, it can be difficult to differentiate bland thrombus from a tumoral clot or acute thrombi from residual lesions [242].

For V/Q scintigraphy, ventilation can be assessed using radiolabeled agents like ^{99m}Tc-labeled aerosols, DTPA, and Technegas®, ^{133}Xenon, or ^{81m}Krypton gases. For perfusion scintigraphy, ^{99m}Tc-MAA can be administered intravenously [13, 354, 449]. Compared to two-dimensional planar imaging, V/Q SPECT enables three-dimensional visualization, enabling better characterization and localization of filling defects [294]. When used in combination with a low-dose CT, SPECT/CT provides detailed anatomical and functional information and may provide confirmatory evidence of PE, like a hyperattenuating clot or differential vessel size, or identify an alternate cause of the patient's symptoms [104]. The basis of the lung perfusion scan interpretation is determined by its arterial anatomy. The end-artery supply of the lung is the reason for its

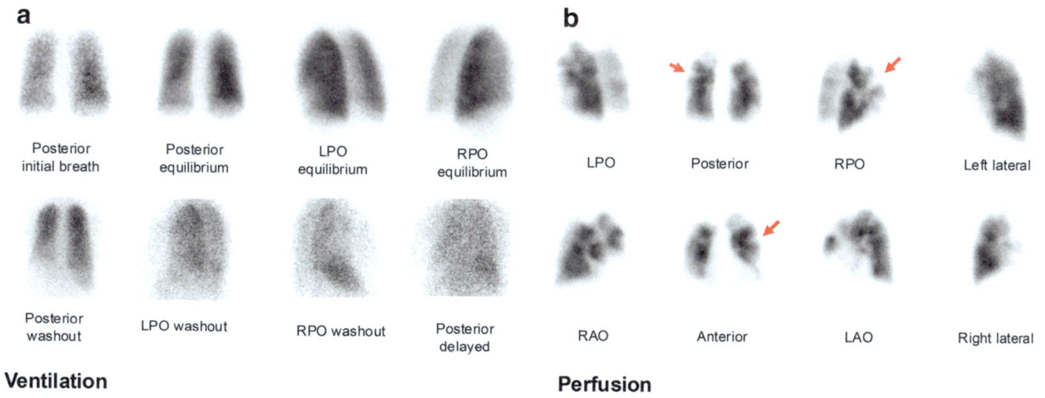

Fig. 25.7 High probability of pulmonary embolism on V/Q scan. Xenon gas ventilation (**a**) and MAA perfusion (**b**) images. No focal defect was noted on ventilation. On perfusion, there are multifocal segmental defects in the bilateral lungs noted on multiple views, with examples noted with red arrows. This appearance is highly concerning for pulmonary embolism

wedge-shaped defects (narrow in the center and wide in the periphery) seen on perfusion scans as perfusion defects. Therefore, it is suggested that the first step to evaluating V/Q studies is to check the lung peripherally; a continuous and expected contour effectively excludes PE, regardless of other findings in the study. If the perfusion images are abnormal, further evaluation is warranted [104, 299]. A high-probability scan for acute PE is defined as one segmental or two subsegmental perfusion defects with a normally ventilated region (Fig. 25.7) [104]. Note that V/Q scans cannot differentiate between chronic and acute PE; therefore, reviewing prior studies, if available, is necessary. Mismatch defects are not specific to PE and can be caused by other conditions such as cancer, congenital vascular abnormalities, veno-occlusive disease, vasculitis, and mediastinal lymphadenopathy.

Other etiologies can cause perfusion defects with different patterns. For example, during a hypoxic event, blood is normally shunted away from poorly ventilated areas by vasoconstriction, resulting in a ventilation-perfusion match. The presence of matched defects on V/Q scan can suggest an alternate diagnosis, such as COPD or airway disease. The presence of a matched V/Q defect with a corresponding radiographic abnormality is indicative of a "triple match" and is typically seen in pneumonia, pleural effusion, and lung mass. PE is more likely to occur in the lower lobes of the lungs due to increased blood flow. In some cases, it may be complicated by pulmonary infarction. Therefore, triple matches in the lower lobes pose a greater concern as they are more likely to indicate PE compared to triple matches in the upper lobes [104, 456]. Another type of defect is a reverse mismatched defect—this represents a ventilation defect with less severe or normal perfusion, which may represent a functional right-to-left shunt [334].

The size of the defect can be calculated as large (greater than 75% of the segment), moderate (25–75% of the segment), and small (less than 25% of the segment) [334]. Different semi-quantitative diagnostic criteria based on the visualization of defects have been suggested to categorize the probability of PE. The most commonly used are the Prospective Investigation of Pulmonary Embolism Diagnosis (PIOPED) criteria and the subsequently revised modified PIOPED II to reduce the high rate of nondiagnostic reports [444]. When the ventilation scan is not performed, the perfusion-only modified PIOPED II (pPIOPED II) and PISAPED criteria can be employed for the interpretation of the perfusion scan [293, 387]. The key diagnostic criteria are presented in Table 25.1. According to the PIOPED II criteria, V/Q scans have a specificity of 93% and a sensitivity of 85%, while the

Table 25.1 Modified PIOPED II and PISAPED criteria

Interpretation	Modified PIOPED II	PIASPED
PE present	High probability (two or more large segmental mismatched defects, or one large and two moderate defects)	One or more wedge-shaped perfusion defects with or without abnormal chest X-ray
PE absent	Normal perfusion	Normal perfusion
	Very low probability One to three small segmental defects Nonsegmental perfusion defects Perfusion defect smaller than corresponding chest X-ray findings Two or more matched defects with normal chest X-ray Stripe sign (evidence of peripheral perfusion in a defect) Pleural effusion in at least one third of pleural cavity in the absence of any other perfusion defect in either lung Single matched defect in the mid and upper lung zone	Near normal Non-wedge-shaped perfusion defect Counter defect caused by: enlarged aorta and mediastinum; cardiomegaly; elevated diaphragm; blunted costophrenic angle and pleural thickening
Nondiagnostic	All other findings	Cannot classify as PE-positive or PE-negative

PIASPED criteria yield a specificity of 97% and a sensitivity of 80%. These are comparable to CTPA values, which have a specificity of 98% and a sensitivity of 86% [350]. Recent V/Q SPECT studies have been conducted on more than 5000 cases, with a reported negative predictive value of 97–99%, sensitivities of 96–99%, and specificities of 96–98% for diagnosis of PE. The rates of nondiagnostic results ranged from 1% to 4% [35, 118, 156, 199]. V/Q SPECT is well-suited for tracking the course of PE since it can identify emboli of varying sizes (Fig. 25.8), enabling a detailed assessment of the progression or regression of the thrombotic condition. Furthermore, the low radiation dose allows for repeated studies, which is suitable for both diagnosis and follow-up [34, 36, 328], including in the pregnant patient [21].

V/Q SPECT/CT demonstrates similar sensitivity as V/Q SPECT but slightly higher specificity for detecting PE [241]. An interesting study by [163] showed that the application of breathing synchronization software can improve conformity between lung perfusion SPECT and lung CT. The lung volume calculated from lung CT and lung perfusion SPECT without using the breathing synchronization software was 3749 ± 788 ml and 3091 ± 610 ml, respectively. There was a significant difference between lung volume calculated from CT and the original lung perfusion SPECT ($P < 0.01$). On the other hand, by using the breathing synchronization software, the lung volume calculated from lung perfusion SPECT and CT was similar. The visual score improved with the use of breathing synchronization software (without software; 1.9 ± 0.6 vs. with software; 3.4 ± 0.7, $P < 0.001$).

Quantitative PET has also been used to evaluate PE. Some studies suggest that FDG-PET can aid in diagnosing PE in patients with cancer, given the common use of FDG in oncological practices. FDG-PET/CT has been found to detect PE as a lesion with focal FDG uptake incidentally. Although the precise physiologic mechanism is still unclear, it is believed that metabolically active cells, particularly neutrophils, at the site of embolism are responsible for the FDG uptake [22, 148, 208]. According to a retrospective study of 13 oncology patients with acute PE, FDG-PET detected greater FDG uptake in regions with thrombi than regions without thrombi, showing focal or curvilinear uptake patterns. The areas of higher FDG uptake, which appeared as focal or curvilinear abnormality in the PET scan, were consistent with the contrast-enhanced CT abnormality identified as PE [454].

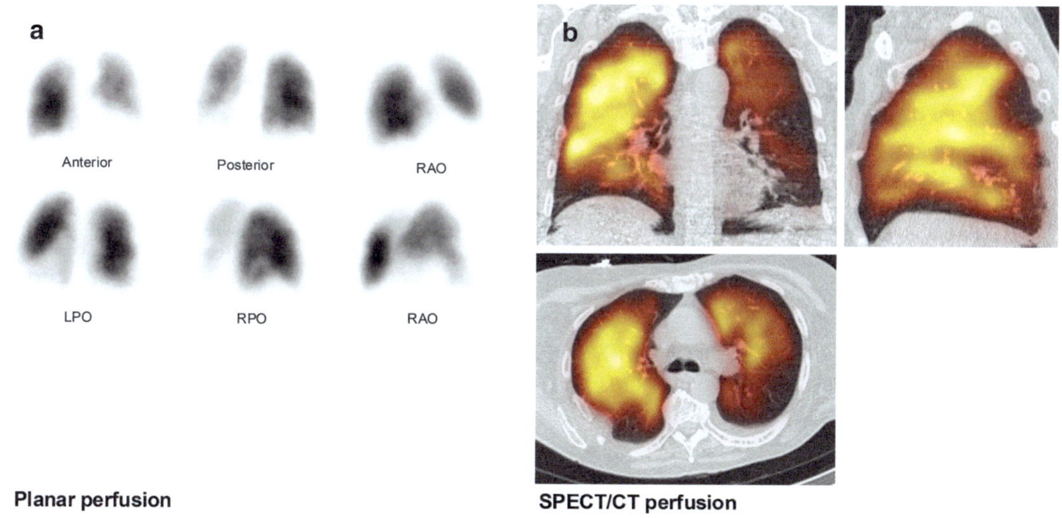

Fig. 25.8 SPECT/CT evaluation of pulmonary embolism. (**a**) Planar imaging shows a possible defect in the posterior left upper lobe. (**b**) SPECT/CT performed immediately after confirms this finding. (Courtesy M. Robertson, BWH)

In another retrospective study [134], a total of 65 cancer patients at an increased risk of PE underwent ^{18}F-FDG PET/CT scans. Among them, 59 cases with PE were discovered for the first time, resulting in an incidental PE rate of 0.32%. The findings similarly demonstrated a higher concentration of FDG uptake within the pulmonary artery involved in or close to the PE compared to normal arteries. Additionally, FDG avidity can also be seen in pulmonary infarcts.

FDG-PET uptake may differentiate PE from other pulmonary artery diseases, such as pulmonary sarcoma [10]. Lee et al. undertook a retrospective study involving 18 subjects, observing that malignant pulmonary artery lesions exhibited higher uptake compared to PE (SUV_{max} 10.2 ± 10.8 vs. 1.7 ± 0.3, $p < 0.001$) [245]. Caution needs to be taken when using uptake values, however, as numerous studies have shown that pulmonary artery sarcoma can have a low FDG uptake [171, 243, 442].

^{68}Gallium V/Q PET/CT is another promising imaging modality for PE detection. A recent study conducted on 24 cancer patients compared the interobserver agreement in the interpretation of ^{68}Gallium V/Q PET/CT with CTPA for the diagnosis of acute PE. In this study, ^{68}Gallium was used as a substitute for Technegas ("Galligas") as well as for MAA labeling. The interobserver agreement in the interpretation of V/Q PET/CT was high compared to CTPA (kappa coefficient of 0.79 vs. 0.39). The researchers attributed the main discrepancies in CTPA findings to detecting clots in the subsegmental arteries [239]. Additionally, a cohort study with 100 subjects similarly found near-perfect interobserver agreement in V/Q SPECT interpretation. In contrast, previous interobserver agreement studies of CTPA showed low interobserver variability among radiologists in interpreting subsegmental PE [89, 145, 338]. Based on the European Society of Cardiology guidelines for the diagnosis and management of acute PE [217], if the CTPA report suggests a single subsegmental PE, a high probability of false-positive results should be considered. To avoid misdiagnosis and unnecessary anticoagulation, the findings should be reviewed again with the radiologist or another reader. Nonetheless, additional studies with larger sample sizes are needed to fully investigate and establish the capacity of V/Q PET/CT for detecting and diagnosing PE.

Acute Respiratory Distress Syndrome

Acute respiratory distress syndrome (ARDS) is the leading cause of death among patients in the critical care setting. According to recent studies, ARDS accounts for 10.4% of admissions to ICUs, and only 60.2% of all patients with ARDS can be properly recognized by clinicians, indicating the need for better diagnosis and management strategies [38, 286]. In ARDS, diffuse endothelial damage occurs alongside the presence of macro- and microthrombi, which can progress to fibrocellular intimal proliferation and subsequent obstruction of small vessels, causing pulmonary hypertension. The lung scintigraphy findings can be variable, as different areas may show either low or high ventilation-perfusion ratios. Multiple bilateral mismatched defects have been reported in ARDS patients [349].

In recent years, PET has been frequently used to study the pathophysiology of ARDS in both clinical and experimental settings. Previously explored tracers include

- ^{15}O oxygen-labeled water ($H_2{}^{15}O$) as a measure of regional perfusion and lung water [305].
- ^{13}N nitrogen ($^{13}N_2$): $^{13}N_2$ infusion to measure regional perfusion, shunt, ventilation of perfused alveoli, and gas trapping followed by $^{13}N_2$ inhalation scans to measure regional aeration and ventilation (including dead-space ventilation) [305, 308].
- ^{11}C: in the form of carbon monoxide (^{11}CO) [337], to derive extravascular lung water from $H_2{}^{15}O$ measurements of lung water, as ^{11}C-methylalbumin [376] to measure vascular permeability, ^{11}C-TSPO for macrophage infiltration [70], or 11C-labeled agents for neutrophil imaging [345].
- ^{68}Ga-transferrin: used to measure vascular permeability [376].
- ^{68}Ga-albumin aggregates: used to assess the regional distribution of pulmonary perfusion in research trials [374].

PET is a versatile imaging modality that can quantify various parameters relevant to ARDS, including regional perfusion, ventilation, aeration, lung vascular permeability, edema, enzyme activity, and pulmonary gene expression [37]. PET imaging offers additional insights into morphological imaging. For example, a CT scan has revealed a mixture of normally aerated and derecruited lung tissue, which is predominant in dependent areas. However, PET has shown that the increase in pulmonary vascular permeability is uniform throughout the lungs in ARDS patients, even in normally aerated areas. This indicates that the disease process affects even the well-aerated regions of the lungs [367].

Moreover, PET measurements of regional perfusion have also found an inverse relationship between the fraction of pulmonary blood flow that perfuses dependent regions of the lung and the patient's PaO_2/FiO_2 ratio [375]. This implies that patients with similar amounts and patterns of lung opacities on CT or chest X-ray images, depending on how effectively their perfusion redistributes away from non-aerated regions, may show significantly different levels of ARDS severity. Combined PET measurements of perfusion and shunt have also shown that redistribution of perfusion toward derecruited areas is a responsible mechanism for the worsening oxygenation after recruitment maneuvers [137, 307] or PEEP [306]. Therefore, clinicians should be careful when using PaO_2 as an index of ARDS severity or the response to treatments, especially if the perfusion distribution is unknown.

Serial PET scans have provided a better understanding of the temporal evolution in disease processes associated with ARDS. In experimental studies, the use of PET with ^{68}Ga-albumin aggregates revealed a biphasic response to acid aspiration, a common cause of ARDS. In the first hour after aspiration, blood flow rises in affected areas, suggesting a hyperemic response. However, by 2 h, perfusion is lower in regions with aspiration than in the spared regions (may be due to hypoxic pulmonary vasoconstriction or vascular compression by the exudate) [191]. The pathophysiology of ARDS is closely linked to hyaluronic acid (HA) or hyaluronan, a type of glycosaminoglycan that is an important component of the extracellular matrix and is widely distributed in the human lung parenchyma [136]. The exudative phase of ARDS is initiated by low-molecular-weight HA, which acts as a sensor of lung tissue damage [255]. Additionally, HA is a powerful water-binding molecule that contributes to interstitial and alveolar edema, leading to the formation of "hyaline membranes" observed in COVID-19 patients [32]. Radioisotopes suitable for SPECT (^{123}I, ^{99m}Tc, and ^{111}In) and PET (^{124}I) imaging can be used to label HA fragments [223, 238, 289]. A recent study by Zhao et al. investigated the efficacy of using radiolabeled HA10 for quantitative imaging of mouse models of ARDS via a high-resolution iQID camera. Dynamic imaging of ^{99m}Tc-HA10 in the mouse models of ARDS revealed a significant increase in uptake and prolonged activity in the lungs, indicative of prominent inflammatory changes. Postmortem biodistribution assessment of ^{99m}Tc-HA10 (%ID/g) was 11.0 ± 3.9 vs. 1.3 ± 0.3 in the ARDS mice and controls, respectively ($P < 0.001$), consistent with an increase in HA10 expression. The researchers suggested that the rate of ^{99m}Tc-HA10 clearance from injured lungs using rapid iQID imaging may offer a functional template for timely evaluation and quantification of ARDS [471].

Acute Lung Injury

As inflammatory cells, especially neutrophils, have higher glucose metabolism than other pulmonary cells, using PET/CT imaging to measure the uptake rate (K_i) of ^{18}F-FDG is a valuable method to evaluate the pulmonary inflammatory response in acute lung injury (ALI) [73, 137]. The Patlak K_i value, a dynamic index reflecting ^{18}F-FDG uptake over time, has been evaluated in-depth for the quantification of animal and human models of ALI [71, 73, 74, 88]. Some experts aimed to compare different quantification methods for dynamic ^{18}F-FDG PET data in human lungs and evaluate their potential in the clinical setting.

In a study by Grecchi et al. [154], 11 patients with ALI and 5 healthy controls underwent a dynamic ^{18}F-FDG PET/CT scan. Four different approaches were used for the quantification of glucose metabolism, including SUV, ratio, Patlak, and spectral analysis iterative filter (SAIF), which were applied at both regional and voxel levels. Compared to the ratio, SUV showed a weaker correlation with the net tracer uptake, whereas both Patlak and SAIF analysis showed no significant spatial or quantitative differences. These findings were in accordance with previous studies that exhibited the superiority of the ratio model in explaining tracer kinetics compared to SUV [428, 434]. Full kinetic modeling presents a multiparametric description of glucose metabolism in the lungs. This technique enables analysis of the spatial distribution of lung inflammation and functional state of the tissues [154].

In contrast to K_i, static indices like standardized uptake ratio (SUR) measure the amount of ^{18}F-FDG in a region of interest (ROI) compared to a reference region [428]. The ability of SUV and SUR_{stat} (static ^{18}F-FDG PET/CT) metrics to estimate K_i (dynamic ^{18}F-FDG PET/CT) has been previously examined. An experimental study on 14 anesthetized pigs with ALI showed a weaker K_i–SUV and a strong K_i–SUR_{stat} correlation at different levels of lung inflammation. They attributed the strong relation between K_i and SUR_{stat} to the shape invariance of the arterial input function of ^{18}F-FDG across all time points and animals [15]. Similarly, another experimental ALI study on dogs showed a strong correlation between K_i and tissue-to-plasma activity ratios, while K_i-SUV association was weak [73]. Additionally, Mannes and colleagues performed FDG-PET in a preclinical model of lipopolysaccharide-induced ALI. The researchers observed a significant increase in lung uptake of ^{18}F-FDG during the induction of ALI and a decrease in ^{18}F-FDG concentration following dexamethasone treatment. Furthermore, the protein expression of inflammatory biomarkers as well as the activity of glycolytic enzymes and neutrophil elastase were found to be augmented in the lungs of affected mice and were associated with higher ^{18}F-FDG uptake. It can be concluded that ^{18}F-FDG PET/CT noninvasively detects lung inflammation and evaluates treatment response to dexamethasone therapy [279].

Chronic Pulmonary Conditions

Chronic Vascular Disease

Chronic Thromboembolic Pulmonary Hypertension

Pulmonary hypertension (PH) is characterized by increased pressure in the pulmonary artery, leading to dyspnea, limited exercise capacity, reduced quality of life, and early death due to right ventricular dysfunction. Chronic thromboembolic pulmonary hypertension (CTEPH) is classified as WHO Group 4 of PH caused by persistent obstruction of the pulmonary artery due to thrombi [99, 211]. The exact incidence of CTEPH is unknown, but it is estimated to affect approximately 0.5–9% of individuals with a history of PE [232]. Thus, CTEPH is a rare but life-threatening condition, which, if left untreated, can be fatal.

Diagnostic algorithms [141, 277] suggest that V/Q lung imaging is an essential initial step in evaluating CTEPH patients [300]. Although V/Q SPECT/CT scans may have higher sensitivity than planar scans in detecting perfusion defects, both modalities can be used for initial screening. The presence of persistent mismatched perfusion defects is a hallmark feature of CTEPH (Fig. 25.9). Normal V/Q scans have a high sensitivity (96–97%) and specificity (90–95%) for excluding CTEPH [309]. However, in non-occlusive disease, V/Q scans may not accurately estimate the degree of pulmonary vascular obstruction. Therefore, even a single segmental perfusion defect should raise suspicion for CTEPH [361]. CTPA can assess lung parenchyma and evaluate for conditions that may mimic CTEPH, but it is not recommended as the initial test [100]. Studies have reported the sensitivity of CTPA in diagnosing CTEPH ranges from 51% to 92% [346]. In a prospective study by He J. et al. involving 114 subjects with CTEPH, the researchers observed a sensitivity of 100% with V/Q scans, which was quantitatively superior to CTPA's sensitivity of 92.2%. Nonetheless, the authors concluded that the results were comparable, and both V/Q scans and CTPA demonstrated excellent efficacy [211, 309].

There is a growing interest in using a pulmonary vascular obstruction index (PVOI) as a quantification method in patients with PE or CTEPH. This index indicates the percentage of the total lung volume with perfusion defects [138, 231]. Although the Meyer score has been used as the reference method for quantifying the PVOI on planar lung V/Q scintigraphy in numerous studies, it is hard to implement in daily practice due to its subjectivity, complexity, and time-consuming nature. In contrast, the segmental visual scoring (SVS) method is commonly used by nuclear medicine physicians. This method assigns a score by adding 5% for each segmental perfusion defect or its equivalent (two subsegments = one segment). The obtained score corresponds to the mean percent volume of a segment in a 20-segment model (100 divided by 20) [240]. Recently, Pennec et al. assessed the valid-

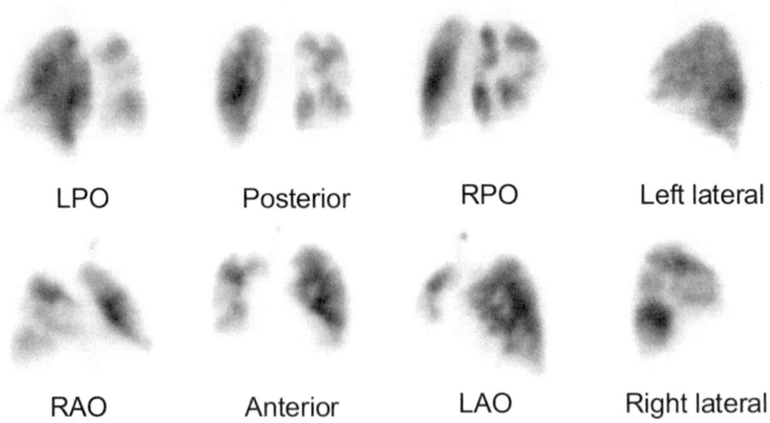

Fig. 25.9 CTEPH on V/Q scan. Perfusion images of CTEPH show similar findings as acute pulmonary embolism with multifocal segmental type defects

ity of the SVS method in their pioneering study by comparing it to the Meyer score for quantifying PVOI on planar V/Q lung scintigraphy. The SVS revealed a strong correlation and low differences in PVOI quantification compared to the Meyer score, making it a more practical and time-efficient option for everyday clinical practice [240].

Several studies have reviewed the feasibility of using V/Q SPECT/CT to provide quantitative information on the extent of perfusion defects in CTEPH [249, 309, 404]. In a recent study, 30 patients with CTEPH underwent ^{99m}Tc–MAA lung perfusion SPECT/CT, and different approaches were used to quantify perfusion defects. Researchers revealed the feasibility of using semiquantitative visual scoring and quantitative volumetric approaches to analyze SPECT images in CTEPH. These methods provide more information than the traditional clinical approach of detecting perfusion defects and may enhance the assessment of perfusion abnormalities. Therefore, a quantitative analysis of threshold-based segmentation of perfused lung volumes using SPECT images can provide a direct measure of the severity and correlates well with established clinical parameters in patients with CTEPH [106]. A prospective assessment [249] of 208 patients, 69 of whom had pulmonary angiography that confirmed CTEPH showed that V/Q planar imaging, V/Q SPECT alone, and perfusion SPECT/CT were all highly effective for diagnosing CTEPH (sensitivity/specificity: planar, 94.2/92.8%; SPECT, 97.1/91.4%; perfusion SPECT/CT, 95.7/90.7%), although planar imaging and SPECT may be more specific (SPECT, 79.2%; planar imaging, 75.84% [$P = 0.012$]; perfusion SPECT/CT, 74.9% [$P < 0.001$]) and sensitive (planar imaging, 54.1%; SPECT, 46.1% [$P < 0.001$]; perfusion SPECT, 46.1% [$P = 0.001$]), respectively, for identifying defects in individual segments.

Several studies have investigated the use of lung perfusion scans to evaluate the response to balloon pulmonary angioplasty (BPA). Hashimoto et al. assessed the efficacy of BPA in patients with CTEPH for the first time using lung perfusion SPECT/CT. Twenty cases diagnosed with CTEPH underwent lung perfusion SPECT/CT before and after BPA. The study analyzed the correlation between functional lung volume obtained from lung perfusion SPECT and other clinical parameters. BPA resulted in improvement in different hemodynamic, clinical, and functional measures, including the functional volume of lung calculated from lung perfusion SPECT (FVL-LPSPECT). There was a notable correlation between FVL-LPSPECT and mean pulmonary artery pressure (mPAP) at baseline ($r = -0.728$, $P < 0.001$). According to their findings, FVL-LPSPECT has the ability to be used as an indicator of BPA effectiveness in CTEPH patients [162]. Similarly, [284] reported that a quantitative index of pulmonary perfusion scintigraphy using three-dimensional fractal analysis could predict therapeutic success following BPA in patients with CTEPH. In their study, patients in the high-mPAP group who had a poor response to BPA showed a substantial decrease in total uptake volume and a greater increase in post-BPA fractal dimension compared to those with low-mPAP group. These findings suggest that persistent image heterogenicity and a smaller total uptake volume increase on ^{99m}Tc-MAA SPECT after BPA may indicate the need for further treatment.

Metabolic imaging is being explored for its potential utility in CTEPH. In a recent study, elevated glucose (measured by ^{18}F-FDG) and fatty acid (β-methyl-p-^{123}I-iodophenyl-pentadecanoic acid (BMIPP)) uptake were observed in the right ventricle of patients with CTEPH. The study further showed reduced uptake following pulmonary endarterectomy [364]. BMIPP deposition in the right ventricle has also been strongly correlated with pulmonary hemodynamics [365]. Although these findings are interesting, the primary role of PET in CTEPH is to differentiate it from other conditions that can mimic the disease, prevent misdiagnosis, and minimize treatment delays.

Hepatopulmonary Syndrome

Identification and quantification of right-to-left shunts is a common indication for quantitative V/Q scans. These shunts can be divided into both cardiac causes, most commonly congenital heart disease (CHD), and noncardiac causes (or intrapulmonary shunts). The role of quantitative V/Q scans in CHD will be discussed separately in the pediatric section, while this section will be limited to noncardiac right-to-left shunts, specifically hepatopulmonary syndrome (HPS). HPS is an uncommon complication that can develop in patients with liver cirrhosis, portal hypertension, and/or congenital portosystemic shunts. While the precise mechanisms underpinning HPS are unknown, it is generally thought that there is an overproduction of vasoactive mediators, such as nitric oxide, resulting in pulmonary angiogenesis and vasodilation [204]. Intrapulmonary vascular dilatations (IPVDs) and similar alterations in the pulmonary microvasculature result in the impairment of gas exchange through mechanisms of ventilation-perfusion mismatch, oxygen diffusion limitation, and anatomic shunting [422].

Quantitative lung perfusion scans can be helpful in the diagnosis of HPS, which requires confirmation of both oxygenation impairment and the presence of shunting from IPVDs. Oxygenation impairment or hypoxemia is established through arterial blood gas (ABG) analysis with an elevated alveolar–arterial oxygen gradient ≥15 mmHg (≥20 mmHg in those 64 years or older) [222, 355]. Pulse oximetry may be used as a screening tool for hypoxemia in patients with chronic liver disease and dyspnea but is not considered sufficient for diagnosis [222]. Lung perfusion scintigraphy represents one of two methods, the other being contrast-enhanced echocardiography (CEE), which can identify the presence of shunting from IVPDs.

As previously mentioned, ^{99m}Tc-MAA particles are trapped in pre-capillary alveolar arterioles following intravenous injection in healthy patients. By contrast, the abnormally dilated pulmonary vessels in patients with HPS are unable to adequately hold the radiolabeled particles, giving them free passage to the systemic circulation.

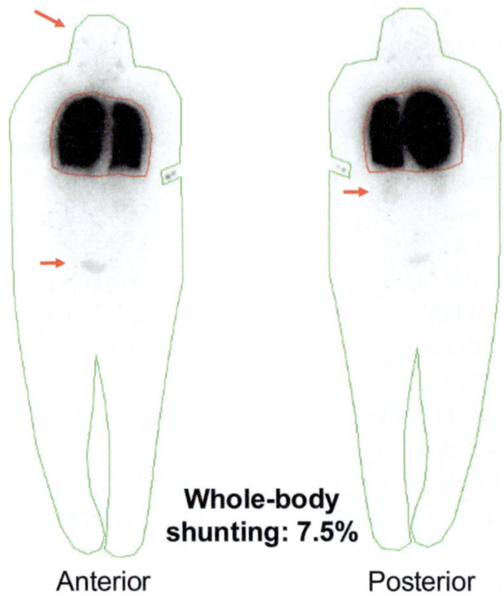

Fig. 25.10 Quantification of systemic shunting in a patient with cirrhosis and hypoxemia. Anterior and posterior ^{99m}Tc-MAA perfusion planar whole-body images reveal homogeneous intense radiotracer uptake within the lungs with mild extrapulmonary uptake, predominantly within the brain, kidneys, and bladder (red arrows). Regions of interest are drawn around the whole body (green outline) and lungs (red outline) on both the anterior and posterior projections for quantification of systemic shunting, calculated as 7.5%. While the shunting was presumed to represent hepatopulmonary syndrome (HPS) in this patient, a patent foramen ovale (PFO) with associated right-to-left shunting was subsequently identified on echocardiogram and confirmed as the cause. This case highlights a potential downside of perfusion scintigraphy in HPS in that it cannot differentiate intracardiac and intrapulmonary shunts

The particles subsequently become lodged in nondilated, highly vascular systemic end-organ capillaries, such as those located in the brain and kidneys [142]. Visualization of radiotracer uptake within the brain and kidneys is diagnostic of right-to-left shunting (Fig. 25.10). Comparison of extrapulmonary counts relative to the total number of counts on whole-body images allows for accurate quantification of the shunt fraction with use of the following formula [143]:

$$\text{R}-\text{L shunt}(\%)=\left[\begin{array}{l}(\text{total body geometric mean counts}-\text{total lung geometric mean counts})\\ /\text{total body geometric mean counts}\end{array}\right]\times 100.$$

^{99m}Tc-MAA scans can underestimate the intrapulmonary shunt fraction in cases of severe liver disease due to the presence of renal and cerebral arterial vasoconstriction, which increases with the progression of liver disease [197]. It is for this reason that whole-body uptake is utilized more commonly for shunt quantification than kidney or brain uptake alone [473]. A shunt fraction greater than 6% is typical for HPS [4].

While ^{99m}Tc-MAA scintigraphy can help in the diagnosis of HPS, it is not considered the initial test of choice. Rather, CEE is considered the gold standard as it is more sensitive and can differentiate between intracardiac and intrapulmonary shunts, unlike ^{99m}Tc-MAA scintigraphy [4, 222]. Despite these drawbacks, ^{99m}Tc-MAA scintigraphy still has utility in this patient population and can be considered complementary to CEE. Specifically, this type of scan is valuable in patients with concomitant lung disease, helping to determine the contribution of shunt versus lung disease to a patient's hypoxemia [121, 283]. Furthermore, quantitative ^{99m}Tc-MAA scans can have prognostic value. In patients planning to undergo liver transplantation, a shunt fraction greater than or equal to 20% is associated with higher perioperative mortality [18]. Finally, it can serve as an alternative imaging option in patients with a nondiagnostic CEE.

Chronic Lung Disease

Chronic Obstructive Pulmonary Dis ease

Chronic obstructive pulmonary disease (COPD) is a heterogeneous lung condition characterized by abnormalities of the airways [chronic bronchitis and/or alveoli (emphysema)] that result in persistent, often progressive airflow obstruction. These pathophysiologic lung changes can be visually represented on V/Q scans as heterogeneous ventilation with multifocal ventilation defects [189]. These defects typically demonstrate corresponding matched perfusion defects but rarely are more pronounced relative to the perfusion defects—referred to as a reverse mismatch [30]. Focal deposition of radiolabeled aerosols in central or peripheral airways is another frequent finding in patients with COPD, more commonly seen with DTPA compared with Technegas [190]. Relative to radio aerosols, xenon tends to be more sensitive to obstructive airway disease, with regions of air trapping manifesting as retention of radiotracer on washout phase images (Fig. 25.11) [104].

This pattern, however, is not specific to COPD. While V/Q scans cannot definitively diagnose COPD, they can suggest early disease prior to the development of anatomic imaging changes, as well as global changes in pulmonary function tests [323]. V/Q scans can additionally be used to grade disease severity [29]. A statistically significant correlation has been reported between the degree of abnormalities seen on aerosol ventilation imaging and pulmonary function tests [394]. Visual interpretation of V/Q scans is typically adequate for these specific applications.

While more limited in scope, quantitative analysis does have a critical role to play in this patient population. Specifically, it is invaluable for the preoperative evaluation of those who plan to undergo lung volume reduction surgery (LVRS), which includes surgical resection and bronchoscopic methods via placement of one-way endobronchial valves [301]. LVRS allows for a reduction in the volume of hyperinflated dysfunctional lung while remaining functioning tissue can re-expand, altogether leading to improved gas exchange [421]. Quantitative V/Q scans enable appropriate target lobe selection. Lung regions with poor perfusion are specifically selected as targets, as higher perfusion in the untreated ipsilateral lobe is a strong predictor of exercise capacity improvement following valve placement [413, 421].

Asthma

Several studies have examined the application of ^{99m}Tc-Technegas for evaluating asthmatic patients. For instance, Farrow et al. established a notable correlation between severe airway hyperresponsiveness and airway closure observed during ventilation SPECT/CT scans [130]. In a separate study involving 14 patients with asthma, the same group of researchers showed that ventilation is decreased in areas affected by bronchoconstriction and that the extent of reduction can

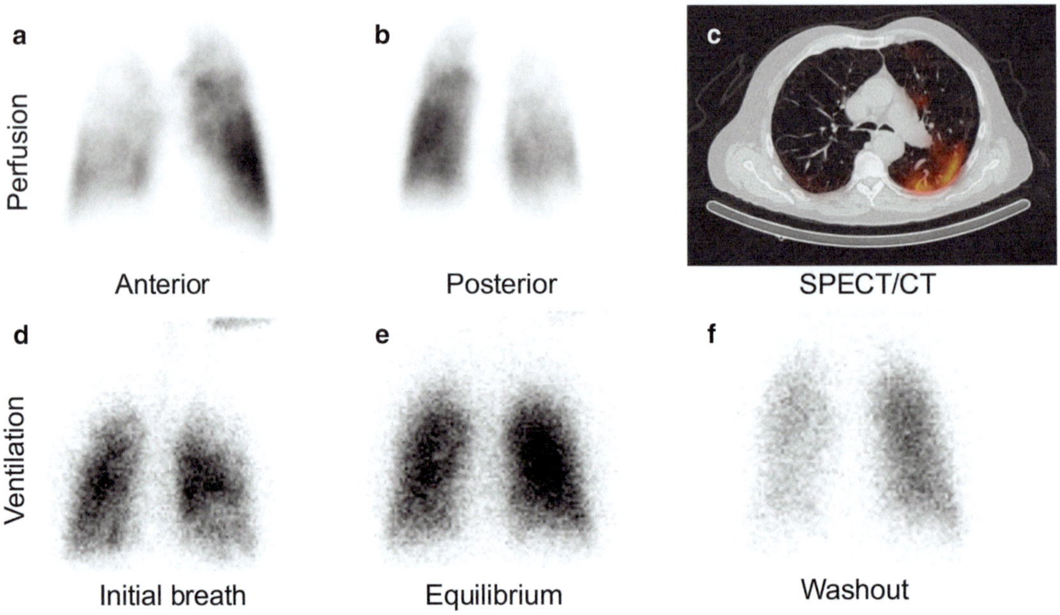

Fig. 25.11 Quantitative ventilation/perfusion scan in a patient with COPD prior to endobronchial valve placement. (**a**) Anterior and (**b**) posterior planar ^{99m}Tc-MAA perfusion images of the lungs demonstrate relatively decreased perfusion in the right compared to the left lung. Within the right lung, there is relatively decreased perfusion in the upper and mid lung zones, with relatively preserved perfusion within the dependent portion of the lower lung zone, while there is relatively decreased perfusion in the upper lung zone in the left lung. (**c**) Axial fused SPECT/CT image of the chest mirrors planar findings with decreased perfusion in the right greater than the left lung due to the presence of severe emphysema. (**d**) Single-breath, (**e**) equilibrium, and (**f**) washout posterior Xe-133 ventilation images of the lungs exhibit matched ventilation defects in the bilateral upper lung zones and right lung base. Air trapping within the right greater than the left lungs can be identified on the washout images. Quantitative analysis (not pictured) confirmed poor perfusion within the right upper and middle lobes. The patient subsequently underwent endobronchial valve placement within the right upper and middle lobes

be predicted by acinar ventilation heterogeneity [131].

In a cohort of 84 patients, ^{99m}Tc-DTPA facilitated the differentiation of individuals with non-smoker COPD from asthmatic patients. The mucociliary clearance, measured as $T_{½}$ using ^{99m}Tc-DTPA, was significantly higher in patients with asthma than in nonsmoking COPD patients [200]. The importance of macrophages in COPD and asthma is well-established, particularly in relation to pulmonary inflammation. Jones et al. studied a radiolabeled form of PK11195, an agent targeting the translocator protein in macrophages. ^{11}C-PK11195 was used to examine patients with COPD, asthma, and healthy individuals [193]. The development of molecular imaging agents specific to matrix metalloproteases (MMPs) released by inflammatory cells, primarily macrophages, has been investigated in asthma and COPD with the goal of early detection and monitoring of disease activity [149].

The role of inflammatory cells, including neutrophils, has been well-established in COPD and asthma. Considering the observed positive correlation between FDG uptake and neutrophil activation, ^{18}F-FDG PET imaging holds immense potential to offer additional information specific to inflammation. However, it is important to note that FDG-PET reflects relative glucose metabolism and is not a direct indicator of neutrophils. To assess the potential utility of ^{18}F-FDG PET/CT as an indicator of pulmonary neutrophilic inflammation, a study involving 30 patients divided into healthy, alpha1-antitrypsin deficiency, and COPD groups was conducted. The study revealed significantly higher FDG uptake in the upper lungs of COPD patients compared to the healthy controls ($P = 0.009$), which was also found to be associated with markers of disease severity. In patients with alpha1-antitrypsin deficiency, there were no significant differences detected between baseline and on-treatment measurements, highlighting the potential of FDG-PET to differentiate among these three study groups [397]. The K_{iN} parameter has been established as the primary metric for quantifying ^{18}F-FDG uptake in COPD and asthma [193, 397]. The K_{iN} of the upper lung zone correlates negatively with pulmonary function and positively with the severity of emphysema as determined by CT scans [397]. However, K_{iN} remains unchanged in patients with stable asthma compared to healthy individuals [193]. Asthma and COPD exacerbations are often provoked by both infections and allergens. Studies suggest that K_{iN} is likely to increase in response to both triggers, as seen in lung transplant recipients with infections [192] and in individuals with asthma after allergen challenge test [161, 408]. Hence, ^{18}F-FDG PET scans should be obtained during periods of clinical stability to examine the accuracy of different quantitative parameters for assessing the specific inflammatory processes associated with lung diseases [72].

Lung Transplant

Quantitative V/Q scans play an important role in patients with chronic lung diseases that are severe enough to warrant lung transplantation. These scans are routinely ordered in the preoperative setting for surgical planning. In those undergoing single-lung transplant, the lung with better perfusion and/or ventilation, as demonstrated on the quantitative V/Q scan, is typically retained while the lung with worse function is replaced [342]. In patients planning to undergo bilateral lung transplants, the surgeon can use the quantitative V/Q scan to determine which lung should be resected first during the surgery. The less functional lung is typically resected first to help decrease the likelihood of needing cardiac bypass during the procedure [342].

While less commonly employed in clinical practice, there is a potential role for quantitative perfusion scans in the postoperative transplant setting for the early identification of chronic lung allograft dysfunction (CLAD) [393, 458]. CLAD typically manifests as a reversal of perfusion toward the native lung in cases of single-lung transplant and a shift in perfusion toward the unaffected lung in bilateral lung transplant [458]. Quantitative lung perfusion scintigraphy 1–3 months following single-lung transplantation was found to predict chronic transplant rejection with higher sensitivity and specificity than FEV_1 (83% and 88% versus 80% and 67%, respectively) [160].

Interstitial Lung Disease

Interstitial lung disease (ILD) is an umbrella term used for a diverse group of diseases that cause pulmonary inflammation and/or fibrosis. ^{18}F-FDG has been extensively studied in the context of ILD [55]. Inflammatory-predominant and metabolically active ILDs are the most intuitive candidates for FDG-PET imaging (Fig. 25.12). For example, Tateishi et al. showed that the SUV of FDG is associated with lymphocyte activity in 22

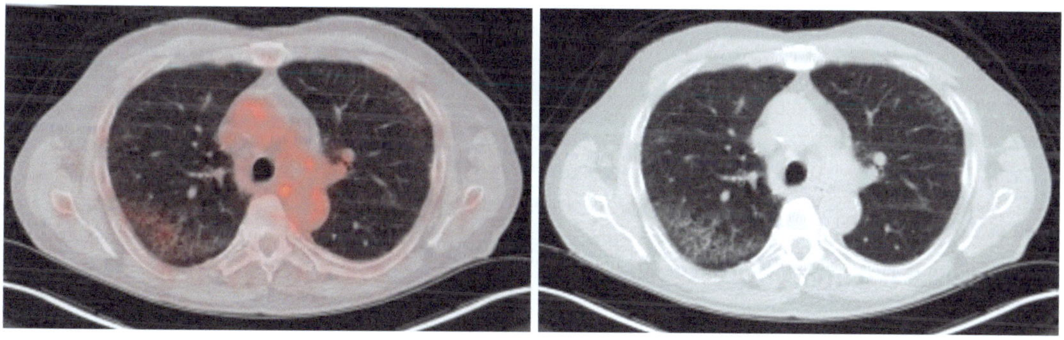

Fig. 25.12 FDG-PET in interstitial lung disease. Subpleural reticulation in the right lower lobe with uptake

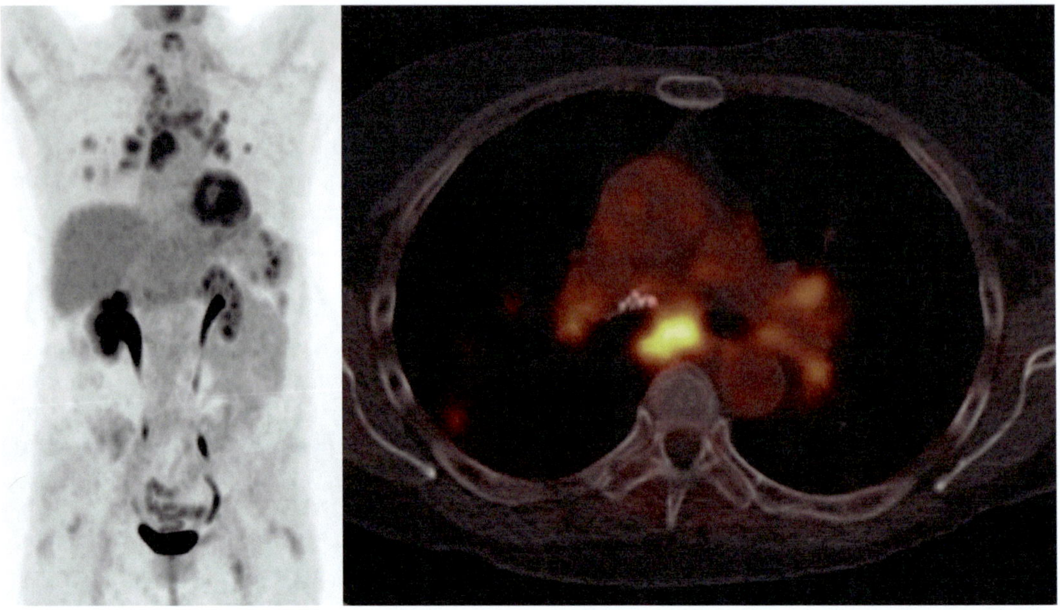

Fig. 25.13 Thoracic manifestation of sarcoidosis on FDG-PET. Multistation FDG-avid mediastinal adenopathy, lung opacities are present on maximum intensity (left) and axial (right) images in a patient with biopsy-proven sarcoidosis. Note is made of FDG-avid splenic manifestations of sarcoid as well

patients diagnosed with organizing pneumonia (OP) [406]. Furthermore, PET activity in metabolically active pulmonary sarcoidosis is correlated with serological evidence of inflammation and loss of pulmonary function (Fig. 25.13) [302].

FDG PET/CT can be particularly useful in sarcoidosis with radiographic stage IV with fibrosis, as the presence of metabolic activity indicates active disease potentially responsive to treatment. In addition, PET/CT can detect active parenchymal disease in radiographic stages 0 and 1 [206, 409]. A major limitation of FDG-PET is its inability to differentiate between benign and malignant causes of ILD. ^{11}C-methionine is a radiotracer used in molecular imaging of amino acid metabolism. This tracer is particularly valuable in tumor imaging because it can detect the increased metabolic activity of amino acids in tumor cells. When combined with FDG, it can help to differentiate inflammation from malignancy, thereby facilitating the diagnosis of sarcoidosis [202]. Increased uptake of ^{18}F-FDG in ILD is primarily due to the high expression of surface GLUT 1–4 receptors on macrophages, neutrophils, and lymphocytes, indicating inflammation. However, subsequent research has shown that the uptake of ^{18}F-FDG reflects overall cellular metabolism and can also be increased in fibrotic areas [117].

^{18}F-FDG PET assessment can distinguish ILD from healthy lung in systemic sclerosis (SSc) patients, suggesting that it may be used as a novel biomarker for evaluating disease activity in SSc-ILD. Peelen et al. reported that the SUV_{mean} values were increased in SSc patients with ILD compared to those without ILD. Moreover, the higher uptake of ^{18}F-FDG in the lungs of SSc patients corresponded to the radiographic findings of ground-glass opacities and reticulation on high-resolution CT imaging [336]. Additionally, Jacqelin et al. conducted a study on 18 patients with cellular and fibrotic nonspecific interstitial pneumonia (NSIP). They found that consolidation, ground-glass opacity, honeycombing, and reticulation exhibited uptake in 90%, 89%, 85%, and 76% of the areas, respectively [182]. Groves et al. showed SUV raised in interstitial pulmonary fibrosis (IPF) and noted higher FDG metabolism in areas of reticulation and honeycombing compared to ground-glass areas [155]. Interestingly, there is also evidence of elevated FDG uptake in seemingly unaffected lung tissue of ILD patients identified by visual inspection and CT density analysis, raising the question of whether SUV is identifying subclinical disease [452]. Conducting additional dual-time-point studies would be useful to determine if these areas undergo significant fibrotic changes on structural images, preferably using formal CT registration tools.

Drug-induced ILD occurs when exposure to a drug causes inflammation and fibrosis of the pulmonary interstitium. In a recent study, 677 patients with lymphoma who underwent multi-cycle chemotherapy were analyzed. FDG-PET/CT imaging revealed increased FDG uptake lung background, thickened septa, reticulation, multiple ground-glass opacities, and grid-shaped blur shadows, observed predominantly in the peripheral lung regions near the pleura. The SUV_{max} in the lung was 2.45 ± 0.52 [272]. Several studies have demonstrated that pulmonary FDG uptake is a predictor of mortality and ILD progression. For instance, in a study by Win and colleagues involving a large cohort of 113 patients, the target-to-background ratio, determined by dividing the SUV_{max} by SUV_{min}, emerged as an independent prognostic indicator for mortality during a mean 29-month follow-up [450].

Recently, some novel PET tracers have been established to diagnose ILD. So far, ^{68}Ga-FAPI-04 (FAP-α) [5, 14, 198], ^{68}Ga-pentixafor (CXCR4) [105], ^{64}Cu-DOTA-ECL1i (CCR2) [54], and ^{68}Ga-CBP8 (collagen type 1) [297] have emerged as the most promising tracers with the potential to improve patient management. Further research is warranted to implement molecular imaging into the clinical management of patients with ILD.

Vascular Conditions

Vasculitides are a heterogeneous group of immune-mediated diseases marked by systemic inflammation targeting blood vessels, leading to ischemic or hemorrhagic complications. Because of the unspecific symptoms, vasculitis may not be initially suspected in the clinical presentation. Therefore, when patients exhibit nonspecific symptoms, the underlying reason may not be detected via biopsy and histopathologic evaluation until vasculitis is identified as a potential factor. For example, vasculitis may present as a fever of unknown origin (FUO) [216]. Identification of FUO remains a challenge. Both the labeled WBC technique [140] and FDG-PET can be used in FUO [303]. Some prefer WBC scan over PET/CT as the primary imaging modality in patients with a high pretest probability for infection [384]. However, FDG-PET has proven to be more sensitive than other imaging modalities [124, 221]. Lung involvement is commonly observed in small-vessel antineutrophil cytoplasmic autoantibody (ANCA)-associated vasculitides. Pulmonary arteries can also be involved in large-vessel vasculitis, such as Takayasu arteritis and giant-cell arteritis, which predominantly target the aorta and its major branches [64]. The radiologic manifestations of pulmonary vasculitis are variable and may include vessel wall thickening, nodules or ground-glass opacities, cavitary lesions, and consolidations [65]. Clinical manifestations such as hemoptysis and chest pain, along with scintigraphic findings of multiple segmental mismatched perfusion defects, may cause clinical overlap between PE and vasculitis. CTPA is valuable in differentiating between these two entities: PE demonstrates intravascular filling defects, whereas vasculitis exhibits vessel wall abnormalities rather than intraluminal abnormalities [164]. FDG-PET/CT is also now commonly used for vasculitis evaluation (Fig. 25.14), with quantitative SUV metrics more of use for monitoring treatment response than initial diagnosis [39].

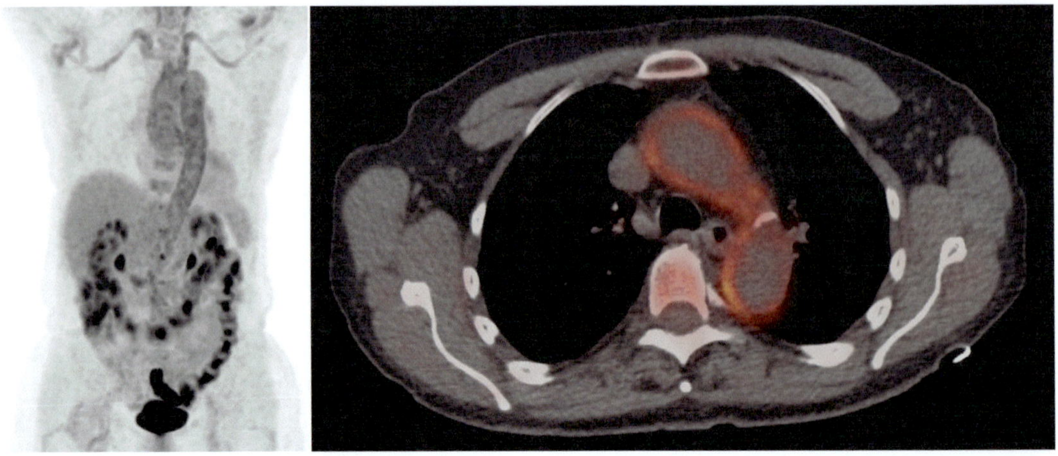

Fig. 25.14 Metabolically active aortitis on FDG-PET. Maximum intensity (left) and axial (right) images in a patient showing diffuse intense uptake along the ascending and descending aorta in keeping with inflammatory aortitis

IgG4-related disease is an immune-mediated chronic fibrotic inflammation affecting multiple organs, including the pulmonary arteries. Pulmonary lesions with low SUV on PET initially raise suspicion of PE or pulmonary thromboembolism. However, most cases have multiple organ involvement, mostly with elevated serum concentrations of IgG4 [103, 475].

Inflammation/Infection

Pneumonitis, or pulmonary inflammation, is a fundamental immune response triggered by harmful stimuli, including exposure to airborne toxins or irritants, respiratory infections, and preexisting lung conditions such as asthma or chronic bronchitis. Inflammation plays a crucial role in the pathogenesis of infection. While not used typically to monitor pneumonia, elevated FDG uptake in lung consolidations is often incidentally found as a sequela of evolving infection and other types of pneumonitis [320].

Antimicrobial peptides (AMPs) labeled with either SPECT (^{99m}Tc) or PET (^{67}Ga) radiotracers have emerged as more specific agents for the localization of infections since they specifically bind to bacterial cell membranes. Studies have demonstrated promising results, particularly in distinguishing bacterial infections from lesions caused by other pathogens [237, 448]. For example, ^{99m}Tc-ethambutol planar and SPECT/CT scintigraphy is effective in tuberculosis as it demonstrates high sensitivity and specificity in detecting pulmonary and extrapulmonary disease [201]. AMPs may be used as a complementary approach in the future, following ^{18}F-FDG, to enhance the specificity of the diagnostic process [8]. However, in translating results from animal models to humans, the process may not be fully comprehensive due to biases associated with animal selection and the index test [20].

Manifestations of COVID-19 are especially pronounced in the thorax. While nuclear medicine is likely not the first line for evaluating this disease at the current time, it is important to recognize imaging manifestations of COVID-19 and associated conditions in nuclear medicine studies [432]. Of special note, awareness of axillary lymphadenopathy after vaccinations on various PET studies should be recognized, especially in oncologic patient follow-up (Fig. 25.15).

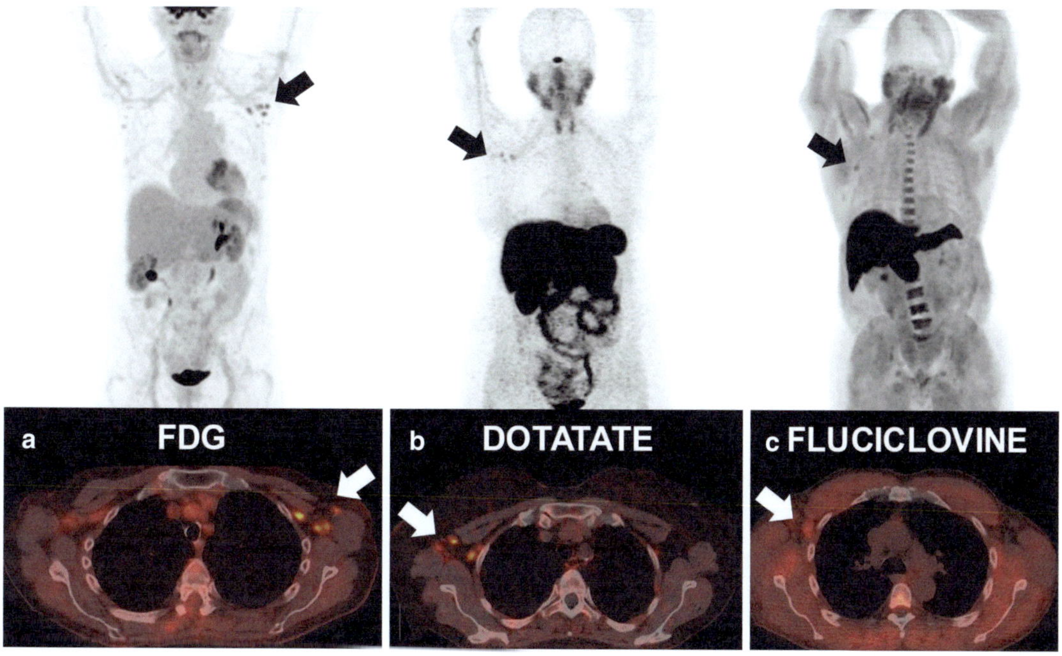

Fig. 25.15 Hypermetabolic lymphadenopathy following COVID vaccination. (**a**) MIP and axial fused images of a 73-year-old woman with lung adenocarcinoma demonstrating ^{18}F-FDG-avid left axillary lymphadenopathy 3 days after receiving the second mRNA-1273 vaccine dose on the left arm. (**b**) MIP and axial fused images of a 57-year-old woman with well-differentiated appendiceal neuroendocrine tumor and ^{68}Ga-DOTATATE-avid right axillary lymphadenopathy 7 days after receiving the second BNT162b2 mRNA vaccine dose on the right arm. (**c**) MIP and axial fused images of a 63-year-old man with recently diagnosed prostate cancer presenting with ^{18}F-fluciclovine-avid right axillary lymphadenopathy 3 days after receiving the third dose of mRNA-1273 vaccine in the right arm. (Reprinted with permission from Vaz et al. [432])

Pediatrics

Congenital Heart Disease (CHD)

By far, the most common indication for quantitative V/Q scans in the pediatric population relates to CHD. Being able to assess for differential lung perfusion in this patient population is crucial, as asymmetric lung perfusion is not only a common downstream effect in patients with complex CHD but also a predictor of long term patient outcomes and exercise capacity [351]. In patients with CHD-associated pulmonary vascular abnormalities, the differential lung perfusion reflects their hemodynamic impact, which in turn helps guide treatment [433]. Current guidelines recommend intervention in cases of relative flow discrepancy between the two lungs ≥35/65%, as this indicates severe underlying pulmonary arterial stenosis [133]. Consequently, multiple major societies have rated this imaging modality as appropriate or may be appropriate following repair or palliation in patients with a variety of CHDs, including single-ventricle heart disease, D-transposition of the great arteries (D-TGA), truncus arteriosus (TA), double-outlet right ventricle (DORV), total anomalous pulmonary venous connection (TAPVC), pulmonary atresia with intact ventricular septum (PA/IVS), and patent ductus arteriosus (PDA) [362].

In patients with CHD-associated right-to-left shunting, quantitative lung perfusion scans have the added benefit of accurate shunt fraction calculation (Fig. 25.16). Right-to-left intracardiac

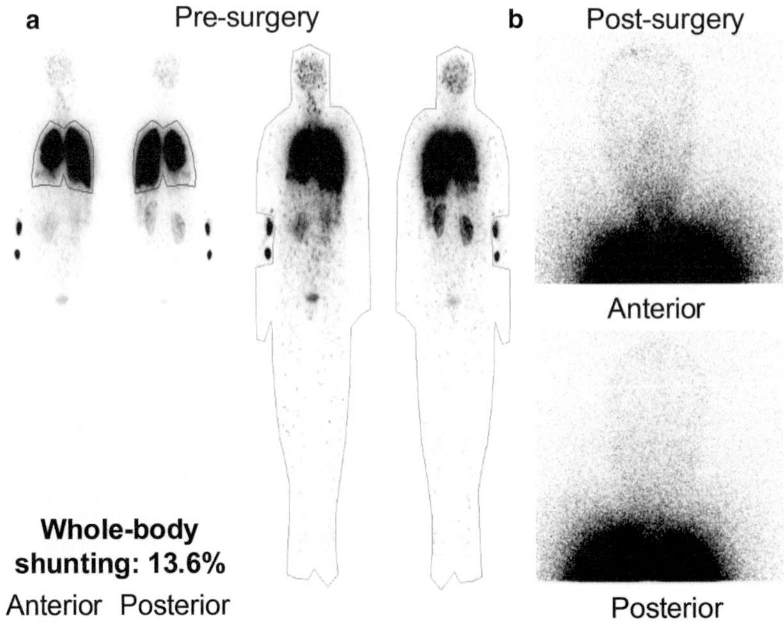

Fig. 25.16 Quantification of whole-body shunting before and after successful closure of a patent foramen ovale (PFO) with associated right-to-left shunting. (**a**) Anterior and posterior ^{99m}Tc-MAA perfusion planar whole-body images demonstrate intense pulmonary and moderate extrapulmonary radiotracer uptake. The presence of extrapulmonary radiotracer, specifically within the brain and kidneys, with shunting greater than 10% confirms the presence of a right-to-left shunt. Regions of interest are drawn around the whole body (green outline) and lungs (red outline) on both the anterior and posterior projections for quantification of systemic shunting, which was determined to be 13.6% for this patient with a PFO in the pre-surgical setting. (**b**) Anterior and posterior planar images of the brain on a follow-up ^{99m}Tc-MAA perfusion study following PFO closure without any detectable brain uptake, confirming successful intervention

shunting occurs in patients with cyanotic CHD, which includes tetralogy of Fallot (TOF), TGA, TA, hypoplastic right heart, TAPVC, and Eisenmenger syndrome [132]. A whole-body scan, using regions of interest over the entire body and the lungs, allows for the accurate estimation of systemic activity, which is proportional to the size and severity of the shunt. Greater than 10% is typically considered abnormal. The process for quantification is similar to that described above for HPS.

While quantitative lung perfusion scintigraphy is simple and widely available, it does have some limitations. Lung scintigraphy is unable to accurately assess perfusion in patients with congenital unilateral absence of the pulmonary artery and bilateral pulmonary artery stenosis if the severity is relatively symmetric [132, 433]. Injection site—upper or lower extremities—can have a large impact on the relative lung perfusion ratio and may over- or underestimate lung perfusion in patients with certain surgical shunts or who have undergone certain palliative procedures, including those with Fontan circulation and surgical SVC-RPA (Glenn) shunts [403]. Knowing a patient's anatomy and surgical history with careful selection of injection sites are thus critical for avoiding interpretation errors.

Cystic Fibrosis

Another common indication for quantitative V/Q scans in the pediatric population relates to the management of patients with cystic fibrosis (CF). Similar to other chronic lung diseases, CF manifests on V/Q scans as heterogeneous ventilation with multifocal ventilation defects and corresponding matching perfusion defects. Given the lack of specificity of these findings, lung scintigraphy is not recommended for the diagnosis of CF. However, it can help monitor disease severity and progression as the degree of abnormalities on ventilation imaging tends to correlate with pulmonary function tests in more advanced disease and better reflects underlying lung damage than clinical status and corresponding chest radiographs, particularly earlier in the disease [126, 183]. These abnormalities may additionally be predictive of the need for further treatment modification and patient outcomes [183, 340]. In a retrospective study of 50 children with CF, 65% of patients with abnormal lung ventilation scans underwent subsequent treatment modification compared with 23% of those with normal scans [183].

In patients with severe disease, quantitative V/Q scans may help in guiding decisions regarding lung transplant. A perfusion disparity >30% between lungs on pre-transplant lung perfusion scintigraphy was shown to be predictive of decreased survival in patients with CF awaiting lung transplant [392]. This would suggest that earlier transplantation, if feasible, may be particularly beneficial for these high-risk patients. Finally, quantitative V/Q scans may be used for preoperative planning and postoperative evaluation in transplant patients, similar to that described above for adult populations.

Congenital Diaphragmatic Hernia

Less common indications for quantitative V/Q scans in the pediatric population include structural abnormalities of the chest, including congenital diaphragmatic hernia (CDH). Isolated CDH is a developmental anomaly characterized by a diaphragmatic defect that permits herniation of abdominal viscera/contents into the thorax. It most commonly occurs on the left side but rarely can be right-sided or bilateral [335]. CDH causes malformation of airway architecture as well as dysfunctional pulmonary microvasculature with fewer arterial branches and abnormally thickened arterial walls [322]. Altogether, these pathophysiologic changes cumulate as pulmonary hypoplasia and secondary pulmonary hypertension, which are associated with significant morbidity and mortality [322]. Hypoplasia is most severe within the lung that is ipsilateral to the defect. Contralateral pulmonary hypoplasia, however, may occur if there is an associated mediastinal shift, compressing the contralateral lung.

Lung perfusion scans in CDH patients demonstrate decreased ipsilateral perfusion and ventilation. The degree of ventilation/perfusion abnormalities tends to reflect the severity of lung hypoplasia and correlates well with changes in pulmonary function tests and other clinical markers of disease [47]. A few studies have suggested that quantitative V/Q scans are able to predict patient outcomes. For example, in a retrospective study of 31 patients with CDH, initial ventilation and perfusion of the ipsilateral lung were not only significantly lower in patients with pulmonary morbidity compared to those without but also were strongly correlated with nutritional status at 1 and 2 years (ventilation: $R = 0.503$, $P < 0.01$; perfusion: $R = 0.760$, $P < 0.0001$) [327]. Following surgical repair, ventilation abnormalities tend to progressively improve and eventually normalize, while perfusion impairment may persist in a subset of patients [185, 395]. As expected, those with persistent abnormalities following surgical repair are more likely to have greater pulmonary morbidity and are at higher risk for poor growth and worse nutritional status compared to those with recovered pulmonary vascular function [95, 333, 395].

Esophageal Transit Scintigraphy

Esophageal transit scintigraphy is an uncommon nuclear medicine scan that can evaluate esophageal motility disorders, dysphagia, and neurodegenerative disorders [287, 369]. For a liquid phase study, the patient ingests a mixture of water and ^{99m}Tc-sulfur colloid or ^{99m}Tc-DTPA as a bolus [287]. Images of the chest, including the oral cavity, are obtained in the posterior projection and acquired at a rapid framing rate (Figs 25.17 and 25.18) [81, 369]. Multiple techniques have been described for the optimization of this scan. At our institution, we have the

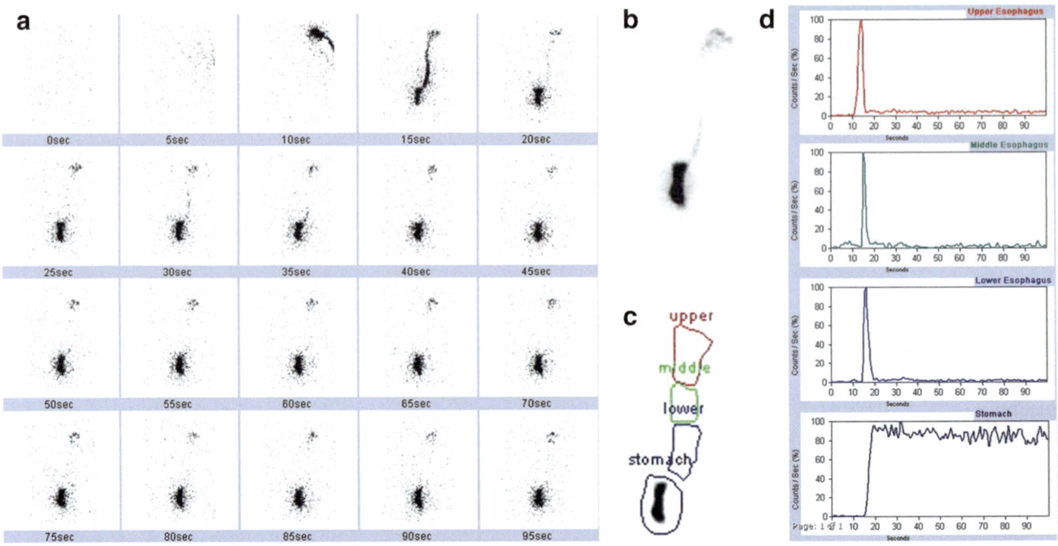

Fig. 25.17 Normal esophageal transit scintigraphy study performed in a 14-year-old girl with dysphagia. (**a**) Posterior upright dynamic images of the esophagus after swallowing water containing ^{99m}Tc-sulfur colloid showing prompt passage of radiotracer through the esophagus. (**b**) Posterior upright composite image depicts the esophagus over the course of the study. (**c**) Regions of interest (ROI) are drawn around the upper, mid, and lower esophagus, and the stomach. (**d**) Time–activity curve generated for each ROI demonstrates prompt passage of radiotracer through each portion of the esophagus (a sharp, discrete spike in sequential order). (Images adapted from Sarma et al. [369])

patient do one swallow while supine and a second one while erect. Two phases of imaging are performed per swallow. For the first phase, the patient swallows once and dynamic images are obtained for 30 s following the initial swallow at 0.25 s per frame for 120 frames. The second phase consists of dynamic images obtained for 10 min at 30 s per frame while the patient "dry swallows" every 30 s during the acquisition.

Following image acquisition, the esophagus is divided into three equal regions of interest (ROIs): proximal, middle, and distal. Time activity curves are created for each ROI, allowing for quantitative analysis. Various quantitative parameters have been validated for clinical use, which include the esophageal transit time and percentage of esophageal transit and retention at specified time points. Esophageal transit time is the time (in seconds) required to clear 90% of the peak activity, where time zero equals the initial swallow. In normal healthy volunteers, a normal transit time is defined as less than 15 s (range of 6–15 s) [16]. Therefore, patients who clear less than 90% of the bolus at 15 s following the initial swallow are considered to have delayed transit. Percentage transit or clearance is measured as the decrease in esophageal activity that occurs from its peak over a specified time point, typically 10 s; it can be calculated using the following formula:

$$\left(\left(\text{number of counts at peak activity minus number of counts at time } t\right) / \text{maximal counts}\right) \times 100\%.$$

A percentage of esophageal transit or clearance that exceeds 83% at 10 s is considered normal [16]. Percentage esophageal retention represents the percentage of the total number of counts that remain in the esophagus at a specified time point, typically 10 min, which represents the

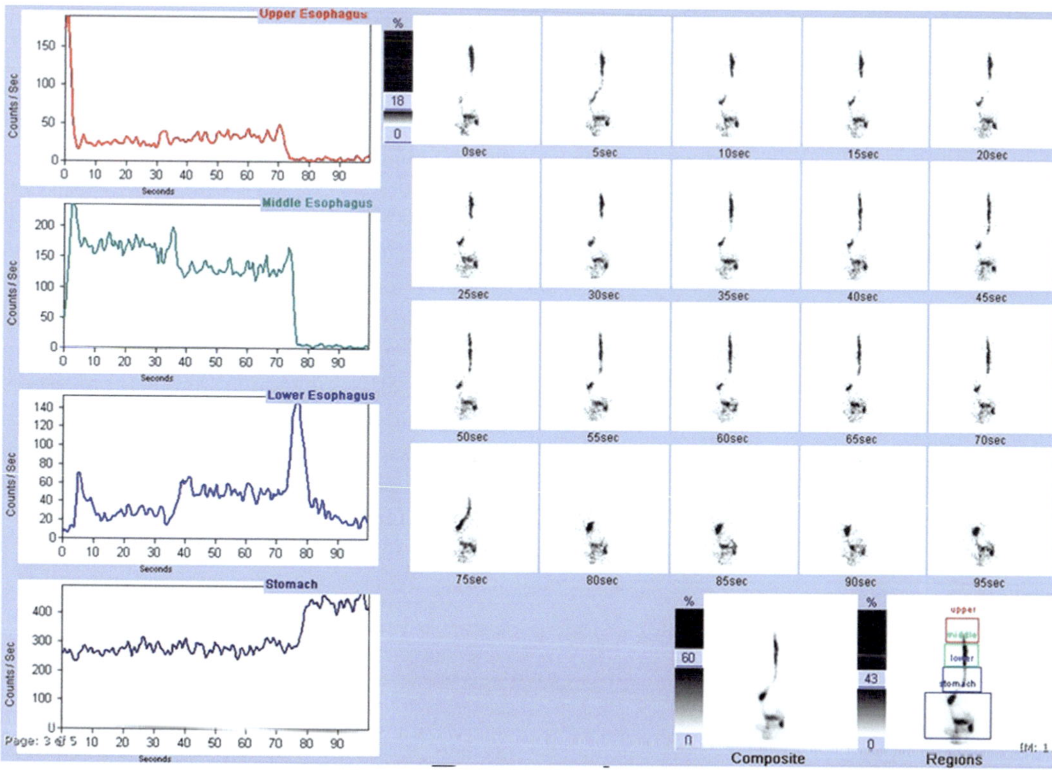

Fig. 25.18 Esophageal transit scintigraphy in a 16-year-old boy with a history of dysphagia. Posterior upright dynamic images demonstrate delayed clearance of scrambled eggs labeled with ^{99m}Tc-sulfur colloid from the mid and distal esophagus, with eventual passage into the stomach at 75–80 s, consistent with nonspecific dysmotility disorder. Manometry showed a large proportion of swallows with ineffective peristalsis. (Images adapted from Sarma et al. [369])

end of the study. Esophageal retention of less than 18% at 10 min has been established as normal in healthy subjects [16].

Through the use of these validated parameters, esophageal scintigraphy can help identify patients with esophageal dysmotility with a similar sensitivity to that of the more commonly utilized techniques of barium swallow and manometry [81, 108, 282]. It, furthermore, provides a more accurate, objective measure of response to intervention or therapy for esophageal stricture.

Lymphoscintigraphy

Malformation of the lymphatic system in the thorax can manifest as chylothorax with multiple congenital, traumatic/iatrogenic, or obstructive secondary to mass effect, among other etiologies [227]. Similar to evaluation of the lymphatics in the extremities, lymphoscintigraphy can be performed with dynamic imaging of ^{99m}Tc-sulfur colloid injected intradermally and following the passage of the radiopharmaceutical across the lymphatic system into systemic circulation followed. Delayed passage and/or atypical distribution of the radiopharmaceutical can be correlated with anatomic imaging to gain insights into the etiology of lymphatic malfunction.

Oncologic Conditions

Quantitative V/Q Scintigraphy

Oncologic indications for quantitative perfusion and ventilation scintigraphy consist of preoperative and radiation therapy planning predominantly in patients with primary lung malignancies. Current guidelines recommend the use of preoperative quantitative lung perfusion and ventilation scintigraphy in patients with borderline lung function—defined as a $FEV_1 > 1$ L but <2–2.5 L in those planning to undergo pneumonectomy—to evaluate their candidacy for lung resection, specifically pneumonectomy [53]. Preoperative evaluation of a patient's pulmonary reserve allows one to predict if the expected postoperative loss of function for that patient will place him/her at an unacceptable risk for perioperative mortality and morbidity and/or long-term disability. While quantitative V/Q scans can accurately predict postoperative lung function in patients undergoing lobectomy or segmentectomy, they have not been shown to add any value or advantage over the simpler segment counting method and thus are not as routinely utilized for this indication [19, 398].

Surgical resection is typically contraindicated in patients with a preoperative $FEV_1 < 1$ L, and thus scintigraphy has little role to play in patients with poor preoperative lung function [360]. In those with borderline pulmonary reserve, lung scintigraphy can be used to predict postoperative lung function by combining spirometry measures with quantitative measurements of the differential ventilation or perfusion. Specifically, a postoperative FEV_1 can be calculated with the following formula [360]:

$$\text{Pre-operative } FEV_1 \times \left(1 - \text{fraction of total perfusion or ventilation for the target region}\right).$$

A postoperative DLCO is similarly calculated by substituting preoperative DLCO for FEV_1. The postoperative FEV_1 can additionally be compared to a predicted FEV_1—corrected for the patient's height, sex, and age—to obtain a percentage of the predicted postoperative value (%PPO), where

$$\begin{aligned}\%\text{PPO } FEV_1 &= \text{computed PPO } FEV_1 \\ &\quad \times 100 / \text{predicted normal } FEV_1.\end{aligned}$$

Again, a %PPO DLCO can be obtained in a similar manner through the substitution of DLCO for FEV_1 in the above equation. Postoperative FEV_1, DLCO, $\%PPO_{FEV1}$, and $\%PPO_{DLCO}$ all represent complementary methods for estimating postoperative lung function. Current American College of Chest Physicians (ACCP) guidelines recommend the use of both $\%PPO_{FEV1}$ and $\%PPO_{DLCO}$ for accurate postoperative lung function prediction [57]. To be considered for surgery, patients must, at a minimum, have a postoperative $FEV_1 > 0.8$–1 L in those undergoing pneumonectomy and >1.5 L for lobectomy as well as a %PPO FEV_1 and DLCO >30% regardless of resection type [53, 57, 360]. If lung scintigraphy predicts a lower postoperative FEV_1 and/or %PPO in a patient, she/he would unlikely have an adequate pulmonary reserve to undergo lung resection safely.

Various studies have evaluated the accuracy of lung scintigraphy in the prediction of postoperative lung function. Overall, the correlation between actual and predicted postoperative lung function using quantitative V/Q scans is quite variable, in part stemming from the heterogeneity that exists among imaging protocols. The literature is mixed with regard to the optimal imaging protocol that would allow for the most accurate prediction of postoperative lung function [19, 331, 339, 451]. Investigators have specifically evaluated the use of SPECT and SPECT/CT over scintigraphy and combined V/Q versus perfusion- or ventilation-only scans with contradictory findings. For example, a prospective study of 32 patients with non-small cell lung cancer who underwent pneumonectomy found that the correlation between preoperative and postoperative lung function was highest for ventilation-only scans ($r = 0.7$ for FEV_1 and 0.73 for %PPO) over both perfusion-only scans ($r = 0.58$ for FEV_1 and 0.60 for %PPO) and combined ventilation/perfusion scans (r = 0.54 for FEV_1 and 0.62 for %PPO), though the differences were not statistically significant [451]. Despite having the highest correlation, lung ventilation scintigraphy generally underestimated postoperative lung function. This study additionally noted that the correlation was higher with SPECT/CT relative to that with scintigraphy. By contrast, other studies have cited a similar accuracy for planar and SPECT or SPECT/CT imaging in predicting postoperative lung function [19, 339].

The other major oncologic indication for quantitative perfusion and ventilation lung scintigraphy is radiation therapy planning. A newer paradigm in radiation therapy is functional lung avoidance radiotherapy, in which functional imaging is used to generate a radiation treatment plan that minimizes dose delivery to normal or highly functional portions of the lung in the hopes that it reduces the probability of radiation-induced pulmonary toxicity [119]. Quantitative ventilation and perfusion imaging provide a spatially oriented map of ventilation and perfusion function, allowing the treating radiation oncologist to adjust the dose delivered to various lung regions based on relative lung function. Following radiation therapy completion, quantitative perfusion/ventilation scintigraphy may additionally allow for the early identification of radiation-induced lung injury [470].

^{18}F-FDG PET/CT

^{18}F-FDG PET/CT is foundational to oncologic imaging. Visual interpretation or qualitative analysis is a mainstay for image interpretation in routine clinical practice for many of its indications, particularly staging, and restaging. While currently more limited in scope, quantitative PET/CT has become increasingly important for study interpretation as it allows for a more objective and accurate measure of a patient's disease compared with visual inspection alone.

Various semi-quantitative and quantitative metabolic and volumetric parameters can be derived from ^{18}F-FDG PET/CT studies. SUV is a ubiquitous semi-quantitative parameter defined as the decay-corrected tissue concentration of a radiotracer in a specific region of interest divided by the injected activity that, in turn, is divided by body weight. Of the various SUV-based parameters, SUV_{max} is the most widely reported in clinical practice; it represents the most intense FDG uptake within a volume of interest, Other SUV-based parameters include SUV_{peak} and SUV_{mean}. Calculating ratios of SUV-based parameters as well as changes in SUV-based parameters from baseline may be reported as well. For example, ΔSUV_{max} measures the change in tumoral glycolytic metabolism over time and is calculated as follows:

$$\left(\text{Baseline SUV}_{max} - \text{follow} - \text{up PET SUV}_{max}\right) / \text{ baseline SUV}_{max} \times 100\%.$$

While SUV-based parameters are convenient and easy to calculate, they are readily influenced by a variety of biological and technical factors, including uptake time and blood glucose levels, which can lead to changes in values up to 10–20% despite there being no accompanying change in the underlying lesion. Normalization with physiologic hepatic and blood-pool uptake is therefore often used for longitudinal lesion comparison in daily clinical practice.

Volumetric parameters are increasingly utilized. Metabolic tumor volume (MTV) is the volume of a tumor that displays FDG uptake above a certain predefined threshold, typically ≥40–60% SUV_{max} or ≥2.5 SUV_{max}. In other words, it represents the volume of the tumor that is metabolically active. Total lesion glycolysis (TLG) is the product of the SUV_{mean} and MTV. In general, volumetric parameters may have greater prognostic and predictive value compared with SUV_{max} [169]. However, the requirement for dedicated software to measure MTV and TLG, the need for strict adherence to protocols for accurate quantification, and the lack of standardization of methods for obtaining these parameters currently limits the wider adoption of these parameters in daily practice. The following discussion will lay out the role and added capabilities of quantitative PET/CT for various primary intrathoracic malignancies as well as discuss their shortcomings and controversies.

Lung Cancer

Primary lung cancers consist of a diverse group of pathologies that are histologically divided into small cell (SCLC) (15%) and non-small cell cancer (NSCLC) subtypes (85%) [420]. The latter is further subdivided into lung adenocarcinoma, squamous cell carcinoma, large cell carcinoma, and other minor variants in order of decreasing incidence. FDG-PET/CT is critical in the management of all subtypes of lung cancer, with important roles in staging, restaging, therapy planning, treatment response assessment, and prognostication [312, 313]. Visual interpretation of images alone is typically sufficient for many of these indications, particularly staging and restaging. Comparatively, quantitative PET analysis operates in a more secondary role in daily clinical practice, complementing but not necessarily replacing visual interpretation. While its exact role has not been clearly defined, there is a growing body of research that suggests quantitative PET analysis has the capacity to provide clinically relevant data at various stages in the management of patients with lung cancer beyond that which can be ascertained from visual interpretation alone.

Current guidelines recommend the use of FDG-PET/CT for evaluation of solitary pulmonary nodules (SPNs, Fig. 25.19), which are defined as round or oval pulmonary parenchymal lesions that are equal to or smaller than 30 mm in diameter, surrounded by pulmonary parenchyma and/or visceral pleura, and are not associated with lymphadenopathy, atelectasis, or pneumo-

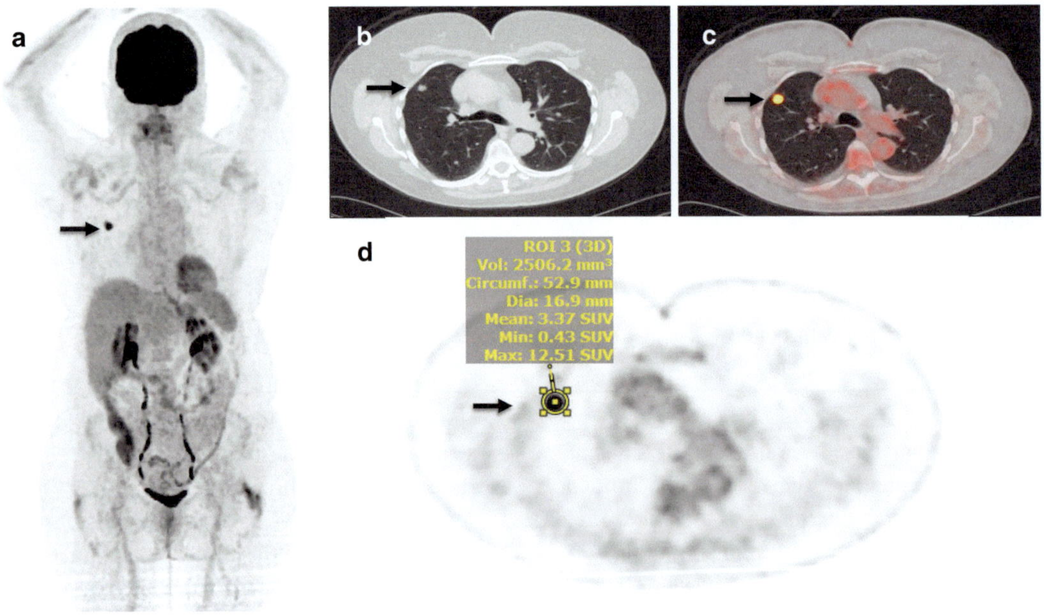

Fig. 25.19 ^{18}F-FDG PET/CT in a patient referred for evaluation of an enlarging solitary pulmonary nodule. (**a**) Whole-body maximum intensity projection (MIP), (**b**) axial co-registered CT, (**c**) fused PET/CT, and (**d**) PET images of the chest display an intensely FDG-avid 10 × 7 mm right upper lobe spiculated solid nodule with SUV_{max} 12.6 (black arrow). While false-positive findings are possible, particularly within endemic regions, the intensity of uptake is suggestive of malignancy. Pathology subsequently returned as a moderately differentiated, acinar-predominant invasive adenocarcinoma with lymphovascular invasion and spread of tumor through airspaces (pT1bN0Mx)

nia [453]. According to the Fleischner Society guidelines, any patient in which a single solid pulmonary nodule greater than 8 mm is found incidentally on chest CT should undergo further evaluation with at least one of the following: FDG-PET/CT, repeat CT at 3 months, or tissue sampling [278]. FDG-PET/CT or biopsy should also be considered for solitary part-solid pulmonary nodules if the solid component is ≥6 mm [278]. This indication for PET/CT is commonly accomplished through visual analysis—with uptake greater than that of background constituting a positive scan—with high sensitivity but variable specificity [152].

Investigators have questioned whether a more quantitative approach can help increase this specificity. Early PET studies suggested a SUV_{max} cutoff of 2.5 can be utilized for this indication with high accuracy [270]. Later studies, however, were unable to corroborate these findings. In comparing semi-quantitative methods to visual interpretation, a meta-analysis demonstrated no difference in accuracy for diagnosing malignant pulmonary lesions [152]. This study concluded that regardless of the method utilized, PET/CT has an overall high sensitivity but intermediate specificity for diagnosis. Part of the issue stems from that while malignant pulmonary nodules tend to have higher FDG uptake relative to benign etiologies, there are many exceptions. False negatives are common among smaller nodules (<1 cm) below the resolution of PET, lesions of low cellularity like mucinous adenocarcinomas, and lesions that are generally less FDG-avid, including lepidic predominant adenocarcinomas and pulmonary carcinoids [312]. Similarly, inflammatory and infectious nodules/lesions are common false-positive findings, particularly within endemic regions [312]. Consequently, it is unlikely that a specific SUV_{max} or other quantitative PET parameter cutoff can definitively differentiate benign from malignant lesions and thus should not be used in isolation to determine a patient's need for biopsy, particularly in high-risk patients.

Baseline PET parameters may offer insights into certain features of the primary tumor, such as histology, grading, and phenotype [60, 123, 271, 415, 441]. While no single semi-quantitative or quantitative PET parameter can be used in isolation to determine any of the features definitively, there are various trends that have been noted. For example, in a retrospective study of 419 patients with stage IA-IIIA lung adenocarcinoma, SUV_{max}, background subtracted volume (BSV), and background-subtracted lesion activity (BSL) on baseline FDG-PET/CT were significantly higher in invasive adenocarcinoma relative to minimally invasive adenocarcinoma (MIA) and adenocarcinoma in situ (AIS) [60]. These same parameters were also able to differentiate MIA from AIS with high sensitivity and specificity. Furthermore, SUV_{max} and BSL strongly or moderately correlated with Ki67 proliferative index in most subtypes, except for micropapillary and solid predominant groups. Other studies have shown that SUV_{max} tends to be lower in lung adenocarcinomas relative to squamous cell carcinomas, particularly in those with lepidic-predominant growth patterns, which are, on average, less FDG-avid than other growth patterns [123, 271, 441]. Lower FDG uptake can also be associated with the presence of EGFR mutations among NSCLCs, while higher FDG uptake is generally seen among tumors with greater PDL-1 expression [113, 415]. A meta-analysis of 15 studies demonstrated an intermediate pooled sensitivity (70%) and specificity (59%) for baseline SUV_{max} in predicting EGFR status in patients with NSCLC [113]. A similar sensitivity and specificity were found for predicting PDL-1 expression [381]. Many efforts have been made to improve this prediction efficacy, including the incorporation of volumetric parameters, radiomics approaches, and artificial intelligence, but this requires further study and may be the direction of future research [415].

Baseline semi-quantitative and quantitative PET parameters may have additional prognostic and predictive value. An early meta-analysis found baseline SUV-based parameters were predictive of patient outcomes in 11 out of 13 studies, with higher SUV being a poor prognostic factor in patients with NSCLC [42]. However, the authors noted that it was unclear if SUV was an independent prognostic factor independent from the clinical stage or performance status. Later studies have suggested that baseline volumetric parameters may hold greater promise over traditional SUV-based parameters for predicting patient outcomes [75, 256]. A consensus regarding these parameters, however, has not been reached.

Another increasingly common role for baseline quantitative FDG-PET/CT is therapy—specifically, radiation therapy planning. FDG-PET/CT complements CT imaging in defining and delineating radiation treatment target volumes for patients with both NSCLC and SCLC. Segmentation is typically accomplished through visual analysis, but quantitative methods are increasingly available. Beyond target volume delineation, quantitative PET has more of an experimental role in radiation therapy planning. It, however, shows great potential for this indication, particularly with newer techniques like molecular imaging-based dose painting. Dose painting delivers a nonuniform radiation dose distribution to the target volume based upon functional or molecular imaging [41]. Dose can be prescribed to tumor subvolumes (subvolume boosting) or to individual voxels (dose painting by numbers) [41]. As FDG-PET/CT provides a quantitative spatiotemporal map of tumor biology, it was hypothesized that it could be utilized to steer and optimize radiation dose distribution in dose painting. As regions within the primary tumor displaying higher metabolism on baseline PET/CT are more likely to represent future locations of local recurrence and less likely to respond to treatment, they are reasonable targets for subvolume boosting.

A few randomized trials have evaluated FDG-PET/CT-based dose painting strategies in NSCLC. The Netherlands randomized phase II PET-boost trial (NCT01024829) assessed a PET-based integrated boosting strategy in 107 patients with inoperable, stage II–III NSCLC [87, 429]. Patients were randomized to receive dose-escalation to either the entire primary tumor (arm A) or intratumoral subvolumes with high FDG uptake (>50% SUV_{max}) (arm B). Interim analysis of the first 20 patients demonstrated the feasibility of this approach while maintaining predefined dose constraints [429]. The dose was safely escalated to at least 72 Gy in 75% of patients without increasing the dose to the organs at risk (OAR). Final results of the study, however, were less promising with reported toxicity rates higher in patients who received subvolume boosting compared to those who received conventional chemoradiation, though within predefined stopping rules [87].

NCT02788461 is an ongoing multicenter phase II randomized trial that is investigating the utility of PET-based subvolume boosting in 78 patients with stage III NSCLC [347]. Patients are randomized to receive either conventional chemoradiation (60 Gy in 30 fractions) or PET-based dose escalation. With the latter, patients receive an integrated boost dose to tumor subvolumes with high FDG uptake (>50% SUV_{max}) to a maximum of 85 Gy in 30 fractions. Initial analysis demonstrates the feasibility of this approach, but results are still pending as to whether this approach can reduce the local regional failure rate and ultimately improve patient outcomes while maintaining a good toxicity profile.

Following radiation, chemotherapy, and/or chemoradiation treatment, FDG-PET/CT can help assess response. In contrast to staging and restaging, NCCN guidelines do not recommend the routine use of FDG-PET/CT for this indication in patients with lung cancer [312, 313]. Despite being considered a second-line imaging modality for this indication, it still offers important clinical information. Following treatment initiation, there is a progressive decrease in the high glycolytic activity of tumor cells, stemming from treatment-directed tumor cell killing and inhibition of tumor cell growth and proliferation. These metabolic changes tend to occur earlier than corresponding morphologic decreases in tumor size on conventional anatomic imaging. This metabolic response to treatment is represented by a reduction in tumoral FDG uptake on PET/CT and typically correlates with major pathologic response (<10% residual tumor) and can be seen earlier than morphologic decreases in tumor size on conventional anatomic imaging [167]. Having a metabolic response on post-treatment PET/CT typically correlates with major pathologic response (<10% residual tumor). While visual interpretation can be utilized for this indication, semi-quantitative and quantitative analyses are crucial for an accurate and objective assessment of treatment response.

Two major PET criteria exist for response assessment in patients with solid tumors, both of which employ quantitative changes in SUV parameters as the index of response. EORTC criteria were the first of the two major PET response criteria to be published, though is now less commonly used. SUV_{max} is used to assess index of response with a reduction of at least 25% in SUV_{max} determining tumor response [462]. PET response criteria in solid tumors (PERCIST) are the more commonly used PET response criteria, which employs SUV_{peak} normalized to lean body mass (SUL) to determine treatment response. An absolute drop of 0.8 SUV_{peak} units and/or 30% change in SUV_{peak} delineates tumor response [436]. Despite the existence of these guidelines, there is still no consensus on the optimal quantitative PET parameter and cutoff for response assessment in patients with lung cancer. Investigators have reported variable cutoff values for post-treatment SUV_{max} and ΔSUV_{max}, with the latter ranging from ≥15% to ≥60% [383]. In addition to these SUV-based parameters, other metabolic and volumetric parameters have been put forth as potential indicators of response. MTV and TLG are particularly promising parameters that may be predictive of patient outcomes, but still require further validation and standardization [298, 388].

While treatment response is more commonly assessed following therapy completion, some have advocated for assessing response earlier. While this approach has not yet been validated, there is some evidence that PET/CT scans obtained during treatment may have some utility. Studies have shown that changes in metabolic and volumetric parameters can occur as early as the end of the second week of treatment in patients with locally advanced NSCLC and may be predictive of end-of-treatment response and patient outcomes [51, 292, 464]. This opens the possibility for quantitative PET response-adapted treatment strategies, which use objective information extracted from the mid-treatment or interim PET/CT to guide or alter the treatment strategy in individual patients. In other words, these strategies permit the identification of poor responders early in treatment who may benefit from treatment modification to ensure improved outcomes.

A small number of prospective studies have evaluated this approach in patients with lung cancer. NEOSCAN is a phase II, prospective trial that evaluated quantitative FDG-PET/CT in guiding chemotherapy regimen in 40 patients with resectable stage IB-IIIA lung cancers [184]. Following a pretreatment PET/CT, patients underwent two cycles of cisplatin plus gemcitabine (in those with squamous cell carcinoma) or pemetrexed (adenocarcinoma). Patients then underwent a repeat PET/CT, which stratified them into responders ($SUV_{peak} \geq 35\%$) and nonresponders ($SUV_{peak} < 35\%$). PET responders continued the initial chemotherapy regimen while nonresponders were switched to vinorelbine plus docetaxel. An additional PET/CT was performed after two cycles of the alternative regimen, again for response assessment. Following initial therapy, 63% of patients ($n = 25/40$) were determined to be metabolic responders. The remaining 38% ($n = 15/40$) of patients were metabolic nonresponders and thus were assigned to receive the alternative chemotherapy regimen. Intention-to-treat analysis demonstrated that 67% (95% CI, 42–85%) of these initial metabolic nonresponders who subsequently switched regimens went on to have partial or complete metabolic response on follow-up PET/CT and 73% had R0 resection at surgery. While this study met its primary endpoint of PET response to the alternative chemotherapy regimen, it was not powered to determine if this strategy could increase the rate of pathologic response or prolong survival in patients. Further studies are therefore required to determine if this is a clinically relevant strategy.

NCT02773238 is an ongoing prospective phase II trial that is investigating a radiotherapy approach known as FLARE RT that combines strategies of functional lung avoidance, a quantitative V/Q scan strategy that was described in a previous section, and PET response-adaptive dose escalation [467]. A precursor study in eight patients with NSCLC by the trial investigators demonstrated the clinical feasibility of the FLARE RT approach and further optimized it by specifically using proton pencil beam scanning for functional lung avoidance versus volumetric modulated arc therapy (VMAT) for FDG-PET dose escalation [244]. This allowed their small subset of patients to receive a mean dose of 70–74 Gy to the FDG-PET-defined biological target volume without violating normal tissue constraints. Fifty-six patients with stage IIB-IIIB NSCLC are currently enrolled for FLARE-RT clinical trial. After baseline FDG-PET/CT and ^{99m}Tc-MAA and ^{99m}Tc-sulfur colloid SPECT/CT scans, patients will undergo functional lung avoidance radiation therapy for 3 weeks, followed by a mid-treatment PET/CT scan for response assessment. Metabolic responders will continue to receive a standard radiation dose that incorporates functional lung avoidance strategies for the remaining fractions. In contrast, nonresponders will receive a nonuniform radiation dose with escalation to radioresistant regions within the GTV based on SUV parameters using a dose-painting-by-numbers approach. The primary objective of this trial is to demonstrate a statistically significant improvement in the 2-year OS for patients in the FLARE RT patient cohort relative to that for patients in the 60 Gy cohort in the RTOG 0617 trial (57% 2-year OS), which would serve as a historical control [52]. Data is still pending for this trial. While PET-adaptive radiation therapy is not currently practiced outside of clinical trials and requires further validation, it holds significant promise.

Pleural Mesothelioma

Mesothelioma is a relatively rare malignancy that arises from the cells of the serosal lining of body cavities. Approximately 85% of these malignancies arise from the pleura [420]. Pleural mesothelioma can be localized or diffuse, with the latter subdivided into three histologic subtypes: biphasic, sarcomatoid, and epithelioid [371]. Epithelioid is the most common subtype, comprising 50–60% of MPM cases, and is associated with a better prognosis than biphasic and sarcomatoid subtypes [371].

^{18}F-FDG PET/CT is considered a second-line imaging modality in patients with malignant pleural mesothelioma (MPM, Fig. 25.20). Yet, it still has critical roles to play in the assessment of this disease at various stages. For example, it is currently recommended as part of the initial staging of MPM in surgical candidates [314]. While PET/CT has little role in T staging, which is determined by the extent of local tumor invasion, its strength lies in its ability to identify distal metastases [135, 314]. It remains unclear as to the specific role that quantitative PET/CT has in the management of MPM patients. Studies are mixed and sometimes contradictory regarding the utility of this approach as it relates to diagnosis, tumor biology, treatment response, and prognostication at both baseline and following treatment, each of which will be further detailed below.

A small number of studies have evaluated the ability of PET parameters to aid in the diagnosis of MPM, specifically as to whether they can help distinguish benign from malignant pleural disease. MPM generally displays a higher SUV_{max} compared with benign etiologies of pleural disease [1, 385, 410]. For example, a retrospective study in 37 patients with primary pleural disease found that a SUV_{max} cutoff of >4.0 differentiated patients with MPM from those with benign asbestos-related pleural thickening with a sensitivity of 88.0%, specificity of 83.3%, positive predictive value of 91.7%, and negative predictive value of 76.9% [385]. While other studies have supported this trend, they each report a different cutoff value, ranging from 2 to 4 [1, 385, 410]. Furthermore, there can be significant overlap in SUV_{max}, resulting in both false negative and positive findings, the latter being particularly common among patients previously having undergone talc pleurodesis, which can cause a localized inflammatory reaction that is FDG-avid.

Quantitative PET/CT has additionally been explored as a tool for better characterizing MPM tumor biology. In a retrospective analysis of 78 patients, Kadota et al. demonstrated that epitheli-

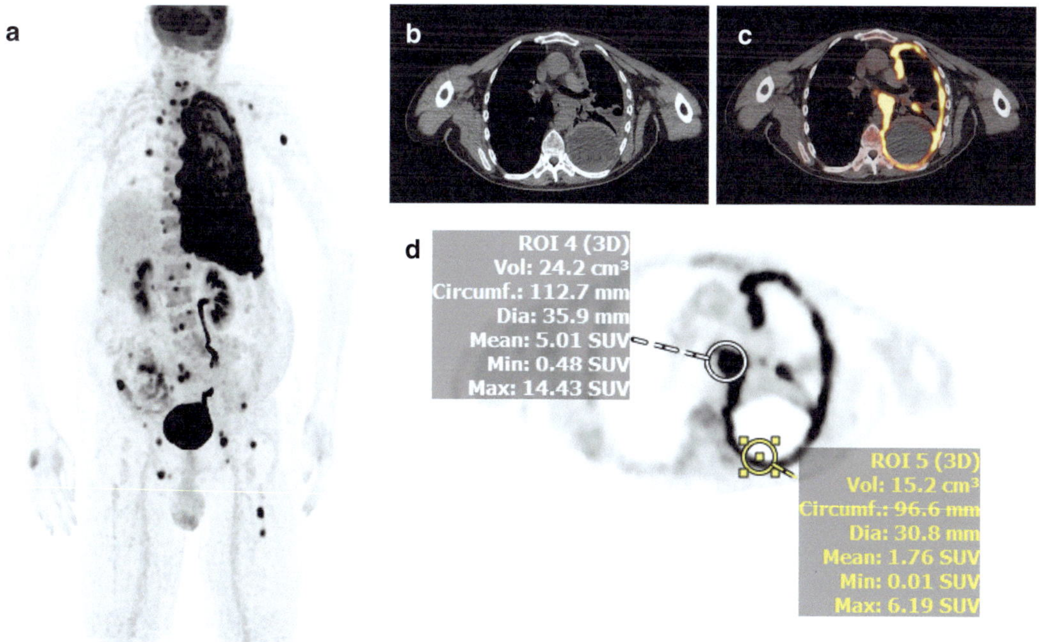

Fig. 25.20 Staging ^{18}F-FDG PET/CT in a patient with biphasic pleural mesothelioma. (**a**) Whole-body maximum intensity projection (MIP) image demonstrates diffuse intense FDG uptake within the left hemithorax along the pleura, consistent with the patient's biopsy-proven mesothelioma. Multifocal extrapleural FDG uptake within the mediastinal lymph nodes and axial and appendicular skeleton, consistent with locoregional and metastatic disease, respectively. (**b**) Axial co-registered CT, (**c**) fused, and (**d**) PET PET/CT images of the chest show confluent intense FDG uptake within a diffusely thickened left pleura. The intensity of pleural uptake is variable with a SUV_{max} 14.4 along the ipsilateral mediastinal pleural surface. Having a higher SUV_{max} on staging PET/CT is generally considered a poor prognostic indicator as is having a biphasic histologic subtype. A region of photopenic loculated left pleural effusion is additionally noted

oid tumors with pleomorphic subtype had a higher baseline SUV_{max} compared to that of non-pleomorphic epithelioid subtypes (n = 57; 6.5 ± 3.2; p = 0.050). While non-epithelioid MPM was noted to have higher SUV_{max} relative to epithelioid tumors, the difference was not statistically significant (9.1 ± 4.8 vs. 7.1 ± 3.9; p = 0.160) [196]. Higher mitotic counts and amount of necrosis were also associated with higher SUV_{max}. This study, however, found no association between SUV_{max} and TNM stage. Overall, the literature tends to be mixed regarding the utility of quantitative PET/CT in differentiating epithelioid versus non-epithelioid subtypes. Only a limited number of studies have shown a statistically significant difference in SUV_{max} for patients with epithelioid versus non-epithelioid MPM [258, 266]. For example, a retrospective analysis by Lim et al. found a significantly lower SUV_{max} in patients with epithelioid subtype (5.5) than those with sarcomatoid/biphasic subtypes (11.7) or mesothelioma, NOS (13.3) (p = 0.003) [258]. In comparison, a much larger number of studies have reported no statistical difference [196, 215, 248].

The largest and most frequently studied role for quantitative PET/CT in patients with MPM relates to its prognostic and predictive value. While the literature tends to be heterogeneous, it generally supports the prognostic value of quantitative PET parameters in the pretreatment setting [213, 258, 405]. In a meta-analysis performed by Taralli et al., metabolic tumor information derived from baseline PET imaging was prognostic in 17 of 19 included studies [405]. Higher tumor uptake was shown to predict worse patient outcomes, with volumetric PET parameters more commonly outperforming SUV-based parameters. However, these PET parameters were not confirmed as independent prognostic factors in seven of these studies, with histology and prior talc pleurodesis as examples of confounding factors. Furthermore, each study reported its own cutoff values for various PET parameters, limiting the ability to apply these findings to a larger population of patients.

Studies evaluating the role of quantitative PET/CT during treatment or in the post-treatment setting are less common. In general, major PET treatment response criteria, specifically EORTC, PERCIST, and imPERCIST, have been shown to outperform modified RECIST criteria for CT in accurately differentiating metabolic responders and nonresponders in patients with MPM [214]. Despite the advantages of PET/CT over conventional imaging for this indication, the use of PET treatment response criteria has not yet been validated in clinical trials for this patient population. Further work is needed to understand the role of quantitative PET/CT in the post-treatment setting and whether it can help guide treatment.

Esophageal Cancer

Esophageal cancer is the eighth most common malignancy worldwide [455]. The principal histopathologic subtypes are squamous cell carcinoma (ESCC) and adenocarcinoma (EAC). While ESCC is the most common histology worldwide, EACs have a higher incidence in the United States [3].

Current guidelines recommend ^{18}F-FDG PET/CT as part of a multimodality strategy for clinical staging of patients with newly diagnosed esophageal cancer [315]. PET/CT has superior detection of distant metastases compared to other noninvasive imaging modalities like CT and EUS [212, 416]. While FDG-PET/CT can also detect locoregional nodal disease, it does so with less sensitivity than EUS, limiting its role in N staging [187]. Similarly, PET/CT typically can delineate the location of the primary tumor, but it does not have the resolution to differentiate among the various layers of the esophageal wall required for accurate T staging [91, 304]. This limitation, however, does not necessarily apply to quantitative PET analysis. A small number of retrospective studies have shown a positive correlation between the intensity of FDG uptake within the primary tumor and cT category [91, 203, 329], though this association is weak and the values and cutoffs published by various studies are inconsistent, making them difficult to apply on a larger scale.

Looking beyond metabolic T staging, numerous studies have shown that baseline PET parameters, typically SUV_{max}, can suggest certain features about the primary tumor, including histology, presence of high-risk features, and grading [257, 391] (Fig. 25.21). While there are no specific parameters that can be universally adopted at this time to determine any of these features in individual patients definitively, the literature has noted various trends. For example, EACs are generally less FDG-avid than ESCCs and tend to display more heterogeneous avidity. EACS that are poorly differentiated or demonstrate diffuse type, signet cell, or mucinous patterns and display more heterogeneous avidity [391]. Furthermore, higher FDG uptake can be associated with the presence of high-risk features. In a retrospective study of 220 patients with ESCC, higher tumor SUV_{max} correlated with greater tumor invasion depth ($p < 0.001$), positive nodal disease ($P < 0.001$), presence of lymphatic and perineural invasion ($p < 0.001$), higher ki-67 index ($P = 0.025$), and greater tumor dedifferentiation ($P = 0.039$) [257]. Despite the existence of these trends, there is significant variation among studies for proposed cutoffs, suggesting that more work is required before considering application to the general population. Quantitative parameters should be considered complementary to other methods in helping to characterize tumor biology and possibly identifying patients who are at higher risk for advanced disease, which in turn can have implications for treatment planning.

A specific aspect of treatment planning that has seen growing interest in recent years is the use of quantitative PET/CT for initial radiation therapy planning. Fan et al. describe one of these radiation therapy approaches in which the dose is selectively boosted to the more metabolically active regions in the gross tumor volume (GTV) that surpass a certain SUV threshold [129]. This

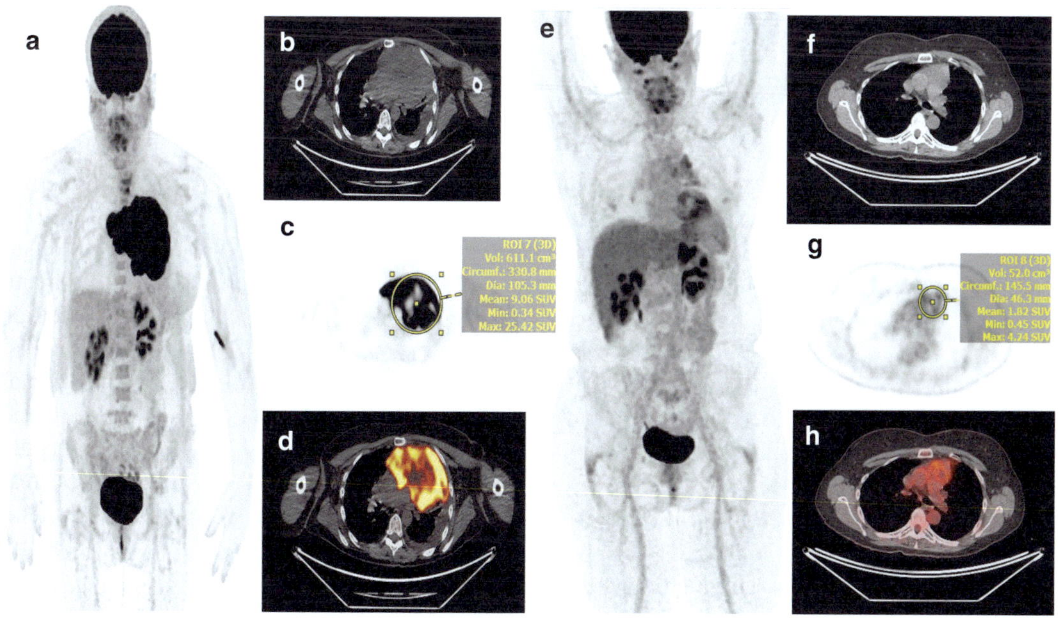

Fig. 25.21 Baseline and post-treatment ^{18}F-FDG PET/CT in a patient with thymic carcinoma. (**a**) Whole-body maximum intensity projection (MIP), (**b**) axial co-registered CT, (**c**) PET, and (**d**) fused PET/CT images of the chest display a large soft tissue anterior mediastinal mass that measures 11.7 × 7.7 cm. The mass is heterogeneous with regions of central photopenia indicative of cystic change and intense peripheral FDG uptake (SUV_{max} 25.4), which is typical for thymic carcinomas. (**e**) Whole-body MIP, (**f**) axial co-registered CT, (**g**) PET, and (**h**) fused PET/CT images of the chest following four cycles of carboplatin/paclitaxel chemotherapy demonstrate a significant interval decrease in size and avidity of the anterior mediastinal mass. The residual mass measures 5.6 × 4.8 cm with a SUV_{max} 4.2, which represents an 83% reduction in FDG uptake compared to baseline, indicative of treatment response

approach is another example of dose painting, specifically subvolume boosting, as described above in the section on lung cancers. A threshold value of 50% SUV_{max} is specifically chosen for this study based upon evidence from an earlier study by the same authors [128]. While this study demonstrates the feasibility of this approach, further investigation is required to specifically evaluate whether it has a clinically significant effect on patient outcomes.

Other uses of FDG-PET/CT in esophageal cancer include the evaluation for recurrent disease and treatment response. While CT can be used as an alternative to PET/CT for the former indication, FDG-PET/CT is the only imaging modality currently recommended for the latter [12, 315]. FDG PET/CT is a highly sensitive indicator of treatment response, displaying changes in tumor metabolism earlier than corresponding decreases in tumor size on anatomic imaging. While specificity also tends to be high in this setting, inflammation from radiotherapy can result in false positives. Post-treatment FDG-PET/CT scans are thus delayed for 5–8 weeks following completion of radiation, improving specificity.

Unlike with staging and restaging, visual interpretation alone is not always adequate to assess for treatment response [425]. This, in addition to the growing need for more accurate, objective measures of disease activity, particularly in the setting of clinical trials, has placed quantitative analysis at the forefront of response assessment. As mentioned above, the most widely used PET criteria for response assessment in solid tumors is PERCIST, which has been validated for use in patients with esophageal cancer [283, 326]. Beyond PERCIST, other quantitative parameters as well as other cutoff values for changes in SUV_{max} to distinguish metabolic responders from nonresponders have been described in the literature with varying sensitivities and specificities [56, 228, 446].

The identification of metabolic response on PET generally correlates with pathologic response to treatment [49, 440]. This correlation holds true in the setting of various neoadjuvant chemotherapy and immunotherapy regimens as well as radiation therapy. Quantitative PET parameters may additionally have prognostic or predictive value beyond the prediction of pathologic response. While there is significant heterogeneity among studies and often contradictory findings, they generally support the prognostic value of quantitative PET analysis on both baseline and post-treatment scans and its ability to predict treatment response and patient outcomes. Numerous studies suggest volumetric parameters, such as TLG, MTV, and their percentage changes from baseline, may be particularly helpful for predicting patient outcomes [69, 159, 169, 219, 324, 389]. However, the exact individual parameters and specific cutoffs that are best for predicting patient outcomes remain unclear.

A few prospective clinical trials have investigated quantitative PET response-adapted treatment strategies in patients with esophageal cancer. MUNICON II is a single-center exploratory phase II prospective clinical trial that evaluated one of these strategies in 110 patients with locally advanced esophageal and esophagogastric junction adenocarcinoma in the neoadjuvant setting [269]. Following a baseline PET/CT, all patients received 2 weeks of platinum and fluorouracil-based induction chemotherapy. A repeat PET/CT was performed on day 14 at the completion of neoadjuvant chemotherapy. A decrease of SUV_{max} from baseline of 35% or more was used to differentiate metabolic responders from nonresponders. Metabolic responders continued to receive neoadjuvant chemotherapy for 12 weeks followed by surgery while metabolic nonresponders discontinued chemotherapy, instead proceeding directly to surgery. Forty-nine percent of patients ($N = 54$) were determined to be metabolic responders on follow-up PET/CT scans. After a median follow-up of 2.3 years, median overall survival (OS) was not reached in metabolic responders, whereas median OS was 25.8 months (19.4–32.2) in nonresponders (HR 2.13, 95% CI, 1.14–3.99; $p = 0.015$). Median event-free survival (EFS) was significantly higher in metabolic responders (29.7 months, 95% CI 7.5–20.6) compared with nonresponders (14.1 months, 95% CI 7.5–20.6) with a hazard ratio of 2.18 (95% CI 1.32–3.62; $p = 0.002$). Furthermore, while major histological remissions (<10% residual tumor) were noted in 29 of 50 metabolic responders (58%, 95% CI 48–67), none were demonstrated in metabolic nonresponders ($p = 0.001$). In summary, MUNICON II bolstered findings from prior retrospective studies, providing concrete evidence that quantitative PET measures as early as two weeks into treatment allow for the accurate identification of nonresponsive tumors, which has important implications for patient outcomes.

CALGB 80803 is a phase II randomized trial that evaluated a different PET response-adapted therapy strategy in 225 patients with locally advanced esophageal and esophagogastric junction adenocarcinomas following induction chemotherapy [150]. All patients underwent a baseline PET/CT followed by random allocation to one of two induction chemotherapy arms: modified oxaliplatin, leucovorin, and fluorouracil (FOLFOX) or carboplatin-paclitaxel (CP). A repeat PET/CT scan was performed 36–42 days following completion of induction chemotherapy. A change in SUV_{max} from baseline was measured for each patient and used to stratify patients into PET responders and non-responders. PET responders—defined as those with a decrease in SUV_{max} greater than or equal to 35%—continued with the same chemotherapy regimen for subsequent neoadjuvant chemoradiation therapy. Contrastingly, PET non-responders—those with a decrease in SUV_{max} from a baseline less than 35%—were switched to the alternative chemotherapy regimen. Metabolic nonresponders who switched to CP following induction FOLFOX or FOLFOX following CP induction were found to have pathologic complete response (pCR) rates of 18% (95% CI, 7.5–33.5) and 20% (95% CI, 10–33.7), respectively, which is significantly higher than the 4% reported in earlier studies among PET nonresponders who continued the same regimen [269]. With the improvement in pCR rates, there was an accompanying increase in overall survival (OS) rates among PET nonresponders. After a median follow-up of 5.2 years, median OS was 27.4 months (95% CI, 19.4 months to not estimable) for PET responders, which not only compared favorably to historic controls but also was not that dissimilar to that for PET responders.

Overall, these studies suggest a possible role for PET-adapted strategies that either escalate or switch therapy based upon interim or early PET/CT scans during neoadjuvant treatment. In contrast, the literature does not currently support the application of de-escalation strategies in this patient population. Numerous studies, including MUNICON II, have shown that neither qualitative nor quantitative PET is sensitive enough to detect residual microscopic disease [98, 269, 425]. Thus, current guidelines do not recommend utilizing PET as a tool to determine if a patient should undergo subsequent esophagectomy [315].

Thymic Epithelial Tumors

Thymic epithelial tumors (TETs) are rare malignancies that arise from the thymus, representing approximately 0.2–1.5% of all malignancies [357]. The fifth edition of the World Health Organization (WHO) classification of thoracic tumors classifies TETs as thymomas, thymic carcinomas, and thymic neuroendocrine tumors (TNETs) [285]. This section will specifically focus on thymomas and thymic carcinomas. Thymomas are further divided into types A, AB, and B, with the latter subdivided into B1, B2, and B3 [285]. The prognosis of patients with thymomas progressively worsens from type A to B3, and those with thymic carcinomas tend to have a worse prognosis than those with thymomas [285]. While not recognized in the WHO classification, some have advocated for the use of a simplified histologic classification, dividing TETs into low-risk thymomas (types A, AB, and B1), high-risk thymomas (types B2 and B3), and thymic carcinomas [281]. Surgery is the mainstay of treatment for patients with TETs, with additional management dependent on TET subtype.

^{18}F-FDG PET/CT is commonly obtained for the preoperative planning and staging of TETs. Visual interpretation allows for the identification of locoregional disease and distant metastases with high sensitivity [316]. Quantitative PET/CT analysis, on the other hand, has a less well-defined role in the management of TETs. Various studies have evaluated its utility in relation to diagnosis and tumor biology, staging, and prognostication/predictive value with mixed results.

A noninvasive study that could aid in the accurate diagnosis of TETs would be invaluable since surgical biopsy is not typically recommended in patients with suspected resectable thymoma due to the substantial potential for tumor seeding [316]. A handful of studies have investigated whether quantitative PET can help differentiate benign pathologies like thymic hyperplasia from TETs. Thymic hyperplasia generally tends to have a lower SUV_{max} relative to high-grade thymomas and thymic carcinomas, rarely demonstrating a SUV_{max} greater than 3 [78, 116, 224, 443]. There remains, however, significant overlap in SUV_{max} for thymic hyperplasia and low-risk thymomas. While the added morphologic evaluation of findings on the CT portion of the exam allows for improved characterization and identification, FDG-PET/CT alone cannot always reliably differentiate between these two entities.

Other studies have explored the use of quantitative PET/CT parameters in differentiating among the various TET histologic subtypes, as their identification in the preoperative setting could have important implications for management, particularly the need for chemoradiation (Fig. 25.22). The totality of these studies supports the general trend that SUV_{max} is significantly higher in thymic carcinomas relative to thymomas [158, 179, 210, 407, 419]. However, there is significant heterogeneity in the reported SUV_{max} cutoff values, ranging from 4.6 to 6.3, thereby limiting its application to the larger population. Similarly, while not necessarily diagnostic, SUV_{max} and other PET parameters have been shown to be higher on average in high risk thymomas and thymic carcinomas than in low-risk thymomas [158, 179, 210, 419].

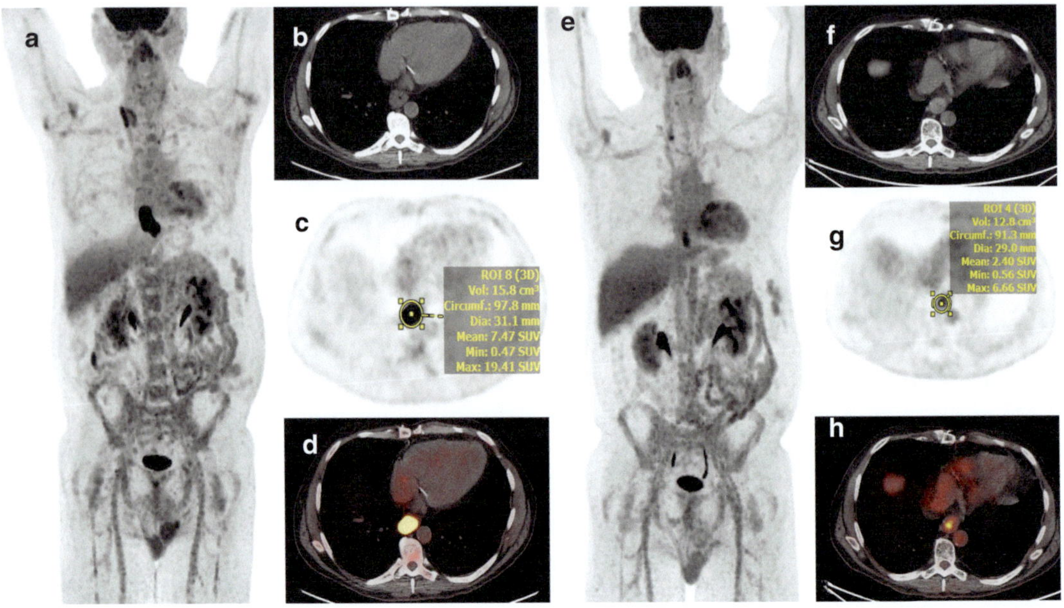

Fig. 25.22 Baseline and post-treatment ^{18}F-FDG PET/CT in a patient with moderately differentiated distal esophageal adenocarcinoma. (**a**) Whole-body maximum intensity projection (MIP), (**b**) axial co-registered CT, (**c**) PET, and (**d**) fused PET/CT images of the chest exhibit an intensely FDG-avid circumferential mass in the distal esophagus (SUV_{max} 19.4). (**e**) Whole-body MIP, (**f**) axial co-registered CT, (**g**) PET, and (**h**) fused PET/CT images of the chest following completion of neoadjuvant carboplatin/paclitaxel chemotherapy and radiation therapy show an interval decrease in size and avidity of the esophageal mass. Compared to baseline, there has been a 65% reduction in FDG uptake (SUV_{max} 6.7), indicative of a partial metabolic treatment response. Pathology from the patient's subsequent esophagectomy confirmed partial response through noting residual intramucosal tumor measuring approximately 15 mm

Quantitative and semi-quantitative PET parameters at baseline and following treatment may have utility for prognostication in patients with TETs [158, 179, 379, 412]. For example, in a retrospective study of 114 patients with TETs, baseline SUV_{max} was shown to be an independent prognostic factor for patient outcomes ($p < 0.001$) [158]. Similar to the malignancies described above, however, there remains significant controversy as to the optimal PET parameter and cutoff value for this indication. Further work is required to understand the utility of PET/CT for this indication.

DOTATATE PET/CT

Most neuroendocrine tumors (NETs), particularly if well-differentiated, express high levels of somatostatin receptors (SSTRs) on their cell surface, specifically subtype 2, allowing for SSTR-based imaging with ^{68}Ga or ^{64}Cu-(DOTA)-peptide PET/CT [170]. DOTATATE PET/CT has rapidly become widespread in the clinical arena and is now considered routine for the diagnosis and staging of patients with well-differentiated neuroendocrine tumors and patient selection for peptide receptor radionuclide therapy (PRRT) [172]. Visual analysis is the cornerstone of DOTATATE PET/CT interpretation and has been standardized with the adoption of criteria like the modified Krenning score [170, 220]. Semi-quantitative and quantitative DOTATATE PET/CT, in contrast, is not common in daily practice. Unlike with FDG-PET/CT, SUV_{max} and other PET parameters have not yet been validated for DOTATATE PET/CT. This may, in part, stem from the fact that SUV-based parameters have different meanings and interpretations for DOTATATE compared with FDG-PET/

CT. DOTATATE SUV-based parameters are representative of receptor density rather than tumor metabolism as is the case with FDG-PET, which in turn has implications for the interpretation of response assessment. Unlike with FDG-PET/CT, decreases in SUV-based parameters on DOTATATE do not necessarily indicate response and could rather represent dedifferentiation.

Despite this limitation, studies are increasingly evaluating the utility and applicability of various semi-quantitative and quantitative DOTATATE PET parameters for the study of NETs, though the majority of these studies have primarily focused on the more common gastroenteropancreatic (GEP) NETs. The application to intrathoracic NETs, specifically pulmonary neuroendocrine tumors (PNETs), on the other hand, has not been as well documented and will be explored below. Thymic neuroendocrine tumors (TNETs) fit within this category as well but are not specifically addressed, given the dearth of literature on this indication.

Pulmonary Neuroendocrine Tumors (PNETs)

PNETs—as well as TNETs—represent a spectrum of neuroendocrine neoplasms that range from low/intermediate grade, such as DIPNECH and carcinoids, to higher grade neoplasms, like large cell neuroendocrine carcinoma and small cell carcinoma. Classification into these tumor subtypes is based on morphologic features, presence of necrosis, and mitotic counts. Unlike with GEP NETs, Ki-67 labeling index is not integrated into the current WHO grading scheme for PNETs or TNETs [352]. Well- to intermediate differentiated NETs that originate from the enterochromaffin or Kulchitsky cells in the respiratory tract are called pulmonary or bronchial carcinoids, which account for 1–2% of all pulmonary malignancies [352]. They are further subdivided into the more prevalent typical (low grade) and less common atypical pulmonary carcinoids (intermediate grade) based upon the number of mitoses present and the extent of necrosis.

A small number of studies have specifically investigated quantitative DOTATATE PET/CT in patients with PNETs, particularly as it relates to characterizing tumor biology and histology. Despite there being limitations with small sample sizes and retrospective studies, the literature overall suggests that certain PET parameters tend to correlate well with tumor grading and can suggest histology [9, 102, 188, 205]. A retrospective analysis of 18 patients with PNETs demonstrated that typical pulmonary carcinoids have significantly higher ^{68}Ga-DOTATATE uptake compared with PNETs of higher grade (median $SUV_{max} = 33$ vs. 2.8, respectively; $p = 0.002$) [205]. These same patients exhibited significantly less ^{18}F-FDG uptake compared to those with PNETs of higher grade (median SUV_{max} 4.9 vs. 16, respectively; $p = 0.005$) with 36% of patients showing little to no FDG uptake. A more recent meta-analysis corroborated these findings, demonstrating a higher mean SUV_{max} on ^{68}Ga-DOTATATE PET/CT for typical pulmonary carcinoids (SUV_{max} range 8.2–118, mean SUV_{max} 36.5 ±21.6) compared with atypical carcinoids (SUV_{max} range 1.1–18.5; mean SUV_{max} 9 ± 5.6; $p < 0.002$) [188]. In addition to higher SUV_{max}, typical pulmonary carcinoids were found to have higher ratios of SUV_{max} on ^{68}Ga-DOTATATE PET relative to that on ^{18}F-FDG PET/CT (1.22–30, mean 13.1 ± 7.3) compared with atypical carcinoids (0.19–3.97, mean 1.7 ± 1.5; $p < 0.001$). Other studies have supported the use of SUV_{max} ratio over individual SUV_{max} values [169].

The role of DOTATATE PET/CT in the assessment of treatment response remains unclear. While there are no studies to date that have restricted their patient population solely to those with PNETs to evaluate this application, there are a few studies that have included them as part of a larger group of patients with NETs. For example, Ortega et al. performed a prospective, multicenter single-arm study in 91 patients with well-differentiated NETs (6 with bronchopulmonary NETs) to determine whether quantitative PET parameters on baseline ^{68}Ga-DOTATATE PET/CT and early PET after one cycle of PRRT were predictive of treatment response and progression-free survival (PFS) [330]. The following metrics were evaluated on baseline and interim PET: lesion-based measures (mean SUV_{max} and ratio of mean lesion SUV_{max} to SUV_{max} in reference organ), segmented DOTATATE tumor volumes (DTTVs), and heterogeneity parameters (coefficient of variation, kurtosis, and skewness). In agreement with prior visual analysis studies, a higher degree of SSTR expression and lower tumor heterogeneity on baseline and interim PET were predictive of PRRT response. Some of the baseline PET parameters were additionally prognostic of clinical outcomes. On multivariate analysis, mean SUV_{max} ($p = 0.019$), ratio of mean lesion SUV_{max} to SUV_{max} in the liver ($p = 0.018$) and spleen ($p = 0.041$), DTTV SUV_{mean} obtained with the liver ($p = 0.0052$), and skewness ($p = 0.048$) correlated with PFS. Changes in PET parameters after 1 cycle of PRRT, on the other hand, were not predictive of clinical outcomes.

Further work is needed to determine PET parameters specific to DOTATATE PET/CT that can be used to both appropriately differentiate responders from nonresponders and that have prognostic/predictive value.

Theranostics

The main role of quantitative thoracic nuclear medicine imaging for theranostics and dosimetry relates to toxicity assessment.

Liver MAA

Transarterial radioembolization (TARE), also known as selective internal radiotherapy (SIRT), is a well-established interventional radiology technique that delivers ^{90}Y-loaded microspheres to target lesions in the liver for treatment of unresectable primary tumors and metastases. Currently, there are two types of microspheres that are FDA approved for clinical use in the United States: SIR-Spheres (Sirtex Medical, North Sydney, Australia) and TheraSpheres (Nordion, Ottawa, Ontario, Canada). SIR-Spheres are nondegradable ^{90}Y-loaded resin microspheres that vary in diameter from 20 to 60 mm. TheraSpheres are ^{90}Y-incorporated glass microspheres that are 20–30 mm in diameter [423]. The microspheres are injected directly into the hepatic artery branches perfusing the target lesion(s), which, because of malignancy-induced vascular alterations, are preferentially taken up by the tumor relative to normal liver parenchyma. This technique allows for a more selective delivery of high-dose internal radiation.

Prior to treatment with ^{90}Y-microspheres, patients undergo simulation for therapy planning. The simulation phase consists of a diagnostic angiography performed in the interventional radiology suite primarily for vascular mapping. At the end of the angiography, ^{99m}Tc-MAA particles are injected intra-arterially into the feeding hepatic vessels. The patient is subsequently transferred to the nuclear medicine department for additional imaging that consists of static anterior and posterior planar images of the thorax and abdomen followed by SPECT/CT. The pretreatment ^{99m}Tc-MAA scan serves a trifold purpose: (1) identification of excessive hepatopulmonary shunting, (2) evaluation for extrahepatic uptake that could lead to nontargeted delivery of microspheres, and (3) dose calculation [235, 445]. As the topic of this chapter is thoracic imaging, we will restrict our discussion to hepatopulmonary shunting.

This procedure applies a theranostic approach by using similar radiopharmaceutical agents for both the therapy planning and treatment phases. MAA particles are considered a surrogate for therapeutic microspheres. MAA particles were specifically chosen for their size and diameter, which closely match those of the microspheres, on the order of 10–100 microns [445]. There are, however, some key differences in their physical characteristics that have the potential to cause discrepancies in their biodistributions. For example, MAA particles are more variable in shape, injected in smaller numbers, and slightly differ in their size distribution with an overall lower mean size compared with microspheres [93, 120]. The latter, in part, helps explain the marginally higher overall risk of pulmonary shunting associated with MAA particles relative to the microspheres [120].

High pulmonary shunting places the patient at risk for radiation-induced pneumonitis and fibrosis following the administration of ^{90}Y microspheres [250]. The ^{99m}Tc-MAA pretreatment scan helps reduce this risk of pulmonary toxicity by identifying patients with excessive pulmonary shunting that may preclude them from undergoing SIRT or require dose modulation. Quantification of hepatopulmonary shunting is expressed with a lung shunt fraction (LSF) (Fig. 25.23). To obtain this value, regions of interest are manually drawn around the lungs and liver on the static anterior and posterior planar images. ROIs for each lung are drawn separately to exclude uptake within the mediastinum and heart. Total liver and lung counts are each obtained through a simple geometric mean of counts in which the square root is taken of the quotient of anterior and posterior counts. The LSF is then calculated using the following equation: ((total lung counts)/ (total lung counts + total liver counts)) × 100%. Assuming a lung mass of 1 kg, the mean lung dose can then be calculated from the LSF using the following simplified MIRD formula [445]:

$$D_{Lung}(Gy) = \text{injected activity}(GBq) \times LSF \times 50.$$

While planar imaging is more commonly utilized to estimate LSF, there is data suggesting this approach likely overestimates pulmonary shunting [111, 144, 147]. Dittman et al. found that planar imaging-derived estimation of LSF was significantly higher than SPECT/CT-derived estimation ($p < 0.0001$), resulting in an average LSF that was 3.6 times higher with the former compared to the latter [111]. The discrepancy was highest in patients with lower LSFs, likely related to liver activity spillover into the basal lungs. While these discrepancies are unlikely to be clinically significant for most patients, they

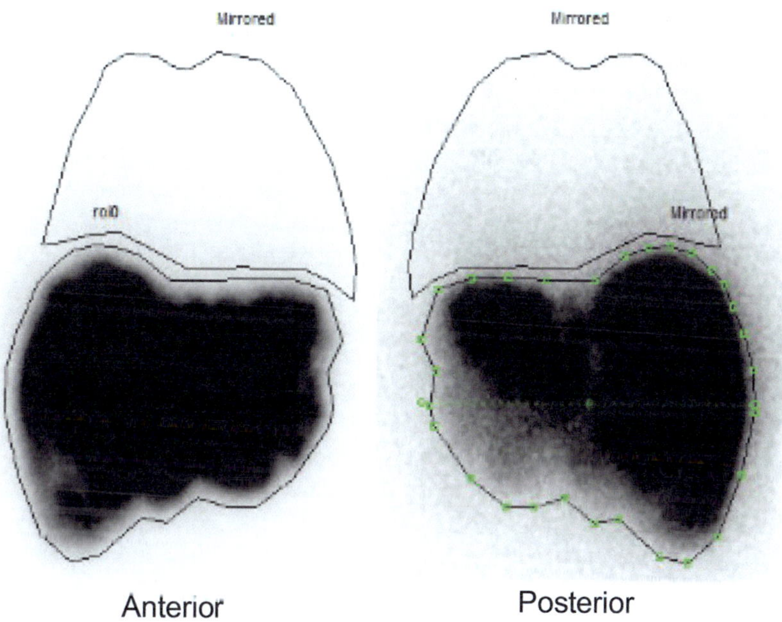

Fig. 25.23 Hepatopulmonary shunt quantification. (**a**) Anterior and (**b**) posterior planar ^{99m}Tc-MAA perfusion images of the chest and abdomen are displayed for a patient with extensive hepatic metastases from atypical pulmonary carcinoid prior to Y-90 radioembolization. To quantify the lung shunt fraction (LSF), regions of interest are drawn, outlining the lungs and liver on both the anterior and posterior images. The hepatopulmonary shunt is 2.9% in this case

can have implications for those with relatively high LSFs who may be contraindicated for SIRT and/or require dose modulation to prevent pulmonary toxicity. Consequently, an increasing number of authors are advocating for the use of SPECT/CT in cases where the planar imaging-derived LSF exceeds 10%, which would allow for a more accurate estimation [79, 111, 445].

LSF has important implications for both the suitability of SIRT as well as dose determination. Specifically, the manufacturer has recommended dose reductions for patients with an LSF greater than 10% who are to receive resin microspheres [59]. In patients who are to be injected with SIRspheres, an LSF of 10–15% should result in a 20% dose reduction, while a 40% dose reduction is recommended in those with an LSF of 16–20%. SIRT with SIRspheres is contraindicated in patients with an LSF above 20% [463]. These values stem from the dose constraint of 30 Gy for a single treatment, as previously established for external beam radiation and a cumulative dose of 50 Gy for multiple treatments [366]. Patients with high LSFs also have the option of undergoing shunt-reducing treatment, including bland embolization and chemoembolization, to become eligible for radioembolization [139, 229, 358, 411]. Repeat ^{99m}Tc-MAA scans may be performed in these patients to determine if the treatment was adequate in reducing the pulmonary shunt to an acceptable level for radioembolization.

In addition to its ability to predict risk for pulmonary toxicity, LSF may also be an independent prognostic indicator of survival in patients treated with SIRT [101, 274, 311, 457]. In a large retrospective study of 606 patients with metastatic colorectal cancer who underwent SIRT, a high LSF, defined as greater than 10%, was predictive of poor overall survival (HR = 1.6; $p < 0.001$) [311]. Interestingly, LSF was only shown to have a weak correlation with serum CEA levels and tumor-to-liver volume ratio and no correlation to prior treatment or presence of extrahepatic metastatic disease, including lung metastases.

Recently, ^{99m}Tc-MAA has been pioneered to guide dosimetry of ^{90}Y-radioembolization of pulmonary malignancies introduced via the bronchial artery. Judicious use of Monte Carlo simulations based on SPECT/CT demonstrates the feasibility of this approach with tolerable toxicity [447].

Targeted Radionuclide Therapies

Radionuclide therapies established for neuroendocrine tumors (NET) have been explored for use in the lung. The safety and efficacy of ^{177}Lu-DOTATATE for the treatment of advanced lung NET and small cell lung cancer have been observed. DOTATATE-PET/CT was used to identify patients amenable to this treatment, with initial signs of good tolerability and response [209, 477]. Recent alpha-emitter-based DOTATATE agents have shown promise in animal models of small-cell lung cancer, motivating further exploration of these agents in clinical trials [157] (NCT05142696, NCT04665739, NCT05130255).

Future Directions in Molecular Imaging of the Thorax

Rapid advances in molecular imaging promise to expand the armamentarium to evaluate systemic physiologic processes noninvasively. Many show promise for evaluating thoracic conditions [476]. Here, we highlight multiple approaches with near clinical translational potential.

Hypoxia Imaging

Tumor hypoxia has been associated with increased aggressive phenotypes and metastatic potential and portends poor clinical prognosis [151], motivating efforts for its evaluation. Multiple nitroimidazole analogs (e.g., ^{18}F-FMISO [186], ^{18}F-FETNIM [459], ^{18}F-HX4 [114], and ^{18}F-FAZA [63]) and the redox agent diacetyl-bis(N4-methylthiosemicarbazone (^{64}Cu-ATSM) [225] have been developed for hypoxic imaging. Several of these agents have shown good correlation with histochemical measures of hypoxia in preclinical models [40], although this can vary depending on the pharmacokinetic properties of the agent (Fig. 25.24) [151]. Furthermore, imaging correlations with patient samples post-surgical resection can be heterogeneous [414]. Nevertheless, studies have shown the potential of these agents to prognosticate patients on therapy [341, 363] and predict overall survival [253].

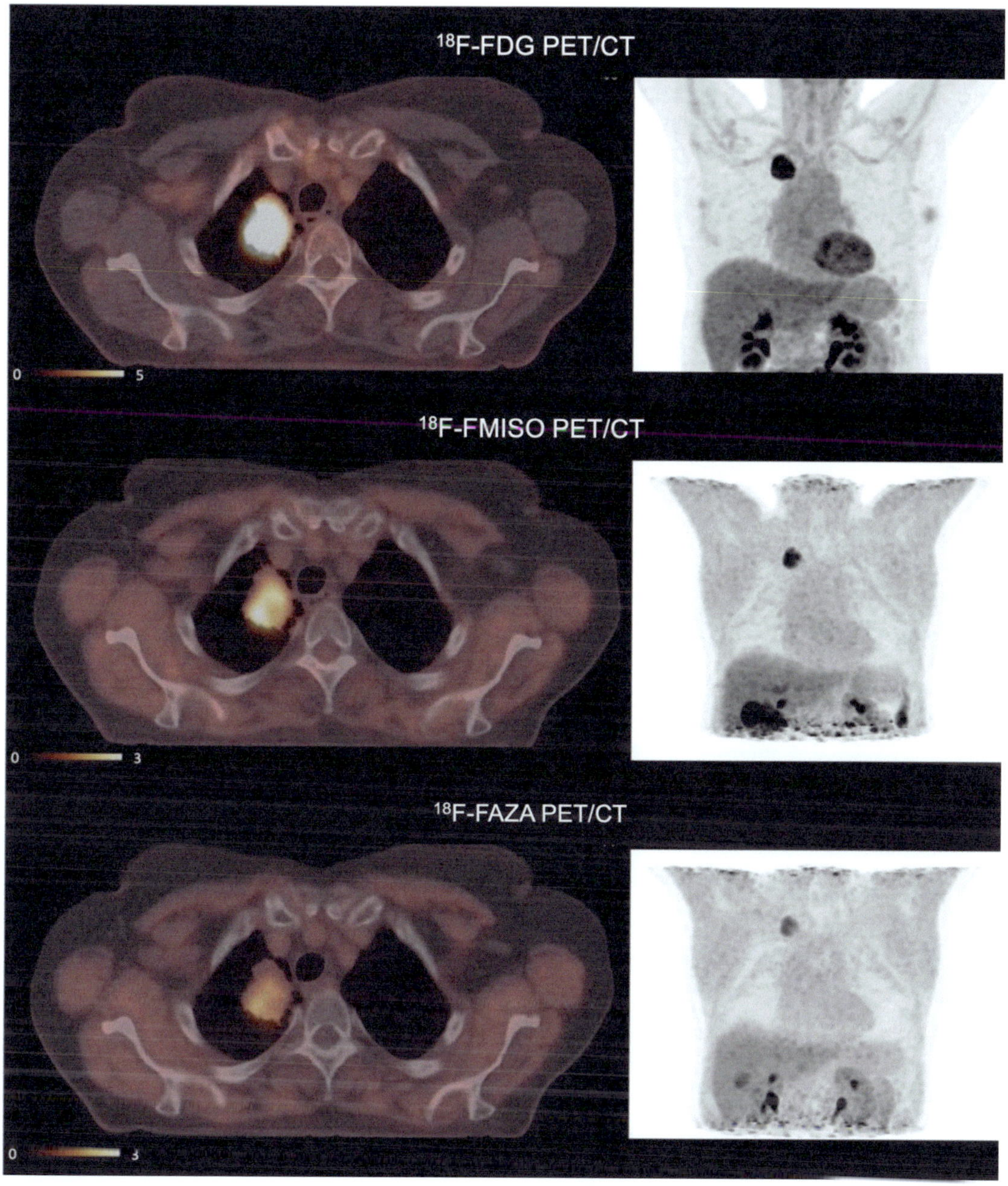

Fig. 25.24 An example of PET scan with ^{18}F-FDG, ^{18}F-FMISO, and ^{18}F-FAZA in a non-small cell lung cancer patient. Hypoxic zones can be seen using FMISO and FAZA, while hypermetabolic regions can be seen using FDG. While uptake to the lesion can be seen with all tracers, SUV was highest with FDG. Moreover, intratumoral distribution of tracer is spatially heterogeneous and not directly concordant between tracers. Furthermore, FMISO has lower uptake than FAZA. (Adapted from Gouel et al. [151])

Imaging Amino Acid Transporter

Amino acid metabolism is important for cancer cell proliferation and can be upregulated in multiple cancer types, including brain [310], prostate [319], and bladder malignancies [317], motivating clinical applications in these settings. This has motivated investigations in amino acid PET imaging in lung cancer. ^{11}C-methionine PET has shown promise for detecting lung cancer brain metastases compared to FDG. L-[3-^{18}F]-alpha-methyltyrosine (^{18}F-FMT) has been shown to correlate to LAT1 amino acid transporters, cell proliferation, and angiogenesis in lung cancers. ^{18}F-labeled (S)-4-(3- -fluoropropyl)-l-glutamic acid shows similar performance to FDG-PET (Fig. 25.25) for staging and evaluation of indeterminate pulmonary nodules [23, 332]. Investigations are ongoing for these agents in the clinic (NCT03824535).

Imaging Angiogenesis

Tumor neoangiogenesis has been implicated as a critical therapeutic and imaging target [275], including in lung cancer [321]. In particular, factors related to the vascular endothelial growth factor (VEGF) pathway, including $\alpha_v\beta_3$ integrin, have been explored as imaging targets with multiple modalities [112, 173]. Vascular perfusion of tumors can be probed with ^{15}O-water [267], but its short half-life likely precludes widespread clinical adoption. Radio-labeled antibodies [25, 276], peptides [236, 474], and small molecules targeting the VEGF or $\alpha_v\beta_3$ integrins have been evaluated in both animal models and humans. In particular, peptides based on the arginine–glycine–aspartic acid (RGD) sequence have been extensively examined [252], with early clinical studies implicating their potential to predict early treatment response to chemotherapy and radiation in non-small cell lung cancer [273].

Prostate-specific membrane antigen (PSMA) PET has revolutionized prostate cancer management [319]. The increased sensitivity of this agent means that prostate cancer metastases to the lung are increasingly visualized. Although most evaluated for prostate cancer, other malignancies can express PSMA. Moreover, PSMA is also expressed in neovasculature [427] and lung cancers [439]—therefore, these lesions can be incidentally found on PSMA-PET imaging (Fig. 25.26). Inflammatory and infectious conditions can also demonstrate PSMA uptake (Fig. 25.27). Integration with clinical history and tissue sampling is therefore imperative for definitive diagnosis [97].

Targeted Receptor and Pathways Imaging

The advent of molecular genotyping, large-scale transcriptomics, and rapid pathologic analytical assays has identified druggable pathways in lung cancer [166]. In particular, tumor receptor tyrosine kinases have been implicated as

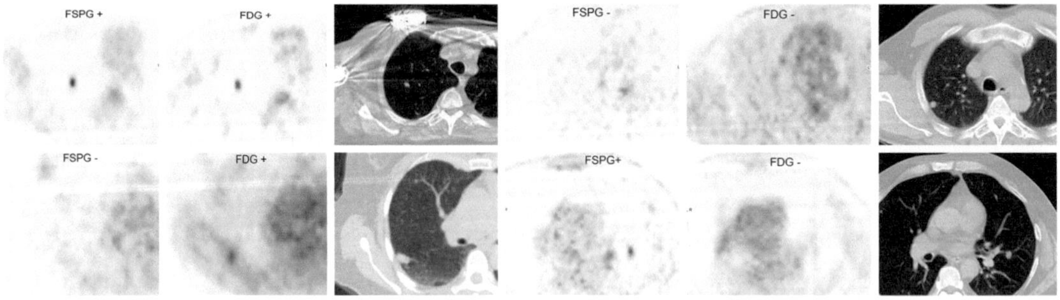

Fig. 25.25 Spectrum of ^{18}F-FSPG PET and ^{18}F-FDG PET findings across different tumors shows that lung tumors can demonstrate marked different amino acid and glucose metabolic profiles. This highlights the potential of multi-isotope phenotyping with PET. (Adapted from Paez et al. [332])

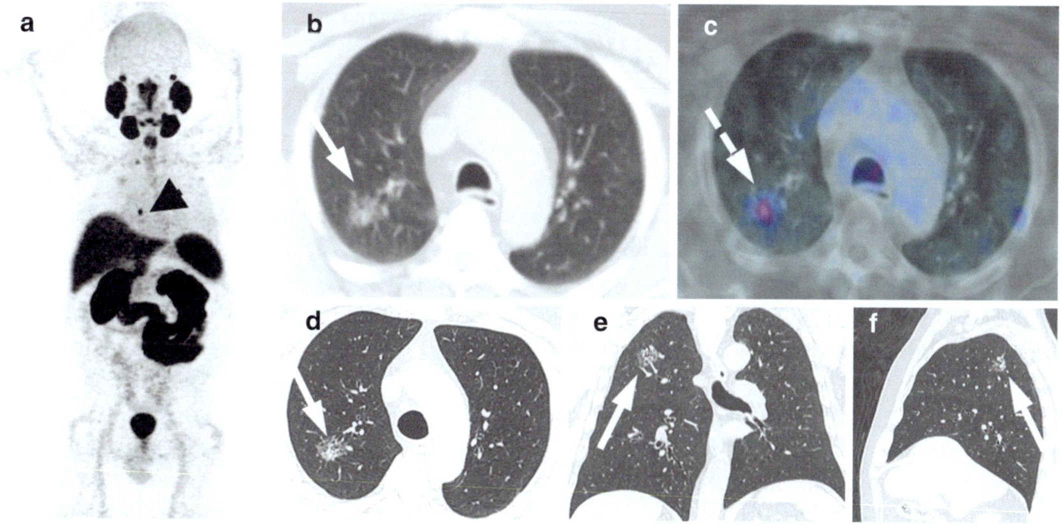

Fig. 25.26 Lung adenocarcinoma with PSMA uptake. ^{68}Ga-PSMA-PET MIP (**a**), axial CT (**b**) and axial PET/CT (**c**), and diagnostic lung CT (**d**–**f**) show a slight uptake (dashed arrow) in a peribronchial subsolid pulmonary nodule in the posterior segment of the right upper lobe (arrows). Biopsy revealed primary lung adenocarcinoma. A confirmed prostate cancer metastatic right pulmonary hilar lymph node with intense uptake was also noted (arrowhead in (**a**)). (Adapted from de Galiza Barbosa et al. [97])

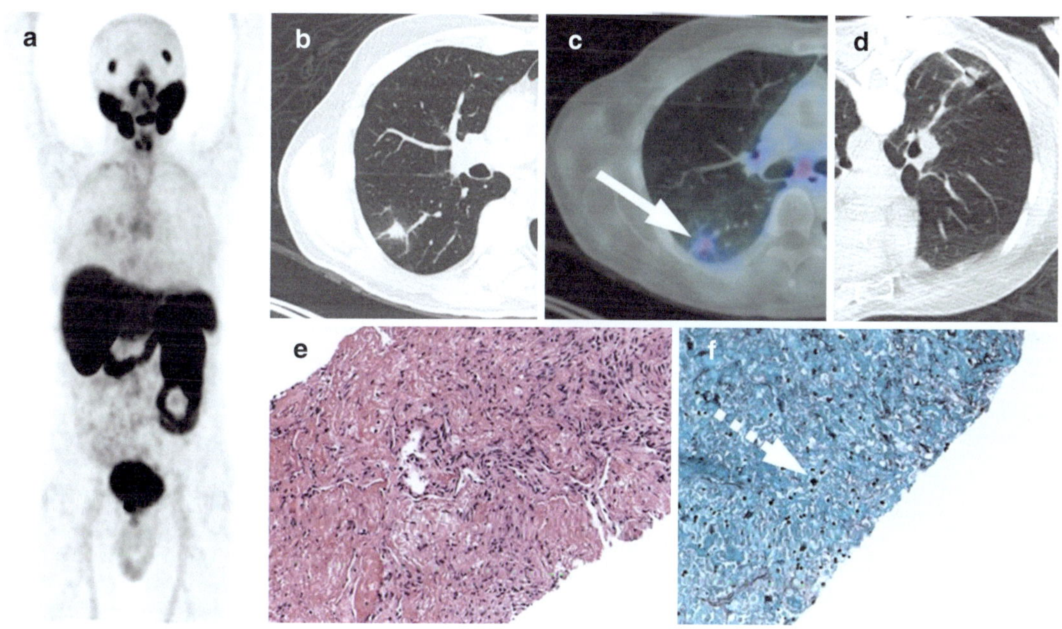

Fig. 25.27 Pulmonary histoplasmosis on PSMA. A 70-year-old patient under staging of prostate cancer (iPSA = 7.0 ng/mL, Gleason 8 = 4 + 4). ^{68}Ga-PSMA-PET MIP (**a**), axial CT (**b**), axial PET/CT (**c**), and CT-guided biopsy (**d**) images show a pulmonary nodule with faint uptake (arrow). Pathology (**e**, **f**) shows a positive Grocott stain with multiple yeasts (dashed arrow) and areas of focal neutrophil conglomerates, consistent with histoplasmosis. (Adapted from de Galiza Barbosa et al. [97])

key regulators of lung cancer pathogenesis, including EGFR [254, 295], c-MET [438], RET [325], and ALK [373]. The ability to identify patients amenable to these therapies, and subsequent response assessment, would be invaluable. Imaging analogs of many of these drug targets have been developed, both with antibody-based and small molecular approaches. ^{89}Zr-cetuximab PET has shown promise in multiple cancer types, including lung cancer, showing increased uptake compared to bloodpool [268]. Small-molecule agents confer more favorable kinetics for imaging, and multiple tyrosine kinase inhibitor probes have been developed. For example, an ^{11}C-labeled EGFR targeting probe was able to identify patients with better progression-free and overall survival to erlotinib [291]. This drug has also been directly labeled with ^{11}C, with initial clinical studies identifying focal uptake in non-small cell lung cancer lesions and adjacent metastatic nodes [290]. ^{18}F probes are more favorable for clinical use, and several ^{18}F-labeled EGFR-TKI have also been explored with promising results [26, 396, 399, 460, 461]. Crizotinib is a dual c-MET/ALK inhibitor, and several efforts have developed imaging analogs of this drug [61, 259]. Other promising agents include the ^{11}C and ^{18}F-isotopologues ROS1/ALK inhibitor lorlatinib, which has been explored for use in brain lesions [85, 86].

Cellular proliferation in lung neoplasms has also been a key biomarker being probed by novel nuclear medicine agents [11]. In particular, 3′-deoxy-3′- [^{18}F]fluorothymidine (FLT) is an agent that proves the activity of thymidine kinase and reflects the cellular proliferation status of cells. Although not routinely used clinically, FLT has shown promise, especially in combination with FDG-PET for identifying early response to chemoradiation and relapse lung cancer [82, 83, 127, 168] (Fig. 25.28). Additional studies are underway to assess its role in the immunotherapy setting [370].

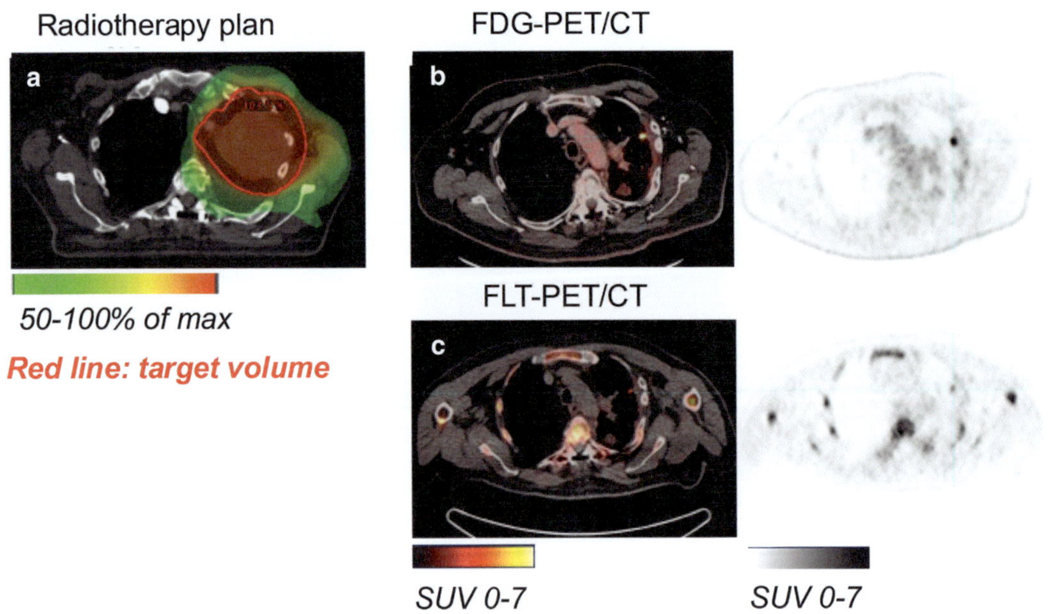

Fig. 25.28 FDG/FLT PET can evaluate for recurrent lung cancer post-radiation. (**a**) Radiotherapy plan from a patient who received 2 Gy × 33 fractions to the left upper lobe lesion. 7 months post radiotherapy, FDG-PET/CT (**b**) and FLT-PET/CT (**c**) of the residual opacity in the left upper lobe both demonstrated high SUV, compatible with relapsed disease. (Adapted from Christensen et al. [82])

Fibroblast Imaging

More than 90% of epithelial cancers, including lung cancer, have high levels of fibroblast activation protein (FAP), a type II transmembrane serine protease, which is strongly linked to different tumor invasion, metastasis, and prognosis [67]. FAP inhibitors have been optimized for PET imaging, with highly promising results for the detection of various malignancies. FAP-targeting probes using antibodies and small molecules, labeled with both ^{18}F and radiometals, have been evaluated for multiple malignancies and are currently in phase 2 trials. Optimized ^{68}Ga-FAPI-04 (Fig. 25.29) [67] and ^{18}F-FAPI-74 have been able to identify non-small cell lung cancer in patients and offer an opportunity for radioligand therapy with the same target [146, 260].

Beyond oncologic applications, targeted imaging agents for characterizing lung fibrosis may offer vital prognostic information for patients with interstitial lung disease. ^{68}Ga-FAPI-04 PET in patients with systemic sclerosis-associated ILD correlated with fibrotic activity and disease progression [43] and has been correlated with pathologic markers of fibrosis in humans [356]. Another agent, ^{68}Ga-CBP8, targets type 1 collagen in fibrotic extracellular matrix and has the potential to identify fibrotic lung regions [297]. Other agents, such as DOTATATE, may also nonspecifically uptake in these locales as part of the inflammatory response [296].

Fibrin Imaging

Fibrin clot formation is an important part of the thromboembolic pathway. Direct visualization would complement the current assessment of pulmonary emboli, as discussed earlier. Fibrin-targeted PET probes have been developed and are in clinical trial assessment [66, 84, 181]. Most recently, the fibrin targeting ^{64}Cu-FBP8 was shown to identify thrombus in the left atrial appendage, with pathologic confirmation [181] and is actively being explored for pulmonary embolism assessment (NCT04022915).

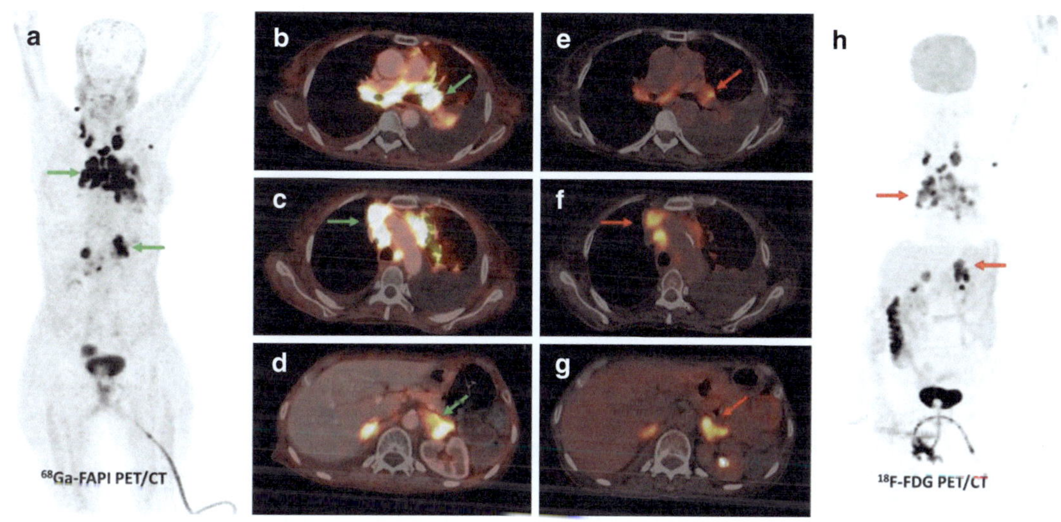

Fig. 25.29 ^{68}Ga-FAPI-04 and FDG-PET/CT images in a 59-year-old woman with biopsy-proven metastatic left lung adenocarcinoma. FAPI-04 PET/CT images revealed intensely tracer-avid left hilar mass lesion [(**b**) green arrow], multistation mediastinal lymphadenopathy [(**a**, **c**) green arrows], and bilateral adrenal metastases [(**a**, **d**) green arrows depicting left adrenal lesion]. Of note, FAPI uptake in these sites was more conspicuous than FDG [(**e**–**h**) red arrows]. (Adapted from Chandekar et al. [67])

Immunotherapy Response Imaging

Systemic immunotherapy is being actively pursued for lung cancer applications [6, 234]. The ability to assess immune cell subsets, phenotype tumors amenable to immune checkpoint blockade, and track delivery of chimeric antigen-receptor T-cells (CAR-T) would facilitate the assessment and translation of these therapies. The reader is referred to recent reviews of nuclear medicine's role in this arena [318, 320], including the ability of imaging to identify the early onset of immune-related toxicities.

Advances in Lung Infection Imaging

Recent advances have explored the use of PET to differentiate bacterial infection from other causes of inflammation in the chest. Of particular note for lung applications, Sellmeyer et al. have developed targeted probes based on the antibiotic trimethoprim and demonstrated its ability to uptake in bacterial lung infections and differentiate them from sterile inflammation or neoplasm [246, 380].

Artificial Intelligence and Computer-Assisted Molecular Imaging

Extensive research is ongoing to apply artificial intelligence (AI) and other computer-aided techniques for chest imaging. Improving image quality through AI-enhanced image reconstruction has improved PET imaging's spatial resolution and noise profiles [348]. Beyond image quality alone, the functional information provided by nuclear medicine studies lends itself to integration into radiomic analysis and deep-learning workflows [46]. Seminal works have applied neural network analyses on V/Q scans, demonstrating the potential of AI for aiding the clinical diagnosis of PE [378]. These have been developed to recognize lung infection and PE patterns, for example, in COVID-19 patients [24]. The most exciting applications of AI and radiomics for lung molecular imaging are the phenotypic and molecular characterization and prognostication of lung cancer [92]. Promising studies, primarily based on FDG-PET/CT, have demonstrated the potential to identify lesions [377] and predict metastasis and treatment response of multiple lung cancer subtypes [50, 174, 437, 472, 478]. Translating these techniques in the clinic will require robust clinical trials to establish value and robust characterization of these approaches [80, 207, 468].

Summary

This chapter reviewed critical considerations for applying nuclear medicine and molecular imaging for thoracic imaging. Quantitative nuclear medicine of the thorax requires the integration of novel instrumentation and medical physics principles, established and novel imaging probes, molecular biology/physiology, and a clear understanding of the applicability of these techniques to address the clinical question at hand.

Acknowledgments T.S.C.N. is supported by a Thrall Innovation Grant (Massachusetts General Hospital), the Lee Family Foundation, and a Department of Defense Physician Research Award (W81XWH-22-1-0061).

Competing Interests The authors have no conflicts of interest to declare that are relevant to the content of this chapter.

References

1. Abe Y, Tamura K, Sakata I, et al. Clinical implications of 18F-fluorodeoxyglucose positron emission tomography/computed tomography at delayed phase for diagnosis and prognosis of malignant pleural mesothelioma. Oncol Rep. 2012;27:333–8. https://doi.org/10.3892/or.2011.1520.
2. Abgral R, Bourhis D, Salaun P-Y. Clinical perspectives for the use of total body PET/CT. Eur J Nucl Med Mol Imaging. 2021;48:1712–8. https://doi.org/10.1007/s00259-021-05293-4.
3. Abnet CC, Arnold M, Wei W-Q. Epidemiology of esophageal squamous cell carcinoma. Gastroenterology. 2018;154:360–73. https://doi.org/10.1053/j.gastro.2017.08.023.
4. Abrams GA, Jaffe CC, Hoffer PB, et al. Diagnostic utility of contrast echocardiography and lung per-

fusion scan in patients with hepatopulmonary syndrome. Gastroenterology. 1995;109:1283–8. https://doi.org/10.1016/0016-5085(95)90589-8.
5. Acharya PS, Zukas A, Chandan V, et al. Fibroblast activation protein: a serine protease expressed at the remodeling interface in idiopathic pulmonary fibrosis. Hum Pathol. 2006;37:352–60. https://doi.org/10.1016/j.humpath.2005.11.020.
6. Ahrens ET, Bulte JWM. Tracking immune cells in vivo using magnetic resonance imaging. Nat Rev Immunol. 2013;13:755–63. https://doi.org/10.1038/nri3531.
7. Aide N, Lasnon C, Kesner A, et al. New PET technologies – embracing progress and pushing the limits. Eur J Nucl Med Mol Imaging. 2021;48:2711–26. https://doi.org/10.1007/s00259-021-05390-4.
8. Akhtar MS, Imran MB, Nadeem MA, Shahid A. Antimicrobial peptides as infection imaging agents: better than radiolabeled antibiotics. Int J Pept. 2012;2012:1–19. https://doi.org/10.1155/2012/965238.
9. Albano D, Dondi F, Bauckneht M, et al. The diagnostic and prognostic role of combined [18F]FDG and [68Ga]-DOTA-peptides PET/CT in primary pulmonary carcinoids: a multicentric experience. Eur Radiol. 2023;33:4167–77. https://doi.org/10.1007/s00330-022-09326-w.
10. Al-Mehisen R, Al-Halees Z, Alnemri K, et al. Primary pulmonary artery sarcoma: a rare and overlooked differential diagnosis of pulmonary embolism. Clues to diagnosis. Int J Surg Case Rep. 2019;65:15–9. https://doi.org/10.1016/j.ijscr.2019.10.014.
11. Alwadani B, Dall'Angelo S, Fleming IN. Clinical value of 3'-deoxy-3'-[(18)F]fluorothymidine-positron emission tomography for diagnosis, staging and assessing therapy response in lung cancer. Insights Imaging. 2021;12:90. https://doi.org/10.1186/s13244-021-01026-1.
12. American College of Radiology. ACR appropriateness criteria® staging and follow-up of Esophageal cancer. 2022, 2023. https://acsearch.acr.org/docs/3163055/Narrative/. Accessed 10 Jul 2023
13. Anderson DR, Kahn SR, Rodger MA, et al. Computed tomographic pulmonary angiography vs ventilation-perfusion lung scanning in patients with suspected pulmonary Embolisma randomized controlled trial. JAMA. 2007;298:2743–53. https://doi.org/10.1001/jama.298.23.2743.
14. Angelina J, Lay MDG, Hui E, Zhang G, McCaughan W. Fibroblast activation protein in liver fibrosis. FBL. 2019;24:1–17. https://doi.org/10.2741/4706.
15. Braune A, Hofheinz F, Bluth T, et al. Comparison of static and dynamic ^{18}F-FDG PET/CT for quantification of pulmonary inflammation in acute lung injury. J Nucl Med. 2019;60:1629. https://doi.org/10.2967/jnumed.119.226597.
16. Antoniou AJ, Raja S, El-Khouli R, et al. Comprehensive radionuclide esophagogastrointestinal transit study: methodology, reference values, and initial clinical experience. J Nucl Med. 2015;56:721–7. https://doi.org/10.2967/jnumed.114.152074.
17. Arabi H, AkhavanAllaf A, Sanaat A, et al. The promise of artificial intelligence and deep learning in PET and SPECT imaging. Phys Medica PM Int J Devoted Appl Phys Med Biol. 2021;83:122–37. https://doi.org/10.1016/j.ejmp.2021.03.008.
18. Arguedas MR, Abrams GA, Krowka MJ, Fallon MB. Prospective evaluation of outcomes and predictors of mortality in patients with hepatopulmonary syndrome undergoing liver transplantation. Hepatol Baltim Md. 2003;37:192–7. https://doi.org/10.1053/jhep.2003.50023.
19. Arnon-Sheleg E, Haberfeld O, Kremer R, et al. Head-to-head prospective comparison of quantitative lung Scintigraphy and segment counting in predicting pulmonary function in lung cancer patients undergoing video-assisted thoracoscopic lobectomy. J Nucl Med. 2020;61:981–9. https://doi.org/10.2967/jnumed.119.234526.
20. Auletta S, Varani M, Horvat R, et al. PET radiopharmaceuticals for specific bacteria imaging: a systematic review. J Clin Med. 2019;8:197. https://doi.org/10.3390/jcm8020197.
21. Azdaki N, Maleki MH, Kazemi T, et al. V/Q scans and computerized tomography pulmonary angiography in pulmonary emboli in pregnancy: Superiority for fetal or mother. J Res Med Sci. 2014;19:683–4.
22. Badr A, Joyce JM, Durick J. Rim of FDG uptake around a pulmonary infarct on PET/CT in a patient with unsuspected pulmonary embolism. Clin Nucl Med. 2009;34:285. https://doi.org/10.1097/RLU.0b013e31819e52bc.
23. Baek S, Choi C-M, Ahn SH, et al. Exploratory clinical trial of (4 S)-4-(3-[18F] fluoropropyl)-l-glutamate for imaging xC- transporter using positron emission tomography in patients with non–small cell lung or breast cancer. Clin Cancer Res. 2012;18:5427–37.
24. Baeza S, Gil D, Garcia-Olivé I, et al. A novel intelligent radiomic analysis of perfusion SPECT/CT images to optimize pulmonary embolism diagnosis in COVID-19 patients. EJNMMI Phys. 2022;9:84. https://doi.org/10.1186/s40658-022-00510-x.
25. Bahce I, Huisman MC, Verwer EE, et al. Pilot study of (89)Zr-bevacizumab positron emission tomography in patients with advanced non-small cell lung cancer. EJNMMI Res. 2014;4:35. https://doi.org/10.1186/s13550-014-0035-5.
26. Bahce I, Yaqub M, Smit EF, et al. Personalizing NSCLC therapy by characterizing tumors using TKI-PET and immuno-PET. Lung Cancer Amst Neth. 2017;107:1–13. https://doi.org/10.1016/j.lungcan.2016.05.025.
27. Bailey DL, Willowson KP. An evidence-based review of quantitative SPECT imaging and potential clinical applications. J Nucl Med. 2013;54:83–9. https://doi.org/10.2967/jnumed.112.111476.
28. Bailey DL, Willowson KP. Quantitative SPECT/CT: SPECT joins PET as a quantitative imag-

ing modality. Eur J Nucl Med Mol Imaging. 2014;41(Suppl 1):S17–25. https://doi.org/10.1007/s00259-013-2542-4.

29. Bajc M, Lindqvist A. Ventilation/perfusion SPECT imaging-diagnosing other cardiopulmonary diseases beyond pulmonary embolism. Semin Nucl Med. 2019;49:4–10. https://doi.org/10.1053/j.semnuclmed.2018.10.012.
30. Bajc M, Neilly JB, Miniati M, et al. EANM guidelines for ventilation/perfusion scintigraphy: part 1. Pulmonary imaging with ventilation/perfusion single photon emission tomography. Eur J Nucl Med Mol Imaging. 2009;36:1356–70. https://doi.org/10.1007/s00259-009-1170-5.
31. Bajc M, Schümichen C, Grüning T, et al. EANM guideline for ventilation/perfusion single-photon emission computed tomography (SPECT) for diagnosis of pulmonary embolism and beyond. Eur J Nucl Med Mol Imaging. 2019;46:2429–51. https://doi.org/10.1007/s00259-019-04450-0.
32. Barton LM, Duval EJ, Stroberg E, et al. COVID-19 Autopsies, Oklahoma, USA. Am J Clin Pathol. 2020;153:725–33. https://doi.org/10.1093/ajcp/aqaa062.
33. Beekman FJ, de Jong HWAM, van Geloven S. Efficient fully 3-D iterative SPECT reconstruction with Monte Carlo-based scatter compensation. IEEE Trans Med Imaging. 2002;21:867–77. https://doi.org/10.1109/TMI.2002.803130.
34. Begic A, Jögi J, Hadziredzepovic A, et al. Tomographic ventilation/perfusion lung scintigraphy in the monitoring of the effect of treatment in pulmonary embolism: serial follow-up over a 6-month period. Nucl Med Commun. 2011;32:508. https://doi.org/10.1097/MNM.0b013e328344dfd5.
35. Begic A, Opanković E, Begović-Hadžimuratović S, et al. Ventilation/perfusion tomography – V/P--SPECT vs planar technique. Case Rep Intern Med. 2014;1 https://doi.org/10.5430/crim.v1n2p205.
36. Begic A, Opankovic E, Cukic V, et al. Impact of ventilation/perfusion single-photon emission computed tomography on treatment duration of pulmonary embolism. Nucl Med Commun. 2015;36:162. https://doi.org/10.1097/MNM.0000000000000224.
37. Bellani G, Guerra L, Musch G, et al. Lung regional metabolic activity and gas volume changes induced by tidal ventilation in patients with acute lung injury. Am J Respir Crit Care Med. 2011;183:1193–9. https://doi.org/10.1164/rccm.201008-1318OC.
38. Bellani G, Laffey JG, Pham T, et al. Epidemiology, patterns of care, and mortality for patients with acute respiratory distress syndrome in intensive care units in 50 countries. JAMA. 2016;315:788. https://doi.org/10.1001/jama.2016.0291.
39. Ben Shimol J, Amital H, Lidar M, et al. The utility of PET/CT in large vessel vasculitis. Sci Rep. 2020;10:17709. https://doi.org/10.1038/s41598-020-73818-2.
40. Bentzen L, Keiding S, Horsman MR, et al. Feasibility of detecting hypoxia in experimental mouse tumours with 18F-fluorinated tracers and positron emission tomography--a study evaluating [18F]Fluoro-2-deoxy-D-glucose. Acta Oncol Stockh Swed. 2000;39:629–37. https://doi.org/10.1080/028418600750013320.
41. Bentzen SM, Gregoire V. Molecular imaging-based dose painting: a novel paradigm for radiation therapy prescription. Semin Radiat Oncol. 2011;21:101–10. https://doi.org/10.1016/j.semradonc.2010.10.001.
42. Berghmans T, Dusart M, Paesmans M, et al. Primary tumor standardized uptake value (SUVmax) measured on fluorodeoxyglucose positron emission tomography (FDG-PET) is of prognostic value for survival in non-small cell lung cancer (NSCLC): a systematic review and meta-analysis (MA) by the European Lung Cancer Working Party for the IASLC Lung Cancer Staging Project. J Thorac Oncol. 2008;3:6–12. https://doi.org/10.1097/JTO.0b013e31815e6d6b.
43. Bergmann C, Distler JHW, Treutlein C, et al. 68Ga-FAPI-04 PET-CT for molecular assessment of fibroblast activation and risk evaluation in systemic sclerosis-associated interstitial lung disease: a single-centre, pilot study. Lancet Rheumatol. 2021;3:e185–94. https://doi.org/10.1016/S2665-9913(20)30421-5.
44. Berker Y, Li Y. Attenuation correction in emission tomography using the emission data—A review. Med Phys. 2016;43:807–32. https://doi.org/10.1118/1.4938264.
45. Beyer T, Townsend DW, Brun T, et al. A combined PET/CT scanner for clinical oncology. J Nucl Med. 2000;41:1369–79.
46. Bianconi F, Palumbo I, Spanu A, et al. PET/CT radiomics in lung cancer: an overview. Appl Sci. 2020;10:1718.
47. Björkman KC, Kjellberg M, Bergström SE, et al. Postoperative regional distribution of pulmonary ventilation and perfusion in infants with congenital diaphragmatic hernia. J Pediatr Surg. 2011;46:2047–53. https://doi.org/10.1016/j.jpedsurg.2011.06.042.
48. Boellaard R. Standards for PET image acquisition and quantitative data analysis. J Nucl Med. 2009;50(Suppl 1):11S–20S. https://doi.org/10.2967/jnumed.108.057182.
49. Borggreve AS, Goense L, van Rossum PSN, et al. Preoperative prediction of pathologic response to neoadjuvant chemoradiotherapy in patients with esophageal cancer using 18F-FDG PET/CT and DW-MRI: a prospective multicenter study. Int J Radiat Oncol Biol Phys. 2020;106:998–1009. https://doi.org/10.1016/j.ijrobp.2019.12.038.
50. Borrelli P, Ly J, Kaboteh R, et al. AI-based detection of lung lesions in [18F]FDG PET-CT from lung cancer patients. EJNMMI Phys. 2021;8:32. https://doi.org/10.1186/s40658-021-00376-5.
51. Bowen SR, Hippe DS, Thomas HM, et al. Prognostic value of early Fluorodeoxyglucose-positron emission tomography response imaging and peripheral immunologic biomarkers: substudy of a phase II

trial of risk-adaptive chemoradiation for unresectable non-small cell lung cancer. Adv Radiat Oncol. 2022;7:100857. https://doi.org/10.1016/j.adro.2021.100857.
52. Bradley JD, Paulus R, Komaki R, et al. Standard-dose versus high-dose conformal radiotherapy with concurrent and consolidation carboplatin plus paclitaxel with or without cetuximab for patients with stage IIIA or IIIB non-small-cell lung cancer (RTOG 0617): a randomised, two-by-two factorial phase 3 study. Lancet Oncol. 2015;16:187–99. https://doi.org/10.1016/S1470-2045(14)71207-0.
53. British Thoracic Society, Society of Cardiothoracic Surgeons of Great Britain and Ireland Working Party. BTS guidelines: guidelines on the selection of patients with lung cancer for surgery. Thorax. 2001;56:89–108. https://doi.org/10.1136/thorax.56.2.89.
54. Brody SL, Gunsten SP, Luehmann HP, et al. Chemokine Receptor 2–targeted molecular imaging in pulmonary fibrosis. A clinical trial. Am J Respir Crit Care Med. 2021;203:78–89. https://doi.org/10.1164/rccm.202004-1132OC.
55. Broens B, Duitman J-W, Zwezerijnen GJC, et al. Novel tracers for molecular imaging of interstitial lung disease: a state of the art review. Autoimmun Rev. 2022;21:103202. https://doi.org/10.1016/j.autrev.2022.103202.
56. Brücher BLDM, Weber W, Bauer M, et al. Neoadjuvant therapy of Esophageal squamous cell carcinoma: response evaluation by positron emission tomography. Ann Surg. 2001;233:300–9.
57. Brunelli A, Kim AW, Berger KI, Addrizzo-Harris DJ. Physiologic evaluation of the patient with lung cancer being considered for resectional surgery: diagnosis and management of lung cancer, 3rd ed: American College of Chest Physicians evidence-based clinical practice guidelines. Chest. 2013;143:e166S–90S. https://doi.org/10.1378/chest.12-2395.
58. Bruyant PP. Analytic and iterative reconstruction algorithms in SPECT. J Nucl Med. 2002;43:1343–58.
59. BTG International Inc. TheraSphere® Yttrium-90 glass microspheres. London, UK; 2022.
60. Bu L, Tu N, Wang K, et al. Relationship between 18F-FDG PET/CT semi-quantitative parameters and International Association for the Study of Lung Cancer, American Thoracic Society/European Respiratory Society Classification in Lung Adenocarcinomas. Korean J Radiol. 2022;23:112–23. https://doi.org/10.3348/kjr.2021.0455.
61. Buck JR, Saleh S, Claus T, et al. N-[(18)F]-Fluoroacetylcrizotinib: a potentially potent and selective PET tracer for molecular imaging of non-small cell lung cancer. Bioorg Med Chem Lett. 2020;30:127257. https://doi.org/10.1016/j.bmcl.2020.127257.
62. Burkett BJ, Bartlett DJ, McGarrah PW, et al. A review of theranostics: perspectives on emerging approaches and clinical advancements. Radiol Imaging Cancer. 2023;5:e220157. https://doi.org/10.1148/rycan.220157.
63. Busk M, Horsman MR, Jakobsen S, et al. Cellular uptake of PET tracers of glucose metabolism and hypoxia and their linkage. Eur J Nucl Med Mol Imaging. 2008;35:2294–303. https://doi.org/10.1007/s00259-008-0888-9.
64. Castañer E, Alguersuari A, Andreu M, et al. Imaging findings in pulmonary vasculitis. Semin Ultrasound CT MR. 2012;33:567–79. https://doi.org/10.1053/j.sult.2012.05.001.
65. Castañer E, Alguersuari A, Gallardo X, et al. When to suspect pulmonary vasculitis: radiologic and clinical clues. Radiogr Rev Publ Radiol Soc N Am Inc. 2010;30:33–53. https://doi.org/10.1148/rg.301095103.
66. Chae SY, Kwon T-W, Jin S, et al. A phase 1, first-in-human study of 18F-GP1 positron emission tomography for imaging acute arterial thrombosis. EJNMMI Res. 2019;9:3. https://doi.org/10.1186/s13550-018-0471-8.
67. Chandekar KR, Prashanth A, Vinjamuri S, Kumar R. FAPI PET/CT imaging—an updated review. Diagnostics. 2023;13:2018.
68. Chandra R, Rahmim A. Nuclear medicine physics: the basics. Lippincott Williams & Wilkins; 2017.
69. Chang S, Kim S-J. Prediction of recurrence and mortality of locally advanced Esophageal cancer patients using pretreatment F-18 FDG PET/CT parameters: intratumoral heterogeneity, SUV, and volumetric parameters. Cancer Biother Radiopharm. 2016;31:1–6. https://doi.org/10.1089/cbr.2015.1932.
70. Chen DL, Agapov E, Wu K, et al. Selective imaging of lung macrophages using [11C]PBR28-based positron emission tomography. Mol Imaging Biol. 2021;23:905–13. https://doi.org/10.1007/s11307-021-01617-w.
71. Chen DL, Bedient TJ, Kozlowski J, et al. [18F]fluorodeoxyglucose positron emission tomography for lung antiinflammatory response evaluation. Am J Respir Crit Care Med. 2009;180:533–9. https://doi.org/10.1164/rccm.200904-0501OC.
72. Chen DL, Cheriyan J, Chilvers ER, et al. Quantification of lung PET images: challenges and opportunities. J Nucl Med. 2017;58:201–7. https://doi.org/10.2967/jnumed.116.184796.
73. Chen DL, Mintun MA, Schuster DP. Comparison of methods to quantitate 18F-FDG uptake with PET during experimental acute lung injury. J Nucl Med. 2004;45:1583–90.
74. Chen DL, Schuster DP. Positron emission tomography with [18F]fluorodeoxyglucose to evaluate neutrophil kinetics during acute lung injury. Am J Physiol Lung Cell Mol Physiol. 2004;286:L834–40. https://doi.org/10.1152/ajplung.00339.2003.
75. Chen HHW, Chiu N-T, Su W-C, et al. Prognostic value of whole-body total lesion glycolysis at pretreatment FDG PET/CT in non-small cell lung

cancer. Radiology. 2012;264:559–66. https://doi.org/10.1148/radiol.12111148.
76. Chen X, Zhou B, Xie H, et al. Direct and indirect strategies of deep-learning-based attenuation correction for general purpose and dedicated cardiac SPECT. Eur J Nucl Med Mol Imaging. 2022;49:3046–60. https://doi.org/10.1007/s00259-022-05718-8.
77. Chevalier E, Boursier C, Claudin M, et al. Feasibility of 177Lu therapy monitoring using fast whole-body SPECT recordings provided by a high-speed 360° CZT camera. Clin Nucl Med. 2020;45:e493–4. https://doi.org/10.1097/RLU.0000000000003169.
78. Chiappetta M, Mendogni P, Cattaneo M, et al. Is PET/CT able to predict histology in thymic epithelial tumours? a narrative review. Diagnostics. 2023;13:98. https://doi.org/10.3390/diagnostics13010098.
79. Chiesa C, Sjogreen-Gleisner K, Walrand S, et al. EANM dosimetry committee series on standard operational procedures: a unified methodology for 99mTc-MAA pre- and 90Y peri-therapy dosimetry in liver radioembolization with 90Y microspheres. EJNMMI Phys. 2021;8:77. https://doi.org/10.1186/s40658-021-00394-3.
80. Choi Y, Yu W, Nagarajan MB, et al. Translating AI to clinical practice: overcoming data shift with explainability. Radiographics. 2023;43:e220105. https://doi.org/10.1148/rg.220105.
81. Chojnowski M, Kobylecka M, Olesińska M. Esophageal transit scintigraphy in systemic sclerosis. Reumatologia. 2016;54:251–5. https://doi.org/10.5114/reum.2016.63666.
82. Christensen TN, Langer SW, Persson G, et al. Impact of [(18)F]FDG-PET and [(18)F]FLT-PET-parameters in patients with suspected relapse of irradiated lung cancer. Diagn Basel Switz. 2021;11 https://doi.org/10.3390/diagnostics11020279.
83. Christensen TN, Langer SW, Persson GF, et al. 18F-FLT-PET/CT adds value to 18F-FDG-PET/CT for diagnosing relapse after definitive radiotherapy in patients with lung cancer. Results of a prospective clinical trial. J Nucl Med. 2020; https://doi.org/10.2967/jnumed.120.247742.
84. Ciesienski KL, Yang Y, Ay I, et al. Fibrin-targeted PET probes for the detection of thrombi. Mol Pharm. 2013;10:1100–10. https://doi.org/10.1021/mp300610s.
85. Collier TL, Maresca KP, Normandin MD, et al. Brain Penetration of the ROS1/ALK Inhibitor Lorlatinib Confirmed by PET. Mol Imaging. 2017a;16:1536012117736669. https://doi.org/10.1177/1536012117736669.
86. Collier TL, Normandin MD, Stephenson NA, et al. Synthesis and preliminary PET imaging of 11C and 18F isotopologues of the ROS1/ALK inhibitor lorlatinib. Nat Commun. 2017b;8:15761. https://doi.org/10.1038/ncomms15761.
87. Cooke SA, de Ruysscher D, Reymen B, et al. 18F-FDG-PET guided vs whole tumour radiotherapy dose escalation in patients with locally advanced non-small cell lung cancer (PET-Boost): results from a randomised clinical trial. Radiother Oncol J Eur Soc Ther Radiol Oncol. 2023;181:109492. https://doi.org/10.1016/j.radonc.2023.109492.
88. Costa ELV, Musch G, Winkler T, et al. Mild Endotoxemia during mechanical ventilation produces spatially heterogeneous pulmonary neutrophilic inflammation in sheep. Anesthesiology. 2010;112:658–69. https://doi.org/10.1097/ALN.0b013e3181cbd1d4.
89. Costantino G, Norsa AH, Amadori R, et al. Interobserver agreement in the interpretation of computed tomography in acute pulmonary embolism. Am J Emerg Med. 2009;27:1109–11. https://doi.org/10.1016/j.ajem.2008.08.019.
90. Couch P, Webb C, Botkin C, et al. Added value of SPECT/CT in post Lu-177 Dotatate treatment for neuroendocrine tumors. J Nucl Med. 2019;60:2044.
91. Cuellar SLB, Carter BW, Macapinlac HA, et al. Clinical staging of patients with early esophageal adenocarcinoma: does FDG-PET/CT have a role? J Thorac Oncol. 2014;9:1202–6. https://doi.org/10.1097/JTO.0000000000000222.
92. Currie G, Hawk KE, Rohren E. The transformational potential of molecular radiomics. J Med Radiat Sci. 2023;70:77–88. https://doi.org/10.1002/jmrs.626.
93. d'Abadie P, Walrand S, Lhommel R, et al. A theranostic approach in SIRT: value of pre-therapy imaging in treatment planning. J Clin Med. 2022;11:7245. https://doi.org/10.3390/jcm11237245.
94. Visvikis D, et al. CT-based attenuation correction in the calculation of semi-quantitative indices of [18F]FDG uptake in PET. Eur J Nucl Med Mol Imaging. 2003;30 https://doi.org/10.1007/s00259-002-1070-4.
95. Dao DT, Kamran A, Wilson JM, et al. Longitudinal analysis of ventilation perfusion mismatch in congenital diaphragmatic Hernia survivors. J Pediatr. 2020;219:160–166.e2. https://doi.org/10.1016/j.jpeds.2019.09.053.
96. Dash A, Pillai MRA, Knapp FF. Production of (177) Lu for targeted radionuclide therapy: available options. Nucl Med Mol Imaging. 2015;49:85–107. https://doi.org/10.1007/s13139-014-0315-z.
97. de Galiza BF, Queiroz MA, Nunes RF, et al. Nonprostatic diseases on PSMA PET imaging: a spectrum of benign and malignant findings. Cancer Imaging. 2020;20:23. https://doi.org/10.1186/s40644-020-00300-7.
98. de Gouw DJJM, Klarenbeek BR, Driessen M, et al. Detecting pathological complete response in Esophageal cancer after neoadjuvant therapy based on imaging techniques: a diagnostic systematic review and meta-analysis. J Thorac Oncol. 2019;14:1156–71. https://doi.org/10.1016/j.jtho.2019.04.004.
99. de Perrot M, Gopalan D, Jenkins D, et al. Evaluation and management of patients with chronic thromboembolic pulmonary hypertension-consensus state-

ment from the ISHLT. J Heart Lung Transplant. 2021;40:1301–26.
100. Gopalan D, Delcroix M, Held M. Diagnosis of chronic thromboembolic pulmonary hypertension. Eur Respir Rev. 2017;26:160108. https://doi.org/10.1183/16000617.0108-2016.
101. Deipolyi AR, Iafrate AJ, Zhu AX, et al. High lung shunt fraction in colorectal liver tumors is associated with distant metastasis and decreased survival. J Vasc Interv Radiol JVIR. 2014;25:1604–8. https://doi.org/10.1016/j.jvir.2014.06.019.
102. Deleu A-L, Laenen A, Decaluwé H, et al. Value of [68Ga]Ga-somatostatin receptor PET/CT in the grading of pulmonary neuroendocrine (carcinoid) tumours and the detection of disseminated disease: single-centre pathology-based analysis and review of the literature. EJNMMI Res. 2022;12:28. https://doi.org/10.1186/s13550-022-00900-3.
103. Deng H, Zhao S, Yue Y, et al. IgG4-related disease of pulmonary artery causing pulmonary hypertension. Medicine (Baltimore). 2018;97:e10698. https://doi.org/10.1097/MD.0000000000010698.
104. Derenoncourt P-R, Felder GJ, Royal HD, et al. Ventilation-perfusion scan: a primer for practicing radiologists. Radiographics. 2021;41:2047–70. https://doi.org/10.1148/rg.2021210060.
105. Derlin T, Jaeger B, Jonigk D, et al. Clinical molecular imaging of pulmonary CXCR4 expression to predict outcome of Pirfenidone treatment in idiopathic pulmonary fibrosis. Chest. 2021;159:1094–106. https://doi.org/10.1016/j.chest.2020.08.2043.
106. Derlin T, Kelting C, Hueper K, et al. Quantitation of perfused lung volume using hybrid SPECT/CT allows refining the assessment of lung perfusion and estimating disease extent in chronic thromboembolic pulmonary hypertension. Clin Nucl Med. 2018:43, e170.
107. Desmonts C, Bouthiba MA, Enilorac B, et al. Evaluation of a new multipurpose whole-body CzT-based camera: comparison with a dual-head Anger camera and first clinical images. EJNMMI Phys. 2020;7:18. https://doi.org/10.1186/s40658-020-0284-5.
108. Di Battista M, Grosso M, Da Rio M, et al. Is oropharyngoesophageal scintigraphy the method of choice for assessing dysphagia in systemic sclerosis? A single center experience. Esophagus. 2023;20:567–72. https://doi.org/10.1007/s10388-023-00995-0.
109. DiCarli M. Nuclear cardiology and multimodal cardiovascular imaging. 1st ed. Philadelphia: Elsevier, Inc; 2021.
110. Dickson J, Ross J, Vöö S. Quantitative SPECT: the time is now. EJNMMI Phys. 2019;6:4. https://doi.org/10.1186/s40658-019-0241-3.
111. Dittmann H, Kopp D, Kupferschlaeger J, et al. A prospective study of quantitative SPECT/CT for evaluation of lung shunt fraction before SIRT of liver tumors. J Nucl Med. 2018;59:1366–72. https://doi.org/10.2967/jnumed.117.205203.
112. Dobrucki LW, Dione DP, Kalinowski L, et al. Serial noninvasive targeted imaging of peripheral angiogenesis: validation and application of a semiautomated quantitative approach. J Nucl Med. 2009;50:1356–63. https://doi.org/10.2967/jnumed.108.060822.
113. Du B, Wang S, Cui Y, et al. Can 18F-FDG PET/CT predict EGFR status in patients with non-small cell lung cancer? A systematic review and meta-analysis. BMJ Open. 2021;11:e044313. https://doi.org/10.1136/bmjopen-2020-044313.
114. Dubois LJ, Lieuwes NG, Janssen MHM, et al. Preclinical evaluation and validation of [18F]HX4, a promising hypoxia marker for PET imaging. Proc Natl Acad Sci U S A. 2011;108:14620–5. https://doi.org/10.1073/pnas.1102526108.
115. Ehman EC, Johnson GB, Villanueva-Meyer JE, et al. PET/MRI: where might it replace PET/CT? J Magn Reson Imaging JMRI. 2017;46:1247–62. https://doi.org/10.1002/jmri.25711.
116. El-Bawab H, Al-Sugair AA, Rafay M, et al. Role of flourine-18 fluorodeoxyglucose positron emission tomography in thymic pathology. Eur J Cardiothorac Surg. 2007;31:731–6. https://doi.org/10.1016/j.ejcts.2007.01.024.
117. El-Chemaly S, Malide D, Yao J, et al. Glucose Transporter-1 distribution in fibrotic lung disease: association with [18F]-2-Fluoro-2-Deoxyglucose-PET scan uptake, inflammation, and neovascularization. Chest. 2013;143:1685–91. https://doi.org/10.1378/chest.12-1359.
118. Elf JE, Jögi J, Bajc M. Home treatment of patients with small to medium sized acute pulmonary embolism. J Thromb Thrombolysis. 2015;39:166–72. https://doi.org/10.1007/s11239-014-1097-y.
119. Elojeimy S, Cruite I, Bowen S, et al. Overview of the novel and improved pulmonary ventilation-perfusion imaging applications in the era of SPECT/CT. AJR Am J Roentgenol. 2016;207:1307–15. https://doi.org/10.2214/AJR.15.15071.
120. Elschot M, Nijsen JFW, Lam MGEH, et al. (^{99}m) Tc-MAA overestimates the absorbed dose to the lungs in radioembolization: a quantitative evaluation in patients treated with ^{166}Ho-microspheres. Eur J Nucl Med Mol Imaging. 2014;41:1965–75. https://doi.org/10.1007/s00259-014-2784-9.
121. El-Shabrawi MH, Omran S, Wageeh S, et al. (99m) Technetium-macroaggregated albumin perfusion lung scan versus contrast enhanced echocardiography in the diagnosis of the hepatopulmonary syndrome in children with chronic liver disease. Eur J Gastroenterol Hepatol. 2010;22:1006–12. https://doi.org/10.1097/MEG.0b013e328336562e.
122. Emond EC, Groves AM, Hutton BF, Thielemans K. Effect of positron range on PET quantification in diseased and normal lungs. Phys Med Biol. 2019;64:205010. https://doi.org/10.1088/1361-6560/ab469d.
123. Ercelep O, Alan O, Telli TA, et al. Differences in PET/CT standardized uptake values involvement

and survival compared to histologic subtypes of lung adenocarcinoma. Tumori. 2021;107:231–7. https://doi.org/10.1177/0300891620950475.
124. Ergül N, Çermik TF. FDG-PET or PET/CT in fever of unknown origin: the diagnostic role of underlying primary disease. Int J Mol Imaging. 2011;2011:318051. https://doi.org/10.1155/2011/318051.
125. Erlandsson K, Buvat I, Pretorius PH, et al. A review of partial volume correction techniques for emission tomography and their applications in neurology, cardiology and oncology. Phys Med Biol. 2012;57:R119–59. https://doi.org/10.1088/0031-9155/57/21/R119.
126. Evans I, Hambleton G, Mann N, Brown J. The distribution of lung damage in children with cystic fibrosis and its relationship to colonisation with Pseudomonas aeruginosa. Eur J Nucl Med. 1987;12:620–2. https://doi.org/10.1007/BF00284539.
127. Everitt SJ, Ball DL, Hicks RJ, et al. Differential 18F-FDG and 18F-FLT uptake on serial PET/CT imaging before and during definitive chemoradiation for non–small cell lung cancer. J Nucl Med. 2014;55:1069–74. https://doi.org/10.2967/jnumed.113.131631.
128. Fan B, Fan P, Kong L, et al. 18F-deoxyglucose positron emission tomography/computed tomography to predict local failure in esophageal squamous cell carcinoma. Oncotarget. 2017;8:34498–506. https://doi.org/10.18632/oncotarget.15606.
129. Fan B, Li C, Mu F, et al. Dose escalation guided by 18F-FDG PET/CT for esophageal cancer. Radiat Med Prot. 2021;2:55–60. https://doi.org/10.1016/j.radmp.2021.04.002.
130. Farrow CE, Salome CM, Harris BE, et al. Airway closure on imaging relates to airway hyperresponsiveness and peripheral airway disease in asthma. J Appl Physiol. 2012;113:958–66. https://doi.org/10.1152/japplphysiol.01618.2011.
131. Farrow CE, Salome CM, Harris BE, et al. Peripheral ventilation heterogeneity determines the extent of bronchoconstriction in asthma. J Appl Physiol Bethesda Md 1985. 2017;123:1188–94. https://doi.org/10.1152/japplphysiol.00640.2016.
132. Fathala A. Quantitative lung perfusion scintigraphy in patients with congenital heart disease. Heart Views. 2010;11:109–14. https://doi.org/10.4103/1995-705X.76802.
133. Feltes TF, Bacha E, Beekman RH, et al. Indications for cardiac catheterization and intervention in pediatric cardiac disease. Circulation. 2011;123:2607–52. https://doi.org/10.1161/CIR.0b013e31821b1f10.
134. Flavell RR, Behr SC, Brunsing RL, et al. The incidence of pulmonary embolism and associated FDG-PET findings in IV contrast-enhanced PET/CT. Acad Radiol. 2014;21:718–25. https://doi.org/10.1016/j.acra.2014.02.013.
135. Flores RM, Akhurst T, Gonen M, et al. Positron emission tomography defines metastatic disease but not locoregional disease in patients with malignant pleural mesothelioma. J Thorac Cardiovasc Surg. 2003;126:11–6. https://doi.org/10.1016/s0022-5223(03)00207-1.
136. Fraser JR, Laurent TC, Laurent UB. Hyaluronan: its nature, distribution, functions and turnover. J Intern Med. 1997;242:27–33. https://doi.org/10.1046/j.1365-2796.1997.00170.x.
137. Musch G, et al. Regional gas exchange and cellular metabolic activity in ventilator-induced lung injury. Anesthesiology. 2007;106 https://doi.org/10.1097/01.anes.0000264748.86145.ac.
138. Picart G, et al. Predictors of residual pulmonary vascular obstruction after pulmonary embolism: results from a prospective cohort study. Thromb Res. 2020;194 https://doi.org/10.1016/j.thromres.2020.06.004.
139. Gaba RC, Vanmiddlesworth KA. Chemoembolic hepatopulmonary shunt reduction to allow safe yttrium-90 radioembolization lobectomy of hepatocellular carcinoma. Cardiovasc Intervent Radiol. 2012;35:1505–11. https://doi.org/10.1007/s00270-012-0371-7.
140. Gaeta GB, Fusco FM, Nardiello S. Fever of unknown origin: a systematic review of the literature for 1995–2004. Nucl Med Commun. 2006;27:205.
141. Galiè N, Humbert M, Vachiery J-L, et al. 2015 ESC/ERS Guidelines for the diagnosis and treatment of pulmonary hypertension: The Joint Task Force for the Diagnosis and Treatment of Pulmonary Hypertension of the European Society of Cardiology (ESC) and the European Respiratory Society (ERS) Endorsed by: Association for European Paediatric and Congenital Cardiology (AEPC), International Society for Heart and Lung Transplantation (ISHLT). Eur Heart J. 2016;37:67–119. https://doi.org/10.1093/eurheartj/ehv317.
142. Gandhi SJ, Babu S, Subramanyam P, Shanmuga Sundaram P. Tc-99m macro aggregated albumin scintigraphy - indications other than pulmonary embolism: a pictorial essay. Indian J Nucl Med IJNM. 2013;28:152–62. https://doi.org/10.4103/0972-3919.119546.
143. Gates GF, Orme HW, Dore EK. Measurement of cardiac shunting with technetium-labeled albumin aggregates. J Nucl Med. 1971;12:746–9.
144. Georgiou MF, Kuker RA, Studenski MT, et al. Lung shunt fraction calculation using 99mTc-MAA SPECT/CT imaging for 90Y microsphere selective internal radiation therapy of liver tumors. EJNMMI Res. 2021;11:96. https://doi.org/10.1186/s13550-021-00837-z.
145. Ghanima W, Nielssen BE, Holmen LO, et al. Multidetector computed tomography (MDCT) in the diagnosis of pulmonary embolism: interobserver agreement among radiologists with varied levels of experience. Acta Radiol Stockh Swed 1987. 2007;48:165–70. https://doi.org/10.1080/02841850601100859.
146. Giesel FL, Heussel CP, Lindner T, et al. FAPI-PET/CT improves staging in a lung cancer patient

with cerebral metastasis. Eur J Nucl Med Mol Imaging. 2019;46:1754–5. https://doi.org/10.1007/s00259-019-04346-z.
147. Gill H, Hiller J. Systematic review of lung shunt fraction quantification comparing SPECT/CT and planar scintigraphy for yttrium 90 radioembolization planning. Clin Transl Imaging. 2021;9:181–8. https://doi.org/10.1007/s40336-021-00417-0.
148. Goethals I, Smeets P, De Winter O, Noens L. Focally enhanced F-18 Fluorodeoxyglucose (FDG) uptake in incidentally detected pulmonary embolism on PET/CT scanning. Clin Nucl Med. 2006;31:497. https://doi.org/10.1097/01.rlu.0000227496.51081.9e.
149. Golestani R, Razavian M, Ye Y, et al. Matrix Metalloproteinase–targeted imaging of lung inflammation and remodeling. J Nucl Med. 2017;58:138–43. https://doi.org/10.2967/jnumed.116.176198.
150. Goodman KA, Ou F-S, Hall NC, et al. Randomized phase II study of PET response-adapted combined modality therapy for esophageal cancer: mature results of the CALGB 80803 (Alliance) trial. J Clin Oncol. 2021;39:2803–15. https://doi.org/10.1200/JCO.20.03611.
151. Gouel P, Decazes P, Vera P, et al. Advances in PET and MRI imaging of tumor hypoxia. Front Med. 2023;10:1055062.
152. Gould MK, Maclean CC, Kuschner WG, et al. Accuracy of positron emission tomography for diagnosis of pulmonary nodules and mass lesions: a meta-analysis. JAMA. 2001;285:914–24. https://doi.org/10.1001/jama.285.7.914.
153. Grant AM, Deller TW, Khalighi MM, et al. NEMA NU 2-2012 performance studies for the SiPM-based ToF-PET component of the GE SIGNA PET/MR system. Med Phys. 2016;43:2334. https://doi.org/10.1118/1.4945416.
154. Grecchi E, Veronese M, Moresco RM, et al. Quantification of dynamic [18F]FDG pet studies in acute lung injurY. Mol Imaging Biol. 2016;18:143–52. https://doi.org/10.1007/s11307-015-0871-3.
155. Groves AM, Win T, Screaton NJ, et al. Idiopathic pulmonary fibrosis and diffuse Parenchymal lung disease: implications from initial experience with 18F-FDG PET/CT. J Nucl Med. 2009;50:538–45. https://doi.org/10.2967/jnumed.108.057901.
156. Grüning T, Drake BE, Farrell SL, Nokes T. Three-year clinical experience with VQ SPECT for diagnosing pulmonary embolism: diagnostic performance. Clin Imaging. 2014;38:831–5. https://doi.org/10.1016/j.clinimag.2014.04.003.
157. Han G, Hwang E, Lin F, et al. Abstract 5042: anti-tumor activity of RYZ101 (Ac-225 DOTATATE) in somatostatin receptor-expressing preclinical models of small-cell lung cancer. Cancer Res. 2023;83:5042. https://doi.org/10.1158/1538-7445.AM2023-5042.
158. Han S, Kim Y-I, Oh JS, et al. Diagnostic and prognostic values of 2-[18F]FDG PET/CT in resectable thymic epithelial tumour. Eur Radiol. 2022;32:1173–83. https://doi.org/10.1007/s00330-021-08230-z.
159. Han S, Kim YJ, Woo S, et al. Prognostic value of volumetric parameters of pretreatment 18F-FDG PET/CT in Esophageal cancer: a systematic review and meta-analysis. Clin Nucl Med. 2018;43:887–94. https://doi.org/10.1097/RLU.0000000000002291.
160. Hardoff R, Steinmetz AP, Krausz Y, et al. The prognostic value of perfusion lung scintigraphy in patients who underwent single-lung transplantation for emphysema and pulmonary fibrosis. J Nucl Med. 2000;41:1771–6.
161. Harris RS, Venegas JG, Wongviriyawong C, et al. 18F-FDG uptake rate is a biomarker of eosinophilic inflammation and airway response in asthma. J Nucl Med. 2011;52:1713–20. https://doi.org/10.2967/jnumed.110.086355.
162. Hashimoto H, Oka T, Nakanishi R, et al. Evaluation of balloon pulmonary angioplasty using lung perfusion SPECT in patients with chronic thromboembolic pulmonary hypertension. J Nucl Cardiol. 2022a;29:3392–400. https://doi.org/10.1007/s12350-022-02971-0.
163. Hashimoto H, Soma T, Mizumura S, et al. Evaluation of lung perfusion by using lung perfusion SPECT and lung CT with breathing synchronization software. Eur J Hybrid Imaging. 2022b;6:32. https://doi.org/10.1186/s41824-022-00154-1.
164. Haydar AA, Goldsmith DJA. Pulmonary embolism— or vasculitis? J R Soc Med. 2004;97:27–8.
165. Heller GV, Hendel R, editors. Nuclear cardiology: practical applications. 4th ed. New York: McGraw Hill; 2022.
166. Herrera-Juárez M, Serrano-Gómez C, Bote-de-Cabo H, Paz-Ares L. Targeted therapy for lung cancer: beyond EGFR and ALK. Cancer. 2023;129:1803.
167. Hicks RJ. Role of 18F-FDG PET in assessment of response in non-small cell lung cancer. J Nucl Med. 2009;50(Suppl 1):31S–42S. https://doi.org/10.2967/jnumed.108.057216.
168. Hiniker SM, Sodji Q, Quon A, et al. FLT-PET-CT for the detection of disease recurrence after stereotactic ablative radiotherapy or hyperfractionation for thoracic malignancy: a prospective pilot study. Front Oncol. 2019;9:467. https://doi.org/10.3389/fonc.2019.00467.
169. Hofheinz F, Li Y, Steffen IG, et al. Confirmation of the prognostic value of pretherapeutic tumor SUR and MTV in patients with esophageal squamous cell carcinoma. Eur J Nucl Med Mol Imaging. 2019;46:1485–94. https://doi.org/10.1007/s00259-019-04307-6.
170. Hofman MS, Lau WFE, Hicks RJ. Somatostatin receptor imaging with 68Ga DOTATATE PET/CT: clinical utility, normal patterns, pearls, and pitfalls in interpretation. Radiogr Rev Publ Radiol Soc N Am Inc. 2015;35:500–16. https://doi.org/10.1148/rg.352140164.
171. Hoiczyk M, Iliodromitis K, Bauer S, et al. Intimal sarcoma of the pulmonary artery with unusual findings:

a case report. Clin Res Cardiol. 2012;101:397–401. https://doi.org/10.1007/s00392-012-0425-5.
172. Hope TA, Bergsland EK, Bozkurt MF, et al. Appropriate use criteria for Somatostatin Receptor PET imaging in neuroendocrine tumors. J Nucl Med. 2018;59:66–74. https://doi.org/10.2967/jnumed.117.202275.
173. Hua J, Dobrucki LW, Sadeghi MM, et al. Noninvasive imaging of angiogenesis with a 99mTc-labeled peptide targeted at alphavbeta3 integrin after murine hindlimb ischemia. Circulation. 2005;111:3255–60. https://doi.org/10.1161/CIRCULATIONAHA.104.485029.
174. Huang B, Sollee J, Luo Y-H, et al. Prediction of lung malignancy progression and survival with machine learning based on pre-treatment FDG-PET/CT. EBioMedicine. 2022;82:104127.
175. Hutton BF. The origins of SPECT and SPECT/CT. Eur J Nucl Med Mol Imaging. 2014;41(Suppl 1):S3–16. https://doi.org/10.1007/s00259-013-2606-5.
176. Hutton BF, Buvat I, Beekman FJ. Review and current status of SPECT scatter correction. Phys Med Biol. 2011;56:R85–112. https://doi.org/10.1088/0031-9155/56/14/R01.
177. Hutton BF, Erlandsson K, Thielemans K. Advances in clinical molecular imaging instrumentation. Clin Transl Imaging. 2018;6:31–45. https://doi.org/10.1007/s40336-018-0264-0.
178. Ichihara T, Ogawa K, Motomura N, et al. Compton scatter compensation using the triple-energy window method for single- and dual-isotope SPECT. J Nucl Med. 1993;34:2216–21.
179. Ito T, Suzuki H, Sakairi Y, et al. 18F-FDG-PET/CT predicts grade of malignancy and invasive potential of thymic epithelial tumors. Gen Thorac Cardiovasc Surg. 2021;69:274–81. https://doi.org/10.1007/s11748-020-01439-7.
180. Izquierdo-Garcia D, Catana C. MR imaging-guided attenuation correction of PET data in PET/MR imaging. PET Clin. 2016;11:129–49. https://doi.org/10.1016/j.cpet.2015.10.002.
181. Izquierdo-Garcia D, Désogère P, Philip AL, et al. Detection and characterization of thrombosis in humans using fibrin-targeted positron emission tomography and magnetic resonance. JACC Cardiovasc Imaging. 2022;15:504–15. https://doi.org/10.1016/j.jcmg.2021.08.009.
182. Jacquelin V, Mekinian A, Brillet PY, et al. FDG-PET/CT in the prediction of pulmonary function improvement in nonspecific interstitial pneumonia. A Pilot Study. Eur J Radiol. 2016;85:2200–5. https://doi.org/10.1016/j.ejrad.2016.10.001.
183. Jaffé A, Hamutcu R, Dhawan RT, et al. Routine ventilation scans in children with cystic fibrosis: diagnostic usefulness and prognostic value. Eur J Nucl Med. 2001;28:1313–8. https://doi.org/10.1007/s002590100573.
184. Je C, et al. Adaptive neoadjuvant chemotherapy guided by (18)F-FDG PET in resectable non-small cell lung cancers: the NEOSCAN Trial. J Thorac Oncol. 2016;11 https://doi.org/10.1016/j.jtho.2015.12.104.
185. Jeandot R, Lambert B, Brendel AJ, et al. Lung ventilation and perfusion scintigraphy in the follow up of repaired congenital diaphragmatic hernia. Eur J Nucl Med. 1989;15:591–6. https://doi.org/10.1007/BF00256935.
186. Jerabek PA, Patrick TB, Kilbourn MR, et al. Synthesis and biodistribution of 18F-labeled fluoronitroimidazoles: potential in vivo markers of hypoxic tissue. Int J Rad Appl Instrum A. 1986;37:599–605.
187. Jiang C, Chen Y, Zhu Y, Xu Y. Systematic review and meta-analysis of the accuracy of 18F-FDG PET/CT for detection of regional lymph node metastasis in esophageal squamous cell carcinoma. J Thorac Dis. 2018;10:6066–76. https://doi.org/10.21037/jtd.2018.10.57.
188. Jiang Y, Hou G, Cheng W. The utility of 18F-FDG and 68Ga-DOTA-Peptide PET/CT in the evaluation of primary pulmonary carcinoid: a systematic review and meta-analysis. Medicine (Baltimore). 2019;98:e14769. https://doi.org/10.1097/MD.0000000000014769.
189. Jögi J, Ekberg M, Jonson B, et al. Ventilation/perfusion SPECT in chronic obstructive pulmonary disease: an evaluation by reference to symptoms, spirometric lung function and emphysema, as assessed with HRCT. Eur J Nucl Med Mol Imaging. 2011;38:1344–52. https://doi.org/10.1007/s00259-011-1757-5.
190. Jögi J, Jonson B, Ekberg M, Bajc M. Ventilation-perfusion SPECT with 99mTc-DTPA versus Technegas: a head-to-head study in obstructive and nonobstructive disease. J Nucl Med. 2010;51:735–41. https://doi.org/10.2967/jnumed.109.073957.
191. Jones HA, Clark RJ, Rhodes CG, et al. In vivo measurement of neutrophil activity in experimental lung inflammation. Am J Respir Crit Care Med. 1994;149:1635–9. https://doi.org/10.1164/ajrccm.149.6.7516252.
192. Jones HA, Donovan T, Goddard MJ, et al. Use of 18FDG-pet to discriminate between infection and rejection in lung transplant recipients. Transplantation. 2004;77:1462–4. https://doi.org/10.1097/01.tp.0000121767.05724.33.
193. Jones HA, Marino PS, Shakur BH, Morrell NW. In vivo assessment of lung inflammatory cell activity in patients with COPD and asthma. Eur Respir J. 2003;21:567–73. https://doi.org/10.1183/09031936.03.00048502.
194. Jones T, Townsend D. History and future technical innovation in positron emission tomography. J Med Imaging Bellingham Wash. 2017;4:011013. https://doi.org/10.1117/1.JMI.4.1.011013.
195. Jung N, Aga N, Lu M, et al. Whole body and SPECT/CT imaging for Dosimetry of 177Lu-labeled radiopharmaceutical therapies: a technologist's perspective. J Nucl Med. 2022;63:4103.

196. Kadota K, Kachala SS, Nitadori J-I, et al. High SUVmax on FDG-PET indicates pleomorphic subtype in epithelioid malignant pleural mesothelioma: supportive evidence to reclassify pleomorphic as nonepithelioid histology. J Thorac Oncol. 2012;7:1192–7. https://doi.org/10.1097/JTO.0b013e3182519d96.
197. Kalambokis G, Tsianos EV. Pitfalls in the assessment of intrapulmonary shunt using lung perfusion scintigraphy in patients with cirrhosis. Liver Int. 2011;31:138–9.; author reply 139-140. https://doi.org/10.1111/j.1478-3231.2010.02330.x.
198. Kalluri R, Zeisberg M. Fibroblasts in cancer. Nat Rev Cancer. 2006;6:392–401. https://doi.org/10.1038/nrc1877.
199. Kan Y, Yuan L, Meeks JK, et al. The accuracy of V/Q SPECT in the diagnosis of pulmonary embolism: a meta-analysis. Acta Radiol. 2015;56:565–72. https://doi.org/10.1177/0284185114533682.
200. Karacavus S, Intepe YS. The role of Tc-99m DTPA aerosol scintigraphy in the differential diagnosis of COPD and asthma. Clin Respir J. 2015;9:189–95. https://doi.org/10.1111/crj.12123.
201. Kartamihardja AHS, Kurniawati Y, Gunawan R. Diagnostic value of 99mTc-ethambutol scintigraphy in tuberculosis: compared to microbiological and histopathological tests. Ann Nucl Med. 2018;32:60–8. https://doi.org/10.1007/s12149-017-1220-1.
202. Kashefi A, Kuo J, Shelton DK. Molecular imaging in pulmonary diseases. AJR Am J Roentgenol. 2011;197:295–307. https://doi.org/10.2214/AJR.11.6675.
203. Kato H, Kuwano H, Nakajima M, et al. Comparison between positron emission tomography and computed tomography in the use of the assessment of esophageal carcinoma. Cancer. 2002;94:921–8.
204. Kawut SM, Krowka MJ, Forde KA, et al. Impact of hepatopulmonary syndrome in liver transplantation candidates and the role of angiogenesis. Eur Respir J. 2022;60:2102304. https://doi.org/10.1183/13993003.02304-2021.
205. Kayani I, Conry BG, Groves AM, et al. A comparison of 68Ga-DOTATATE and 18F-FDG PET/CT in pulmonary neuroendocrine tumors. J Nucl Med. 2009;50:1927–32. https://doi.org/10.2967/jnumed.109.066639.
206. Keijsers RGM, Grutters JC. In Which Patients with Sarcoidosis Is FDG PET/CT Indicated? J Clin Med. 2020;9:890. https://doi.org/10.3390/jcm9030890.
207. Kelly CJ, Karthikesalingam A, Suleyman M, et al. Key challenges for delivering clinical impact with artificial intelligence. BMC Med. 2019;17:195. https://doi.org/10.1186/s12916-019-1426-2.
208. Khandelwal AR, Li G, Takalkar AM. Incidental detection of unsuspected pulmonary embolism on oncologic FDG PET/CT imaging. Clin Nucl Med. 2011;36:720. https://doi.org/10.1097/RLU.0b013e318219b102.
209. Kim C, Liu SV, Subramaniam DS, et al. Phase I study of the (177)Lu-DOTA(0)-Tyr(3)-Octreotate (lutathera) in combination with nivolumab in patients with neuroendocrine tumors of the lung. J Immunother Cancer. 2020;8 https://doi.org/10.1136/jitc-2020-000980.
210. Kim K, Jeong J-H, Kim S-J. Diagnostic test accuracy of 18F-FDG PET or PET/CT for characterization of histologic type of thymic epithelial tumor: a meta-analysis. Clin Nucl Med. 2022;47:36–42. https://doi.org/10.1097/RLU.0000000000003921.
211. Kim NH, Delcroix M, Jais X, et al. Chronic thromboembolic pulmonary hypertension. Eur Respir J. 2019;53:1801915. https://doi.org/10.1183/13993003.01915-2018.
212. Kim TJ, Kim HY, Lee KW, Kim MS. Multimodality assessment of esophageal cancer: preoperative staging and monitoring of response to therapy. Radiogr Rev Publ Radiol Soc N Am Inc. 2009;29:403–21. https://doi.org/10.1148/rg.292085106.
213. Kitajima K, Doi H, Kuribayashi K, et al. Prognostic value of pretreatment volume-based quantitative 18F-FDG PET/CT parameters in patients with malignant pleural mesothelioma. Eur J Radiol. 2017;86:176–83. https://doi.org/10.1016/j.ejrad.2016.11.019.
214. Kitajima K, Maruyama M, Yokoyama H, et al. Response to Immune Checkpoint Inhibitor Therapy in Patients with Unresectable Recurrent Malignant Pleural Mesothelioma Shown by FDG-PET and CT. Cancer. 2021;13:1098. https://doi.org/10.3390/cancers13051098.
215. Klabatsa A, Chicklore S, Barrington SF, et al. The association of 18F-FDG PET/CT parameters with survival in malignant pleural mesothelioma. Eur J Nucl Med Mol Imaging. 2014;41:276–82. https://doi.org/10.1007/s00259-013-2561-1.
216. Knockaert DC, Vanneste LJ, Bobbaers HJ. Fever of Unknown Origin in Elderly Patients. J Am Geriatr Soc. 1993;41:1187–92. https://doi.org/10.1111/j.1532-5415.1993.tb07301.x.
217. Konstantinides SV, Meyer G, Becattini C, et al. 2019 ESC Guidelines for the diagnosis and management of acute pulmonary embolism developed in collaboration with the European Respiratory Society (ERS). Eur Heart J. 2020;41:543–603. https://doi.org/10.1093/eurheartj/ehz405.
218. Koral KF, Dewaraja Y, Li J, et al. Update on hybrid conjugate-view SPECT tumor dosimetry and response in 131I-tositumomab therapy of previously untreated lymphoma patients. J Nucl Med. 2003;44:457–64.
219. Krengli M, Ferrara E, Guaschino R, et al. 18F-FDG PET/CT as predictive and prognostic factor in esophageal cancer treated with combined modality treatment. Ann Nucl Med. 2022;36:450–9. https://doi.org/10.1007/s12149-022-01733-9.
220. Krenning EP, Bakker WH, Breeman WA, et al. Localisation of endocrine-related tumours with radioiodinated analogue of somatostatin. Lancet

Lond Engl. 1989;1:242–4. https://doi.org/10.1016/s0140-6736(89)91258-0.
221. Królicki L. "To be or not to be" for PET in rheumatology. A marriage of love or of convenience? Reumatologia. 2017;55:1–3. https://doi.org/10.5114/reum.2017.66679.
222. Krowka MJ, Fallon MB, Kawut SM, et al. International Liver Transplant Society practice guidelines: diagnosis and management of hepatopulmonary syndrome and portopulmonary hypertension. Transplantation. 2016;100:1440–52. https://doi.org/10.1097/TP.0000000000001229.
223. Kuehl C, Zhang T, Kaminskas LM, et al. Hyaluronic acid molecular weight determines lung clearance and biodistribution after instillation. Mol Pharm. 2016;13:1904–14. https://doi.org/10.1021/acs.molpharmaceut.6b00069.
224. Kumar A, Regmi SK, Dutta R, et al. Characterization of thymic masses using (18)F-FDG PET-CT. Ann Nucl Med. 2009;23:569–77. https://doi.org/10.1007/s12149-009-0283-z.
225. Kurihara H, Honda N, Kono Y, Arai Y. Radiolabelled agents for PET imaging of tumor hypoxia. Curr Med Chem. 2012;19:3282–9. https://doi.org/10.2174/092986712801215964.
226. Kuttner S, Lassen ML, Øen SK, et al. Quantitative PET/MR imaging of lung cancer in the presence of artifacts in the MR-based attenuation correction maps. Acta Radiol Stockh Swed 1987. 2020;61:11–20. https://doi.org/10.1177/0284185119848118.
227. Kwatra NS, Grant FD, Lim R, Lee EY. Up-to-date review of nuclear medicine applications in pediatric thoracic imaging. Eur J Radiol. 2017;95:418–27. https://doi.org/10.1016/j.ejrad.2016.04.007.
228. Kwee RM. Prediction of tumor response to neoadjuvant therapy in patients with esophageal cancer with use of 18F FDG PET: a systematic review. Radiology. 2010;254:707–17. https://doi.org/10.1148/radiol.09091324.
229. Kwok N, Irani Z, Sheth R, Arellano RS. Hepatopulmonary shunt reduction with bland embolization for yttrium-90 radioembolization. Diagn Interv Imaging. 2016;97:369–70. https://doi.org/10.1016/j.diii.2015.12.005.
230. Kyme AZ, Fulton RR. Motion estimation and correction in SPECT, PET and CT. Phys Med Biol. 2021;66:18TR02. https://doi.org/10.1088/1361-6560/ac093b.
231. Raj L, et al. Predictors for residual pulmonary vascular obstruction after unprovoked pulmonary embolism: implications for clinical practice-The PADIS-PE Trial. Thromb Haemost. 2019;119 https://doi.org/10.1055/s-0039-1692424.
232. Valerio L, et al. Chronic thromboembolic pulmonary hypertension and impairment after pulmonary embolism: the FOCUS study. Eur Heart J. 2022;43 https://doi.org/10.1093/eurheartj/ehac206.
233. Ladefoged CN, Law I, Anazodo U, et al. A multicentre evaluation of eleven clinically feasible brain PET/MRI attenuation correction techniques using a large cohort of patients. Neuroimage. 2017;147:346–59. https://doi.org/10.1016/j.neuroimage.2016.12.010.
234. Lahiri A, Maji A, Potdar PD, et al. Lung cancer immunotherapy: progress, pitfalls, and promises. Mol Cancer. 2023;22:40. https://doi.org/10.1186/s12943-023-01740-y.
235. Lambert B, Mertens J, Sturm EJ, et al. 99mTc-labelled macroaggregated albumin (MAA) scintigraphy for planning treatment with 90Y microspheres. Eur J Nucl Med Mol Imaging. 2010;37:2328–33. https://doi.org/10.1007/s00259-010-1566-2.
236. Lang L, Li W, Guo N, et al. Comparison study of [18F]FAl-NOTA-PRGD2, [18F]FPPRGD2, and [68Ga]Ga-NOTA-PRGD2 for PET imaging of U87MG tumors in mice. Bioconjug Chem. 2011;22:2415–22. https://doi.org/10.1021/bc200197h.
237. Lawal I, Zeevaart J, Ebenhan T, et al. Metabolic Imaging of Infection. J Nucl Med. 2017;58:1727–32. https://doi.org/10.2967/jnumed.117.191635.
238. Laznicek M, Laznickova A, Cozikova D, Velebny V. Preclinical pharmacokinetics of radiolabelled hyaluronan. Pharmacol Rep PR. 2012;64:428–37. https://doi.org/10.1016/s1734-1140(12)70784-3.
239. Le Pennec R, Iravani A, Woon B, et al. Gallium-68 ventilation/perfusion PET-CT and CT pulmonary angiography for pulmonary embolism diagnosis: an interobserver agreement study. Front Med. 2021;7:599901.
240. Le Pennec R, Tromeur C, Orione C, et al. Quantification of the pulmonary vascular obstruction index on ventilation/perfusion lung scintigraphy: comparison of a segmental visual scoring to the Meyer score. Front Med. 2022;9:970808.
241. Le Roux P-Y, Robin P, Delluc A, et al. Additional value of combining low-dose computed tomography to V/Q SPECT on a hybrid SPECT-CT camera for pulmonary embolism diagnosis. Nucl Med Commun. 2015;36:922. https://doi.org/10.1097/MNM.0000000000000351.
242. Le Roux P-Y, Robin P, Salaun P-Y. New developments and future challenges of nuclear medicine and molecular imaging for pulmonary embolism. Thromb Res. 2018;163:236–41. https://doi.org/10.1016/j.thromres.2017.06.031.
243. Lee D-H, Jung T-E, Lee J-H, et al. Pulmonary artery intimal sarcoma: poor 18F-fluorodeoxyglucose uptake in positron emission computed tomography. J Cardiothorac Surg. 2013a;8:40. https://doi.org/10.1186/1749-8090-8-40.
244. Lee E, Zeng J, Miyaoka RS, et al. Functional lung avoidance and response-adaptive escalation (FLARE) RT: multimodality plan dosimetry of a precision radiation oncology strategy. Med Phys. 2017;44:3418–29. https://doi.org/10.1002/mp.12308.
245. Lee EJ, Moon SH, Choi JY, et al. Usefulness of fluorodeoxyglucose positron emission tomography in malignancy of pulmonary artery mimicking pul-

monary embolism. ANZ J Surg. 2013b;83:342–7. https://doi.org/10.1111/j.1445-2197.2012.06205.x.
246. Lee IK, Jacome DA, Cho JK, et al. Imaging sensitive and drug-resistant bacterial infection with [11C]-trimethoprim. J Clin Invest. 2023;132 https://doi.org/10.1172/JCI156679.
247. Lee JS. A review of deep-learning-based approaches for attenuation correction in positron emission tomography. IEEE Trans Radiat Plasma Med Sci. 2021;5:160–84. https://doi.org/10.1109/TRPMS.2020.3009269.
248. Lee ST, Ghanem M, Herbertson RA, et al. Prognostic value of 18F-FDG PET/CT in patients with malignant pleural mesothelioma. Mol Imaging Biol. 2009;11:473–9. https://doi.org/10.1007/s11307-009-0203-6.
249. Wang L, Wang M, Yang T, et al. A prospective, comparative study of ventilation–perfusion planar imaging and ventilation–perfusion SPECT for chronic thromboembolic pulmonary hypertension. J Nucl Med. 2020;61:1832. https://doi.org/10.2967/jnumed.120.243188.
250. Leung TW, Lau WY, Ho SK, et al. Radiation pneumonitis after selective internal radiation treatment with intraarterial 90yttrium-microspheres for inoperable hepatic tumors. Int J Radiat Oncol Biol Phys. 1995;33:919–24. https://doi.org/10.1016/0360-3016(95)00039-3.
251. Levin CS, Maramraju SH, Khalighi MM, et al. Design features and mutual compatibility studies of the time-of-flight PET capable GE SIGNA PET/MR system. IEEE Trans Med Imaging. 2016;35:1907–14. https://doi.org/10.1109/TMI.2016.2537811.
252. Li L, Chen X, Yu J, Yuan S. Preliminary clinical application of RGD-containing peptides as PET radiotracers for imaging tumors. Front Oncol. 2022;12:837952. https://doi.org/10.3389/fonc.2022.837952.
253. Li L, Hu M, Zhu H, et al. Comparison of 18F-Fluoroerythronitroimidazole and 18F-fluorodeoxyglucose positron emission tomography and prognostic value in locally advanced non-small-cell lung cancer. Clin Lung Cancer. 2010;11:335–40. https://doi.org/10.3816/CLC.2010.n.042.
254. Li Y, Mao T, Wang J, et al. Toward the next generation EGFR inhibitors: an overview of osimertinib resistance mediated by EGFR mutations in non-small cell lung cancer. Cell Commun Signal. 2023;21:71.
255. Liang J, Jiang D, Noble PW. Hyaluronan as a therapeutic target in human diseases. Adv Drug Deliv Rev. 2016;97:186–203 https://doi.org/10.1016/j.addr.2015.10.017.
256. Liao S, Penney BC, Wroblewski K, et al. Prognostic value of metabolic tumor burden on 18F-FDG PET in nonsurgical patients with non-small cell lung cancer. Eur J Nucl Med Mol Imaging. 2012;39:27–38. https://doi.org/10.1007/s00259-011-1934-6.
257. Lim CH, Park Y-J, Shin M, et al. Tumor SUVs on 18F-FDG PET/CT and aggressive pathological features in Esophageal squamous cell carcinoma. Clin Nucl Med. 2020a;45:e128–33. https://doi.org/10.1097/RLU.0000000000002926.
258. Lim JH, Choi JY, Im Y, et al. Prognostic value of SUVmax on 18F-fluorodeoxyglucose PET/CT scan in patients with malignant pleural mesothelioma. PloS One. 2020b;15:e0229299. https://doi.org/10.1371/journal.pone.0229299.
259. Lin Q, Zhang Y, Fu Z, et al. Synthesis and evaluation of (18)F labeled crizotinib derivative [(18)F]FPC as a novel PET probe for imaging c-MET-positive NSCLC tumor. Bioorg Med Chem. 2020;28:115577. https://doi.org/10.1016/j.bmc.2020.115577.
260. Lindner T, Altmann A, Giesel F, et al. 18F-labeled tracers targeting fibroblast activation protein. EJNMMI Radiopharm Chem. 2021;6:26. https://doi.org/10.1186/s41181-021-00144-x.
261. Ljungberg M. Handbook of nuclear medicine and molecular imaging for physicists: instrumentation and imaging procedures, vol. I. CRC Press; 2022a.
262. Ljungberg M. Handbook of nuclear medicine and molecular imaging for physicists: modelling, dosimetry and radiation protection, vol. II. CRC Press; 2022b.
263. Ljungberg M. Handbook of nuclear medicine and molecular imaging for physicists: radiopharmaceuticals and clinical applications, vol. III. CRC Press; 2022c.
264. Ljungberg M, Celler A, Konijnenberg MW, et al. MIRD Pamphlet No. 26: Joint EANM/MIRD guidelines for quantitative 177Lu SPECT applied for dosimetry of radiopharmaceutical therapy. J Nucl Med. 2016;57:151–62. https://doi.org/10.2967/jnumed.115.159012.
265. Lloyd JJ, Shields RA, Taylor CJ, et al. Technegas and Pertechnegas particle size distribution. Eur J Nucl Med. 1995;22:473–6. https://doi.org/10.1007/BF00839062.
266. Lococo F, Rena O, Torricelli F, et al. 18F-fluorodeoxyglucose positron emission tomography in malignant pleural mesothelioma: diagnostic and prognostic performance and its correlation to pathological results. Interact Cardiovasc Thorac Surg. 2020;30:593–6. https://doi.org/10.1093/icvts/ivz303.
267. Lodge MA, Jacene HA, Pili R, Wahl RL. Reproducibility of tumor blood flow quantification with 15O-water PET. J Nucl Med. 2008;49:1620–7. https://doi.org/10.2967/jnumed.108.052076.
268. van Loon J, Even AJG, Aerts HJWL, et al. PET imaging of zirconium-89 labelled cetuximab: a phase I trial in patients with head and neck and lung cancer. Radiother Oncol. 2017;122:267–73. https://doi.org/10.1016/j.radonc.2016.11.020.
269. Lordick F, Ott K, Krause B-J, et al. PET to assess early metabolic response and to guide treatment of adenocarcinoma of the oesophagogastric

junction: the MUNICON phase II trial. Lancet Oncol. 2007;8:797–805. https://doi.org/10.1016/S1470-2045(07)70244-9.
270. Lowe VJ, Hoffman JM, DeLong DM, et al. Semiquantitative and visual analysis of FDG-PET images in pulmonary abnormalities. J Nucl Med. 1994;35:1771–6.
271. Lu P, Yu L, Li Y, Sun Y. A correlation study between maximum standardized uptake values and pathology and clinical staging in nonsmall cell lung cancer. Nucl Med Commun. 2010;31:646–51.
272. Lu T, Yang G. 18F-FDG PET/CT imaging in the diagnosis of drug-induced lung disease and pulmonary infection in lymphoma. Medicine (Baltimore). 2021;100:e27107. https://doi.org/10.1097/MD.0000000000027107.
273. Luan X, Huang Y, Gao S, et al. (18)F-alfatide PET/CT may predict short-term outcome of concurrent chemoradiotherapy in patients with advanced non-small cell lung cancer. Eur J Nucl Med Mol Imaging. 2016;43:2336–42. https://doi.org/10.1007/s00259-016-3505-3.
274. Ludwig JM, Ambinder EM, Ghodadra A, et al. Lung shunt fraction prior to Yttrium-90 radioembolization predicts survival in patients with neuroendocrine liver metastases: single-center prospective analysis. Cardiovasc Intervent Radiol. 2016;39:1007–14. https://doi.org/10.1007/s00270-016-1323-4.
275. Lugano R, Ramachandran M, Dimberg A. Tumor angiogenesis: causes, consequences, challenges and opportunities. Cell Mol Life Sci CMLS. 2020;77:1745–70. https://doi.org/10.1007/s00018-019-03351-7.
276. Luo H, England CG, Graves SA, et al. PET imaging of VEGFR-2 expression in lung cancer with 64Cu-labeled Ramucirumab. J Nucl Med. 2016;57:285–90. https://doi.org/10.2967/jnumed.115.166462.
277. Delcroix M, et al. ERS statement on chronic thromboembolic pulmonary hypertension. Eur Respir J. 2021;57 https://doi.org/10.1183/13993003.02828-2020.
278. MacMahon H, Naidich DP, Goo JM, et al. Guidelines for management of incidental pulmonary nodules detected on CT images: from the Fleischner Society 2017. Radiology. 2017;284:228–43. https://doi.org/10.1148/radiol.2017161659.
279. Mannes PZ, Barnes CE, Latoche JD, et al. 2-deoxy-2-[18F]fluoro-D-glucose positron emission tomography to monitor lung inflammation and therapeutic response to Dexamethasone in a Murine Model of acute lung injury. Mol Imaging Biol. 2023;1–11 https://doi.org/10.1007/s11307-023-01813-w.
280. Mannheim JG, Schmid AM, Schwenck J, et al. PET/MRI hybrid systems. Semin Nucl Med. 2018;48:332–47. https://doi.org/10.1053/j.semnuclmed.2018.02.011.
281. Marchevsky AM, Gupta R, McKenna RJ, et al. Evidence-based pathology and the pathologic evaluation of thymomas: the World Health Organization classification can be simplified into only 3 categories other than thymic carcinoma. Cancer. 2008;112:2780–8. https://doi.org/10.1002/cncr.23492.
282. Mariani G, Boni G, Barreca M, et al. Radionuclide gastroesophageal motor studies. J Nucl Med. 2004;45:1004–28.
283. Martinez G, Barberà JA, Navasa M, et al. Hepatopulmonary syndrome associated with cardiorespiratory disease. J Hepatol. 1999;30:882–9. https://doi.org/10.1016/s0168-8278(99)80143-3.
284. Maruoka Y, Nagao M, Baba S, et al. Three-dimensional fractal analysis of 99mTc-MAA SPECT images in chronic thromboembolic pulmonary hypertension for evaluation of response to balloon pulmonary angioplasty: association with pulmonary arterial pressure. Nucl Med Commun. 2017;38:480. https://doi.org/10.1097/MNM.0000000000000673.
285. Marx A, Chan JKC, Chalabreysse L, et al. The 2021 WHO classification of tumors of the thymus and Mediastinum: what is new in Thymic epithelial, germ cell, and mesenchymal tumors? J Thorac Oncol. 2022;17:200–13. https://doi.org/10.1016/j.jtho.2021.10.010.
286. Matthay MA, Zemans RL, Zimmerman GA, et al. Acute respiratory distress syndrome. Nat Rev Dis Primers. 2019;5:1–22. https://doi.org/10.1038/s41572-019-0069-0.
287. Maurer AH. Gastrointestinal motility, part 1: esophageal transit and gastric emptying. J Nucl Med. 2015;56:1229–38. https://doi.org/10.2967/jnumed.112.114314.
288. McMillan AB, Bradshaw TJ. Artificial intelligence-based data corrections for attenuation and Scatter in position emission tomography and single-photon emission computed tomography. PET Clin. 2021;16:543–52. https://doi.org/10.1016/j.cpet.2021.06.010.
289. Meléndez-Alafort L, Nadali A, Zangoni E, et al. Biokinetic and dosimetric studies of 188Re-hyaluronic acid: a new radiopharmaceutical for treatment of hepatocellular carcinoma. Nucl Med Biol. 2009;36:693–701. https://doi.org/10.1016/j.nucmedbio.2009.04.006.
290. Memon AA, Weber B, Winterdahl M, et al. PET imaging of patients with non-small cell lung cancer employing an EGF receptor targeting drug as tracer. Br J Cancer. 2011;105:1850–5. https://doi.org/10.1038/bjc.2011.493.
291. Meng X, Loo BWJ, Ma L, et al. Molecular imaging with 11C-PD153035 PET/CT predicts survival in non-small cell lung cancer treated with EGFR-TKI: a pilot study. J Nucl Med. 2011;52:1573–9. https://doi.org/10.2967/jnumed.111.092874.
292. Mileshkin L, Hicks RJ, Hughes BGM, et al. Changes in 18F-fluorodeoxyglucose and 18F-fluorodeoxythymidine positron emission tomography imaging in patients with non-small cell lung cancer treated with erlotinib. Clin Cancer Res.

2011;17:3304–15. https://doi.org/10.1158/1078-0432.CCR-10-2763.
293. Miniati M, Pistolesi M, Marini C, et al. Value of perfusion lung scan in the diagnosis of pulmonary embolism: results of the Prospective Investigative Study of Acute Pulmonary Embolism Diagnosis (PISA-PED). Am J Respir Crit Care Med. 1996;154:1387–93. https://doi.org/10.1164/ajrccm.154.5.8912753.
294. Mirza H, Hashmi MF. Lung ventilation perfusion scan (VQ Scan). In: StatPearls. Treasure Island: StatPearls Publishing; 2023.
295. Monaco SE, Nikiforova MN, Cieply K, et al. A comparison of EGFR and KRAS status in primary lung carcinoma and matched metastases. Hum Pathol. 2010;41:94–102. https://doi.org/10.1016/j.humpath.2009.06.019.
296. Montesi SB, Désogère P, Fuchs BC, Caravan P. Molecular imaging of fibrosis: recent advances and future directions. J Clin Invest. 2019a;129:24–33. https://doi.org/10.1172/JCI122132.
297. Montesi SB, Izquierdo-Garcia D, Désogère P, et al. Type I Collagen–targeted positron emission tomography imaging in idiopathic pulmonary fibrosis: first-in-human studies. Am J Respir Crit Care Med. 2019;200:258–61. https://doi.org/10.1164/rccm.201903-0503LE.
298. Moon SH, Cho S-H, Park LC, et al. Metabolic response evaluated by 18F-FDG PET/CT as a potential screening tool in identifying a subgroup of patients with advanced non-small cell lung cancer for immediate maintenance therapy after first-line chemotherapy. Eur J Nucl Med Mol Imaging. 2013;40:1005–13. https://doi.org/10.1007/s00259-013-2400-4.
299. Moore AJE, Wachsmann J, Chamarthy MR, et al. Imaging of acute pulmonary embolism: an update. Cardiovasc Diagn Ther. 2018;8:225–43. https://doi.org/10.21037/cdt.2017.12.01.
300. Moradi F, Morris TA, Hoh CK. Perfusion scintigraphy in diagnosis and management of thromboembolic pulmonary hypertension. Radiographics. 2019;39:169–85. https://doi.org/10.1148/rg.2019180074.
301. Mortensen J, Berg RMG. Lung scintigraphy in COPD. Semin Nucl Med. 2019;49:16–21. https://doi.org/10.1053/j.semnuclmed.2018.10.010.
302. Mostard RLM, Verschakelen JA, Kroonenburgh MJPG van, et al. Severity of pulmonary involvement and 18F-FDG PET activity in sarcoidosis. Respir Med. 2013;107:439–47. https://doi.org/10.1016/j.rmed.2012.11.011.
303. Mulders-Manders C, Simon A, Bleeker-Rovers C. Fever of unknown origin. Clin Med (Lond). 2015;15:280–4. https://doi.org/10.7861/clinmedicine.15-3-280.
304. Munden RF, Macapinlac HA, Erasmus JJ. Esophageal cancer: the role of integrated CT-PET in initial staging and response assessment after preoperative therapy. J Thorac Imaging. 2006;21:137–45. https://doi.org/10.1097/00005382-200605000-00005.
305. Musch G. Molecular imaging of inflammation with PET in acute and ventilator-induced lung injury. Front Physiol. 2023;14:1177717.
306. Musch G, Bellani G, Vidal Melo MF, et al. Relation between shunt, aeration, and perfusion in experimental acute lung injury. Am J Respir Crit Care Med. 2008;177:292–300. https://doi.org/10.1164/rccm.200703-484OC.
307. Musch G, Harris RS, Vidal Melo MF, et al. Mechanism by which a sustained inflation can worsen oxygenation in acute lung injury. Anesthesiology. 2004;100:323–30. https://doi.org/10.1097/00000542-200402000-00022.
308. Musch G, et al. A window on the lung: molecular imaging as a tool to dissect pathophysiologic mechanisms of acute lung disease. Contrast Media Mol Imaging. 2019;2019:1510507.
309. Tunariu N, Gibbs SJR, Win Z, Gin-Sing W, Graham A, Gishen P, et al. Ventilation-perfusion scintigraphy is more sensitive than multidetector CTPA in detecting chronic thromboembolic pulmonary disease as a treatable cause of pulmonary hypertension. J Nucl Med. 2007;48 https://doi.org/10.2967/jnumed.106.039438.
310. Najjar AM, Johnson JM, Schellingerhout D. The emerging role of amino acid PET in neuro-oncology. Bioeng Basel Switz. 2018;5 https://doi.org/10.3390/bioengineering5040104.
311. Narsinh KH, Van Buskirk M, Kennedy AS, et al. Hepatopulmonary shunting: a prognostic indicator of survival in patients with metastatic colorectal Adenocarcinoma treated with 90Y radioembolization. Radiology. 2017;282:281–8. https://doi.org/10.1148/radiol.2016152100.
312. National Comprehensive Cancer Network. Non-small cell lung cancer (Version 3.2023), 2023. https://www.nccn.org/professionals/physician_gls/pdf/nscl.pdf.
313. National Comprehensive Cancer Network. Small cell lung cancer (Version 3.2023), 2022. https://www.nccn.org/professionals/physician_gls/pdf/sclc.pdf.
314. National Comprehensive Cancer Network. Mesothelioma: Pleural (Version 1.2023), 2023. https://www.nccn.org/professionals/physician_gls/pdf/meso_pleural.pdf.
315. National Comprehensive Cancer Network. Esophageal and Esophagogastric junction cancers (Version 2.2023), 2023. https://www.nccn.org/professionals/physician_gls/pdf/esophageal.pdf.
316. National Comprehensive Cancer Network. Thymomas and thymic carcinomas (Version 1.2023), 2023. https://www.nccn.org/professionals/physician_gls/pdf/thymic.pdf.
317. Ng T, Konik A, Harrington K, et al. Fluciclovine-PET assessment of amino-acid transporter kinetics for primary staging of muscle-invasive

bladder cancer. J Nucl Med. 2022a;63(supplement 2):3053.
318. Ng TSC, Allen HH, Rashidian M, Miller MA. Probing immune infiltration dynamics in cancer by in vivo imaging. Curr Opin Chem Biol. 2022b;67:102117. https://doi.org/10.1016/j.cbpa.2022.102117.
319. Ng TSC, Gao X, Salari K, et al. Incorporating PSMA-targeting theranostics into personalized prostate cancer treatment: a multidisciplinary perspective. Front Oncol. 2021;11:722277. https://doi.org/10.3389/fonc.2021.722277.
320. Ng TSC, Miller MA. Chapter Thirteen - Image-guided cancer immunotherapy. In: Amiji MM, Milane LS, editors. Engineering technologies and clinical translation. Academic Press; 2022. p. 427–67.
321. Ng TSC, Seethamraju RT, Bueno R, Gill RR. Clinical implementation of a free-breathing, motion-robust dynamic contrast-enhanced MRI protocol to evaluate pleural tumors. AJR Am J Roentgenol. 2020;215:94–104. https://doi.org/10.2214/AJR.19.21612.
322. Nobuhara KK, Wilson JM. Pathophysiology of congenital diaphragmatic hernia. Semin Pediatr Surg. 1996;5:234–42.
323. Norberg P, Persson HL, Schmekel B, et al. Does quantitative lung SPECT detect lung abnormalities earlier than lung function tests? Results of a pilot study. EJNMMI Res. 2014;4:39. https://doi.org/10.1186/s13550-014-0039-1.
324. Nose Y, Makino T, Tatsumi M, et al. Risk stratification of oesophageal squamous cell carcinoma using change in total lesion glycolysis and number of PET-positive lymph nodes. Br J Cancer. 2023;128:1879–87. https://doi.org/10.1038/s41416-023-02151-y.
325. Novello S, Califano R, Reinmuth N, et al. RET fusion-positive non-small cell lung cancer: the evolving treatment landscape. Oncologist. 2023;28:402–13.
326. Odawara S, Kitajima K, Katsuura T, et al. Tumor response to neoadjuvant chemotherapy in patients with esophageal cancer assessed with CT and FDG-PET/CT - RECIST 1.1 vs. PERCIST 1.0. Eur J Radiol. 2018;101:65–71. https://doi.org/10.1016/j.ejrad.2018.02.009.
327. Okuyama H, Kubota A, Kawahara H, et al. Correlation between lung scintigraphy and long-term outcome in survivors of congenital diaphragmatic hernia. Pediatr Pulmonol. 2006;41:882–6. https://doi.org/10.1002/ppul.20466.
328. Olsson C-G, Bitzén U, Olsson B, et al. Outpatient tinzaparin therapy in pulmonary embolism quantified with ventilation/perfusion scintigraphy. Med Sci Monit Int Med J Exp Clin Res. 2006;12:PI9–13.
329. Omloo JMT, Sloof GW, Boellaard R, et al. Importance of fluorodeoxyglucose-positron emission tomography (FDG-PET) and endoscopic ultrasonography parameters in predicting survival following surgery for esophageal cancer. Endoscopy. 2008;40:464–71. https://doi.org/10.1055/s-2008-1077302.
330. Ortega C, Wong RKS, Schaefferkoetter J, et al. Quantitative 68Ga-DOTATATE PET/CT parameters for the prediction of therapy response in patients with progressive metastatic neuroendocrine tumors treated with 177Lu-DOTATATE. J Nucl Med. 2021;62:1406–14. https://doi.org/10.2967/jnumed.120.256727.
331. Oswald NK, Halle-Smith J, Mehdi R, et al. Predicting postoperative lung function following lung cancer resection: a systematic review and meta-analysis. EClinicalMedicine. 2019;15:7–13. https://doi.org/10.1016/j.eclinm.2019.08.015.
332. Paez R, Shah C, Cords AJ, et al. 18F-FSPG PET imaging for the evaluation of indeterminate pulmonary nodules. PloS One. 2022;17:e0265427. https://doi.org/10.1371/journal.pone.0265427.
333. Pal K, Gupta DK. Serial perfusion study depicts pulmonary vascular growth in the survivors of non-extracorporeal membrane oxygenation-treated congenital diaphragmatic hernia. Neonatology. 2010;98:254–9. https://doi.org/10.1159/000278820.
334. Parker JA, Coleman RE, Grady E, et al. SNM practice guideline for lung Scintigraphy 4.0. J Nucl Med Technol. 2012;40:57–65. https://doi.org/10.2967/jnmt.111.101386.
335. Partridge EA, Peranteau WH, Herkert L, et al. Right- versus left-sided congenital diaphragmatic hernia: a comparative outcomes analysis. J Pediatr Surg. 2016;51:900–2. https://doi.org/10.1016/j.jpedsurg.2016.02.049.
336. Peelen DM, Zwezerijnen BGJC, Nossent EJ, et al. The quantitative assessment of interstitial lung disease with positron emission tomography scanning in systemic sclerosis patients. Rheumatology (Oxford). 2020;59:1407–15. https://doi.org/10.1093/rheumatology/kez483.
337. Pees A, Chassé M, Lindberg A, Vasdev N. Recent developments in carbon-11 chemistry and applications for first-in-human PET studies. Molecules. 2023;28:931.
338. Pena E, Kimpton M, Dennie C, et al. Difference in interpretation of computed tomography pulmonary angiography diagnosis of subsegmental thrombosis in patients with suspected pulmonary embolism. J Thromb Haemost JTH. 2012;10:496–8. https://doi.org/10.1111/j.1538-7836.2011.04612.x.
339. Piai DB, Quagliatto R, Toro I, et al. The use of SPECT in preoperative assessment of patients with lung cancer. Eur Respir J. 2004;24:258–62. https://doi.org/10.1183/09031936.04.00123503.
340. Piepsz A, Wetzburger C, Spehl M, et al. Critical evaluation of lung scintigraphy in cystic fibrosis: study of 113 patients. J Nucl Med. 1980;21:909–13.
341. Piert M, Machulla H-J, Picchio M, et al. Hypoxia-specific tumor imaging with 18F-fluoroazomycin arabinoside. J Nucl Med. 2005;46:106–13.

342. Pinho DF, Banga A, Torres F, Mathews D. Ventilation perfusion pulmonary scintigraphy in the evaluation of pre-and post-lung transplant patients. Transplant Rev (Orlando). 2019;33:107–14. https://doi.org/10.1016/j.trre.2018.10.003.
343. Pratt EC, Lopez-Montes A, Volpe A, et al. Simultaneous quantitative imaging of two PET radiotracers via the detection of positron–electron annihilation and prompt gamma emissions. Nat Biomed Eng. 2023; https://doi.org/10.1038/s41551-023-01060-y.
344. Prenosil GA, Sari H, Fürstner M, et al. Performance characteristics of the biograph vision Quadra PET/CT system with a long axial field of view using the NEMA NU 2-2018 standard. J Nucl Med. 2022;63:476–84. https://doi.org/10.2967/jnumed.121.261972.
345. Puuvuori E, Chiodaroli E, Estrada S, et al. PET imaging of neutrophil elastase with 11C-GW457427 in acute respiratory distress syndrome in pigs. J Nucl Med. 2023;64:423–9.
346. Raisinghani A, Ben-Yehuda O. Echocardiography in chronic thromboembolic pulmonary hypertension. Semin Thorac Cardiovasc Surg. 2006;18:230–5. https://doi.org/10.1053/j.semtcvs.2006.09.006.
347. Raman S, Bissonnette J-P, Warner A, et al. Rationale and protocol for a Canadian Multicenter Phase II randomized trial assessing selective metabolically adaptive radiation dose escalation in locally advanced non-small-cell lung cancer (NCT02788461). Clin Lung Cancer. 2018;19:e699–703. https://doi.org/10.1016/j.cllc.2018.05.002.
348. Reader AJ, Schramm G. Artificial intelligence for PET image reconstruction. J Nucl Med. 2021;62:1330–3. https://doi.org/10.2967/jnumed.121.262303.
349. Reed MD, Markov G, Finlay MD, et al. Unusual ventilation-perfusion scintigraphy in adult respiratory distress syndrome secondary to acute lupus myocarditis. Clin Nucl Med. 2004;29:831–3. https://doi.org/10.1097/00003072-200412000-00020.
350. Reinartz P, Wildberger JE, Schaefer W, et al. Tomographic imaging in the diagnosis of pulmonary embolism: a comparison between V/Q lung scintigraphy in SPECT technique and multislice spiral CT. J Nucl Med. 2004;45:1501–8.
351. Rhodes J, Dave A, Pulling MC, et al. Effect of pulmonary artery stenoses on the cardiopulmonary response to exercise following repair of tetralogy of Fallot. Am J Cardiol. 1998;81:1217–9. https://doi.org/10.1016/s0002-9149(98)00095-2.
352. Rindi G, Mete O, Uccella S, et al. Overview of the 2022 WHO classification of neuroendocrine neoplasms. Endocr Pathol. 2022;33:115–54. https://doi.org/10.1007/s12022-022-09708-2.
353. Ritt P. Recent developments in SPECT/CT. Semin Nucl Med. 2022;52:276–85. https://doi.org/10.1053/j.semnuclmed.2022.01.004.
354. Roach PJ, Bailey DL, Schembri GP, Thomas PA. Transition from planar to SPECT V/Q scintigraphy: rationale, practicalities, and challenges. Semin Nucl Med. 2010;40:397–407. https://doi.org/10.1053/j.semnuclmed.2010.07.004.
355. Rodríguez-Roisin R, Krowka MJ. Hepatopulmonary syndrome--a liver-induced lung vascular disorder. N Engl J Med. 2008;358:2378–87. https://doi.org/10.1056/NEJMra0707185.
356. Röhrich M, Leitz D, Glatting FM, et al. Fibroblast activation protein-specific PET/CT imaging in fibrotic interstitial lung diseases and lung cancer: a translational exploratory study. J Nucl Med. 2022;63:127–33. https://doi.org/10.2967/jnumed.121.261925.
357. Rosai J, Sobin LH. Histological typing of tumours of the thymus. Berlin/Heidelberg: Springer; 1999.
358. Rose SC, Hoh CK. Hepatopulmonary shunt reduction using chemoembolization to permit yttrium-90 radioembolization. J Vasc Interv Radiol JVIR. 2009;20:849–51. https://doi.org/10.1016/j.jvir.2009.03.010.
359. Roth D, Gustafsson J, Sundlöv A, Sjögreen Gleisner K. A method for tumor dosimetry based on hybrid planar-SPECT/CT images and semiautomatic segmentation. Med Phys. 2018;45:5004–18. https://doi.org/10.1002/mp.13178.
360. Roy PM. Preoperative pulmonary evaluation for lung resection. J Anaesthesiol Clin Pharmacol. 2018;34:296–300. https://doi.org/10.4103/joacp.JOACP_89_17.
361. Ryan KL, Fedullo PF, Davis GB, et al. Perfusion scan findings understate the severity of angiographic and hemodynamic compromise in chronic thromboembolic pulmonary hypertension. Chest. 1988;93:1180–5. https://doi.org/10.1378/chest.93.6.1180.
362. Sachdeva R, Valente AM, Armstrong AK, et al. ACC/AHA/ASE/HRS/ISACHD/SCAI/SCCT/SCMR/SOPE 2020 appropriate use criteria for multimodality imaging during the follow-up care of patients with congenital heart disease: a report of the American College of Cardiology Solution Set Oversight Committee and Appropriate Use Criteria Task Force, American Heart Association, American Society of Echocardiography, Heart Rhythm Society, International Society for Adult Congenital Heart Disease, Society for Cardiovascular Angiography and Interventions, Society of Cardiovascular Computed Tomography, Society for Cardiovascular Magnetic Resonance, and Society of Pediatric Echocardiography. J Am Coll Cardiol. 2020;75:657–703. https://doi.org/10.1016/j.jacc.2019.10.002.
363. Saga T, Inubushi M, Koizumi M, et al. Prognostic value of 18F-fluoroazomycin arabinoside PET/CT in patients with advanced non-small-cell lung cancer. Cancer Sci. 2015;106:1554–60.
364. Sakao S, Daimon M, Voelkel NF, et al. Right ventricular sugars and fats in chronic thromboembolic pulmonary hypertension. Int J Cardiol.

2016;219:143–9. https://doi.org/10.1016/j.ijcard.2016.06.010.
365. Sakao S, Miyauchi H, Voelkel NF, et al. Increased right ventricular fatty acid accumulation in chronic thromboembolic pulmonary hypertension. Ann Am Thorac Soc. 2015;12:1465–72. https://doi.org/10.1513/AnnalsATS.201504-236LE.
366. Salem R, Lewandowski RJ, Gates VL, et al. Research reporting standards for radioembolization of hepatic malignancies. J Vasc Interv Radiol JVIR. 2011;22:265–78. https://doi.org/10.1016/j.jvir.2010.10.029.
367. Sandiford P, Province MA, Schuster DP. Distribution of regional density and vascular permeability in the adult respiratory distress syndrome. Am J Respir Crit Care Med. 1995;151:737–42. https://doi.org/10.1164/ajrccm/151.3_Pt_1.737.
368. Sari H, Reaungamornrat J, Catalano OA, et al. Evaluation of deep learning-based approaches to segment bowel air pockets and generate pelvic attenuation maps from CAIPIRINHA-accelerated Dixon MR images. J Nucl Med. 2022;63:468–75. https://doi.org/10.2967/jnumed.120.261032.
369. Sarma A, Grant FD, Kwatra NS. Esophageal transit scintigraphy in children: a user's guide and pictorial review. Pediatr Radiol. 2019;49:663–77. https://doi.org/10.1007/s00247-018-4301-y.
370. Sato M, Umeda Y, Tsujikawa T, et al. Predictive value of 3'-deoxy-3'-18F-fluorothymidine PET in the early response to anti-programmed death-1 therapy in patients with advanced non-small cell lung cancer. J Immunother Cancer. 2021;9 https://doi.org/10.1136/jitc-2021-003079.
371. Sauter JL, Dacic S, Galateau-Salle F, et al. The 2021 WHO classification of tumors of the Pleura: advances since the 2015 classification. J Thorac Oncol. 2022;17:608–22. https://doi.org/10.1016/j.jtho.2021.12.014.
372. Schaefferkoetter JD, Osman M, Townsend DW. The importance of quality control for clinical PET imaging. J Nucl Med Technol. 2017;45:265–6. https://doi.org/10.2967/jnmt.117.198465.
373. Schneider JL, Lin JJ, Shaw AT. ALK-positive lung cancer: a moving target. Nat Cancer. 2023;4:330–43.
374. Schuster DP. The evaluation of lung function with PET. Semin Nucl Med. 1998;28:341–51. https://doi.org/10.1016/s0001-2998(98)80037-8.
375. Schuster DP, Anderson C, Kozlowski J, Lange N. Regional pulmonary perfusion in patients with acute pulmonary edema. J Nucl Med. 2002;43:863–70.
376. Schuster DP, Markham J, Welch MJ. Positron emission tomography measurements of pulmonary vascular permeability with Ga-68 transferrin or C-11 methylalbumin. Crit Care Med. 1998;26:518–25.
377. Schwyzer M, Martini K, Benz DC, et al. Artificial intelligence for detecting small FDG-positive lung nodules in digital PET/CT: impact of image reconstructions on diagnostic performance. Eur Radiol. 2020;30:2031–40. https://doi.org/10.1007/s00330-019-06498-w.
378. Scott JA, Palmer EL. Neural network analysis of ventilation-perfusion lung scans. Radiology. 1993;186:661–4. https://doi.org/10.1148/radiology.186.3.8430170.
379. Seki N, Sakamoto S, Karube Y, et al. ^{18}F-fluorodeoxyglucose positron emission tomography for evaluation of thymic epithelial tumors: utility for World Health Organization classification and predicting recurrence-free survival. Ann Nucl Med. 2014;28:257–62. https://doi.org/10.1007/s12149-014-0804-2.
380. Sellmyer MA, Lee I, Hou C, et al. Bacterial infection imaging with [18F]fluoropropyl-trimethoprim. Proc Natl Acad Sci. 2017;114:8372–7. https://doi.org/10.1073/pnas.1703109114.
381. Seol HY, Kim YS, Kim S-J. Predictive value of 18F-fluorodeoxyglucose positron emission tomography/computed tomography for PD-L1 expression in non-small cell lung cancer: a systematic review and meta-analysis. Thorac Cancer. 2020;11:3260–8. https://doi.org/10.1111/1759-7714.13664.
382. Shao L, Freifelder R, Karp JS. Triple energy window scatter correction technique in PET. IEEE Trans Med Imaging. 1994;13:641–8. https://doi.org/10.1109/42.363104.
383. Sheikhbahaei S, Mena E, Yanamadala A, et al. The value of FDG PET/CT in treatment response assessment, follow-up, and surveillance of lung cancer. AJR Am J Roentgenol. 2017;208:420–33. https://doi.org/10.2214/AJR.16.16532.
384. Signore A, Jamar F, Israel O, et al. Clinical indications, image acquisition and data interpretation for white blood cells and anti-granulocyte monoclonal antibody scintigraphy: an EANM procedural guideline. Eur J Nucl Med Mol Imaging. 2018;45:1816–31. https://doi.org/10.1007/s00259-018-4052-x.
385. Simsek FS, Cakmak M, Kuslu D, et al. How can we use positron emission tomography/computed tomography more accurately for characterization of asbestos-related pleural thickening? Arch Med Sci. 2021;19:385–91. https://doi.org/10.5114/aoms/111529.
386. Song H, Ferri V, Duan H, et al. SPECT at the speed of PET: a feasibility study of CZT-based whole-body SPECT/CT in the post 177Lu-DOTATATE and 177Lu-PSMA617 setting. Eur J Nucl Med Mol Imaging. 2023;50:2250–7. https://doi.org/10.1007/s00259-023-06176-6.
387. Sostman HD, Miniati M, Gottschalk A, et al. Sensitivity and specificity of perfusion scintigraphy combined with chest radiography for acute pulmonary embolism in PIOPED II. J Nucl Med. 2008;49:1741–8. https://doi.org/10.2967/jnumed.108.052217.
388. Soussan M, Chouahnia K, Maisonobe J-A, et al. Prognostic implications of volume-based measurements on FDG PET/CT in stage III non-small-cell lung cancer after induction chemotherapy. Eur J

Nucl Med Mol Imaging. 2013;40:668–76. https://doi.org/10.1007/s00259-012-2321-7.
389. Soydal Ç, Yüksel C, Küçük NÖ, et al. Prognostic value of metabolic tumor volume measured by 18F-FDG PET/CT in esophageal cancer patients. Mol Imaging Radionucl Ther. 2014;23:12–5. https://doi.org/10.4274/Mirt.07379.
390. Spencer BA, Berg E, Schmall JP, et al. Performance evaluation of the uEXPLORER total-body PET/CT scanner based on NEMA NU 2-2018 with additional tests to characterize PET scanners with a long axial field of view. J Nucl Med. 2021;62:861–70. https://doi.org/10.2967/jnumed.120.250597.
391. Stahl A, Ott K, Weber WA, et al. FDG PET imaging of locally advanced gastric carcinomas: correlation with endoscopic and histopathological findings. Eur J Nucl Med Mol Imaging. 2003;30:288–95. https://doi.org/10.1007/s00259-002-1029-5.
392. Stanchina ML, Tantisira KG, Aquino SL, et al. Association of lung perfusion disparity and mortality in patients with cystic fibrosis awaiting lung transplantation. J Heart Lung Transplant. 2002;21:217–25. https://doi.org/10.1016/s1053-2498(01)00376-x.
393. Starobin D, Shitrit D, Steinmetz A, et al. Quantitative lung perfusion following single lung transplantation. Thorac Cardiovasc Surg. 2007;55:48–52. https://doi.org/10.1055/s-2006-924709.
394. Stavngaard T, Mortensen J. Assessment of ventilation inhomogenity with Krypton SPECT and planar imaging. Clin Physiol Funct Imaging. 2005;25:106–12. https://doi.org/10.1111/j.1475-097X.2004.00598.x.
395. Stefanutti G, Filippone M, Tommasoni N, et al. Cardiopulmonary anatomy and function in long-term survivors of mild to moderate congenital diaphragmatic hernia. J Pediatr Surg. 2004;39:526–31. https://doi.org/10.1016/j.jpedsurg.2003.12.006.
396. Su H, Seimbille Y, Ferl GZ, et al. Evaluation of [(18)F]gefitinib as a molecular imaging probe for the assessment of the epidermal growth factor receptor status in malignant tumors. Eur J Nucl Med Mol Imaging. 2008;35:1089–99. https://doi.org/10.1007/s00259-007-0636-6.
397. Subramanian DR, Jenkins L, Edgar R, et al. Assessment of pulmonary neutrophilic inflammation in emphysema by quantitative positron emission tomography. Am J Respir Crit Care Med. 2012;186:1125–32. https://doi.org/10.1164/rccm.201201-0051OC.
398. Suga K, Kawakami Y, Iwanaga H, et al. Automated breath-hold perfusion SPECT/CT fusion images of the lungs. AJR Am J Roentgenol. 2007;189:455–63. https://doi.org/10.2214/AJR.06.1290.
399. Sun X, Xiao Z, Chen G, et al. A PET imaging approach for determining EGFR mutation status for improved lung cancer patient management. Sci Transl Med. 2018;10:eaan8840. https://doi.org/10.1126/scitranslmed.aan8840.
400. Sundlöv A, Gustafsson J, Brolin G, et al. Feasibility of simplifying renal dosimetry in 177Lu peptide receptor radionuclide therapy. EJNMMI Phys. 2018;5 https://doi.org/10.1186/s40658-018-0210-2.
401. Surti S, Karp JS. Update on latest advances in time-of-flight PET. Phys Med. 2020;80:251–8. https://doi.org/10.1016/j.ejmp.2020.10.031.
402. Surti S, Pantel AR, Karp JS. Total body PET: why, how, what for? IEEE Trans Radiat Plasma Med Sci. 2020;4:283–92. https://doi.org/10.1109/trpms.2020.2985403.
403. Talwar S, Sankhyan L, Patel C, et al. Evaluation of differential pulmonary perfusion using 99mTc macroaggregated albumin after the Fontan procedure. Interact Cardiovasc Thorac Surg. 2018;26:651–9. https://doi.org/10.1093/icvts/ivx377.
404. Tan TH, Ismail R. Utility of lung perfusion SPECT/CT in detection of pulmonary thromboembolic disease: outcome analysis. Nucl Med Mol Imaging. 2023;57:1–8. https://doi.org/10.1007/s13139-021-00726-2.
405. Taralli S, Giancipoli RG, Caldarella C, et al. The prognostic value of 18F-FDG PET imaging at staging in patients with malignant pleural mesothelioma: a literature review. J Clin Med. 2021;11:33. https://doi.org/10.3390/jcm11010033.
406. Tateishi U, Hasegawa T, Seki K, et al. Disease activity and 18F-FDG uptake in organising pneumonia: semi-quantitative evaluation using computed tomography and positron emission tomography. Eur J Nucl Med Mol Imaging. 2006;33:906–12. https://doi.org/10.1007/s00259-006-0073-y.
407. Tatematsu T, Okuda K, Saito Y, et al. The usefulness of fluorodeoxyglucose-positron emission tomography as a preoperative diagnostic tool for thymic epithelial tumors. Gland Surg. 2021;10:690–6. https://doi.org/10.21037/gs-20-718.
408. Taylor IK, Hill AA, Hayes M, et al. Imaging allergen-invoked airway inflammation in atopic asthma with [18F]-fluorodeoxyglucose and positron emission tomography. Lancet Lond Engl. 1996;347:937–40. https://doi.org/10.1016/s0140-6736(96)91416-6.
409. Teirstein AS, Machac J, Almeida O, et al. Results of 188 whole-body fluorodeoxyglucose positron emission tomography scans in 137 patients with sarcoidosis. Chest. 2007;132:1949–53. https://doi.org/10.1378/chest.07-1178.
410. Terada T, Tabata C, Tabata R, et al. Clinical utility of 18-fluorodeoxyglucose positron emission tomography/computed tomography in malignant pleural mesothelioma. Exp Ther Med. 2012;4:197–200. https://doi.org/10.3892/etm.2012.572.
411. Theysohn JM, Schlaak JF, Müller S, et al. Selective internal radiation therapy of hepatocellular carcinoma: potential hepatopulmonary shunt reduction after sorafenib administration. J Vasc Interv Radiol JVIR. 2012;23:949–52. https://doi.org/10.1016/j.jvir.2012.04.007.
412. Thomas A, Mena E, Kurdziel K, et al. 18F-Fluorodeoxyglucose positron emission

tomography in the management of patients with thymic epithelial tumors. Clin Cancer Res. 2013;19:1487–93. https://doi.org/10.1158/1078-0432.CCR-12-2929.
413. Thomsen C, Theilig D, Herzog D, et al. Lung perfusion and emphysema distribution affect the outcome of endobronchial valve therapy. Int J Chron Obstruct Pulmon Dis. 2016;11:1245–59. https://doi.org/10.2147/COPD.S101003.
414. Thureau S, Piton N, Gouel P, et al. First comparison between [18f]-FMISO and [18f]-Faza for preoperative pet imaging of hypoxia in lung cancer. Cancer. 2021;13:4101.
415. Tien Cong B, Cam Phuong P, Thai P-V, et al. Prognostic significance of PD-L1 expression and standardized uptake values in the primary lesions of stage IV adenocarcinoma lung cancer. Front Med. 2022;9:895401. https://doi.org/10.3389/fmed.2022.895401.
416. Tirumani H, Rosenthal MH, Tirumani SH, et al. Esophageal carcinoma: current concepts in the role of imaging in staging and management. Can Assoc Radiol J J Assoc Can Radiol. 2015;66:130–9. https://doi.org/10.1016/j.carj.2014.08.006.
417. Tohme MS, Qi J. Iterative image reconstruction for positron emission tomography based on a detector response function estimated from point source measurements. Phys Med Biol. 2009;54:3709. https://doi.org/10.1088/0031-9155/54/12/007.
418. Torbicki A, Perrier A, Konstantinides S, et al. Guidelines on the diagnosis and management of acute pulmonary embolism: the Task Force for the Diagnosis and Management of Acute Pulmonary Embolism of the European Society of Cardiology (ESC). Eur Heart J. 2008;29:2276–315. https://doi.org/10.1093/eurheartj/ehn310.
419. Treglia G, Sadeghi R, Giovanella L, et al. Is (18) F-FDG PET useful in predicting the WHO grade of malignancy in thymic epithelial tumors? A meta-analysis. Lung Cancer Amst Neth. 2014;86:5–13. https://doi.org/10.1016/j.lungcan.2014.08.008.
420. Tsao M-S, Nicholson AG, Maleszewski JJ, et al. Reprint of "Introduction to 2021 WHO classification of thoracic tumors". J Thorac Oncol. 2022;17:337–40. https://doi.org/10.1016/j.jtho.2022.01.008.
421. Tulchinsky M, Fotos JS, Wechalekar K, Dadparvar S. Applications of ventilation-perfusion scintigraphy in surgical management of chronic obstructive lung disease and cancer. Semin Nucl Med. 2017;47:671–9. https://doi.org/10.1053/j.semnuclmed.2017.08.001.
422. Tumgor G. Cirrhosis and hepatopulmonary syndrome. World J Gastroenterol. 2014;20:2586–94. https://doi.org/10.3748/wjg.v20.i10.2586.
423. Uliel L, Royal HD, Darcy MD, et al. From the angio suite to the γ-camera: vascular mapping and 99mTc-MAA hepatic perfusion imaging before liver radioembolization--a comprehensive pictorial review. J Nucl Med. 2012;53:1736–47. https://doi.org/10.2967/jnumed.112.105361.
424. Umutlu L, Herrmann K. Current and emerging applications. In: PETMR Imaging Curr Emerg Appl; 2018. p. 1–8.
425. Valkema MJ, Noordman BJ, Wijnhoven BPL, et al. Accuracy of 18F-FDG PET/CT in predicting residual disease after neoadjuvant chemoradiotherapy for esophageal cancer. J Nucl Med. 2019;60:1553–9. https://doi.org/10.2967/jnumed.118.224196.
426. Van Audenhaege K, Van Holen R, Vandenberghe S, et al. Review of SPECT collimator selection, optimization, and fabrication for clinical and preclinical imaging. Med Phys. 2015;42:4796–813. https://doi.org/10.1118/1.4927061.
427. Van de Wiele C, Sathekge M, de Spiegeleer B, et al. PSMA expression on neovasculature of solid tumors. Histol Histopathol. 2020;35:919–27. https://doi.org/10.14670/HH-18-215.
428. van den Hoff J, Oehme L, Schramm G, et al. The PET-derived tumor-to-blood standard uptake ratio (SUR) is superior to tumor SUV as a surrogate parameter of the metabolic rate of FDG. EJNMMI Res. 2013;3:77. https://doi.org/10.1186/2191-219X-3-77.
429. van Elmpt W, De Ruysscher D, van der Salm A, et al. The PET-boost randomised phase II dose-escalation trial in non-small cell lung cancer. Radiother Oncol J Eur Soc Ther Radiol Oncol. 2012;104:67–71. https://doi.org/10.1016/j.radonc.2012.03.005.
430. Vandenberghe S, Moskal P, Karp JS. State of the art in total body PET. EJNMMI Phys. 2020;7:35. https://doi.org/10.1186/s40658-020-00290-2.
431. Vandervoort E, Sossi V. An analytical scatter correction for singles-mode transmission data in PET. IEEE Trans Med Imaging. 2008;27:402–12. https://doi.org/10.1109/TMI.2007.909851.
432. Vaz N, Franquet E, Heidari P, et al. COVID-19: findings in nuclear medicine from head to toe. Clin Imaging. 2023;99:10–8. https://doi.org/10.1016/j.clinimag.2023.04.003.
433. Venet M, Friedberg MK, Mertens L, et al. Nuclear imaging in pediatric cardiology: principles and applications. Front Pediatr. 2022;10:909994.
434. Veronese M, Rizzo G, Aboagye EO, Bertoldo A. Parametric imaging of ^{18}F-fluoro-3-deoxy-3-L-fluorothymidine PET data to investigate tumour heterogeneity. Eur J Nucl Med Mol Imaging. 2014;41:1781–92. https://doi.org/10.1007/s00259-014-2757-z.
435. Vija AH, Massanes F, Platsch G, et al. Lu177-PSMA treatment monitoring with 20-minute total acquisition time for eye-to-thigh quantitative SPECT/CT. J Nucl Med. 2021;62 (supplement 1):1001.
436. Wahl RL, Jacene H, Kasamon Y, Lodge MA. From RECIST to PERCIST: evolving considerations for PET response criteria in solid tumors. J Nucl Med. 2009;50(Suppl 1):122S–50S. https://doi.org/10.2967/jnumed.108.057307.
437. Wallis D, Soussan M, Lacroix M, et al. An [18F] FDG-PET/CT deep learning method for fully automated detection of pathological mediastinal lymph nodes in lung cancer patients. Eur J Nucl Med Mol

Imaging. 2022;49:881–8. https://doi.org/10.1007/s00259-021-05513-x.
438. Wang C, Lu X. Targeting MET: discovery of small molecule inhibitors as non-small cell lung cancer therapy. J Med Chem. 2023;66:7670.
439. Wang H, Wang S, Song W, et al. Expression of prostate-specific membrane antigen in lung cancer cells and tumor neovasculature endothelial cells and its clinical significance. PloS One. 2015a;10:e0125924. https://doi.org/10.1371/journal.pone.0125924.
440. Wang X, Yang W, Zhou Q, et al. The role of 18F-FDG PET/CT in predicting the pathological response to neoadjuvant PD-1 blockade in combination with chemotherapy for resectable esophageal squamous cell carcinoma. Eur J Nucl Med Mol Imaging. 2022;49:4241–51. https://doi.org/10.1007/s00259-022-05872-z.
441. Wang Y, Ma S, Dong M, et al. Evaluation of the factors affecting the maximum standardized uptake value of metastatic lymph nodes in different histological types of non-small cell lung cancer on PET-CT. BMC Pulm Med. 2015b;15:20. https://doi.org/10.1186/s12890-015-0014-2.
442. Watanabe K, Shinkai M, Kaneko T. Autopsy case of pulmonary artery sarcoma forming aneurysm without FDG uptake. Arch Bronconeumol. 2016;52:535–6. https://doi.org/10.1016/j.arbres.2016.02.014.
443. Watanabe T, Shimomura H, Mutoh T, et al. Positron emission tomography/computed tomography as a clinical diagnostic tool for anterior mediastinal tumors. Surg Today. 2019;49:143–9. https://doi.org/10.1007/s00595-018-1712-1.
444. Webber MM, Gomes AS, Roe D, et al. Comparison of Biello, McNeil, and PIOPED criteria for the diagnosis of pulmonary emboli on lung scans. AJR Am J Roentgenol. 1990;154:975–81. https://doi.org/10.2214/ajr.154.5.2108571.
445. Weber M, Lam M, Chiesa C, et al. EANM procedure guideline for the treatment of liver cancer and liver metastases with intra-arterial radioactive compounds. Eur J Nucl Med Mol Imaging. 2022;49:1682–99. https://doi.org/10.1007/s00259-021-05600-z.
446. Weber WA, Ott K, Becker K, et al. Prediction of response to preoperative chemotherapy in adenocarcinomas of the esophagogastric junction by metabolic imaging. J Clin Oncol. 2001;19:3058–65. https://doi.org/10.1200/JCO.2001.19.12.3058.
447. Wehrenberg-Klee E, An T, Heidari P, et al. SPECT/CT Dosimetry of Bronchial Artery (99m)Tc Macroaggregated Albumin injection in pulmonary malignancies: feasibility evaluation of Bronchial Artery (90)Y radioembolization. Radiology. 2025;314:e240331. https://doi.org/10.1148/radiol.240331.
448. Welling MM, Hensbergen AW, Bunschoten A, et al. An update on radiotracer development for molecular imaging of bacterial infections. Clin Transl Imaging. 2019;7:105–24. https://doi.org/10.1007/s40336-019-00317-4.
449. Wiener RS, Schwartz LM, Woloshin S. Time trends in pulmonary embolism in the United States: evidence of overdiagnosis. Arch Intern Med. 2011;171:831–7. https://doi.org/10.1001/archinternmed.2011.178.
450. Win T, Screaton NJ, Porter JC, et al. Pulmonary 18F-FDG uptake helps refine current risk stratification in idiopathic pulmonary fibrosis (IPF). Eur J Nucl Med Mol Imaging. 2018;45:806–15. https://doi.org/10.1007/s00259-017-3917-8.
451. Win T, Tasker AD, Groves AM, et al. Ventilation-perfusion scintigraphy to predict postoperative pulmonary function in lung cancer patients undergoing pneumonectomy. AJR Am J Roentgenol. 2006;187:1260–5. https://doi.org/10.2214/AJR.04.1973.
452. Win T, Thomas BA, Lambrou T, et al. Areas of normal pulmonary parenchyma on HRCT exhibit increased FDG PET signal in IPF patients. Eur J Nucl Med Mol Imaging. 2014;41:337–42. https://doi.org/10.1007/s00259-013-2514-8.
453. Winer-Muram HT. The solitary pulmonary nodule. Radiology. 2006;239:34–49. https://doi.org/10.1148/radiol.2391050343.
454. Wittram C, Scott JA. 18F-FDG PET of pulmonary embolism. AJR Am J Roentgenol. 2007;189:171–6. https://doi.org/10.2214/AJR.06.0640.
455. World Health Organization. International Agency for Research on Cancer. In: Estim. Number new cases 2020 world sexes ages Excl NMSC. https://gco.iarc.fr/today/online-analysis-table?v=2020&mode=cancer&mode_population=continents&population=900&populations=900&key=asr&sex=0&cancer=39&type=0&statistic=5&prevalence=0&population_group=0&ages_group%5B%5D=0&ages_group%5B%5D=17&group_cancer=1&include_nmsc=0&include_nmsc_other=1.
456. Worsley DF, Kim CK, Alavi A, Palevsky HI. Detailed analysis of patients with matched ventilation-perfusion defects and chest radiographic opacities. J Nucl Med. 1993;34:1851–3.
457. Xing M, Lahti S, Kokabi N, et al. 90Y radioembolization lung shunt fraction in primary and metastatic liver cancer as a biomarker for survival. Clin Nucl Med. 2016;41:21–7. https://doi.org/10.1097/RLU.0000000000000915.
458. Yamamoto H, Sugimoto S, Kurosaki T, et al. Lung perfusion scintigraphy to detect chronic lung allograft dysfunction after living-donor lobar lung transplantation. Sci Rep. 2020;10:10595. https://doi.org/10.1038/s41598-020-67433-4.
459. Yang DJ, Wallace S, Cherif A, et al. Development of F-18-labeled fluoroerythronitroimidazole as a PET agent for imaging tumor hypoxia. Radiology. 1995;194:795–800. https://doi.org/10.1148/radiology.194.3.7862981.
460. Yeh HH, Ogawa K, Balatoni J, et al. Molecular imaging of active mutant L858R EGF receptor (EGFR) kinase-expressing nonsmall cell lung carcinomas using PET/CT. Proc Natl Acad Sci U

S A. 2011;108:1603–8. https://doi.org/10.1073/pnas.1010744108.
461. Yeh SH-H, Lin C-F, Kong F-L, et al. Molecular imaging of nonsmall cell lung carcinomas expressing active mutant EGFR kinase using PET with [(124)i]-morpholino-IPQA. Biomed Res Int. 2013;2013:549359. https://doi.org/10.1155/2013/549359.
462. Young H, Baum R, Cremerius U, et al. Measurement of clinical and subclinical tumour response using [18F]-fluorodeoxyglucose and positron emission tomography: review and 1999 EORTC recommendations. European Organization for Research and Treatment of Cancer (EORTC) PET Study Group. Eur J Cancer Oxf Engl 1990. 1999;35:1773–82. https://doi.org/10.1016/s0959-8049(99)00229-4.
463. Yttrium S-S. Microspheres package Insert, SIRTeX Medical. Lane Cove; 2004.
464. Zander T, Scheffler M, Nogova L, et al. Early prediction of nonprogression in advanced non-small-cell lung cancer treated with erlotinib by using [(18)F]fluorodeoxyglucose and [(18)F]fluorothymidine positron emission tomography. J Clin Oncol. 2011;29:1701–8. https://doi.org/10.1200/JCO.2010.32.4939.
465. Zanzonico P. Routine quality control of clinical nuclear medicine instrumentation: a brief review. J Nucl Med. 2008;49:1114–31. https://doi.org/10.2967/jnumed.107.050203.
466. Zeimpekis KG, Kotasidis FA, Huellner M, et al. NEMA NU 2-2018 performance evaluation of a new generation 30-cm axial field-of-view discovery MI PET/CT. Eur J Nucl Med Mol Imaging. 2022;49:3023–32. https://doi.org/10.1007/s00259-022-05751-7.
467. Zeng J, Patel S, Rengan R, Bowen SR. FLARE RT for patients with stage IIB-IIIB non-small cell lung cancer: personalizing radiation therapy using PET/CT and SPECT/CT imaging. Clin GovGoogle Sch; 2020.
468. Zhang J, Budhdeo S, William W, et al. Moving towards vertically integrated artificial intelligence development. Npj Digit Med. 2022;5:143. https://doi.org/10.1038/s41746-022-00690-x.
469. Zhang L, Ren Z, Xu C, et al. Influencing factors and prognostic value of (18)F-FDG PET/CT metabolic and volumetric parameters in non-small cell lung cancer. Int J Gen Med. 2021;14:3699–706. https://doi.org/10.2147/IJGM.S320744.
470. Zhang W, Wang J, Tang M, et al. Quantitative study of lung perfusion SPECT scanning and pulmonary function testing for early radiation-induced lung injury in patients with locally advanced non-small cell lung cancer. Exp Ther Med. 2012;3:631–5. https://doi.org/10.3892/etm.2012.468.
471. Zhao F, Barber CJ, Sammani S, et al. Use of radiolabeled hyaluronic acid for preclinical assessment of inflammatory injury and acute respiratory distress syndrome. Nucl Med Biol. 2022;114–115:86–98. https://doi.org/10.1016/j.nucmedbio.2022.10.002.
472. Zhao H, Su Y, Lyu Z, et al. Non-invasively discriminating the pathological subtypes of non-small cell lung cancer with pretreatment 18F-FDG PET/CT using deep learning. Acad Radiol. 2024; https://doi.org/10.1016/j.acra.2023.03.032.
473. Zhao H, Tsauo J, Zhang X-W, et al. Technetium-99m-labeled macroaggregated albumin lung perfusion scan for diagnosis of hepatopulmonary syndrome: a prospective study comparing brain uptake and whole-body uptake. World J Gastroenterol. 2020;26:1088–97. https://doi.org/10.3748/wjg.v26.i10.1088.
474. Zheng K, Liang N, Zhang J, et al. 68Ga-NOTA-PRGD2 PET/CT for Integrin imaging in patients with lung cancer. J Nucl Med. 2015;56:1823–7. https://doi.org/10.2967/jnumed.115.160648.
475. Zhou Y, Shao L, Ruan W, et al. Pulmonary vascular involvement of IgG4-related disease: case series with a PRISMA-compliant systemic review. Medicine (Baltimore). 2019;98:e14437. https://doi.org/10.1097/MD.0000000000014437.
476. Zhu J, Pan F, Cai H, et al. Positron emission tomography imaging of lung cancer: an overview of alternative positron emission tomography tracers beyond F18 fluorodeoxyglucose. Front Med. 2022;9 https://doi.org/10.3389/fmed.2022.945602.
477. Zidan L, Iravani A, Oleinikov K, et al. Efficacy and safety of 177Lu-DOTATATE in lung neuroendocrine tumors: a bi-center study. J Nucl Med. 2021; https://doi.org/10.2967/jnumed.120.260760.
478. Zukotynski KA, Gaudet VC, Uribe CF, et al. Clinical applications of artificial intelligence in positron emission tomography of lung cancer. PET Clin. 2022;17:77–84.
479. IAEA quality control atlas for scintillation camera systems. International Atomic Energy Agency, Vienna, 2003.
480. PET/CT atlas on quality control and image artefacts. International Atomic Energy Agency, Vienna, 2014.

Quantitative Imaging of Sarcopenia

26

Eddy D. Zandee van Rilland
and Aparna Komarraju

Background

Sarcopenia is broadly defined as abnormally low muscle strength with associated reduction in skeletal muscle mass, quality, and function. While initially described in elderly patients, sarcopenia can occur in the setting of various pathologic conditions in both older and younger individuals, including disuse, hormonal abnormalities, malabsorption, inflammatory conditions, cancer, chronic illness, and neurodegenerative disease [1–3]. Importantly, sarcopenia is associated with various adverse clinical outcomes including falls, fractures, physical disability, hospitalization, and death [1]. As of 2010, approximately 50 million people worldwide were estimated to have sarcopenia with its prevalence expected to rise to 200 million by 2050 [4]. Furthermore, the estimated total annual cost of hospitalizations in patients with sarcopenia in the United States in 2014 was USD $40.4 billion [5]. With the population of people over 60 projected to double by 2050, the clinical and economic impact of sarcopenia is expected to be substantial [6, 7]. Therefore, sarcopenia has become an important healthcare issue worldwide and remains an area of robust clinical and radiological research.

The diagnosis of sarcopenia includes the evaluation of muscle mass, function, and physical performance. While muscle function and physical performance can be determined through clinical exams including grip strength devices to test muscle function and gait speed tests to evaluate physical performance, muscle mass is commonly measured on imaging [8]. Quantitative data on muscle mass can be obtained using various imaging studies, including whole-body dual x-ray absorptiometry (DXA), ultrasound (US), magnetic resonance imaging (MRI), and computed tomography (CT). The objective of this book chapter is to provide a modality-based review of the quantitative imaging methods currently used to diagnose sarcopenia.

Dual-Energy X-Ray Absorptiometry

DXA is the most common imaging modality to evaluate body composition in the clinical setting. It is already widely used for the evaluation of bone mineral density. For the evaluation of muscle mass, a whole-body scan is performed with a

The original version of the chapter has been revised. A correction to this chapter can be found at https://doi.org/10.1007/978-3-032-14103-3_28

E. D. Zandee van Rilland
Department of Radiology, Stanford University Medical Center, Palo Alto, CA, USA

A. Komarraju (✉)
Department of Radiology, Beth Israel Deaconess Medical Center, Harvard Medical School, Boston, MA, USA
e-mail: akomarra@bidmc.harvard.edu

R. Gill, P. Rajiah (eds.), *Quantitative Imaging in the Thorax*,
https://doi.org/10.1007/978-3-032-14103-3_26

source emitting two different energy-level x-rays to concurrently measure lean mass and fat mass. The measured lean mass values of the upper and lower limbs are summed and indexed to the patient's height to determine the appendicular lean mass index (ALMI). The ALMI has been validated and accepted in various disease states [3]. In patients with suspected sarcopenia, the European Working Group on Sarcopenia in Older People (EWGSOP) guidelines use ALMI cut-off values of <5.5 kg/m^2 in women and <7.0 kg/m^2 in men to define low muscle mass [5]. Similar to the evaluation of osteoporosis with DXA, ALMI cut-offs are also based on the T-score defining sarcopenia as two standard deviations below young normal reference ($T < -2.0$) [2]. In conjunction with clinical data, the ALMI ultimately can help confirm the diagnosis of low muscle mass in patients with suspected sarcopenia [8].

There are several advantages to DXA. First, DXA is widely available and a relatively affordable imaging study. DXA measurements are also accurate and reproducible, and the overall radiation dose for a DXA study is low (<1 mrem). Additionally, the lean mass and fat mass measurements on DXA have been shown to strongly correlate with the amount of adipose and lean tissue on CT and MRI [9, 10]. As a result, the EWGSOP guidelines currently recommend DXA as the first-line imaging modality for the evaluation of muscle mass in patients with suspected sarcopenia [11].

However, DXA has a few limitations. First, DXA provides bi-dimensional data without the ability to assess the muscle quality. Additionally, DXA measurements may be influenced by the hydration status of the patient, potentially providing inaccurately elevated lean mass measurements in hypervolemic cardiac or nephropathic patients. There is also reported variability in measurements between different densitometer brands, which makes standardized values and reference standards more challenging to implement [12].

Radiography

Radiographs are not routinely used in quantitative assessment of the muscle mass or sarcopenia; however, they can be useful in assessing the overall muscle bulk and volume due to the differences in densities of structures. Radiography is widely available and accessible and relatively inexpensive compared to other modalities, although it does involve a small amount of radiation. Obtaining bilateral radiographs can be helpful particularly in patients with muscular dystrophy or polio for comparison. Further imaging can be obtained as needed clinically. Figures 26.1 and 26.2 illustrate an example of a patient with polio who has asymmetric loss of muscle bulk as seen on the radiographs (right worse than left).

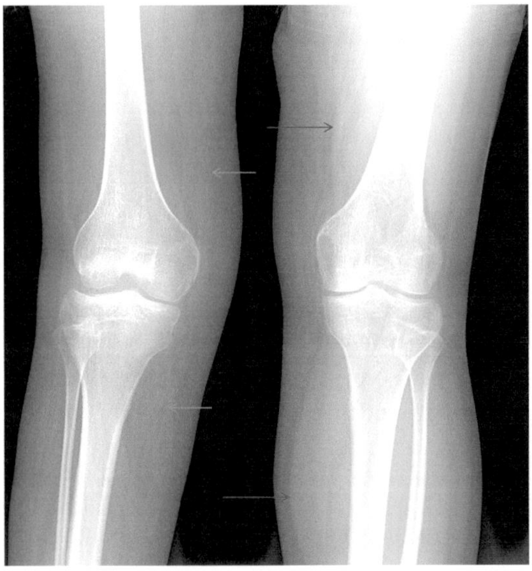

Fig. 26.1 Frontal radiographs of the bilateral knees, with loss of muscle bulk and volume within the right distal thigh and proximal calf (green arrows) and relatively preserved muscle bulk in the left distal thigh and proximal calf (blue arrows)

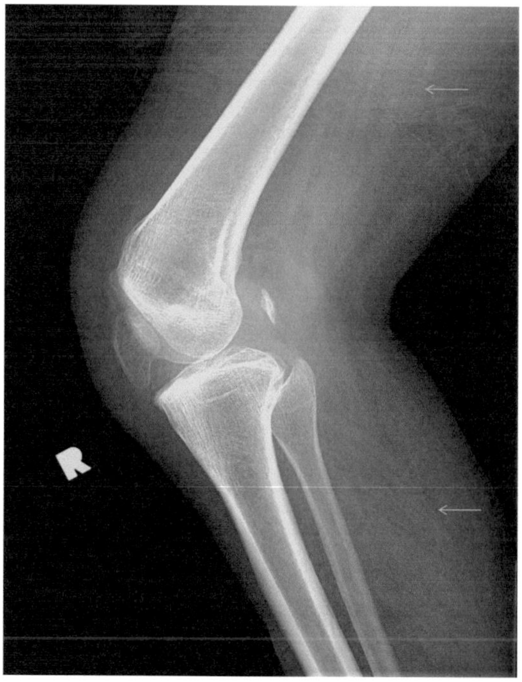

Fig. 26.2 Lateral radiograph of the right knee on the same patient with loss of normal muscle bulk in the distal thigh and proximal calf (green arrows)

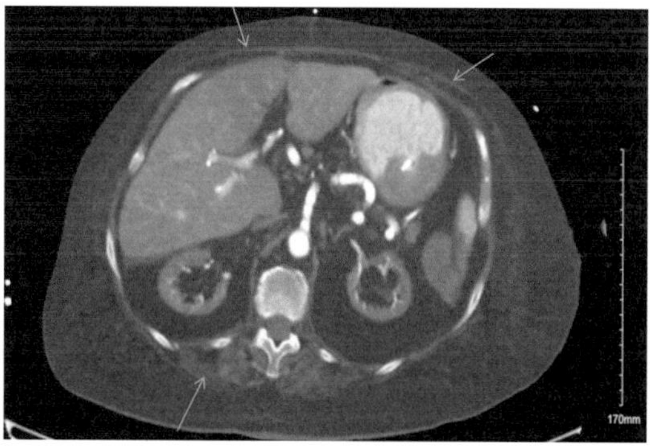

Fig. 26.3 Axial CT image of the abdomen in a 64-year-old patient with end-stage renal disease on dialysis demonstrates a significant loss of muscle bulk, including the rectus abdominis and bilateral paraspinous muscles (arrows)

Computed Tomography

CT is effective in assessing both muscle bulk and quality (e.g., degree of myosteatosis). Unlike DXA, which estimates whole-body lean mass, CT measures muscle size (e.g., cross-sectional area [CSA]) and quality (e.g., average Hounsfield unit attenuation) in specific areas of the body. These measurements have been shown to be highly accurate in estimating muscle mass and overall body composition [1, 13]. Currently, abdominal CT is generally preferred for the evaluation of sarcopenia with a region of interest (ROI) drawn around both psoas muscles (at either the L3 or L4 vertebral body levels) or around all muscles (paraspinous, psoas, and abdominal muscles) on a single slice of the abdomen at the L3 vertebral body level to obtain the CSA [14, 15]. Other approaches include segmentation of the thigh muscles at the level of the mid-thigh or the paraspinous muscles in the cervical spine at C3 [16, 17]. In terms of thoracic imaging, prior studies have evaluated the efficacy of paraspinous muscle segmentation in the thoracic spine at T12 in patients undergoing chest CTs for lung cancer imaging [18, 19] or transcatheter aortic valve replacement planning [20]. In a study evaluating patients with chronic obstructive pulmonary disease, CSA of the erector spinae muscles were measured on chest CT to determine optimal cut-off measurements for sarcopenia [21]. Similarly, a study evaluating 347 patients with non-small cell lung cancer found a correlation between low muscle index (muscle area/ body mass index) of the pectoralis muscle on CT and poor long-term health outcomes [22].

Currently, segmentation of muscles can be performed manually with a ROI tool on a Picture Archiving and Communication System (PACS) or with specialized segmentation software that allows for standardized thresholding of muscle (−29 to 150 HU) and fat (−30 to −190 HU). The CSA is indexed for height (CSA/height^2) to obtain the skeletal muscle index (SMI) with reported values for the L3 SMI of <52.4 cm^2/m^2 for men and <38.5 cm^2/m^2 for women as diagnostic criteria for sarcopenia [23]. Figure 26.3 illustrates an example of a patient with significant muscle volume loss and fatty infiltration as seen on CT. Figure 26.4 illustrates an example of a patient with a history of previous rectus muscle trauma and subsequent calcification and fatty infiltration of the rectus muscle.

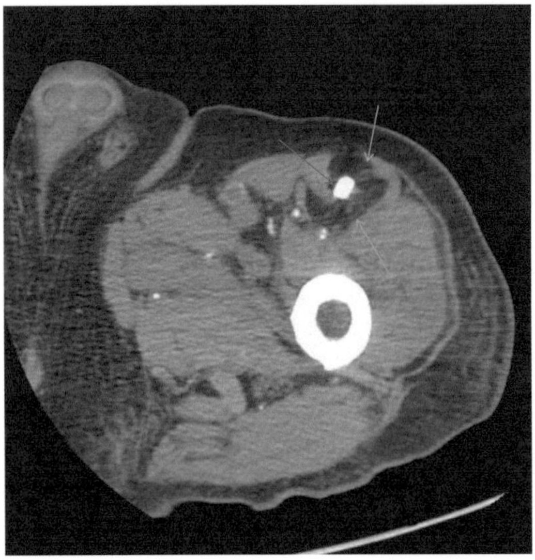

Fig. 26.4 Axial CT image of the proximal left thigh in a 53-year-old patient with a history of old rectus femoris muscle tear demonstrates calcification (blue arrow) within the muscle with associated surrounding muscle atrophy and fatty infiltration, as indicated by the green arrows

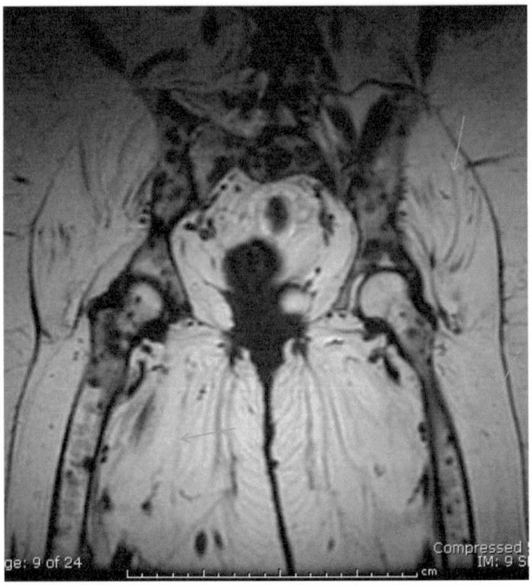

Fig. 26.5 Coronal T1-weighted MRI image of the pelvis and proximal thighs demonstrates diffuse osseous lesions and severe atrophy and fatty infiltration of all imaged pelvic and proximal thigh musculature bilaterally (arrows)

The main advantage of CT for the evaluation of muscle mass is the ability to both quantitatively and qualitatively assess the muscle with cross-sectional imaging. CT measurements using CSA and SMI are accurate and reproducible [8]. Additionally, CT is commonly performed for various indications, allowing for the opportunistic assessment for sarcopenia. A study by Yao et al. found that opportunistic CT-derived metrics, specifically skeletal muscle density, correlated with clinical features of sarcopenia as reflected by validated questionnaires for sarcopenia [24].

The main limitation of CT is the relatively high costs and radiation dose. However, these limitations do not apply in the opportunistic setting when CT scans are being performed for other indications. Artifacts, such as metallic streak artifact, are another major limitation to CT and may invalidate attenuation measurements of the muscles. Additionally, variability in tube current or the administration of intravenous contrast can directly influence muscle attenuation values, limiting evaluation of muscle mass and quality [25]. Lastly, there are currently no validated thresholds or established guidelines with CT to establish a diagnosis of sarcopenia.

Magnetic Resonance Imaging

Similar to CT, MRI can accurately measure CSA on cross-sectional images. Due to high contrast resolution, MRI can assess muscle quality and identify the presence of muscular fat, edema, and fibrosis [1]. On conventional MRI sequences, qualitative grading of regional muscle edema, fatty infiltration, and atrophy are commonly performed. Additional MRI techniques using proton density fat-fraction with Dixon sequences and chemical shift-based water-fat separation sequences allow for quantitative evaluation of myosteatosis [26–28]. Additionally, diffusion tensor imaging, fractional anisotropy, and T2 mapping sequences have also recently been used to evaluate fatty infiltration of the muscle in sarcopenic patients, although largely in the research setting [29–31]. Figures 26.5 and 26.6 illustrate an example of a patient with diffuse osseous lesions under treatment with near-complete fatty

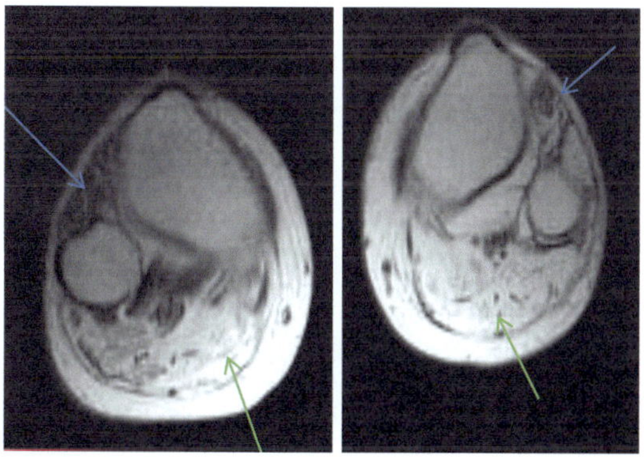

Fig. 26.6 Axial T1-weighted MRI image of the bilateral calves demonstrates severe atrophy and fatty infiltration of the calf musculature, most prominent in the posterior compartment (green arrows) with relative sparing of the anterolateral compartment muscles (blue arrows)

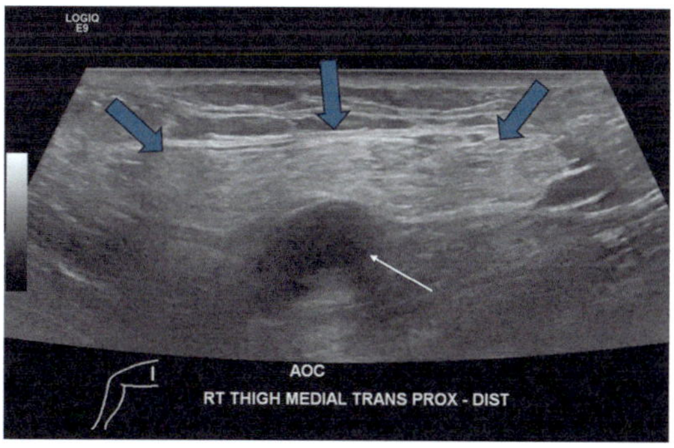

Fig. 26.7 70M presenting with muscle weakness. Ultrasound image at the level of the mid-thigh medially demonstrates diffusely echogenic appearance of the sartorius muscle, compatible with diffuse fatty infiltration (blue block arrows). The hypoechoic structure in the center is the Superficial Femoral Artery (arrow)

infiltration and atrophy of the muscles around the pelvis, proximal thighs, and calves bilaterally.

Like CT, MRI provides the ability to both quantitatively and qualitatively assess the muscle with the use of cross-sectional imaging. MRI measurements are highly accurate and reproducible and can identify the presence of muscle edema and steatosis [8]. Unlike CT or DXA, there is no associated radiation.

The main limitation of MRI is the high costs and lower availability relative to the other imaging modalities. Additionally, some patients may have contraindications to MRI including non-compatible hardware/implanted devices or severe claustrophobia. Scanning and post-processing times are longer. Similar to CT, reference cut-off points for low muscle mass are not well established. Lastly, there is heterogeneity in imaging protocols and sequences across different MRI systems, vendors, and institutions.

Ultrasound

Ultrasound can reliably assess muscle mass and quality by measuring CSA, muscle thickness, and muscle volume with good reproducibility of measurements [32, 33]. Additionally, US can provide information on muscle quality by demonstrating the presence of fat echogenicity within the muscle tissue. The most well-established findings of sarcopenia on US have been decreased muscle thickness, decreased cross-sectional area, and increased echogenicity. Additional metrics have been studied, including muscle volume, stiffness, and fascicle length [34]. Figure 26.7 illustrates an example of a patient with muscle atrophy and fatty infiltration of the sartorius muscle.

US is readily accessible in most parts of the world and is relatively inexpensive. Unlike CT or DXA, there is no associated radiation, and images are obtained dynamically. US machines are also portable, allowing for greater mobility of imaging to patients in intensive care units and nursing homes. Additionally, US plays an overall important role in developing countries where access to CT or MRI may be more limited.

The main limitation of ultrasound is the highly operator-dependent nature of scanning and image acquisition. As a result, US measurements may have relatively lower accuracy and reproducibility.

Future Directions

With continued increase in imaging volumes annually, opportunistic screening of sarcopenia remains an area of increasing interest and active research. Although opportunistic imaging can be done with several imaging modalities, CT has been specifically studied due to the prevalence of CT scans in clinical practice. Additionally, CT measurements are generally easy to perform with high reproducibility. Given that quantitative measurements of muscle quantity and quality are not routinely performed on CT, further research to establish and validate imaging guidelines on opportunistic evaluation for sarcopenia is needed.

Similarly, there has been a substantial increase in interest in the role of artificial intelligence in the imaging evaluation of sarcopenia. Several recent studies have evaluated deep learning-based approaches to automate CT segmentation of the muscle, fatty tissue, and bone to assist in the evaluation of body composition and sarcopenia [35, 36–38]. Ultimately, further research into the role and clinical impact of these automated segmentation and deep learning-based models is needed in the evaluation of patients with sarcopenia.

References

1. Boutin RD, Yao L, Canter RJ, Lenchik L. Sarcopenia: current concepts and imaging implications. AJR Am J Roentgenol. 2015;205:[web] W255–66.
2. Marty E, Liu Y, Samuel A, Or O, Lane J. A review of sarcopenia: enhancing awareness of an increasingly prevalent disease. Bone. 2017;105:276–86.
3. Brioche T, Pagano AF, Py G, Chopard A. Muscle wasting and aging: experimental models, fatty infiltrations, and prevention. Mol Asp Med. 2016;50:56–87.
4. Cruz-Jentoft AJ, Baeyens JP, Bauer JM, et al. European Working Group on Sarcopenia in older people. Sarcopenia: European consensus on definition and diagnosis: report of the EuropeanWorking Group on Sarcopenia in Older People. Age Ageing. 2010;39(04):412–23.
5. Goates S, Du K, Arensberg MB, Gaillard T, Guralnik J, Pereira SL. Economic impact of hospitalizations in US adults with sarcopenia. J Frailty Aging. 2019;8(2):93–9.
6. Janssen I, Shepard DS, Katzmarzyk PT, Roubenoff R. The healthcare costs of sarcopenia in the United States. J Am Geriatr Soc. 2004;52(1):80–5.
7. Bruyère O, Beudart C, Locquet M, et al. Sarcopenia as a public health problem. Eur Geriatr Med. 2016;7:272–5.
8. Albano D, Messina C, Vitale J, Sconfienza LM. Imaging of sarcopenia: old evidence and new insights. Eur Radiol. 2020;30(4):2199–2208.
9. Kullberg J, Brandberg J, Angelhed JE, et al. Whole-body adipose tissue analysis: comparison of MRI, CT and dual energy X-ray absorptiometry. Br J Radiol. 2009;82(974):123–30.
10. Guglielmi G, Ponti F, Agostini M, Amadori M, Battista G, Bazzocchi A. The role of DXA in sarcopenia. Aging Clin Exp Res. 2016;28(6):1047–1060.
11. Cruz-Jentoft AJ, Bahat G, Bauer J, et al. Sarcopenia: revised European consensus on definition and diagnosis. Age Ageing. 2019;48(1):16–31.
12. Park SS, Lim S, Kim H, Kim KM. Comparison of Two DXA Systems, Hologic Horizon W and GE Lunar Prodigy, for Assessing Body Composition in Healthy Korean Adults. Endocrinol Metab (Seoul). 2021 Dec;36(6):1219-1231.
13. Shen W, Punyanitya M, Wang Z, et al. Total body skeletal muscle and adipose tissue volumes: estimation from a single abdominal cross-sectional image. J Appl Physiol (1985). 2004;97:2333–8.
14. Lenchik L, Boutin RD. Sarcopenia: beyond muscle atrophy and into the new frontiers of opportunistic imaging, precision medicine, and machine learning. Semin Musculoskelet Radiol 2018;22:307–22.
15. Amini B, Boyle SP, Boutin RD, Lenchik L. Approaches to Assessment of Muscle Mass and Myosteatosis on Computed Tomography: A Systematic Review. J Gerontol A Biol Sci Med Sci. 2019;74(10):1671–78.
16. Santanasto AJ, Goodpaster BH, Kritchevsky SB, et al. Body composition remodeling and mortality: the Health Aging and Body Composition Study. J Gerontol A Biol Sci Med Sci 2017;72(04):513–19.
17. Swartz JE, Pothen AJ, Wegner I, Smid EJ, Swart KM, de Bree R, Leenen LP, Grolman W. Feasibility of using head and neck CT imaging to assess skeletal muscle mass in head and neck cancer patients. Oral Oncol. 2016;62:28–33.
18. Kim EY, Kim YS, Park I, et al. Evaluation of sarcopenia in small-cell lung cancer patients by routine chest CT. Support Care Cancer 2016;24(11):4721–26.
19. Yang M, Tan L, Xie L, Hu S, Liu D, Wang J, Li W. Factors That Improve Chest Computed Tomography-Defined Sarcopenia Prognosis in Advanced Non-Small Cell Lung Cancer. Front Oncol. 2021 Oct 1;11:754975.
20. Nemec U, Heidinger B, Sokas C, Chu L, Eisenberg RL. Diagnosing Sarcopenia on Thoracic Computed Tomography: Quantitative Assessment of Skeletal Muscle Mass in Patients Undergoing Transcatheter Aortic Valve Replacement. Acad Radiol. 2017;24(9):1154–61.
21. Sato S, Muro S, Aoyama T, Hirai T. Quantitative computed tomography-based evaluation of skeletal muscle and presence of sarcopenia in patients with chronic obstructive pulmonary disease. Respir Investig. 2022;60(5):709–12.

22. Sun C, Anraku M, Kawahara T, et al. Prognostic significance of low pectoralis muscle mass on preoperative chest computed tomography in localized non-small cell lung cancer after curative-intent surgery Lung Cancer. 2020;147:71–76.
23. Prado CM, Lieffers JR, McCargar LJ, et al. Prevalence and clinical implications of sarcopenic obesity in patients with solid tumours of the respiratory and gastrointestinal tracts: a population-based study. Lancet Oncol 2008;9(07):629–35.
24. Yao L, Petrosyan A, Fuangfa P, Lenchik L, Boutin RD. Diagnosing sarcopenia at the point of imaging care: analysis of clinical, functional, and opportunistic CT metrics. Skeletal Radiol. 2021;50(3):543–50.
25. Boutin RD, Kaptuch JM, Bateni CP, Chalfant JS, Yao L. Influence of IV Contrast Administration on CT Measures of Muscle and Bone Attenuation: Implications for Sarcopenia and Osteoporosis Evaluation. AJR Am J Roentgenol. 2016;207(5):1046–54.
26. Grimm A, Meyer H, Nickel MD, et al. Repeatability of Dixon magnetic resonance imaging and magnetic resonance spectroscopy for quantitative muscle fat assessments in the thigh. J Cachexia Sarcopenia Muscle. 2018;9(6):1093–100.
27. Fischer MA, Pfirrmann CWA, Espinosa N, Rapti DA, Buck FM. Dixon-based MRI for assessment of muscle-fat content in phantoms, healthy volunteers and patients with achillodynia: comparison to visual assessment of calf muscle quality. Eur Radiol 2014; 24:1366–37.
28. Alizai H, Nardo L, Karampinos DC, et al. Comparison of clinical semi-quantitative assessment of muscle fat infiltration with quantitative assessment using chemical shift-based water/fat separation in MR studies of the calf of post-menopausal women. Eur Radiol 2012; 22:1592–600.
29. Melville DM, Mohler J, Fain M, Muchna AE, Krupinski E, Sharma P, Taljanovic MS. Multiparametric MR imaging of quadriceps musculature in the setting of clinical frailty syndrome. Skeletal Radiol. 2016;45(5):583–9.
30. Azzabou N, Hogrel JY, Carlier PG. NMR based biomarkers to study age-related changes in the human quadriceps. Exp Gerontol. 2015;70:54–60.
31. Codari M, Zanardo M, di Sabato ME, et al. MRI derived biomarkers related to sarcopenia: a systematic review. J Magn Reson Imaging 2020;51(4):1117 27.
32. Scott JM, Martin DS, Ploutz-Snyder R, et al. Reliability and validity of panoramic ultrasound for muscle quantification. Ultrasound Med Biol. 2012;38(9):1656–61.
33. Ticinesi A, Meschi T, Narici MV, Lauretani F, Maggio M. Muscle Ultrasound and Sarcopenia in Older Individuals: A Clinical Perspective. J Am Med Dir Assoc. 2017 Apr 1;18(4):290–300.
34. Perkisas S, Bastijns S, Baudry S, et al. Application of ultrasound for muscle assessment in sarcopenia: 2020 SARCUS update. Eur Geriatr Med 2021; 12(1):45–59.
35. Pickhardt PJ, Perez AA, Garrett JW, Graffy PM, Zea R, Summers RM. Fully Automated Deep Learning Tool for Sarcopenia Assessment on CT: L1 Versus L3 Vertebral Level Muscle Measurements for Opportunistic Prediction of Adverse Clinical Outcomes. AJR Am J Roentgenol. 2022;218(1):124–31.
36. Tsai KJ, Chang CC, Lo LC, Chiang JY, Chang CS, Huang YJ. Automatic segmentation of paravertebral muscles in abdominal CT scan by U-Net: The application of data augmentation technique to increase the Jaccard ratio of deep learning. Medicine (Baltimore). 2021;100(44):e27649
37. Yao N, Li X, Wang L, Cheng X, Yu A, Li C, Wu K. Deep learning for automatic segmentation of paraspinal muscle on computed tomography. Acta Radiol. 2023;64(2):596–604.
38. Somasundaram E, Castiglione JA, Brady SL, Trout AT. Defining Normal Ranges of Skeletal Muscle Area and Skeletal Muscle Index in Children on CT Using an Automated Deep Learning Pipeline: Implications for Sarcopenia Diagnosis. AJR Am J Roentgenol. 2022 Aug;219(2):326–36.

27 Applications of Artificial Intelligence in Quantitative Imaging

Raúl San José Estépar, Ariel Hernán Curiale, and Pietro Nardelli

Artificial Intelligence Principles in Medical Imaging

AI is a field of computer science dedicated to devising systems capable of performing tasks that typically require human intelligence. These tasks include, but are not limited to, visual perception, speech recognition, decision-making, and language translation. Among its many subsets, deep learning has emerged as a promising technique that employs multi-layer artificial neural networks that learn from vast amounts of data in ways that mimic the human brain's own methods [4]. Deep learning gained importance in computer vision when neural networks, particularly convolutional neural networks (CNNs), outperformed traditional methods in several visual recognition tasks [5]. Convolutional neural networks have become the backbone of image recognition tasks, demonstrating performance that can match human accuracy in different diagnostic tasks [6].

AI's evolution within medical imaging has been particularly dramatic, mainly driven by the dual advancements in data availability and computational power. Initially, medical imaging AI systems heavily relied on rule-based algorithms and manual feature extraction. These early systems, though pioneering, were limited in scalability and performance, struggling with the complexity and variability inherent in medical data. The advent of deep learning marked a significant shift by automatically extracting and learning complex patterns directly from raw data. This ability makes deep learning particularly suited for tasks such as image segmentation, registration, and quantitative analysis, which are central to medical imaging. The predictive capabilities of these systems extend beyond mere image analysis, aiding in diagnosis, prognostication, and risk stratification with unprecedented precision.

Frameworks and Architectures in Medical Imaging AI

The AI frameworks currently used in thoracic imaging falls under one of the following deep learning categories as illustrated in Fig. 27.1:

- *CNNs*: These networks are foundational to the application of deep learning in image analysis, including medical imaging. Designed specifically to process pixel data, CNNs mimic the receptive fields of neurons by applying filters to input images, creating feature maps that highlight the presence of specific features at different locations in the image [7]. This pro-

R. San José Estépar (✉) · A. H. Curiale · P. Nardelli
Applied Chest Imaging Laboratory, Department of Radiology, Brigham and Women's Hospital, Harvard Medical School, Boston, MA, USA
e-mail: rsanjose@bwh.harvard.edu

R. Gill, P. Rajiah (eds.), *Quantitative Imaging in the Thorax*,
https://doi.org/10.1007/978-3-032-14103-3_27

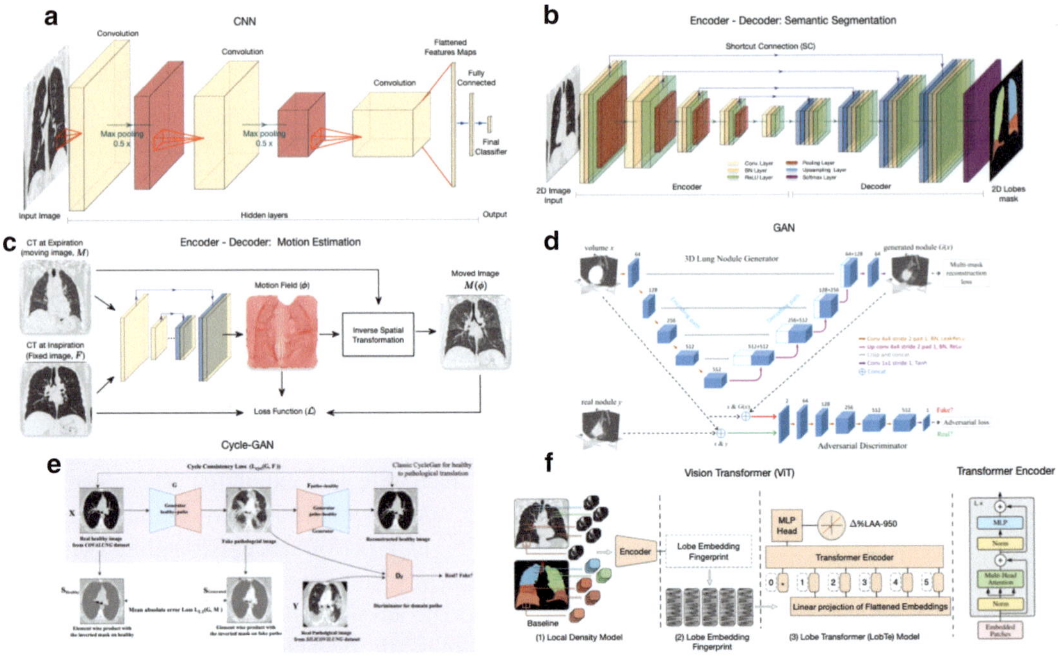

Fig. 27.1 Schematic representation of key AI architectures applied in thoracic imaging, illustrating data flow through the neural networks for image analysis, registration, and segmentation tasks. (**a**) CNN for image quantification, (**b**) encoder-decoder workflow for semantic segmentation, (**c**) encoder-decoder approach for motion estimation, (**d**) generative adversarial networks for lung segmentation [1, 8], (**e**) CycleGAN workflow for lung segmentation, and (**f**) vision transformer workflow to predict emphysema progression in COPD

cess allows the network to learn hierarchical representations of features from the input images, making CNNs exceptionally good at tasks like image classification, object detection, and segmentation in medical imaging. CNNs are constructed from units of compact kernels of neurons that slide across an image to produce an output image map. These neurons function like logistic regressors, generating a response at each image location as a weighted sum of the image intensities. The kernels determine the weight of each location, and these neural kernels are assembled in multiple channels to create a CNN convolutional layer. Several such layers, each functioning differently yet complementarily, make up the CNN (Fig. 27.1a). Information flows forward through these layers, with deeper layers aggregating it in a non-linear manner. The remarkable success of CNNs in medical imaging inspired the development of other deep learning paradigms designed to exploit various aspects of the information flowing through the network.

- *Generative approaches*: Generative AI encompasses a class of machine learning models that can generate new data, such as images or text, based on patterns learned from the existing data. In thoracic imaging, generative AI techniques have the potential to enhance various aspects of medical image analysis and clinical decision-making. Key applications of generative AI in this field include image synthesis, image enhancement, image-to-image translation, and anomaly detection and deep feature extraction (Table 27.1). Some of the most relevant generative architectures used in the context of medical and thoracic imaging are:
  - *Encoder-Decoder Architectures*: Encoder-decoder architectures are specialized neural networks designed to transform an input into an output while maintaining a certain level of contextual information from the input (Fig. 27.1b–c). In medical imaging,

Table 27.1 Generative AI applications

Generative AI task	Description	Application
Image synthesis	Create synthetic medical images that resemble real patient scans	Data augmentation to train deep learning models improving their performance and robustness
Image enhancement	Improvement of the quality of thoracic images using generative approaches for denoising or image deconvolution	Reduction of noise, artifacts, improvement in resolution, and enhancement of specific features
Image-to-image translation	These models can translate images from one domain to another, such as converting low-dose CT scans to high-dose scans or converting MRI images to CT-like images	Modality synthesis Cross-modality applications for functional imaging Reduction of radiation exposure by workflow simplification
Anomaly detection	Recognition of normal patterns in thoracic images and identify regions that deviate from these patterns	Flagging areas of interest for further radiological evaluation
Deep features	Generative approaches can be used to extract quantitative features from pathological regions	Data-driven radiomics Risk assessment and early diagnosis Disease monitorization

these architectures are often employed for image segmentation, where each pixel of an image is classified into various categories (e.g., different types of tissue or abnormalities). The encoder compresses the input into a lower-dimensional representation, capturing essential features, while the decoder reconstructs the output from this representation, focusing on specific tasks like detailing a segmentation map. The U-Net architecture is a notable example [9], renowned for its efficiency in medical image segmentation due to its ability to use context effectively by connecting corresponding encoder and decoder layers at several spatial resolutions (Fig. 27.1b).

- *Generative Adversarial Networks (GANs)*: These models consist of a dual-network architecture—the generator and the discriminator—that compete against each other [10]. The generator creates images, typically using an encoder-decoder architecture, while the discriminator evaluates their authenticity, determining whether they are real or produced by the generator. This framework is highly beneficial in medical imaging for synthesizing realistic medical images for training models, especially when actual medical data are scarce or difficult to obtain. GANs can also enhance image quality, generate missing data, or translate images from one modality to another (e.g., magnetic resonance imaging (MRI) to computed tomography (CT)) [11, 12], which can be extremely useful for training purposes and cross-modal diagnostics (Fig. 27.1d–e).
- *Transformers*: Originally designed for natural language processing, transformers have recently been adapted for image analysis tasks through architectures like vision transformers (ViT) [13, 14]. These models utilize global self-attention mechanisms to weigh the importance of different parts of the input data, allowing the model to focus on relevant features regardless of their position in the sequence or image. This approach is particularly promising for medical imaging tasks that require analysis of large, complex images, where relevant features might be widely dispersed and complement each other (Fig. 27.1f).
- *Diffusion Models*: Diffusion models are a newer class of generative models that learn to generate data by reversing a gradual process of adding noise to real images [15]. In medical imaging, diffusion models hold potential for generating high-quality, realistic images for purposes such as training data augmentation and anomaly detection.

These models can create detailed and accurate synthetic medical images, useful for training diagnostic models without privacy concerns or logistical issues associated with using real patient data.

Learning Approaches in Medical Imaging

Machine learning approaches in medical imaging can be classified into four major categories, each tailored to different problem types and characteristics of the data used for training:

- *Supervised Learning*: This is the most prevalent method in medical imaging AI, where models are meticulously trained using labeled datasets to solve specific tasks. These datasets contain images annotated or classified according to specific criteria, such as disease markers or diagnostic outcomes. This approach is used in tasks requiring high accuracy and specificity, including tumor detection, disease progression monitoring, and therapeutic efficacy assessment [16].
- *Unsupervised Learning*: Unlike supervised learning, unsupervised learning algorithms operate without labeled data. These algorithms are designed to identify inherent patterns and structures within the data, making them ideal for exploratory analysis or generating new insights where the data may not be comprehensively labeled. Applications in thoracic imaging include anomaly detection or the identification of novel imaging biomarkers [17].
- *Semi-supervised Learning*: This method combines elements of both supervised and unsupervised learning. It is particularly advantageous in situations where labeled data are limited—a common scenario in medical imaging due to the expense and complexity of data annotation. Semi-supervised learning can significantly enhance learning accuracy and efficiency by using a large amount of unlabeled data alongside a smaller set of labeled examples [18].
- *Reinforcement Learning*: This type of learning allows an AI system to learn and improve its performance through trial-and-error interactions with an environment. An "agent," typically a neural model, learns and makes decisions within a given setting or context, receiving feedback based on rewards and penalties that guide its learning. One key advantage of this approach is that it can learn complex patterns and decision-making strategies without requiring extensive manual labeling of training data, making it a promising approach for medical imaging applications. Additionally, it is effective in integrating human feedback during training to fine-tuned models. Reinforcement learning has been explored in abnormality detection tasks like lung nodule recognition [19].

Model Implementation and Training

The adoption of deep learning in medical imaging has been significantly advanced through various neural network training techniques. A key development was the introduction of the rectified linear unit (ReLU) as an activation function [20], replacing sigmoid functions. ReLU addressed issues related to the vanishing gradient problem, maintaining a steady gradient flow through deep architectures and enabling the training of deeper networks.

Pooling techniques have also been crucial. By aggregating the outputs of neuron clusters at one layer into a single neuron in the next, pooling reduces the spatial size of the representation. This makes feature detection invariant to scale and orientation. Additionally, strategies such as dropout [21] and batch normalization [22] have addressed the challenges like overfitting and internal covariate shift, respectively. Dropout randomly omits a fraction of the neurons at each training stage, forcing the network to learn more robust features, reducing the overfitting and enhancing its ability to generalize to unseen data. Batch normalization addresses the vanishing gradient problem and internal covariate shift by normalizing the inputs of each layer to have a consistent distribution. This stabilizes and accelerates the training process, enabling the use of higher learning rates and reducing sensitivity to initialization. Recent strategies based on the attention mechanism [13], popularized by the transformer architecture, is a powerful method that enables models to selectively focus on different parts of the input data when making decisions, akin to how humans pay attention to specific details in a complex task. This allows the model to dynamically prioritize relevant information, regardless of its position in the sequence, which is particularly advantageous in tasks like natural language processing and image recognition.

Proper sampling of data population distribution is essential for training AI models, ensuring that the model generalizes well for the condition of interest. In scenarios with limited data for imaging applications, transfer learning is an effective technique. Layer-wise unsupervised pre-training can be utilized to prepare the network by learning general features without labeled data, which can then be fine-tuned using supervised learning to adjust these features for specific tasks [23]. This approach has been pivotal in utilizing unlabeled datasets effectively, enhancing the versatility and applicability of deep learning models.

These advancements collectively have facilitated the training of increasingly complex neural networks with multiple layers and millions of parameters, thus broadening the scope and efficacy of deep learning applications in medical imaging applications.

Advances in Image Reconstruction

Recent advancements in image reconstruction for CT and MRI have significantly improved the quality of thoracic imaging. These improvements, particularly in enhanced contrast and resolution, are crucial for accurately diagnosing and managing thoracic conditions.

Deep Learning In CT Reconstruction

The application of deep learning techniques in CT reconstruction represents a significant advancement in medical imaging [24]. These methods leverage CNNs and other machine learning models to enhance image quality, reduce noise, and lower radiation doses. This is particularly beneficial for thoracic imaging, where clarity in differentiating tissue types and detecting minute lesions is critical. These advancements not only enhance diagnostic image quality but also play a crucial role in minimizing patient exposure to ionizing radiation, aligning with ongoing efforts to improve patient safety in medical imaging:

- *Enhancing Image Quality and Reducing Noise*: Deep learning-based image reconstruction (DLIR) techniques are particularly useful for improving the signal-to-noise ratio and enhancing image contrast [25, 26]. Traditional CT scanners can produce noisy images, especially at lower doses. DLIR addresses this by learning optimal noise reduction strategies from large datasets of high-quality images acquired in optimal conditions. The result is more detailed images, essential for accurately diagnosing thoracic pathologies such as small lung nodules or subtle interstitial lung changes.
- *Dose Reduction*: A significant advantage of deep learning in CT reconstruction is its potential to reduce the radiation dose required for diagnostic-quality images [27]. By efficiently processing lower-dose scans to enhance clarity and detail, DLIR minimizes the patient radiation exposure. This is particularly important in thoracic imaging, where patients, such as those with chronic respiratory conditions or lung cancer, may require frequent scans over their treatment course. Lower radiation doses make CT scans safer for these vulnerable populations.
- *Speed and Efficiency*: Deep learning algorithms can also speed up the reconstruction process, a crucial factor when quick diagnosis is needed [24]. For emergencies such as pulmonary embolisms or traumatic injuries, DLIR can rapidly process images, allowing for faster clinical decision-making. Furthermore, the efficiency of DLIR supports larger-scale screening programs, such as those

for lung cancer, by handling high volumes of scans without compromising image quality.

- *Integration with Other Imaging Modalities:* DLIR advancing standalone CT imaging and enhancing the integration of CT with other imaging modalities. For instance, in PET/CT imaging used for cancer staging, DLIR can improve the CT component, thereby enhancing the overall image quality and diagnostic accuracy of the combined modality [28]. This integration is crucial in thoracic oncology, where precise imaging guides targeted therapies and surgical interventions.

MRI Enhancements Through Deep Learning

Traditional MRI techniques have been limited by inherent challenges, such as long scan times, sensitivity to motion artifacts, and low proton density in specific organs like the lungs. Deep learning is revolutionizing MRI by addressing these challenges, enhancing image quality, and reducing scan duration, which is especially beneficial in the dynamic environment of thoracic imaging [29].

One of the most significant impacts of deep learning on MRI is the reduction in scan times. Deep learning techniques such as CNNs and recurrent neural networks have played a significant role in enhancing static and dynamic MRI reconstruction by learning the spatio-temporal dependencies in heavily under-sampled k-space data [30–32]. This is particularly advantageous in thoracic imaging, where patient comfort and reducing motion artifacts are crucial. Faster scans mean less time for patient movement, which is often problematic in respiratory or cardiac-related imaging.

Deep learning is also expanding the capabilities of MRI in dynamic and functional imaging. Techniques like ultrashort echo time (UTE) and hyperpolarized gas MRI benefit from deep learning algorithms that can handle the complex, rapid changes in signal associated with breathing and heartbeats [33, 34]. For example, Fourier decomposition MRI for V/Q imaging relies heavily on registration techniques as a crucial step in its reconstruction paradigm. Deep learning registration provides a low computational cost alternative during the inference stage once the models are trained [35, 36]. These advancements also allow for real-time visualization of lung ventilation and perfusion, critical for assessing conditions such as chronic obstructive pulmonary disease (COPD), interstitial diseases, asthma, and pulmonary hypertension (PH).

A significant challenge in thoracic MRI is motion artifacts, which can compromise the diagnostic quality of the images. Thanks to deep learning advancements, more robust methods for motion correction, essential for accurate imaging of the lungs and heart, have been introduced. These algorithms adaptively learn from variations in patient movement to predict and correct distortions in the image, ensuring higher accuracy and consistency in diagnostic performance [37, 38]. Finally, deep learning is also facilitating the shift from qualitative to quantitative MRI by enabling the automated detection and quantification of biomarkers within the thoracic region. Techniques such as MRI fingerprinting, facilitated by deep learning, allow for the precise quantification of tissue properties [39]. This capability is invaluable for early disease detection, treatment monitoring, and tailored therapeutic strategies based on measurable physiological changes.

Super-Resolution and Small Structure Imaging

Super-resolution techniques in thoracic imaging are enabling the visualization of small structures, such as pulmonary nodules (PN) and intricate vascular networks, with high fidelity [40–42]. These techniques overcome the limitations of conventional imaging resolutions, enabling detailed examination of thoracic anatomy and pathology [43].

Clinical applications of super-resolution imaging include the detailed assessment of lung nodules, characterization of interstitial lung diseases (ILD), and evaluation of coronary arteries.

By providing high-resolution images, these techniques facilitate early detection and accurate characterization of thoracic diseases, which is essential for timely and effective treatment.

Emerging Clinical Applications Enabled by Advanced Reconstruction

The integration of advanced imaging reconstruction technologies, particularly those utilizing deep learning, has catalyzed a series of promising clinical applications in thoracic imaging. Some of the imaging applications that are benefiting from improvements in quality are summarized in Table 27.2.

These technologies refine the existing diagnostic and therapeutic approaches while introducing novel applications that enhance clinical outcomes. Here, we explore several key areas where these advancements based on deep-learning approaches are setting new standards in patient care.

- *Photon-Counting Detector (PCD) CT*: PCD CT stands out as one of the most significant technological advancements in CT imaging. Unlike conventional energy-integrating detectors, PCDs count individual photons, resulting in images with higher spatial resolution and contrast. This technology offers notable advantages in thoracic imaging, improving the visualization of complex anatomical structures such as the bronchial tree, vascular systems, and small nodules. Enhanced image quality facilitates more accurate diagnoses and improves the detection of subtle pathological changes, particularly crucial for conditions like early-stage lung cancer or vascular diseases [44].
- *Cinematic Rendering and 3D Modeling*: Cinematic rendering, a novel visualization technique, uses advanced algorithms to produce photorealistic images from CT and MRI data [45]. This technique allows for a more intuitive understanding of complex anatomical relationships by providing lifelike depictions of the thoracic anatomy. In clinical practice, cinematic rendering aids surgeons and clinicians in planning intricate procedures such as tumor resections or vascular surgeries [46]. Moreover, it enhances communication with patients, helping them understand their medical conditions and planned interventions more clearly.
- *Real-Time Image-Guided Interventions*: Advancements in image reconstruction have also facilitated the development of real-time image-guided intervention systems, particularly in the context of minimally invasive thoracic surgeries and biopsies. These systems leverage ultra-fast image reconstruction to deliver real-time feedback during procedures, which is crucial for reducing the risk of complications and improving surgical outcomes. Significant progress in cone-beam CT reconstruction techniques, for instance, has enabled high-fidelity imaging, providing essential

Table 27.2 Clinical application of AI-driven advance reconstruction and post-processing techniques

Lung cancer screening and nodule characterization	High-resolution, low-dose CT scans facilitated by deep learning reconstruction can improve the detection and characterization of pulmonary nodules, aiding in early lung cancer diagnosis and monitoring
Cardiovascular imaging	Super-resolution reconstruction techniques can enhance the visualization of coronary arteries, enabling better assessment of stenosis, plaque composition, and other cardiovascular abnormalities
Pulmonary vascular imaging	Improved contrast and resolution in CT angiography can aid in the evaluation of pulmonary vascular diseases, such as pulmonary embolism and pulmonary hypertension
Airway imaging	HRCT reconstructions can provide detailed visualization of the airways, facilitating the assessment of airway diseases, such as asthma, COPD, and bronchiectasis. Improved monitorization of airway changes in novel therapeutics targeting airway remodeling

guidance for navigating the intricate structures of the thoracic region during complex interventions [47, 48].

- *Pediatric Imaging*: The application of advanced reconstruction techniques in pediatric imaging represents a critical advancement. Children are particularly sensitive to ionizing radiation. Therefore, reducing exposure while maintaining diagnostic quality is paramount. Techniques such as DLIR in low-dose CT protocols have proven effective in achieving this balance. Moreover, the use of PCD CT can further reduce doses by optimizing photon utilization [49]. These advancements are particularly beneficial for chronic conditions requiring multiple imaging sessions over time, such as congenital heart diseases or chronic pulmonary disorders.

Screening and Diagnostic Applications of AI

Plain Film Radiographs

The automatic interpretation of X-rays by AI algorithms has revolutionized the diagnostic process. AI models are trained to recognize patterns and abnormalities in X-ray images, enabling the identification and reporting of thoracic diseases with high accuracy [50]. These AI-assisted interpretations can serve as a second opinion for radiologists, enhancing diagnostic accuracy and reducing the likelihood of oversight [51].

Recent developments in AI have transformed the interpretation of chest X-rays (CXR) by employing deep convolutional neural networks to detect and diagnose conditions such as tuberculosis and pneumonia with remarkable accuracy [52]. For instance, techniques developed by Lakhani et al. utilized models like AlexNet and GoogLeNet to achieve a 96% accuracy rate in identifying tuberculosis from CXR images [53]. This level of precision highlights AI's potential to significantly enhance the diagnostic process in primary and emergency medicine [54]. AI models are trained to recognize patterns and abnormalities that might be overlooked in manual interpretations. By automating the detection process, AI serves as a reliable second opinion for radiologists, thereby improving diagnostic accuracy and reducing the likelihood of oversight in emergency situations [55]. However, evaluations of currently available commercial systems reveal certain limitations, including performance gaps related to false positives and reduced accuracy in complex cases with multiple findings, indicating that further refinement is necessary to fully realize the potential of AI in clinical practice [56].

AI's ability to enhance the detection and localization of lung nodules represents another significant advancement [57]. AI-powered systems, especially those based on CNNs, are adept at identifying subtle patterns in CXR images that may indicate the presence of nodules. These systems not only detect nodules but also accurately pinpoint their locations within the lung fields, thereby aiding in precise diagnostic follow-up [58]. In a randomized controlled trial comparing expert performance with and without AI-assisted computer-aided detection (CAD) for lung nodule detection, the group using AI demonstrated higher detection rates without an increase in false referral rates, underscoring the potential of AI to enhance clinical outcomes while maintaining diagnostic accuracy [59].

Augmentation of CXR with AI has shown to be useful in prognostication of patient in inpatient settings. Those applications were particularly catalyzed in the early phases of the COVID-19 pandemic [60]. In a retrospective study of patients hospitalized with COVID-19, incorporating CXR with clinical information was effective in predicting severe illness and acute respiratory distress syndrome (ARDS) [61]. Further research underscores the potential of AI-enhanced X-ray imaging in accurately detecting ARDS, highlighting its value as a critical tool in managing respiratory crises [62].

AI algorithms also play a crucial role in ensuring that patients with urgent conditions receive immediate attention, enhancing workflow within radiology departments [51]. This capability is particularly beneficial in high-volume clinical settings, where timely diagnosis can drastically affect patient outcomes. For example, AI systems can be used to identify abnormal X-rays, flagging these cases for prompt review [63], or the identification of unremarkable cases that could be staged for automatic reporting [64]. Such prioritization is crucial in managing patient flow and treatment efficacy in busy medical facilities.

Deep learning approaches utilizing X-rays have also demonstrated potential in predicting long-term mortality and opportunistic detection of chronic conditions within retrospective cohorts [65–67]. While these tools are still in the early stages of development, they hold a significant promise for risk stratification and population management, especially in value-based healthcare settings where the efficient allocation of scarce resources is crucial.

Computed Tomography

Based on the NLST and NELSON trial results, lung cancer screening programs in the USA and other European countries have advanced their implementation as effective tools for early lung cancer detection [68, 69]. CT-based lung cancer detection and prognostication have significantly advanced with the integration of deep learning technologies. These advancements have enhanced the accuracy and efficiency of lung cancer screening, which is crucial for early detection and improved patient outcomes.

CAD systems for nodule detection have seen a significant improvement since adopting a deep learning approach with remarkable consistency across imaging protocol and scanning parameters [70]. Multi-scale CNN models have been developed to capture nodule heterogeneity and achieved an 88.84% accuracy for nodule classification against noisy backgrounds [71]. Retrospective analyses of deep learning methodologies developed in a public competition for the detection of lung cancer in low-dose CT scans have shown performance comparable to that of radiologists [72]. These findings highlight the potential of AI to complement human expertise and enhance diagnostic efficiency in demanding clinical environments. This is especially true in high-volume screening scenarios, where the risk of radiologist burnout due to heavy workloads is significant.

Deep learning also extends to risk stratification and prognostication, with models like Sybil leading the way [73]. Utilizing deep learning techniques, Sybil predicts future lung cancer risk from a single low-dose CT scan. This approach enables personalized screening schedules and early interventions, aligning with the principles of precision medicine. By predicting lung cancer risk, Sybil facilitates a proactive approach to lung health, potentially transforming screening methodologies. Other studies using serial CT imaging data have also shown promising results in estimating the 3-year malignancy risk of pulmonary nodules [74]. Such predictive capabilities underscore the shift toward customized healthcare that AI and thoracic imaging could have, where treatment plans and screening intervals are tailored to individual risk profiles, enhancing the effectiveness of lung cancer prevention strategies.

Computed Tomography: Obstructive and Diffuse Lung Diseases

The diagnosis and prognosis of COPD and ILD remain complex, despite established diagnostic criteria and guidelines that emphasize the role of CT imaging. While spirometry remains the clinical standard for diagnosing obstructive and diffuse lung diseases, it often falls short in defining the full extent and nature of the pathology. CNNs have emerged as powerful tools for automating diagnosis and improving disease prognostication in these conditions. For instance, Gonzalez et al. demonstrated that a three-layer CNN applied to chest CT scans could predict COPD GOLD status with a 74.0% one-class-off accuracy while also forecasting mortality (C-index = 0.72) and acute exacerbations (C-index = 0.61) [75]. Similarly, Tang and colleagues used residual neural networks to effectively diagnose COPD, achieving an area under the curve (AUC) of 0.88 in the PanCan cohort, with stable replication results in the ECLIPSE study based on a subset of CT slices [76].

Artificial intelligence has also catalyzed the quantitative characterization of various COPD phenotypes by providing robust estimates of emphysema and gas trapping [77, 78]. For example, a deep learning model utilizing multi-slice CT readings offers automated visual subtyping of emphysema according to the Fleischner Society grading criteria. These AI-driven assessments have been shown to enhance mortality prediction compared to traditional visual evaluations performed by experts [79, 80]. Additionally, attention-based approaches have demonstrated improved accuracy in detecting emphysema even in low-dose CT scans, further highlighting the potential of AI to refine diagnostic precision in COPD [81].

The application of AI in identifying and classifying fibrotic lung disease, particularly usual interstitial pneumonia (UIP), has shown a significant clinical impact [140]. Currently, the diagnosis of UIP relies heavily on subjective interpretation of high-resolution CT (HRCT) scans, which can vary between radiologists. AI systems like SOFIA, which utilizes a deep learning approach, have demonstrated the capability to provide automated diagnoses of UIP based on a four-slice image montage [82]. Patient-level UIP probabilities were strongly associated with transplant-free survival and 12-month disease progression. Interestingly, SOFIA was able to reclassify a substantial proportion of visually indeterminate UIP cases, and this reclassification correlated with improved transplant-free survival, highlighting the utility of deep learning models in detecting subtle fibrotic patterns and enhancing diagnostic accuracy, particularly in challenging indeterminate cases.

More advanced machine learning techniques, such as multi-instance learning using weakly labeled CT patches, have further refined the detection of histologic UIP compared to traditional visual assessments (AUC = 0.79 vs. 0.71) [18]. Individuals identified as UIP-positive by these algorithms exhibited a significantly greater annual decline in forced vital capacity (FVC) than those classified as UIP-negative reflecting the prognostic value of automated detection.

Computed Tomography: Cardiovascular Diseases

CT has significantly enhanced the ability to diagnose various cardiovascular conditions such as pulmonary embolism (PE), coronary artery calcium (CAC) scoring, and aortic aneurysms. However, the interpretation of CT images is complex and time-consuming, often requiring highly specialized expertise. The integration of AI into diagnostic workflows enables more efficient, accurate, and standardized interpretations of vascular conditions in CT scans:

- *Pulmonary Embolism*: Recent developments in CNNs have introduced automated PE detection in CT pulmonary angiography (CTPA) scans, which has the potential to reduce diagnosis time, minimize errors, and improve patient outcomes. For instance, a 3D CNN technique that combines imaging information from CTPA scans with clinical patient data to automatically classify PE cases achieved an impressive AUROC of 0.95, significantly outperforming single-modality models [83]. A two-stage 3D CNN trained on a large dataset of 28,000 CTPAs from nine clinical centers to first segment PE and then classify the regions of interest reported a sensitivity of 92.7% and a specificity of 95.5%, with central emboli showing the highest detection rates (95.7%), followed by segmental (93.3%) and subsegmental emboli (85.7%) [84].
  Beyond enhancing diagnosis, AI algorithms play a critical role in quality improvement. Hahn et al. developed an AI tool to segment the main pulmonary trunk and assess contrast enhancement levels in CT pulmonary angiograms, facilitating systematic and timely analyses across multiple scanners and time points [85]. By automating these processes, AI ensures efficient and consistent quality checks, which are vital in busy clinical environments.
- *Coronary Artery Calcium Scoring:* AI has shown a great promise in automating and improving the accuracy of CAC scoring. For example, Chao et al. developed a deep learning system to automatically calculate calcium scores from CT scans, which are critical for cardiovascular risk assessment [86]. Alternative approaches using two consecutive CNNs are able to detect CAC, thoracic aorta calcifications, and cardiac valve calcifications

across the entire CT scans [87]. This method demonstrated excellent detection performance and high agreement in risk categorization on a large, diverse dataset of low-dose chest CT scans. Further supporting AI's efficacy in CAC scoring, van Velzen et al. conducted a study involving 7240 scans across various protocols and patient demographics, developing a CNN-based deep learning technique that demonstrated improved agreement with manual scoring (ICC 0.84–0.99) [88]. This approach led to more consistent risk stratification when additional protocol-specific CT scans were included. Deep learning approaches have shown high concordance between automated and manual scores [89], emphasizing AI's role in reliable risk assessment [3].

- *Aortic Aneurysms*: AI models have been developed to enhance the detection and segmentation of aortic aneurysms from CT images. CNNs can accurately segment and measure aortic aneurysms, highlighting the potential of AI to mitigate underdiagnosis in clinical studies not originally intended for aneurysm detection [90]. Additionally, CNNs have shown greater consistency and reproducibility in assessing thoracic aortic diameters compared to traditional methods in patients with various aortic abnormalities, identifying factors that impact the algorithm's performance [91]. Understanding these factors is crucial for the safe integration of AI into clinical practice. Chung et al. further illustrated deep learning is also effective in predicting biomechanical wall stresses in abdominal aortic aneurysms, significantly streamlining the process compared to conventional manual methods [92]. This advancement paves the way for large-scale studies to deepen our understanding of aneurysm behavior and rupture risk. Finally, AI can enhance the efficiency of thoracic aortic aneurysm CT follow-ups, ensuring diagnostic accuracy while improving reporting speed without compromising quality [93].

MRI

AI is contributing to the automated post-processing of MRI imaging to enable better quantification of lung diseases. These advancements collectively enhance the diagnostic capabilities of MRI in pulmonary medicine, making it a more reliable and comprehensive tool for clinicians. One example is the use of a 2D U-Net to perform volumetric lung segmentation from UTE proton MRI in a multiplane fashion [94]. Increased robustness in UTE MRI lung segmentation can be achieved by combining adaptive machine learning strategies like k-mean after the initial U-Net segmentation for further robustness [95]. Robust lung segmentation in MRI is essential for quantitative analysis of functional parameters and its use in clinical studies. Notable examples are also the application of advanced deep learning segmentation in the quantification of neonatal lung diseases using MRI [96].

Quantitative Imaging and Disease Monitorization

Radiomics

Radiomics is a rapidly evolving field in quantitative imaging that uses advanced imaging features to objectively and quantitatively describe tumor phenotypes [97]. Although the term is not strictly defined, radiomics generally focuses on extracting quantitative metrics, known as radiomic features, from various types of medical images, such as CT scans or MRIs. These features essentially capture detailed characteristics of tissues and lesions, including texture, shape, and distinctions from the surrounding tissue [98]. The integration of radiomic features with demographic, histologic, genomic, or proteomic data holds the potential to enhance clinical problem-solving capabilities, providing clinicians with comprehensive diagnostic and prognostic information [2].

What makes radiomic features particularly powerful is their ability to offer valuable insights into disease processes. For instance, radiomics enables the quantification of tumor heterogeneity—variations in appearance and behavior among tumor cells [99, 100]. This comprehensive approach to medical decision-making facilitates personalized and effective treatments.

In the context of lung cancer, radiomics offers a non-invasive means to characterize tumors and assess their heterogeneity. By analyzing subtle patterns and textures within radiographic images that may not be discernible to the human eye, radiomics enables clinicians to glean insights into tumor biology, tumor staging, and treatment response. For example, Rios Velazquez et al. demonstrated that CT radiomics could predict somatic mutations, EGFR and KRAS, in pulmonary nodules with an AUC of 0.8 [101]. A similar study demonstrated that a hybrid approach, combining radiomic features and deep learning, achieved an area under the curve (AUC) of 0.7 for detecting EGFR mutations in patients with non-small cell lung cancer (NSCLC) [102].

Selection of radiomics features can be done using machine learning approach to find radiographic biomarkers for specific diagnostic tasks. For example, a radiomics prediction model based on only two features from an initial set of 103 could be used to detect PN malignancy early with an accuracy of 84.6% [71]. Yang et al. demonstrated the effectiveness of radiomic signatures derived from pre-treatment CT images in predicting the tumor responses of NSCLC patients undergoing first-line chemotherapy, targeted therapy, or a combination of both with and AUC of 0.721 [103]. Similar studies using various analysis and imaging techniques have corroborated these findings [104–107]. Ultimately, this technology may enable not only the identification but also the confirmation of diagnosis and planning of lung cancer treatment without the need for invasive tissue sampling.

Radiomics, particularly when combined with machine learning, offers a more detailed and accurate approach to staging and classifying COPD compared to traditional methods. A lobe-based radiomics method has proven effective in classifying COPD severity based on the GOLD criteria, especially in distinguishing between milder and more severe stages [108]. Additionally, integrating radiomic features with quantitative CT measures and demographic data further enhances the accuracy of models for classifying COPD status and severity [109].

Despite its immense potential, the widespread clinical adoption of radiomics in lung cancer and other respiratory conditions still faces challenges related to standardization, reproducibility, and validation across different imaging platforms and patient cohorts [110]. However, ongoing research efforts and technological advancements continue to drive progress in this field, paving the way for personalized care for patients with lung cancer.

Airway Characterization

Advancements in AI have significantly enhanced the quantitative imaging of the airway tree from chest CT scans, particularly for assessing complex structures like airway walls. This imaging involves measuring airway dimensions, wall thickness, and lumen area—key metrics for diagnosing and monitoring respiratory conditions such as COPD, asthma, and bronchiectasis. While traditional methods are time-consuming and subject to inter-observer variability, AI-driven techniques enable more accurate and automated assessments, offering valuable insights into disease severity and progression.

Several studies have introduced innovative techniques that use deep learning to automatically segment the bronchial tree from CT images, achieving high accuracy and low false-positive rates compared to conventional methods [111–113]. Generative approaches that combined a CNN to automatically measure bronchial lumen and wall thickness from chest CT scans have been proposed showing good precision to different reconstruction protocols [114].

Bronchiectasis, a chronic condition characterized by the abnormal widening of the bronchi, can be challenging to diagnose and monitor effectively using traditional imaging methods. Recent advancements in artificial intelligence and deep learning have significantly improved the accuracy and efficiency of CT-based assessments of bronchiectasis by assessing airway tapering [115]. AI techniques have been used to separate pulmonary arteries and veins [116] and match them with the corresponding airways, enabling precise measurements of airway lumen and artery diameters. These measurements are essential for calculating the airway-to-artery diameter ratio, which is a key marker for diagnosing and monitoring bronchiectasis [117]. This approach has shown that AI-based CT measures are associated with increased exacerbations in COPD patients over time [117]. Furthermore, deep learning has enhanced the identification of air trapping in lung CT scans [118], aiding in the early detection and clinical management of pulmonary conditions such as cystic fibrosis, asthma, and COPD.

Vascular Characterization

Vascular characterization using chest CT scans involves the assessment of blood vessel structures, including the pulmonary arteries and veins. This process is particularly important for diagnosing and managing diseases such as pulmonary embolism, PH, and pulmonary vascular disease (PVD). PH is characterized by elevated blood pressure within the pulmonary arteries, while PVD encompasses various disorders affecting the blood vessels in the lungs. In the context of pulmonary diseases, several studies have demonstrated the effectiveness of deep learning-based approaches for automatic segmentation and quantification of the pulmonary vasculature volumes of small vessels in CT scans [119, 120]. Separation of the arterial and venous tree has been enabled by deep learning coupled with graph-cut optimization to enforce topological consistency that has shown high classification accuracy (96% to 98%) [116, 121]. These methods are enabling the characterization of pre-capillary and post-capillary diseases.

Improved vascular reconstruction of the small vessel reconstruction combined with arterial/venous differentiation has paved the way for large-scale clinical quantification of changes in the pulmonary vasculature and the definition of new biomarkers for accurate analysis of PVD, specifically in the phenotyping of pulmonary arterial hypertension [122]. The characterization of the vascular tree is enabling the study of the relationship among distal pulmonary arterial pruning, emphysema, and right ventricular size in patients with PH and COPD (Fig. 27.2) [123].

Advances in Functional Imaging Using AI

In functional imaging, accurate lung segmentation is essential for localizing and quantifying regional data. Deep learning, especially using CNNs like U-Nets, has significantly improved lung segmentation by offering more precise and consistent results across various imaging modalities and functional parameters of perfusion and ventilation [124, 125].

Deformable image registration (DIR) is another critical tool in functional imaging, particularly for assessing ventilation and perfusion by mapping images across different respiratory phases. While traditional DIR methods are effective, they are computationally intensive and often struggle with the complexities of lung imaging. Deep learning-based DIR approaches offer a more efficient alternative, using CNNs to model complex deformation fields with less computational demand and improved accuracy [36, 126, 127].

Multiparametric imaging, which integrates structural and functional data, benefits significantly from DIR, enabling more comprehensive assessments of lung pathophysiology. Techniques like multiparametric response maps, which combine CT and hyperpolarized MRI data, were able to reveal emphysema and small airway disease not otherwise identified with CT or MRI, reflecting the power of multimodal approaches in disease characterization [128]. The incorporation of deep learning into these multiparametric approaches is poised to advance clinical applications, offering more detailed and actionable insights into disease characterization and patient management. Multi-resolution U-Net architectures have been proposed for robust lobar segmentation in CT images to enable regional quantification of dynamic CT series [129, 130].

AI is also playing a crucial role in the development and assessment of fractional flow reserve computed tomography (FFR-CT), which has emerged as a valuable tool in cardiac imaging by providing both anatomical and functional information about coronary artery disease [131]. This advanced imaging technique enhances decision-making processes for invasive coro-

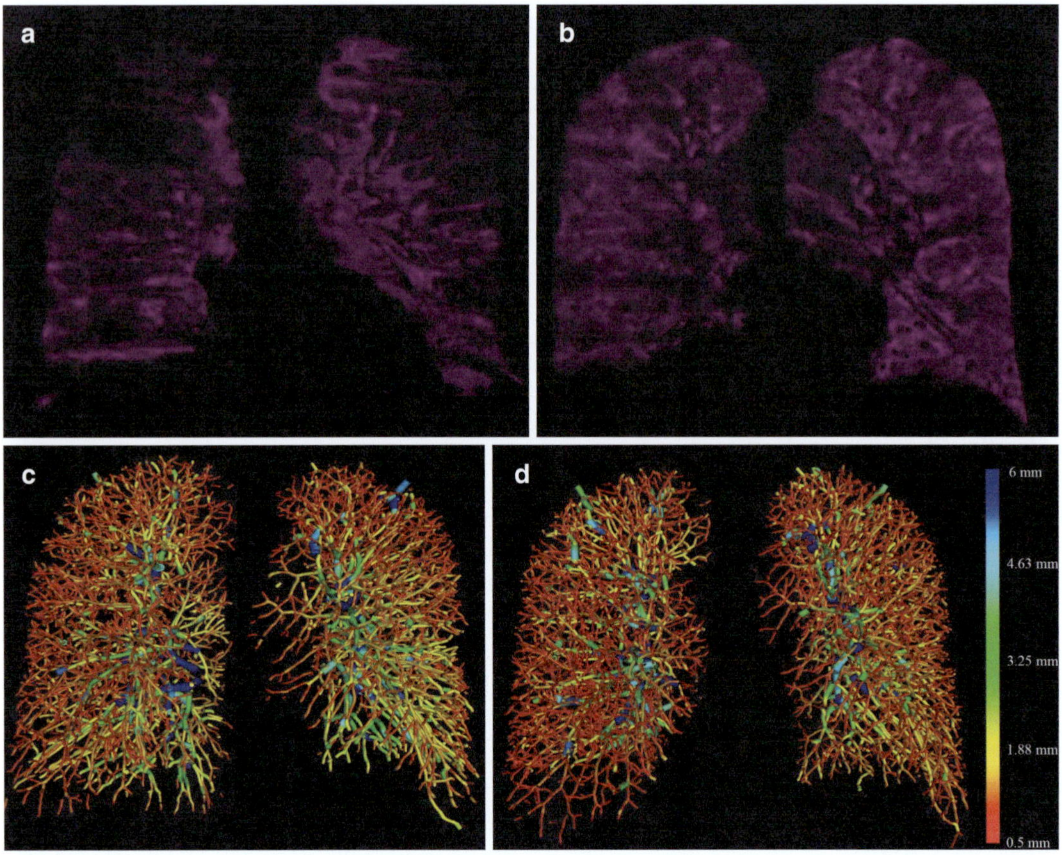

Fig. 27.2 Interplay between vascular structure using AI reconstruction approaches and pulmonary perfusion using dual-energy CT. Top row: (**a**) A 3D iodine map illustrating a significant perfusion defect. (**b**) Follow-up imaging demonstrating the resolution of this perfusion defect. Bottom row: (**c**) Vascular tree reconstruction from the same patient. (**d**) Subsequent imaging reveals an increase in small vessel volume (indicated in red/orange)

nary angiography and revascularization interventions, ultimately reducing the number of unnecessary invasive procedures [132]. By integrating AI-driven analysis with traditional CT imaging, FFR-CT offers a non-invasive means to evaluate the physiological impact of coronary artery lesions.

Generative AI is playing an increasingly important role in advancing synthetic functional imaging, where it facilitates the creation of functional imaging data from simpler or more readily available structural modalities like CT. This approach, often referred to as image-to-image translation, harnesses advanced generative deep learning techniques like GANs and diffusion models to establish and exploit relationships between different imaging modalities.

In particular, GANs, especially in their semi-supervised variants, significantly enhance the stability and accuracy of synthetic functional imaging. For instance, conditional CycleGANs have been utilized to generate dual-energy CT-derived iodine perfusion maps from single-energy CT scans, effectively eliminating the need for paired datasets (Fig. 27.3) [11]. Additionally, the use of 3D attention residual neural networks to estimate blood perfusion from chest CT scans holds a promise for improving the diagnosis and management of vascular-related diseases such as PE and PH [133]. ViT have also been proposed to perform synthetic expiratory imaging from inspiratory imaging, enabling the assessment of gas trapping using only an inspiratory protocol [134]. Alternative generative approaches using regres-

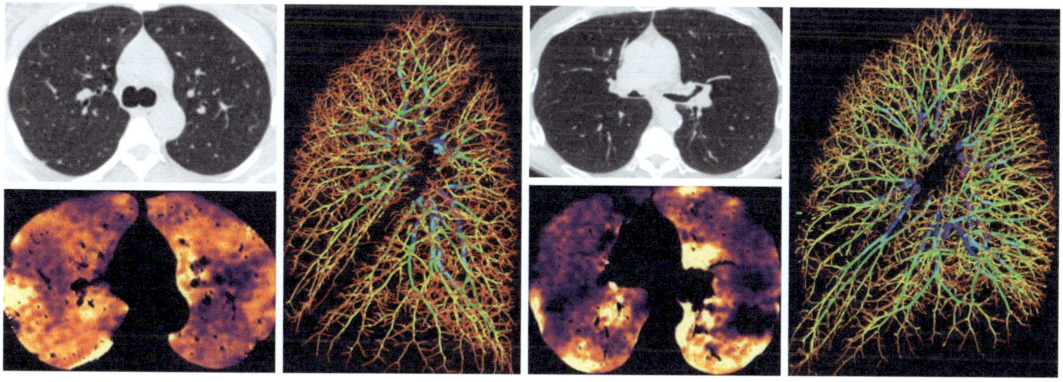

Fig. 27.3 Examples of synthetic iodine perfusion maps obtained with a generative approach from single-energy CT scans and reconstructed vascular trees for a control subject (left) and a subject with vascular pruning (right). The control subject's iodine perfusion map shows normal perfusion throughout the lung, with the corresponding vascular tree reconstruction displaying a well-distributed network of vessels. The color coding of the vascular reconstruction indicates vessel radius, where red represents smaller vessels (0–1 mm), and blue represents larger vessels (5–6 mm). In contrast, the subject with vascular pruning exhibits reduced perfusion in certain lung regions, as seen on the synthetic iodine perfusion map. The corresponding vascular tree reconstruction reveals a notable reduction in smaller vessels (red, 0–1 mm), indicative of vascular pruning

sion CNNs have demonstrated the potential to directly estimate local tissue volume changes and lung ventilation from a single chest CT scan, whether acquired at TLC or FRC, opening new avenues for functional lung imaging with simplified protocols [12].

Future Directions in AI-Enhanced Thoracic Imaging

Looking forward, the ongoing evolution of image reconstruction technologies holds the promise of even broader applications. Artificial intelligence models are currently being trained to predict patient outcomes based on imaging data, potentially integrating image-derived biomarkers into routine clinical practice. Furthermore, advancements such as dual-energy CT and advanced PET imaging will enhance functional assessments and molecular imaging, offering deeper insights into disease mechanisms.

Foundation models represent a transformative shift in AI, with the potential to reshape thoracic imaging by offering a unified model that spans across multiple applications. Unlike the narrow, task-specific models currently in use, foundation models could integrate various imaging modalities and clinical data, creating a comprehensive framework for thoracic radiology. Drawing inspiration from advances in fields like genomics and digital pathology [135–137], where large, versatile models have already shown promise, thoracic imaging could benefit from a similar convergence. For instance, a foundation model trained in a vast amount of diverse imaging data could streamline diagnosis, prognostication, and treatment planning across a wide range of pulmonary diseases, improving both accuracy and efficiency. However, early evidence suggests that thoracic X-ray foundation models may be sensitive to biases, leading to uneven performance across different patient subgroups [138]. This concern underscores the need for further research as these generalist models are developed and implemented.

The integration of radiology and digital pathology through AI presents an exciting frontier in thoracic imaging. As digital pathology continues to advance, particularly in lung diseases, there is a growing opportunity to create a unified diagnostic approach that combines imaging and histopathological data. According to the state-of-the-art review by Viswanathan et al. [139], AI has already demonstrated a significant potential in lung digital pathology. By aligning this progress with radiological data, clinicians could achieve a more comprehensive understanding of disease processes, facilitating earlier and more accurate diagnoses. AI-driven integration could also enhance the correlation between radiological findings and histopathological outcomes, ultimately leading to better patient management and personalized treatment strategies.

Radiologists and clinicians frequently face significant barriers when integrating AI into practice, including the difficulty of analyzing and comparing outcomes generated by various algorithms. Identifying the optimal network or model for specific thoracic conditions remains a substantial challenge due to the complexity and the "black-box" nature of these models. This lack of transparency can hinder trust and reliance on AI tools, as the decision-making process of the models is often obscure and difficult to comprehend. Establishing validation frameworks that continuously monitor AI-based systems will be essential for a smooth and safe integration into the clinical workflow.

Moreover, while data scientists and researchers may report promising algorithmic performances, translating these results into clinical settings requires rigorous validation and testing. Assessing the optimal network for a specific condition requires not only evaluating its performance metrics but also validating its ability to seamlessly integrate into clinical workflows while adhering to medical standards and practices.

Advancing AI-driven radiomics and deep learning in medical imaging faces the challenge of limited large, clinically rich datasets, particularly evident in specialized modalities such as MRI. Collaborative efforts among healthcare institutions to develop standardized, diverse datasets, encompassing a wide range of patient demographics and disease stages, are essential for enhancing AI model training and generalizability. Furthermore, while the Food and Drug Administration's twenty-first Century Cures Act supports the use of real-world data in drug evaluations, the heterogeneity and quality concerns of such data necessitate careful consideration to safeguard the reproducibility and reliability of AI applications in clinical settings.

Conclusion

Overall, deep learning has revolutionized the field of thoracic image analysis by providing powerful tools for automating tasks that were once labor-intensive or challenging for traditional computer vision algorithms. As the field continues to evolve, we can expect to see further advancements in the accuracy, robustness, and interpretability of AI systems for medical imaging applications. Advanced imaging reconstruction technologies are transforming thoracic imaging, enabling higher image quality and safer, faster, and more precise diagnostics. As these technologies continue to evolve and integrate with clinical workflows, they promise to significantly improve patient care outcomes across a wide range of thoracic conditions.

AI is not only augmenting the role of traditional imaging techniques but also catalyzing their evolution into more quantitative and precise diagnostic tools. As AI technologies continue to evolve, their integration into highly available modalities like chest X-ray analysis is expected to expand, further improving the efficacy of medical diagnostics and personalized patient care. Additionally, more sophisticated modalities like CT and MRI can benefit from advanced radiomics enabled by deep learning, paving the way for personalized diagnostic and prognostic tools. Areas like lung cancer screening management have enabled early detection of lung cancer, and AI-based second readings are enabling improved detection and prognostication.

While generative AI holds a great promise in thoracic imaging, it is important to acknowledge that these techniques are still in developmental stages and require rigorous validation to enable their clinical implementation. Ongoing research aims to improve reliability, interpretability, and clinical utility of generative AI models in thoracic imaging applications. Looking ahead, the field is likely to see more sophisticated AI models that incorporate a broader range of data inputs and offer more comprehensive diagnostic insights. There is also a growing interest in developing AI systems that can explain their decision-making processes, thereby increasing their acceptability among clinicians. Moreover, as AI technology continues to evolve, its integration into personalized medicine approaches is likely to become increasingly prevalent. These approaches tailor treatment plans to individual patients based on a combination of genetic, environmental, and imaging data, promising to further optimize patient care and outcomes in the field of thoracic medicine.

References

1. Wang S, Cao G, Wang Y, Liao S, Wang Q, Shi J, Li C, Shen D. Review and prospect: artificial intelligence in advanced medical imaging. Front Radiol. 2021;1:781868.
2. Mei X, Lee HC, Diao KY, Huang M, Lin B, Liu C, Xie Z, Ma Y, Robson PM, Chung M, Bernheim A, Mani V, Calcagno C, Li K, Li S, Shan H, Lv J, Zhao T, Xia J, Long Q, Steinberger S, Jacobi A, Deyer T, Luksza M, Liu F, Little BP, Fayad ZA, Yang Y. Artificial intelligence-enabled rapid diagnosis of patients with COVID-19. Nat Med. 2020;26:1224–8.
3. Miller RJH, Killekar A, Shanbhag A, Bednarski B, Michalowska AM, Ruddy TD, Einstein AJ, Newby DE, Lemley M, Pieszko K, Van Kriekinge SD, Kavanagh PB, Liang JX, Huang C, Dey D, Berman DS, Slomka PJ. Predicting mortality from AI cardiac volumes mass and coronary calcium on chest computed tomography. Nat Commun. 2024;15:2747.
4. Choi RY, Coyner AS, Kalpathy-Cramer J, Chiang MF, Campbell JP. Introduction to machine learning, neural networks, and deep learning. Transl Vis Sci Technol. 2020;9:14.
5. Cheng PM, Montagnon E, Yamashita R, Pan I, Cadrin-Chenevert A, Perdigon Romero F, Chartrand G, Kadoury S, Tang A. Deep learning: an update for radiologists. Radiographics. 2021;41:1427–45.
6. Esteva A, Kuprel B, Novoa RA, Ko J, Swetter SM, Blau HM, Thrun S. Dermatologist-level classification of skin cancer with deep neural networks. Nature. 2017;542:115–8.
7. LeCun YB, Léon, Bengio Y, Haffner P. Handwritten digit recognition with a back-propagation network. In: Touretzky DS, editor. Advances in neural information processing systems 2. Denver: Morgan Kaufmann; 1990. p. 396–404.
8. Jin D, Xu Z, Tang Y, Harrison AP. and Mollura DJ, 2018. CT-realistic lung nodule simulation from 3D conditional generative adversarial networks for robust lung segmentation. In Medical Image Computing and Computer Assisted Intervention–MICCAI 2018. 21st International Conference, Granada, Spain, September 16–20, 2018, Proceedings, Part II 11 (pp. 732–740). Springer International Publishing.
9. Ronneberger OF, Philipp, Brox T. U-Net: convolutional networks for biomedical image segmentation. In: Navab NH, Joachim, Wells WM, Frangi AF, editors. Medical image computing and computer-assisted intervention (MICCAI) 2015. Cham: Springer; 2015. p. 234–41.
10.
11. Goodfellow IP-A, Jean, Mirza M, Xu B, Warde-Farley D, Ozair S, Courville A, Bengio Y. Generative adversarial nets. In: Advances in neural information processing systems (NeurIPS). Montreal, Canada; 2014. p. 2672–80.
12. Nardelli P, Estepar RSJ, Rahaghi FN, Estepar RSJ. Functional-consistent CycleGAN for CT to iodine perfusion map translation. Thorac Image Anal. 2020;2020(12502):109–17.
13. Gerard SE, Chaudhary MFA, Herrmann J, Christensen GE, San Jose Estepar R, Reinhardt JM, Hoffman EA. Direct estimation of regional lung volume change from paired and single CT images using residual regression neural network. Med Phys. 2023;50:5698–714.
14. Vaswani AS, Noam, Parmar N, Uszkoreit J, Jones L, Gomez AN, Kaiser Ł, Polosukhin I. Attention is all you need. In: Advances in neural information processing systems (NeurIPS). Long Beach, CA; 2017. p. 5998–6008.
15. Dosovitskiy AB, Lucas, Kolesnikov A, Weissenborn D, Zhai X, Unterthiner T, Dehghani M, Minderer M, Heigold G, Gelly S, Uszkoreit J, Houlsby N. An image is worth 16x16 words: transformers for image recognition at scale. arXiv preprint arXiv:201011929 2020.
16. Ho JJ, Ajay, Abbeel P. Denoising diffusion probabilistic models. In: Advances in neural information processing systems (NeurIPS); 2020. p. 6840–51.
17. Chen X, Wang X, Zhang K, Fung KM, Thai TC, Moore K, Mannel RS, Liu H, Zheng B, Qiu Y. Recent advances and clinical applications of deep learning in medical image analysis. Med Image Anal. 2022;79:102444.
18. Nakao T, Hanaoka S, Nomura Y, Murata M, Takenaga T, Miki S, Watadani T, Yoshikawa T, Hayashi N, Abe O. Unsupervised deep anomaly detection in chest radiographs. J Digit Imaging. 2021;34:418–27.
19. Humphries SM, Thieke D, Baraghoshi D, Strand MJ, Swigris JJ, Chae KJ, Hwang HJ, Oh AS, Flaherty KR, Adegunsoye A, Jablonski R, Lee CT, Husain AN, Chung JH, Strek ME, Lynch DA. Deep learning classification of usual interstitial pneumonia predicts outcomes. Am J Respir Crit Care Med. 2024;209:1121–31.
20. Ali I, Hart GR, Gunabushanam G, Liang Y, Muhammad W, Nartowt B, Kane M, Ma X, Deng J. Lung nodule detection via deep reinforcement learning. Front Oncol. 2018;8:108.
21. Nair VH, Geoffrey E. Rectified linear units improve restricted Boltzmann machines. In: Proceedings of the 27th international conference on machine

learning (ICML). Haifa, Israel: Omnipress; 2010. p. 807–14.
22. Srivastava NH, Geoffrey, Krizhevsky A, Sutskever I, Salakhutdinov R. Dropout: a simple way to prevent neural networks from overfitting. J Mach Learn Res. 2014;15:1929–58.
23. Ioffe SS, Christian. Batch normalization: accelerating deep network training by reducing internal covariate shift. In: Proceedings of the 32nd international conference on machine learning (ICML); 2015. p. 448–56.
24. Erhan DB, Yoshua, Courville A, Manzagol P-A, Vincent P, Bengio S. Why does unsupervised pre-training help deep learning? J Mach Learn Res. 2010;11:625–60.
25. Koetzier LR, Mastrodicasa D, Szczykutowicz TP, van der Werf NR, Wang AS, Sandfort V, van der Molen AJ, Fleischmann D, Willemink MJ. Deep learning image reconstruction for CT: technical principles and clinical prospects. Radiology. 2023;306:e221257.
26. Nam JG, Ahn C, Choi H, Hong W, Park J, Kim JH, Goo JM. Image quality of ultralow-dose chest CT using deep learning techniques: potential superiority of vendor-agnostic post-processing over vendor-specific techniques. Eur Radiol. 2021;31:5139–47.
27. Shan H, Padole A, Homayounieh F, Kruger U, Khera RD, Nitiwarangkul C, Kalra MK, Wang G. Competitive performance of a modularized deep neural network compared to commercial algorithms for low-dose CT image reconstruction. Nat Mach Intell. 2019;1:269–76.
28. Wang H, Li LL, Shang J, Song J, Liu B. Application of deep learning image reconstruction in low-dose chest CT scan. Br J Radiol. 2022;95:20210380.
29. Pain CD, Egan GF, Chen Z. Deep learning-based image reconstruction and post-processing methods in positron emission tomography for low-dose imaging and resolution enhancement. Eur J Nucl Med Mol Imaging. 2022;49:3098–118.
30. Gassenmaier S, Kustner T, Nickel D, Herrmann J, Hoffmann R, Almansour H, Afat S, Nikolaou K, Othman AE. Deep learning applications in magnetic resonance imaging: has the future become present? Diagnostics (Basel). 2021;11:2181.
31. Duan C, Deng H, Xiao S, Xie J, Li H, Sun X, Ma L, Lou X, Ye C, Zhou X. Fast and accurate reconstruction of human lung gas MRI with deep learning. Magn Reson Med. 2019;82:2273–85.
32. Wang S, Su Z, Ying L, Peng X, Zhu S, Liang F, Feng D, Liang D. Accelerating magnetic resonance imaging via deep learning. Proc IEEE Int Symp Biomed Imaging. 2016;2016:514–7.
33. Lin DJ, Johnson PM, Knoll F, Lui YW. Artificial intelligence for MR image reconstruction: an overview for clinicians. J Magn Reson Imaging. 2021;53:1015–28.
34. Torres L, Kammerman J, Hahn AD, Zha W, Nagle SK, Johnson K, Sandbo N, Meyer K, Schiebler M, Fain SB. Structure-function imaging of lung disease using ultrashort echo time MRI. Acad Radiol. 2019;26:431–41.
35. Kruger SJ, Nagle SK, Couch MJ, Ohno Y, Albert M, Fain SB. Functional imaging of the lungs with gas agents. J Magn Reson Imaging. 2016;43:295–315.
36. de Vos BD, Berendsen FF, Viergever MA, Sokooti H, Staring M, Isgum I. A deep learning framework for unsupervised affine and deformable image registration. Med Image Anal. 2019;52:128–43.
37. Tian LG, Hastings, Vialard F-X, Kwitt R, Estépar SJ, Raúl, Rushmore RJ, Makris N, Bouix S, Niethammer M. GradICON: approximate diffeomorphisms via gradient inverse consistency. In: IEEE/CVF conference on computer vision and pattern recognition. Vancouver, BC, Canada; 2023. p. 18084–94.
38. Usman M, Latif S, Asim M, Lee BD, Qadir J. Retrospective motion correction in multishot MRI using generative adversarial network. Sci Rep. 2020;10:4786.
39. Oksuz I, Clough JR, Ruijsink B, Anton EP, Bustin A, Cruz G, Prieto C, King AP, Schnabel JA. Deep learning-based detection and correction of cardiac MR motion artefacts during reconstruction for high-quality segmentation. IEEE Trans Med Imaging. 2020;39:4001–10.
40. Lundervold AS, Lundervold A. An overview of deep learning in medical imaging focusing on MRI. Z Med Phys. 2019;29:102–27.
41. Masutani EM, Bahrami N, Hsiao A. Deep learning single-frame and multiframe super-resolution for cardiac MRI. Radiology. 2020;295:552–61.
42. You C, Li G, Zhang Y, Zhang X, Shan H, Li M, Ju S, Zhao Z, Zhang Z, Cong W, Vannier MW, Saha PK, Hoffman EA, Wang G. CT super-resolution GAN constrained by the identical, residual, and cycle learning ensemble (GAN-CIRCLE). IEEE Trans Med Imaging. 2020;39:188–203.
43. Li Y, Iwamoto Y, Lin L, Xu R, Tong R, Chen YW. VolumeNet: a lightweight parallel network for super-resolution of MR and CT volumetric data. IEEE Trans Image Process. 2021;30:4840–54.
44. Qiu D, Cheng Y, Wang X, Zhang X. Multi-window back-projection residual networks for reconstructing COVID-19 CT super-resolution images. Comput Methods Prog Biomed. 2021;200:105934.
45. Nehra AK, Rajendran K, Baffour FI, Mileto A, Rajiah PS, Horst KK, Inoue A, Johnson TF, Diehn FE, Glazebrook KN, Thorne JE, Weber NM, Shanblatt ER, Gong H, Yu L, Leng S, McCollough CH, Fletcher JG. Seeing more with less: clinical benefits of photon-counting detector CT. Radiographics. 2023;43:e220158.
46. Mahmood F, Chen R, Sudarsky S, Yu D, Durr NJ. Deep learning with cinematic rendering: fine-tuning deep neural networks using photorealistic medical images. Phys Med Biol. 2018;63:185012.
47. Brookmeyer C, Chu LC, Rowe SP, Fishman EK. Clinical implementation of cinematic rendering. Curr Probl Diagn Radiol. 2024;53:313–28.

48. Lu K, Ren L, Yin FF. A geometry-guided deep learning technique for CBCT reconstruction. Phys Med Biol. 2021;66:10.1088/1361-6560/ac145b.
49. Thummerer A, Seller Oria C, Zaffino P, Visser S, Meijers A, Guterres Marmitt G, Wijsman R, Seco J, Langendijk JA, Knopf AC, Spadea MF, Both S. Deep learning-based 4D-synthetic CTs from sparse-view CBCTs for dose calculations in adaptive proton therapy. Med Phys. 2022;49:6824–39.
50. Tsiflikas I, Thater G, Ayx I, Weiss J, Schaefer J, Stein T, Schoenberg SO, Weis M. Low dose pediatric chest computed tomography on a photon counting detector system - initial clinical experience. Pediatr Radiol. 2023;53:1057–62.
51. Yu F, Endo M, Krishnan R, Pan I, Tsai A, Reis EP, Fonseca E, Lee HMH, Abad ZSH, Ng AY, Langlotz CP, Venugopal VK, Rajpurkar P. Evaluating progress in automatic chest X-ray radiology report generation. Patterns (N Y). 2023;4:100802.
52. Gefter WB, Prokop M, Seo JB, Raoof S, Langlotz CP, Hatabu H. Human-AI symbiosis: a path forward to improve chest radiography and the role of radiologists in patient care. Radiology. 2024;310:e232778.
53. Hwang EJ, Park S, Jin KN, Kim JI, Choi SY, Lee JH, Goo JM, Aum J, Yim JJ, Cohen JG, Ferretti GR, Park CM. Development D, Evaluation G. Development and validation of a deep learning-based automated detection algorithm for major thoracic diseases on chest radiographs. JAMA Netw Open. 2019;2:e191095.
54. Lakhani P, Sundaram B. Deep learning at chest radiography: automated classification of pulmonary tuberculosis by using convolutional neural networks. Radiology. 2017;284:574–82.
55. van Beek EJR, Ahn JS, Kim MJ, Murchison JT. Validation study of machine-learning chest radiograph software in primary and emergency medicine. Clin Radiol. 2023;78:1–7.
56. Hwang EJ, Goo JM, Nam JG, Park CM, Hong KJ, Kim KH. Conventional versus artificial intelligence-assisted interpretation of chest radiographs in patients with acute respiratory symptoms in emergency department: a pragmatic randomized clinical trial. Korean J Radiol. 2023;24:259–70.
57. Lind Plesner L, Muller FC, Brejnebol MW, Laustrup LC, Rasmussen F, Nielsen OW, Boesen M, Brun AM. Commercially available chest radiograph AI tools for detecting airspace disease, pneumothorax, and pleural effusion. Radiology. 2023;308:e231236.
58. Yoo H, Kim KH, Singh R, Digumarthy SR, Kalra MK. Validation of a deep learning algorithm for the detection of malignant pulmonary nodules in chest radiographs. JAMA Netw Open. 2020;3:e2017135.
59. Kim JY, Ryu WS, Kim D, Kim EY. Better performance of deep learning pulmonary nodule detection using chest radiography with pixel level labels in reference to computed tomography: data quality matters. Sci Rep. 2024;14:15967.
60. Nam JG, Hwang EJ, Kim J, Park N, Lee EH, Kim HJ, Nam M, Lee JH, Park CM, Goo JM. AI improves nodule detection on chest radiographs in a health screening population: a randomized controlled trial. Radiology. 2023;307:e221894.
61. Hwang EJ, Kim KB, Kim JY, Lim JK, Nam JG, Choi H, Kim H, Yoon SH, Goo JM, Park CM. COVID-19 pneumonia on chest X-rays: performance of a deep learning-based computer-aided detection system. PLoS One. 2021;16:e0252440.
62. Lee HW, Yang HJ, Kim H, Kim UH, Kim DH, Yoon SH, Ham SY, Nam BD, Chae KJ, Lee D, Yoo JY, Bak SH, Kim JY, Kim JH, Kim KB, Jung JI, Lim JK, Lee JE, Chung MJ, Lee YK, Kim YS, Lee SM, Kwon W, Park CM, Kim YH, Jeong YJ, Jin KN, Goo JM. Deep learning with chest radiographs for making prognoses in patients with COVID-19: retrospective cohort study. J Med Internet Res. 2023;25:e42717.
63. Sjoding MW, Taylor D, Motyka J, Lee E, Co I, Claar D, McSparron JI, Ansari S, Kerlin MP, Reilly JP, Shashaty MGS, Anderson BJ, Jones TK, Drebin HM, Ittner CAG, Meyer NJ, Iwashyna TJ, Ward KR, Gillies CE. Deep learning to detect acute respiratory distress syndrome on chest radiographs: a retrospective study with external validation. Lancet Digit Health. 2021;3:e340–8.
64. Schalekamp S, van Leeuwen K, Calli E, Murphy K, Rutten M, Geurts B, Peters-Bax L, van Ginneken B, Prokop M. Performance of AI to exclude normal chest radiographs to reduce radiologists' workload. Eur Radiol. 2024;34:7255.
65. Plesner LL, Muller FC, Brejnebol MW, Krag CH, Laustrup LC, Rasmussen F, Nielsen OW, Boesen M, Andersen MB. Using AI to identify unremarkable chest radiographs for automatic reporting. Radiology. 2024;312:e240272.
66. Weiss J, Raghu VK, Bontempi D, Christiani DC, Mak RH, Lu MT, Aerts H. Deep learning to estimate lung disease mortality from chest radiographs. Nat Commun. 2023;14:2797.
67. Lu MT, Ivanov A, Mayrhofer T, Hosny A, Aerts H, Hoffmann U. Deep learning to assess long-term mortality from chest radiographs. JAMA Netw Open. 2019;2:e197416.
68. Pyrros A, Borstelmann SM, Mantravadi R, Zaiman Z, Thomas K, Price B, Greenstein E, Siddiqui N, Willis M, Shulhan I, Hines-Shah J, Horowitz JM, Nikolaidis P, Lungren MP, Rodriguez-Fernandez JM, Gichoya JW, Koyejo S, Flanders AE, Khandwala N, Gupta A, Garrett JW, Cohen JP, Layden BT, Pickhardt PJ, Galanter W. Opportunistic detection of type 2 diabetes using deep learning from frontal chest radiographs. Nat Commun. 2023;14:4039.
69. National Lung Screening Trial Research T, Aberle DR, Adams AM, Berg CD, Black WC, Clapp JD, Fagerstrom RM, Gareen IF, Gatsonis C, Marcus PM, Sicks JD. Reduced lung-cancer mortality with low-dose computed tomographic screening. N Engl J Med. 2011;365:395–409.

70. de Koning HJ, van der Aalst CM, de Jong PA, Scholten ET, Nackaerts K, Heuvelmans MA, Lammers JJ, Weenink C, Yousaf-Khan U, Horeweg N, van 't Westeinde S, Prokop M, Mali WP, Mohamed Hoesein FAA, van Ooijen PMA, Aerts J, den Bakker MA, Thunnissen E, Verschakelen J, Vliegenthart R, Walter JE, Ten Haaf K, Groen HJM, Oudkerk M. Reduced lung-cancer mortality with volume CT screening in a randomized trial. N Engl J Med. 2020;382:503–13.
71. D'Hondt L, Kellens PJ, Torfs K, Bosmans H, Bacher K, Snoeckx A. Absolute ground truth-based validation of computer-aided nodule detection and volumetry in low-dose CT imaging. Phys Med. 2024;121:103344.
72. Choi W, Oh JH, Riyahi S, Liu CJ, Jiang F, Chen W, White C, Rimner A, Mechalakos JG, Deasy JO, Lu W. Radiomics analysis of pulmonary nodules in low-dose CT for early detection of lung cancer. Med Phys. 2018;45:1537–49.
73. Jacobs C, Setio AAA, Scholten ET, Gerke PK, Bhattacharya H, Brink M, Ranschaert E, de Jong PA, Silva M, Geurts B, Chung K, Schalekamp S, Meersschaert J, Devaraj A, Pinsky PF, Lam SC, van Ginneken B, Farahani K. Deep learning for lung cancer detection on screening CT scans: results of a large-scale public competition and an observer study with 11 radiologists. Radiol Artif Intell. 2021;3:e210027.
74. Mikhael PG, Wohlwend J, Yala A, Karstens L, Xiang J, Takigami AK, Bourgouin PP, Chan P, Mrah S, Amayri W, Juan YH, Yang CT, Wan YL, Lin G, Sequist LV, Fintelmann FJ, Barzilay R. Sybil: a validated deep learning model to predict future lung cancer risk from a single low-dose chest computed tomography. J Clin Oncol. 2023;41:2191–200.
75. Venkadesh KV, Aleef TA, Scholten ET, Saghir Z, Silva M, Sverzellati N, Pastorino U, van Ginneken B, Prokop M, Jacobs C. Prior CT improves deep learning for malignancy risk estimation of screening-detected pulmonary nodules. Radiology. 2023;308:e223308.
76. Gonzalez G, Ash SY, Vegas-Sanchez-Ferrero G, Onieva Onieva J, Rahaghi FN, Ross JC, Diaz A, San Jose Estepar R, Washko GR, Copdgene, Investigators E. Disease staging and prognosis in smokers using deep learning in chest computed tomography. Am J Respir Crit Care Med. 2018;197:193–203.
77. Tang LYW, Coxson HO, Lam S, Leipsic J, Tam RC, Sin DD. Towards large-scale case-finding: training and validation of residual networks for detection of chronic obstructive pulmonary disease using low-dose CT. Lancet Digit Health. 2020;2:e259–67.
78. Castaldi PJ, San Jose Estepar R, Mendoza CS, Hersh CP, Laird N, Crapo JD, Lynch DA, Silverman EK, Washko GR. Distinct quantitative computed tomography emphysema patterns are associated with physiology and function in smokers. Am J Respir Crit Care Med. 2013;188:1083–90.
79. Pompe E, Galban CJ, Ross BD, Koenderman L, Ten Hacken NH, Postma DS, van den Berge M, de Jong PA, Lammers JJ, Mohamed Hoesein FA. Parametric response mapping on chest computed tomography associates with clinical and functional parameters in chronic obstructive pulmonary disease. Respir Med. 2017;123:48–55.
80. Humphries SM, Notary AM, Centeno JP, Strand MJ, Crapo JD, Silverman EK, Lynch DA. Genetic epidemiology of CI. Deep learning enables automatic classification of emphysema pattern at CT. Radiology. 2020;294:434–44.
81. Lynch DA, Moore CM, Wilson C, Nevrekar D, Jennermann T, Humphries SM, Austin JHM, Grenier PA, Kauczor HU, Han MK, Regan EA, Make BJ, Bowler RP, Beaty TH, Curran-Everett D, Hokanson JE, Curtis JL, Silverman EK, Crapo JD. Genetic epidemiology of CI. CT-based visual classification of emphysema: association with mortality in the COPDGene study. Radiology. 2018;288:859–66.
82. Fuhrman J, Yip R, Zhu Y, Jirapatnakul AC, Li F, Henschke CI, Yankelevitz DF, Giger ML. Evaluation of emphysema on thoracic low-dose CTs through attention-based multiple instance deep learning. Sci Rep. 2023;13:1187.
83. Walsh SLF, Mackintosh JA, Calandriello L, Silva M, Sverzellati N, Larici AR, Humphries SM, Lynch DA, Jo HE, Glaspole I, Grainge C, Goh N, Hopkins PMA, Moodley Y, Reynolds PN, Zappala C, Keir G, Cooper WA, Mahar AM, Ellis S, Wells AU, Corte TJ. Deep learning-based outcome prediction in progressive fibrotic lung disease using high-resolution computed tomography. Am J Respir Crit Care Med. 2022;206:883–91.
84. Huang SC, Pareek A, Zamanian R, Banerjee I, Lungren MP. Multimodal fusion with deep neural networks for leveraging CT imaging and electronic health record: a case-study in pulmonary embolism detection. Sci Rep. 2020;10:22147.
85. Weikert T, Winkel DJ, Bremerich J, Stieltjes B, Parmar V, Sauter AW, Sommer G. Automated detection of pulmonary embolism in CT pulmonary angiograms using an AI-powered algorithm. Eur Radiol. 2020;30:6545–53.
86. Hahn LD, Hall K, Alebdi T, Kligerman SJ, Hsiao A. Automated deep learning analysis for quality improvement of CT pulmonary angiography. Radiol Artif Intell. 2022;4:e210162.
87. Chao H, Shan H, Homayounieh F, Singh R, Khera RD, Guo H, Su T, Wang G, Kalra MK, Yan P. Deep learning predicts cardiovascular disease risks from lung cancer screening low dose computed tomography. Nat Commun. 2021;12:2963.
88. Lessmann N, van Ginneken B, Zreik M, de Jong PA, de Vos BD, Viergever MA, Isgum I. Automatic calcium scoring in low-dose chest CT using deep neural networks with dilated convolutions. IEEE Trans Med Imaging. 2018;37:615–25.
89. van Velzen SGM, Lessmann N, Velthuis BK, Bank IEM, van den Bongard D, Leiner T, de Jong PA,

Veldhuis WB, Correa A, Terry JG, Carr JJ, Viergever MA, Verkooijen HM, Isgum I. Deep learning for automatic calcium scoring in CT: validation using multiple cardiac CT and chest CT protocols. Radiology. 2020;295:66–79.

90. Zeleznik R, Foldyna B, Eslami P, Weiss J, Alexander I, Taron J, Parmar C, Alvi RM, Banerji D, Uno M, Kikuchi Y, Karady J, Zhang L, Scholtz JE, Mayrhofer T, Lyass A, Mahoney TF, Massaro JM, Vasan RS, Douglas PS, Hoffmann U, Lu MT, Aerts H. Deep convolutional neural networks to predict cardiovascular risk from computed tomography. Nat Commun. 2021;12:715.

91. Macruz FBC, Lu C, Strout J, Takigami A, Brooks R, Doyle S, Yun M, Buch V, Hedgire S, Ghoshhajra B. Quantification of the thoracic aorta and detection of aneurysm at CT: development and validation of a fully automatic methodology. Radiol Artif Intell. 2022;4:e210076.

92. Monti CB, van Assen M, Stillman AE, Lee SJ, Hoelzer P, Fung GSK, Secchi F, Sardanelli F, De Cecco CN. Evaluating the performance of a convolutional neural network algorithm for measuring thoracic aortic diameters in a heterogeneous population. Radiol Artif Intell. 2022;4:e210196.

93. Chung TK, Liang NL, Vorp DA. Artificial intelligence framework to predict wall stress in abdominal aortic aneurysm. Appl Eng Sci. 2022;10:100104.

94. Rueckel J, Reidler P, Fink N, Sperl J, Geyer T, Fabritius MP, Ricke J, Ingrisch M, Sabel BO. Artificial intelligence assistance improves reporting efficiency of thoracic aortic aneurysm CT follow-up. Eur J Radiol. 2021;134:109424.

95. Zha W, Fain SB, Schiebler ML, Evans MD, Nagle SK, Liu F. Deep convolutional neural networks with multiplane consensus labeling for lung function quantification using UTE proton MRI. J Magn Reson Imaging. 2019;50:1169–81.

96. Guo F, Capaldi DP, McCormack DG, Fenster A, Parraga G. Ultra-short echo-time magnetic resonance imaging lung segmentation with under-annotations and domain shift. Med Image Anal. 2021;72:102107.

97. Mairhormann B, Castelblanco A, Hafner F, Koliogiannis V, Haist L, Winter D, Flemmer A, Ehrhardt H, Stocklein S, Dietrich O, Forster K, Hilgendorff A, Schubert B. Automated MRI lung segmentation and 3D morphologic features for quantification of neonatal lung disease. Radiol Artif Intell. 2023;5:e220239

98. Yip SS, Aerts HJ. Applications and limitations of radiomics. Phys Med Biol. 2016;61:R150–66.

99. Mayerhoefer ME, Materka A, Langs G, Haggstrom I, Szczypinski P, Gibbs P, Cook G. Introduction to radiomics. J Nucl Med. 2020;61:488–95.

100. Moon SH, Kim J, Joung JG, Cha H, Park WY, Ahn JS, Ahn MJ, Park K, Choi JY, Lee KH, Kim BT, Lee SH. Correlations between metabolic texture features, genetic heterogeneity, and mutation burden in patients with lung cancer. Eur J Nucl Med Mol Imaging. 2019;46:446–54.

101. Choi ER, Lee HY, Jeong JY, Choi YL, Kim J, Bae J, Lee KS, Shim YM. Quantitative image variables reflect the intratumoral pathologic heterogeneity of lung adenocarcinoma. Oncotarget. 2016;7:67302–13.

102. Rios Velazquez E, Parmar C, Liu Y, Coroller TP, Cruz G, Stringfield O, Ye Z, Makrigiorgos M, Fennessy F, Mak RH, Gillies R, Quackenbush J, Aerts H. Somatic mutations drive distinct imaging phenotypes in lung cancer. Cancer Res. 2017;77:3922–30.

103. Kim S, Lim JH, Kim CH, Roh J, You S, Choi JS, Lim JH, Kim L, Chang JW, Park D, Lee MW, Kim S, Heo J. Deep learning-radiomics integrated noninvasive detection of epidermal growth factor receptor mutations in non-small cell lung cancer patients. Sci Rep. 2024;14:922.

104. Yang F, Zhang J, Zhou L, Xia W, Zhang R, Wei H, Feng J, Zhao X, Jian J, Gao X, Yuan S. CT-based radiomics signatures can predict the tumor response of non-small cell lung cancer patients treated with first-line chemotherapy and targeted therapy. Eur Radiol. 2022;32:1538–47.

105. Gevaert O, Echegaray S, Khuong A, Hoang CD, Shrager JB, Jensen KC, Berry GJ, Guo HH, Lau C, Plevritis SK, Rubin DL, Napel S, Leung AN. Predictive radiogenomics modeling of EGFR mutation status in lung cancer. Sci Rep. 2017;7:41674.

106. Liu Y, Kim J, Balagurunathan Y, Li Q, Garcia AL, Stringfield O, Ye Z, Gillies RJ. Radiomic features are associated with EGFR mutation status in lung adenocarcinomas. Clin Lung Cancer. 2016;17(441–448):e446.

107. Yip SS, Kim J, Coroller TP, Parmar C, Velazquez ER, Huynh E, Mak RH, Aerts HJ. Associations between somatic mutations and metabolic imaging phenotypes in non-small cell lung cancer. J Nucl Med. 2017;58:569–76.

108. Zou J, Lv T, Zhu S, Lu Z, Shen Q, Xia L, Wu J, Song Y, Liu H. Computed tomography and clinical features associated with epidermal growth factor receptor mutation status in stage I/II lung adenocarcinoma. Thorac Cancer. 2017;8:260–70.

109. Zhao M, Wu Y, Li Y, Zhang X, Xia S, Xu J, Chen R, Liang Z, Qi S. Learning and depicting lobe-based radiomics feature for COPD severity staging in low-dose CT images. BMC Pulm Med. 2024;24:294.

110. Makimoto K, Hogg JC, Bourbeau J, Tan WC, Kirby M, Can CCRG. Enhancing COPD classification using combined quantitative computed tomography and texture-based radiomics: a CanCOLD cohort study. ERJ Open Res. 2024;10:00968.

111. Chetan MR, Gleeson FV. Radiomics in predicting treatment response in non-small-cell lung cancer: current status, challenges and future perspectives. Eur Radiol. 2021;31:1049–58.

112. Garcia-Uceda A, Selvan R, Saghir Z, Tiddens H, de Bruijne M. Automatic airway segmentation

from computed tomography using robust and efficient 3-D convolutional neural networks. Sci Rep. 2021;11:16001.

113. Zhang M, Wu Y, Zhang H, Qin Y, Zheng H, Tang W, Arnold C, Pei C, Yu P, Nan Y, Yang G, Walsh S, Marshall DC, Komorowski M, Wang P, Guo D, Jin D, Wu Y, Zhao S, Chang R, Zhang B, Lu X, Qayyum A, Mazher M, Su Q, Wu Y, Liu Y, Zhu Y, Yang J, Pakzad A, Rangelov B, Estepar RSJ, Espinosa CC, Sun J, Yang GZ, Gu Y. Multi-site, multi-domain airway tree modeling. Med Image Anal. 2023;90:102957.
114. Wang P, Guo D, Zheng D, Zhang M, Yu H, Sun X, Ge J, Gu Y, Lu L, Ye X, Jin D. Accurate airway tree segmentation in CT scans via anatomy-aware multiclass segmentation and topology-guided iterative learning. IEEE Trans Med Imaging. 2024;43:4294.
115. Nardelli P, Ross JC, San Jose Estepar R. Generative-based airway and vessel morphology quantification on chest CT images. Med Image Anal. 2020;63:101691.
116. Kuo W, Perez-Rovira A, Tiddens H, de Bruijne M. Normal Chest CTsg. Airway tapering: an objective image biomarker for bronchiectasis. Eur Radiol. 2020;30:2703–11.
117. Nardelli P, Jimenez-Carretero D, Bermejo-Pelaez D, Washko GR, Rahaghi FN, Ledesma-Carbayo MJ, San Jose Estepar R. Pulmonary artery-vein classification in CT images using deep learning. IEEE Trans Med Imaging. 2018;37:2428–40.
118. Diaz AA, Nardelli P, Wang W, San Jose Estepar R, Yen A, Kligerman S, Maselli DJ, Dolliver WR, Tsao A, Orejas JL, Aliberti S, Aksamit TR, Young KA, Kinney GL, Washko GR, Silverman EK, Jose S, Estepar R. Artificial intelligence-based CT assessment of bronchiectasis: the COPDGene study. Radiology. 2023;307:e221109.
119. Ram S, Hoff BA, Bell AJ, Galban S, Fortuna AB, Weinheimer O, Wielputz MO, Robinson TE, Newman B, Vummidi D, Chughtai A, Kazerooni EA, Johnson TD, Han MK, Hatt CR, Galban CJ. Improved detection of air trapping on expiratory computed tomography using deep learning. PLoS One. 2021;16:e0248902.
120. Estepar RS, Kinney GL, Black-Shinn JL, Bowler RP, Kindlmann GL, Ross JC, Kikinis R, Han MK, Come CE, Diaz AA, Cho MH, Hersh CP, Schroeder JD, Reilly JJ, Lynch DA, Crapo JD, Wells JM, Dransfield MT, Hokanson JE, Washko GR, Study CO. Computed tomographic measures of pulmonary vascular morphology in smokers and their clinical implications. Am J Respir Crit Care Med. 2013;188:231–9.
121. Nam JG, Witanto JN, Park SJ, Yoo SJ, Goo JM, Yoon SH. Automatic pulmonary vessel segmentation on noncontrast chest CT: deep learning algorithm developed using spatiotemporally matched virtual noncontrast images and low-keV contrast-enhanced vessel maps. Eur Radiol. 2021;31:9012–21.
122. Pu J, Leader JK, Sechrist J, Beeche CA, Singh JP, Ocak IK, Risbano MG. Automated identification of pulmonary arteries and veins depicted in non-contrast chest CT scans. Med Image Anal. 2022;77:102367.
123. Rahaghi FN, Nardelli P, Harder E, Singh I, Sanchez-Ferrero GV, Ross JC, San Jose Estepar R, Ash SY, Hunsaker AR, Maron BA, Leopold JA, Waxman AB, San Jose Estepar R, Washko GR. Quantification of arterial and venous morphologic markers in pulmonary arterial hypertension using CT imaging. Chest. 2021;160:2220–31.
124. Washko GR, Nardelli P, Ash SY, Vegas Sanchez-Ferrero G, Rahaghi FN, Come CE, Dransfield MT, Kalhan R, Han MK, Bhatt SP, Wells JM, Aaron CP, Diaz AA, Ross JC, Cuttica MJ, Labaki WW, Querejeta Roca G, Shah AM, Young K, Kinney GL, Hokanson JE, Agusti A, San Jose Estepar R. Arterial vascular pruning, right ventricular size, and clinical outcomes in chronic obstructive pulmonary disease. A longitudinal observational study. Am J Respir Crit Care Med. 2019;200:454–61.
125. Schiwek M, Triphan SMF, Biederer J, Weinheimer O, Eichinger M, Vogelmeier CF, Jorres RA, Kauczor HU, Heussel CP, Konietzke P, von Stackelberg O, Risse F, Jobst BJ, Wielputz MO, group Cs. Quantification of pulmonary perfusion abnormalities using DCE-MRI in COPD: comparison with quantitative CT and pulmonary function. Eur Radiol. 2022;32:1879–90.
126. Triphan SMF, Bauman G, Konietzke P, Konietzke M, Wielputz MO. International workshop for pulmonary functional I. Magnetic resonance imaging of lung perfusion. J Magn Reson Imaging. 2024;59:784–96.
127. Fu Y, Lei Y, Wang T, Higgins K, Bradley JD, Curran WJ, Liu T, Yang X. LungRegNet: an unsupervised deformable image registration method for 4D-CT lung. Med Phys. 2020;47:1763–74.
128. Cai N, Chen H, Li Y, Peng Y, Guo L. Registration on DCE-MRI images via multi-domain image-to-image translation. Comput Med Imaging Graph. 2023;104:102169.
129. MacNeil JL, Capaldi DPI, Westcott AR, Eddy RL, Barker AL, McCormack DG, Kirby M, Parraga G. Pulmonary imaging phenotypes of chronic obstructive pulmonary disease using multiparametric response maps. Radiology. 2020;295:227–36.
130. Gerard SE, Herrmann J, Kaczka DW, Musch G, Fernandez-Bustamante A, Reinhardt JM. Multi-resolution convolutional neural networks for fully automated segmentation of acutely injured lungs in multiple species. Med Image Anal. 2020;60:101592.
131. Gerard SE, Patton TJ, Christensen GE, Bayouth JE, Reinhardt JM. FissureNet: a deep learning approach for pulmonary fissure detection in CT images. IEEE Trans Med Imaging. 2019;38:156–66.
132. Peters B, Paul JF, Symons R, Franssen WMA, Nchimi A, Ghekiere O. Invasive fractional-flow-reserve prediction by coronary CT angiography using artificial intelligence vs. computational fluid

dynamics software in intermediate-grade stenosis. Int J Cardiovasc Imaging. 2024;40:1875.
133. Becker LM, Peper J, Verhappen B, Swart LA, Dedic A, van Dockum WG, van der Ent M, Royaards KJ, Niezen A, Hensen JJ, van Kuijk JP, Mohamed Hoesein FAA, Leiner T, Bruning TA, Swaans MJ. Real world impact of added FFR-CT to coronary CT angiography on clinical decision-making and patient prognosis - IMPACT FFR study. Eur Radiol. 2023;33:5465–75.
134. Ren G, Zhang J, Li T, Xiao H, Cheung LY, Ho WY, Qin J, Cai J. Deep learning-based computed tomography perfusion mapping (DL-CTPM) for pulmonary CT-to-perfusion translation. Int J Radiat Oncol Biol Phys. 2021;110:1508–18.
135. Chaudhary MFA, Gerard SE, Christensen GE, Cooper CB, Schroeder JD, Hoffman EA, Reinhardt JM. LungViT: ensembling cascade of texture sensitive hierarchical vision transformers for cross-volume chest CT image-to-image translation. IEEE Trans Med Imaging. 2024;43:2448–65.
136. Theodoris CV, Xiao L, Chopra A, Chaffin MD, Al Sayed ZR, Hill MC, Mantineo H, Brydon EM, Zeng Z, Liu XS, Ellinor PT. Transfer learning enables predictions in network biology. Nature. 2023;618:616–24.
137. Vorontsov E, Bozkurt A, Casson A, Shaikovski G, Zelcchowski M, Severson K, Zimmermann E, Hall J, Tenenholtz N, Fusi N, Yang E, Mathieu P, van Eck A, Lee D, Viret J, Robert E, Wang YK, Kunz JD, Lee MCH, Bernhard JH, Godrich RA, Oakley G, Millar E, Hanna M, Wen H, Retamero JA, Moye WA, Yousfi R, Kanan C, Klimstra DS, Rothrock B, Liu S, Fuchs TJ. A foundation model for clinical-grade computational pathology and rare cancers detection. Nat Med. 2024;30:2924.
138. Lu MY, Chen B, Williamson DFK, Chen RJ, Liang I, Ding T, Jaume G, Odintsov I, Le LP, Gerber G, Parwani AV, Zhang A, Mahmood F. A visual-language foundation model for computational pathology. Nat Med. 2024;30:863–74.
139. Glocker B, Jones C, Roschewitz M, Winzeck S. Risk of bias in chest radiography deep learning foundation models. Radiol Artif Intell. 2023;5:e230060.
140. Viswanathan VS, Toro P, Corredor G, Mukhopadhyay S, Madabhushi A. The state of the art for artificial intelligence in lung digital pathology. J Pathol. 2022;257:413–29.
141. Humphries SM, Mackintosh JA, Jo HE, Walsh SLF, Silva M, Calandriello L, Chapman S, Ellis S, Glaspole I, Goh N, Grainge C, Hopkins PMA, Keir GJ, Moodley Y, Reynolds PN, Walters EH, Baraghoshi D, Wells AU, Lynch DA, Corte TJ. Quantitative computed tomography predicts outcomes in idiopathic pulmonary fibrosis. Respirology. 2022;27:1045–53.

Correction to: Quantitative Imaging of Sarcopenia

Eddy D. Zandee van Rilland
and Aparna Komarraju

Correction to:
Chapter 26 in: R. Gill, P. Rajiah (eds.), *Quantitative Imaging in the Thorax*, https://doi.org/10.1007/978-3-032-14103-3_26

The original version of Chap. 26 was recently published with errors on pages 545 and 547. The errors have been corrected as listed below:

- **Page 545, section "Computed Tomography"**: "CSA/heigh2" in sentence "The CSA is indexed for height (CSA/heigh2) to…" has been now corrected to "CSA/height^2"
- **Page 547**:

➢ In Fig. 26.6 legend, the comma "," in "green arrows" has been removed.
➢ Fig. 26.7 has now been replaced with a revised figure (new figure is given below).
➢ In Fig. 26.7 legend, "Sartorius" was corrected to "sartorius."
➢ In the "Ultrasound" section, the phrase "in the setting of massive rotator cuff tear" has been now corrected to "of the sartorius muscle." The updated version now reads as follows:

"Figure 26.7 illustrates an example of a patient with muscle atrophy and fatty infiltration of the sartorius muscle."

The updated version of this chapter can be found at
https://doi.org/10.1007/978-3-032-16112-3_26

R. Gill, P. Rajiah (eds.), *Quantitative Imaging in the Thorax*,
https://doi.org/10.1007/978-3-032-14103-3_28

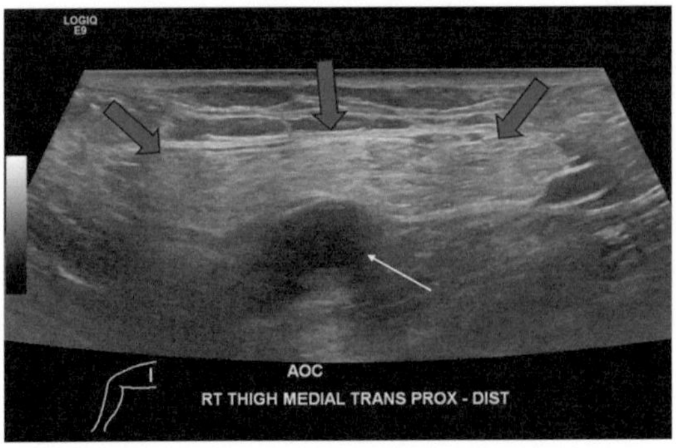

Fig. 26.7 70M presenting with muscle weakness. Ultrasound image at the level of the mid-thigh medially demonstrates diffusely echogenic appearance of the sartorius muscle, compatible with diffuse fatty infiltration (blue block arrows). The hypoechoic structure in the center is the Superficial Femoral Artery (arrow)

Index

R. Gill, P. Rajiah (eds.), *Quantitative Imaging in the Thorax*,
https://doi.org/10.1007/978-3-032-14103-3

D

Q

R

U

V

W

X

MIX
Papier aus verantwortungsvollen Quellen
Paper from responsible sources
FSC® C105338

If you have any concerns about our products,
you can contact us on
ProductSafety@springernature.com

In case Publisher is established outside the EU,
the EU authorized representative is:
Springer Nature Customer Service Center GmbH
Europaplatz 3, 69115 Heidelberg, Germany

Printed by Libri Plureos GmbH
in Hamburg, Germany